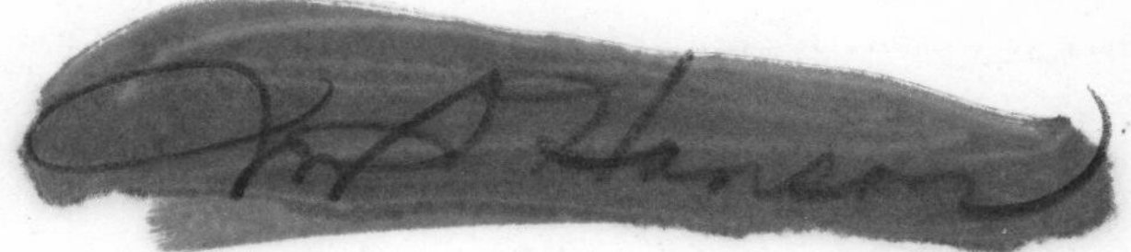

1978
CURRENT THERAPY
1978

CONSULTING EDITORS:

W. B. SAUNDERS COMPANY / PHILADELPHIA / LONDON / TORONTO

1978
1978
1978
1978
1978
1978

CURRENT THERAPY

LATEST APPROVED METHODS OF TREATMENT FOR THE PRACTICING PHYSICIAN

EDITED BY HOWARD F. CONN, M.D.

1978
1978
1978

W. B. Saunders Company: West Washington Square
Philadelphia, PA 19105

1 St. Anne's Road
Eastbourne, East Sussex BN21 3UN, England

1 Goldthorne Avenue
Toronto, Ontario M8Z 5T9, Canada

Current Therapy ISBN 0-7216-2663-7

Last digit is the print number: 9 8 7 6 5 4 3 2 1

Consulting Editors

THE ENDOCRINE SYSTEM

FREDERIC C. BARTTER, M.D.

Clinical Professor of Medicine, Georgetown University Medical School. Chief, Hypertension-Endocrine Branch, Clinical Center, National Institutes of Health, Bethesda, Maryland.

OBSTETRICS AND GYNECOLOGY

WALTER A. BONNEY, M.D.

Clinical Professor, Obstetrics and Gynecology, West Virginia University School of Medicine, Morgantown, West Virginia.

THE CARDIOVASCULAR SYSTEM

GEORGE E. BURCH, M.D., F.A.C.P.

Emeritus Professor of Medicine, Tulane University School of Medicine, New Orleans, Louisiana.

THE RESPIRATORY SYSTEM

BENJAMIN BURROWS, M.D.

Professor of Internal Medicine, University of Arizona College of Medicine. Staff, Arizona Health Sciences Center; Consultant, Veterans Administration Hospital, Tucson, Arizona.

METABOLIC DISORDERS

JAMES B. FIELD, M.D.

Professor of Medicine, University of Pittsburgh School of Medicine. Director, Clinical Research Unit, Presbyterian-University Hospital, University of Pittsburgh School of Medicine, Pittsburgh, Pennsylvania.

THE UROGENITAL TRACT

WILLARD E. GOODWIN, M.D., F.A.C.S., F.A.A.P.

Professor of Surgery/Urology (Pediatric Urology), University of California School of Medicine, Los Angeles. Staff Urologist, University of California Medical Center, Los Angeles; Senior Consultant in Urology, Wadsworth Veterans Administration Hospital, Los Angeles; Consultant in Urology, Los Angeles County Harbor General Hospital, Torrance; Consultant, St. Francis Hospital, Lynwood; Consulting Staff, Hollywood Presbyterian Hospital, Los Angeles; Honorary Consulting Staff, Santa Monica Hospital, Santa Monica; Courtesy Staff, St. John's Hospital, Santa Monica, and Hospital of the Good Samaritan, Los Angeles; Consulting Staff, The Cedars of Lebanon Hospital and Mount Sinai Hospital, Los Angeles, California.

PSYCHIATRY

LAWRENCE C. KOLB, M.D.

Emeritus Professor of Psychiatry, College of Physicians and Surgeons, Columbia University. Consultant in Psychiatry and Honorary Member, Medical Board, The Presbyterian Hospital in the City of New York, New York.

DISEASES OF THE SKIN AND THE VENEREAL DISEASES

CLARENCE S. LIVINGOOD, M.D.

Chairman Emeritus, Department of Dermatology, Henry Ford Hospital. Clinical Professor of Dermatology, University of Michigan Medical School. Staff Physician, Department of Dermatology, Henry Ford Hospital, Detroit, Michigan.

THE LOCOMOTOR SYSTEM

DANIEL J. McCARTY, M.D.

Professor of Medicine, The Medical College of Wisconsin. Senior Attending Physician and Director of Medical Service, Milwaukee County General Hospital, Milwaukee, Wisconsin.

THE NERVOUS SYSTEM

FRED PLUM, M.D.

Anne Parrish Titzell Professor and Chairman, Department of Neurology, Cornell University Medical College, New York, New York.

THE INFECTIOUS DISEASES

CHARLES H. RAMMELKAMP, M.D., D.Sc.

Professor of Medicine and Professor of Preventive Medicine, Case Western Reserve University Medical School. Director of Medicine, Cleveland Metropolitan General Hospital, Cleveland, Ohio.

THE DIGESTIVE SYSTEM

JAMES L. A. ROTH, M.D., Ph.D., D.Sc. (Hon.), F.A.C.P.

Professor of Clinical Medicine, School of Medicine, University of Pennsylvania. Director, Institute of Gastroenterology, and Chief, Gastroenterology Service, Presbyterian–University of Pennsylvania Medical Center; Consulting Gastroenterologist, U. S. Naval Medical Center, Bethesda, Maryland, and U. S. Naval Hospital, Lankenau Hospital, and Roxborough Memorial Hospital, Philadelphia, Pennsylvania.

THE BLOOD AND SPLEEN

R. WAYNE RUNDLES, Ph.D., M.D.

Professor of Medicine, Duke University Medical School. Hematology-Oncology Staff, Member of Comprehensive Cancer Center, Durham, North Carolina.

DISEASES OF ALLERGY

THOMAS E. VAN METRE, Jr., M.D.

Associate Professor of Medicine, The Johns Hopkins University School of Medicine. Physician-in-Charge, Allergy Clinic, The Johns Hopkins Hospital, Baltimore, Maryland.

NOTICE

Extraordinary efforts have been made by the authors, the editors, and the publisher of this book to insure that dosage recommendations are precise and in agreement with standards officially accepted at the time of publication.

It does happen, however, that dosage schedules are changed from time to time in the light of accumulating clinical experience and continuing laboratory studies. This is most likely to occur in the case of recently introduced products.

It is urged, therefore, that you check the manufacturer's recommendations for dosage, *especially if the drug to be administered or prescribed is one that you use only infrequently or have not used for some time.*

THE PUBLISHERS

Preface

This edition of *Current Therapy* is the thirtieth of an annual series devoted to bringing concise information on current therapeutic methods to the practicing physician.

The authors have been carefully selected not only for their active interest in the specific diseases discussed but also as recognized authorities in the medical world. They have explained their present methods in brief, to-the-point discussions but in sufficient detail for proper management of the illness. All material has been reviewed before publication to assure the inclusion of the latest therapy.

The term "method of" refers to the regimen in use by the author-clinician; it does not imply that the named author was the originator. Present-day treatment is by and large a summation of the work of many clinicians over the years.

This is a new edition rather than a revision of the old. Two hundred and sixty-three or 92 per cent of the articles are by authors new to this edition. Certain deletions and additions of topics have been made in keeping with the changes in the importance of certain diseases and the worldwide distribution of the book.

To the readers, who by their enthusiastic acceptance of the past editions of *Current Therapy* have made this one possible, and to the contributors, who were able to find time in their busy schedules to prepare their articles, the Editor expresses his sincere thanks.

The Editor also wishes to express his appreciation to Mr. C. F. Robinson and Mrs. Franklin Cole for their valuable assistance in the preparation of the book, and to the staff of the W. B. Saunders Company for their thoughtful help and guidance.

HOWARD F. CONN, M.D., F.A.C.P.
Uniontown, Pennsylvania

Contributors

WHITNEY W. ADDINGTON, M.D.

Associate Professor of Medicine, Northwestern University Medical School. Chairman, Division of Pulmonary Medicine, Cook County Hospital; Consultant, Children's Memorial Hospital, Chicago, Illinois.
Tuberculosis and Other Mycobacterial Diseases

DAVID H. ALPERS, M.D.

Professor of Medicine and Chief, Division of Gastroenterology, Washington University School of Medicine. Physician, Barnes Hospital, St. Louis, Missouri.
The Malabsorption Syndrome

I. G. ANCES, M.D.

Professor, University of Maryland School of Medicine. University of Maryland Hospital and Mercy Hospital, Baltimore, Maryland.
Amenorrhea

NANCY C. ANDREASEN, M.D., PH.D.

Associate Professor, Psychiatry, University of Iowa College of Medicine, Iowa City, Iowa.
Affective Disorders

JAY M. ARENA, M.D.

Professor of Pediatrics and Director, Duke Poison Control Center, Duke University Medical Center, Durham, North Carolina.
Acute Miscellaneous Poisoning

JOHN A. ARKINS, M.D.

Professor of Medicine, Medical College of Wisconsin. Allergy-Immunology Section, Milwaukee County Medical Complex, Milwaukee, and Veterans Administration Hospital, Wood, Wisconsin.
Asthma in Adults

DONALD ARMSTRONG, M.D.

Professor of Medicine, Cornell University Medical College. Chief, Infectious Disease Service, Department of Medicine, and Director, Microbiology Laboratory, Memorial Sloan-Kettering Cancer Center, New York, New York.
Bacteremia

LOUIS V. AVIOLI, M.D.

Professor of Medicine and Director, Division of Bone and Mineral Metabolism, Washington University School of Medicine. Jewish Hospital of St. Louis, Barnes Hospital, Children's Hospital, and Shriners Hospital for Crippled Children, St. Louis, Missouri.
Osteoporosis

WILLIAM C. BAILEY, M.D.

Associate Professor of Medicine, University of Alabama in Birmingham School of Medicine. Chief, Pulmonary Disease Section, Veterans Administration Hospital, Birmingham, Alabama.
Silicosis

LYNN H. BANOWSKY, M.D.

Professor of Surgery/Urology and Chief, Renal Transplantation, University of Texas Health Science Center at San Antonio. Bexar County Hospital and Audie Murphy Veterans Administration Hospital, San Antonio, Texas.
Bacterial Infections of the Urinary Tract (Male)

HUGH R. K. BARBER, M.D.

Clinical Professor of Obstetrics and Gynecology, Cornell Medical College. Director, Department of Obstetrics and Gynecology, Lenox Hill Hospital; Attending Surgeon, Gynecology Service, Memorial Hospital; Attending Obstetrician-Gynecologist, New York Hospital, New York, New York.
Cancer of the Uterus

JAMES W. BARD, M.D.

Clinical Associate Professor of Medicine, University of Kentucky Medical Center. Chief, Section of Dermatology, Lexington Clinic, Lexington, Kentucky.
Seborrheic Dermatitis

ROBERT W. BARNES, M.D.

David M. Hume Professor of Surgery, Medical College of Virginia. Attending Surgeon, Medical College of Virginia Hospitals and McGuire Veterans Administration Hospital, Richmond, Virginia.
Degenerative Arterial Disease

JAMES A. BATTS, JR., M.D.

Professor, Obstetrics and Gynecology, Columbia University College of Physicians and Surgeons. Director, Department of Obstetrics and Gynecology, Harlem Hospital Center, New York, New York.
Abortion

SAMUEL Z. BAVLI, M.D.

Research Fellow in Medicine, Harvard Medical School. Fellow in Endocrinology, Peter Bent Brigham Hospital, Boston, Massachusetts.
Hyperthyroidism

WILLIAM B. BEAN, M.D.

Kempner Professor and Director of the Institute for the Medical Humanities and Professor of Medicine, University of Texas Medical Branch; Sir William Osler Professor of Medicine, University of Iowa College of Medicine. Attending, University of Texas Medical Branch Hospitals, Galveston, Texas, and University Hospitals, Iowa City, Iowa.
Pellagra

LEWIS C. BECKER, M.D.

Associate Professor of Medicine, Johns Hopkins University School of Medicine. Director, Coronary Care Unit, Johns Hopkins Hospital, Baltimore, Maryland.
Acute Myocardial Infarction

RICHARD S. BERGER, M.D.

Clinical Associate Professor of Medicine, Rutgers Medical School. Raritan Valley Hospital, Greenbrook, New Jersey.
Spider Bites and Scorpion Stings

WILMA F. BERGFELD, M.D.

Head of Section of Dermatopathology, Departments of Dermatology and Pathology, Cleveland Clinic. Staff Dermatologist, Cleveland Clinic, Cleveland, Ohio.
Cancer of the Skin

IRWIN D. BERNSTEIN, M.D.

Associate Professor in Pediatrics, University of Washington School of Medicine. Attending Physician, Children's Orthopedic Hospital and Medical Center; Associate Member, Fred Hutchinson Cancer Research Center, Seattle, Washington.
Acute Childhood Leukemia

RICHARD O. BICKS, M.D.

Associate Clinical Professor of Medicine, University of Tennessee Center for Health Sciences. Director, Division of Gastroenterology and of Gastrointestinal Training, Baptist Memorial Hospital; Consultant, City of Memphis Hospitals, Memphis, Tennessee.
Nonspecific Ulcerative Colitis

J. THOMAS BIGGER, JR., M.D.

Professor of Medicine and Pharmacology, College of Physicians and Surgeons, Columbia University. Attending Physician, The Presbyterian Hospital, New York, New York.
Premature Beats

W. ARCHIE BLEYER, M.D.

Assistant Professor of Pediatrics and Adjunct Assistant Professor of Medicine, University of Washington School of Medicine. Staff Physician in Hematology/Oncology, Children's Orthopedic Hospital and Medical Center; Assistant Member, Fred Hutchinson Cancer Research Center, Seattle, Washington.
Acute Childhood Leukemia

GIANNI BONADONNA, M.D.

Director, Division of Medical Oncology, Istituto Nazionale Tumori, Milan, Italy.
Hodgkin's Disease: Chemotherapy

JAMES R. BONNER, M.D.

Assistant Professor, Department of Medicine, University of South Alabama Medical School, Mobile, Alabama.
Bacterial Pneumonia

SYLVIA S. BOTTOMLEY, M.D.

Professor of Medicine, University of Oklahoma College of Medicine. Staff Physician, Veterans Administration Hospital, University Hospital, Oklahoma Children's Memorial Hospital, and Presbyterian Hospital, Oklahoma City, Oklahoma.
Anemia Due to Iron Deficiency

WILLIAM T. BOWLES, M.D.

Associate Professor of Urology, Washington University School of Medicine. Associate Surgeon, Barnes Hospital and Affiliated Hospitals and St. Louis Children's Hospital, St. Louis, Missouri, and St. Clement Hospital, Red Bud, Illinois.
Bacterial Infections of the Urinary Tract (Female)

RICHARD J. BOXER, M.D.

Instructor in Urology, University of California, Los Angeles, California
Genitourinary Tuberculosis

JAMES L. BREEN, M.D.

Clinical Professor of Obstetrics and Gynecology, Jefferson Medical College. Director, Department of Obstetrics and Gynecology, St. Barnabas Medical Center, Livingston, New Jersey.
Vulvovaginitis

ROBERT W. BRENNAN, M.D.

Professor of Medicine and Chief, Neurology Division, The Milton S. Hershey Medical Center of The Pennsylvania State University, Hershey, Pennsylvania.
Rehabilitation of the Patient with Hemiplegia

HAROLD BROWN, M.D.

Professor of Medicine, Baylor College of Medicine. Senior Attending, Ben Taub General Hospital and The Methodist Hospital; Consultant, Veterans Administration Hospital, Houston, Texas.
Malignant Carcinoid Syndrome

SUNTHORN BUNYAVIROCH, M.D.

Assistant Clinical Professor of Obstetrics and Gynecology, Columbia University College of Physicians and Surgeons. Assistant Attending and Chief of Abortion Service, Harlem Hospital Center, New York, New York.
Abortion

IRVING BUTERMAN, M.D.

Fellow in Gynecologic Oncology, sponsored by the New York City Division of the American Cancer Society, Lenox Hill Hospital, New York, New York.
Cancer of the Uterus

HUGO A. CABRERA, PH.D.

Hospital Epidemiologist and Director of Microbiology, Mount Carmel Medical Center, Columbus, Ohio.
Gas Gangrene and Similar Anaerobic Soft Tissue Infections

DONALD B. CALNE, M.D.

National Institutes of Health, Bethesda, Maryland.
Parkinson's Disease

GUY D. CAMPBELL, M.D.

Professor of Medicine, University of Mississippi School of Medicine. Chief, Pulmonary Disease Service, Veterans Administration Hospital; Attending Physician, University Hospital, Jackson, Mississippi.
North American Blastomycosis

THOMAS J. CARLOW, M.D.

Assistant Professor of Neurology (Neuro-Ophthalmology), University of New Mexico School of Medicine. Chief, Neuro-Ophthalmology Section, Veterans Administration Hospital, Albuquerque, New Mexico.
Episodic Vertigo

WILLIAM A. CARO, M.D.

Associate Professor of Clinical Dermatology, Northwestern University Medical School. Attending Dermatologist, Northwestern Memorial Hospital, Chicago, Illinois.
Lichen Planus

THOMAS E. CARSON, M.D., F.A.C.P.

Assistant Clinical Professor, Louisiana State University. Captain, Medical Corps, U.S. Navy. Chief of Dermatology, Naval Regional Medical Center, New Orleans, Louisiana.
Chancroid

HUGO F. CARVAJAL, M.D.

Associate Professor of Pediatrics, University of Texas Medical Branch. Chief of Pediatrics, Shriners Burns Institute, Galveston, Texas.
Burns

FRED F. CASTROW II, M.D.

Clinical Associate Professor of Dermatology, University of Texas Medical School at Houston. Academic Chief of Dermatology, Department of Family Practice, Memorial Hospital System, Houston, Texas.
Hidradenitis Suppurativa

THOMAS A. CHAPEL, M.D.

Associate Professor of Dermatology, Wayne State University. Attending Staff, Detroit General, Harper-Grace, Hutzel, and Detroit Memorial Hospitals, Detroit, and Veterans Administration Hospital, Allen Park, Michigan.
Granuloma Inguinale; Lymphogranuloma Venereum

RONALD L. CHARD, JR., M.D.

Clinical Professor of Pediatrics, University of Washington School of Medicine. Associate Director, Hematology-Oncology Division, Children's Orthopedic Hospital and Medical Center; Clinical Associate Member, Fred Hutchinson Cancer Research Center, Seattle, Washington.
Acute Childhood Leukemia

NEIL S. CHERNIACK, M.D.

Professor of Internal Medicine and Director, Pulmonary Division, Case Western Reserve University School of Medicine. Attending Physician, Wade Park Veterans Administration Hospital and University Hospitals, Lakeside Division, Cleveland, Ohio.
Chronic Bronchitis and Emphysema

P. N. CHHUTTANI, M.D., F.A.M.S.

Professor of Internal Medicine, Postgraduate Institute of Medical Education and Research, Chandigarh. Consulting Physician, Nehru Hospital, Postgraduate Institute of Medical Education and Research, Chandigarh, India.
Amebiasis

TADEUSZ P. CHORZELSKI, M.D.

Professor of Dermatology, Department of Dermatology, Warsaw School of Medicine, Warsaw, Poland.
Pemphigus and Bullous Pemphigoid

HARRIS R. CLEARFIELD, M.D.

Professor of Medicine, Hahnemann Medical College. Director, Division of Gastroenterology, Hahnemann Hospital, Philadelphia, Pennsylvania.
Gaseousness

WILLIAM E. CLENDENNING, M.D.

Professor of Clinical Medicine (Dermatology), Dartmouth Medical School. Attending Dermatologist, Dartmouth-Hitchcock Medical Center, Hanover, New Hampshire.
Mycosis Fungoides

THEODORE COHEN, M.D.

Chief Resident, Obstetrics and Gynecology, St. Barnabas Medical Center, Livingston, New Jersey.
Vulvovaginitis

GEORGE F. COLLINS, M.B., CH.B., F.R.C.P.(C.)

Associate Professor, Department of Pediatrics, McGill University. Assistant Director, Department of Cardiology, The Montreal Children's Hospital, Montreal, Quebec, Canada.
Congenital Heart Disease

JOHN J. COLLINS, JR., M.D.

Professor of Surgery, Harvard Medical School. Chief, Division of Thoracic and Cardiac Surgery, Peter Bent Brigham Hospital, Boston, Massachusetts.
Acquired Diseases of the Aorta

MIGUEL COLÓN-MORALES, M.D.

Associate Professor, Clinical Anesthesiology, School of Medicine, University of Puerto Rico. Director, Department of Anesthesiology, Teachers Hospital, San Juan, Puerto Rico.
Obstetric Analgesia and Anesthesia

REX B. CONN, M.D.

Professor of Pathology and Laboratory Medicine, Emory University School of Medicine. Director of Clinical Laboratories, Emory University Hospital, Atlanta, Georgia.
Laboratory Reference Values of Clinical Importance

MARCEL E. CONRAD, M.D.

Professor of Medicine and Director, Division of Hematology and Oncology, University of Alabama in Birmingham. Hematologist and Oncologist, University of Alabama in Birmingham and Veterans Administration Hospital, Birmingham, Alabama.
Hemochromatosis and Hemosiderosis

ALLAN R. COOKE, M.D.

Professor of Medicine, Kansas University Medical Center. Director, Division of Gastroenterology, and Attending Physician, Kansas University Medical Center, Kansas City, Kansas, and Veterans Administration Hospital, Kansas City, Missouri.
Peptic Ulcer

BERNARD A. COOPER, M.D.

Professor of Medicine and Physiology, McGill University. Director, Haematology Division, Royal Victoria Hospital, Montreal, Quebec, Canada.
Pernicious Anemia and Other Forms of Vitamin B_{12} Deficiency

ROBERT J. CORLISS, M.D.

Associate Clinical Professor of Pediatrics, University of Wisconsin Medical School; Co-Director, Biodynamics Laboratory, University of Wisconsin. Chief of Cardiology, Madison General Hospital, Madison, Wisconsin.
Care and Rehabilitation After Myocardial Infarction

RAYMOND L. CORNELISON, JR., M.D.

Clinical Instructor, Department of Dermatology, University of Oklahoma School of Medicine. Attending Dermatologist, University Hospital, Oklahoma City, and Midwest City Memorial Hospital, Midwest City, Oklahoma.
Pityriasis Rosea

MALCOLM COX, M.D.

Assistant Professor of Medicine, University of Pennsylvania School of Medicine. Attending Physician, Philadelphia Veterans Administration Hospital and Hospital of the University of Pennsylvania, Philadelphia, Pennsylvania.
Diabetes Insipidus

TAKEY CRIST, M.D., F.A.C.O.G., F.A.C.S.

Clinical Assistant Professor, University of North Carolina. Obstetrics-Gynecology Department, Onslow Memorial Hospital, Jacksonville, North Carolina.
Postpartum Care

JANET CUTTNER, M.D.

Associate Professor of Medicine and Neoplastic Diseases, Mount Sinai School of Medicine, New York, New York.
Acute Leukemia in Adults

ANGELO E. DAGRADI, M.D.

Professor of Medicine, University of California, Irvine, School of Medicine. Chief, Gastroenterology Section, Veterans Administration Hospital, Long Beach, California.
Gastritis

DAVID C. DALE, M.D.

Associate Professor of Medicine, University of Washington School of Medicine. Attending Physician, University of Washington Hospital, Seattle, Washington.
Neutropenia

MABELLE DORA D'AMODIO, M.D.

Assistant Professor of Pediatrics, New York Medical College. Attending Physician, Metropolitan Hospital, New York, New York.
Normal Infant Feeding

GILBERT H. DANIELS, M.D.

Assistant Professor of Medicine, Harvard Medical School. Assistant Physician, Massachusetts General Hospital, Boston, Massachusetts.
Simple (Nontoxic) Goiter

STUART H. DANOVITCH, M.D.

Associate Clinical Professor of Medicine, George Washington School of Medicine. Attending Gastroenterologist, Veterans Administration Hospital and Washington Hospital Center; Consulting Gastroenterologist, National Children's Medical Center, Washington, D.C.
Acute Pancreatitis

CHARLES H. DART, JR., M.D.

Assistant Clinical Professor, Thoracic Surgery, UCLA Medical School. Chief of Cardiac Surgery, Community Memorial Hospital, Ventura; Chief of Surgery, Saint John's Hospital, Oxnard; Consultant, Wadsworth Veterans Administration Hospital, Los Angeles, California.
Cardiac Arrest

NAND S. DATTA, M.D., M.S., M.CH., F.A.C.S.

Associate Professor of Surgery/Urology, Charles R. Drew Postgraduate Medical School. Acting Chief, Division of Urology, Department of Surgery, Martin Luther King Jr. General Hospital, Los Angeles, California.
Trauma of the Genitourinary System

JEAN DAVIGNON, M.D., M.SC., F.R.C.P.(C.), F.A.C.P.

Professor of Medicine, University of Montreal Faculty of Medicine. Director, Department of Lipid Metabolism and Atherosclerosis Research, Clinical Research Institute of Montreal. Head, Section of Vascular Medicine, Hôtel-Dieu Hospital, Montreal, Quebec, Canada.
The Hyperlipoproteinemias

THOMAS R. DEETZ, M.D.

Instructor of Medicine, Program in Infectious Diseases and Microbiology, The University of Texas Medical School at Houston, Texas.
Rat-Bite Fever

MORGAN D. DELANEY, M.D.

Assistant Professor of Pulmonary Medicine, University of Miami School of Medicine, Miami, Florida.
Acute Respiratory Failure

NICHOLAS D. D'ESOPO, M.D.

Associate Clinical Professor, Yale University School of Medicine. Chief, Pulmonary Disease Section, Veterans Administration Hospital, West Haven, Connecticut.
Primary Lung Abscess

FRANK A. DISNEY, M.D.

Clinical Associate Professor of Pediatrics, University of Rochester School of Medicine. Senior Associate Pediatrician, Strong Memorial Hospital; Chief of Pediatrics Emeritus, Highland Hospital; Consultant Pediatrician, Genesee and Rochester General Hospitals, Rochester, New York.
Streptococcal Pharyngitis

NOBLE DOSS, JR., M.D.

Chief Resident in Obstetrics and Gynecology, Parkland Memorial Hospital, Dallas, Texas.
Toxemia of Pregnancy

GEORGE W. DRACH, M.D.

Professor of Surgery/Urology, University of Arizona. Chief of Urology, Arizona Health Sciences Center, Tucson, Arizona.
Prostatitis

H. BRUCE DULL, M.D., S.M.

Assistant Director for Program, Center for Disease Control. Clinical Associate Professor of Preventive Medicine and Community Health, Department of Preventive Medicine and Community Health, Emory University School of Medicine, Atlanta, Georgia.
Active Immunization for Infectious Diseases

W. CHRISTOPHER DUNCAN, M.D.

Associate Professor, Department of Dermatology, Baylor College of Medicine. Active Staff, The Methodist Hospital and Ben Taub General Hospital; Consultant Staff, Veterans Administration Hospital; Courtesy Staff, St. Luke's Episcopal Hospital, Texas Children's Hospital, Hermann Hospital, and Center Pavilion Hospital, Houston, Texas.
Diseases of the Nails

HENRY G. DUNN, M.B., F.R.C.P. (LOND.), F.R.C.P.(C.)

Professor and Head, Division of Neurology, Department of Paediatrics, University of British Columbia. Senior Active Staff and Head, Division of Paediatric Neurology, Vancouver General Hospital; Active Staff, Children's Hospital, Vancouver, British Columbia, Canada.
Epilepsy in Children

HERBERT L. DUPONT, M.D.

Professor and Director, Program in Infectious Diseases and Clinical Microbiology, The University of Texas Medical School at Houston. Infectious Disease Consultant to M. D. Anderson Hospital and Tumor Institute and St. Joseph Hospital, Houston, Texas.
Foodborne Illness

BRIAN G. M. DURIE, M.D.

Tucson, Arizona.
Multiple Myeloma

RICHARD M. EHRLICH, M.D.

Associate Professor of Surgery and Urology and Co-Chief, Renal Transplantation Service, UCLA School of Medicine. Co-Chief, Urology Division, Wadsworth Veterans Administration Hospital, Los Angeles, California.
Genitourinary Tuberculosis

HANS E. EINSTEIN, M.D.

Clinical Professor of Medicine, University of Southern California School of Medicine. Attending Physician, Memorial, Mercy, and San Joaquin Hospitals, Bakersfield, California.
Coccidioidomycosis

ARTHUR B. EISENBREY, M.D.

Chief of Neurosurgical Service, Children's Hospital of Michigan. Assistant Professor, Wayne State University School of Medicine, Detroit, Michigan.
Head Injuries in Children

JOHN W. ENSINCK, M.D.

Professor of Medicine, University of Washington School of Medicine. University of Washington Affiliated Hospitals, Seattle, Washington.
Reactive Hypoglycemia

WILLIAM L. EPSTEIN, M.D.

Professor, University of California, San Francisco, California.
Poison Ivy Dermatitis

RICHARD EVANS III, M.D., COL MC

Chief, Allergy–Clinical Immunology Service, and Chief, Clinical Investigation Service, Walter Reed Army Medical Center, Washington, D.C.
Allergic Reactions to Insect Stings

ANDREAS FANCONI, M.D.

Professor of Pediatrics, University of Zurich. Head of Pediatric Division, Cantonal Hospital, Winterthur, Switzerland.
Rickets and Osteomalacia

GUIDO FANCONI, M.D.

Honorary Professor of Pediatrics, University of Zurich, Switzerland.
Rickets and Osteomalacia

STEPHEN FLECK, M.D.

Professor of Psychiatry and Public Health, Yale University School of Medicine. Psychiatrist-in-Chief, Yale Psychiatric Institute; Psychiatrist-in-Chief, Connecticut Mental Health Center, New Haven, Connecticut.
Schizophrenia

ROBERT P. FOSNAUGH, M.D.

Adjunct Professor, Department of Dermatology, Wayne State University School of Medicine, Detroit, Michigan.
Herpes Gestationis; Papular Dermatitis of Pregnancy

FRANCIS F. FOUNTAIN, JR., M.D.

Clinical Associate Professor of Medicine, University of Tennessee Center for Health Sciences. Active Staff and Director of Pulmonary Function Laboratory, Methodist Hospital; Staff Physician, University of Tennessee Hospital, Memphis, Tennessee.
Histoplasmosis

IRVING H. FOX, M.D.

Assistant Professor of Biological Chemistry and Associate Professor of Internal Medicine, University of Michigan. Associate Director of the Clinical Research Unit and Attending Rheumatologist, University of Michigan Medical Center, Ann Arbor, Michigan.
Gout

RICHARD A. R. FRASER, M.D.

Associate Professor of Neurosurgery, Cornell University Medical College—New York Hospital. Attending Neurosurgeon, Cornell University Medical College, Memorial Sloan-Kettering Cancer Center, and Hospital for Special Surgery, New York, New York.
Brain Abscess

ROBERT P. FRIEDMAN, M.D.

Associate, Department of Medicine (Dermatology), University of Arizona College of Medicine. Teaching Staff, Tucson Medical Center; Staff, St. Mary's Hospital, St. Joseph's Hospital, and Kino Hospital, Tucson, Arizona.
Pediculosis

EDUARD G. FRIEDRICH, JR., M.D.

Associate Professor of Gynecology and Obstetrics, Medical College of Wisconsin. Director, Outpatient Facilities and Undergraduate Education, Department of Gynecology and Obstetrics, Milwaukee County Medical Complex, Milwaukee, Wisconsin.
Pelvic Inflammatory Disease

WESLEY FURSTE, M.D., F.A.C.S.

Clinical Professor of Surgery, Ohio State University, Columbus, Ohio.
Gas Gangrene and Similar Anaerobic Soft Tissue Infections

WILLIAM H. GAASCH, M.D.

Associate Professor of Medicine, Tufts University School of Medicine. Director, Cardiac Non-Invasive Laboratory, New England Medical Center Hospital, Boston, Massachusetts.
Pericarditis

JOHN T. GALAMBOS, M.D.

Professor of Medicine, Emory University School of Medicine, Atlanta, Georgia.
Cirrhosis

WESLEY K. GALEN, M.D.

Assistant Professor of Dermatology, Tulane University School of Medicine. Tulane Medical Center Hospital and Charity Hospital of New Orleans, Louisiana.
Neurodermatitis

WILSON V. GARRETT, M.D.

Fellow, Peripheral Vascular Surgery, University of Iowa Hospitals and Clinics, Iowa City, Iowa.
Degenerative Arterial Disease

ROBERT GELBER, M.D.

Assistant Clinical Professor of Medicine, University of California, San Francisco, School of Medicine. Chief, Infectious Disease Service, and Chief, Leprosy Pharmacology, United States Public Health Service Hospital, San Francisco, California.
Leprosy

RALPH A. GIANNELLA, M.D.

Associate Professor of Medicine, University of Kentucky School of Medicine. Chief, Gastroenterology Service, Veterans Administration Hospital; Attending Physician, Albert Chandler Medical Center and Veterans Administration Hospital, Lexington, Kentucky.
Acute Viral and Bacterial Dysenteries

JAMES E. GIBBONS, M.D., C.M., F.A.A.P., F.A.C.C.

Associate Professor, Department of Pediatrics, McGill University. Director, Department of Cardiology, The Montreal Children's Hospital, Montreal, Quebec, Canada.
Congenital Heart Disease

ROBERT J. GINSBERG, M.D., F.R.C.S.(C.)

Assistant Professor, Department of Surgery, University of Toronto. Head, Division of Thoracic Surgery, Toronto Western Hospital; Consultant Thoracic Surgeon, Princess Margaret Hospital, Toronto, Ontario, Canada.
Primary Lung Cancer

GERALD A. GLOWACKI, M.D.

Assistant Professor, Department of Obstetrics and Gynecology, Johns Hopkins University. Director, Department of Obstetrics and Gynecology, Franklin Square Hospital, Baltimore, Maryland.
Hemorrhage in Late Pregnancy

ALLAN GOLDBLATT, M.D.

Associate Professor of Pediatrics at the Massachusetts General Hospital, Harvard Medical School. Chief, Pediatric Cardiology, Pediatrician, Assistant Physician, and Assistant in Medicine, Massachusetts General Hospital, Boston, Massachusetts.
Rheumatic Fever

ALVIN F. GOLDFARB, M.D.

Clinical Professor of Obstetrics and Gynecology, University of Pennsylvania School of Medicine. Attending Obstetrician and Gynecologist, The Pennsylvania Hospital, Philadelphia, Pennsylvania.
Primary Dysmenorrhea

MARTIN G. GOLDNER, M.D., F.A.C.P.

Emeritus Professor of Medicine, State University of New York Medical Center at New York. Emeritus Director, Department of Medicine, Jewish Hospital and Medical Center, Brooklyn, New York.
Diabetes Mellitus in the Adult

LOREN E. GOLITZ, M.D.

Assistant Professor of Dermatology and Pathology, University of Colorado Medical School. Chief of Dermatology, Denver General Hospital, Denver, Colorado.
Lupus Erythematosus

JOSEPH H. GOODMAN, M.D.

Assistant Professor of Surgery, The Ohio State University. Attending Neurosurgeon, The Ohio State University Hospital; Provisional, Children's Hospital, Columbus, Ohio.
Acute Head Injuries

HARRY GRABSTALD, M.D.

Associate Professor of Urology, Cornell University Medical College. Attending Surgeon, Memorial Hospital, New York, New York.
Tumors of the Genitourinary Tract

LAMAN A. GRAY, SR., M.D.

Clinical Professor of Obstetrics and Gynecology, University of Louisville School of Medicine and University of Kentucky College of Medicine. Active Staff, Norton Hospital, Louisville, Kentucky.
Endometriosis

WILLIAM B. GREENOUGH III, M.D., F.A.C.P.

Scientific Director for Biomedical Sciences, Cholera Research Laboratory, Dacca, Bangladesh.
Cholera

ALFRED J. GRINDON, M.D.

Associate Professor of Pathology, Emory University School of Medicine. Director, Atlanta Regional Red Cross Blood Program; Pathologist, Grady Memorial Hospital, Atlanta, Georgia.
Untoward Reactions to Blood Transfusion

ROBERT P. GRUNINGER, M.D.

Associate Professor of Medicine and Microbiology, University of Massachusetts Medical School. Director, Division of Infectious Diseases. Saint Vincent Hospital, Worcester, Massachusetts.
Measles

BRUCE W. HALSTEAD, M.D.

Director, International Biotoxicological Center, World Life Research Institute, Colton, California.
Portuguese Man-of-War Stings

JOHN D. HAMILTON, M.D.

Associate Professor, Duke University Medical Center. Attending Physician, Veterans Administration Hospital, Durham, North Carolina.

Rocky Mountain Spotted Fever

CHARLES B. HAMMOND, M.D.

Associate Professor, Department of Obstetrics and Gynecology, Duke University Medical Center. Director, Reproductive Endocrinology Division, Durham, North Carolina.

Dysfunctional Uterine Bleeding

VIRGIL HANSON, M.D.

Professor of Pediatrics, University of Southern California School of Medicine. Head, Division of Rheumatology and Rehabilitation, Childrens Hospital of Los Angeles, Los Angeles, California.

Juvenile Rheumatoid Arthritis

DONALD R. HARKNESS, M.D.

Professor of Internal Medicine, University of Miami School of Medicine. Chief of Hematology, Veterans Administration Hospital, Miami, Florida.

Hemolytic Anemia—Nonimmune

JOHN R. HARTMANN, M.D.

Clinical Professor of Pediatrics, University of Washington School of Medicine. Director, Division of Hematology/Oncology, Children's Orthopedic Hospital and Medical Center; Associate Director for Extramural Affairs, Fred Hutchinson Cancer Research Center, Seattle, Washington.

Acute Childhood Leukemia

WILLIAM K. HASS, M.D.

Professor of Neurology, New York University School of Medicine. Attending Neurologist, University and Bellevue Hospitals; Consultant in Neurology, Veterans Administration Hospital, New York, New York.

Acute Ischemic Cardiovascular Disease

E. E. HEDBLOM, M.D.

Retired Captain, Medical Corps, U.S. Navy, Brunswick, Maine.

Disturbances Due to Cold

BEREL HELD, M.D.

Professor of Obstetrics and Gynecology, The University of Texas Medical School at Houston. Chief, Obstetrics and Gynecology Service, Hermann Hospital; Consultant in Gynecology, M. D. Anderson Hospital and Tumor Institute, Houston, Texas.

Antepartum Care

EVERETT D. HENDRICKS, M.D.

Active Staff, Yavapai Community Hospital; Urologic Consultant, Veterans Administration Hospital, Prescott, Arizona.

Benign Prostatic Hyperplasia

VICTOR HERBERT, M.D., J.D.

Professor and Vice-Chairman of Medicine, State University of New York Downstate Medical Center. Attending Physician, State University Hospital and Kings County Hospital, Brooklyn; Chief, Hematology and Nutrition Laboratory, Veterans Administration Hospital, Bronx, New York.

Scurvy

PABLO HERNANDEZ M, M.D.

Caracas, Venezuela.

Chronic Pancreatitis

JOHN H. HICKS, M.D.

Clinical Professor, Department of Dermatology, University of Miami School of Medicine. Attending, Jackson Memorial Hospital and Mercy Hospital, Miami, Florida.

Creeping Eruption

LADISLAV P. HINTERBUCHNER, M.D.

Clinical Professor of Neurology, State University of New York Downstate Medical Center. Neurologist-in-Chief, The Brooklyn and Cumberland Hospitals, Brooklyn, New York.

Idiopathic Peripheral Facial Paralysis

JULIAN T. HOFF, M.D.

Associate Professor of Neurological Surgery, University of California, San Francisco. Active Attending and Chief of Service, H. C. Moffitt Hospital, San Francisco, California.

Intracerebral Hemorrhage

FREDERICK J. HOFMEISTER, M.D., F.A.C.O.G.

Clinical Professor of Gynecology and Obstetrics, Medical College of Wisconsin. Attending Staff, Department of Obstetrics and Gynecology, Lutheran Hospital of Milwaukee, Milwaukee County General Hospital, and Elmbrook Memorial Hospital; Consulting Staff, West Allis Memorial Hospital, Wisconsin.

Toxemia of Pregnancy

FRANK M. HOWARD, JR., M.D.

Associate Professor of Neurology, Mayo Medical School. Attending Neurologist, Rochester Methodist and St. Marys Hospitals, Rochester, Minnesota.

Myasthenia Gravis

CLARK HUFF, M.D.

Assistant Professor of Dermatology, University of Colorado School of Medicine, Denver, Colorado.

Dermatomyositis-Polymyositis

JAMES M. HUGHES, M.D.

Fellow, Division of Infectious Diseases, University of Virginia School of Medicine, Charlottesville, Virginia.

Bacterial Meningitis

MICHAEL HUME, M.D.

Professor of Surgery, Tufts University School of Medicine. Chief of Surgical Services, Lemuel Shattuck Hospital, Boston, Massachusetts.

Massive Thrombophlebitis of the Lower Extremities

WILLIAM E. HUNT, M.D.

Professor of Surgery, The Ohio State University. Attending Neurosurgeon, The Ohio State University Hospital; Affiliated Teaching, Riverside Methodist Hospital; Consulting, St. Anthony's Hospital and Children's Hospital, Columbus, Ohio.

Acute Head Injuries

SIDNEY HURWITZ, M.D.

Associate Clinical Professor of Pediatrics and Dermatology, Yale University School of Medicine. Attending Physician in Pediatrics and Dermatology, Yale–New Haven Medical Center; Hospital of St. Raphael, New Haven, Connecticut.

Bacterial Infections of the Skin

PETER ERIC HUTCHINSON, M.B., M.R.C.P.

Consultant Dermatologist, Leicester Royal Infirmary and Leicester General Hospital, Leicester, England.

Alopecia

STEFANIA JABLONSKA, M.D.

Professor of Dermatology, Department of Dermatology, Warsaw School of Medicine, Warsaw, Poland.

Pemphigus and Bullous Pemphigoid

ELIZABETH J. JAMES, M.D.

Associate Professor, Departments of Child Health and Obstetrics-Gynecology, University of Missouri. Director of Perinatal Medicine, University of Missouri Medical Center, Columbia, Missouri.

Resuscitation of the Newborn

MICHAEL JARRATT, M.D.

Associate Professor, Department of Dermatology, Baylor College of Medicine. The Methodist Texas Children's, St. Luke's Episcopal, Ben Taub General, and Veterans Administration Hospitals, Houston, Texas.

Herpes Simplex

ROBERT L. JETTON, M.D.

Greenville County Hospital System Affiliated Hospitals. Chief of Dermatology, St. Francis Community Hospital, Greenville, South Carolina.

Precancerous Lesions of the Skin and Mucous Membranes

WILLIAM R. JEWELL, M.D.

Professor of Surgery and Assistant Dean, College of Medicine, University of Kansas Medical Center. Consultant in Surgery, Veterans Administration Hospital, Kansas City, Missouri.

Diseases of the Breast

F. LEONARD JOHNSON, M.B., B.S.

Assistant Professor, Pediatrics, University of Washington. Staff Physician in Hematology/Oncology, Children's Orthopedic Hospital; Assistant Member, Fred Hutchinson Cancer Research Center, Seattle, Washington.

Acute Childhood Leukemia

THEODORE L. JOHNSON, M.D.

Clinical Associate Professor of Medicine, University of Minnesota School of Medicine. Attending Physician, The Duluth Clinic and Miller-Dwan, St. Mary's, and St. Luke's Hospitals, Duluth, Minnesota.

Chronic Renal Failure

RONALD C. JONES, M.D.

Professor of Surgery, The University of Texas Health Science Center at Dallas. Attending General Surgeon, Parkland Memorial Hospital, Children's Medical Center, and Presbyterian Hospital at Dallas, Dallas, Texas.

Rabies

THOMAS C. JONES, M.D.

Associate Professor of Medicine and Public Health, Cornell Medical College. Associate Attending Physician, Division of Infectious Diseases, The New York Hospital, New York, New York.

Trichinellosis

FREDERIC ROSS KAHL, M.D.

Assistant Professor of Medicine, Bowman Gray School of Medicine of Wake Forest University. Attending Cardiologist, North Carolina Baptist Hospital, Winston-Salem, North Carolina.

Tachycardia

RAJYALAKSHMI KAKARLA, M.D.

Chief Resident in Obstetrics and Gynecology, Lenox Hill Hospital, New York, New York.

Cancer of the Uterus

ALAN L. KAPLAN, M.D.

Associate Professor, Baylor College of Medicine. Attending, Methodist, St. Luke's, Texas Children's, Diagnostic Center, and Veterans Administration Hospitals, Houston, Texas.

Thrombophlebitis

GEORGE W. KAPLAN, M.D., M.S., F.A.A.P., F.A.C.S.

Associate Clinical Professor of Surgery, University of California at San Diego. Chief, Pediatric Urology, University of California at San Diego; Chief of Urology, Children's Hospital, San Diego, California.

Bacterial Infections of the Urinary Tract (Female Children)

KAREN L. KAPLAN, M.D., PH.D.

Assistant Professor of Medicine, Columbia University

College of Physicians and Surgeons. Assistant Attending Physician, Presbyterian Hospital, New York, New York.
Disseminated Intravascular Coagulation

HARRY IRVING KATZ, M.D.

Clinical Associate Professor, Department of Dermatology, University of Minnesota.
Dermatitis Herpetiformis

WILLIAM N. KELLEY, M.D.

Professor and Chairman, Department of Internal Medicine, University of Michigan Medical School. Professor of Biological Chemistry, University of Michigan Medical School, Ann Arbor, Michigan.
Gout

WILLIAM A. KELLY, M.D.

Professor, Department of Neurologic Surgery, University of Washington School of Medicine. Attending Physician, University Hospital, Veterans Administration Hospital, and Harborview Medical Center, Seattle, Washington.
Brain Tumors

STEVEN G. KELSEN, M.D.

Assistant Professor of Internal Medicine and Director, Pulmonary Division Fellowship Training Program, Case Western Reserve University School of Medicine. Attending Physician, University Hospitals–Lakeside Division, and Veterans Administration Hospital, Cleveland, Ohio.
Chronic Bronchitis and Emphysema

JOHN A. KENNEY, JR., M.D.

Professor and Chairman, Department of Dermatology, Howard University College of Medicine. Chief of Dermatology, Howard University Hospital; Attending Staff, Children's Hospital National Medical Center, Veterans Administration Hospital of Washington, and District of Columbia General Hospital of Washington; Consultant Staff, Washington Hospital Center; Consultant in Dermatology, U.S. Department of State, Washington, D.C.
Pigmentary Disturbances

GERALD T. KEUSCH, M.D.

Professor of Medicine, Mt. Sinai School of Medicine. Attending Physician, Mt. Sinai Hospital, New York, New York.
Bacillary Dysentery

MOHAMMED Y. KHAN, M.D., PH.D., F.R.C.P.(C.)

Assistant Professor of Internal Medicine, University of Minnesota School of Medicine. Director, Infectious Disease Section, Hennepin County Medical Center, Minneapolis, Minnesota.
Brucellosis

LOWELL R. KING, M.D.

Professor of Urology and Surgery, Northwestern University Medical School. Active Attending Urologist, Surgeon-in-Chief, The Children's Memorial Hospital; Attending Urologist, Northwestern Memorial and Columbus Hospitals, Chicago, Illinois.
Childhood Enuresis

C. THOMAS KISKER, M.D.

Associate Professor, University of Iowa College of Medicine, Department of Pediatrics. Chief, Division of Hematology-Oncology, University of Iowa Hospitals, Iowa City, Iowa.
Vitamin K Deficiency

CARL M. KJELLSTRAND, M.D.

Professor of Medicine and Surgery, University of Minnesota School of Medicine. Chief, Division of Nephrology, University of Minnesota Hospital, Minneapolis, Minnesota.
Chronic Renal Failure

HAROLD L. KLAWANS, M.D.

Professor, Rush University. Associate Chairman, Department of Neurological Sciences, Rush–Presbyterian–St. Luke's Medical Center, Chicago, Illinois.
Parkinson's Disease

RAYMOND S. KOFF, M.D.

Associate Professor of Medicine, Boston University School of Medicine. Chief, Hepatology Section, Veterans Administration Hospital and Boston University Medical Center, Boston, Massachusetts.
Acute Viral Hepatitis

MICHAEL K. KOWALSKI, M.D., MAJ, MC

Fellow, Gynecologic Oncology Service, Department of Obstetrics and Gynecology, Walter Reed Army Medical Center, Washington, D.C.
Preoperative and Postoperative Care for Elective Gynecology Surgery

FRANKLIN KOZIN, M.D.

Assistant Professor of Medicine, The Medical College of Wisconsin. Milwaukee County Medical Complex, Milwaukee, Wisconsin.
Ankylosing Spondylitis

DOROTHY T. KRIEGER, M.D.

Professor of Medicine, Mount Sinai School of Medicine. Attending in Medicine and Director, Division of Endocrinology and Metabolism, Mount Sinai Hospital, New York, New York.
Cushing's Syndrome

NEIL A. KURTZMAN, M.D.

Professor of Medicine, University of Illinois Abraham Lincoln School of Medicine; Professor of Physiology, University of Illinois School of Basic Medical Sciences. Chief, Section of Nephrology, University of Illinois Hospital, Chicago, Illinois.
Parenteral Nutrition in Adults

JOEL M. LAMON, M.D.

Investigator, Metabolism Branch, National Cancer Institute, National Institutes of Health, Bethesda, Maryland.
The Porphyrias

JOHN H. LARAGH, M.D.

Hilda Altschul Master Professor of Medicine, The New York Hospital–Cornell Medical Center. Director of Cardiovascular Center and Chief, Department of Cardiology, Department of Medicine, New York Hospital, New York, New York.
Hypertension

JOHN C. LaROSA, M.D.

Associate Professor of Medicine and Director, Lipid Research Clinic, George Washington University Medical Center, Washington, D.C.
Xanthomas

P. REED LARSEN, M.D.

Associate Professor of Medicine, Harvard Medical School. Investigator, Howard Hughes Medical Institute; Head, Thyroid Unit, and Senior Associate in Medicine, Peter Bent Brigham Hospital, Boston, Massachusetts.
Hyperthyroidism

WALTER G. LARSEN, M.D.

Associate Clinical Professor of Dermatology, University of Oregon Medical School, Portland, Oregon.
Inflammatory Eruptions of the Hands and Feet

DUANE L. LARSON, M.D., F.A.C.S.

Professor of Surgery, Plastic and Maxillofacial, University of Texas Medical Branch. Galveston. Chief of Staff, Shriners Burns Institute, Galveston, Texas.
Burns

DAVID H. LAW, M.D.

Professor of Medicine, University of New Mexico School of Medicine. Chief, Medical Service, Veterans Administration Hospital, Albuquerque, New Mexico.
Crohn's Disease

GLEN A. LEHMAN, M.D.

Assistant Professor of Medicine, Indiana University School of Medicine, Indianapolis, Indiana.
Tumors of the Colon and Rectum

JOHN M. LEONARD, M.D.

Assistant Professor, University of Washington. Chief of Medicine, U.S. Public Health Service Hospital, Seattle; Attending Physician, University Hospital, Seattle, Washington.
Hypopituitarism

RICHARD LEONARDS, M.D.

Assistant Clinical Professor, Pediatrics, University of California School of Medicine, San Francisco. Hospital Epidemiologist, Children's Hospital, San Francisco, California.
Diphtheria

KENNETH B. LEWIS, M.D.

Assistant Professor of Medicine, The Johns Hopkins University. Chairman, Department of Medicine, Franklin Square Hospital, Baltimore, Maryland.
Heart Block

S. M. LEWIS, M.D., F.R.C.Path.

Reader in Haematology, Royal Postgraduate Medical School, London. Consultant Haematologist, Hammersmith Hospital, London, England.
Aplastic Anemia

JAMES J. LEYDEN, M.D.

Assistant Professor of Dermatology, University of Pennsylvania School of Medicine. Chief of Dermatology Clinic, University of Pennsylvania, Philadelphia, Pennsylvania.
Atopic Dermatitis

ROBERT W. LIGHTFOOT, Jr., M.D.

Associate Professor of Medicine, Medical College of Wisconsin. Associate Attending Physician, Milwaukee County Medical Complex; Chief, Rheumatology Service, Wood Veterans Administration Hospital, Milwaukee, Wisconsin.
Osteoarthritis

KARL A. LOFGREN, M.D., M.S. (Surgery)

Associate Professor of Surgery, Mayo Medical School. Head, Section of Peripheral Vein Surgery, Mayo Clinic and Mayo Foundation, Rochester, Minnesota.
Primary Varicose Veins

GERALD LOGUE, M.D.

Assistant Professor, Duke University School of Medicine. Chief, Hematology, Veterans Administration Hospital, Durham, North Carolina.
Hemolytic Anemia—Immune

CHARLES M. LUETJE, M.D., F.A.C.S.

Assistant Professor of Surgery, Otolaryngology Service, University of Missouri. Attending Staff, Otology and Neuro-Otology, Trinity Lutheran, St. Mary's, St. Luke's, Truman Medical Center, and St. Joseph Hospitals, Kansas City, Missouri.
Meniere's Disease

JOHN C. MAIZE, M.D.

Associate Professor of Dermatology, State University of New York at Buffalo. Assistant Attending Dermatologist, Buffalo General Hospital, Buffalo, New York.
Stasis Dermatitis and Ulcers

PHILIP W. MAJERUS, M.D.

Professor of Medicine and Biochemistry, Washington University School of Medicine, St. Louis, Missouri.
Bleeding Disorders Secondary to Platelet Abnormalities

DENNIS G. MAKI, M.D.

Assistant Professor of Medicine, University of Wisconsin. Chief, Infectious Disease Unit, and Ovid O. Meyer Scholar in Medicine, University of Wisconsin Hospitals, Madison, Wisconsin.
Q Fever

DOMENICO J. MANZONE, M.D.

Instructor, Department of Urology, Northwestern University Medical School, Chicago, Illinois.
Childhood Enuresis

ELLIOTT M. MARCUS, M.D.

Professor of Neurology, University of Massachusetts School of Medicine; Lecturer in Neurology, Tufts University School of Medicine. Director, Division of Neurology, St. Vincent Hospital, Worcester, Massachusetts.
Multiple Sclerosis

MERVILLE C. MARSHALL, Jr., M.D.

Clinical Associate, Clinical Endocrinology Branch, National Institute of Arthritis, Metabolism, and Digestive Diseases, National Institutes of Health, Bethesda, Maryland.
Hypothyroidism

DEAN T. MASON, M.D.

Professor of Medicine, Professor of Physiology, and Chief, Cardiovascular Medicine, University of California at Davis School of Medicine and Sacramento Medical Center, Davis and Sacramento, California. President, American College of Cardiology.
Congestive Heart Failure

DONALD MASSARO, M.D.

Sertel Professor of Pulmonary Medicine, University of Miami School of Medicine, Miami, Florida. Medical Investigator, Veterans Administration.
Acute Respiratory Failure

WILLIAM D. MATTERN, M.D.

Associate Professor of Medicine, University of North Carolina. Medical Director, Dialysis Program, North Carolina Memorial Hospital, Chapel Hill, North Carolina.
Acute Renal Failure

WILLIAM McBRIDE, M.D., F.R.C.O.G.

Lecturer in Obstetrics, Universities of Sydney and New South Wales. Senior Obstetrician and Gynaecologist, The Women's Hospital, Sydney, Australia.
Rubella

DONALD S. McLAREN, M.D., Ph.D., D.T.M.&H.

Reader in Physiology, University Medical School, Edinburgh, Scotland.
Beriberi

CHARLES K. McSHERRY, M.D.

Professor of Surgery, Mount Sinai School of Medicine. Director of Surgery, Beth Israel Medical Center, New York, New York.
Cholecystitis and Cholelithiasis

THOMAS A. MEDSGER, Jr., M.D.

Associate Professor of Medicine, University of Pittsburgh School of Medicine. Attending Rheumatologist, University of Pittsburgh, Presbyterian-University, and Veterans Administration Hospitals, Pittsburgh, Pennsylvania.
Bursitis and Calcific Tendinitis

JAMES C. MELBY, M.D.

Professor of Medicine, Boston University School of Medicine. Head, Section of Endocrinology and Metabolism, University Hospital, Boston, Massachusetts.
Adrenal Insufficiency

ROBERT S. MENDELSOHN, M.D.

Associate Professor, Department of Community Health and Preventive Medicine, Abraham Lincoln School of Medicine, University of Illinois. Attending Physician, Michael Reese Hospital, Chicago; Attending Physician, Saint Francis Hospital, Evanston, Illinois.
Care of the Low Birth Weight Infant

ROSCOE E. MILLER, M.D.

Distinguished Professor of Radiology and Chief of Gastrointestinal Radiology, Indiana University School of Medicine, Indianapolis, Indiana.
Tumors of the Colon and Rectum

BERNADETTE MODELL, Ph.D., M.B.B.Chir.

Honorary Lecturer in Paediatrics, University College Hospital Medical School, London, England.
Thalassemia

WILLIAM J. MOGABGAB, M.D.

Professor of Medicine, Tulane University School of Medicine. Consultant, Charity Hospital of Louisiana at New Orleans; Consultant in Infectious Disease, Veterans Administration Hospital, New Orleans, Louisiana.
Epidemic Influenza

ROYAL M. MONTGOMERY, M.D.

Consulting Dermatologist, Hospital for Special Surgery and Roosevelt Hospital; Director of Dermatology, St. Johns Queens Hospital, New York, New York.
Warts

MELVIN R. MOORE, M.D.

Associate Professor of Medicine, Emory University School of Medicine. Director of the Interdepartmental Oncology Ward, Grady Memorial Hospital, Atlanta, Georgia.
Non-Hodgkin's Lymphomas

ALEJANDRO MORALES, M.D.

Staff Physician, Henry Ford Hospital, Detroit, Michigan.
Scabies

KENNETH M. MOSER, M.D.

Professor of Medicine, University of California, San Diego, School of Medicine. Director, Pulmonary Division, University of California, San Diego, Medical Center Hospitals, San Diego, California.
Pulmonary Embolism

MAURICE A. MUFSON, M.D.

Professor of Medicine, Marshall University School of Medicine. Associate Chief of Staff for Research, Veterans Administration Hospital; Associate Attending Physician, Cabell Huntington and St. Mary's Hospital, Huntington, West Virginia.
Viral Respiratory Infections

SIGFRID A. MULLER, M.D., F.A.C.P.

Professor of Dermatology, Mayo Medical School. Consultant, Department of Dermatology, Mayo Clinic and Mayo Foundation, Rochester, Minnesota.
Psoriasis

R. RICHARD MURRAY, M.D.

Assistant Professor, Department of Obstetrics and Gynecology, University of New Mexico School of Medicine. Active Staff, Bernalillo County Medical Center; Consultant, Presbyterian Hospital, Albuquerque, New Mexico.
Uterine Myomas

ALLEN R. MYERS, M.D.

Associate Professor of Medicine, University of Pennsylvania School of Medicine, Philadelphia, Pennsylvania.
Scleroderma

HYMIE L. NOSSEL, CH.B., D.PHIL.

Professor of Medicine, Columbia University College of Physicians and Surgeons. Attending Physician, Presbyterian Hospital, New York, New York.
Disseminated Intravascular Coagulation

G. ROBERT NUGENT, M.D.

Professor of Surgery and Chairman, Division of Neurosurgery, West Virginia University Medical Center, Morgantown, West Virginia.
Trigeminal and Glossopharyngeal Neuralgia

RICHARD H. OI, M.D.

Assistant Professor, Obstetrics and Gynecology, University of California, Davis, School of Medicine, Davis, California.
The Menopause

DAVID ORIEL, M.D.

Honorary Senior Lecturer in Venereology, University College Hospital Medical School. Director, Department of Genito-urinary Medicine, University College Hospital, London, England.
Nongonococcal Urethritis

ROBERT A. O'ROURKE, M.D.

Professor of Medicine and Chief, Division of Cardiology, The University of Texas Health Science Center at San Antonio. Attending Cardiologist, Bexar County Hospital and Audie L. Murphy Memorial Veterans Administration Hospital, San Antonio, Texas.
Atrial Fibrillation

LUIS F. OSPINA, M.D.

Senior Fellow in Endocrinology, U.S. Public Health Service Hospital and University of Washington, Seattle, Washington.
Hypopituitarism

CHARLES N. OSTER, M.D.

Principal Investigator, Rickettsiology Division, U.S. Army Medical Research Institute of Infectious Diseases, Ft. Detrick, Maryland.
Tularemia

LAFAYETTE G. OWEN, M.D.

Executive Director, Dermatology, and Associate in Pathology, University of Louisville School of Medicine, Louisville, Kentucky.
Drug Eruptions

EDDY D. PALMER, M.D.

Clinical Professor of Medicine, New Jersey School of Medicine. Attending, Hackettstown Community Hospital, Hackettstown, New Jersey.
Constipation

ROBERT C. PARK, M.D., COL, MC

Chief, Gynecologic Oncology Service, Department of Obstetrics and Gynecology, Walter Reed Army Medical Center, Washington, D.C.
Preoperative and Postoperative Care for Elective Gynecology Surgery

DONALD H. PARKS, M.D., F.R.C.S.(C.)

Assistant Professor of Surgery, Division of Plastic Surgery, University of Texas Medical Branch, Galveston. Chief of Surgery, Shriners Burns Institute, Galveston, Texas.
Burns

JOHN A. PARRISH, M.D.

Associate Professor of Dermatology, Harvard Medical School. Assistant Dermatologist, Massachusetts General Hospital, Boston, Massachusetts.
Photosensitivity and Sunburn

ROBERT L. PEAKE, M.D.

Associate Professor of Medicine, University of Texas Medical Branch at Galveston. Attending Endocrinologist, University of Texas Medical Branch at Galveston, Texas.
Thyroiditis

PETER L. PERINE, M.D.

Venereal Disease Control Division, Bureau of State Services, Center for Disease Control, Public Health Service, Department of Health, Education, and Welfare, Atlanta, Georgia.
Gonorrhea

ROBERT L. PERKINS, M.D.

Professor of Medicine and Medical Microbiology, School of Medicine, The Ohio State University. Attending Physician and Director, Division of Infectious Diseases, University Hospitals, Columbus, Ohio.
Mumps

M. L. PERNOLL, M.D.

Associate Professor, Department of Obstetrics and Gynecology, and Head, Division of Perinatal Medicine, University of Oregon Health Sciences Center, Portland, Oregon.
Ectopic Pregnancy

J. L. PIPKIN, M.D.

Clinical Professor of Dermatology, University of Texas Medical School. Consultant, Department of Dermatology, Brooke General Hospital, Fort Sam Houston; Chief of Dermatology and Syphilology Service, Robert B. Green Memorial Hospital; Director of Dermatological Clinics, City County Hospital, Robert B. Green Memorial Hospital, University of Texas Medical School, San Antonio, Texas.
Keloids

RONALD L. PITTS, M.D.

Assistant Professor, University of Kansas, Department of Internal Medicine, Kansas City. Staff, Shawnee Mission Hospital, Shawnee Mission, Kansas.
Herpes Zoster

ROBERT T. PLUMB, M.D.

Associate Clinical Professor, University of California, San Diego. Chief of Urology, Sharp Hospital, San Diego, and Coronado Hospital, Coronado; Senior Staff, Mercy and University Hospitals, San Diego, California.
Balanitis and Balanoposthitis

KENNETH A. POPIO, M.D.

Assistant Professor of Medicine, University of Rochester School of Medicine and Dentistry. Co-Director of Cardiac Catheterization Laboratory and Associate Physician, Strong Memorial Hospital, Rochester, New York.
Angina Pectoris

JOSEPH L. POTTER, M.D., PH.D.

Adjunct Professor of Biology, The University of Akron. Director of Biochemistry, The Children's Hospital Medical Center of Akron, Akron, Ohio.
Mucopurulent Bronchitis and Emphysema

DARLEEN F. POWARS, M.D.

Associate Professor of Pediatrics, University of Southern California School of Medicine. Attending, Pediatric Hematology-Oncology, Los Angeles County–USC Medical Center, Los Angeles; Consultant, Pediatric Hematology-Oncology, Long Beach Childrens Hospital, Long Beach, White Memorial Medical Center, Los Angeles, and Huntington Hospital, Pasadena, California.
Sickle Cell Disease

STEVEN EARL PRAWER, M.D.

Clinical Assistant Professor, University of Minnesota, Department of Dermatology, Minneapolis, Minnesota.
Dermatitis Herpetiformis

LEONARD R. PROSNITZ, M.D.

Associate Professor of Therapeutic Radiology, Yale University School of Medicine. Attending Physician, Yale–New Haven Hospital, New Haven, Veterans Administration Hospital, West Haven, and Uncas-on-Thames Hospital, Norwich, Connecticut.
Hodgkin's Disease: Radiation Therapy

KANTI R. RAI, M.D.

Associate Professor of Medicine, School of Medicine, Health Sciences Center, State University of New York at Stony Brook. Attending Hematologist-Oncologist, Long Island Jewish–Hillside Medical Center, New Hyde Park, New York.
The Chronic Leukemias

RAYMOND V. RANDALL, M.D., M.S. (MED.), F.A.C.P.

Senior Consultant, Mayo Clinic, and Professor of Medicine, Mayo Medical School. Consultant in Internal Medicine and Endocrinology, Rochester Methodist Hospital and St. Mary's Hospital, Rochester, Minnesota.
Acromegaly

NEIL H. RASKIN, M.D.

Associate Professor of Neurology, University of California School of Medicine, San Francisco. Attending Physician, University of California Hospitals (Moffitt, San Francisco General, Veterans Administration), San Francisco, California.
Headache

AARON R. RAUSEN, M.D.

Professor of Pediatrics, Mount Sinai School of Medicine of the City University of New York. Director of Pediatrics, Beth Israel Medical Center; Attending Pediatrician, Mount Sinai Hospital, New York, New York.
Hemolytic Disease of the Newborn

SHLOMO RAZ, M.D.

Assistant Professor, Surgery/Urology, UCLA Center for the Health Sciences. Co-Chief, Urology Service, Veterans Administration Hospital, Sepulveda, California.
Urethral Strictures

REES B. REES, M.D.

Clinical Professor of Dermatology, University of California, San Francisco. Consultant, Letterman Army Medical Center, Shriners Hospital for Crippled Children, St. Luke's Hospital and Mount Zion Hospital and Medical Center, San Francisco, California.
Pruritus Ani and Vulvae

CHARLES M. REEVE, D.D.S., M.S. (DENTAL SURGERY)

Assistant Professor of Dentistry, Mayo Medical School. Consultant, Department of Dentistry, Mayo Clinic and Mayo Foundation, Rochester, Minnesota.
Disorders of the Mouth (Benign)

RICHARD B. RESNICK, M.D.

Associate Professor, Department of Psychiatry, New York Medical College. Attending Psychiatrist and Director, Division of Drug Abuse Research and Treatment, New York Medical College, Flower and Fifth Avenue Hospitals, New York, New York.
Narcotic Poisoning

ARTHUR C. RESSMANN, M.D.

Clinical Associate Professor, The University of Texas Health Science Center. Consultant, Brooke Army Medical Center, Fort Sam Houston, Texas.
Keloids

RONALD J. RESSMANN, M.D.

San Antonio, Texas.
Keloids

TELFER B. REYNOLDS, M.D.

Professor of Medicine, University of Southern California School of Medicine. Chief, Hepatology Section, Los Angeles County–University of Southern California Medical Center, Los Angeles, California.
Bleeding Esophageal Varices

JEROME P. RICHIE, M.D.

Assistant Professor, Harvard Medical School. Chief of Urologic Oncology, Peter Bent Brigham Hospital; Consultant, Sidney Farber Cancer Institute, Boston, Massachusetts.
Epididymitis

KARL H. RIECKMANN, M.D., D.P.H.

Director, Malaria Research Program, University of New Mexico, Albuquerque, New Mexico.
Malaria

HARRIS D. RILEY, JR., M.D.

Distinguished Professor of Pediatrics, University of Oklahoma College of Medicine. Chief, Children's Memorial Hospital, University of Oklahoma Health Sciences Center, Oklahoma City, Oklahoma.
Whooping Cough

JOSEPH A. RINALDO, JR., M.D.

Clinical Assistant Professor of Medicine, Wayne State University School of Medicine. Medical Director, Providence Hospital, Southfield, Michigan.
Dysphagia and Esophageal Obstruction

GRANT V. RODKEY, M.D.

Associate Clinical Professor of Surgery, Harvard Medical School. Visiting Surgeon, Massachusetts General Hospital, Boston, Massachusetts.
Diverticula of the Alimentary Canal

ROY S. ROGERS III, M.D., M.S. (DERMATOLOGY)

Assistant Professor of Dermatology, Mayo Medical School. Consultant, Department of Dermatology, Mayo Clinic and Mayo Foundation, Rochester, Minnesota.
Disorders of the Mouth (Benign)

RICHARD E. ROSENFIELD, M.D.

Professor of Pathology, Mount Sinai School of Medicine, of the City University of New York. Director, Department of Blood Bank and Clinical Microscopy, Mount Sinai Hospital, New York, New York.
Hemolytic Disease of the Newborn

ROBERT H. RUBIN, M.D.

Assistant Professor of Medicine, Harvard Medical School. Assistant Physician, Infectious Disease Unit, Massachusetts General Hospital, Boston, Massachusetts.
Salmonellosis (Other Than Typhoid Fever)

ANDREW H. RUDOLPH, M.D.

Associate Professor, Department of Dermatology, Baylor College of Medicine. Chief of Dermatology, Houston Veterans Administration Hospital; Staff, Ben Taub General, Jefferson Davis, Methodist, St. Luke's Episcopal, Texas Children's, and Hermann Hospitals, Houston, Texas.
Superficial Fungus Infections of the Skin

CLARENCE E. RUPE, M.D., F.A.C.P.

Associate Professor, Clinical Faculty, Wayne State University School of Medicine. Chief of Medicine, St. John Hospital, Detroit, Michigan.
Polyarteritis

THOMAS J. RUSSELL, M.D.

Associate Clinical Professor of Dermatology, The Medical College of Wisconsin. Chief of Dermatology, Milwaukee County General Hospital, Milwaukee, Wisconsin.
Rosacea

JOHN F. RYAN, M.D.

Associate Professor of Anaesthesia, Harvard Medical School. Director, Pediatric Anesthesia, Massachusetts General Hospital, Boston, Massachusetts.
Disturbances Due to Heat

HUSSAIN I. SABA, M.D., PH.D.

Assistant Professor of Medicine, College of Medicine, University of South Florida. Attending Hematologist, Veterans Administration Hospital and Tampa General Hospital, Tampa, Florida.
Hemophilia and Allied Conditions

LESTER B. SALANS, M.D.

Associate Professor of Medicine, Dartmouth–Hitchcock Medical Center, Hanover, New Hampshire. Associate Director for Diabetes, Endocrine, and Metabolic Diseases, National Institute of Arthritis, Metabolism, and Digestive Diseases, National Institutes of Health, Bethesda, Maryland.
Obesity

RALPH B. SAMSON, M.D.

Director, Colon and Rectal Residency Program, Grant Hospital, Columbus; Attending, Grant Hospital and Mount Carmel Medical Center, Columbus, Ohio.
Hemorrhoids, Anal Fissure, and Anal Fistula

MERLE A. SANDE, M.D.

Associate Professor of Medicine, Division of Infectious Diseases, University of Virginia School of Medicine. Vice Chairman, Department of Medicine, Charlottesville, Virginia.
Infective Endocarditis

W. EUGENE SANDERS, JR., M.D.

Professor and Chairman, Department of Medical Microbiology, and Professor of Medicine, Creighton University School of Medicine. Attending Physician, Creighton Memorial–St. Josephs and Veterans Administration Hospitals, Omaha, Nebraska.
Relapsing Fever

WILLIAM R. SANDUSKY, M.D.

C. Bruce Morton II Professor of Surgery, University of Virginia School of Medicine. Surgeon, University of Virginia Hospital, Charlottesville, Virginia.
Tetanus

ARTHUR SAWITSKY, M.D.

Professor of Medicine and Clinical Pathology, Schools of of Medicine and Basic Sciences, Health Sciences Center, State University of New York at Stony Brook. Director of Cancer Programs and Chief of Hematology-Oncology, Long Island Jewish–Hillside Medical Center, New Hyde Park, New York.
The Chronic Leukemias

C. GLENN SAWYER, M.D.

Professor of Medicine and Director, Section of Cardiology, Bowman Gray School of Medicine of Wake Forest University. Attending Cardiologist, North Carolina Baptist Hospital, Winston-Salem, North Carolina.
Tachycardia

SAM T. SCALING, M.D.

Chief Resident, Obstetrics and Gynecology, Baylor College of Medicine and Baylor Affiliated Hospitals, Houston, Texas.
Thrombophlebitis

HERBERT H. SCHAUMBURG, M.D.

Professor and Vice-Chairman, Department of Neurology, Albert Einstein College of Medicine, Bronx, New York.
Peripheral Neuropathy

W. MICHAEL SCHELD, M.D.

Fellow, Division of Infectious Diseases, University of Virginia School of Medicine, Charlottesville, Virginia.
Infective Endocarditis

WILLIAM R. SCHILLER

Associate Professor of Surgery, Medical College of Ohio. Medical College Hospital, Toledo, Ohio.
Tumors of the Stomach

ROBERT N. SCHNITZLER, M.D.

Clinical Associate Professor of Medicine, The University of Texas Health Science Center at San Antonio. Attending Cardiologist, Methodist Hospital, San Antonio Community Hospital, and St. Luke's Lutheran Hospital, Texas.
Atrial Fibrillation

ALAN H. SCHRAGGER, M.D.

Clinical Assistant Professor, Hahnemann Medical School. Chief of Dermatology, Allentown General Hospital and Sacred Heart Hospital, Allentown, Pennsylvania.
The Erythemas

ROBERT B. SCHULTZ, M.D.

Associate Attending Pediatrician, Hollywood Memorial Hospital, Hollywood, Florida.
Diabetes Mellitus in Childhood and Adolescence

ROBERT H. SCHWARTZ, M.D.

Associate Professor of Pediatrics, University of Rochester School of Medicine and Dentistry. Senior Associate Pediatrician, Strong Memorial Hospital, Rochester, New York.
Asthma in Childhood

JOHN J. SCIARRA, M.D., PH.D.

Professor and Chairman, Department of Obstetrics and Gynecology, Northwestern University Medical School. Attending Staff, Prentice Women's Hospital and Maternity Center of Chicago, Illinois.

Contraception

CORNELIUS E. SEDGWICK, M.D.

Surgeon, Lahey Clinic Foundation. Associate Clinical Professor of Surgery, Harvard Medical School. Chairman, Department of Surgery, New England Deaconess Hospital, Boston, Massachusetts.

Intestinal Obstruction

WILLIAM E. SEGAR, M.D.

Professor, University of Wisconsin Medical School, Madison, Wisconsin.

Parenteral Fluid Therapy in Children

DONALD SERAFIN, M.D.

Associate Professor, Plastic and Reconstructive Surgery, Duke University Medical Center. Chief, Plastic Surgery, Veterans Administration Hospital; Attending Physician, Durham County General Hospital, Durham, North Carolina.

Disorders of the Mouth (Malignant)

GUY A. SETTIPANE, M.D.

Associate Clinical Professor, Brown University. Physician in Charge, Division of Allergy, Rhode Island Hospital, Providence, Rhode Island.

Adverse Reactions to Drugs: Hypersensitivity

DANIEL J. SEXTON, M.D.

Staff, Oklahoma City Clinic. Attending Physician, Presbyterian Hospital, Oklahoma City, Oklahoma.

Rocky Mountain Spotted Fever

ALAN R. SHALITA, M.D.

Associate Professor and Head, Division of Dermatology, State University of New York, Downstate Medical Center. Chief of Dermatology, State University Hospital, Kings County Hospital Center, and Brookdale Hospital Medical Center, Brooklyn; Consultant Dermatologist, Brooklyn Veterans Administration Hospital and St. John's Hospital, Brooklyn, New York.

Acne Vulgaris

ROBERT S. SHAPIRO, M.D.

Chief Resident in Surgery, Medical College of Ohio, Toledo, Ohio.

Tumors of the Stomach

JOHN T. SHARP, M.D.

Professor of Clinical Science (Medicine), University of Illinois College of Clinical Medicine. Chief, Medical Service, Veterans Administration Hospital, Danville, Illinois.

Rheumatoid Arthritis

THOMAS W. SHEEHY, M.D., M.S.

Professor, University of Alabama School of Medicine. Chief of Medicine, Veterans Administration Hospital; Professor of Medicine, University Hospital, Birmingham, Alabama.

Macrocytic (Megaloblastic) Anemia (Other Than Pernicious Anemia)

PAUL A. SHURIN, M.D.

Assistant Professor, Pediatrics, Case Western Reserve University. Associate Director, Pediatric Ambulatory Service, Cleveland Metropolitan General Hospital, Cleveland, Ohio.

Otitis Media

LOUIS E. SILTZBACH, M.D.

Clinical Professor of Medicine, Emeritus, The Mount Sinai School of Medicine. Consultant Director of Sarcoidosis Laboratory and Clinic, The Mount Sinai Hospital, New York, New York.

Sarcoidosis

CAROL SINGER, M.D.

Associate Professor of Medicine, Cornell University Medical College. Assistant Attending Physician, Infectious Disease Service, Department of Medicine, Memorial Sloan-Kettering Cancer Center, New York, New York.

Bacteremia

FREDERICK R. SINGER, M.D.

Associate Professor of Medicine, University of Southern California School of Medicine. Attending Physician, Los Angeles County–University of Southern California Medical Center, Los Angeles, California.

Hyper- and Hypoparathyroidism

FRANK REES SMITH, M.D.

Associate Professor of Clinical Medicine, Columbia University College of Physicians and Surgeons. Associate Attending Physician, Presbyterian and Harlem Hospitals, New York, New York.

Hypo- and Hypervitaminosis A

J. LAWTON SMITH, M.D.

Professor of Ophthalmology, University of Miami School of Medicine, Miami, Florida. Bascom Palmer Eye Institute, Miami, Florida.

Optic Neuritis

LYNWOOD H. SMITH, M.D.

Professor of Internal Medicine, Mayo Medical School, Rochester, Minnesota. Consultant, Internal Medicine and Nephrology, Mayo Clinic and Foundation, Rochester, Minnesota.

Renal Calculi

AQUILES SOBRERO, M.D.

Professor, Department of Obstetrics and Gynecology, Northwestern University Medical School. Adjunct Attending Staff, Prentice Women's Hospital and Maternity

Center of Northwestern Memorial Hospital, Chicago, Illinois.
Contraception

GAIL E. SOLOMON, M.D.

Clinical Associate Professor of Neurology and Pediatrics, Cornell University Medical College. Associate Attending, Neurology and Pediatrics, and Director of Electroencephalography, The New York Hospital, New York, New York.
Epilepsy in Adolescents and Adults

MICHAEL R. SOULES, M.D.

Assistant Professor, Department of Obstetrics and Gynecology, Division of Reproductive Endocrinology, Duke University Medical Center, Durham, North Carolina.
Dysfunctional Uterine Bleeding

C. RITCHIE SPENCE, M.D.

Assistant Chief, Urology, Brooke Army Medical Center, Fort Sam Houston; Consultant in Urologic Surgery, Veterans Administration Hospital, Kerrville, Texas.
Pyelonephritis

GABRIEL SPERGEL, M.D.

Associate Professor of Internal Medicine, State University of New York Downstate Medical Center. Physician-in-Charge, Metabolic Research Unit, and Chief of Hypertension Service, Jewish Hospital and Medical Center of Brooklyn, Brooklyn, New York.
Pheochromocytoma

FREDERICK T. SPORCK, M.D.

Instructor, West Virginia University. West Virginia University Hospital, Morgantown, West Virginia.
Sinusitis

PHILIP M. SPRINKLE, M.D.

Professor and Chairman, Division of Otolaryngology, West Virginia University. West Virginia University Hospital, Morgantown, West Virginia.
Sinusitis

HUGH E. STEPHENSON, JR., M.D.

Professor of Surgery, University of Missouri School of Medicine. Chief, General Surgery, University of Missouri School of Medicine, Columbia, Missouri.
Empyema Thoracis

JOHN J. STEVENS, M.D.

Assistant Professor of Allergy and Immunology, University of California, San Diego. Director, Allergy Clinic, Mercy Hospital; Consultant, Veterans Administration Hospital and U.S. Naval Hospital, San Diego, California.
Allergic Rhinitis Due to Inhalant Factors

ROGER H. STEWART, M.D.

Assistant Clinical Professor of Dermatology, University of Miami School of Medicine. University of Miami, Holy Cross, Cypress Community, and North Ridge Hospitals, Fort Lauderdale, Florida.
Miliaria

CHARLES W. STRATTON, M.D.

Assistant Professor of Medicine, West Virginia University Medical Center, Charleston Division. Director, Microbiology-Serology Laboratory, Charleston Area Medical Center, Charleston, West Virginia.
Psittacosis

WHEELAN D. SUTLIFF, M.D.

Emeritus Professor of Medicine, University of Tennessee Center for Health Sciences. Senior Staff Physician, University of Tennessee Hospital; Consultant, Veterans Administration Hospital and Baptist Memorial Hospital, Memphis, Tennessee.
Histoplasmosis

GREGORY H. SZEYKO, M.D.

Assistant Professor of Internal Medicine, Texas Tech University School of Medicine. Attending Physician, Infectious Diseases, Texas Tech Regional Academic Health Center, R. E. Thomason Hospital, El Paso, Texas.
Nonbacterial Pneumonia

LARRY H. TABER, M.D.

Associate Professor of Pediatrics, Baylor College of Medicine. Texas Children's Hospital and Ben Taub General Hospital, Houston, Texas.
Chickenpox

JAMES S. TAYLOR, M.D.

Head, Section of Industrial Dermatology, Cleveland Clinic Foundation, Cleveland, Ohio.
Occupational Dermatoses

JAMES I. TENNENBAUM, M.D.

Clinical Professor of Medicine and Director, Division of Allergy, Ohio State University College of Medicine. Director, Division of Allergy, University Hospital; Attending Staff, Grant Hospital, Columbus, and Licking County Memorial Hospital, Newark; Courtesy Staff, Children's Hospital and Mt. Carmel Hospital, Columbus, Ohio.
Anaphylaxis and Serum Sickness

GEORGE B. THEIL, M.D.

Professor and Co-Chairman, Department of Medicine, The Medical College of Wisconsin. Chief of Medical Service, Veterans Administration Center, Wood (Milwaukee), Wisconsin. Supported by the Research Service of the Veterans Administration.
Glomerular Disorders

F. ANTHONY THOMAS, M.D.

North Kansas City Memorial Hospital, North Kansas City, Missouri.
Contact Dermatitis

SUMNER E. THOMPSON III, M.D.

Venereal Disease Control Division, Bureau of State Services, Center for Disease Control, Public Health Service, Department of Health, Education, and Welfare, Atlanta, Georgia.
Gonorrhea

E. GEORGE THORNE, M.D.

Associate Professor of Dermatology, University of Colorado School of Medicine. Chief, Dermatology, Veterans Administration Hospital, Denver, Colorado.
Urticaria and Angioedema

CHARLES S. THURSTON, M.D.P.A.

Clinical Associate Professor, Department of Medicine, The University of Texas Health Science Center at San Antonio, Texas.
Pseudofolliculitis Barbae

PETER A. TOMASULO, M.D.

Associate Medical Director, Milwaukee Blood Center, Inc. Clinical Assistant Professor of Medicine (Hematology), University of Wisconsin. Associate Medical Director (Internal Medicine), Great Lakes Hemophilia Foundation. Attending Hematologist, Sinai Hospital and Deaconess Hospital, Milwaukee, Wisconsin.
Therapeutic Use of Blood Components

WILLIAM N. TOTH, M.D.

Assistant Clinical Professor of Medicine, College of Physicians and Surgeons, Columbia University. Chief, Department of Medicine, Overlook Hospital, Summit; Consultant in Medicine, Fair Oaks Hospital, Summit, New Jersey.
Infectious Mononucleosis

DONALD P. TSCHUDY, M.D.

Senior Investigator, Metabolism Branch, National Cancer Institute, National Institutes of Health, Bethesda, Maryland.
The Porphyrias

JERROLD A. TURNER, M.D.

Associate Professor of Medicine and Microbiology and Immunology, UCLA School of Medicine. Assistant Medical Director and Chief, Section of Parasitic Diseases, Los Angeles County Harbor General Hospital, Torrance, California.
Intestinal Parasites

PAUL B. UNDERWOOD, JR., M.D.

Professor, Obstetrics and Gynecology, and Director, Gynecologic Oncology, Medical University of South Carolina, Charleston, South Carolina.
Carcinoma of the Vulva

JOE R. UTLEY, M.D.

Professor of Surgery, University of California, San Diego, School of Medicine. Chief, Division of Cardiothoracic Surgery, University Hospital, San Diego, California.
Atelectasis

ANDRE J. VAN HERLE, M.D.

Associate Professor of Medicine, UCLA School of Medicine, Los Angeles, California.
Thyroid Gland Malignancies

WILLIAM H. WAINWRIGHT, M.D.

Attending Psychiatrist, The Roosevelt Hospital, New York, New York.
Delirium

KENNETH W. WARREN, M.D.

Lecturer in Surgery, Harvard Medical School. Surgeon, New England Baptist Hospital and New England Deaconess Hospital, Boston, Massachusetts.
Chronic Pancreatitis

LOUIS R. WASSERMAN, M.D.

Distinguished Service Professor, Mount Sinai School of Medicine. Attending Hematologist, The Mount Sinai Hospital, New York, New York. Chairman, The Polycythemia Vera Study Group.
Polycythemia Vera

FREDERICK D. WAX, M.D.

Resident in Dermatology, Dartmouth-Hitchcock Medical Center, Hanover, New Hampshire.
Mycosis Fungoides

PEYTON E. WEARY, M.D.

Professor and Chairman, Department of Dermatology, University of Virginia School of Medicine. Attending Staff, University of Virginia Hospital, Charlottesville, Virginia.
Nevi

MICHAEL A. WEBER, M.D.

Assistant Professor of Medicine, The New York Hospital–Cornell Medical Center, New York, New York.
Hypertension

STEPHEN B. WEBSTER, M.D.

Clinical Assistant Professor, University of Minnesota Medical School and University of Wisconsin Medical School. Gundersen Clinic and Lutheran Hospital, La Crosse, Wisconsin.
Pruritus

NEAL J. WEINREB, M.D.

Assistant Professor of Medicine, Mount Sinai School of Medicine. Assistant Attending Physician, The Mount Sinai Hospital, New York, New York. Executive Officer, The Polycythemia Vera Study Group.
Polycythemia Vera

BRUCE D. WEINTRAUB, M.D.

Senior Investigator, Clinical Endocrinology Branch, National Institute of Arthritis, Metabolism, and Digestive Diseases, National Institutes of Health, Bethesda, Maryland.
Hypothyroidism

CHARLES E. WELLS, M.D.

Professor of Psychiatry and Neurology and Vice-Chairman, Department of Psychiatry, Vanderbilt University School of Medicine, Nashville, Tennessee.
Psychoneurosis

CHRISTIAN WERTENBAKER, M.D.

Fellow in Neuro-ophthalmology, Columbia-Presbyterian Medical Center, New York, New York.
Peripheral Neuropathy

CHRISTOF WESTENFELDER, M.D.

Assistant Professor of Medicine, University of Illinois Abraham Lincoln School of Medicine. Director of Dialysis Unit, University of Illinois Hospital; Attending in Nephrology, Veterans Administration West Side Hospital, Chicago, Illinois.
Parenteral Nutrition in Adults

JAMES A. WHITAKER, M.D.

Fellow in Gastroenterology, Kansas University Medical Center, Kansas City, Kansas.
Peptic Ulcer

PAUL J. WIESNER, M.D.

Chief, Operational Research Branch, VD Control Division, Center for Disease Control, Atlanta, Georgia.
Syphilis

KENNETH H. WILLIAMS, M.D.

Assistant Professor of Psychiatry and Internal Medicine, University of Pittsburgh School of Medicine. Director, Alcohol–Drug Abuse Clinic, Western Psychiatric Institute and Clinic, Pittsburgh, Pennsylvania.
Alcoholism

CHARLES L. WISSEMAN, Jr., M.D.

Professor and Chairman, Department of Microbiology, University of Maryland School of Medicine, Baltimore, Maryland.
Typhus Fever

JERRY S. WOLINSKY, M.D.

Assistant Professor of Neurology, University of California, San Francisco. Research Associate in Neurology, Veterans Administration Hospital, San Francisco, California.
Viral Meningoencephalitis

FREDERICK J. WRIGHT, M.A., M.D., F.R.C.P., F.R.C.P.E., D.T.M.&H.

Retired Senior Lecturer in Diseases of Tropical Climates, University of Edinburgh, Scotland.
Typhoid Fever

JESS R. YOUNG, M.D.

Head, Department of Peripheral Vascular Disease, Cleveland Clinic Foundation, Cleveland, Ohio.
Decubitus Ulcer

NORMAN R. ZINNER, M.D., M.S., F.A.C.S.

Clinical Professor of Urology, Charles R. Drew Postgraduate Medical School, Los Angeles. Attending Urologist, Martin Luther King Jr. General Hospital, Los Angeles; Attending Surgeon (Urology), Torrance Memorial Hospital, Torrance, California.
Trauma of the Genitourinary System

Contents

SECTION 1. THE INFECTIOUS DISEASES

SECTION 2. THE RESPIRATORY SYSTEM

SECTION 3. THE CARDIOVASCULAR SYSTEM

SECTION 4. THE BLOOD AND SPLEEN

SECTION 5. THE DIGESTIVE SYSTEM

SECTION 6. METABOLIC DISORDERS

SECTION 7. THE ENDOCRINE SYSTEM

SECTION 8. THE UROGENITAL TRACT

SECTION 9. THE VENEREAL DISEASES

SECTION 10. DISEASES OF ALLERGY

SECTION 11. DISEASES OF THE SKIN

SECTION 12. THE NERVOUS SYSTEM

SECTION 13. THE LOCOMOTOR SYSTEM

SECTION 14. OBSTETRICS AND GYNECOLOGY

SECTION 15. PSYCHIATRY

SECTION 16. PHYSICAL AND CHEMICAL INJURIES

SECTION 17. APPENDICES AND INDEX

SECTION 1

The Infectious Diseases

AMEBIASIS

method of
P. N. CHHUTTANI, M.D.
Chandigarh, India

Amebiasis—infection with *Entamoeba histolytica*—may be asymptomatic, may be associated with mild to severe colonic symptoms, or may produce a liver abscess which may extend into contiguous territory. Rarely *E. histolytica* may even invade tissues other than and remote from colon and liver. Diagnosis can be easy, as for example in acute amebic dysentery when the stool microscopically may be teeming with motile trophozoite forms; and yet the diagnosis of amebic liver abscess may be divulged only on the autopsy table. Improvement in serologic diagnosis as well as availability of liver scans has altered the situation to the patient's advantage, but a high degree of suspicion is the most important aid in detecting invasive amebiasis of any tissue. A large number of effective drugs are available, and a clinical as well as a parasitic cure can be expected as a rule if the drugs are chosen wisely and treatment is given in time. Failures of treatment are due to either erroneous diagnosis or a reinfection in an endemic area. In serious forms of the disease, such as colonic perforation and peritonitis or an extensive hepatic amebiasis with complications, even the specific agents available may not succeed if their use has been delayed too long.

EMETINE HYDROCHLORIDE

This is a powerful trophocidal amebicide of established value in management of hepatic amebiasis and amebic dysentery. However, in the case of colonic amebiasis, clinical relief is often not followed by a parasitic cure. The drug has a cumulative effect, and the dose should be reduced at the extremes of age, during pregnancy, or when nutritional status is poor. The drug is best avoided in myocardial failure with hypotension, Addison's disease, and polyneuritis. In the United States of America, the use of emetine hydrochloride is contraindicated in pregnancy and in children.

Toxicity and Tolerance. The drug is well tolerated as a rule, and its toxic effects tend to be exaggerated. Its effects on the myocardium, leading to hypotension, tachycardia, and nonspecific electrocardiographic changes, are well established and are seen in only a minority of patients. Injections are often painful. There may be nausea, vomiting, abdominal cramps, or diarrhea. Rarely, muscle cramps or a peripheral neuropathy may occur. Direct injection into a main nerve can produce permanent paralysis.

Dosage. Emetine is given intramuscularly or deep subcutaneously in the dose of 1.0 mg. per kg. per day for 6 to 10 days. Combination therapy enables one to keep total dosage on the lower side. The daily dose must not exceed 65 mg., and the drug should not be used if the systolic blood pressure falls well below 100 mm. of Hg. A modified rest regimen (with toilet facilities) is a good routine precaution during its use.

Dehydroemetine (investigational in the United States; may be available from the Parasitic Disease Drug Service, Atlanta, Georgia)

This synthetic variant of emetine is just as effective but enjoys the advantage of being less cumulative and less toxic. Indications and contraindications are identical.

Dosage. The daily dose is 1.5 mg. per kg., with an upper limit of 90 mg. It is given as an intramuscular or deep subcutaneous injection.

Chloroquine (Nivaquine, Aralen, Resochin)

This drug is a direct amebicide and is concentrated in the liver. Its chief value lies in the fact that in combination with emetine it gives more satisfactory response than either drug alone. For many years there was no alternative to emetine, and the advent of chloroquine was a distinct advance in therapeutics, although with the further addition of metronidazole (and allied compounds) the position has further improved. There are clinical situations in the tropics in which antimalarial and amebicidal actions are desired simultaneously, i.e., in a therapeutic test in management of a pyrexia of uncertain origin. Here chloroquine is a very useful drug in spite of its activity being second to that of emetine or metronidazole.

Toxicity and Tolerance. Apart from nausea and vomiting and occasionally headache, there is as a rule no manifest toxicity in 3 to 4 weeks' use of the drug. Visual disturbances are uncommon and are usually associated with long-term use of the drug. Convulsions have been described, and the drug is contraindicated in porphyria.

Dosage. The dose is 300 mg. of chloroquine base taken orally twice daily for the first 2 days, and then 150 mg. twice daily for 3 weeks.

Metronidazole (Flagyl)

This drug, used extensively for less than a decade in amebiasis, appeared to approach an ideal amebicidal in that it was effective in all forms and manifestations of amebiasis and also had not presented any major toxic effects. However, the original promise has been qualified by a definite failure rate.

Toxicity and Tolerance. Metallic taste in the mouth, dizziness, nausea, and diarrhea may occur. Discoloration of urine and leukopenia can be seen. Antabuse-like action may take place when used in association with intake of alcohol. The drug should be avoided in such a situation and also in patients with blood dyscrasias.

Dosage. Oral administration of 400 to 800 mg. of metronidazole thrice a day for 5 days suffices as a rule for all manifestations of amebiasis. However, a repeat course can be given safely, and the drug can also be combined with other amebicides.

Intestinal Amebicides

Their choice is wide, their utility less than ideal, and their use confined to asymptomatic as well as symptomatic intestinal forms of the disease, excluding ameboma. They are of adjuvant value when combined with emetine or chloroquine, as these latter two agents have poor intestinal luminal action.

Diiodohydroxyquinoline. The dose is 600 mg. orally thrice daily for 21 days. Iodism may occur.

Iodochlorhydroxyquin (not available in the United States of America). The dose is 250 mg. orally thrice daily for 21 days. Iodism or diarrhea may occur. Its association with subacute myelo-optic neuropathy remains unproved.

5,7-Dichloro-hydro-8-hydroxyquinaldine (Sios-teran) (not available in the United States). The dose is 200 mg. orally thrice daily for 21 days. Iodism does not occur.

Diloxanide Furoate (Furamide) (not available in the United States). The dose is 0.5 gram orally thrice a day for 10 days. It may sometimes produce mild gastrointestinal symptoms.

Antibiotics

These act mostly by modifying the bowel flora and therefore are useful in intestinal forms of the disease. If the liver abscess is secondarily infected, these drugs are indicated. Oxytetracycline (Terramycin), tetracycline (Achromycin), and chlortetracycline (Aureomycin) are regarded as superior to demethylchlortetracycline (Declomycin, Ledermycin).

Toxicity, Tolerance, and Dosage. Oxytetracycline or tetracycline given orally 250 mg. thrice daily for 7 to 10 days is well tolerated, and no serious ill effects are seen as a rule. It is worth combining their use with oral administration of vitamin B complex.

MANAGEMENT OF AMEBIASIS

Given a correct diagnosis, clinical as well as parasitic cure is the rule after use of the therapy outlined here. Amebiasis is endemic in wide areas of the world, commonly involves many members of the family, and may be present undetected in the staffs of eating houses. A reinfection therefore can easily take place and may pass off as a relapse.

A test of cure is three negative stool examinations, one of which should be performed after administration of a purgative. This should be done for all forms of amebiasis 1 to 3 months after treatment.

A working classification of amebic infection from the point of view of its therapy would be (1) asymptomatic amebiasis, (2) mild dysenteric or nondysenteric symptomatic amebiasis, (3) acute amebic dysentery, and (4) extraintestinal amebiasis.

Symptomless Amebiasis

The controversy about the wisdom of treating "symptomless cyst passers" is an academic luxury of those in temperate climates; the argument loses much of its force in the tropics where the ravages of amebiasis are seen at first hand. A significant number of amebic liver abscess patients do not give a history of intestinal symptoms. In other words, a symptomless cyst passer, given adverse environment, may go on to develop serious forms of the disease.

1. Metronidazole, 400 mg. given orally thrice daily for 5 days, has given excellent results.

2. Diloxanide furoate, diiodohydroxyquinoline, or iodochlorhydroxyquin is given as a 3-week course as indicated earlier. These drugs give good results.

Chronic Intestinal Amebiasis

The clinical distinction of acute amebic dysentery from chronic intestinal amebiasis is not always sharp. When the symptoms are at all marked, the same course of treatment as outlined for acute amebic dysentery should be given. When the symptoms are mild and there is no diarrhea, the treatment required would be the same as outlined for asymptomatic amebiasis.

Whenever symptoms persist after treatment and parasitic cure, a thorough search for alternative etiologic factors must be made. It is not uncommon for the irritable colon syndrome to be diagnosed as amebiasis. Similarly, other serious colonic diseases such as carcinoma must not be lost sight of.

Acute Amebic Dysentery

1. The patient is placed on a modified rest regimen with bathroom facilities until the acute symptoms subside. Rarely the dysentery in amebiasis may be as severe as acute bacillary dysentery, accompanied by fever, severe diarrhea, griping, tenesmus, and dehydration. Hospitalization and parenteral therapy are required in such patients.

2. A bland, nonresidual high protein diet is given.

3. Metronidazole, 400 to 800 mg. orally thrice daily for 5 days, is highly effective.

4. Tetracycline or oxytetracycline, 250 mg. orally four times a day, should be added if there is fever or the symptoms are at all marked.

OR:

1. Dehydroemetine (investigational in the United States), 90 mg. (or emetine, 60 mg.) deep subcutaneously or intramuscularly daily for 6 to 10 days.

2. A diiodohydroxyquinoline course for 21 days or a diloxanide furoate course for 10 days, and/or a course of tetracyclines.

Local complications of severe amebic colonic ulceration are not rare. Localized or generalized peritonitis may follow a perforation that may be so slight as not to be visible at autopsy or may be of fairly large size. Apart from specific therapy, the general principles of treatment—e.g., correction of fluid and electrolyte imbalance, parenteral therapy, surgical drainage, and use of suitable antibiotics—are important. Surgical interference such as exteriorization of the bowel and colectomy has at times been resorted to with benefit.

Ameboma should be treated exactly the same as acute amebic dysentery. We have found metronidazole effective for this condition. In our tropical practice a patient with a colonic mass awaiting investigation is routinely advised to take such a course unless a thorough search for parasites and serologic exclusion of invasive amebiasis can be carried out.

Acute amebic dysentery may occur in association with idiopathic ulcerative colitis. When a course of treatment for the former only partially clears up symptoms, treatment for ulcerative colitis must be given. Rarely the colonic ulceration in acute amebic dysentery may take several weeks to heal even after specific treatment has produced a parasitic cure. Therefore associated ulcerative colitis should not be diagnosed without sufficient observation.

Acute amebic dysentery may also occur in association with colonic carcinoma. Therefore any persistent signs and symptoms after specific treatment must lead to investigation of the patient for this possibility.

If there is ulceration of the skin around the genitalia or in the area of a drainage tube draining an appendicular abscess, direct smears must be taken for a search for *E. histolytica.* Failure to treat this sort of complication can be catastrophic.

Hepatic Amebiasis

1. Emetine or dehydroemetine* (60 and 90 mg., respectively), given deep subcutaneously or intramuscularly once daily for 10 days.

2. Chloroquine, 300 mg. of base twice daily orally for 2 days, and then 150 mg. twice daily for 3 weeks.

3. A course of an intestinal amebicide. This may be diiodohydroxyquinoline, 600 mg. orally thrice daily for 21 days, or diloxanide furoate, 0.5 gram thrice daily for 10 days. All three drugs can be given simultaneously, or the first two given together followed by the third.

OR:

Metronidazole, 400 to 800 mg. orally thrice daily for 5 days, is effective. The course can be

*Investigational for this use in the United States.

repeated or prolonged to 10 days if the clinical condition so indicates.

OR:

1. Emetine (as above) for 6 days.
2. Metronidazole (as above) for 5 days.
3. Chloroquine (as above) for 21 days.

All three drugs can be given simultaneously if required.

If a liver abscess is secondarily infected, a course of tetracyclines should be given. However, when the microorganism has been identified, the antibiotic required will be indicated by sensitivity tests.

Aspiration of Liver Abscess

1. If there is significant liver enlargement (above or below the costal margin) or edema of the chest wall that does not rapidly respond to treatment, a wide-bore needle should be used for closed aspiration.

2. The site of aspiration should be (a) in the area of localized swelling, (b) at the point of maximum tenderness, or (c) in the ninth intercostal space in the midaxillary line if neither (a) nor (b) is present.

3. As much pus as possible should be removed.

Open surgical drainage is required only when the abscess cavity is secondarily infected and closed aspirations as well as specific treatment have not led to its closure.

Rarely an abscess in the left lobe of the liver may have to be aspirated under vision after a laparotomy.

Complications of liver abscess, such as rupture into the pleura (producing empyema), the lung (producing lung abscess), the pericardium (producing pericarditis), or the peritoneum (producing peritonitis), all must be given the specific treatment for liver abscess, as well as being managed along standard surgical lines for these complications. Closed drainage by aspiration and specific drug therapy are as a rule sufficient for empyema, pericarditis, and peritonitis caused by burst amebic abscess. Should a chronic lung abscess result which does not clear up on antiamebic treatment and the use of suitable antibiotics, radical surgical treatment may be required. Fortunately, this is rare.

Rare Miscellaneous Complications

Metastatic pulmonary abscess, brain abscess, ulcerative lesions of the genitalia, and skin ulceration caused by *E. histolytica* do occur rarely and present diagnostic problems. However, treatment with systemic amebicides such as emetine or metronidazole gives satisfactory results.

BACTEREMIA

method of
CAROL SINGER, M.D.,
and DONALD ARMSTRONG, M.D.
New York, New York

Introduction

The rational approach to treating bacteremia involves knowing the factors predisposing to infection in the patient, the source of the infection, and the specific microorganism responsible. Host factors important in the development and prognosis of bacteremia include (1) underlying disease, such as neoplasia, diabetes mellitus, chronic alcoholism, rheumatic heart disease, and others; (2) the immunologic status of the patient, including cellular (polymorphonuclear and mononuclear phagocytes) and humoral (immunoglobulins and complement function) factors, which may be altered by an underlying disease or prescribed medications; and (3) other iatrogenic factors, such as indwelling bladder or intravenous catheters.

In order to promptly initiate treatment for sepsis, it is essential to recognize the signs and symptoms indicating possible bacteremia. In many cases, patients will present with high fever, shaking chills, tachycardia, and tachypnea. Shock and mental changes, including delirium and coma, may or may not be present. However, changes may be more subtle, and the clinician must always be aware of the possibility of sepsis in appropriate clinical settings. In neonates and young children, irritability, poor feeding, or lethargy may be the earliest and only signs of sepsis.

When bacteremia is suspected, rapid and thorough evaluation of the patient is essential. The general clinical status of the patient and the urgency for treatment must be determined. A complete history and physical examination may reveal the source of infection, and therefore guide therapy. Additional information may be obtained by chest and abdominal roentgenograms and other radiologic examinations when indicated, and by microscopic examination of urine, sputum, pleural effusion, spinal fluid, and abscesses or wounds. A Gram stain of the aforementioned body fluids and exudates may provide valuable information in initiating appropriate antibiotic therapy even before culture results are available. If skin lesions are present, material from them should be Gram stained and cultured. Blood cultures should be obtained before initiating antibiotic therapy. At least two blood cultures, preferably from different sites, should be obtained, both to increase yield and to better evaluate the possibility of a blood culture contaminant. Organisms such as *Staphylococcus epidermidis*, *Propionibacterium acnes*, and diphtheroids are frequently contaminants, although in immunosuppressed patients or in patients with prosthetic heart valves, these organisms may represent true infection. If endocarditis is suspected, five or six blood cultures should be obtained.

Specific Therapy

When the microorganism responsible for an episode of bacteremia is known, antibiotic therapy can be specifically directed at that organism. Table 1 lists the microorganisms most frequently encountered as causes of sepsis and the antibiotics preferred in their treatment. Antibiotics should be administered intravenously in doses adequate to eradicate the specific microorganism. Tobramycin and amikacin are new aminoglycosides whose use, we believe, should be restricted to the treatment of infections caused by organisms resistant to gentamicin. Duration of therapy depends on a number of factors, including the source of the infection and the clinical status of the patient. In general, a 2 week course of antibiotics is indicated for proved cases of bacteremia. Longer periods of therapy may be required if drainage of the infected site is poor and signs of infection persist. In bacterial endocarditis, 4 to 6 weeks of therapy are indicated, and in most cases of bacteremia caused by *Staphylococcus aureus,* in which more than two blood cultures are positive, 4 to 6 weeks of therapy are recommended because of the high incidence of endocarditis with multiple positive blood cultures for *S. aureus,* and the tendency for *S. aureus* to cause metastatic abscesses and persist. It should be emphasized that duration of therapy must be individualized to fit the clinical situation.

TABLE 1. **Antimicrobial Agents for the Treatment of Bacteremia**

ORGANISM	DRUGS OF CHOICE	ALTERNATIVES
Gram-positive cocci		
Staphylococcus aureus	Oxacillin or nafcillin	A cephalosporin, clindamycin, vancomycin
Streptococcus pyogenes (Groups A, B, C, G)	Penicillin G	Erythromycin, cephalosporin, clindamycin, vancomycin
Streptococcus, Group D enterococcus	Penicillin G or ampicillin plus streptomycin or gentamicin	Vancomycin plus streptomycin or gentamicin
Streptococcus bovis	Penicillin G plus or minus streptomycin	Cephalosporin, vancomycin
Streptococcus viridans	Penicillin G	Cephalosporin, vancomycin, clindamycin
Anaerobic streptococci	Penicillin G	Cephalosporin, vancomycin, erythromycin, clindamycin
Streptococcus pneumoniae (pneumococcus)	Penicillin G	Erythromycin, cephalosporin, clindamycin
Gram-negative cocci		
Neisseria gonorrhoeae (gonococcus)	Penicillin G	Tetracycline, erythromycin
Neisseria meningitidis	Penicillin G	Chloramphenicol, sulfonamide (only if sulfonamide sensitive)
Gram-positive bacilli		
Clostridium perfringens	Penicillin G	Chloramphenicol, clindamycin, erythromycin
Listeria monocytogenes	Ampicillin	Penicillin, tetracycline, erythromycin
Gram-negative bacilli		
Escherichia coli	Ampicillin, cephalosporin, gentamicin	Chloramphenicol, tobramycin,* amikacin*
Klebsiella pneumoniae	Gentamicin plus or minus cephalosporin	Chloramphenicol, tetracycline, tobramycin, amikacin
Klebsiella enterobacter	Gentamicin	Chloramphenicol, carbenicillin, tobramycin, amikacin
Proteus mirabilis	Ampicillin	Cephalosporin, gentamicin, chloramphenicol, tobramycin, amikacin
Proteus species	Gentamicin	Chloramphenicol, carbenicillin
Pseudomonas aeruginosa	Gentamicin and carbenicillin	Tobramycin, amikacin, colistin
Salmonella	Chloramphenicol	Ampicillin, sulfamethoxazole-trimethoprim
Bacteroides fragilis	Clindamycin or chloramphenicol	Tetracycline
Bacteroides species (oropharynx)	Penicillin G	Clindamycin, chloramphenicol, tetracycline
Serratia species	Gentamicin	Chloramphenicol, carbenicillin
Shigella species	Ampicillin	Chloramphenicol, trimethoprim-sulfamethoxazole
Hemophilus influenzae	Chloramphenicol	Ampicillin, trimethoprim-sulfamethoxazole
Acinetobacter (Mima, Herellea)	Gentamicin	Chloramphenicol, tobramycin

*For enteric gram-negative rod bacteremia, tobramycin or amikacin may be used if organisms are resistant to gentamicin but sensitive to tobramycin and amikacin, or, empirically, if gentamicin resistance is prevalent in the hospital or community.

Table 2 lists the antibiotics most commonly used in treating bacteremia, the recommended dosages in patients with normal renal function, and some of the side effects to be anticipated. In patients with impaired renal function, the serum creatinine and creatinine clearance should be measured and followed carefully during antibiotic therapy. With moderate (creatinine clearance less than 50 ml. per minute) and severe (creatinine clearance less than 10 ml. per minute) renal failure, the dosages of certain antibiotics must be altered to avoid toxic serum levels. Serum antibiotic levels, if available, can be very helpful in determining antibiotic dosage. A number of publications offer guidelines for the adjustment of antibiotic dosage in the presence of renal impairment. Dosages need not be significantly altered in the presence of renal failure with chloramphenicol, erythromycin, and clindamycin. The doses of the penicillins and cephalosporins (e.g., ampicillin, oxacillin, nafcillin, and cephalothin) should be slightly decreased (by about one third) in the presence of uremia. In the presence of renal failure, very high doses of penicillin or carbenicillin may lead to central nervous system toxicity, varying from myoclonus to seizures. In severe renal failure, the dose of carbenicillin should be reduced to 130 to 180 mg. per kg. per day (8 to 10 grams per day) and to 100 mg. per kg. per day (6 grams per day) in anuric individuals. Dosages of all the aminoglycosides must be reduced when renal failure is present, and a variety of nomograms exist to aid in regimens. The "rule of 8's" may be used as a guide to gentamicin administration, whereby the serum creatinine is multiplied by 8 (to yield twice the half-life) and the value obtained used as the interval between doses of 1 mg. per kg. Tetracycline and sulfonamides should be avoided, if possible, in severe renal failure.

Initiation of Antibiotic Therapy

Before the report of a positive blood culture, certain clinical conditions may suggest the offending organism or organisms. In patients with cellulitis, *Streptococcus pyogenes* and *S. aureus* are the most common causes, although gram-negative bacilli and *Clostridium species* may occasionally be responsible. In patients with severe burns, infec-

TABLE 2. **Recommended Doses of Antibiotics Used in Bacteremia and Potential Toxicity**

ANTIBIOTIC	TOTAL DAILY DOSE	INTERVAL BETWEEN DOSES	MAJOR SIDE EFFECTS
Amikacin	15 mg./kg./day	q. 8–12 h.	Ototoxicity, nephrotoxicity
Ampicillin	100–200 mg./kg./day	q. 6 h.	Rash, hypersensitivity, diarrhea
Carbenicillin	500 mg./kg./day	q. 4 h.	Sodium overload, hypokalemia, hypersensitivity, CNS toxicity in uremia, bleeding disorder
Cefazolin	85 mg./kg./day (4–6 grams/day)	q. 6 h.	Hypersensitivity
Cephalothin	100–200 mg./kg./day	q. 4–6 h.	Hypersensitivity, thrombophlebitis, possible renal toxicity with aminoglycosides
Chloramphenicol	40–75 mg./kg./day	q. 6 h.	Hematopoietic toxicity (aplasia rare), gray-baby syndrome
Clindamycin	40 mg./kg./day	q. 6 h.	Diarrhea
Colistimethate	2.5–5.0 mg./kg./day	q. 8 h.	Nephrotoxicity, circumoral paresthesias
Erythromycin	30–60 mg./kg./day (1–4 grams/day)	q. 6 h.	Gastrointestinal disorders, transient deafness (rare)
Gentamicin	3–5 mg./kg./day	q. 6 h.	Nephrotoxicity, ototoxicity (mainly vestibular)
Kanamycin	15 mg./kg./day	q. 8–12 h.	Ototoxicity (mainly hearing loss), nephrotoxicity
Nafcillin	100–200 mg./kg./day	q. 4–6 h.	Hypersensitivity
Oxacillin	100–200 mg./kg./day	q. 4–6 h.	Hypersensitivity
Penicillin G	150,000–300,000 units/kg./day (10–20 million units/day)	q. 4 h.	Hypersensitivity, seizures in uremic patients
Sulfonamides	100 mg./kg./day	q. 6 h.	Rash, nephrotoxicity, blood dyscrasias (hemolytic anemia or neutropenia), Stevens-Johnson syndrome
Tetracycline	15–30 mg./kg./day (1–2 grams/day)	q. 6 h.	Gastrointestinal disorders, nephrotoxicity, hepatotoxicity
Tobramycin	3–5 mg./kg./day	q. 6 h.	Nephrotoxicity, ototoxicity
Trimethoprim-sulfamethoxazole	4 tabs. P.O./day or up to 9 ampules (400 mg. sulfamethoxazole and 80 mg. trimethoprim per ampule) per day*	q. 12 h.	As for sulfonamides, plus toxic pancytopenia
Vancomycin	30 mg./kg./day (2 grams/day)	q. 6 h.	Nephrotoxicity, thrombophlebitis, ototoxicity (hearing loss)

*Intravenous preparation available on investigational basis at this time.

tions with *S. aureus* and *Streptococcus pyogenes* have largely been replaced by gram-negative aerobic bacteria, such as *Pseudomonas aeruginosa* or *Serratia marcescens,* and, more recently, by *Candida* and *Aspergillus species.* Urinary tract infections are most often caused by gram-negative bacilli, especially *Escherichia coli,* and, less commonly, by *Proteus mirabilis* or other gram-negative rods. In some hospitals, up to 50 per cent of *E. coli* isolates are resistant to ampicillin. A Gram stain of the urine can be very valuable in indicating whether a urinary tract infection is due to a gram-negative rod or to the enterococcus or Staphylococcus.

Infections of the female genital tract may lead to bacteremia and shock. Severe postpartum and postabortal sepsis, sometimes accompanied by peritonitis, are frequently mixed infections, and include anaerobic streptococci, *Bacteroides fragilis,* enteric gram-negative rods, *Clostridium sp.,* and, less commonly, *Neisseria gonorrhoeae.* Therapy must be directed against these multiple organisms, usually including clindamycin or chloramphenicol and gentamicin, and often requires surgical removal of devitalized tissue. In infections following gastrointestinal surgery, or when perforation of the bowel has occurred, infections are also frequently mixed, and surgical drainage is usually necessary. This is particularly crucial when *Clostridium perfringens* is involved. Cellulitis of the flanks and abdomen, with or without crepitation, may be the earliest indication of Clostridium sepsis. Aspiration of the cellulitis may reveal the large gram-positive rods. Infection of the hepatobiliary tract usually involves *E. coli, Klebsiella sp.,* enterococcus, and occasionally *Salmonella sp.*

Patients with pulmonary infections may or may not have accompanying bacteremia. Gram stain of the sputum may give valuable information as to the causative organism. *Streptococcus pneumoniae* (pneumococcus) is still the most common cause of community-acquired bacterial pneumonias. However, pneumonia complicating influenza may be caused by *Staphylococcus aureus* or gram-negative organisms, and initial antibiotic therapy must cover these organisms as well. Patients with chronic lung disease may have pneumonia caused by *Hemophilus influenzae* or *Klebsiella pneumoniae,* and aspiration pneumonias may be caused by a variety of oropharyngeal flora, most of which are sensitive to penicillin. In hospital-acquired pneumonias, and in patients who are severely neutropenic, gram-negative pneumonias are common. Therefore initial treatment depends to a great extent on the type of patient and the setting in which the pneumonia develops.

If endocarditis is suspected, multiple blood cultures are usually positive, and the causative organism can usually be identified quickly. *Streptococcus viridans,* enterococci, and *Streptococcus bovis* are common causes of subacute bacterial endocarditis. Treatment can usually await identification of the organism. In acute bacterial endocarditis, in which *S. aureus, Streptococcus pneumoniae,* or gram-negative bacilli may be the cause, empirical treatment may be necessary before cultural results are available. Such acute endocarditis or endarteritis may occur in drug addicts, in patients with prosthetic heart valves, or in patients with underlying cardiac valve abnormalities.

Infections of bones and joints are often hematogenous in origin, and are most often caused by *S. aureus, Streptococcus pyogenes,* and gram-negative bacilli. However, a variety of organisms, including Salmonella in patients with sickle cell anemia and *N. gonorrhoeae* in patients with disseminated gonococcemia, may be responsible. A specific microbiologic diagnosis is essential for adequate treatment.

Newborn infants and neonates are particularly susceptible to Group B streptococcal infection, as well as gram-negative bacteremia, especially *E. coli.* As mentioned before, signs and symptoms of sepsis in infants may be subtle and minimal at first.

The immunosuppressed host, particularly the severely neutropenic patient (polymorphonuclear leukocyte count less than 500 per cu. mm.) who is febrile, should be considered septic and treated appropriately. Frequently, there is no obvious source of infection, and the patient may appear relatively well or severely toxic. In either case, early empirical therapy with broad-spectrum antibiotics is indicated.

Table 3 lists the antibiotic combinations which may be used in the patient presumed to be bacteremic. Delay in treatment may prove lethal. It should be noted that if bacteremia with *Salmonella sp.* is suspected, chloramphenicol or ampicillin should be included in the antibiotic regimen.

TABLE 3. **Empirical Therapy of Presumed Bacteremia**

If no obvious source:
  Oxacillin or nafcillin and gentamicin*
    or
  Cephalosporin and gentamicin
If severe neutropenia:
  Oxacillin or cephalosporin plus gentamicin and carbenicillin
If gastrointestinal or genital source:
  Chloramphenicol or clindamycin plus gentamicin
If clostridium is suspected:
  Penicillin and gentamicin

*If gentamicin resistance is prevalent, it should be replaced by tobramycin or amikacin.

General Measures in the Treatment of Bacteremia

In addition to the appropriate use of antibiotics, certain basic measures may be equally important in terminating bacteremia. Foley catheters, intravenous catheters, parenteral nutrition catheters, and other foreign bodies may be the source of infection, and their removal may result in rapid improvement. Similarly, debridement of infected wounds or decubiti, drainage of abscesses or empyemas, relief of urinary tract obstruction or gastrointestinal obstruction, and surgical removal of devitalized bowel are essential to successful therapy.

The septic patient must be carefully monitored during therapy. Mortality in bacteremia associated with shock is very high, as high as 80 per cent in some series. In such patients, fluid and electrolyte balance, urinary output, daily weights, and coagulation factors must be measured frequently. Urinary output via a Foley catheter is one of the most important parameters to measure, and it should be maintained at 40 to 75 ml. per hour. Disseminated intravascular coagulation may occur and may require treatment with heparin. A central venous pressure (CVP) catheter may be helpful in the administration of fluids. If there is any doubt as to the validity of the CVP readings, or if left ventricular dysfunction is suspected, a Swan-Ganz catheter, which measures pulmonary capillary wedge pressure (PCWP), may be helpful. If the CVP and PCWP are low, volume expansion with plasma, albumin, saline, or blood, if indicated, should be initiated, until the CVP reaches 13 to 15 cm. of water, or the PCWP is 15 to 18 mm. Hg. If volume expansion does not raise the blood pressure to levels necessary to maintain blood flow to the brain, heart, and kidneys, pressor agents may be required. A variety of pressors have been used in septic shock, each with advantages and disadvantages. Levarterenol (Levophed) causes marked vasoconstriction, and may cause increased cardiac output. However, renal vasoconstriction also occurs, and this may offset the advantages of the increase in blood pressure. Four to 8 mg. is placed in 1000 ml. 5 per cent dextrose in water (D5-W) or dextrose and saline (D/S), and the infusion monitored to raise systolic blood pressure to 90 or 100 mm. Hg. Isoproterenol (Isuprel) is a beta-adrenergic stimulator, and increases cardiac output by both inotropic and chronotropic effects. Peripheral vascular resistance is lowered. Cardiac arrhythmias, especially premature ventricular contractions, may occur. One mg. of isoproterenol is placed in 500 ml. D5-W and infused at a rate of less than 10 micrograms per minute. Dopamine, a newer agent in the treatment of shock, has a positive inotropic effect, but less of a chronotropic effect on the heart. Its main advantage is that it causes dilatation of the renal and mesenteric arteries and decreases coronary vascular resistance. It does, however, cause peripheral vascular constriction, and may cause premature ventricular contractions. Infusion is usually begun at a rate of 2 to 5 micrograms per kg. per minute, with most patients responding to 20 micrograms per kg. per minute. Occasionally, infusions of greater than 50 micrograms per kg. per minute have been effective.

Other adjunctive measures in the treatment of septic shock are still controversial. The use of high doses of corticosteroids (100 to 1000 mg. of methylprednisolone) every 4 to 6 hours over 8 to 48 hours is advocated by some. Recently, the use of white blood cell transfusions in septic neutropenic patients has been studied, and may be of value in those patients with prolonged neutropenia.

Although prompt treatment of bacteremia is essential, the patient's clinical course and cultural results should be regularly re-evaluated, as new infections with other bacteria or fungi may emerge during treatment.

BRUCELLOSIS

method of
MOHAMMED Y. KHAN, M.D.
Minneapolis, Minnesota

Brucellosis is an infectious disease of mammals that is transmitted to human beings by contact with infected animals or their products. The disease has been commonly found in goats *(Brucella melitensis)*, dairy cattle *(B. abortus)*, swine *(B. suis)*, sheep and hares *(B. ovis)*, desert wood rats *(B. neotomae)*, and dogs *(B. canis)*. Pregnant animals are particularly susceptible and often abort. As a result of control measures in the United States, human brucellosis has declined from a peak of about 6000 cases in 1947 to 328 cases in 1975. The majority of these cases have occurred in people working in the meat processing industry. Dairy farmers, veterinarians, and bacteriology laboratory workers are also at increased risk of contacting this infection. Epidemics of human brucellosis have been traced to the ingestion of unpasteurized dairy products, especially imported cheese.

General Measures

Patients with brucellosis may wish to rest in bed as long as they are febrile. Dehydrated patients should receive glucose and electrolyte solutions intravenously. The diet should be liberal with calories and carbohydrates to prevent starvation acidosis.

Antimicrobial Therapy

The keystone of therapy is the early use of specific antimicrobial agents. Patients with uncomplicated infection should be treated with tetracycline hydrochloride, given orally on an empty stomach in a dose of 0.5 gram every 6 hours for 3 to 4 weeks. Tetracycline should be avoided in young children and pregnant patients. Streptomycin may be given with tetracycline to seriously ill patients and those with abscesses. The dose of streptomycin should be 0.5 gram injected intramuscularly every 12 hours for 2 to 3 weeks. Streptomycin dosage should be modified in patients with renal insufficiency or discontinued if there is evidence of vestibular dysfunction. Streptomycin alone is ineffective in brucellosis. Patients who are intolerant of the aforementioned antibiotics may be effectively treated with trimethoprim-sulfamethoxazole (co-trimoxazole), given orally in a dose of 2 tablets three times daily for 2 to 3 weeks. Each tablet of co-trimoxazole contains 80 mg. of trimethoprim and 400 mg. of sulfamethoxazole. (This use of trimethoprim-sulfamethoxazole is not listed in the manufacturer's official directive.)

Relapse

All treated patients should be followed for 6 months with monthly blood cultures and agglutination tests. When tetracycline is used alone, relapses of symptoms and bacteremia may occur in half of the patients. The relapses are rarely due to bacterial resistance to tetracycline. Poor penetration by tetracycline into the macrophages, where some Brucella organisms persist, may explain relapses of brucellosis. A favorable clinical response usually follows a second course of tetracycline treatment. The incidence of relapse can be further reduced by concurrent use of streptomycin or by increasing the dose of tetracycline to 3 to 4 grams daily. (This tetracycline dose is outside the range approved by the Food and Drug Administration.)

Corticosteroids

Antimicrobial therapy may initially provoke high fever, delirium, or shock. Such Herxheimer-like reactions may be prevented by simultaneous administration of a glucosteroid. Prednisone, 20 mg. orally, or hydrocortisone sodium succinate, 100 mg. parenterally, may be given every 8 hours for 3 to 4 days. Glucosteroids should be given only together with adequate doses of an effective antimicrobial agent.

Complications

Accessible abscesses should be drained surgically. Abscesses of the spleen or of one kidney are cured by the removal of the organ. Spondylitis can be cured with appropriate antimicrobics, bed rest, and braces without surgical drainage. Patients with Brucella endocarditis who develop intractable cardiac decompensation need prompt replacement of the diseased valves. All surgical procedures should be performed under appropriate antimicrobial coverage.

Prevention

There is no safe and effective Brucella vaccine available for human use at this time. Pasteurization of dairy products will prevent infections induced by ingestion.

CHICKENPOX
(Varicella-Zoster)

method of
LARRY H. TABER, M.D.
Houston, Texas

The same virus (varicella-zoster, VZ) causes both chickenpox and herpes zoster; the different manifestations represent primary infection and reactivation, respectively. The primary infection (chickenpox) is usually a mild illness characterized by disseminated cutaneous vesicular lesions. Varicella (chickenpox) is most commonly seen in children, primarily between the ages of 2 and 8 years (90 per cent of cases). It is highly contagious, and a secondary attack rate of 87 per cent has been observed among susceptible siblings in a household following a primary case. The illness is communicable through direct contact with an infected person 1 to 2 days preceding eruption of lesions. The incubation period ranges from 10 to 21 days, with the usual time interval being 14 to 15 days.

Varicella in the Normal Host

General Considerations. Varicella is a self-limited disease. Successive lesions usually appear over a 3 day period. Crusting of lesions occurs within 5 days in mild cases and within 10 days in severe cases. Patients are infectious until lesions have crusted and should remain home until that time.

Crusted lesions do not contain infectious virus. Contacts are not quarantined, and no isolation procedures need be carried out in the home unless there is a susceptible, immunocompromised person in the household.

Prevention of this disease is not necessary for a well child, and therefore no attempt at prophylaxis is indicated for well children.

Pruritus. Relief may be achieved by the local application of calamine-antihistamine lotions and/or oral antihistamines. Antihistamines should be used judiciously in patients with vomiting, as they may mask involvement of the central nervous system occasionally seen in varicella.

Fever. Acetaminophen is preferable for fever control and relief of any constitutional symptoms.

Skin Infections. Bacterial superinfection is a rather common occurrence in chickenpox and is usually due to *Staphylococcus aureus* and/or Group A beta-hemolytic Streptococcus. The skin may become involved with impetiginous lesions, pustules, and/or cellulitis. These lesions should be treated with an appropriate antibiotic, the selection of which should be guided by cultures for bacteria and antibiotic susceptibility studies.

The fingernails of patients with chickenpox should be kept short and the hands clean. This may minimize secondary skin infections caused by scratching.

Complications of Varicella in the Normal Host

Encephalitis. Symptoms of encephalitis may occur in patients before the vesicular eruption, but occur more frequently 5 to 7 days after onset of the eruption. Symptoms include fever, confusion, vomiting, and altered state of consciousness. Encephalitis occurs in approximately 1 per 1000 patients with varicella. A lumbar puncture should be performed, but cautiously in those patients with clinical evidence of increased intracranial pressure. Patients with encephalitis require (1) maintenance of good airway, (2) monitoring of vital signs, (3) strict intake and output records, and (4) daily examination for evidence of secondary bacterial infections in the lung, skin, or urinary tract.

Raised intracranial pressure is the most serious threat to the patient. In patients with cerebral edema, fluid intake is restricted. The patient should be in an upright position. The administration of dexamethasone sodium phosphate has been used for reduction of increased intracranial pressure. The dosage employed is an initial intravenous dose of 10 mg., followed by 4 mg. intramuscularly or intravenously every 6 hours. An initial effect may be seen within 12 hours. This drug is gradually discontinued as soon as cerebral edema has subsided. In small children (<20 kg.), 1 mg. per kg. per day in four divided doses is used. One half of the total daily dose may be given as an initial dose.

Some authorities also use osmotically hypertonic agents such as mannitol or glycerol. Mannitol is given intravenously in a 20 per cent solution in an amount of 1.0 to 2 grams per kg. over 30 to 45 minutes. This dosage may be repeated. (See manufacturer's official directive for use in children under 12 years of age.) When mannitol is used, *careful attention* to fluid intake and output is needed. Glycerol is more effective in treating chronic cerebral edema than acute cerebral edema. Hypotonicity of body fluids should be prevented.

Other Neurologic Complications of Varicella. Rarely optic neuritis, Guillain-Barré syndrome, or transverse myelitis may occur. Acute cerebellar ataxia may be present without signs of encephalitis. Reye's syndrome, usually sudden in onset with vomiting and altered state of consciousness, may occur in children after chickenpox.

Varicella Pneumonia. This complication is recognized chiefly in adults (or compromised hosts). It may be mild or potentially fatal. In patients with evidence of pneumonia, sputum or tracheal aspirate specimens should be obtained for Gram stain and bacterial cultures. Cytology of respiratory cells in the sputum may reveal intranuclear inclusions, and this finding would be indicative of varicella pneumonia. Of course, bacterial superinfection may occur in patients with varicella pneumonia, and antibiotics should not be withheld in severely ill patients before bacterial culture results are available. There is no specific therapy for varicella pneumonia. In patients who have a severe pulmonary diffusion defect, a *short* course of a pharmacologic dosage of steroid may be tried. Careful attention should be given to the maintenance of a good airway in these patients. Assisted ventilation may be required.

Other Complications of Varicella. Rarer complications include hepatitis, uveitis and orchitis, arthritis, and purpura fulminans.

Varicella-Zoster Infections in the Compromised Host

General Considerations. Primary varicella in the susceptible compromised host may cause severe hemorrhagic chickenpox with multiple organ system involvement. Zoster in the same group of patients may disseminate and involve multiple organ systems. The patients at highest risk from varicella are those with incompetence of their cell-mediated immunity. These would include athymic children, children with Wiskott-Aldrich syndrome, and patients receiving corticosteroids, antimetabolites, alkylating agents, or ionizing radiation as therapy. These patients often have leukemia, Hodgkin's disease, or lymphomas, or have been on long-term corticosteroid therapy for some chronic illness.

Physicians participating in the medical care of these patients should make every effort by history and serologic evaluation of each patient to determine his "immune status" for varicella-zoster virus.

Certainly parents with susceptible, immunosuppressed children should be cautioned to prevent exposure of their children to either varicella or zoster and, if exposure occurs, to notify their physician immediately.

Susceptible patients who are receiving corticosteroids and are exposed to varicella should have their steroid dosage reduced to one to one and a half times physiologic levels over a time period which is consistent with safety. In immunosuppressed patients on steroids who develop varicella or zoster, the adjustment of the steroid dosage must be individualized, with primary consideration given to the basic disease process for which the patient is being treated.

Prophylaxis—Passive Immunization. ZOSTER IMMUNE GLOBULIN (ZIG). Susceptible patients at high risk from varicella (as defined above) should be passively immunized after intimate contact with a patient with infectious chickenpox. Passive immunization has been shown to decrease the severity of the disease or make it clinically inapparent. *Zoster immune globulin* (ZIG), which contains high titers of antibody against varicella-zoster virus, is presently available for use in the *susceptible immunocompromised host.* Zoster immune globulin should be given within 72 hours after exposure. The recommended prophylactic dosage is 1.25 ml. per 10 kg. of body weight. This preparation is available by request directed to one of the regional ZIG consultants shown in Table 1.

IMMUNE SERUM GLOBULIN (ISG). Immune serum globulin (ISG) has been used for passive immunization in susceptible high risk patients. It is less effective than ZIG, but at times is the only material available. In the susceptible immunocompromised patient, a dosage of 1.2 ml. per kg. has been given.

ZOSTER IMMUNE PLASMA. Zoster immune plasma obtained from a convalescent donor has also been used for passive immunization. Its antibody titer is variable. If convalescent zoster HbsAg free plasma is available for administration, it may be given to an exposed susceptible high-risk patient in a maximum dosage of 10 ml. per kg. Results of prophylaxis with this material have been variable, but its use is warranted when ZIG is not available.

Treatment of Varicella Zoster Infection

The Compromised Host. There is no specific treatment modality for the immunocompromised host with a varicella-zoster infection. For this reason prevention of varicella in the susceptible compromised host should be emphasized as optimal management of these patients.

Recently antiviral chemotherapy has been utilized in immunosuppressed patients with varicella-zoster infections. Controlled studies are being undertaken for evaluation of the effectiveness of vidarabine (adenine arabinoside) in the treatment of immunosuppressed patients who have varicella-zoster infection. Vidarabine is a purine nucleoside which possesses antiviral activity against members of the herpes family. This drug seems to have low or no toxicity for humans in the dosage employed for antiviral chemotherapy.

Two other antiviral chemotherapeutic agents, idoxuridine (IDU) and cytosine arabinoside (Ara-C), have been employed with little success in the therapy of severe herpetic disease in the immunosuppressed. In both cases the toxicity of these drugs outweighs any beneficial antiviral effects, and for this reason administration of these two drugs cannot be recommended for use in patients with varicella-zoster infections.

The use of zoster immune plasma in the compromised host with varicella is controversial. If used, plasma should be obtained from a convalescent donor and should be HbsAg free. The dosage employed is 10 ml. per kg.

Varicella Infection in the Pregnant Female and the Newborn Infant. Maternal infection with varicella in the first months of pregnancy may result in congenital abnormalities in the newborn infant. Severe or fatal varicella may occur in 5 to 10 day old infants when their mothers have lesions of varicella 4 days or less prior to delivery. At this time interval, it is unlikely that passively acquired varicella-zoster antibody will be present to modify the infection. In infants who contract the disease, the mortality rate is about 35 per cent.

ZIG has been approved for use in the newborn infant whose mother develops varicella within 4 days prior to delivery or 24 hours after delivery of her infant. To obtain ZIG for administration, one of the listed ZIG consultants should be contacted. If the mother develops the lesion of varicella beyond 24 hours after delivery or if the neonate has intimate exposure to varicella in the first weeks of life, ISG, 1.2 ml. per kg., is recommended by some authorities.

Hospital Exposure

It is important to try to minimize the elective hospital admissions of children with varicella to prevent the exposure of the high-risk patient population to this infection. Routine attempts to elicit a history of exposure to varicella prior to actual hospital admission may be helpful. The child who is incubating varicella and develops lesions in the hospital usually exposes other per-

TABLE 1. **1977 Regional ZIG Consultants**

Region	Consultants
New England:	Adolf W. Karchmer, M.D. Martin S. Hirsch, M.D. Massachusetts General Hospital, Boston 02114 Office 617-726-3812 Residence 617-891-8358 (Dr. Karchmer) 617-969-2587 (Dr. Hirsch) John F. Modlin, M.D. Children's Hospital and Medical Center, Boston 02115 Office 617-734-6000 Ext. 3531
Mid-Atlantic:	Anne A. Gershon, M.D. Department of Pediatrics New York University Medical Center, New York 10016 Office 212-561-3612 Residence 212-369-5126
Mideast:	Richard G. Judelsohn, M.D. 857 Delaware Avenue, Buffalo 14209 Office 716-634-0744 Residence 716-688-5579
Southeast and National:	Neal A. Halsey, M.D. Walter A. Orenstein, M.D. Gregory F. Hayden, M.D. David L. Heymann, M.D. J. Lyle Conrad, M.D. Alan R. Hinman, M.D. Center for Disease Control Immunization Division, Atlanta 30333 Office 404-633-3311 Ext. 3736 Residence 404-876-6428 (Dr. Halsey) 404-633-2727 (Dr. Orenstein) 404-874-6703 (Dr. Hayden) 404-633-9017 (Dr. Heymann) 404-636-3902 (Dr. Conrad)
Southeast:	Robert L. Rosenberg, M.D. University of Tennessee College of Medicine, Memphis 38103 Office 901-528-5774 Residence 901-754-6896
Midwest:	Richard Hong, M.D. Sheldon Horowitz, M.D. University of Wisconsin Medical Center, Madison 53706 Office 608-262-6954 Residence 608-836-8189 (Dr. Hong) 608-238-5218 (Dr. Horowitz)
Mountain:	Brian Lauer, M.D. C. Henry Kempe, M.D. University of Colorado Medical Center, Denver 80220 Office 303-394-8501 (Dr. Lauer) 303-394-7576 (Dr. Kempe) Residence 303-320-4013 (Dr. Lauer) 303-377-6563 (Dr. Kempe)
Pacific:	Moses Grossman, M.D. Delmer Pascoe, M.D. San Francisco General Hospital, San Francisco 94110 Office 415-565-8361 (Dr. Grossman) 415-565-8376 (Dr. Pascoe) Residence 415-681-0475 (Dr. Grossman) 415-562-3242 (Dr. Pascoe) Joel D. Meyers, M.D. Hutchinson Cancer Research Center Seattle, Washington 98104 Office 206-292-2892 Residence 206-232-3003

sons prior to the eruption of definable vesicles. The susceptible contacts in a hospital setting then have a chance of contracting disease. When recognized, the child with varicella is isolated and discharged home as soon as is compatible with good medical management. A history of previous varicella should be obtained and recorded in the charts of exposed children. All those who are susceptible by history and who are in the high risk groups enumerated above should receive ZIG as soon as possible after exposure. If ZIG cannot be obtained, ISG should be used. All normal children so exposed should be discharged as soon as is consistent with good medical management, in an attempt to prevent secondary cases from developing in the hospital. Quarantine of susceptible exposed contacts who cannot be discharged from the hospital is also appropriate from 7 to 21 days after their exposure to minimize the threat of contact with immunocompromised patients. The parents should be advised of the exposure of their children to varicella.

CHOLERA

method of
WILLIAM B. GREENOUGH III, M.D.
Dacca, Bangladesh

Diarrhea caused by infection with *Vibrio cholerae* results in the rapid loss of large volumes of fluid from the body. This loss leads to a decreased volume of circulating blood and reduced perfusion of vital organs. Untreated, the majority of patients who present with clinical cholera die. This is due to hypovolemic shock and can occur within 2 hours of the first symptom. With proper treatment survival without complications is assured.

The disease is produced when organisms are ingested in water or food. They multiply in the small intestine, where a protein toxin is produced. This toxin attaches to specific receptor sites on the cells which line the gut. A cell membrane associated enzyme, adenylate cyclase, is stimulated, leading to increased levels of cyclic AMP. This event produces a secretory state in the intestinal tract as well as decreasing the absorption of sodium. When the net transfer of salts and water from the mesenteric circulation into the gut lumen exceeds the absorptive capacity of both small and large intestines, diarrhea occurs. The rate of fluid loss in cholera can reach more than 1 liter per hour, with maximum losses of 30 liters over a 24 hour period when replacement is adequate. More commonly, losses are 300 to 400 ml. per hour, with a total output of 5 to 10 liters in the first 36 hours. The stool is not fecal and has a somewhat "fishy" odor. It is white to yellow and opalescent with flecks of mucus, giving the "rice-water" characteristic.

Other gram-negative bacteria, particularly *Escherichia coli* and noncholera vibrios, also produce diarrhea which is mediated by toxins that are very similar to the cholera toxin. During initial stages the clinical presentation of patients with diarrhea caused by such bacteria may be indistinguishable from that of disease caused by *V. cholerae*. In such cases, however, the diarrhea tends not to be sustained for as long. All bacteria causing cholera-like diarrhea may be readily grown from stool or rectal swab specimens on standard media. Tests for the presence of enterotoxins are becoming more available but are not yet routine. Direct examination of stool by darkfield or specific fluorescent antisera, if available, permits a rapid, specific diagnosis of cholera. It should be emphasized that correct treatment of the individual patient does not in any way depend on a bacteriologic diagnosis. The importance of correct etiologic diagnosis lies in recognizing the presence of an epidemic in a community, particularly among mild cases and carriers, so that the spread of disease may be checked.

The composition of fluid lost in stool depends on the rate of loss and is similar or identical for all infections which cause diarrhea in the same way as *V. cholerae*. At rates of loss of more than 200 ml. per hour the concentration of sodium in the stool approaches that of plasma (140 mEq. per liter). As the rate of fluid and electrolyte loss increases, the concentrations of all components except bicarbonate approach their respective plasma values. At lower rates both potassium and bicarbonate increase in concentration, whereas that of sodium decreases. The stool is isosmotic with respect to plasma. The goals of treatment are entirely determined by the amount and composition of fluid loss, and all symptoms and signs appear to be secondary to the physiologic consequences of these losses.

Objectives of Treatment

1. Initiate treatment early with oral glucose-electrolyte solutions in all possible cases of severe diarrhea in order to prevent hypovolemia leading to shock.
2. Correct hypovolemic shock rapidly with intravenous fluids, once extensive losses have occurred.
3. Maintain a normally hydrated state by replacing losses on a volume-for-volume basis. This may be done cheaply and effectively with oral glucose-electrolyte solutions. Intravenous replacement must be used only if losses are not effectively replenished by mouth.

4. Be sure adequate potassium and bicarbonate are given to avoid complications of hypokalemia and acidosis.

5. Give an antibiotic that kills *V. cholerae* to shorten the duration of diarrhea.

6. Be alert for and treat hypoglycemia should it occur, particularly in children who have poor nutritional status.

Evaluation of Patients

When seen, patients should be rapidly evaluated. It requires only seconds to (1) feel for carotid, femoral, and radial pulses; (2) observe for flat neck veins, poor skin turgor, sunken eyes with soft eyeballs, cold wrinkled fingers, and muscle cramps; and (3) observe respirations for rate and amount of ventilation, and listen to lung bases. Weighing the patient is very useful if the situation permits. An arrangement is essential whereby stool can flow freely into a bucket such that a collapsed or semicomatose patient is not expected to move onto a commode. Bedpans are insufficient to accommodate the volumes passed, and bedding soaked with rice-water stool may be a vehicle for noscocomial spread of cholera.

When 8 to 12 per cent of body weight has been lost, there will be an absent or barely palpable radial pulse and no measurable blood pressure by a cuff manometer. Muscle cramps are likely to be severe, the eyes sunken, and skin turgor poor. In this situation fluid should be replaced to the extent of 10 per cent of the body weight as rapidly as possible intravenously through a large bore needle in the most accessible veins. Such patients represent severe volume depletion. Moderate depletion results from a loss of 4 to 8 per cent of body weight. These patients will have postural hypotension, diminished skin turgor, decreased pulse volume, and flat neck veins. When volume loss is less than 4 per cent of body weight, there will be few signs of depletion, but thirst will be prominent. All conscious patients with volume depletion caused by cholera will be thirsty roughly in proportion to the amount of their losses.

Pitfalls in Diagnosis

There are several important traps that can be avoided by an observer who is aware of them.

1. In populations with endemic severe atherosclerosis, volume depletion shock can precipitate infarction of vital organs such as the heart, brain, kidneys, or intestinal tract. Early recognition of this may lead to special precautions such as placement of a central venous line to monitor volume replacement and avoid overhydration, or closer monitoring of potassium replacement should renal failure ensue.

2. Failure to regain consciousness in children may be due to hypoglycemia. Early recognition and treatment can be lifesaving.

3. The presence of partial intestinal obstruction or other surgical conditions can occasionally lead to severe volume depletion mimicking cholera.

4. Certain neoplasms such as medullary carcinoma of the thyroid, pancreatic adenomas, or neural tumors of the gut can lead to cholera-like diarrhea.

5. Excessive use of laxatives, particularly those containing phenolphthalein, can masquerade as cholera.

Electrolyte Replacement Solutions

Both oral and intravenous solutions are effective in treating cholera. When shock is not present, nearly all patients can be treated by mouth. It is particularly important to know this when confronted with large numbers of patients and few health workers to give care or when the disease occurs in areas where intravenous fluids are not available. In such situations early recognition and early initiation of oral replacement may save many lives.

Intravenous Solutions. An ideal replacement solution would duplicate in composition what has been lost in the stool. The most widely available commercial preparations are (1) Ringer's lactate, which has as its composition (in mEq. per liter) sodium, 130; potassium, 4; lactate, 28; and chloride, 109; (2) 2:1 saline:lactate, using isotonic sodium chloride and 1/6 M sodium lactate; this solution has (in mEq. per liter) sodium, 154; chloride, 97; and lactate, 57. Neither of these solutions contains glucose or potassium; thus potassium chloride should be added at 10 mEq. per liter. If hypoglycemia is suspected, additional glucose must be given.

Intravenous solutions that can be specially prepared and more closely approximate the ideal composition include the following: (1) Diarrheal Treatment Solution (DTS), prepared in grams per liter: NaCl, 4; Na acetate, 6.5 (or Na lactate, 5.4); KCl, 1; and glucose, 8. This contains (in mEq. or mM. per liter) Na, 118; K, 13; Cl, 83; HCO_3 (as acetate or lactate), 48; and glucose, 50. (2) "Dacca Solution." This contains (in grams per liter) NaCl, 5; Na acetate, 6.5; KCl, 1; and (in mEq. or mM. per liter) Na, 134; K, 13; Cl, 99; and HCO_3 (as acetate), 48.

Each of these four solutions has been used extensively in the treatment of cholera and other severe diarrheal disease, with mortality rates of less than 1 per cent in epidemic situations in which there were large numbers of patients and limited medical personnel. The choice of fluid depends primarily upon availability; DTS, if available, is the most universally applicable.

If none of the aforementioned fluids are available, isotonic saline can be given to correct the initial hypovolemia; replacement of base and potassium must then be done orally as described below.

Oral Solutions. Although a variety of solutions have been successfully employed, there is one currently recommended by the World Health Organization, by a consensus of those with the most experience. Glucose is essential to facilitate absorption of sodium in the small intestine. Sucrose can be substituted if glucose is not available, although the concentration should be doubled (in order to supply the same amount of glucose following hydrolysis in the intestine).

The oral solution contains (in mEq. or mM. per liter) Na, 90; K, 20; Cl, 80; HCO_3, 30; glucose, 111; and (in grams per liter) sodium chloride, 3.5; sodium bicarbonate, 2.5; potassium chloride, 1.5; and glucose, 20.

Although available commercially in some countries, this oral solution is not yet available in the United States. Measured amounts of salts and glucose can be mixed and stored in moisture-proof plastic or foil packets and mixed as needed (enough for 1 liter gives a small, easily dispensable packet). Ordinary clean drinking water at room temperature can be used for making the solution; it should be prepared fresh daily to avoid bacterial contamination that may occur with storage. Using standard household measuring spoons, the following proportions should be used in 1 liter: sodium chloride, ½ teaspoon; sodium bicarbonate, ½ teaspoon; potassium chloride, ¼ teaspoon; glucose, 2 tablespoons.

The solution has a slightly salty taste, but is well tolerated; flavorings have been advocated to make the fluid more palatable, but these are not critical in its acceptability by the patient.

Oral fluids can be given by mouth or, when necessary, through a nasogastric tube. Patients drinking from a glass or cup should be told to drink a measured amount of fluid over a certain time period. This must equal stool losses.

Vomiting, although frequently present, does not prevent the use of oral fluids. If vomiting occurs, the fluid should be given in smaller amounts more frequently. In most patients this simple modification will obviate the problem. Occasionally vomiting is so severe that it precludes the use of oral fluids, in which case intravenous fluid must be given. Oral fluids may again be instituted after normal hydration has been restored.

Rarely, if there is glucose malabsorption, the oral fluid will not be well absorbed, and a marked increase in diarrhea will occur. In this situation, a large amount of glucose is found in the stool. This can be quickly verified by testing. Stopping the oral fluid will decrease diarrhea; these persons will require intravenous replacement.

Initial Replacement

Patients admitted with hypotension must be treated immediately with intravenous fluids. When this is the case, approximately 10 per cent of body weight has been lost in fluids. One can easily approximate the fluid requirement if the body weight is known; if not known, it can be estimated.

For *adults*, a large bore intravenous needle (No. 18) should be placed in an arm vein or, if this is impossible, in a femoral vein. (In the latter case the needle may have to be held manually in place while the first liter of fluid is given.) The intravenous replacement solution should be infused as rapidly as possible, so that approximately 2 liters is given over the first 30 minutes. It may be necessary to start a second intravenous line if the infusion cannot be given rapidly enough through one line. Usually after this amount of fluid has been given, the patient is no longer in shock and one can fix a more permanent needle in an arm vein for further intravenous therapy if necessary.

Intravenous therapy is most easily begun in *children* using scalp vein needles; the external jugular vein is often the most convenient site for initial rehydration. Children in shock should receive intravenous fluids at a rate of about 40 ml. per kg. of body weight over the first 30 minutes.

Following the correction of shock, one may decide to give the remaining replacement therapy by continuing the intravenous infusion or may at that point begin oral therapy. This decision will depend on the severity of vomiting and alertness of the patient. Regardless of the route, the remaining replacement fluid should be given over the next 2 to 3 hours in adults, and 6 to 8 hours in children. Additional losses must also be replaced on a volume-for-volume basis during the early period and throughout the course of the illness.

By the end of 4 hours the adult patient should have no physical evidence of dehydration, a normal pulse, and a feeling of well-being. Children may remain lethargic for up to 12 to 18 hours. When this is the case, blood glucose should be checked or, if this is not possible, additional glucose administered. Urine output is a good index of adequate hydration but may not begin for 8 to 12 hours.

Patients with moderate or mild dehydration on admission may be started directly on oral fluids for correction of estimated deficits during the first 4 hours.

Maintenance Therapy

This aspect of therapy involves the replacement of diarrheal fluid losses that occur from the beginning of hospitalization until significant diarrhea ceases. This period rarely lasts beyond 48 hours when antibiotics are used; the majority of the fluid losses are in the first 24 hours.

Early in the course of treatment diarrhea may be minimal; once shock is corrected, however, volume loss may be rapid.

All the diarrheal fluid lost may be replaced orally with glucose-electrolyte solution. The only exceptions would be the rare patient with marked vomiting or the one who cannot absorb glucose. Occasionally patients with prolonged very high stool rates (greater than 1 liter per hour in adults) cannot drink fast enough to keep up with losses. In that case intravenous fluids may be necessary temporarily until the stool rate decreases. In about 10 per cent of patients, it may be desirable to give some of the maintenance requirements by the intravenous route.

Estimates of how much fluid must be given to maintain normal hydration are based on some estimate of diarrheal fluid lost. This is most easily accomplished by the use of a cholera bed, whereby all diarrheal output is collected into a calibrated bucket placed under a bed in which a hole has been made to accommodate the buttocks of the patient. A rubber sheet with a sleeve leading into the bucket ensures complete collection of stool. This is most convenient and comfortable for the patient and permits simple recording of diarrheal output. An input-output chart should be kept on each patient; urinary output should be collected separately.

Oral replacement should be given at a rate of 1.5 times the stool output; this will ensure equal replacement of all stool losses, and will supply adequate free water requirements of the patient. Drinking water should also be made available.

The patient should be evaluated during this period at least once every 2 to 4 hours, and the amount of required fluid calculated on the output of the previous 4 hour period. During the first 4 hours, when the output is not yet known, approximately 15 ml. per kg. per hour on the average can be given.

If oral therapy is not adequately replacing fluid losses, one will detect an increase in heart rate and a decrease in skin turgor; this can be confirmed by a rising hematocrit or measure of plasma protein (such as plasma specific gravity). Intravenous fluids can then be given to correct this deficit. Intravenous fluids for maintenance are given on a volume-for-volume basis.

A normal diet for age should be started as soon as the patient is hungry. There is no reason to withhold food while diarrhea is occurring. In the same manner, feeding may be resumed in breast-fed infants after correction of the initial dehydration and when sufficient time has elapsed to permit tetracycline to eliminate vibrios. Milk chelates this antibiotic and renders it inactive, and this should be kept in mind when it is used.

Antibiotics

Oral tetracycline remains the drug of choice in cholera; it eliminates the vibrios usually within 24 hours, and significant diarrhea by 48 hours. The drug can be started at the time oral fluids are started; there is no advantage to giving it parenterally. *V. cholerae* has shown no significant resistance to tetracycline, even though this drug has been widely used in cholera treatment for the past 12 years. The doses are, for adults, 500 mg. every 6 hours for 48 hours; and for children, 50 mg. per kg. per day in four 6-hourly doses for 48 hours. (See manufacturer's official directive before using tetracycline in children under the age of 8 years.)

Other drugs that can be used if tetracycline is not available include furazolidone: for adults, 100 mg. every 6 hours for 3 days; and for children, 5 mg. per kg. per day in four divided doses. Chloramphenicol may also be used: for adults, 500 mg. every 6 hours for 3 days; and for children, 75 mg. per kg. per day in four divided doses.

Some antibiotics such as the aminoglycosides, although effective in vitro, have little therapeutic effect.

Complications of Cholera

Complications occurring during therapy for cholera are uniformly prevented by adequate replacement of fluid and electrolytes and glucose. If those replacements are inadequate, the following complications can be seen:

1. Persistence or recurrence of hypovolemic shock. This is always the result of inadequate fluid replacement unless a cardiac infarct or other vascular complication has occurred. In populations with severe atherosclerosis, volume depletion has a much higher risk and can lead to infarction of vital organs and irreversible damage.

2. Acute renal failure. This usually means that prolonged or recurrent episodes of hypotension have occurred secondary to inadequate fluid replacement. If the initial shock is treated correctly and the patient is maintained adequately, acute renal failure will not develop.

3. Persistence of nausea or vomiting. This usually indicates uncorrected acidosis or saline depletion.

4. Hypokalemia. In children this may lead to cardiac arrhythmias and possibly paralytic ileus. In adults it is rarely symptomatic. Potassium replacement should be given as part of the initial replacement therapy, without waiting for urinary

flow to begin except when there is a known history of previous renal failure.

5. Overhydration. This results from excessive intravenous fluid replacement. It may be manifest by puffiness of the eyes in children, and occasionally by pulmonary edema, particularly in the setting of uncorrected acidosis. Prolonged acidosis in neglected patients can lead to pulmonary edema and shock in the presence of normal hydration. In this situation isotonic sodium bicarbonate may be used sufficiently to correct the acidosis.

6. Hypoglycemia. This may be manifest by seizures in a small percentage of children, usually those with significant malnutrition; it is thought to be due to poor liver glycogen stores. Addition of glucose to the initial intravenous replacement solution should prevent this.

7. Abortion. This is seen in women in the third trimester of pregnancy, and is secondary to severe saline depletion.

Useless Treatment Measures

The previously mentioned therapeutic measures are entirely adequate to treat cholera. Some treatment measures that may inadvertently be employed are useless and may even be detrimental to the patient. These include the following:

1. Vasopressors such as levarterenol (L-norepinephrine). Patients with hypovolemic shock are already maximally vasoconstricted and need only volume replacement (as intravenous electrolyte solutions).

2. Steroids. There is no clinical rationale for their use.

3. Cardiotonics, such as nikethamide (Coramine).

4. Oxygen. Cyanosis implies only the need for correction of the hypovolemic shock.

5. Blood or plasma transfusions. Water and electrolyte replacement only if necessary.

6. Oral antidiarrheal medication, such as kaolin, pectin, bismuth, charcoal, or paregoric. These do not influence the course of the disease and may interfere with the effectiveness of tetracycline by binding it in the gut lumen.

DIPHTHERIA

method of
RICHARD LEONARDS, M.D.
San Francisco, California

Two hundred to 300 cases of diphtheria have been reported annually in the United States during the last decade. Within this time the mortality has decreased from approximately 10 per cent to less than 5 per cent. This is not due to better diagnosis or therapy, which has not changed appreciably, but to clustering of cases and a shift in age to the older patient, mortality being greater in the young child. In 1975, 246 of 307 total cases in the United States occurred in the state of Washington, and of these, 201 patients were between 20 and 60 years of age.

General Management

The patient with confirmed or suspected diphtheria should be hospitalized. Strict isolation, including handwashing, masks, gowns, and fomite control, should be strictly enforced until two negative cultures have been obtained after antibiotics have been discontinued for at least 48 hours. Absolute bed rest is essential during the critical phase of the illness; this is much more important in the management of diphtheria than in many other illnesses. In uncomplicated cases 14 days may suffice; in severe cases several weeks may be necessary. There are no special dietary considerations other than that the food contain the usual essential nutritional factors and that it be of a consistency easy to swallow. Pharyngeal discomfort may be relieved by aspirin with or without codeine in appropriate dose for weight. Exceptionally, hot irrigations with isotonic saline or 30 per cent glucose solutions may be helpful.

Use of Antitoxin

Antitoxin is the most important aspect of therapy and must be given to all patients in whom diphtheria cannot be excluded by physical examination. Although definitive diagnosis can be made by cultural isolation with virulence tests, it is not prudent to delay treatment pending bacteriologic confirmation. Also, there is no justification for withholding antitoxin in an advanced stage of the disease. The amount of toxin in the circulation at any given time is really quite small. The role of antitoxin is to (1) neutralize this circulating toxin, (2) bind any toxin subsequently produced, and (3) neutralize as much as possible the toxin not yet irreversibly bound to tissue.

Tests for Hypersensitivity. The use of horse serum (the only diphtheria antitoxin available) for any purpose occasionally results in mild reactions and, less commonly, in severe reactions. It is mandatory to test for hypersensitivity to horse serum before diphtheria antitoxin is injected. A syringe containing 1 ml. of 1:1000 aqueous epinephrine must be in readiness, for fatal reactions, although rare, have been precipitated by skin tests.

Both the two tests in current use are recommended. The skin test is performed by the intradermal injection of 0.1 ml. of 1:1000 dilution of diphtheria antitoxin in saline solution. A positive reaction reaches its maximum in 15 to 20 minutes and is characterized by induration, erythema, and pseudopod formation. The positive test is usually unmistakable, but if there is any doubt, a second test should be done with a slightly higher concentration, such as 0.1 ml. of a 1:200 dilution. A control injection of 0.1 ml. of isotonic saline solution should be done at the same time. In the ophthalmic test, 1 drop of a 1:10 saline dilution of antitoxin is instilled into the conjunctival sac of one eye and 1 drop of isotonic saline into the other eye as a control. Suffusion, itching, tearing, and edema appearing within 30 minutes in the test eye constitute a positive test. This reaction may be neutralized by the instillation of 1 drop of 1:1000 epinephrine solution. The clinical history is of equal or greater importance than the skin and eye test. The patient should be questioned regarding asthma, vasomotor rhinitis, and urticaria, especially in relation to horses. Previous use of horse serum increases the likelihood of reaction.

Dosage. In general the amount of antitoxin used is proportional to the extent of involvement (size of membrane) and the duration of illness. Weight or size of the patient is of less importance. Early, patients with small membranes can be treated with 20,000 units, increasing to 80,000 units on the third day of illness or for those with extensive membranes.

Route. The intravenous route is preferred in nonhypersensitive patients. The serum should be diluted 1:10 in isotonic saline and infused in an extremity over a 30 minute period. If volume is a problem, one half of the dose may be given intramuscularly. If the clinical history or the skin or ophthalmic tests are suggestive of hypersensitivity, antitoxin should be given with extreme caution. Antitoxin should never be given intravenously in this situation. Serial dilutions of antitoxin should be utilized as outlined in the brochure supplied by the manufacturer.

Antibiotics

The use of erythromycin or penicillin is routine. Although the drugs have no effect on the clinical course of diphtheria, they are necessary in the treatment of associated infections, e.g., beta-hemolytic streptococcal pharyngitis, and in the rapid clearing of the carrier state. If intravenous solutions are required for other reasons, aqueous penicillin may be incorporated in a dose of 2.4 million units over 24 hours. Procaine penicillin, 600,000 units intramuscularly every 12 hours for 10 to 14 days, is also suitable. Erythromycin is more active in vitro and has also been effective in clearing the carrier state in some patients when penicillin has failed. The dose orally is 25 to 50 mg. per kg. in divided doses every 6 hours. For intravenous use in the patient allergic to penicillin, the gluceptate salt is used, 3 to 5 mg. per kg. in the same divided doses. Chemical thrombophlebitis is a problem.

Steroids

Prednisone, 2 mg. per kg. in divided doses every 6 hours, is recommended by several authorities who feel it may modify or prevent the subsequent development of severe myocarditis. It is given for 5 days, followed by weaning over another 5 days. The effectiveness of this treatment remains to be proved.

Management of Complications

Serum Sickness. Serum sickness, fever, rash, and arthralgia may follow the administration of horse serum despite negative hypersensitivity tests, and are more likely to occur in those patients who received large amounts of antitoxin. The prophylactic use of cyproheptadine (Periactin) has been shown to be helpful in modifying or preventing this complication. From day 4 through 16, cyproheptadine should be administered according to the following schedule, which is greater than that recommended in the pharmaceutical label:

Less than 20 kg.	12 mg.
20 to 39 kg.	0.7 mg. per kg.
40 to 59 kg.	0.6 mg. per kg.
Over 60 kg.	0.5 mg. per kg.

The total dose should be divided and administered at 4 to 6 hour intervals.

Myocarditis. Patients who have a toxin-induced amegakaryocytic thrombocytopenia as an early manifestation of diphtheria are particularly likely to develop the toxemic complications of myocarditis—renal failure, shock, polyneuritis, and death. Cardiac complications are responsible for most diphtheritic deaths, as conduction defects, myocarditis with failure, or both. In early mild diphtheria serial electrocardiograms (ECG) are useful and are replaced by external cardiac monitoring if significant cardiac abnormality develops. A transvenous right ventricular pacemaker may be useful in those patients with a conduction problem and mild myocarditis. Failure is managed by careful fluid and salt restriction, along with monitoring central venous pressure. Digoxin, if necessary, should be used in half the recommended dose, or 0.6 mg. per square meter orally as a digitalizing dose, with 0.12 mg. per square meter as a maintenance dose. Furosemide, 1 mg. per kg., may be used as a diuretic. Should a vasopressor be needed, isoproterenol is probably preferred over metaraminol or levarterenol. Dopamine is probably contraindicated because of its association with ventricular arrhythmias. Should ventricular or atrial tachycardia develop, the prognosis is grim. Lidocaine hydrochloride, 1 mg. per kg., may be given in a rapid infusion.

Laryngotracheal Obstruction. Should the patient show signs of significant laryngeal obstruction, i.e., stridor, dyspnea, retractions, and tachypnea, tracheostomy is indicated and should be done before the patient is exhausted and cyanotic. Attempts to aspirate or remove part of a laryngotracheal membrane with forceps under direct vision may be made first by a skilled operator, but it is unwise to attempt to strip the pseudomembrane away from the underlying mucous membrane.

Neurologic Complications. Palatal paralysis is not uncommon and may occur 7 to 10 days after the onset of the disease. This is felt to be a result of the local effect of toxin on the peripheral nerves. Regurgitation through the nose and a nasal voice are signs of this difficulty, which may be treated by feeding through a nasogastric tube. More extensive paralysis may develop 2 to 4 weeks after onset with a picture clinically similar to that of the Guillain-Barré syndrome. Albuminocytologic dissociation may be present. Although severe involvement of muscles of deglutition is infrequent, it may develop, requiring tracheostomy as well as tube feedings to avoid drowning in oral secretions and, rarely, gastrostomy. Diaphragmatic paralysis may occur, requiring artificial respiratory assistance. The iron lung was originally developed for this condition. Ocular palsies may occur as late as 6 weeks after onset of the disease, with diplopia and difficulty with accommodation.

Other Complications. Acute otitis media, bronchopneumonia, and acute streptococcal pharyngitis may appear during the course of diphtheria and are treated by conventional methods. Proteinuria and occasionally microscopic hematuria are not uncommon findings during the acute phase of the disease. Although diphtheria is a severe illness, after recovery the patient rarely has permanent sequelae in any organ system.

Prophylaxis of Contacts

Persons who have been immunized actively with diphtheria toxoid should be given an immediate recall booster of fluid toxoid. They should be cultured for the presence of *Corynebacterium diphtheriae* at least twice in the first week after contact. Should organisms appear, antibiotic therapy should be promptly instituted. Penicillin or erythromycin may be used as in the therapy for the acute disease. For persons not previously immunized, serial cultures are taken during the first week and antibiotic treatment is instituted.

Management of the Carrier State

Isolation of *C. diphtheriae* from the respiratory tract does not per se indicate a clinically significant carrier state. The organism must be studied for virulence. Treatment is instituted only if toxigenic bacteria are present. The use of antibiotics in the same dosage as in the acute phase of the clinical disease is by far the most effective method of managing the situation. Readministration of larger doses of an antibiotic agent is usually successful in the few instances in which the first course of therapy fails. Very rarely, tonsillectomy may be indicated.

Prevention

The best time for immunization is during infancy, and the potency of the diphtheria toxoid is enhanced by the addition of other vaccines, particularly pertussis vaccine. In the United States the diphtheria toxoid is generally given in combination with tetanus toxoid and pertussis vaccine. Three doses of 0.5 ml. are given intramuscularly, starting when the child is 2 or 3 months of age and at intervals of 6 to 8 weeks. Booster injections should be given at approximately 18 months of age, prior to starting school, and at 5 to 10 year intervals thereafter. Preparations containing pertussis vaccine should not be used after 5 years of age because of the increasing severity of reactions to this product. Adult diphtheria-tetanus toxoid may be used for primary immunization or recall immunizations in persons over 10 years of age throughout life.

BACILLARY DYSENTERY

method of

GERALD T. KEUSCH, M.D.
New York, New York

Bacillary dysentery is one of the clinical presentations of acute shigellosis; it is not the only form, nor indeed is it the most common manifestation. The dysentery syndrome, characterized by exceedingly frequent passage (30 to 40 times per day) of scanty, bloody, mucoid stools, with severe abdominal cramps and tenesmus, can also be caused by certain serotypes of *Escherichia coli* (but not those included in the group known as enteropathogenic *E. coli*) and occasionally by Salmonella species, which all possess in common with shigellae the ability to invade the intestinal mucosa. The more common clinical presentation is that of watery diarrhea accompanied by moderate to high fever. When dysentery develops, it is ordinarily preceded by a recognizable period of watery diarrhea lasting a few hours to a day or more. Recent investigations show that diarrhea is due to excessive secretion of water and electrolytes by proximal small bowel, whereas dysentery is the result of an ulcerating, inflammatory colitis. This anatomic separation explains the temporal sequence of clinical symptoms following oral inoculation of the organism. *S. sonnei*, now the most prevalent Shigella species in the United States, is more likely to produce watery diarrhea alone, whereas *S. dysenteriae* 1, which recently was epidemic in Mexico and Central America and occasionally is recovered here from travelers to those countries, is more likely to cause a telescoped clinical course with prominent dysentery. *S. flexneri*, the second common Shigella species in the United States, can cause either clinical form of disease.

Because of their invasive properties, very few Shigella organisms are required to cause illness. As few as 10 to 100 *S. dysenteriae* 1 comprise an infectious dose; for the other species, between 1000 and 10,000 will suffice. This is a tiny inoculum (for even 10 million bacteria per ml. of water will not produce a visibly turbid solution) and therefore easily transmitted from person to person. Household spread of infection after introduction by the index case, usually a school-age child, is thus very common. In addition to the discomfort of clinical shigellosis, prevention of intrafamilial transmission constitutes a second reason for specific therapy. Fortunately, the inflammation resulting from intestinal invasion by shigellae provides a clue to their presence before results of bacteriologic investigation are available. A simple examination of the stool under the microscope will show an army of leukocytes, whereas virtually none are found in that from toxigenic *E. coli* or viral diarrhea.

Therapy

Treatment may be divided into nonspecific (supportive) and specific (antimicrobial) measures. A few general comments are appropriate.

1. Dehydration should be managed by replacement therapy and acidosis corrected quickly.
2. Febrile seizures, most often seen in older children, should be controlled acutely with barbiturates and rapid lowering of temperature by rubbing the skin with warm water and a Turkish towel. Temperature can be maintained thereafter in the 100 to 101°F. (37.8 to 38.3°C.) range by small regular doses of aspirin every 4 hours, according to the age and size of the child.
3. Lactase deficiency may occur during acute shigellosis so that inclusion of milk in the diet, although not contraindicated, should be carefully observed.
4. Analgesics for intestinal cramps are not helpful.
5. Inhibitors of bowel mobility, including tincture of opium (DTO), paregoric, and diphenoxylate, are reported to worsen symptoms of shigellosis, presumably by prolonging the contact between the bacteria and intestinal mucosa, thereby facilitating bacterial invasion. This situation has not been observed in my experience; however, there is also no convincing evidence of efficacy from controlled clinical trial. Therefore, there appears to be little or no reason to prescribe these drugs, particularly for children. Adults with mild to moderate symptoms may be made happier at times, perhaps no better, and usually no worse by their use.

Rehydration. Because the proximal small bowel seems to be the site of major fluid loss, oral rehydration, taking advantage of the mechanism of glucose-facilitated sodium absorption, appears to be efficacious. Prerequisites for oral therapy of shigellosis are the same as for other diarrheal diseases: (1) first or second degree dehydration, (2) bowel sounds present, and (3) patient conscious and able to drink. The principle is to provide an actively transported sugar, such as glucose, and sodium together in the lumen of the bowel. This may be achieved by feeding Coke syrup in water, the beverage Gatorade, or packaged pharmaceutical preparations (Lytren, Pedialyte). A simple solution can also be made at home or in the doctor's office by mixing simple chemicals according to Hirschhorn et al.: ½ teaspoon of salt, ½ teaspoon of bicarbonate of soda, ¼ teaspoon of KCl (if available), and 2 tablespoons of glucose (or 4 tablespoons of table sugar) to 1 liter of water. Young children appear to regulate their intake when offered such fluids ad libitum each hour to correct dehydration without excessive salt intake and precipitation of a hyperosmotic state. Oral therapy may increase total stool output, whereas net absorption is increased. The state of hydration of the patient, and not stool volume, must be monitored.

Parenteral fluid administration is required for severe dehydration or if oral ingestion is not possible because of intractable vomiting. When these have been corrected by initial intravenous fluids, rehydration may be continued by the oral route. Weight regain, in fact, appears to be more rapid in children treated with oral glucose-electrolye solution and early refeeding than in those maintained without oral feeding and given intravenous fluids.

Antimicrobials. Controlled clinical trials have clearly demonstrated two critical points regarding antimicrobial therapy of shigellosis: (1) agents to which the organism is sensitive shorten the clinical course as well as eradicate the pathogen from the stool; and (2) oral nonabsorbable drugs are no more effective than placebo, presumably because they fail to reach the population of bacteria within the lamina propria. A major problem, however, has been development of resistance caused by transferable extrachromosomal DNA R-factors (a phenomenon ironically first demonstrated in *S. flexneri* by Watanabe in 1957 in Japan). Furthermore, although treatment of patients with drugs to which the infecting organism is resistant in vitro is without effect, in vitro sensitivity is no guarantee of clinical efficacy. Thus neither cephalexin nor amoxicillin is recommended, although shigellae are, in general, susceptible. Resistance to antimicrobial agents is much more common in *S. sonnei* than in *S. flexneri* and is both time and locale specific. There is, therefore, no one optimal choice for initial therapy; the decision must be based on a knowledge of the sensitivity of strains being isolated *at the time* in each physician's area. The following agents are clinically effective when given for 5 days for susceptible strains: ampicillin, tetracycline, chloramphenicol, and trimethoprim-sulfamethoxazole combinations. When the organism is sensitive, ampicillin is the drug of choice in a dose of 100 mg. per kg. or 2 grams per day for children and adults, respectively. Tetracycline is not recommended for children under 8 years of age, because it is deposited in bone and teeth and may interfere with bone growth and normal deposition of enamel. Adults, however, may be treated with 2 grams per day for 5 days, or a single bolus dose of 2.5 grams. In contrast, chloramphenicol is not recommended for either children or adults except for severe illness caused by isolates resistant to all other available agents. Trimethoprim (10 mg. per kg. per day) in combination with sulfamethoxazole (50 mg. per kg. per day) (TMP-SMX) has recently been shown to be as effective as ampicillin. It is at present the drug of choice when isolates are ampicillin resistant. Because shigellosis is not currently a Food and Drug Administration–approved indication for use of TMP-SMX, it is recommended that informed consent be obtained prior to its administration. In the event that TMP-SMX cannot be used either, nalidixic acid (55 mg. per kg. per day) may be tried, although it is less effective than both ampicillin and TMP-SMX. (This use of nalidixic acid is not listed in the manufacturer's official directive.) *Candida albicans* often overgrows the bowel flora in ampicillin-treated patients, but only rarely is clinical thrush seen. Thus Candida should not be treated unless specific lesions are found.

Convalescent carriage of Shigella is usually short lived and does not require antimicrobial therapy. In fact, there is no evidence that antimicrobics can eradicate the carrier state in the unusual situation of prolonged excretion of the organism. By the same token, effective antimicrobial therapy of acute disease does not lead to a longer duration of post-treatment positive stool cultures, as in the case with Salmonella infection. Lactulose, pushed to the threshold of tolerance (diarrhea), can convert positive stools to negative *during the period of its administration,* presumably through an effect on stool pH (decrease) and short chain fatty acid content (increase). The organisms reappear when lactulose is discontinued.

Because the infection is usually self-limited and acquired drug resistance is a problem, the decision to treat acute shigellosis with antimicrobials must include several factors, among them severity of the clinical disease, the likelihood of intrafamilial spread because of the presence of young children who cannot be expected to maintain strict standards of personal hygiene, and the pattern of antimicrobial resistance of the organism. When used, administration of antimicrobials early in the course of the illness is most likely to prove effective.

GAS GANGRENE AND SIMILAR ANAEROBIC SOFT TISSUE INFECTIONS

method of
WESLEY FURSTE, M.D.,
and HUGO CABRERA, PH.D.
Columbus, Ohio

Many of the great men of medicine have been interested in gas gangrene as a complication of wounds because of its spectacular nature, fulminating course, profound toxemia, mutilating effects, and high mortality. During the past few decades, gas gangrene has become a general term which has been loosely applied to a number of conditions.

Clinical Picture

Clostridial myositis of the spreading or diffuse type represents true gas gangrene resulting from trauma. It may be manifested clinically as the crepitant type, the noncrepitant or edematous type, the mixed type, or the profound toxemic type. Diffuse clostridial myositis is essentially an affection of the muscles, and, comparatively, at first, connective tissues may be little affected.

Three distinct zones in gas gangrene can be recognized:

1. A central or dead zone which consists of distintegrated muscle destroyed by trauma, organized clot, and a vast number of organisms.

2. A second or dying zone which contains devitalized muscle fibers covered by masses of bacteria and the products of infection. The anatomic arrangement of these muscle fibers remains undisturbed even though the fibers become separated by an exudate which is or is not packed with leukocytes, according to the type of infection. Local leukocytosis usually is associated with mixed infections.

TABLE 1. **Gas Gangrene and Similar Anaerobic Soft Tissue Infections***

I. Deep infections with muscle involvement
  A. Gas gangrene
    1. Gas gangrene resulting from soft tissue trauma; clostridial myositis; clostridial myonecrosis
    2. Abdominal wall gas gangrene; postoperative clostridial sepsis of the abdominal wall; clostridial myonecrosis of the abdominal wall
    3. Uterine clostridial infections
    4. Gas gangrene of the heart
  B. Streptococcal myositis; anaerobic streptococcal myonecrosis; anaerobic streptococcal myositis
  C. Infected vascular gas gangrene; nonclostridial gas gangrene; nonclostridial myositis
II. Superficial infections
  A. Hemolytic streptococcal gangrene
  B. Acute infectious staphylococcal gangrene
  C. Anaerobic cellulitis; crepitant phlegmon; clostridial cellulitis
  D. Necrotizing fasciitis
  E. Synergistic necrotizing cellulitis
III. Simple clostridial contamination of wounds
IV. Infiltration or injection of gas into wounds
  A. Battle wounds
  B. Pranksters' jokes
  C. Self-inflicted wounds (malingering)
V. Gas in tissues after industrial accidents
  A. Magnesiogenous pneumagranuloma
VI. Gas in tissues after injections of chemicals
  A. Injection of drugs
  B. Accidental injection of a foreign agent
    1. Benzene

*This table consists of diagnoses which have been reported in the literature or to the authors. Closely related diagnoses are grouped together.

3. A third or normal zone in which the muscle is normal, except for some cellular infiltration.

The *incubation period* between the occurrence of the injury and the onset of gas gangrene varies from a few hours to a few days.

Prophylaxis

Prophylaxis of gas gangrene in wounds requires the best type of surgical technique and the indicated use of antibiotics.

Surgical Wound Care. The most effective means of preventing these anaerobic conditions continues to be early and adequate care of wounds. Such surgical care includes wide incision, thorough debridement of all devitalized and potentially devitalized tissues, removal of contaminating dirt and all foreign bodies, and effective drainage as required. Adequate debridement is especially important in irregular deep wounds in which there are loculations and recesses which favor anaerobic bacterial growth. Dead and devitalized tissue and foreign bodies must be removed at the time of initial operation. In war wounds, in wounds in which treatment has been inordinately delayed, and in all wounds other than on the face and in which there has been some trauma to the soft tissues, such thorough debridement should be coupled with delayed suture of the wound. The wound should be left open for 4 to 7 days following the debridement, and then delayed suture should be accomplished if the wound has remained clean and shows no evidence of infection.

Similar surgical principles should be observed when elective surgical procedures are performed for lesions of any of the body cavities or of the extremities.

Antibiotics. Antibiotic therapy is of some prophylactic value when combined with proper surgical procedures. Experimental and clinical experience affirms this principle, but indicates that antibiotic therapy alone cannot be relied upon to prevent the occurrence of clostridial myositis.

TABLE 2. **Microorganisms Which May Produce Gas in Human Tissues**

GRAM STAIN RESULT	AEROBES	ANAEROBES
Gram-positive microorganisms		
Cocci	*Staphylococcus aureus (Staphylococcus pyogenes)* Group A Streptococcus (*Streptococcus pyogenes;* beta-hemolytic Streptococcus)	Peptostreptococcus (anaerobic Streptococcus)
Bacilli		*Clostridium perfringens* *Clostridium novyi* *Clostridium septicum* *Clostridium histolyticum* *Clostridium sporogenes* *Clostridium tertium* and other clostridia species which may be responsible for gas gangrene
Gram-negative microorganisms		
Bacilli	*Escherichia coli* *Klebsiella pneumoniae* Enterobacter species	*Bacteroides fragilis*

Penicillin, cephalothin, clindamycin, and chloramphenicol are reported to be effective against over 80 per cent of tested strains of *Cl. perfringens*.

Penicillin administered intravenously in doses of 1,000,000 to 3,000,000 units every 4 to 8 hours is the chemotherapeutic agent of choice to be used in conjunction with adequate surgery for the prevention of gas gangrene. Massive doses of penicillin can prolong the period during which surgical intervention short of amputation can be effective.

Antitoxin. Gas gangrene antitoxins have no place in the prophylaxis of gas gangrene. There may be multiple species of gas gangrene clostridia involved, each of which requires a specific antitoxin for neutralization of its exotoxin. Moreover, the antitoxin cannot be distributed to neutralize the exotoxin being produced in the nonviable, avascular tissue involved. In addition, not infrequently there are significant reactions to the large amounts of gas gangrene antitoxin which have been recommended. Furthermore, large series of cases have not unequivocally proved the desirability of prophylactic gas gangrene antitoxin.

Hyperbaric Oxygen Therapy. Hyperbaric oxygen therapy remains experimental and unproved as a prophylactic therapeutic measure in gas gangrene. The experimental evidence indicates that it has little value without adequate surgical debridement.

Therapy

For proper treatment, there must be an accurate diagnosis with respect to the tissues involved and to the types of bacteria involved and their drug sensitivities. The deep and spreading infections may require mutilating operations; the superficial and localized infections may require only multiple incisions; and the pure gas infiltrations and contaminations may require only diagnostic incisions. The extent and depth of a gas infection is easily—and relatively safely—determined by longitudinal incisions of the skin, superficial fascia, and deep fascia. The type of bacteria can be quickly determined to some extent by an immediate Gram stain. Culture, identification, and sensitivity tests can be completed later to determine the most appropriate antibiotic for therapy.

Radical Surgical Wound Care. Such care should be effected as soon after diagnosis as possible. Optimally, it consists of multiple incisions for decompression and drainage of the fascial compartments, excision of the involved muscles, or open amputation when necessary, followed by adequate immobilization of the affected part. *Early and adequate operation is the primary and most effective means of treating clostridial myositis.* If the diagnosis is made early, while the gangrene is relatively localized, radical decompression of the involved fascial compartments by extensive longitudinal incisions and excision of infected muscle usually arrest the progress and eliminate the need for amputation. If the diagnosis is reached when the process is extensive and has caused irreversible gangrenous changes, open amputation of the guillotine type becomes necessary.

Gas gangrene of the abdominal wall or perineum presents special problems; but, again, the same surgical principles apply. *Multiple incisions, fasciotomy*, and *extirpation of* as much *involved tissue* as is technically feasible should be undertaken.

Marlex, Mersilene, or Prolene mesh may be used for temporary and permanent containment of abdominal viscera after extensive clostridial myonecrosis of the abdominal wall. Debridement is carried out through parallel incisions with maximum preservation of skin and subcutaneous tissue. Mesh is used temporarily until the infection is completely controlled. The mesh is then removed, and the skin and subcutaneous tissue are reapproximated. This procedure gives excellent wound coverage and markedly shortens the hospital stay.

On occasion, a postabortal infection may be caused by *Cl. perfringens*. Women infected with this organism may be critically ill with general sepsis, shock, and renal failure. Massive doses of antibiotics and heroic measures, such as peritoneal dialysis or hemodialysis, may not suffice. *Hysterectomy* is also indicated.

In contrast to the deep and more serious anaerobic infections, for the *superficial* and *less serious infections, debridement of the wound* involved may be all that is necessary. Devitalized tissue must be excised. When the infection extends along fascial planes beyond the traumatized area of the wound, long incisions must be made to open these areas and to excise the necrotic fascia. Following debridement, the wounds should be copiously irrigated with isotonic solutions before a dressing is applied. Such wounds are obviously not closed primarily.

Antibiotics. These drugs, as already indicated, may add much to the successful care of gas infections. Major considerations in anaerobic bacteriology are proper specimen collection, immediate transportation to the laboratory, and prompt inoculation and placement of specimen under anaerobic conditions. Special collection and transport methods, such as the following, may be used to ensure the survival of the most fastidious anaerobic organisms:

1. The syringe technique can be effectively used in the case of abscess. The skin is decontami-

nated, and pus is removed with a needle and syringe. All air is eliminated, the needle is inserted into a cork or rubber stopper, and the specimen is carried promptly to the laboratory, where it must be immediately processed.

2. Specimens can be collected in rubber-stoppered tubes that have been gassed out with oxygen-free CO_2.

3. Anaerobic culturettes containing reduced transport medium are presently commercially available, and are good transport systems.

Although the management of anaerobic soft tissue infections is mainly surgical, antibiotic therapy is a vital adjunct. Patients with anaerobic soft tissue infections should be given antibiotics in high dosage and—whenever possible—by the intravenous route.

The initial choice of antibiotic is based on the findings of the Gram stain of the exudate, but should eventually be modified as indicated by the results of the culture and sensitivity tests.

A very important fact to keep in mind in the interpretation of the smear and the culture is that the *presence of gram-positive rods* or other organisms in either smear or culture does *not necessarily* indicate that *an infection* is present. Colonization of uninfected wounds by microorganisms is not an uncommon occurrence. The clinical picture should be taken into account before the institution of what could be unnecessary antimicrobial therapy. Although occasionally an infection does develop in these contaminated lesions, in many cases a thorough cleaning and debridement will suffice.

Patients with infections from which a Gram stain reveals large gram-positive rods or gram-positive small to tiny cocci, or both, can be treated with 1,000,000 to 3,000,000 units of penicillin every 3 to 4 hours intravenously. Sodium penicillin is preferred to potassium penicillin to avoid administration of large amounts of potassium. Cultures from these lesions will in most cases grow *Cl. perfringens* and anaerobic Streptococcus. Patients who are allergic to penicillin can receive either 2 grams of cephalothin every 4 hours or 600 mg. of clindamycin every 6 to 8 hours intravenously. These last two antibiotics will also be effective against any pencillinase-producing staphylococci that may be present.

For patients from whom a gram-stained smear of the exudate shows pleomorphic gram-negative bacilli or gram-negative rods with tapered ends, either 600 mg. of clindamycin every 6 to 8 hours or 1 gram of chloramphenicol every 6 hours intravenously is recommended. Cultures from these lesions will often grow *Bacteroides fragilis* or some other Bacteroides species. Carbenicillin in doses of 24 to 30 grams per 24 hours may also be used for these organisms.

In multimicrobial infections, especially infections in which the Gram stain demonstrates both gram-positive and gram-negative organisms, a combination of 3,000,000 units of penicillin every 4 hours and 1 gram of chloramphenicol every 6 hours intravenously is very effective. This is the most effective combination that can be used against all anaerobes. It should be remembered that the use of chloramphenicol may be associated

TABLE 3. **Antibiotic Treatment of Gas Infections Based on Gram Stain Results, Cultures, and Sensitivity Tests**

GRAM STAIN RESULT	PRESUMPTIVE MICROORGANISM	ANTIBIOTICS
Gram-positive cocci	Anaerobic Streptococcus	Penicillin Cephalosporins Clindamycin Chloramphenicol
Gram-positive bacilli	Clostridium species	Penicillin Cephalosporins Clindamycin Chloramphenicol
Gram-negative bacilli	Bacteroides species	Clindamycin Chloramphenicol Carbenicillin
	Coliforms	Cephalosporins Ampicillin Gentamicin Tobramycin Amikacin Chloramphenicol Carbenicillin

with very serious side effects. If the cultures eventually grow enteric organisms that are resistant to chloramphenicol, such as Pseudomonas or Proteus, a combination of 60 to 80 mg. of gentamicin every 8 hours and 600 mg. of clindamycin every 6 hours intravenously is excellent therapy.

If gentamicin-resistant strains of Pseudomonas are present, 500 mg. of amikacin every 12 hours intramuscularly can be used instead of gentamicin. As with other aminoglycosides, amikacin serum levels should be monitored both to ensure adequate serum levels and to decrease the chances of toxicity. Such determinations should be routine in desperately ill patients in whom adequate therapy is important for survival. Carbenicillin, 4 to 5 grams every 6 hours intravenously, is effective against most enteric organisms, with the exception of Klebsiella. Carbenicillin is also effective against Pseudomonas and *Bacteroides fragilis*. In patients with severe renal impairment and when serum levels cannot be adequately monitored, carbenicillin can be substituted for gentamicin. Awareness of the high sodium load of carbenicillin must be kept in mind, especially in patients with cardiac disease, and signs of overload must be carefully monitored.

Antitoxin. Antitoxin therapy is controversial. The most compelling indications are (1) shock and (2) hemolytic anemia which may be caused by circulating alpha-toxin. The commercially available polyvalent product contains antitoxin for *Cl. perfringens, Cl. septicum, Cl. histolyticum, Cl. novyi,* and *Cl. bifermentans*. Suggested dosage is 50,000 units every 6 hours for 1 to 2 days intravenously. If antitoxin is administered, proper precautions—before, during, and after administration—are to be effected. At present, we are not convinced of the value of the therapeutic use of antitoxin in view of (1) multiple Clostridium species being responsible causative microorganisms, (2) inability of the body to deliver the antitoxin to the avascular gangrenous tissue, (3) the reactions produced by the heterologous antitoxin, and (4) a lack of noncontroversial evidence that antitoxin has been of value in the treatment of human gas gangrene.

Hyperbaric Oxygen. The administration of hyperbaric oxygen, too, is controversial. Good results have been reported in certain medical centers. The following factors, however, must be considered: (1) oxygen penetrates poorly into necrotic tissue; (2) there are certain associated hazards, such as oxygen toxicity with disorientation and convulsions; (3) seriously ill patients are difficult to manage in a chamber; and (4) the apparatus is frequently not available. When used, recommended treatment is 100 per cent oxygen at 3 atmospheres pressure for 1 to 2 hours at 8 hour intervals. One salient advantage of hyperbaric oxygen is that the involved tissue quickly becomes demarcated so that the extent of resection is readily apparent. Hyperbaric oxygen may be worthwhile for a patient with gas gangrene prior to radical excisional surgery—provided the apparatus is reasonably convenient and provided there is no undue delay in the indicated and necessary surgical intervention.

Tetanus Prophylaxis. For all wounds, the best possible type of tetanus prophylaxis—including, when indicated, the administration of adsorbed tetanus toxoid and/or tetanus immune globulin (human)—is to be effected. Such prophylaxis is described in this and previous editions of *Current Therapy*. Although gas gangrene is a complication primarily of severe wounds, it is emphasized that tetanus may occur after wounds of any size and even in patients in whom no wound can be demonstrated.

Adequate Supportive Therapy. The general supportive measures of value in the management of gas gangrene include frequent or daily whole blood, packed erythrocytes, or plasma transfusions; maintenance of the fluid and electrolyte balance; adequate immobilization of the infected and injured parts; pulmonary oxygen therapy; and the relief of pain. Frequent blood transfusions are necessary to correct the profound anemia with which this condition is frequently associated, and are one of the mainstays of postoperative management. Plasma is usually reserved for the correction of persistent hemoconcentration in selected cases of the "wet" type of clostridial infection. Acidosis is corrected with appropriate therapy.

Exchange Transfusions. Exchange transfusion is another technique advocated for patients who have hemolysis caused by the alpha-toxemia. This approach has been used in uterine and abdominal wall gas gangrene. It is a desperation measure, however, and has not been proved in controlled trials.

Control of Renal Failure. Hemodialysis or peritoneal dialysis may be needed to control renal insufficiency.

Steroids. The use of steroids in the treatment of gas gangrene is debatable, even though these agents might well be of some help in treating the bacteremic shock. It would seem that they might also depress the known resistance that the body maintains to infection of any kind. There are no adequate criteria at present to draw conclusions. Individual criteria for each patient must be exercised regarding the possible use of steroids.

Secondary Operative Procedures. Secondary operative procedures to facilitate healing of the wound or function of the extremity should be performed as indicated. They should obviously be postponed until after the infection has been brought completely under control, however.

Hypothermia. It would seem that reduction of the fever, which in a few patients rises to an alarming level, might be beneficial. On the assumption that this idea is correct, hypothermia has been employed throughout several areas of the world.

Concluding Comments

Early and adequate surgical wound care is still the *best method* for both the prevention and the treatment of gas gangrene and similar anaerobic soft tissue infections. *Antibiotic therapy* has been shown to be a valuable adjunct to surgical intervention, and penicillin in massive doses appears to be the agent of choice for the clostridia. *General supportive measures*, including frequent *blood transfusions*, are most important for these virulent anaerobic soft tissue infections.

In view of the many persons—such as the patients themselves, their families and friends, nursing staffs, hospital administrators, public health officers, government officials, and lawyers—who can be involved in the care of patients with anaerobic soft tissue infections, it is strongly recommended that *physicians* and other *medical scientists,* who are held medically, morally, and legally accountable, *document in writing their observations, decisions, and care of these patients.*

FOODBORNE ILLNESS

method of
HERBERT L. DuPONT, M.D.
Houston, Texas

The general ubiquity of bacterial, viral, and parasitic agents as well as toxic substances in nature assures that we have a recurrent exposure to them. Food serves as an excellent medium for growth of microbial agents, and development of symptomatic disease after ingestion of contaminated food correlates with at least one of four factors:

TABLE 1. **Chemical Foodborne Disease**

ETIOLOGY	VEHICLE	INCUBATION PERIOD	CLINICAL ASPECTS	DIAGNOSIS	TREATMENT
Heavy metals (tin, antimony, copper, etc.)	Characteristic container for food	3 min.–3 hrs.	Gastrointestinal (GI) symptoms, metallic taste	Detection of metal in food	Symptomatic
Paralytic shellfish poisoning	Mollusks	10–60 min.	Paresthesias of lips, mouth, face; GI symptoms	Detection of toxin in mollusks, history of dinoflagellates in water where gathered	Symptomatic
Ciguatera poisoning	Fish, oysters, clams	30 min.–24 hrs.	GI symptoms, dry mouth paresthesias, pain in teeth	Detection of toxin in food	Symptomatic
Puffer fish poisoning	Blowfish	10 min.–4 hrs.	Paresthesias, numbness, "floating" sensation	Detection of toxin in food	Symptomatic
Scombroid poisoning	Tuna, mackerel, etc.	5 min.–1 hr.	Flushing, headache, dizziness, GI symptoms, pruritus	Elevated histamine levels in fish	Antihistamines
"Chinese restaurant syndrome"	Monosodium glutamate (MSG)	5–30 min.	Burning sensation in chest, neck, abdomen, extremities; sweating, tachycardia	Heavy concentrations of MSG in foods	Symptomatic
Mushroom poisoning	*Amanita muscaria*	1–3 hrs.	GI symptoms, perspiration, salivation, bradycardia	Detection of toxin in mushroom or ingestion of specific mushroom	Gastric lavage (induce vomiting), atropine for muscarinic effects
	Other mushrooms	1–18 hrs.	GI symptoms, confusion, delirium, visual disturbance	Detection of toxin in mushroom or ingestion of specific mushroom	Symptomatic

1. The level of contamination or number of viable cells per gram of food.

2. The presence of an aggressive (virulent) agent which is capable of toxin production or invading the intestinal mucosa.

3. Presence of a host factor which enhances susceptibility (e.g., achlorhydria, prior gastric resection, agammaglobulinemia, protein caloric malnutrition, newborn, aged). Here an inoculum size too low to induce illness in the healthy may be sufficient to result in illness.

4. Presence in food of a toxic chemical.

Foodborne illness can be divided into two general forms: infection and intoxication (or poisoning). The two forms can usually be separated by determining the incubation period of the illness. In an intoxication there is a shorter incubation period which in all but botulism is generally less than 4 hours after ingesting the food. Infection from ingestion of contaminated food will have an incubation period greater than 5 hours, as the organisms must proliferate to high numbers in the gut.

Foodborne disease is suggested when two or more persons experience a similar illness after ingestion of a common meal. A single case of botulism or chemical food poisoning is sufficient to make the diagnosis.

Treatment of foodborne illness depends upon the diagnosis and can be divided into general and specific forms. Tables 1 through 4 offer a partial list of diseases which can be transmitted by ingestion of contaminated food and indicate their treatment. Other foodborne agents not mentioned in the tables are mycotoxins (aflatoxin) from *Aspergillus flavus* (contaminating cereal grains and peanut products), alkyl mercury poisoning, insecticides and fungicidal agents, nitrite contamination of meats, cholera, and tuberculosis.

Many of the foodborne illnesses are associated with fluid and electrolyte losses which may result in dehydration. Therapy in these situations is directed toward symptomatic measures and replacement of fluid and electrolytes. Diarrhea and abdominal discomfort usually can be controlled with an agent such as bismuth subsalicylate (Pepto-Bismol) given 30 ml. each half hour for eight doses. Oral electrolyte and fluid therapy in many patients can be replaced by bottled soft drinks, although some patients may require hospitalization and intravenous fluids.

TABLE 2. **Bacterial Foodborne Disease—Absence of Fever**

ETIOLOGY	INCUBATION PERIOD	CLINICAL ASPECTS	DIAGNOSIS	TREATMENT
Staphylococcal food poisoning	1–5 hrs.	Prostration, vomiting, diarrhea	Characteristic incubation period, vomiting out of proportion to diarrhea	Symptomatic, intravenous fluids
Clostridium perfringens	8–22 hrs.	Diarrhea with systemic symptoms or vomiting	Organisms in stool or food	Symptomatic
Toxigenic *Escherichia coli*	8–96 hrs.	Diarrhea (which may be profuse) without systemic symptoms	Isolation of agent in stool or food; serologic response to infection	Symptomatic, intravenous fluids
Bacillus cereus	8–20 hrs.	Abdominal cramps, diarrhea, nausea	Detection of organism in food	Symptomatic
Clostridium botulinum —"botulism"	5–36 hrs.	Malaise, weakness, cranial nerve paralysis, blurred vision, ptosis, dysarthria, dysphagia (GI symptoms may be seen with type E disease)	Detection of botulinal toxin in stool, serum, or food, or when food is epidemiologically incriminated	1. Gastric lavage, or induce vomiting with ipecac, 30–45 ml. 2. Cathartic—Mg citrate or $MgSO_4$ 3. Botulinal antitoxin (obtained from CDC (404-633-3311 or 404-633-2176), trivalent ABE if type is unknown, or AB or E if type is known—1 ml. (one vial) I.V. plus 1 ml. I.M., followed by two similar injections in 2–4 hrs. if symptoms persist 4. In severe cases, guanidine hydrochloride, 14–50 mg./kg./day P.O. (investigational) until symptoms improve

TABLE 3. **Bacterial Foodborne Disease with Fever**

ETIOLOGY	INCUBATION PERIOD	CLINICAL ASPECTS	DIAGNOSIS	TREATMENT
Shigella	7–120 hrs.	Abdominal pain (cramps), fecal urgency, tenesmus, diarrhea with or without blood and mucus in stools	Isolation of Shigella from stool	*Children:* Ampicillin, 100 mg./kg./day in three or four divided doses (P.O., I.M., or I.V.) for 5 days *or* Trimethoprim (TM), 10 mg., and sulfamethoxazole (SMX), 50 mg./kg./day for 5 days* *Adults:* Tetracycline, 2.5 grams in a single dose *or* TM, 160 mg., and SMX, 800 mg., b.i.d. for 5 days*
E. coli (invasive type)	8–24 hrs.	Same as Shigella	Isolation of invasive *E. coli* from stool or food	Symptomatic; antibiotics have not been evaluated, but should be similar to Shigella in response to treatment
Salmonella				
Gastroenteritis	8–24 hrs.	Abdominal pain, diarrhea, nausea, vomiting	Isolation of Salmonella from stool or food	Symptomatic (treat as typhoid if clinical course suggests bacteremia)
Typhoid fever	6–14 days	Headache, abdominal pain, constipation, or diarrhea	Isolation of Salmonella from stool, blood, or food	Ampicillin, 100 mg./kg./day in three or four divided doses (I.V.) for 2 wks., or *for children:* TM, 10 mg., and SMX, 50 mg./kg./day for 2 wks., or *for adults:* TM, 160 mg., and SM, 800 mg., q. 12 hrs. for 2 wks.* (Chloramphenicol may be preferred if organism is known to be sensitive)
Vibrio parahemolyticus	12–24 hrs.	Diarrhea, occasionally blood or mucus in stool	Isolation of vibrio from stool or food or illness traced to seafood	Symptomatic

*This use of these agents is not listed in the manufacturer's official directive.

TABLE 4. **Miscellaneous Foodborne Disease**

ETIOLOGY	INCUBATION PERIOD	CLINICAL ASPECTS	DIAGNOSIS	TREATMENT
Group A Streptococcus	2–4 days	Febrile upper respiratory infection	Isolation of organism from pharynx and food	*Children:* Phenoxymethyl penicillin, 25–50 mg./kg./day for 10 days, or benzathine penicillin, 25,000 units/kg. in a single injection *Adults:* Phenoxymethyl penicillin, 250 mg. q.i.d. for 10 days, or benzathine penicillin, 1.2 million units in a single injection
Brucella	5–30 days	Protracted febrile illness	Serologic response to infection; isolation of agent from blood	Tetracycline, 500 mg. P.O. q. 6 hrs. for 3 to 6 wks.
Trichinella spiralis	3–28 days	GI symptoms followed by fever, eosinophilia, periorbital edema, and myalgias	Serologic response or demonstration of larvae in food or muscle	Symptomatic; in severe cases thiabendazole, 25 mg./kg. twice daily for 5–7 days (daily dose not to exceed 3 grams with or without corticosteroids)
Giardiasis	4–15 days	Diarrhea	Protozoa seen in stool or in small bowel fluid or "touch prep" using duodenal biopsy	Metronidazole,* 250 mg. q.i.d. for 10 days *or* Quinacrine (Atabrine), 100 mg. t.i.d. for 10 days
E. histolytica	More than 7 days	Diarrhea	Unidirectionally motile trophozoites with ingested red blood cells	Metronidazole, 750 mg. t.i.d. for 10 days *plus* Diiodohydroxyquin, 650 mg. t.i.d. for 21 days
Hepatitis A or B	10–50 days	GI symptoms, jaundice	Liver function abnormalities; serologic confirmation in hepatitis B	Symptomatic

*This use of metronidazole is not listed in the manufacturer's official directive.

EPIDEMIC INFLUENZA

method of
WILLIAM J. MOGABGAB, M.D.
New Orleans, Louisiana

Infection with influenza A virus occurs in epidemic proportions every 2 to 3 years and with influenza B virus every 3 to 6 years during the winter or early spring. The incidence is low during the intervening periods, but sporadic illnesses or localized outbreaks can usually be found. Because of the variation in degree of illness in individuals and because the disease is relatively milder in children, it may be difficult to recognize isolated cases of influenza or a large proportion of cases in epidemics. The occurrence of asymptomatic infections and afebrile upper respiratory illnesses is quite common. When there is a frequent appearance of sicknesses with sudden onset accompanied by chills or chilliness, fever, headache, backache, muscular aching, anorexia, malaise, and symptoms referable to the respiratory tract, it is likely that the virus is prevalent in the population. In a locality outbreaks last for several weeks with highest incidence in school children, but illnesses develop in all age groups. An increase in deaths from all causes occurs during the period of prevalence, chiefly among persons with chronic illnesses and in the aged.

Influenza viruses A and B are antigenically distinct members of the myxovirus group. Their size is 80 to 120 nm.; they have an inner nucleoprotein containing ribonucleic acid surrounded by an ether-sensitive envelope. The virus has toxic properties but the hemagglutinin (H) of the protein coat is nontoxic and can be separated for preparation of vaccine. An enzyme, neuraminidase (N), assists the invasive properties of these viruses. They can be readily inactivated by disinfectants, temperatures of 56°C. (132.8°F.) for a few minutes, and acid or alkaline solutions.

Influenza A viruses cause more severe illnesses, larger-scale epidemics, and higher death rates than influenza B virus. Lack of extreme antigenic change of the latter virus results in considerable immunity in the adult population. Pandemics have been caused by influenza A virus only. The last, caused by a new antigenic variant, designated A-2 (H2N2), appeared in 1957, and it was replaced in 1968 by the Hong Kong (H3N2) variant. A change in influenza B virus occurred in 1962.

Definitive Diagnosis

Definitive diagnosis of influenza rests upon laboratory evidence. It is very important to confirm the presence of the virus in several typical early cases in the community in order to be alerted. This can be readily accomplished by ultraviolet microscopic examination of cells from a nasopharyngeal smear after reaction with fluorescein-conjugated antiserum. Next, the virus should be recovered and characterized as to type and subtype in each area so that vaccine effectiveness can be predicted and evaluated. Pharyngeal washings should be collected with solutions buffered to pH 7.0 to 7.4 and containing protein, i.e., bacterial culture broths or boiled skim milk, or special solutions from the virus laboratory. These specimens should be transported on ice without freezing. For serologic diagnosis by the hemagglutination-inhibition or complement-fixation test a blood sample should be obtained during the first few days of illness and a second 2 to 3 weeks later.

Pathogenesis

The pathogenesis of influenza provides the best insight into therapy and prevention of complications. The viruses have toxic properties, and, although there is no evidence of dissemination or multiplication beyond the respiratory tract, the clinical disease has many systemic manifestations. Cyanosis, bradycardia or tachycardia arrhythmia, or hypotension may be found in patients without previously known cardiovascular disease. Delirium may be extreme. Obviously, the patient with severe influenza should be examined carefully and frequently. Parenteral fluids and oxygen may be needed, as well as other measures that become indicated. Postinfluenzal asthenia might be a result of the same mechanism. Patients with influenza may experience fever of 101 to 104°F. (38.3 to 40°C.) for 1 to 5 days and considerable aching. Bed rest, analgesics, and aspirin are all that is needed for these, but the patient should be kept quiet for a day after the fever has subsided.

Invasion and destruction of focal areas of the ciliated epithelium of the nasopharynx, trachea, and bronchi cause the respiratory signs and symptoms. Thus, tracheobronchitis, manifested by substernal burning and deep cough that frequently becomes productive, is common toward the end of the febrile phase. Since reparative processes require 2 weeks or longer, the cough may persist even without secondary bacterial invasion. Antitussive agents are needed for severe cough. A throat culture at the onset of illness and smears and cultures of sputum when productive cough appears will contribute to prevention of pneumonia by indicating the need for therapy of bacterial infection of the bronchi. Antibiotics should not be administered prior to demonstration of purulent sputum containing bacteria, because this will only foster invasion by organisms that are more difficult to treat. *Streptococcus pneumoniae* (pneumococcus) and, secondly, *Staphylococcus aureus* are the most common bacterial invaders. In some areas and in patients with chronic lung disease, *Haemophilus influenzae* or other gram-negative bacilli are the cause.

Reye's syndrome, characterized by encephalopathy and fatty liver with high mortality, has been associated with influenza and other virus infections in children, but the pathogenesis remains obscure. Guillain-Barré syndrome also may rarely occur following influenza or vaccination.

Pneumonia

Pneumonia constitutes the most important of the complications. Pneumonia that begins during the height of the febrile stage is frequently fulminating. It may be due to a combination of viral and bacterial infections in which rapid spread is made possible by the preceding viral injury to bronchioles and alveoli with resulting hyperemia, edema, and exudate. Delay in recognition frequently occurs because a febrile illness is already present. Increased dyspnea, chest pain, and cough productive of purulent, rusty, or blood-tinged sputum are indications of onset. Extensive bilateral pneumonia may be present. In this instance vigorous measures are necessary. Appropriate antibiotics, adrenocorticosteroids, oxygen with or without mechanical ventilation, removal of excess secretions, and adequate control of respiratory exchange are all indicated. Similar therapeutic problems are caused by primary influenza virus pneumonia. This is more common and more likely to be fatal in persons with heart disease, especially mitral stenosis. Chest x-rays reveal fanning perihilar infiltrate of a diffuse and nodular nature. Since it is difficult to exclude the presence of concomitant bacterial invasion in these patients, antibiotics should be administered, along with any available anti-influenza virus drug.

Pneumonias that occur near the end of the febrile phase or shortly thereafter are not difficult therapeutic problems unless there is predisposing chest disease, complicating chronic illness, or an antibiotic-resistant organism as the etiologic agent. Delay in therapy of a staphylococcal pneumonia will result in permanent bronchial damage.

Vaccination

Vaccination is the most satisfactory means of preventing and controlling influenza. At present all vaccines are prepared with virus propagated in the embryonated egg and, consequently, contain egg protein. Hypersensitivity is rare, but it can be readily determined and avoided by questioning potential recipients regarding this common food item. Other reactions are inconsequential and are usually confined to soreness at the site of injection. Occasional brief febrile episodes respond to aspirin. "Whole-virus" vaccines are considerably refined and purified, which helps to reduce unpleasant reactions. "Split-virus" vaccines, produced by chemical disruption of the virus particle, are still less toxic, especially in children, but are also less immunogenic. Only inactivated virus vaccine is licensed in the United States, but attenuated live virus vaccine is used intranasally in many other countries.

Efficacy of influenza vaccine has been repeatedly demonstrated by controlled studies of the Commission on Influenza of the Armed Forces Epidemiological Board and by the low rates of this disease in annually vaccinated military personnel. Undoubtedly greater challenges to immunization occur in civilian populations because of large numbers of unvaccinated people, especially children, who are excreting considerable amounts of virus. Since secretory antibody in the respiratory tract is apparently necessary for protection, titers of serum antibody must be adequate because the secretory antibody is usually in proportion to the serum antibody but in lesser concentration. At present the best method of enhancing effectiveness of influenza vaccine is annual immunization of all persons, including children.

Vaccine should be administered in the fall of each year to provide maximum protection during the usual season in which influenza occurs. The annual recommendations of the Public Health Service Advisory Committee on Immunization Practices should be reviewed for the current year. Intramuscular administration of 0.5 ml. to adults, 0.25 ml. to children 3 to 5 years of age, and 0.15 ml. to those 6 to 35 months of age is recommended. Only "split-virus" vaccines should be given to persons less than 18 years of age. Those below age 6 are given two doses 4 or more weeks apart. Intradermal administration of 0.1 ml. of vaccine as a substitute for 1.0 ml. in adults is not recommended, because the amount of antigen inoculated determines the degree of antibody response. In children it is more painful than intramuscular administration.

Most of the deaths from influenza occur in persons with cardiovascular or pulmonary disease of all types, those with metabolic diseases, and those 65 years of age or older. Besides the risk of death, these people are the most susceptible to serious complications of influenza. Accordingly, annual vaccination is imperative. To avoid community or industrial paralysis, vaccination is recommended for those in essential occupations. Medical personnel and the armed forces must be included.

Chemoprophylaxis

Chemoprophylaxis may be indicated during the epidemic period if vaccination has been neglected in people in the high risk categories and an outbreak of A-2 influenza is recognized in the community. Amantadine hydrochloride (Symmetrel) can be given by mouth for 10 to 30 days or periods as long as 90 days if necessary in the following dosages: adults, 200 to 400 mg. daily; children 1 year to 9 years of age, 2 to 4 mg. per pound of body weight per day (but not to exceed 150 mg. per day) given in two or three equal portions; children 9 years to 12 years of age, total daily dose of 200 mg. given as 100 mg. twice a day. Central nervous system effects, especially in elderly persons, may occur. It should not be given to pregnant women or nursing mothers and should not be used as a substitute for vaccination.

LEPROSY

method of
ROBERT GELBER, M.D.
San Francisco, California

Introduction

Leprosy is a chronic disease resulting from intracellular infection with *Mycobacterium leprae*. It is only rarely fatal, but as a result of being the only human bacterial disease in which peripheral nerves are invaded, denervation, trauma, and secondary infection may result in disability and deformity. Though leprosy is not endemic in the United States or Western Europe, it is estimated that throughout the world 12 million people are affected. In many cultures leprosy patients are still ostracized, and diagnosis and treatment are frequently hindered by lack of facilities, fear, and prejudice. It has only been in recent years that the scientific foundations for rational therapy of leprosy have begun to emerge.

Leprosy encompasses a wide spectrum of manifestations, ranging from the polar tuberculoid through the borderline to the polar lepromatous. The various forms of leprosy have a distinct clinical appearance, which correlates well with a particular bacteriology, morphology, and pathophysiology. Classification of the type of leprosy present in a particular patient is important both as a guideline to appropriate antimicrobial therapy and as a means of predicting the various "reactions" which may appear and require special treatment.

Initial Evaluation

The initial evaluation of the leprosy patients should be sufficiently thorough so that clinical evolution, which may be both slow and subtle, can be objectively measured. In addition to a complete history and physical examination, when possible, patients should have a urinalysis, complete blood count (CBC), blood urea nitrogen (BUN), creatinine, liver function tests, chest x-rays, at least one skin biopsy for hematoxylin-eosin and acid-fast staining, a complete set of clinical photographs, and ophthalmologic and neurologic consultation to include objective sensory testing, voluntary muscle testing, and assessment of nerve conduction velocities. Patients should be fitted with specially molded shoes to prevent plantar ulcers and specifically counseled on how to avoid trauma to anesthetic parts. Smokers should be provided with cigarette holders. Physical therapy for weakened extremities and contractions should begin immediately so as to improve strength and maintain joint mobility. Patients should be oriented to their disease process from the outset so that they understand the normal clinical response to therapy and learn to recognize signs of drug toxicity and reactions. Both upon initial evaluation and upon follow-up, consideration of the fears of patients and prejudices of others must be an integral part of the successful management of the leprosy patient.

In the United States, initial evaluation and follow-up may be obtained without cost at the United States Public Health Service (USPHS) Hospitals at Carville, Louisiana, Staten Island, New York, and San Francisco, California, where there are established experience and expertise with this disease, as well as access to experimental drugs. Because lepromatous leprosy has an incubation period of at least a few years and a low order of contagion, and since patients are rendered noninfectious soon after the initiation of therapy, hospitalization for initial evaluation need not be mandatory but, in many instances, may prove useful in expediting the evaluation and orienting the patient to the disease process.

Chemotherapy

Because of the sheer bacterial numbers and the lack of cell-mediated immunity, the lepromatous form of leprosy presents the greater therapeutic difficulty. Dapsone (4,4′-diaminodiphenylsulfone, or DDS) is the agent of choice for treating all forms of leprosy; although certain other antimicrobials are available through the previously mentioned Public Health Service Hospitals, it is the only agent approved for general use as treatment of leprosy in the United States. It has the virtues of being relatively safe, effective, and inexpensive. In lepromatous leprosy dapsone should be initiated and maintained as a single daily adult dose of 100 mg. for lifetime. Although previously leprologists had built up to this maintenance dose slowly and discontinued dapsone during reaction, particularly erythema nodosum leprosum (ENL), these measures no longer appear reasonable. Lesions do not begin to show noticeable improvement for a few months, and it is important that both clinician and patient understand these expectations. Dapsone is cross-allergenic with sulfonamides and should not be initiated in patients with a history of sulfa allergy. It may cause a hemolytic anemia, particularly in G-6-PD–deficient patients, and may result in a dose-related methemoglobinemia and sulfhemoglobinemia in certain patients.

Although primary dapsone resistance has not yet been reported, extrapolating from tuberculosis chemotherapy, it is not surprising that dapsone monotherapy of lepromatous leprosy may result in the development of dapsone-resistant relapse. This becomes clinically apparent with the development of new lesions despite continued dapsone administration at a minimum of 5 years after the initiation of dapsone therapy. The risks of developing dapsone-resistant relapse vary between 2.5 and 40 per cent in different series. It appears that lower dosage regimens and intermittent adherence to therapy predispose to such relapse. Furthermore, even after 10 or more years of dapsone therapy, lepromatous leprosy patients harbor viable dapsone-sensitive *M. leprae* "persisters," capable of causing clinical relapse if therapy is discontinued; hence, the recommendation for lifetime therapy of lepromatous disease.

In certain remote regions where patients do not have access to medical facilities and cannot be expected to take medication regularly, the repository sulfone DADDS, 225 mg. intramuscularly every 77 days, might be substituted for dapsone in the treatment of all forms of leprosy. However, resulting plasma levels of DDS are sufficiently low and the potential for developing dapsone resistance is of sufficient magnitude that treatment of the lepromatous form of the disease with this agent alone should be avoided if at all possible.

Because of the dual problems of bacterial resistance and persistence, lepromatous leprosy ideally should be treated with at least two agents. On the other hand, tuberculoid and borderline leprosy patients, in whom neither dapsone resistance nor persisters are problems, require only monotherapy with dapsone. Tuberculoid leprosy should be treated with dapsone, 50 mg. twice weekly for just 5 years, and borderline leprosy with 100 mg. daily for 10 years.

Rifampin has proved both in animal and human studies to be significantly more potent than dapsone against *M. leprae*. A single daily adult dose of 600 mg. is recommended in lepromatous leprosy. (This use of rifampin is not listed in the manufacturer's official directive.) Indeed, nodules appear to begin flattening in weeks with rifampin rather than the months required for dapsone. There is no available information on what duration of rifampin together with dapsone will prevent drug-resistant relapse, and whether such combination chemotherapy for any duration will allow discontinuation of therapy without subsequent relapse from "persisters." Furthermore, the cost of rifampin, about $300 per patient-year, is prohibitively expensive in most developing nations where leprosy is a problem. At present, then, it is recommended that in lepromatous leprosy rifampin be administered for at least a few months up to several years, depending on local financial resources, together with dapsone, which should be continued indefinitely. It should be stressed that discontinuation of rifampin followed by reinstitution has been associated with severe and even fatal episodes of thrombocytopenia and renal failure.

Particularly because of allergy to sulfones and in the therapy of sulfone resistance, other second-line antimicrobial agents may be necessary to treat leprosy:

Clofazimine (B663 or Lamprene) appears as potent as dapsone against *M. leprae* (investigational). One hundred mg. orally twice or three times weekly is an effective alternative to dapsone administration. Its administration is unfortunately associated with a red-black discoloration which may be unnoticeable in blacks and other dark-skinned persons but is cosmetically unacceptable to many people with lighter complexions.

Thiambutosine has been used in the treatment of leprosy but is only weakly bacteriostatic. It is poorly absorbed from the gastrointestinal tract, and hence, when utilized, should be given in the intramuscularly repository form at 1 to 2 grams weekly. Thiambutosine when utilized as monotherapy for lepromatous leprosy regularly results in drug-resistant relapse after only 2 to 4 years of therapy. Hence, the only utility of this agent in the therapy of leprosy is in combination with another agent so as to prevent drug resistance.

Streptomycin in a daily dose of 1 gram intramuscularly is as potent as dapsone against *M. leprae*. (This use of streptomycin is not listed in the manufacturer's official directive.) However, because of its potential for nephrotoxicity and eighth nerve damage, no more than 1 year's therapy can be recommended. Hence, streptomycin should be used only with another agent that can be administered on a longer-term basis.

Ethionamide is even more active than dapsone against *M. leprae* and when utilized should be given in a once daily dosage of 500 mg. (This use of ethionamide is not listed in the manufacturer's official directive.) Unfortunately, ethionamide is expensive and, because of gastrointestinal upset and other toxicity, is not well tolerated.

Reactions and Their Treatment

About 50 per cent of patients with lepromatous leprosy, generally within the first few years of antimicrobial therapy, may develop the syndrome of erythema nodosum leprosum (ENL). This syndrome may consist of one or a number of the following manifestations: crops of erythematous painful skin nodules that remain a few days and are most commonly found on the extensor surface of the extremities, fever that may be as high as 105°F. (40.5°C.), painful neuritis which may result in further nerve damage, lymphadenitis, uveitis, orchitis, and occasionally large joint arthritis and glomerulonephritis. Histopathologically, this syndrome is secondary to a vasculitis and is probably the result of immune complexes. The clinical manifestations may be mild and evanescent or severe, recurrent, and occasionally fatal. Therapy must be individualized. Thalidomide is most effective and indeed the agent of choice for both treatment of ENL, and, if repeated episodes occur, prophylaxis, in a single evening dose of 100 to 400 mg. In the United States, it is available only through the Public Health Services Hospitals previously mentioned. Because of thalidomide's potential for causing severe birth defects, including phocomelia, it should not be administered to women in the child-bearing years. Side effects include tranquilization to which tolerance generally develops rapidly.

Corticosteroids are equally effective against ENL but because of their toxicities are not the preferred agent. Generally even the most severe ENL can be controlled with 60 mg. of prednisolone per day and tapered over a 3 or 4 week period. If breakthrough ENL occurs as with thalidomide, the dose of steroids may be increased, and some patients may require maintenance corticosteroids to prevent further flares, for which generally 10 to 15 mg. of prednisolone per day is sufficient. Clofazimine (investigational), although slow in onset and only moderately effective in doses of 300 mg. per day, may enable one to reduce the steroid requirement for therapy of ENL.

Patients with borderline leprosy may develop signs of inflammation, usually within previous skin lesions, and painful neuritis which may cause further nerve damage and occasionally fever; these are called nonlepromatous lepra reactions. If occurring prior to therapy, they are termed "downgrading reactions"; if occurring during therapy, usually within a few weeks or months of the start of treatment, they are termed "reversal reactions." Therapy is required in the presence of neuritis, in skin inflammation of a sufficient extent that ulceration appears likely, or for cosmetic reasons, especially if lesions involve the face. Thalidomide is of no value for lepra reactions. Corticosteroids are usually effective in controlling these reactions at about 20 to 30 mg. prednisolone per day, but generally must be maintained for a few months prior to tapering. Clofazimine may be of some value in decreasing the steroid requirement in these reactions in the same dose as for treating ENL, but is not as effective in nonlepromatous lepra reactions.

Prophylaxis

Family contacts of patients with leprosy should have annual physical examinations. Because the incubation period in leprosy may be from 5 to 10 years, long-term observation is indicated. Although the exact role of chemoprophylaxis has not been defined, it is our policy to treat adult family contacts of lepromatous leprosy patients with dapsone, 50 mg. twice weekly, or DADDS, 225 mg. intramuscularly every 77 days for 2 years. Children are given smaller doses, according to weight.

Rehabilitation

Follow-up visits should always include examination of the feet, and ulcers must be vigorously treated with specific antibiotics, debridement, and plaster of Paris until healed. Tendon transplants to permit substitution of innervated for denervated muscles may provide patients with more functional use of hands and enable them to close their eyes so that corneal trauma and its sequelae will not lead to blindness. Reconstructive surgery should not be initiated until patients have received at least 6 months of therapy directed against *M. leprae* and at least 6 months after signs of reaction have abated if maximal results are to be expected. When possible, mechanical devices may help the severely deformed, and job retraining may be necessary to prevent trauma and further disability.

MALARIA

method of
KARL H. RIECKMANN, M.D.
Albuquerque, New Mexico

Adequate treatment of malaria depends on accurate identification of the Plasmodium causing the infection—*P. falciparum, P. vivax, P. ovale,* or

P. malariae. This can be done only by thorough examination of thick and thin blood films. Prompt diagnosis and early treatment of acute falciparum malaria are essential, because it is a potentially lethal disease. Before starting treatment, the most likely geographic origin of the infection should be determined, because certain areas of the world harbor drug-resistant strains of *P. falciparum.* The initial therapeutic objective is to eliminate asexual erythrocytic parasites, the forms responsible for the symptoms and pathologic complications of the infection. If gametocytes persist or appear after onset of treatment, local epidemiologic conditions may necessitate the administration of another drug to prevent the transmission of the disease to susceptible anopheline mosquitoes. Infections caused by one of the other species, *P. vivax, P. ovale,* or *P. malariae,* are not usually fatal; but because of a tendency to long-term relapses caused by intermittent reinvasion of the bloodstream by exoerythrocytic parasites, treatment should include medication which is effective against persisting tissue schizonts in the liver. As relapses are observed only in patients with mosquito-induced infections, tissue schizonticidal drugs are not required for treating patients who have acquired their infections through blood transfusions or, in drug addicts, through sharing needles or syringes.

Patients with mixed infections involving more than one species (e.g., *P. falciparum* and *P. vivax*) require special consideration. Some of them may develop a clinical attack of falciparum malaria, and subsequently, after elimination of the asexual erythrocytic parasites of *P. falciparum* by appropriate treatment, they may suffer another acute episode of malaria caused by the release of exoerythrocytic parasites of *P. vivax* into the bloodstream. Careful attention to identification of the species will exclude the possibility of a recurring falciparum infection and will enable appropriate treatment to be instituted for radical cure of the vivax infection.

Chemotherapy

The recommended therapeutic regimens employ drugs which are currently available in the United States. If parenteral preparations of quinine or chloroquine are not available locally, they may be obtained from the Parasitic Diseases Drug Service, Center for Disease Control (CDC), Atlanta, Georgia; telephone: (404) 633-3311.

The drug doses listed are those usually recommended for adults. Proportionately lower doses are used in the treatment of children.

Treatment of Patients Infected with P. falciparum. Treatment will vary according to the geographic origin of the causative organism and the severity of the infection. It should be instituted immediately after the diagnosis has been made. Any modifications in therapy, based upon the results of in vitro drug susceptibility tests, can be introduced within 1 or 2 days after the start of treatment.

Infections Originating in Areas with No Chloroquine Resistance. Chloroquine or amodiaquine is still effective in curing falciparum malaria acquired in Africa, Central America (excluding Panama), and Western Asia. A total of 1500 mg. of chloroquine or amodiaquine base is administered orally over a period of 3 days. This is equivalent to 2500 mg. of chloroquine diphosphate or 1960 mg. of amodiaquine dihydrochloride. The initial dose of 600 mg. base is followed by administration of 300 mg. base of the drug at 6, 24, and 48 hours. If the patient is vomiting, treatment is initiated by parenteral administration of chloroquine dihydrochloride. Single doses of 200 mg. of chloroquine base may be repeated every 6 hours for no more than 24 hours and should be discontinued as soon as the patient is able to tolerate oral medication. Parenteral preparations of chloroquine should be given only in intramuscular injections (not intravenously, unless administered by slow infusion), and the dosage for children should not exceed 5 mg. per kg. of body weight.

The course of the infection after initiation of treatment should be monitored closely. Parasite counts are performed at least twice a day for 2 days to determine whether the infection is responding to treatment. An increase in the number of asexual parasites 24 hours after onset of treatment may indicate drug resistance, and alternative treatment should be considered (see below). The recommended treatment usually results in disappearance of parasitemia, as judged by examination of 0.1 microliter of blood, within 3 to 5 days after the start of treatment.

Persistence of asexual parasites for a week after onset of treatment or recrudescence of parasitemia within a month of treatment (in United States or other areas where reinfection can be excluded) suggests the presence of a chloroquine-resistant infection. The presence of gametocytes, the nonpathogenic sexual stages of the parasite infective to mosquitoes, does not indicate drug resistance. If the attending physician is reasonably certain that the prescribed drug was taken, blood and urine specimens should be collected to confirm drug absorption. The discovery of drug-resistant infections acquired in areas from which chloroquine resistance had not been observed previously should be publicized and reported to the Center for Disease Control. This will alert physicians to the extension of resistant strains and to the need of modifying the treatment of infections acquired in those areas.

Infections Originating in Areas with Chloroquine Resistance. Falciparum malaria acquired in Panama, South America, and Asia east of Pakistan should not be treated with chloroquine. This drug should also not be used for treating blood-induced infections, the origin of which is obscure, or chloroquine-treated infections in which a recrudescence of parasitemia has been observed.

The standard treatment of such infections is the administration of quinine sulfate, 650 mg. every 8 hours for 10 to 14 days, in combination with pyrimethamine, 25 mg. twice daily for 3 days, and sulfadiazine, 500 mg. every 6 hours for 5 days. Although this regimen is very effective in controlling the infection, an occasional patient may suffer a subsequent recrudescence of parasitemia. The cinchonism caused by quinine administration is seldom severe enough to require discontinuation of drug therapy. However, determination of the plasma quinine levels is useful in adjusting the intake of quinine. In patients with impaired renal or hepatic function, considerably less quinine may be required to maintain plasma levels within the therapeutic range of 5 to 10 mg. per liter.

Another effective treatment regimen involves the administration of quinine sulfate for 3 days (650 mg. every 8 hours) and, starting concurrently, tetracycline hydrochloride for 10 days (250 mg. every 6 hours). If quinine is not immediately available, the standard 3 day course of amodiaquine may be used instead of quinine. Although the latter regimen has been highly effective against chloroquine-resistant infections, the course of parasitemia should be watched very closely in the event that an infection with a marked degree of resistance to amodiaquine is encountered.

In areas where anopheline mosquitoes are present, special care should be taken to avoid the introduction of drug-resistant strains of *P. falciparum.* Consequently, any patient showing gametocytes within 6 weeks after the acute clinical episode has subsided should receive a single oral dose of 30 to 45 mg. of primaquine base to render the gametocytes noninfective to mosquitoes.

"SEVERE" OR "COMPLICATED" FALCIPARUM INFECTIONS. Immediate treatment with intravenous quinine should be instituted in patients with >100,000 parasites per microliter of blood or with cerebral, renal, or pulmonary complications. Quinine dihydrochloride, 600 mg. dissolved in 500 ml. of isotonic saline solution, should be infused *slowly* over a period of 8 hours. This may be repeated once every 8 hours until the patient is able to tolerate oral medication. Patients with renal failure should receive considerably less quinine, possibly 600 mg. every 24 hours; the actual quantity administered would depend on the findings obtained by close monitoring of plasma quinine levels and electrocardiographic QRS complexes.

The management of patients who have developed renal, pulmonary, or cerebral complications is similar to that usually employed for such an occurrence in other disease entities. Comatose patients with cerebral malaria, for example, may benefit by administration of dexamethasone sodium phosphate, 3 to 10 mg. every 8 hours, for reducing cerebral edema and by administration of dextran 75, 500 ml. every 12 hours, for minimizing intravascular sludging.

Treatment of Patients Infected with P. vivax, P. ovale, or P. malariae. Chloroquine or amodiaquine is the drug of choice for terminating acute attacks in patients infected with these species. A conventional 3 day course with one of these drugs, administered in doses as noted previously, will eliminate asexual blood forms. It will not, however, eliminate exoerythrocytic hepatic forms of *P. vivax* or *P. ovale.* Additional treatment with primaquine is needed to prevent subsequent relapses. Primaquine diphosphate is given orally, once a day, for 14 days at a daily dose of 15 mg. base (26 mg. salt). The drug may induce hemolysis in patients whose erythrocytes are deficient in glucose-6-phosphate dehydrogenase (G-6-PD). Although hemolysis may be severe in some patients, conventional doses of primaquine often do not produce more than a transient and mild anemia.

Relapses sometimes occur despite primaquine administration. In such instances, the standard 14 day course may be repeated or, alternatively, the drug may be administered once a week for 8 weeks at a weekly dose of 45 mg. base (79 mg. salt). The latter drug regimen may be both more effective and less hemolytic than the administration of smaller daily doses of primaquine for 2 weeks. If primaquine administration is associated with severe hemolysis or failure to produce radical cure, treatment and suppression of the infection with chloroquine or amodiaquine may have to be continued for several months or years until the exoerythrocytic tissue forms have been exhausted.

Supportive Treatment. During the administration of antimalarial chemotherapy, supportive measures should be undertaken to relieve symptoms associated with acute attacks of malaria. Headaches and generalized discomfort related to high fever are relieved by administration of salicylates, sponging with tepid water, and fanning. The maintenance of adequate hydration is important, but precautions must be taken not to precipitate pulmonary or cerebral edema by administration of excessive fluids. Patients with a mild anemia usually recover spontaneously after institution of antimalarial chemotherapy, but patients with severe anemia should be given transfusions of packed red blood cells. Splenic enlargement is common during and following an acute attack of malaria, and slight tenderness under the left costal margin is no reason for concern. Evidence of peritoneal or diaphragmatic irritation, on the other hand, may indicate rupture of the spleen (especially in vivax infections) and the need for urgent surgical intervention.

Chemoprophylaxis

The risk of acquiring malaria in endemic areas of the world varies widely from one locality to another and depends on local conditions such as weather, altitude, prevalence of disease, and mosquito control activities. Although the disease is generally more prevalent in rural areas, contact with mosquitoes between dusk and dawn should also be avoided in urban centers. Exposure to malaria vectors can be reduced by wearing clothes which cover most of the body, by applying mosquito repellants such as N,N–diethyltoluamide (OFF, DEET) to exposed areas of the skin, and by sleeping in screened rooms or under mosquito netting. In addition to such general protective measures, it is usually advisable to start a regular chemoprophylactic drug regimen 1 or 2 weeks before arriving in a malarious area and to continue it for 8 weeks after the last possible exposure to malaria.

The weekly ingestion of 300 mg. of chloroquine base or 400 mg. of amodiaquine base prevents the development of falciparum infections sensitive to chloroquine. In addition, it actively suppresses vivax and ovale infections. As these drugs exert no activity against persisting tissue forms, primaquine should be taken by persons (with *no* G-6-PD deficiency) who are returning from an area in which they were probably exposed to mosquitoes infected with *P. vivax* or *P. ovale.* This can be done conveniently by simply including a weekly dose of 45 mg. of primaquine base during the last 8 weeks of chemoprophylaxis with chloroquine or amodiaquine. Alternatively, a daily dose of 15 mg. primaquine base can be taken for 14 days after leaving an endemic area. For persons with G-6-PD deficiency, the prophylactic use of primaquine is usually contraindicated; the drug should be given only under close medical supervision to prevent relapses following an acute attack of malaria. Gastrointestinal disturbances, which are sometimes observed after taking chloroquine or primaquine, can be minimized by taking the drugs after meals.

In some areas overseas, chlorguanide (100 to 200 mg. daily) or pyrimethamine (25 mg. weekly) is used as a malaria prophylactic. The major drawback in using these compounds is the presence of strains of *P. falciparum, P. vivax,* and *P. malariae* in parts of Africa, Asia, and Oceania which are resistant to these drugs.

The chemoprophylactic regimens referred to so far will not always protect persons against chloroquine-resistant infections of *P. falciparum.* Although amodiaquine may be somewhat superior to chloroquine in suppressing such infections, adequate protection cannot be expected after the use of either one of these drugs. Sulfonamide-pyrimethamine or sulfone-pyrimethamine combinations have been advocated as prophylactics in areas with chloroquine resistance. The combination of 500 mg. of sulfadoxine and 25 mg. of pyrimethamine (Fansidar), taken once a week, has proved effective in many areas with chloroquine-resistant malaria. Although this drug combination is not available within the United States, it may be obtained overseas. Since chronic toxicity studies during long-term drug administration have not yet been carried out, it is advisable not to take it continuously for more than a few months. Physicians should also be alert to allergic reactions or toxic side effects, such as the Stevens-Johnson syndrome, which have been associated with other sulfonamides. It should be noted that sulfonamide-pyrimethamine combinations do not provide adequate protection against *P. vivax* infections in areas where blood stages of this species are resistant to pyrimethamine and that, as with chloroquine, they exert no effect against relapsing tissue stages.

Current prophylactic regimens are not uniformly effective against different plasmodial species and strains, and they do not always prevent the development of malaria infections. Recipients of antimalarial drugs should therefore be informed of this possibility and urged to seek medical advice if they develop any symptoms during or after chemoprophylaxis.

MEASLES
(Rubeola)

method of
ROBERT P. GRUNINGER, M.D.
Worcester, Massachusetts

Measles is due to a single antigenic type RNA-containing paramyxovirus. There is no treatment for the specific illness. Supportive measures during the primary illness or during the complications of measles are beneficial. Antibiotics are indicated only in the treatment of complications caused by bacteria. Effective attenuated (live) measles virus vaccine and human immune serum globulin (ISG) make preventive measures the most important initial approach to this disease. The failure to implement immunization either on an individual patient basis or in a community-wide program has been associated with the resurgence of incidence of both the disease and its complications. The latter may be a cause of death or latent neurologic illness such as subacute sclerosing panencephalitis or possibly multiple sclerosis. Unless a worldwide immunization program essentially eliminates the virus from man (the only source), increased case rates will occur in unprotected populations.

Prevention

Active Immunization. A single subcutaneous injection of an attenuated (live) measles vaccine is recommended at 15 months of age, because all maternal transplacental antibody has disappeared by then. Earlier vaccination, between 6 months and 15 months of age, is unpredictable in its efficacy, and it should only be done if measles commonly occurs in the area in children less than 1 year old or if there is an outbreak of measles. A vaccination should be given to any child 15 months old or over if not previously immunized, if previously immunized with inactive (killed) vaccine, or if immunized with attenuated (live) vaccine before 13 months of age. The vaccine may be given any time up to and including the day of exposure to measles. When in doubt about the details of the measles immunization history, an inoculation of the vaccine should be given. No deleterious effects have been observed following reimmunization of previously vaccinated or naturally immune persons. Vaccination generally is not indicated in adults. The exception would be to vaccinate the adult who has no previous immunization and no previous exposure. As measles is worldwide, lack of previous exposure is unlikely, although an occasional community of people is recognized where measles has not occurred.

Deferred and/or Contraindicated Immunization. Vaccination should be deferred for 8 or more weeks in a child who has received immune serum globulin (ISG) (also called gamma globulin), whole blood, or plasma as therapy or prophylaxis related to another illness. It is contraindicated in any child with primary or secondary cell-mediated (T-cell lymphocyte) deficiency. Several examples are children with leukemia, lymphoma, or combined immunodeficiency (Swiss-type agammaglobulinemia), or those who have received immunosuppressive therapy such as steroids, antimetabolites, alkalating agents, or irradiation. Vaccination is also contraindicated in those with active tuberculosis, in pregnancy, or in an acute febrile illness.

Vaccines. There are several attenuated measles vaccines available either as a separate vaccine or combined with other attenuated virus vaccines. The separate vaccines include attenuated Edmonston B strain propagated in either chick embryo or canine renal cell culture and the Schwarz strain and the Moraten strain each propagated in chick cell tissue culture. The combined vaccines include rubella and/or mumps with the measles vaccine. Because of the 90 per cent probability of side effects (fever, minor toxicity, and faint rash occurring 5 to 10 days postvaccination) associated with the Edmonston B strain, ISG may be given to ameliorate these effects. The ISG should be given at the same time in a different site. It is optional with the Edmonston B strain propagated in chick embryo but should be given with the Edmonston B strain propagated in canine renal cell. Either the Schwarz strain or the Moraten strain, which are further attenuated Edmonston strains, may be given cautiously to the patient with allergy to egg, and neither requires simultaneous ISG to ameliorate the vaccine side effects. These latter two vaccines are readily available. Most other separate measles vaccines have been or will be discontinued.

Administration of combined vaccine or simultaneous administration of two or more separate vaccines is possible. Individual circumstances, such as age, disease prevalence, and socioeconomic conditions, will dictate appropriateness, as any of the following appear to be effective: measles plus rubella; measles, rubella, and mumps; measles plus smallpox (probably ill advised in the United States); separate Schwarz strain and "Cendehill" rubella strain; or measles, rubella, and mumps combination with the third or fourth trivalent oral polio vaccine. A practical and possibly sounder immunologic approach would be measles vaccination at 15 months and rubella and mumps vaccinations at preschool age.

Special Considerations. The tuberculosis skin test may be falsely negative up to 3 months after the measles vaccine. Thus if there is a history or reasonable probability of exposure to tuberculosis, a skin test should be done before or at the time of measles vaccination. If the skin test is positive and there is no active tuberculosis, isoniazid (INH) prophylaxis should be given after the vaccine. If there is active tuberculosis, it should be arrested before measles vaccination.

Passive Immunization (Postexposure). Passive immunization with human ISG is not necessary in any child with a past history of measles or previously immunized with attenuated virus unless the vaccine was given before 13 months of age. In the patient unimmunized or immunized with inactivated (killed) vaccine (no longer available), ISG is given in separate sites, 0.04 ml. per kg. intramuscularly. Attenuated vaccine may be given subcutaneously in a different site along with the ISG if given on the day of exposure to measles. Thereafter, only ISG should be given. Alternatively, a "preventive" dose, 0.25 mg. per kg. of ISG, may be given intramuscularly. This should be followed by immunization with the attenuated vaccine in about 2 months unless clinical measles occurs. If the exposed unimmunized child has leukemia, is receiving immunosuppressive therapy, or has any T-cell deficiency disease, 20 to 30 ml. of ISG should be given intramuscularly immediately.

Active Disease

Uncomplicated. Measles, in the majority of patients, is uncomplicated. The patients require no specific therapy other than symptomatic use of bed rest, fluids, antipyretics for high fever, analgesics, antitussives, skin lotion for itching, and a darkened room for photophobia. Isolation of the patient is recommended, if possible, during the catarrhal stage (4 to 5 days before rash) and through the third day of rash. The catarrhal stage or prodromal stage begins about 9 to 10 days after measles exposure. The patient with measles should be kept from all high-risk persons such as hospitalized patients, pregnant females, and immunosuppressed patients with leukemia or lymphoma.

Thrombocytopenia and lymphocytopenia may occur. The former, of itself, does not warrant aggressive therapy. Often the platelet count will have stabilized or in fact have started to rise at the time petechiae or purpura are most pronounced. A lymphocyte count of less than 2000 per cu. mm. during the rash of measles is a bad prognostic sign.

Complicated Measles. Less than 10 per cent of patients with measles develop complications. The most common is otitis media, which most often occurs in the younger child. This frequently requires appropriate antibiotic treatment, which should be based upon well known age-related bacterial cause. Croup is another common complication of the younger patient. Supportive therapy, including humidification, bed rest, and observation for more serious respiratory infection, is indicated. Pneumonia is the most serious respiratory complication. It most often occurs in the child between 10 and 14 years old. Pneumonia may be interstitial of the giant cell type caused by the measles virus alone, in which case only supportive therapy (oxygen, antipyretic) is indicated. If the pneumonia is caused by a bacterial suprainfection such as *Streptococcus pneumoniae* or *Staphylococcus aureus* coagulase (+), specific antibiotic treatment is indicated. Tuberculosis should be considered, especially if history of exposure to active tuberculosis and the pneumonia is protracted. Neurologic complications are varied. Encephalitis is an early complication. It occurs following the appearance of the rash and is a major cause of death. Only supportive therapy is available, as no antiviral agent has demonstrated beneficial effect. Steroids, except as a consideration for cerebral edema, are *not* indicated. Late complications include subacute sclerosing panencephalitis and, doubtfully, multiple sclerosis. A variety of other complications have been associated with measles. Perhaps the most feared, although extremely rare, is so-called "black or hemorrhagic measles" or purpura fulminans, which occurs prior to the characteristic rash. Therapy must be directed to defects in coagulation.

BACTERIAL MENINGITIS

method of
JAMES M. HUGHES, M.D.
Charlottesville, Virginia

Bacterial meningitis is a life-threatening infection. Prior to the antibiotic era, most patients died; those who survived often had severe neurologic sequelae. With prompt diagnosis, selection of the appropriate antibiotic regimen, and provision of excellent supportive care, both the case-fatality rate and the frequency of neurologic sequelae can be dramatically reduced.

In order to make a prompt diagnosis, the physician must maintain a high index of suspicion of bacterial meningitis in any patient with fever and altered mental status; meningeal signs are usually but not invariably present. If such a patient has no evidence of either increased intracranial pressure or focal neurologic disease, a lumbar puncture should be performed as soon as possible; if the patient has evidence of increased intracranial pressure or focal neurologic disease, an emergency brain scan or computerized tomography should be performed to rule out the presence of a mass lesion prior to the lumbar puncture. Although a bacteriologic diagnosis may be suggested by clinical features (e.g., petechial rash associated with meningococcal disease), the patient's age (e.g., group B streptococci or *Escherichia coli* in the neonate, *Hemophilus influenzae* in the older child, meningococcus in the teenager or young adult, pneumococcus in the older adult), or other epidemiologic features (e.g., *Staphylococcus aureus* or Enterobacteriaceae following head trauma or neurosurgery, *Staphylococcus epidermidis* or *S. aureus* in association with a ventriculoatrial or ventriculoperitoneal shunt infection), a Gram stain of the sediment obtained after centrifugation of cerebrospinal fluid may guide the selection of an antimicrobial regimen. Therapy may have to be modified when the identification of the responsible organism and determination of its antibiotic sensitivity are complete.

Successful therapy of bacterial meningitis requires delivery of an appropriate antibiotic into contact with organisms in the cerebrospinal fluid. It cannot be assumed that a drug effective against an organism in vitro will necessarily be successful in eradicating the infection. Additional factors such as protein-binding of the antibiotic and permeability of the blood-brain barrier to the drug must also be considered. For evaluation of therapeutic efficacy, follow-up lumbar punctures are usually indicated 1 to 2 days after therapy is initiated and, if the patient responds, 1 to 2 days after completion of therapy. In addition, particularly if the patient does not respond as expected, serum and spinal fluid antibiotic levels and bactericidal levels may be useful in verifying that an appropriate drug is being administered in an adequate dose by an appropriate route.

Antibiotic Therapy

Pneumococcal Meningitis. The drug of choice is penicillin in large doses, as indicated in Table 1. For the penicillin-allergic patient, chloramphenicol is the recommended alternative (Table 2). Parenteral therapy should be continued for 10 to 14 days.

Meningococcal Meningitis. The drug of choice is penicillin (Table 1), and the alternative in the allergic patient is chloramphenicol. The patient should be treated parenterally for 10 to 14 days or for 5 days after fever has resolved, whichever is longer.

Hemophilus Influenzae Meningitis. Because of the recent emergence of beta-lactamase producing strains of *H. influenzae*, chloramphenicol has replaced ampicillin as the drug of choice for *H. influenzae* meningitis when the antibiotic sensitivity of the responsible organism is unknown. Either a combination of ampicillin and chloramphenicol or chloramphenicol alone should be used initially (Table 1). If the organism is found to be sensitive to ampicillin, the chloramphenicol can be discontinued and ampicillin

TABLE 1. **Parenteral Antibiotic Therapy of Bacterial Meningitis***

		DAILY PEDIATRIC DOSAGE		
ANTIBIOTIC	DAILY ADULT DOSAGE	*<1 Week of Age*	*1–4 Weeks of Age*	*>4 Weeks of Age*†
Penicillin G	20–24 million units I.V. (continuous infusion or 12 doses)	100,000 units/kg. I.V. (2 doses)	300,000 units/kg. (6 doses)	300,000 units/kg. (12 doses)
Semisynthetic penicillins (methicillin, nafcillin, oxacillin)	12 grams I.V. (6 doses)	100 mg./kg. I.V. (2 doses)	200 mg./kg. I.V. (4 doses)	200 mg./kg. I.V. (6 doses)
Ampicillin	12 grams I.V. (6 doses)	100 mg./kg. I.V. (3 doses)	200 mg./kg. I.V. (4 doses)	200 mg./kg. I.V. (6 doses)
Carbenicillin	30 grams I.V. (6 doses)	300 mg./kg. I.V. (3 doses)	400 mg./kg. I.V. (4 doses)	600 mg./kg. I.V. (6 doses)
Chloramphenicol	4 grams I.V. (4 doses)	Not used	Not used	100 mg./kg. I.V. (4 doses)
Vancomycin‡	2 grams I.V. (4 doses)	Not used	Not used	40 mg./kg. I.V. (3 doses)
Kanamycin‡	Not used	15 mg./kg. I.M. (2 doses)	15 mg./kg. I.M. (3 doses)	15 mg./kg. I.M. (3 doses)
Gentamicin‡	5 mg./kg. I.V. (3 doses)	5 mg./kg. I.V. (2 doses)	5 mg./kg. I.V. (3 doses)	5 mg./kg. I.V. (3 doses)
Tobramycin‡	5 mg./kg. I.V. (3 doses)	4 mg./kg. I.V. (2 doses)	5 mg./kg. I.V. (3 doses)	5 mg./kg. I.V. (3 doses)
Amikacin‡	15 mg./kg. I.V. (3 doses)	15 mg./kg. I.V. (2 doses)	15 mg./kg. I.V. (2 doses)	15 mg./kg. I.V. (2 doses)

*Assumes normal renal function.
†Total dose should not exceed recommended adult dose.
‡Dosage and/or interval must be altered if even mild renal insufficiency exists.

TABLE 2. **Antibiotic of Choice, Alternative, and Duration of Therapy in Bacterial Meningitis**

PATHOGEN	ANTIBIOTIC OF CHOICE*	ALTERNATIVE*†	DURATION OF THERAPY
Pneumococcus	Penicillin G	Chloramphenicol	10–14 days
Meningococcus	Penicillin G	Chloramphenicol	10–14 days or 5 afebrile days§
H. influenzae	Ampicillin*	Chloramphenicol	10–14 days
Enterobacteriaceae (adults)	Gentamicin or tobramycin and carbenicillin	Chloramphenicol	14 days
Enterobacteriaceae (neonates)	Ampicillin or aminoglycoside	None	21 days
Group B Streptococcus	Penicillin G	Vancomycin	14–21 days
S. aureus	Semisynthetic penicillin‡	Vancomycin	21–28 days
S. epidermidis	Semisynthetic penicillin‡	Vancomycin	21–28 days
L. monocytogenes	Penicillin G or ampicillin	Chloramphenicol	14 days (adults) 14–21 days (neonates)
Unknown:			
Neonate	Ampicillin and aminoglycoside	None	21 days
Child	Chloramphenicol	None	14 days
Adult	Penicillin G	Chloramphenicol	14 days
Head trauma or neurosurgery	Semisynthetic penicillin and aminoglycoside	Vancomycin and aminoglycoside	21–28 days
Shunt	Semisynthetic penicillin	Vancomycin	21–28 days

*Assumes that organism is sensitive in vitro.
†In patients allergic to the antibiotic of choice.
‡Penicillin G is preferred if the organism is sensitive.
§Whichever is longer.

substituted if it was not also used initially. The duration of therapy is 10 to 14 days.

Gram-Negative Meningitis (Adults). The initial selection of an antimicrobial agent is influenced by local antibiotic sensitivity patterns. Therapy should be initiated with both an aminoglycoside and carbenicillin (Table 1). Because of their relatively poor penetration into spinal fluid, the aminoglycoside should be administered both intravenously and intrathecally* into the lumbar space initially in dosages indicated (Table 3); gentamicin or tobramycin should be used in areas where gram-negative rods are not resistant to these drugs. Amikacin should be substituted in areas where gentamicin and tobramycin resistance is encountered. Once antibiotic sensitivity data are available, either gentamicin or tobramycin may be substituted for amikacin if the organism is sensitive. Carbenicillin should be discontinued if the organism is resistant.

Spinal fluid chemistries, Gram stain, and culture should be performed daily on fluid obtained at the time of intralumbar administration of the antibiotic. If no clinical or bacteriologic improvement occurs in the first 48 to 72 hours of therapy, the possibility of ventriculitis should be entertained and confirmed by a ventricular tap. If ventriculitis is present, insertion of a subcutaneous reservoir should be considered for intraventricular administration of the aminoglycoside. Therapy should be continued for 2 weeks or 7 days after spinal fluid cultures become sterile, whichever is longer. Intralumbar or intraventricular therapy should be continued until the spinal fluid is sterile and cell counts and chemistries are approaching normal.

*The intrathecal use of aminoglycosides is not listed in the manufacturer's official directive.

TABLE 3. **Intrathecal Therapy of Gram-Negative Bacterial Meningitis**

ANTIBIOTIC	ADULT DOSAGE*	PEDIATRIC DOSAGE*†
Kanamycin	Not used	1–4 mg. by intraventricular route every 24 hours
Gentamicin‡ Tobramycin‡	5 mg. by intralumbar or intraventricular route every 24 hours	
Amikacin†‡	5–10 mg. by intralumbar or intraventricular route every 24 hours	

*Administered in a concentration of 2 to 5 mg. per ml. in isotonic saline solution or cerebrospinal fluid.
†Data on efficacy and appropriate dose are limited or nonexistent; both serum and spinal fluid antibiotic and bactericidal levels should be closely monitored.
‡The intrathecal use of these agents is not listed in the manufacturer's official directive.

Neonatal Meningitis. In children less than 2 months of age, the most common causes of meningitis are *Escherichia coli* and group B streptococci. Initial therapy of meningitis in this age group should include ampicillin and either kanamycin or gentamicin (depending on local experience with antibiotic resistance of gram-negative rods) in the dosages indicated (Table 1). Recent evidence indicates that combined intravenous and intralumbar administration of the aminoglycoside is no more efficacious than parenteral administration alone in this age group. If the patient fails to respond to parenteral therapy, administration of the aminoglycoside intraventricularly may be considered (Table 3); a study to evaluate the efficacy of this mode of therapy in neonates is currently in progress.

Antibiotic therapy can be modified once the responsible organism has been identified and, in the case of the gram-negative rod, its sensitivity pattern determined. If group B streptococci are identified, the aminoglycoside may be discontinued and penicillin G substituted for ampicillin. If gram-negative rods are identified, the aminoglycoside may be discontinued if the organism is sensitive to ampicillin. Duration of therapy is 14 to 21 days for group B streptococcal meningitis and 21 days for gram-negative meningitis.

Staphylococcal Meningitis. The drug of choice for the therapy of *S. aureus* meningitis, which occurs most often following head trauma or a neurosurgical procedure, is a semisynthetic penicillin in the dosage indicated (Table 1). If the organism is sensitive to penicillin, this drug should be substituted. In the penicillin-allergic patient, vancomycin should be used; in this case, because of limited information on the permeability of the blood-brain barrier to vancomycin, it is very important to follow spinal fluid vancomycin and bactericidal levels as well as chemistries, Gram stain, and culture initially every 1 to 2 days to document therapeutic efficacy. The appropriate duration of therapy is not well established, but treatment should be continued for at least 3 weeks or at least 10 days after spinal fluid has returned to normal chemically and microbiologically, whichever is longer.

In cases of meningitis caused by *S. epidermidis*, which are usually associated with the presence of a foreign body, the organism is often resistant to semisynthetic penicillins. Initial therapy should be vancomycin until antibiotic sensitivity data are available (Table 1). When antibiotic sensitivities are known, a semisynthetic penicillin or penicillin G may then be substituted. Duration of therapy is similar to that for *S. aureus* meningitis.

Listeria Meningitis. Meningitis caused by *Listeria monocytogenes* is relatively uncommon but may be encountered in neonates and immunocompromised patients and should be suspected whenever a spinal fluid bacteriology report states that "diphtheroids" were isolated. The antibiotic of choice for this infection is either ampicillin or penicillin G in the dosage shown (Table 1); chloramphenicol is a suitable alternative in allergic persons. Duration of therapy is 14 to 21 days.

Cerebrospinal Fluid Shunt Infection. The most common organisms causing meningitis in the presence of ventriculoatrial and ventriculoperitoneal shunts inserted for the relief of hydrocephalus are *S. aureus* and *S. epidermidis*. Antibiotic therapy of these infections is the same as that outlined for staphylococcal meningitis. In addition, the shunt should be removed, if possible, when therapy is initiated.

Meningitis of Unknown Cause. Not infrequently, patients have an illness and spinal fluid findings compatible with bacterial meningitis, but have negative Gram stains and cultures. A history of recent antibiotic therapy should be sought, and these patients should be carefully evaluated for evidence of a parameningeal focus of infection and tuberculous and fungal meningitis. Initial antibiotic therapy in this setting is determined by the age of the patient and the clinical setting. Neonates should be treated with ampicillin and an aminoglycoside. Older children should be treated either with ampicillin and chloramphenicol or with chloramphenicol alone. Adults should be treated with penicillin or ampicillin. In the patient with a history of open head trauma or who acquires meningitis in the hospital, therapy should include a semisynthetic penicillin (vancomycin if the patient is allergic to penicillin) and an aminoglycoside (gentamicin, tobramycin, or amikacin); the aminoglycoside should be administered by both the intravenous and either the intralumbar or intraventricular routes.

General Measures

All patients with suspected or proved bacterial meningitis should be hospitalized in an intensive care unit. Vital signs and intake and output should be monitored, and patients should not be given anything orally until they are sufficiently alert to eat without aspirating. Intravenous catheters should be changed every 48 to 72 hours, and care should be taken to avoid the development of decubitus ulcers. Urinary catheterization should be avoided if possible to reduce the risk of nosocomial urinary tract infection.

Respiratory and circulatory status should be closely monitored. In the comatose or obtunded patient, care should be taken to prevent aspiration. If shock occurs, a central venous or Swan-Ganz catheter should be inserted to monitor fluid replacement. Use of vasoactive agents such as dopamine or isoproterenol may also be required. In addition, if shock accompanies possible or proved meningococcal meningitis, the possibility of adrenal insufficiency (the Waterhouse-Friderichsen syndrome) should be immediately considered. If there is evidence of adrenal insufficiency, glucocorticoids should be administered after prompt evaluation of adrenal function.

Disseminated intravascular coagulation (DIC) is another potential complication of bacterial meningitis, especially when meningococci are responsible. The role of heparin in the management of this syndrome is controversial; blood loss should be replaced while the underlying bacterial cause is being treated with antibiotics.

Cerebral edema may occur and can be managed with mannitol and controlled hyperventilation. Because of uncertainty regarding the effect of glucocorticoids on the underlying meningitis, these agents should probably not be used unless there is evidence of adrenal insufficiency. Seizures may be controlled with phenytoin or phenobarbital. Diazepam may be used acutely if necessary.

The syndrome of inappropriate antidiuretic hormone (ADH) secretion may occur; serum electrolytes should be monitored to detect it early, and free water should be restricted if the syndrome develops.

Sterile subdural effusions may be recognized during therapy of meningitis in infants. If these effusions are accompanied by focal neurologic signs, fluid should be aspirated daily in 10 to 15 ml. volumes until resolution.

Failure to Respond to Appropriate Therapy

When patients have persistent positive spinal fluid cultures or prolonged fever in the face of appropriate antibiotic therapy (i.e., the organism is sensitive to the antibiotic in vitro), a number of possible explanations should be considered. In the case of persistent positive cultures, the patients may have failed to respond because an error in the laboratory sensitivity testing led to the selection of the wrong drug, because a drug active in vitro is inactive in vivo, or because an active drug has not gained access to the site of infection because of failure to cross the blood-brain barrier or to enter an infected ventricle. Additional possible explanations include the existence of a parameningeal focus of infection (e.g., brain abscess, subdural empyema, epidural abscess, sinusitis, or mastoiditis), the presence of a foreign body (e.g., ventriculoatrial or ventriculoperitoneal shunt or sutures), and the emergence during therapy of a clone of organisms resistant to the antibiotic regimen. Such patients should be evaluated with these possibilities in mind; repeat antibiotic sensitivity testing and spinal fluid antibiotic and bactericidal levels should be performed and skull x-rays and a brain or computerized tomography scan considered.

In the case of persistent fever in the face of sterilization of the spinal fluid, other possibilities should be considered. These include infection elsewhere (nosocomial urinary tract, pulmonary, and bloodstream infections are especially common in these very ill patients), infected decubitus ulcers, thrombophlebitis, and drug fever.

Public Health Considerations

Antibiotic prophylaxis is recommended for close contacts of patients with meningococcal meningitis. Close contacts include residents of the same household, roommates, and anyone with a history of direct exposure to oral secretions (e.g., through mouth-to-mouth resuscitation or kissing). The drug of choice is rifampin; the dose is 600 mg. orally twice a day for adults, 10 mg. per kg. orally twice a day for children aged 1 to 12 years, and 5 mg. per kg. orally twice a day for children less than 1 year of age. Therapy should be continued for 2 days. If the strain of meningococcus is known to be sensitive to sulfonamides, one of these drugs should be used. The dosage of the sulfonamide (sulfisoxazole, sulfamethoxazole) is 1 gram orally twice a day for adults, 500 mg. orally twice a day for children 1 to 12 years of age, and 500 mg. orally once a day for children over 2 months of age but less than 1 year of age. Antibiotic prophylaxis should be initiated as soon as the diagnosis is made. Therapy should not be delayed pending results of antibiotic sensitivity testing; nasopharyngeal cultures play no role in determining candidates for prophylaxis.

Cases of meningococcal meningitis should be promptly reported to local public health authorities so that a search for secondary cases can be conducted. Hospitalized patients with suspected or confirmed meningococcal disease should be isolated for the first 24 to 48 hours of therapy.

INFECTIOUS MONONUCLEOSIS

method of
WILLIAM N. TOTH, M.D.
Summit, New Jersey

Infectious mononucleosis is an acute infectious disease of the reticuloendothelial system caused by the Epstein-Barr (E-B) virus. The classic clinical presentation of fever, sore throat, and lymphadenopathy, especially involving the posterior cervical nodes, is well recognized. Variations, however, are common, and at times complications may be the first presenting feature. The relative and absolute lymphocytosis and the presence of heterophile antibody complete the diagnostic criteria. Occasionally heterophile negative cases are seen, and a fluorescent antibody technique is available to prove the presence of the IgM antibody specific for the E-B virus. The incidence of infectious mononucleosis is about 50 per 100,000 and thereby qualifies it as one of the most common illnesses of young adults. The disease is almost always transmitted by direct oral contact, hence the name "kissing disease." It can also be transmitted by drinking glasses, straws, and food utensils. Very rarely infectious mononucleosis reportedly has been transmitted via blood transfusion. The incubation period of this disease is approximately 42 days.

Treatment

General Principles. ACUTE PHASE—FIRST TO TWENTY-FIRST DAY. Fever is virtually always present and can be from very low grade to as high as 105°F. (40.5°C.). It usually lasts 4 to 14 days and rarely up to 3 to 4 weeks. During this acute phase of the illness, rest is the most important treatment, but absolute bed rest is not necessary or indicated. Fever is controlled easily by acetaminophen or aspirin. Once the fever has subsided for 24 to 48 hours, the patient should be encouraged to resume sedentary activity—for example, academic studies and sit-down hobbies. Restriction of physical activity is necessary for approximately 21 days because of the risk of splenic rupture up to that time.

Sore throat associated with marked dysphagia is very common. Severe pharyngeal pain, as well as heavy exudate and edema, is often seen. Symptomatic management in the form of warm saline gargles and/or carbamide peroxide and anhydrous glycerol (Gly-Oxide) gargles can be helpful, especially if carried out prior to taking nourishment. Analgesics of varying potency, including narcotics, may be necessary. Corticosteroids should be used promptly if more than mild pain or dysphagia is present. There is usually a dramatic response to corticosteroids, and prompt use precludes progressive debilitation and pharyngeal obstruction. A dosage schedule for corticosteroids is given in a subsequent paragraph. Antibiotics are not indicated unless throat cultures are taken and a significant organism is grown. About 20 to 25 per cent of patients with infectious mononucleosis will have a concurrent beta-hemolytic streptococcal infection proved by culture. Penicillin or erythromycin should be used in the routine dosage for beta-hemolytic streptococci, namely, 250 mg. of either drug four times daily for a 10 day course. Parenteral antibiotics can be given if necessary. In patients with a history of rheumatic fever and glomerulonephritis, a full course of penicillin or its substitute should be administered. Ampicillin should be avoided in patients with infectious mononucleosis, as there is an unusual sensitivity to this drug for some unknown reason. Approximately 80 per cent of patients will develop skin rashes when given ampicillin.

Asthenia may be produced to the point of stuporousness in the acute phase of illness. This symptom may respond dramatically to corticosteroids when it is due to the toxicity of the infection per se. Malaise and fatigue are rarely prolonged beyond 4 to 6 weeks of illness. Headache responds to routine analgesic therapy and is a minor symptom in this illness if complications are absent. Anorexia and dysphagia can lead to significant weight loss of up to 10 to 15 pounds, as well as dehydration, and the usual supportive measures must be employed to prevent profound debilitation. Corticosteroids once again will prevent unnecessary debilitation. There are no dietary restrictions for patients with infectious mononucleosis, but liquids and soft food are recommended initially. All neurologic complications, as well as hemolytic anemia, prominent hepatic inflammation, or pharyngeal obstruction, must be treated promptly with corticosteroid therapy. Once the diagnosis has been clearly established, there is little need for continued laboratory testing with regard to either blood counts or liver function tests. Certainly repeated determination of the heterophile titer is useless.

CONVALESCENT PHASE—FOURTEENTH TO FORTY-SECOND DAY. During the convalescent phase, a gradual return to normal activity is encouraged once the temperature has normalized for a 24 to 48 hour period. Physical reconditioning should be gradual and should begin after the twenty-first day of illness when the risk of splenic rupture has passed. Any overlimitation of patients regarding physical activity leads to deconditioning and a sense of invalidism. In fact, over-restricting patients frequently leads them to exaggerate symptoms for the purposes of secondary gain. By the end of the fourth to the sixth week of illness, even contact sports can be permitted, as long as a serious complication has not been present. Common sense in avoidance of fatigue and maintaining good nutrition is essential in this phase of the disease.

Corticosteroid Therapy. I use corticosteroids in all but the mild clinical forms of the disease. Once the diagnosis is firmly established, steroids should be utilized in all other cases. It has been clearly demonstrated that corticosteroids reduce the duration and severity of the illness, thereby limiting the degree of debilitation and loss of time from normal endeavors. In addition, corticosteroids will prevent complications and even progression of the usual course of the disease. Corticosteroid therapy has not been shown to interfere with the immunity conferred by the disease. In patients who are treated with corticosteroids, their symptomatic relief is dramatic in all parameters. A course of corticosteroids should be individualized depending on the clinical picture and whether or not complications are present. In severely ill patients, or with complications, I use prednisone or its equivalent dosage form, giving 80 mg. in four divided doses for 2 days, 60 mg. in four divided doses for 2 days, 40 mg. in four divided doses for 2 days, 20 mg. in two divided doses for 2 days, and 10 mg. in two divided doses for 2 days. In a more moderate form of illness, I use prednisone, 40 mg. in four divided doses for 3 days, 20 mg. in four divided doses for 3 days, and 10 mg. in two divided doses for 3 days. Parenteral steroids may be utilized if the clinical situation warrants and will produce a very prompt and dramatic effect.

Surgery. Very rarely tracheostomy is indicated in a patient with severe pharyngeal inflammation causing a respiratory obstructive syndrome. Steroids used promptly as outlined above preclude the need for intubation and/or tracheostomy. Splenectomy must be done for the life-threatening complication of splenic rupture. The exact incidence of this complication is not known and is fortunately very infrequent. The mere development of abdominal pain should alert the physician to the complication of possible or impending splenic rupture, whether the pain be in the left upper quadrant or elsewhere in the abdomen. Scrupulous observation for confirmatory signs and symptoms of splenic rupture is mandatory. Abdominal symptoms may well preclude actual rupture by hours or even days. All patients who have infectious mononucleosis deserve close observation for any of the complications which can occur.

Isolation. It is not necessary to isolate patients with infectious mononucleosis, because the disease is transmitted with great difficulty even in the ways already mentioned. The patient does remain infected for a very long period of time after the illness has cleared, perhaps a year or more. A carrier state has been established for as long as 2 years by virtue of the persistent presence of the E-B virus in pharyngeal tissue and lymphocytes. The E-B virus has also been recovered from vaginal and urethral sources; however, venereal routes of transmission have not been proved. Gamma globulin has no therapeutic use to either patient or contacts. The cleansing of eating and drinking objects should be by standard hygienic means, preferably using an automatic dishwasher.

Prognosis

Virtually all patients will return to their normal preillness state of health and activity within 4 to 6 weeks of the onset of the disease. Deaths are extremely rare and when reported are due to splenic rupture. Rarely residuals may persist in patients who have had neurologic complications of this disease. Infectious mononucleosis has been shown to exacerbate very infrequently. This could occur in the early months following the acute phase of the disease. So few cases are clearly documented that it is difficult to know the reasons for exacerbation. In patients who show exacerbation, the acute phase seems to recur in its entirety, with the physical and laboratory features again present. Infectious mononucleosis is said to have recurred in rare instances. However, such cases found in the literature certainly do not preclude other possibilities and frequently are based on a positive heterophile test. Once a patient has had infectious mononucleosis, immunity to the disease is established.

MUMPS

method of
ROBERT L. PERKINS, M.D.
Columbus, Ohio

Mumps (Epidemic Parotitis)

No specific treatment is available for mumps parotitis or complications. For parotitis, seasoned or spicy food and drink which might excessively stimulate salivary secretions should be avoided so as to minimize pain. Similarly, atropine-like medications should not be given in an attempt to reduce parotid secretions, because inspissation and obstruction of ductal flow could cause added pain or secondary infection.

Analgesics may be given for pain of salivary origin. For pain in children or adults, acetylsalicylic acid usually suffices in doses of 40 to 80 mg. per kg. per 24 hours in six divided doses; however, larger doses causing salicylism or gastric irritation may result in confusing symptoms in patients who have undetected pancreatitis or meningoencephalitis.

Patients of all ages should be restricted to bed rest during the acute phase of illness, because the prevailing but unproved clinical opinion persists that excessive activity may cause complications or extension of infection.

Mumps virus has been found in saliva as long as 7 days before and 4 to 9 days after appearance of parotitis, and consequently patients should ideally have respiratory isolation until swelling of parotid or submandibular salivary glands subsides.

Complications of Mumps

Orchitis. Orchitis and/or epididymitis occurs in 18 to 43 per cent of postpubertal males; although commonly unilateral, 37 per cent bilateral involvement has been observed in an epidemic. For pain, oral acetylsalicylic acid in the aforementioned doses may be tried before resorting to a narcotic. Children may be given codeine, 3 mg. per kg. per 24 hours, and adults, 3 to 6 mg. per kg. per 24 hours, orally or subcutaneously, in six divided doses. With massive testicular swelling, extreme discomfort may occur, justifying meperidine hydrochloride, 1 mg. per kg. intramuscular single doses in children and 1 to 1.4 mg. per kg. in adults; doses may be repeated every 4 to 6 hours provided respiratory depression or other side effects do not occur. Morphine sulfate may be required by some patients for pain relief but may possibly be contraindicated in those with pancreatitis, as the effect on smooth muscle may cause spasm of biliary and pancreatic sphincters; the resultant increase in intraductal pressure may be associated with elevation of plasma amylase and lipase.

Bed rest and support of the scrotum with a suspensory may afford some relief, but the additional use of continuous ice bags combined with an analgesic is often more effective. Surgical incision of the tunica albuginea to relieve swelling should not be performed.

Meningoencephalitis. The aseptic meningitis syndrome or meningoencephalitis may appear in 0.5 to 23 per cent of patients, including a significant number without parotitis. Treatment is symptomatic. Severe neurologic deficit is rare but may require additional supportive measures. Myelitis may require urinary bladder intubation because of sphincter dysfunction. Lumbar puncture may give significant relief from headache but should not be repeated except for diagnostic purposes. Narcotics for pain relief should be used only with caution. Seizures should be treated with major anticonvulsant drugs.

Other Complications. The incidence of other clinically significant complications is relatively low, but each may on occasion cause severe illness. Pancreatitis, arthritis, mastitis, thyroiditis, nephritis, myocarditis, oophoritis, and thrombocytopenia may require individualized supportive therapy.

Adrenocorticosteroid Therapy. Hydrocortisone and derivatives and ACTH have been employed for various complications of mumps, particularly orchitis, often with equivocal results. In addition, serious questions exist regarding possible facilitation of spread of virus caused by steroids. However, favorable subjective responses have frequently been described, with lessening of testicular swelling, lysis of fever, decrease in headache, and abeyance of symptoms of pancreatitis. Spread of infection to an uninvolved parotid gland or testes during steroid treatment and resurgence of fever and other symptoms with early or rapid reduction of dosage have also been noted. Thus the decision to employ high dosage corticosteroid therapy depends upon the severity and nature of the complication, keeping in mind that further extension of the infection during treatment and relapse after discontinuation may occur. In addition, corticosteroid treatment may be associated with serious secondary infections. Guidelines are lacking for dosages in the few instances in which such treatment may be indicated. Preference probably should be given to a short-term high dosage regimen with tapering as rapid as permitted by clinical response.

Preventive Measures

Postexposure Prophylaxis. The relative risk of infection in persons exposed to active mumps can be assessed in part by obtaining serologic tests; the presence of antibody is a reasonable indicator of immunity, even in those who give no history of mumps. If serologic tests are not readily available, a mumps skin test may be useful; a large reaction (≥1.5 cm. erythema at 24 to 36 hours) has been found by some investigators to correlate with immunity. However, if the immune status of the exposed person remains in doubt, mumps hyperimmune human gamma globulin (4.5 ml. intramuscularly) may be employed in an attempt to prevent serious complications, especially orchitis in postpubertal males. Standard pooled immune human gamma globulin has no apparent value for mumps prophylaxis.

Vaccines. An available attenuated (live) virus mumps vaccine produces solid longlasting immunity (>4 years) in greater than 95 per cent of vaccinees. Adverse effects have been infrequent, and the viable vaccine should be employed routinely in infants after 12 months of age as part of primary immunizations. Postexposure vaccination is not contraindicated, but immediately subsequent mumps infection could be erroneously attributed to the vaccine. The value of the vaccine during the postexposure period is unknown. The viable vaccine should not be given to patients with impaired host resistance resulting from underlying disease or related immunosuppressive therapy; it should also not be given to those who are febrile, pregnant, or allergic to egg protein or neomycin. An available inactivated (killed) vaccine may be considered in immunosuppressed or pregnant patients but may give short-lived protection.

INTESTINAL PARASITES

method of
JERROLD A. TURNER, M.D.
Torrance, California

Drug Availability

Many drugs that are widely used throughout the world for the treatment of parasitic infections do not have approval of the Food and Drug Administration for general use within the United States. The Parasitic Disease Drug Service of the Center for Disease Control in Atlanta, Georgia, provides certain of these unapproved drugs on investigational protocols to physicians for the treatment of specific diseases. Included with the protocol is complete information on dosages and precautions for administration of the drugs.

In some instances, drugs which have governmental approval for the treatment of specific infections have been found useful in other diseases. When any of these generally available drugs are used for conditions other than those specified by the Food and Drug Administration, they are considered investigational, and the prescribing physician must employ the procedures and precautions, such as informed consent, which are appropriate for the use of an experimental drug.

Pregnancy

The information available for most antiparasitic drugs is inadequate to determine safety in pregnancy. The benefits of treatment must be weighed against the potential hazards to the mother and the fetus. Mild or light infections with many species of intestinal parasites are of little clinical significance, and treatment, if indicated, may be deferred until the patient is delivered.

Multiple Infections

It is common to find that patients are infected with more than one species of intestinal parasite. If all species infecting a patient cannot be effectively treated with a single medication, it is necessary to plan a sequence of therapy. The administration of multiple drugs simultaneously should be avoided.

In general, if the patient with a multiple infection has symptoms which can be attributed to one species of infecting organism, it is best to treat that particular infection first. In an asymptomatic patient, treatment of the infection that has the greatest pathogenic potential usually should take precedence over the less clinically important parasites.

The treatment of intestinal nematodes has been simplified by the advent of mebendazole (Vermox), a drug which is effective in ascariasis, hookworm infection, trichuriasis, and enterobiasis. Recent evidence indicates that it may be highly effective in certain tapeworm infections as well.

Thiabendazole (Mintezol) also has a broad spectrum of activity against intestinal roundworms, but its toxicity limits its use, as a primary drug, to strongyloidiasis. However, if the patient has strongyloidiasis, the clinician should be aware that thiabendazole is also effective for concomitant ascariasis and enterobiasis, and may have a low degree of efficacy in trichuriasis.

Protozoal Infections

Nonpathogenic Protozoa. *Entamoeba coli, Endolimax nana, Iodamoeba bütschlii,* and *Chilomastix mesnili* are not associated with disease and require no treatment. *Entamoeba hartmanni* is considered to be nonpathogenic. It is differentiated from the pathogenic *Entamoeba histolytica* only on the basis of size, and overlap between the two species is possible. Therefore the decision whether or not to initiate treatment should be based on clinical information in addition to the laboratory report. Treatment, if indicated, would be as described for amebiasis.

Giardiasis. Some authorities feel that asymptomatic infections with *Giardia lamblia* do not require treatment. However, it is my firm belief that treatment is always indicated to avoid the potential for illness at some future time and to decrease the possibility of spread of the infection among contacts. Quinacrine (Atabrine, mepacrine) is the drug of choice and is available in 100 mg. tablets. The dosage is 7 mg. per kg. (maximum, 300 mg.) divided into three doses taken daily with meals for 7 days. For small children, it is helpful to have the drug made up in a flavored, sweet syrup to mask the bitter taste. The toxicity of quinacrine is largely gastrointestinal (nausea, vomiting, and abdominal pain) but is uncommon at this dosage. Prolonged courses of quinacrine may result in yellow discoloration of the skin and conjunctiva. Various skin eruptions rarely have been reported. Quinacrine is contraindicated in pregnant women, in conjunction with treatment with 8-aminoquinoline compounds, and in patients with psoriasis. The efficacy of this treatment is high, and marked symptomatic improvement is expected within 4 days. The course may be repeated, if necessary, after a 2 week rest period. Alternative chemotherapy with metronidazole (Flagyl) or furazolidone (Furoxone) probably is somewhat less efficacious. Manufacturer's information should be consulted regarding toxicity and contraindications. Metronidazole is available in 250 mg. tablets and may be given in a dosage of 10 to 15 mg. per kg. (maximum, 750 mg.) in three divided doses daily for 7 days. (*Note*: when used for giardiasis, metronidazole is considered investigational.) Furazolidone is supplied as 100 mg. tablets and as a suspension containing 50 mg. per 15 ml. with kaolin and pectin. It is administered in a dosage of 5 mg. per kg. in four divided doses daily for 5 days.

Dientamoeba Fragilis Infection. Because of the delicate nature of this organism, its prevalence has not been appreciated. The use of preservative techniques in the collection of fecal specimens has helped to reveal this organism as a possible cause of mild to moderate gastrointestinal symptoms.

The infection may be treated with tetracycline, 10 to 20 mg. per kg. (maximum, 1 gram) given in four divided doses daily for 7 days. Tetracycline should not be given to children under 14 years of age. Alternative therapy using diiodohydroxyquin, available in 650 mg. tablets, is given as 30 to 40 mg. per kg. (maximum 1.95 grams) divided into three daily doses for 21 days. Diiodohydroxyquin is no longer available as Diodoquin but is manufactured by several companies under the generic name. The toxicity of diiodohydroxyquin includes various forms of dermatitis, abdominal discomfort, diarrhea, anal pruritus, headache, and hypoesthesia of the hands and feet. Contraindications are hypersensitivity to iodine or to any 8-hydroxyquinoline compound. Because of the occurrence of neurologic damage associated with a similar 8-hydroxyquinoline compound, repetitive or prolonged courses or an increase in the dose above that recommended should be avoided.

Trichomoniasis. Infection with the intestinal flagellate *Trichomonas hominis* is probably of no clinical significance, although there are anecdotes which implicate the organism as a possible cause of diarrhea. It may respond to tetracycline as administered in Dientamoeba infections.

Balantidiasis. Rarely diagnosed in the United States, infection with *Balantidium coli* is usually effectively treated with oxytetracycline (Terramycin), 10 to 20 mg. per kg. (maximum 1 gram) given daily in four divided doses for 10 days. Diiodohydroxyquin used as noted for Dientamoeba infection is also effective.

Helminth Infections

Ascariasis. Even asymptomatic infections with *Ascaris lumbricoides* should always be treated because of the potential for the worms to cause intestinal obstruction, to invade the biliary or pancreatic ducts, or to cause laryngeal or tracheal obstruction.

Mebendazole (Vermox) is highly effective and is supplied as 100 mg. tablets and administered in doses of 100 mg. twice daily for 3 days. This dosage applies to all age groups regardless of weight. The only reported toxicity has been transient abdominal pain and diarrhea associated with the expulsion of massive numbers of worms. Mebendazole is contraindicated in pregnant women because of teratogenicity demonstrated in animals. It should be used with caution in patients under the age of 2 years. Alternative therapy is available using pyrantel pamoate (Antiminth) or piperazine (Antepar). The increased frequency of side effects with pyrantel and the differing doses for variations in body weight for both preparations make mebendazole a more convenient choice.

Thiabendazole (Mintezol) is effective, but its side effects are marked, and it should not be used for ascariasis unless there is concomitant infection with *Strongyloides stercoralis*.

If follow-up examinations in 2 to 4 weeks do not show total absence of Ascaris eggs, retreatment is indicated.

Hookworm Infection. Both common species of hookworm, *Ancylostoma duodenale* and *Necator americanus,* may be successfully treated with mebendazole as for ascariasis. Effective alternative therapy is available using bephenium (Alcopara) as in Trichostrongylus infections or using tetrachloroethylene (Nema worm capsules) as in intestinal fluke infection (this is a veterinary preparation not officially approved for human use). The low toxicity and convenience of mebendazole make it the drug of choice.

Heavy infections with hookworms, particularly in association with a marginal intake of dietary iron, may produce a secondary anemia. Oral iron supplements are indicated in addition to antiparasitic treatment in these patients.

If follow-up fecal examinations in 2 to 4 weeks still show only a few hookworm eggs, this represents a clinically insignificant infection, and retreatment is unnecessary.

Trichuriasis (Whipworm Infection). Most patients with *Trichuris trichiura* infection seen in the United States have light worm loads and are asymptomatic. When gastrointestinal symptoms are associated with a light whipworm infection, it is common to find that they originate from some other abnormality. Mebendazole, used as described for ascariasis, is very effective. Because of its toxicity and the degree of efficacy, thiabendazole is not a primary drug in this infection.

The goal of treatment is a marked reduction

in the worm load. It is not always possible to eliminate all the parasites. A few Trichuris eggs seen on follow-up fecal examinations 2 to 4 weeks after treatment do not indicate a need for further courses of medication.

Enterobiasis. Infections with the pinworm *Enterobius vermicularis* are extremely common. Among school children, prevalence rates of 70 per cent are not unusual. Fortunately, symptoms occur in less than 10 per cent of those infected. Most texts and pharmaceutical companies recommend, in addition to chemotherapy, a long list of hygienic measures which are thought to help in the prevention of reinfection. Available evidence indicates that exceptional efforts directed toward personal hygiene or the environment are futile. Reinfections frequently occur in spite of the most rigorous attempts to rid the household of pinworm eggs. Reintroduction of pinworms into the home from such sources as playmates, school contacts, and visits to other homes is unavoidable. Therefore a major component of therapy is counseling the family concerning the high prevalence of infection, its benign nature, and the ineffective aspect of extraordinary hygienic measures.

Chemotherapy should be directed toward the symptomatic patient. Temporary elimination of sources of infection within the home may be attempted by treating all family members every 2 weeks for three treatments. This approach is expensive and will not prevent reintroduction of infection from outside the household. Mebendazole (Vermox) in the dose of a single 100 mg. tablet for all ages is highly effective, and no significant side effects have been reported. It is contraindicated in pregnant women and should be used with caution in children under the age of 2 years. Alternative single-dose therapy may be carried out with pyrvinium pamoate (Povan) or pyrantel pamoate (Antiminth). Pyrvinium is supplied as 50 mg. tablets and as a flavored suspension containing 10 mg. per ml. It is administered in a single dose of 5 mg. per kg. Nausea, vomiting, abdominal pain, and diarrhea occur in a small number of patients. The drug is a red dye and will stain if spilled. Following treatment, the stool may be colored red; if vomiting occurs, the red color may be mistakenly interpreted as gastrointestinal bleeding. Pyrantel is supplied as a flavored suspension containing 50 mg. base per ml. and is given in a single dose of 11 mg. per kg. (maximum, 1 gram). Complaints of nausea, vomiting, abdominal pain, and diarrhea occur in a small number of patients. Less common are reports of transient serum glutamic oxaloacetic transaminase (SGOT) elevation, headache, dizziness, drowsiness, insomnia, and skin rash.

Follow-up examinations for pinworm infections are unnecessary if the patient's symptoms respond to treatment. Recurrence of symptoms 5 or 6 weeks after treatment usually indicates reinfection. If symptoms persist following treatment, they may represent treatment failure or may indicate some other process which causes anal pruritus. Persisting infection should be confirmed by cellulose tape swabs or by observing adult worms on the perianal skin.

Strongyloidiasis. All infections with *Strongyloides stercoralis* should be treated. This parasite has the ability to autoinfect, and infections may persist for the life of the host. Strongyloidiasis may be fatal in the immunologically compromised patient, and is a particular threat to infected persons who receive high-dose corticosteroids.

The drug of choice, thiabendazole (Mintezol), is highly effective and is available as a flavored suspension containing 125 or 250 mg. per 5 ml., as pediatric drops containing 100 mg. per ml., and as chewable 500 mg. tablets. It is administered as 50 mg. per kg. (maximum, 3 grams) in two divided doses daily for 2 days. Nausea, vomiting, and dizziness are common side effects. Diarrhea, abdominal pain, pruritus, drowsiness, giddiness, and headache may also occur. Rare complications of treatment are a transient rise in serum glutamic oxaloacetic transaminase (SGOT), cholestasis and parenchymal liver damage, numbness, tinnitus, hyperirritability, abnormal sensation in the eyes, visual disturbances, hypotension, collapse, perianal rash, hyperglycemia, hematuria, crystalluria, and malodorous urine. Hypersensitivity reactions are rare but may be severe. Fatal cases of the Stevens-Johnson syndrome have been reported. Other allergic manifestations have been angioedema, anaphylaxis, and skin rashes. The drug is contraindicated in patients with known hypersensitivity to thiabendazole. It should be administered with caution in patients with known hepatic or renal disease.

Follow-up fecal examination 3 to 4 weeks after treatment using special concentration or culture techniques (Baermann or Haradi-Mori) or examination of duodenal contents is more accurate than relying solely upon routine stool examinations.

Trichostrongyliasis. There is no widely accepted standard treatment for infection with species of Trichostrongylus. Outside the United States, levamisole is frequently used. Thiabendazole, as used for strongyloidiasis, is effective, but drugs with less serious potential toxicity are preferred. Bephenium hydroxynaphthoate (Alcopara) is investigational for use in this infection, but may be tried in a dosage of 100 mg. per kg. (maximum, 10 grams) in two divided doses in 1 day. The drug is supplied in packets of 5 grams. It is made more palatable by mixing with chocolate milk, fruit juice, or flavored carbonated beverages. The patient should avoid eating for 2 hours after each dose. Occasionally nausea, vomiting, and mild diarrhea may occur.

Tapeworm Infections. Mild or vague gastrointestinal symptoms have been attributed to all tapeworm infections. However, treatment is often precipitated by the patient's distress at discovering migrating proglottids or passing a chain of tapeworm segments.

Taenia saginata (beef tapeworm) poses little danger to its host and is largely a nuisance. Infection with *Taenia solium* is hazardous because cysticercosis may develop in the host or in others who may accidentally ingest the ova produced by the adult worm. *Diphyllobothrium latum* infections in certain areas of Scandinavia, Finland, and adjacent Russia occasionally produce megaloblastic anemia, but otherwise symptoms of infection are mild or absent. *Hymenolepis nana* infection is usually detected on routine stool examination in the asymptomatic individual. However, these infections should be treated, because the eggs excreted in the stool are infectious for others.

Niclosamide (Yomesan) is the current drug of choice for all tapeworm infections. It is available in the United States through the Parasitic Disease Drug Service, Center for Disease Control, Atlanta, Georgia. Niclosamide is supplied as chewable 500 mg. tablets. For infections with *T. saginata, T. solium* and *D. latum,* a single dose is chewed thoroughly following a light meal. The dosages are as follows: children weighing 25 to 75 lbs. receive 1 gram; children weighing more than 75 lbs. receive 1.5 grams; adults receive 2 grams. Side effects are rare and usually consist of nausea, vomiting, and abdominal pain. Rare instances of dizziness, fever, and urticaria have been reported. The drug should not be used in pregnant women or in children under the age of 2 years. Follow-up consists of requesting patients to observe for proglottids, and stool examinations should be done 3 months after treatment.

In cases of *T. solium* infection there is a theoretical possibility of the release of eggs into the gut lumen and therefore a risk of cysticercosis. This complication has never been reported, but the patient should be informed of this concern prior to treatment.

H. nana infections require more prolonged treatment because of larval stages which occur in the intestinal villi. Niclosamide should be taken following a light meal and the tablets chewed thoroughly before swallowing. It is administered in these dosages: children weighing 25 to 75 lbs., 1 gram on the first day, followed by 500 mg. daily for 6 days; children weighing more than 75 lbs., 1.5 grams initially followed by 1 gram daily for 6 days; adults, 2 grams daily for 7 days. Follow-up consists of fecal examinations 2 weeks and 3 months after completion of treatment.

Intestinal Fluke Infection. Infections with *Fasciolopsis buski, Heterophyes heterophyes,* and *Metagonimus yokogawai* may be treated with tetrachloroethylene. This drug is approved but may be difficult to obtain. It is available only as Nema worm capsules for veterinary use, but this preparation is safe and effective in humans. Tetrachloroethylene is supplied in soft gelatin capsules of 0.2, 1.0, and 2.5 ml. It is administered in the fasting state in a single dose. The dose is 0.10 to 0.12 ml. per kg. (maximum, 5 ml.). Frequent side effects are nausea, vomiting, epigastric burning, and abdominal cramps. Rarely headache, vertigo, inebriation, and somnolence may occur if an excess of the drug is absorbed. Concurrent conditions such as anemia and dehydration should be corrected prior to administering the drug. Relative contraindications exist for very young, severely ill children and for patients with liver disease. Alcohol should be avoided before treatment and for 24 hours after treatment.

Liver Fluke Infection. Chronic *Opisthorchis* (*Clonorchis*) *sinensis* and *Opisthorchis viverrini* infections are usually asymptomatic, and studies of symptomatology and liver function have failed to reveal abnormalities of much clinical significance. This is fortunate, for there is no available effective chemotherapy. Chloroquine has been used in these infections, but it appears only to suppress egg production for a limited period. The course of chloroquine recommended is 500 to 750 mg. daily in two or three divided doses for 6 to 8 weeks.

Fasciola hepatica infections may be treated with bithionol (Lorothidol) or dehydroemetine. Both drugs must be obtained through the Parasitic Disease Drug Service, Center for Disease Control, Atlanta, Georgia. Bithionol has a slight advantage over dehydroemetine in that it is given orally. It is supplied in 500 mg. gelatin capsules, and, because the capsules should not be opened, the drug must be given in 500 mg. increments. The dosage is 30 to 50 mg. per kg. divided into two doses, given on alternate days for 10 to 15 doses. Side effects consisting of diarrhea and abdominal cramps are common but usually subside after 2 or 3 days of treatment. Nausea, vomiting, urticaria, dizziness, headache, and excessive salivation may occur with less frequency. Rarely, toxic hepatitis, cardiac arrhythmias, and proteinuria have been reported. It is contraindicated in those patients with known bithionol sensitivity, and it is not recommended in pregnant women or in children under 8 years of age.

Dehydroemetine (investigational in the

United States of America) is supplied in 2 ml. ampules containing 30 mg. per ml. It is given as a deep intramuscular injection in a schedule of 1 mg. per kg. daily for 10 days. Toxic effects consisting of nausea and diarrhea may occur. Electrocardiographic abnormalities are common, but usually disappear within 2 weeks after the cessation of therapy. Hypotension of some degree may occur. Pain and weakness in muscles in the area of the injection site have been noted. There are reports of polyneuritis with transient paralysis, and neurasthenia may be common and slow to resolve over several months following treatment. Relative contraindications exist in patients with cardiac or neurologic abnormalities. The patient should be at bed rest during treatment and gradually resume activity over a period of several weeks after therapy is completed.

Follow-up for Fasciola infection should consist of three fecal examinations 1 month after treatment.

Schistosomiasis. Adult worms of *Schistosoma mansoni* and *Schistosoma japonicum* parasitize the venules of the intestinal tract and produce ova which are excreted in the feces. The drugs available for the treatment of these infections have significant toxic potential.

Decisions regarding treatment should be individualized. Factors such as the intensity of infection, complications resulting from the schistosome infection, and the presence of other concomitant diseases should be weighed against the toxicity of the drug to be employed.

Although a newer, orally administered compound, niridazole (Ambilhar), is available through the Parasitic Disease Drug Service, it has limited usefulness because of the uncommon, but severe, central nervous system side effects and the need to hospitalize patients during treatment. It has also been found to be carcinogenic in mice.

The antimonial compounds have significant toxicity but usually can be administered safely with careful monitoring.

S. mansoni infection may be treated with stibocaptate (sodium antimony dimercaptosuccinate, Astiban), which is available through the Parasitic Disease Drug Service, Center for Disease Control, Atlanta, Georgia. It is supplied in 5 ml. ampules containing 0.5 gram of white crystalline powder. It is administered intramuscularly in a 10 per cent solution once or twice weekly for a total of five injections. The dosage is 8 mg. per kg. (total, 40 mg. per kg.) for adults and 10 mg. per kg. (total, 50 mg. per kg.) for children.

S. japonicum requires intravenous therapy with antimony potassium tartrate (tartar emetic). This drug is supplied as a crystalline powder containing 36.5 per cent trivalent antimony or as a 0.5 per cent solution. It is administered very slowly intravenously through a fine needle to avoid extravasation. Spasms of coughing and transient pruritus are associated with intravenous injection. Pneumonitis, arthralgias, myalgias, abnormalities in liver function, headache, mild rashes, and electrocardiographic changes may occur. Uncommon side effects are hepatitis, hemolytic anemia, thrombocytopenia, and anaphylactoid reactions. Antimonials are contraindicated in the presence of myocarditis, hepatitis, or severe liver disease and in patients with concurrent bacterial or viral infections. Persistence of arthralgias or rashes or the development of progressive proteinuria requires cessation of treatment. Assessment of platelets should be done periodically during the course of therapy.

Follow-up examinations may be made 2 months after treatment; however, reappearance of viable eggs following unsuccessful treatment may not occur until much later. Negative examinations 6 months after therapy are necessary to consider the patient cured. Dead ova may continue to be excreted after treatment. Therefore the persistence of active infection should be determined by observing for motile flame cells within the miracidia or by performing a hatching test.

PSITTACOSIS

method of
CHARLES W. STRATTON, M.D.
Charleston, West Virginia

Introduction

Psittacosis is an infection of birds caused by the obligate intracellular bacterium, *Chlamydia psittaci*. Over 90 species of birds may contract this illness, which in them commonly produces diarrhea, weakness, and apathy. Transmission to humans occurs when dust particles containing viable organisms are inhaled. In adults the spectrum of disease ranges from a mild influenza-like syndrome through a severe pneumonitis to a fatal illness resembling typhoid fever. Overt clinical infections in children are uncommon.

Human cases have most often been traced to psittacine birds, pigeons, and common barnyard fowl. Poultry workers, petshop employees, and pigeon handlers are thus at increased risk. Human-to-human transmission, although rare, has been documented.

Treatment

The greatest problem in treatment is the early recognition of this entity, at which point antimicrobials are most effective. Psittacosis should be considered in the differential diagnosis of atypical pneumonia, particularly with the syndrome of "viral" pneumonia accompanied by prolonged high fever, severe headache, and relative bradycardia. Any history of contact with birds should be actively sought. Although chlamydiae may be cultured in the yolk sac of fertilized hen's eggs, such isolation can be hazardous and should be attempted only by qualified laboratories. The demonstration of rising complement-fixing antibodies in convalescent serum is diagnostic but also time consuming. Moreover, early therapy with tetracycline may delay antibody rise for months. Initiation of treatment should obviously precede the definite diagnosis and must be based on clinical grounds alone. In such patients strict respiratory isolation is mandatory. Correct procedures may be found in the Center for Disease Control manual, *Isolation Techniques for Use in Hospitals*.

Supportive Therapy. Seriously ill patients will generally put themselves at bed rest. Hospitalization in such patients is usually indicated in order to maintain fluid and electrolyte balance with intravenous therapy. In addition, some patients will have significant hypoxia and may need to be in an intensive care unit, where arterial blood gases may be monitored and respiratory support systems used as indicated. Patients with milder cases may be allowed activity as tolerated.

High fevers of 103 to 104°F. (39.5 to 40°C.) may necessitate either salicylates (600 mg. every 3 to 4 hours) or acetaminophen (650 mg. every 3 to 4 hours) or hypothermic blankets. Antipyretics should be given around the clock to prevent the repeated bouts of rigors that may occur with "prn" doses. Cough and/or headache may occasionally warrant treatment with codeine (15 mg. every 4 to 6 hours).

Specific Therapy. Tetracycline remains the drug of choice for psittacosis. The preferred dose and route is 500 mg. orally every 6 hours for 2 weeks. For those needing intravenous therapy, 250 mg. of tetracycline can be given intravenously every 6 hours. Failure of defervescence in 24 to 48 hours with this regimen should prompt a careful review of other diagnostic possibilities.

Patients with impaired renal function should receive doxycycline (100 mg. orally every 12 hours) instead of tetracycline. Children and pregnant women should not receive tetracyclines. These groups may be treated with either penicillin (1 million units of aqueous penicillin given intravenously every 4 hours) or chloramphenicol (50 mg. per kg. per day in four divided doses).

Relapses after any one of the aforementioned regimens may occur. These can usually be treated with another 2 week course of oral tetracycline at 2 grams per day in divided doses.

Public Health Measures. The incidence of psittacosis in the United States has been decreasing because of the use of tetracycline in poultry and bird feed. Individual cases should be reported to appropriate public health officials, as an investigation of other family members and/or fellow workers may be needed. There are no vaccines available for use in man.

Q FEVER

method of
DENNIS G. MAKI, M.D.
Madison, Wisconsin

Introduction

Q fever is a self-limiting systemic infection caused by *Coxiella burnetii* which is common but frequently undiagnosed. Distributed almost worldwide, the causative organism has a unique ability among the Rickettsiaceae to withstand prolonged periods of desiccation, in association with dust, straw, wool, hides, or clothes, and to resist flash pasteurization and many chemical disinfectants. It infects a wide variety of wild and domestic animals as well as man; asymptomatically infected livestock, particularly dairy cattle and sheep, comprise the major source of human illness. Infected animals pass large numbers of organisms in their milk and excretions, but the membranes of parturition are particularly heavily infected. Although infections in animals may derive from tick-borne spread, human infection almost always results from inhalation of airborne organisms, occasionally from ingestion of contaminated milk. The extraordinary persistence of *C. burnetii* organisms in the environment, for months to years, and their high infectivity account for the many epidemics of Q fever in soldiers and in persons working on farms and ranches, in abattoirs and meat-packing plants, and in research and diagnostic laboratories. Except for laboratory outbreaks, human infection invariably connotes animal contact, which may have been very indirect or transient and frequently is not recalled. Human-to-human transmission is inexplicably rare. Based on seroepidemiologic surveys, Q fever is most often subclinical or undiagnosed. Even the most severe cases rarely end fatally; death ensues from overwhelming pneumonia or refractory endocarditis.

Supportive Therapy

1. Most patients with Q fever can be adequately managed at home. The elderly and patients with serious underlying diseases, respiratory distress, or incapacitating symptoms usually require hospitalization.

2. *Fever* should be suppressed in patients with cardiac disease and children with a history of febrile convulsions, when it is extreme (>40°C. or 104°F.), and when it causes severe discomfort. As-

pirin or acetaminophen is preferably given continuously (for adults, 600 mg. orally every 4 hours) to avert discomforting extremes of temperature and associated chills. Refractory hyperpyrexia is best managed with a hypothermia blanket or by sponging with tepid water rather than with alcohol.

3. The profound *malaise* and *fatigue* which characterize acute Q fever implicitly bring about needed rest. There seems little indication to enforce strict bed rest. During convalescence, ambulation should be encouraged to avert thromboembolic complications.

4. Patients who are *dehydrated* because of severe anorexia or vomiting should receive appropriate fluid and electrolyte repletion and maintenance therapy by intravenous infusion.

5. For patients with severe *chest pain* or *headache*, codeine sulfate, 15 to 45 mg. every 6 hours, usually provides adequate analgesia if aspirin or acetominophen has not brought relief.

6. The same dosage of codeine can be used to suppress severe *cough,* which is uncommon.

7. *Intensive support:* Patients who are severely ill, usually those advanced in age or suffering from underlying diseases, require close monitoring of their ventilatory status, which should include serial determinations of arterial blood gases. Humidified oxygen or even total ventilatory support may be indicated. Even when pneumonia is present, respiratory secretions in Q fever are usually scant; pulmonary physiotherapy or tracheal suctioning is rarely necessary.

Antimicrobial Therapy of Acute Q Fever

Coxiella burnetii strains are susceptible to tetracyclines and chloramphenicol, but resistant to erythromycin, penicillin, and streptomycin. Although most patients with acute Q fever will recover without chemotherapy, treatment with a tetracycline or chloramphenicol, especially within the first 3 days, usually produces defervescence within 48 hours, shortening the duration of illness. Furthermore, treatment may prevent development of chronic infection, specifically endocarditis. Thus all patients with Q fever should probably receive a course of antirickettsial chemotherapy, especially patients with valvular heart disease.

Prophylactic administration of tetracycline at the time of initial exposure will delay but not prevent clinical illness; however, treatment late in the incubation period (9 to 21 days) appears to reliably avert systemic disease.

In vitro, tetracyclines are clearly superior to chloramphenicol, and clinically they appear to be more effective. Tetracycline or oxytetracycline is the drug of choice and, in adults, may be given orally in a dosage of 500 mg. four times daily. A tetracycline analogue, doxycycline, given orally, 100 mg. twice daily for 3 days followed by 50 mg. twice daily, was very effective in experimentally produced infections in adults.

Tetracyclines should be used with great caution, if at all, during pregnancy and, except for doxycycline, in patients with pre-existent renal disease. These states greatly increase the risk of serious drug toxicity. Such patients and patients allergic to tetracycline may be treated with chloramphenicol, 500 mg. every 6 hours. Use of chloramphenicol mandates close surveillance for reversible myelosuppression (hemogram, platelet count, and reticulocyte count three times weekly), which calls for reduction in dosage or discontinuation of the drug.

Because of producing permanent discoloration of teeth, tetracyclines should not be used in children under the age of 8 years unless absolutely necessary medically. Q fever in children is rarely encountered. For children with severe infection, oxytetracycline, 25 mg. per kg., or chloramphenicol, 50 mg. per kg. daily, in four divided doses, may be used. (Oxytetracycline has been associated with the least tooth discoloration of all of the tetracyclines; in several studies, the effects of a single course were cosmetically undetectable.)

Both intravenous and intramuscular injections of tetracycline are very painful. Doxycycline produces much less local inflammation than other tetracyclines, and also can be used safely in full doses in patients with renal insufficiency. For patients who must be treated parenterally, especially those who are critically ill, doxycycline may be given by intravenous injection, 100 mg. every 12 hours for 3 days, followed by 50 mg. every 12 hours. If tetracycline or oxytetracycline is used parenterally, the daily dosage in adults should never exceed 2 grams; 500 mg. every 12 hours will give excellent therapeutic levels. Children may receive 10 mg. per kg. daily in divided doses.

Antimicrobial therapy should be continued until the patient has been fully afebrile for at least 5 days. Relapse is very rare. Retreatment with the same regimen that produced an initial response is usually effective.

Endocarditis

In the past, even when recognized and treated with drugs effective against Q fever, endocarditis caused by *C. burnetii* was rarely cured, and almost inevitably proved fatal due to valvular destruction and refractory heart failure. Neither tetracyclines nor chloramphenicol are rickettsicidal. The first successes with this grave complication of Q fever were achieved by surgically excising the infected valve and replacing it with a prosthesis. An increasing number of patients have now been cured *medically*, with prolonged tetracycline therapy—1 to 5 years. Thus *C. burnetii* endocarditis should be treated with tetracycline or oxytetracycline, 500 mg. four times daily by mouth for 2 months, followed by 1 gram daily in divided doses for at least a year. Patients failing to respond to medical therapy or who show hemodynamic evidence of deteriorating valvular function should undergo valve replacement, followed by a prolonged course of tetracycline. Control of the infection is usually accompanied by a falling titer of antibodies to the phase I antigen.

Prevention of Q Fever

Although interhuman transmission of *C. burnetii* is rare, hospital outbreaks of Q fever, several of considerable magnitude, have been reported. Hospitalized patients with presumed Q fever should have a single room, but more elaborate isolation precautions are not considered necessary. Patients' secretions and urine may contain infectious organisms. Linens and clothing should be autoclaved and clinical specimens labeled as biohazards. Autopsies of fatal cases appear to be particularly hazardous and should be performed only with the most stringent protective measures in effect.

Because of the high endemicity of *C. burnetii* infections in dairy herds in the United States, consumption of unpasteurized milk is best assiduously avoided.

An effective killed vaccine has been developed for persons in high risk occupations, but is associated with a high incidence of local and systemic reactions. These can be markedly reduced by skin-testing recipients prior to immunization to identify and exclude hypersensitive persons. Wide-scale immunization of livestock, currently not economically feasible, would probably reduce the incidence of human illness.

All patients with confirmed Q fever should be reported promptly to the local public health department for epidemiologic follow-up.

RABIES

method of
RONALD C. JONES, M.D.
Dallas, Texas

Introduction

In the United States in 1975, 2674 confirmed cases of animal rabies were reported. Eighty-four per cent of these cases occur in wildlife and 16 per cent in domestic species. Of the major hosts, skunks account for 46 per cent; bats, 19 per cent; foxes, 10 per cent; raccoons, 7 per cent; cattle, 6 per cent; dogs, 5 per cent; and cats, 4 per cent. Florida and Georgia are the only parts of the United States where a cycle of transmission in raccoons has been established. The most common domestic animals reported to have rabies, in order of frequency, were cattle, dogs, cats, horses and mules, sheep and goats, and swine. Bites of the rodents, including squirrels, rabbits, hamsters, gerbils, guinea pigs, chipmunks, rats, and mice, very rarely require specific rabies prophylaxis.

Of the few cases of human rabies which have been reported in the past 10 years, many have resulted from exposure outside the United States. Foreign-acquired disease represents a significant portion of the rabies problem in this country.

Circumstances of the Bite

Circumstances surrounding the attack frequently furnish vital information as to indication for rabies immune globulin, human (RIG), and duck embryo vaccine (DEV). Most bites by domestic animals are provoked attacks, and with this history rabies vaccine can usually be withheld if the animal appears healthy. Children are frequently bitten while attempting to separate fighting animals or while teasing or accidentally hurting the animal. Bites during attempts to feed or handle an apparently healthy wild or domestic animal should generally be regarded as provoked.

The dog that bites without apparent cause or provocation should be considered rabid. Since the rabies vaccine used in dogs is not 100 per cent effective, the fact that the dog has been vaccinated does not rule out the possibility that it may develop rabies; however, when the animal is properly immunized, the risk of rabies is minimal. Each case of possible exposure must be individualized before a conclusion can be reached concerning antirabies therapy.

Type of Exposure

The likelihood that rabies will result from a bite varies with its extent and location. For convenience in approaching management, two categories of exposure are widely accepted: *Severe*—multiple or deep puncture wounds or any bites on the head, face, neck, hands, or fingers. *Mild*—scratches, lacerations, or single bites on areas of the body other than the head, face, neck, hands, or fingers, or open wounds and abrasions suspected of being contaminated with saliva.

An unprovoked attack is more likely to indicate the animal is rabid.

Management of Biting Animals

Most animal bites of human beings are by dogs and cats, and in most instances it is possible to observe the biting animal for signs of rabies. Domestic animals that bite a person should be captured and observed for symptoms of rabies for 10 days; if no symptoms are present, the animal is assumed to be nonrabid. If the animal dies or is killed, the head should not be damaged but should be sent, refrigerated but not frozen, to a public health laboratory for examination. Clinical signs of rabies in wild animals cannot be interpreted reliably; therefore stray or unwanted dogs, cats, or wild animals should be killed immediately and their heads submitted for rabies examination by fluorescent microscopy. Antirabies prophylaxis is usually indicated unless the attack was provoked. If the brain is negative by fluorescent antibody examination for rabies, one can assume that the saliva contains no virus and the bitten person need not be treated.

Presence of Rabies in Region

It is important to learn from the county health department which animals, both domestic and wild, have been reported to be rabid within the past 10 years in the particular area. This gives the physician some idea of the possibility of a specific animal's transmitting rabies.

Incubation Period

It is generally accepted that the incubation period for rabies in humans ranges from 10 days to 1 year, with the majority of cases occurring within 4 months from the time of exposure. In cases of exposure of the head, neck, or upper extremities, the incubation period may be less than 30 days. Therefore an immediate decision of therapy is important.

Postexposure Prophylaxis

Immediate Local Care. Vigorous local treatment may be as important as specific antirabies therapy by removing the rabies virus if present. Free bleeding from the wound should be encouraged. Local care of an animal bite consists of the following measures:

1. Thorough irrigation and cleansing with copious amounts of saline solution and soap solution.
2. Swabbing with a 1 or 2 per cent solution of benzalkonium chloride (all soap should be removed before application of quaternary ammonium compounds, because soap neutralizes the activity of such compounds).
3. Debridement.
4. Administration of tetanus toxoid.
5. Suturing of the wound. Immediate suturing is not generally advised, as it theoretically may contribute to the development of rabies; however, there is no evidence to suggest that, after appropriate treatment, suturing is detrimental.

Effectiveness of Vaccine in Humans. Duck embryo rabies vaccine (DEV) is a killed vaccine prepared from fixed virus. Comparative effectiveness of vaccines can be judged only by reported failures. During the years 1957 through 1968, there were eight rabies deaths among 225,000 patients treated with DEV, or 1:28, 100.

Experience indicates that rabies vaccine is most effective when given immediately after exposure and when the incubation period exceeds 30 days. Human beings may contract rabies after having received 14 or 21 doses of DEV and antirabies serum or RIG, particularly if the incubation period is less than 30 days.

Passive Immunization. Rabies immune globulin, human (RIG), 20 I.U. per kg. of body weight, is recommended for most exposures classified as severe, for all bites by rabid animals or those suspected of having rabies, for unprovoked bites by wild carnivores and bats, and for nonbite exposure by animals suspected of being rabid. A portion of the RIG should be used to infiltrate the wound, and the remainder administered intramuscularly. When indicated, RIG is used instead of equine serum and should be used regardless of the interval between exposure and treatment. RIG is given on one occasion only and as early as possible following exposure. The use of human immune antirabies globulin should be accompanied by 21 doses of vaccine over a 14 day period, giving two doses per day for the first 7 days (Table 1).

TABLE 1. **Postexposure Antirabies Treatment Guide**

The following recommendations are only a guide. They should be applied in conjunction with knowledge of the animal species involved, circumstances of the bite or other exposure, vaccination status of the animal, and presence of rabies in the region.

SPECIES OF ANIMAL	CONDITION OF ANIMAL AT TIME OF ATTACK	TREATMENT OF EXPOSED HUMAN
Skunk, fox, coyote, raccoon, bat	Regard as rabid	RIG + DEV*
Dog / Cat	Healthy	None†
	Unknown (escaped)	RIG + DEV
	Rabid or suspected rabid	RIG + DEV*
Other	Consider individually (see Circumstances of the Bite in text)	

Definitions: RIG—rabies immune globulin, human; DEV—duck embryo vaccine.

*Discontinue vaccine if fluorescent antibody (FA) tests of animal killed at time of attack are negative.

†Begin RIG + DEV at first sign of rabies in biting dog or cat during holding period (10 days).

RIG, in combination with duck embryo vaccine (DEV), is considered the best postexposure prophylaxis. If RIG is not available, the recommended dose of equine antirabies serum is 40 I.U. per kg. of body weight.

Active Immunization. PRIMARY IMMUNIZATION. At least 23 injections of vaccine in the dose recommended by the manufacturer are administered. These are given subcutaneously in the abdomen, lower back, or lateral aspect of the thighs; rotation of sites is recommended.

For severe exposure, 21 doses of vaccine are recommended. These 21 doses are administered as two doses per day for the first 7 days, and then one dose per day for seven daily doses. This method is preferred to detect the slow responder. A shorter course of vaccine is not recommended, as passive immunity induced by serum may limit response to vaccine. The vaccine may be stopped if the animal is proved nonrabid.

BOOSTER DOSES. Two booster doses, one 10 days and the other 20 days after completion of the primary course, are administered. Two booster doses are particularly important if RIG or antirabies serum was used in the initial therapy. A serum antibody titer is drawn at the time of the second booster dose to detect the poor responder, and these poor responders are given additional boosters until an adequate titer is obtained. If two additional booster doses of vaccine do not result in demonstrable antibody, authorities at the State Health Department or Center for Disease Control (CDC) should be consulted to determine if alternative procedures such as the use of experimental vaccine (human diploid rabies vaccine) should be used.

Factors that contribute to a poor antibody response include administration of steroid during postexposure prophylaxis and use of more than 55 I.U. per kg. of equine antirabies serum (Corey, L., Hattwich, M., et al.: Ann. Intern. Med. *85*:170, 1976).

Reactions to Vaccine and Antiserum. DEV should not be given unless there is a definite indication for its use.

1. Local reactions to DEV occur in approximately two thirds of patients. These consist of erythema, pruritus (13 per cent), pain and tenderness at the site of inoculation, or fever, malaise and myalgia (33 per cent), and either regional or systemic lymphadenopathy.

2. Generalized reactions are occasionally observed, usually after 5 to 8 doses. Generalized urticaria may occur in one third of patients receiving DEV alone and in 50 per cent of patients also receiving equine and antirabies serum. (a) Immediate reactions may occur in an individual sensitive to avian tissue. Epinephrine is helpful in anaphylactic reactions. Should a severe complication develop, and if, in the view of the severity of the exposure, the amount of immunization already obtained is considered inadequate, experimental vaccines should be considered. (b) Neurologic reactions to nerve tissue vaccine constitute the principal hazard to its use. They occur in three main types: peripheral neuritis, the spinal form, and the cerebral form with acute encephalitis. Dorsolumbar paralysis may be either flaccid or spastic. Peripheral neuritis may involve facial, oculomotor, glossopharyngeal, or vagal nerves.

Signs and Symptoms of Clinical Rabies. The first sign of clinical rabies may be paresthesia, tingling, or pain near the site of the bite or in the affected extremity. Symptoms noted with the onset of clinical rabies include headaches, stiff neck, malaise, lethargy, and seizures. Severe pulmonary symptoms include wheezing, hyperventilation, and dyspnea.

Instead of only sedation and symptomatic treatment, it is now recognized that intensive supportive care is indicated. There is multiple organ involvement, including brain, heart, and lungs. Strict attention must be given to the management of airway, pulmonary care, cardiac arrhythmias, and seizures. The patient will require tracheostomy, vigorous suctioning, phenytoin (Dilantin) for seizures, close monitoring of blood gases, electrocardiograms, electroencephalograms, and possibly a ventricular shunt. Nursing care is extremely important.

Pre-exposure Prophylaxis

Unimmunized Persons. The relatively low frequency of generalized reactions to DEV has made it more practical to offer pre-exposure immunization to persons in high-risk groups: veterinarians, animal handlers, certain laboratory workers, and those, especially children, who live in areas of the world where rabies is a constant threat. Others whose vocational or avocational pursuits result in frequent contact with dogs, cats, foxes, skunks, or bats should also be considered for pre-exposure prophylaxis.

A significant number of citizens of this country have been and will probably continue to be exposed to rabies in other countries where rabies in dogs is a major problem. Because rabies in animals is widespread in large areas of Asia, Africa, and Latin America, the Foreign Quarantine Program of the United States Public Health Service has recently advised that pre-exposure immunization against rabies with DEV be suggested for Americans traveling in these countries.

1. Two 1.0 ml. injections of DEV given subcutaneously in the deltoid area 1 month apart are followed by a third dose 6 to 7 months after the

second dose. This series of three injections can be expected to have produced neutralizing antibody in 80 to 90 per cent of vaccinees by 1 month after the third dose.

2. For more rapid immunization, three 1.0 ml. injections of DEV are given at weekly intervals with a booster dose 3 months later. This schedule elicits an antibody response in about 80 per cent of the vaccinees. A neutralizing antibody titer is obtained 1 month after the last injection.

3. Rabies antibody titers can be obtained through the State Health Department. If no antibody is detected, booster doses are given until a response is demonstrated. Persons with continuing exposure should receive 1.0 ml. boosters every 2 years.

Exposure to Persons Previously Immunized. 1. For nonbite exposure to rabies in a person who has demonstrated an antibody response to antirabies vaccination received in the past, a single booster dose of vaccine is recommended.

2. In the case of a severe exposure, five daily doses of vaccine, followed by a booster dose 20 days later, should be given. RIG is not given to persons who have previously demonstrated immune response from vaccination, as it may inhibit a rapid anamnestic response.

3. If it is not known whether an exposed person had antibody, the complete postexposure antirabies treatment is given. Because of variation in vaccine potency and individual response, immunization should not be considered complete until antibody is demonstrated in the patient's serum.

RAT-BITE FEVER

method of
THOMAS R. DEETZ, M.D.
Medina, Ohio

Rat-bite fever is the name given to acute infections caused by either *Streptobacillus moniliformis* or *Spirillum minus*. In the United States, *Str. moniliformis* is by far the more common, whereas in Asia the *Sp. minus* infection predominates. Children comprise the majority of cases; others at risk include the urban poor, farmers, laboratory workers, and those with frequent exposure to rats. A history of a rat bite is not always obtainable, and other animals can transmit the disease.

Infection with *Str. moniliformis*, a pleomorphic microaerophilic gram-negative bacterium, is characterized by an incubation period of 2 to 10 days, with little or no reaction at the bite site. The patient characteristically experiences chills, fever, headaches, upper respiratory symptoms, polyarthralgias, and a morbilliform eruption. Complications include septic arthritis, endocarditis, bronchitis, and pneumonia. *Sp. minus* infections are associated with a longer incubation period of 1 to 5 weeks, followed by a local reaction at the site of inoculation, chills, fever, myalgias, arthralgias, headaches, and a red-brown macular eruption.

Treatment

Prophylactic. The wound should be cleansed with a topical antiseptic solution. The incidence of *Str. moniliformis* infection following rat bites appears to be 10 per cent. As such, prophylactic antibiotic therapy is probably indicated only for those patients with cardiac valvular disease. When indicated, phenoxymethyl penicillin, 250 mg. orally four times a day for 3 days, can be used. Other patients should be alerted as to the symptoms and followed through the incubation period.

General Measures. The symptomatic patients should be admitted to the hospital for the purposes of adequate collection of cultures, parenteral antibiotic therapy, and determination of response to therapy. Antipyretics may be used for symptomatic relief, although the response to antibiotics is usually rapid.

Antibiotics. Penicillin is the drug of choice for either infection. Therapy is begun with at least 15 mg. (24,000 units) per kg. per 24 hours of aqueous crystalline penicillin G intravenously, in six divided doses. Alternatively, procaine penicillin G in doses of 600,000 units intramuscularly every 12 hours appears to be effective. Once the patient becomes afebrile, oral therapy with phenoxymethyl penicillin, 500 mg. in four divided doses daily, can be started. Therapy should be continued for 7 to 10 days. For adult patients allergic to penicillin, either tetracycline or erythromycin, in total daily doses of 1.5 to 2.0 grams given in four divided doses, can be used. For penicillin-allergic children, erythromycin, 30 mg. per kg. per 24 hours in four divided doses, should be used. Prior to the parenteral use of these drugs, the potential toxicities, including local thrombophlebitis and hepatic dysfunction, should be reviewed by the physician.

Complicated Infections. Endocarditis should be treated with aqueous crystalline penicillin G, 12 to 20 million units per 24 hours, in six divided doses intravenously for 4 weeks. Repeat blood cultures, serum bactericidal assays, and antibiotic sensitivities should be used to monitor the effectiveness of therapy as well as to detect the emergence of L-forms. Streptomycin, 500 mg. intramuscularly twice daily, or tetracycline, 500 mg. four times daily intravenously, appears to be effective for alternative use when penicillin is absolutely contraindicated. Pneumonia, septic arthritis, and meningitis should be treated as in other bacterial infections in those sites, with the doses of penicillin for meningitis therapy the same as for bacterial endocarditis.

Clinical Course. The response to appropriate therapy is rapid, usually with marked improvement in 48 hours. With adequate therapy no relapses should occur. The mortality in untreated infections with either organism is approximately 10 per cent. Prevention of rat-bite fever is dependent on public health and sanitation measures designed to reduce the rodent population. Occupational exposures can be reduced by proper methods in animal handling. Human-to-human transmission has never been documented.

RELAPSING FEVER

method of
W. EUGENE SANDERS, Jr., M.D.
Omaha, Nebraska

Relapsing fever is an acute systemic infectious disease caused by any one of several species of spirochetes belonging to the genus Borrelia. It may be referred to as "vagabond fever" in Spain, "fowl nest fever" in China, "bilious typhoid" in Egypt, and "gorgoya" in South America. The disease is transmitted to humans by lice or ticks. Louse-borne infections tend to occur in epidemics, especially in the Middle East, Africa, and South America. They are not seen in this country. Tick-borne infections are endemic to the western United States—Oklahoma, Kansas, Texas, Oregon, Washington, and California. They occur primarily in campers, hunters, and fishermen. Small outbreaks have been reported from the area around Lake Tahoe and in the Grand Canyon National Park. Patients may not recall having been bitten by a tick, because the species of Ornithodoros that transmit the disease in the United States often bite without inducing pain and then leave the host after only a brief period of feeding at night.

Treatment

The plan of management should be designed to achieve the following goals: (1) provision of supportive care in the acute phases of illness, (2) control of systemic symptoms, (3) elimination of the spirochetes with appropriate antimicrobial therapy, (4) amelioration of the Jarisch-Herxheimer reaction that accompanies drug therapy, (5) prevention and treatment of complications of the disease, and (6) protection of the hospital staff.

Supportive Care. Hospitalization, bed rest, and close observation are mandatory because most patients are acutely ill. In addition, peripheral vascular collapse, severe dehydration, mental confusion, delirium, or widespread hemorrhage may appear precipitously, and these must be detected immediately. Proper fluid and electrolyte balance must be maintained. Control of nausea, vomiting, and systemic symptoms may facilitate maintenance of adequate hydration and nutrition.

Systemic Symptoms. Fever need not be controlled unless (1) the temperature exceeds 40°C. (104°F.) or (2) the accompanying hypermetabolic state is poorly tolerated by the patient. Use of tepid water sponges and a fan is probably the safest and most reliable means of lowering body temperature. Hypothermic blankets may also be employed with extreme elevations of temperature. Salicylates should be avoided, at least initially.

Nausea and vomiting may be controlled by administration of antiemetics such as promethazine, 25 mg. intramuscularly every 4 to 6 hours. In acutely ill patients, hydration should be maintained by intravenous administration of appropriate fluid and electrolyte solutions. The state of hydration should be monitored by clinical appearance, pulse, blood pressure, and urinary output. In patients with more severe disease, continuous recording of central venous pressure may be prudent.

Pain may be severe and disabling. However, it usually responds to mild, nonsalicylate analgesics. Acetaminophen, 650 mg. orally every 4 hours, is quite effective in most patients.

Antimicrobial Therapy. Tetracycline is the drug of choice for treatment of relapsing fever. For patients who can tolerate oral medication, 30 mg. of tetracycline hydrochloride per kg. of body weight should be administered daily in four equally divided doses. This represents approximately 2.0 grams daily in an adult of average weight. The drug should be continued for approximately 10 days or for 7 days after the patient becomes afebrile. For patients who are prostrate, nauseated, or vomiting, the drug should be administered intravenously in a dosage of 10 mg. per kg. daily in three equally divided doses at 8 hour intervals. Chloramphenicol is equally effective in similar dosages and routes of administration; however, because of the risk of hematologic toxicity, tetracycline is preferred. A single intramuscular injection of 300,000 units of procaine penicillin G, followed 24 hours later by one dose of 500 mg. of tetracycline orally, has been reported to be effective in treatment of louse-borne relapsing fever. Penicillin is not predictably effective in the tick-borne disease because of the prevalence of resistant strains of Borrelia.

Jarisch-Herxheimer Reaction. The Jarisch-Herxheimer reaction is associated with the sudden intravascular destruction of large numbers of spirochetes by antimicrobial agents. It occurs very frequently, if not always, among patients treated appropriately for relapsing fever. The reaction is characterized by four distinctive phases: prodrome, chill, flush, and defervescence. The prodromal or latent phase lasts approximately 1 hour after administration of the first therapeutic dose of tetracycline or other agents with activity against Borrelia. Onset of the chill phase is heralded by increasing blood pressure, pulse, and cardiac output. Rigors are usually severe and last 10 to 30 minutes. Temperature rises abruptly to approximately 38.3°C. (101°F.); however, increases to 41.1 to 43.3°C. (106 to 110°F.) have been observed in some patients. Apprehension, nausea, and vomiting are common. Confusion, delirium, and, rarely, convulsions may supervene. As the rigors subside and the fever approaches its peak, the flush phase begins. Peripheral vasodilatation and a fall in blood pressure ensue. Cardiac output remains high in most patients, but heart failure may occur in the elderly or in the presence of underlying cardiovascular disease. Within 6 to 7 hours the phase of defervescence or recovery begins. Fever subsides gradually. Most patients are afebrile within 18 hours of onset of the reaction. Subsequent doses of the antimicrobial agent do not aggravate the reaction or precipitate recurrences. Although rare, fatalities tend to occur in association with hypotension and cardiac failure during the flush phase.

Many modifications in the basic therapeutic regimen have been advocated in an attempt to prevent or ameliorate the Jarisch-Herxheimer reactions. Unfortunately, most of these have not withstood the test of time or scientific scrutiny. Some have recommended that initial dosages of antimicrobial agents be reduced "prophylactically"; however, it now appears that if the dosage is lowered sufficiently to prevent the reaction, the drug will have no effect upon the infecting microorganisms. Corticosteroids have been shown not to alter the course of the reaction once it has begun. Use of hydrocortisone prior to the institution of antimicrobial therapy also appears to afford little or no protective effect. Thus treatment should be directed toward the systemic symptoms and complications of the reaction. Again, control of fever by sponging with tepid water is necessary only if the temperature exceeds 40°C. (104°F.) or the hypermetabolic state is tolerated poorly. Hypothermic blankets may be used with extreme hyperpyrexia. Patients should be kept recumbent until afebrile and normotensive. Hydration should be maintained and mild hypotension often may be controlled by judicious use of crystalloid solutions intravenously. Central venous pressure should be monitored if severe hypotension is noted during the flush phase. If cardiac failure ensues, the patient must be given oxygen and digitalized rapidly. Initially, 0.5 to 1.0 mg. of digoxin should be given intravenously. Fortunately, the potentially life-threatening cardiovascular abnormalities usually respond promptly to these simple measures.

Complications. The major complications of relapsing fever are disseminated intravascular coagulation (DIC), rupture of the spleen, and thrombophlebitis. Prolonged prothrombin times, low levels of fibrin degradation products, and petechiae are detected in a substantial number of patients; however, they do not necessarily portend appearance of hemorrhagic phenomena. In the few patients with early signs of DIC and hemorrhage, the following measures should be instituted: (1) antimicrobial therapy appropriate for the infecting microorganism; (2) anticoagulation with heparin, 50 to 100 U.S.P. units per kg. of body weight intravenously at once, followed by 10 to 15 units per kg. per hour, which may be administered by slow intravenous infusion; and (3), if indicated, transfusion with fresh blood, platelet-rich plasma, or platelet concentrates. Heparin should be used with extreme caution in patients with profound thrombocytopenia. Prolonged prothrombin times in the absence of DIC may be reversed by the administration of 10 to 20 mg. of vitamin K intramuscularly.

The acute onset of severe abdominal pain should always suggest the possibility of rupture of the spleen. If the pain is initially localized in the left upper quadrant and then becomes generalized with abdominal rigidity and a fall in blood pressure, the diagnosis is strongly suggested. Splenectomy should be performed immediately.

Prevention

Avoidance or control of the arthropod vectors is necessary for the prevention of relapsing fever in endemic or epidemic areas. Hospitalized patients do not require isolation; however, extreme precautions are necessary to prevent accidental inoculation of hospital personnel with even small quantities of the patient's blood.

RHEUMATIC FEVER

method of
ALLAN GOLDBLATT, M.D.
Boston, Massachusetts

The past 50 years have seen a major decline in the incidence and severity of rheumatic fever. Despite this change in the epidemiology of the disease, it behooves us to be alert to this antigen-antibody reaction and its clinical manifestations. The diagnosis must be established by clinical judgment based on the medical history, abnormal physical findings, and appropriate laboratory studies. The long-term implications and the often unfortunate social stigma associated with this disease require each physician to be secure in his diagnosis before so labeling the patient.

The goals of therapy include eradication of the group A streptococcal infection; suppression of the inflammatory symptoms of the disease; control of the cardiac manifestations, especially congestive heart failure; prevention of recurrences of rheumatic fever; and preservation of the emotional and physical integrity of the patient.

Eradication of the Group A Streptococcal Infection

Prior to initiating antibiotic therapy for the streptococcal infection, a throat culture should be obtained. It must be remembered that the culture may be negative either because of the previous administration of antimicrobial agents or because of the spontaneous disappearance of the streptococci during the latent period between the antecedent pharyngitis and the onset of rheumatic symptoms. The absence of a positive culture does not preclude the diagnosis, and the patient should receive penicillin in amounts to maintain therapeutic levels for 10 days. For older children and adults, a single intramuscular injection of 1.2 million units of long-acting benzathine penicillin G is appropriate. Children under 6 years of age should receive 600,000 units of benzathine penicillin G intramuscularly.

Those patients for whom oral penicillin may be appropriate should receive an initial dose of 500,000 units, to be followed by 250,000 units four times per day for 10 days. Patients sensitive to penicillin may use erythromycin in a dosage of 250 mg. four times per day for 10 days.

Immediately upon completion of the 10 day course of antibiotics, a program of antibiotic prophylaxis should be instituted (see Prevention of Recurrences of Rheumatic Fever).

Suppression of the Inflammatory Symptoms

The drugs most commonly utilized in suppression of the inflammatory symptoms of rheumatic fever are salicylates and steroids. Neither is curative, and there is no convincing evidence that they shorten the course of the illness. In fact, there is no scientific evidence that cardiac damage is prevented or minimized by either salicylates or steroids. Their benefits are palliative in reducing the acute inflammatory manifestations of the disease process. Clinical observation, however, suggests that steroid administration may in fact reduce the acute changes more rapidly in those patients in whom carditis is associated with the rheumatic fever process.

Patients With Polyarthritis Without Carditis

Salicylates are the treatment of choice. If, as has been suggested, administration of aspirin does not affect the long-term sequelae of the disease process, a dosage adequate to relieve the symptoms of arthritis, fever, and malaise is appropriate. A dosage of 50 mg. of aspirin per pound (110 mg. per kg.) of body weight administered in six divided doses per day is usually adequate to accomplish relief of symptoms. Within 48 to 72 hours this can be reduced to four divided doses per day in order to avoid awakening the patient during the night hours. The duration of aspirin therapy is 1 week after all clinical signs have subsided, usually resulting in a 2 to 4 week course of treatment. Blood levels are not routinely necessary except in those instances in which there are either toxic reactions (i.e., vomiting, tinnitus, hyperpnea, or bleeding) or inadequate relief of inflammatory symptoms.

Patients usually tolerate aspirin well, and it may be taken after meals or with milk to reduce gastric acidity.

Patients With Carditis With or Without Congestive Heart Failure

Steroids, specifically prednisone, are the drugs of choice, at least initially. In those patients without overt congestive heart failure, prednisone is administered orally in a dosage ranging from 40 to 80 mg. per day in four divided doses. An adequate response will usually occur in 1 to 2 weeks, at which time the steroid can be tapered rapidly. Aspirin should be instituted several days prior to discontinuation of prednisone and should be continued until all clinical and laboratory signs of rheumatic activity have returned to normal. The average duration of this combined therapy is 6 to 8 weeks. A persistent elevation of the sedimentation rate in the absence of other evidence of rheumatic activity is, in itself, not always an indication to continue therapy.

For those patients with associated congestive heart failure, prednisone will have to be continued for 2 to 4 weeks before substitution with salicylates is begun. The weaning process should be more gradual. The duration of the combined therapy in these patients is usually 12 to 16 weeks.

In addition to the use of suppressive medication, anticongestive measures should be instituted to treat the heart failure. These include bed rest, oxygen, digoxin, fluid and sodium restriction, and diuretics. Dietary potassium intake should be increased in those patients receiving diuretics.

Rebound Phenomena

Occasionally when suppression therapy is reduced or discontinued, clinical or laboratory signs of rheumatic activity will reappear. Mild rebounds usually subside spontaneously within a few days and need no further medication. If, however, the rebound is significant and reinstitution of therapy is required, salicylates should be used rather than steroids.

Bed Rest and Physical Activity

In the past, strict bed rest and restriction of physical activities were considered mandatory for the care of children with rheumatic fever. That need has been questioned more recently, especially in those children without carditis. The patient should be placed at rest during the initial phase of treatment. Within 7 days, with abolition of acute symptoms and laboratory evidence of decreasing inflammatory activity, a program of gradual increase in physical activities may be instituted. If no rebound occurs within 2 weeks, the child may return to school. However, full physical activity, especially competitive sports, should be restricted for approximately 1 month.

For those patients with carditis, bed rest should be prolonged until there is no longer any evidence of progressive cardiac dysfunction. Here the duration of bed rest may last for 6 to 8 weeks, rarely longer. During this period of convalescence, a coordinated program of recreational therapy and school instruction should be carried out in an effort to minimize the often associated emotional and intellectual trauma. Physical activities should be introduced gradually dependent upon the patient's cardiac reserve. The majority of these children will recover completely and be able to lead unrestricted lives.

Chorea

Sydenham's chorea (St. Vitus' dance) is an uncommon but major manifestation of rheumatic fever. It may occur alone or be accompanied by other rheumatic fever signs and symptoms. The condition is self-limiting, with recovery of the neuromuscular and emotional abnormalities usually within 2 to 3 months. Treatment is therefore directed primarily at the physical discomfort and psychologic stress imposed upon the patient and his family. Emotional support to the patient and family is extremely important. Rest and a protective environment are beneficial, and removal from school is usually required. In the more severe cases of chorea, precautions must be taken to avoid injury to the patient. Sedatives, tranquilizers, and steroids have all been tried with varying results. No one drug has been shown consistently to be more effective than another. Every patient with chorea should receive a 10 day course of penicillin, followed by institution of an antibiotic prophylactic regimen to prevent subsequent streptococcal infections.

Prevention of Recurrences of Rheumatic Fever

The ability to prevent recurrences of rheumatic fever is based upon appropriate antibiotic prophylaxis to eradicate repeated streptococcal infections in those patients at risk. Prophylactic therapy should be initiated immediately following treatment for the primary streptococcal infection. The drug of choice is penicillin. The most consistently reliable results are obtained with the intramuscular administration of 1.2 million units of benzathine penicillin G every 4 weeks. For those who prefer oral medication, and most do, success will depend upon patient understanding and cooperation. Oral penicillin in the form of buffered penicillin G, 250,000 units twice a day, is adequate for prevention of recurrences. In those patients with a penicillin sensitivity, either oral sulfadiazine, 1 gram once a day for patients over 60 pounds and 0.5 gram per day for those under 60 pounds, *or* erythromycin, 250 mg. twice a day, should be utilized.

When streptococcal infections occur despite the prophylactic regimen, they should be treated promptly and vigorously (see Eradication of Group A Streptococcal Infection).

The duration of antibiotic prophylaxis is a subject of continuing discussion. All agree that those patients with cardiac involvement should continue their prophylaxis indefinitely. The same can be said of those with chorea because of the significant incidence of associated rheumatic mitral valve disease appearing later in life. Patients with rheumatic fever and no cardiac involvement or chorea should be treated with antibiotic prophylaxis through those years of greatest risk—namely, the first 2 decades of life. In the absence of recurrences, prophylaxis may be discontinued but reinstated during periods of increased risk (e.g., for those in military service or boarding schools, mothers of young children, and school teachers).

Special antibiotic prophylaxis to prevent bacterial endocarditis is recommended for those rheumatic patients with cardiac involvement. Transitory bacteremia may result from dental manipulation, oral surgical procedures, tonsillectomy, adenoidectomy, bronchoscopy, incision and drainage of abscesses, dilatation and curettage, and instrumentation of the genitourinary tract. Thus, appropriate antibiotic coverage must be instituted at the time of those procedures to decrease, if not completely prevent, the occurrence of bacterial endocarditis.

The drug of choice is penicillin. Procaine penicillin G, 600,000 units, plus 600,000 units of crystalline penicillin G intramuscularly 1 to 2 hours before the procedure and once daily for 2 days following the procedure, is recommended. If oral penicillin is to be used, at least 250 mg. of alpha-phenoxymethyl penicillin (penicillin V) four times each day should be administered. This should commence preferably the day before and continue for 2 days after the procedure, for a total of 4 days.

For those patients with a sensitivity to penicillin, erythromycin should be used in a dose of 250 mg. four times a day by mouth for older children and adults. Small children's dosage is 20 mg. per pound not to exceed 1 gram per day. Duration of treatment is again 4 days.

Preservation of the Emotional and Physical Integrity of the Patient

Rheumatic fever is a chronic disease prone to recurrences, and thus ongoing education of the natural history of the disease and emotional support are the cornerstones for fulfillment of the patient's potential as a total person. Society in its uncertainty will often place physical and intellectual limitations on these patients, and it is our duty to work wherever possible for the removal of such restrictions.

ROCKY MOUNTAIN SPOTTED FEVER

method of
DANIEL J. SEXTON, M.D.,
Oklahoma City, Oklahoma,
and JOHN D. HAMILTON, M.D.,
Durham, North Carolina

Introduction

Rocky Mountain spotted fever (RMSF) is caused by *Rickettsia rickettsii.* Both the vector and principal reservoir of RMSF are hard-shelled (Ixodid) ticks. The most important tick vectors in the United States are the Rocky Mountain wood tick *(Dermacentor andersoni)*, the American dog tick *(D. variabilis)*, the Lone Star tick *(Amblyomma americanum)*, and the rabbit tick *(Haemaphysalis leporispalustris)*. The rabbit tick does not bite man but is important in the cycling of rickettsial infection among wild animals.

Although RMSF may affect all age groups, more than 75 per cent of cases in the United States occur in people less than 20 years old. Documented cases of RMSF have been reported from 45 of the 50 states, although reported incidence of the disease is highest in the southeastern United States. Because of the ease and rapidity of modern travel facilities, physicians in areas not considered highly endemic for RMSF must be alert for cases of disease "imported" from endemic areas. Risk of infection is higher in rural dwellers and outdoor enthusiasts such as hikers and campers. The disease occurs predominantly during the spring and summer months.

It is axiomatic that the diagnosis of RMSF must be made solely upon clinical grounds. Antimicrobial therapy should never be withheld while awaiting laboratory results. Between one third and one fourth of RMSF cases have no history of tick bite. Thus the absence of a history of tick bite should not in itself dissuade the physician from suspecting RMSF and instituting therapy.

Treatment

The only two drugs effective in the treatment of RMSF are chloramphenicol and tetracycline. The former is potentially toxic to the bone marrow, and the latter can cause dental staining in children and is potentially hepatotoxic in high dosages, especially if given to pregnant women. Both drugs are rickettsiostatic and are equally effective.

Chloramphenicol may be administered to adults either orally or intravenously at 50 mg. per kg. per day in four divided doses. The recommended dose for children is 50 to 100 mg. per kg. per day. It should not be given intramuscularly, as absorption is erratic and unpredictable by this route. Frequent checks of the platelet count, hematocrit, and white blood cell count are mandatory in patients receiving chloramphenicol. Two types of bone marrow toxicity can occur in chloramphenicol-treated patients: one is common, dose-related, and reversible; the other is very rare, is idiosyncratic, and results in usually irreversible aplastic anemia. Because of its potential for hematopoietic toxicity, chloramphenicol is best reserved for patients with severe disease, especially when clinical differentiation between RMSF and meningococcemia is difficult. Total daily doses should not exceed 4 grams. The recommended oral dose of tetracycline for both adults and children is 25 to 40 mg. per kg. every day (see manufacturer's official directive before administration to children under 8 years of age). If tetracycline is given intravenously, daily dosages should not exceed 2 grams in adults. The intravenous dose of tetracycline for children is 10 mg. per kg. every 12 hours. All tetracyclines are excreted by the kidneys; thus patients with impaired renal function may have to be given lower doses. If given orally, tetracycline should be taken between meals and concomitant administration of milk and antacids avoided. Tetracycline is not recommended in pregnant women. No antimicrobial therapy other than tetracycline or chloramphenicol has been shown to be effective in RMSF. Sulfonamides have been shown to have a deleterious effect on the course of the illness. Antimicrobial therapy is usually effective within 48 to 96 hours of starting treatment and should be continued for 3 to 5 days after the patient has become afebrile.

Patients infected with *R. rickettsii* may develop a number of serious complications, including renal failure, hyponatremia and other electrolyte imbalances, hypotension with vascular collapse, stupor, and coma. These complications primarily arise as a result of a generalized Rickettsia-induced vasculitis.

Careful monitoring of blood pressure, pulse, venous pressure, and other parameters of intravascular volume as well as urine output is important. Intravascular volume deficits should be corrected, using either saline or colloid-containing solutions. Rickettsia-induced myocarditis may occur; thus careful observation for signs and symptoms of congestive heart failure is required during administration of fluids.

Hyponatremia may be a prominent laboratory abnormality in patients with RMSF. If there is evidence of volume and salt depletion such as postural hypotension, poor skin turgor, or dry mucous membranes, intravenous therapy with isotonic saline solution is indicated. The syndrome of inappropriate antidiuretic hormone secretion (SIADH) has been reported with *R. rickettsii* infection. If SIADH is suspected, appropriate laboratory tests, including measurements of urine and serum osmolality, should be made. If SIADH is present, water should be restricted.

Thrombocytopenia is relatively common in hospitalized patients with RMSF, and disseminated intravascular coagulation (DIC) may occur in some patients. The efficacy of heparin in Rickettsia-induced DIC has not been demonstrated. DIC in this illness is probably best treated by combating its underlying cause (rickettsemia) with either tetracycline or chloramphenicol.

Central nervous system derangements, ranging from confusion to seizures or coma, are fairly common in RMSF. Lumbar puncture often shows a mild pleocytosis and a slightly elevated spinal fluid protein concentration. These findings may lead to diagnostic confusion with enteroviral or meningococcal disease.

Secondary bacterial infections such as pneumonia or urinary tract infections may occur in patients with RMSF and should be appropriately evaluated and treated.

A variety of supportive measures, such as oxygen, mechanical ventilation, and intensive nursing care, may be necessary in patients with RMSF. *R. rickettsii* infection can produce illnesses ranging from mild to fatal, and the physician must individualize treatment accordingly.

Prevention

Spotted fever group rickettsiae circulate in nature in a tick-animal cycle completely independent of infection in man; therefore traditional vector control methods such as those used in malaria are neither effective nor practical. Persons exposed to ticks and tick-infested areas should regularly inspect their bodies and remove attached ticks promptly and carefully. A period of time must pass from attachment until ticks are capable of transmitting their infection to humans; thus the prompt removal of infected ticks may prevent human disease. Care should be used in removing attached ticks. Disease transmission by either airborne or percutaneous routes may result when ticks are squashed or crushed. Recommended methods of tick removal include use of a tweezers or use of paper or cloth to protect the fingers.

Dogs may develop an asymptomatic or subclinical rickettsemia and thus infect all simultaneously feeding ticks. Care should be taken when removing ticks from pet dogs. Pet dogs in endemic areas should be treated with tick repellants.

The currently available RMSF vaccine is of only limited benefit. Although the incubation period is prolonged in human subjects given RMSF vaccine and then exposed to *R. rickettsii*, a number of deaths from RMSF have been reported in people who received multiple doses of the vaccine. RMSF vaccine is currently recommended only for persons with laboratory exposure to spotted fever group rickettsiae. The vaccine is prepared from embryonated egg yolk sacs and is contraindicated in persons allergic to eggs. The vaccine is given weekly for 3 weeks at a dose of 1.0 ml. subcutaneously. A booster dose is recommended 6 to 12 months after the initial immunization series.

Since a well established cycle of rickettsial infection exists in nature, reduction in morbidity and mortality caused by RMSF is best accomplished by prompt recognition and treatment of human disease. Both physicians and patients living in endemic areas should be periodically reminded of the clinical and epidemiologic features of the disease.

RUBELLA

method of
WILLIAM McBRIDE, M.D., F.R.C.O.G.
Sydney, Australia

Rubella (German measles) is a mild virus infection which usually affects the majority of children during their schoolage years. School children are the principal spreaders of this infection, which is normally endemic but at times reaches epidemic proportions. It is at this time that there is the greatest risk to women of child-bearing age. The infection spreads by the respiratory route.

In adults the clinical manifestations are mild; the host develops lymphadenopathy, particularly of the postauricular and suboccipital nodes. This may be the only sign for several days until coryza, malaise, low grade fever, and conjunctival irritation begin. The rubella rash is generally maculopapular and erythematous, and begins on the face 16 to 18 days after viral inoculation. The rash continues for 2 to 3 days. More serious but less frequent complications are thrombocytopenia, arthralgia, arthritis, and encephalitis.

The treatment required for the infection itself is 2 to 3 days of rest and perhaps aspirin for the discomfort and fever.

Prevention of Rubella

Gregg's 1941 discovery of the rubella embryopathy syndrome makes it imperative that pregnant women be protected against rubella; however, should the infection occur, the correct diagnosis is essential so that the possible sequelae of the infection can be explained to both the woman and her husband.

Although most children are infected with rubella, recent surveys have shown that approximately 25 per cent of women of child-bearing age have no immunity when tested by hemagglutination-inhibition (HI) test. Girls at the age of puberty should be immunized against rubella, using attenuated rubella virus vaccine, and the vaccination should be repeated each 10 years of their reproductive life.

The majority of women plan their families, and they should be encouraged to have an HI test to determine their immunity to rubella before they wish to become pregnant. If they do not have immunity as shown by a satisfactory antibody titer, they should be advised to be vaccinated for rubella at least 3 months before they plan to conceive.

The physician supervising the pregnancy of any woman should have an HI test performed at the time of her first consultation. The majority of pregnant women will exhibit immunity to rubella. HI-positive patients should be told that they are immune to rubella and asked if they know when they had the rubella infection. If they state that the infection was recent, there may be the possibility of fetal infection. However, if they have no immunity, they should be warned to avoid contact with any child or the parent of any child known to have rubella for the first 16 weeks of their pregnancy. They should also be instructed on the dietary needs of pregnancy.

Should a woman present with a history of a probable rubella infection or exposure to rubella in early pregnancy, she should have her HI antibody titer determined and the test repeated 3 weeks later. If there is a significant rise in titer level, she should have her serum tested to determine whether specific rubella IgM antibody is present.

If the serologic tests indicate infection with rubella within the first 16 weeks of pregnancy, the seriousness of the situation must be fully explained to both parents. The spread of the virus to the placenta resulting in infection of the fetus has been estimated as up to 50 per cent in the first gestational month, 30 per cent during the second month, and approximately 10 per cent in the third month and 5 per cent in the fourth month. Rubella embryopathy consists of congenital heart disease, hearing loss, cataract or glaucoma, psychomotor retardation, and neonatal purpura, either singly or in combination. Because of the high risk of serious deformity, the parents should be strongly advised that the pregnancy be terminated; however, the ultimate decision must be made by both parents. The decision of the parents to terminate the pregnancy or allow it to proceed must be given by them in writing so that it can be filed with the mother's records.

The use of gamma globulin by intramuscular injection immediately after exposure to rubella may prevent or alter the clinical signs of rubella. Its efficacy in reducing fetal risk, however, has not been determined with control series. Since affected infants have been born to mothers who receive gamma globulin immediately after exposure, dependence on gamma globulin to prevent fetal abnormalities is ill advised.

Treatment of Congenital Rubella

It is important that the newborn with congenital rubella be isolated in order to prevent the spread of the virus throughout the nursery and the obstetric service. The infant will excrete the virus for up to 2 years.

There is no specific treatment for the rubella-affected child apart from recognition of its disabilities. Defective development of the eye, ear, and heart remain as the classic triad of teratogenesis. The eye and heart defects are usually easily diagnosed, but sensorineural hearing loss, the common defect of congenital rubella, poses the greatest diagnostic difficulties. The problems of assessing auditory acuity in infants is obvious. Reliable testing, especially of unilateral or mild hearing loss, must often be delayed until late childhood. Probably half the children infected in utero will have unilateral or bilateral hearing deficits. The deficit may be mild or severe and may represent the only rubella defect, especially when the infection occurs after the first trimester. As anticipated, defective or absent speech may result from severe hearing loss.

Psychomotor development should be assessed periodically; accurate assessment can be made at the age of 5 years, and follow-up studies should be repeated throughout the school years.

There is little that can be done for the loss of vision, but the heart lesions are often amenable to surgery.

SALMONELLOSIS (OTHER THAN TYPHOID FEVER)

method of
ROBERT H. RUBIN, M.D.
Boston, Massachusetts

An estimated 2 million persons are infected with salmonellae in the United States each year, with more than 99 per cent of these infections being due to one of the more than 1500 nontyphoidal Salmonella serotypes (species). The major source for such infections is infected foodstuffs, particularly inadequately cooked poultry, egg and dairy products, beef, and pork. However, especially within families, among young children, and within institutions for the mentally ill and retarded, person-to-person spread may amplify the epidemiologic effects of a particular exposure.

The clinical effects of human salmonellosis may be divided into four syndromes: *gastroenteritis, bacteremia* with and without *focal* extraintestinal infection, *enteric fever,* and the asymptomatic *carrier state.* Each of these clinical syndromes requires a different diagnostic and therapeutic approach.

Antibiotic therapy of Salmonella infection, *in those patients in whom it is indicated,* is complicated by two factors: an incomplete correlation between in vitro antibiotic sensitivity testing and the clinical efficacy of a drug, and a high rate of plasmid-mediated antibiotic resistance among many Salmonella serotypes. Practically, only four drugs are ever clinically effective against salmonellae: chloramphenicol, ampicillin and its congener amoxicillin, and trimethoprim-sulfamethoxazole. Antibiotic sensitivity testing in vitro is essential to ensure sensitivity of the particular infecting strain to the drug chosen from among these four, as *resistance to a drug in vitro is correlated with clinical failure*. In vitro sensitivity to drugs other than these four, however, is meaningless clinically, as other antibiotics currently available are of no value in the treatment of any form of Salmonella infection. It should be noted that chloramphenicol, although quite effective given orally or intravenously, should never be administered intramuscularly, as presently available preparations are poorly absorbed from this site.

Gastroenteritis

Gastroenteritis caused by nontyphoidal salmonellae is the most common clinically recognized Salmonella syndrome, making up approximately two thirds of all diagnosed Salmonella infections, and accounting for 10 to 15 per cent of all instances of acute food poisoning in the United States each year. Clinical disease usually begins some 8 to 48 hours after ingestion of the organisms, with nausea and vomiting, followed within a few hours by periumbilical and right lower quadrant abdominal cramps, diarrhea, and fever. In healthy persons, the incidence of transient bacteremia during the course of Salmonella gastroenteritis is estimated at 1 to 4 per cent; in patients with profound ileus, underlying inflammatory bowel disease, lymphoproliferative disorders and perhaps other immunosuppressed states, and hemoglobinopathies, the rate of bacteremia is probably significantly higher.

Management. 1. The patient is placed at bed rest, with careful monitoring of vital signs, intake and output, and body weight.

2. Fluid and electrolyte imbalances are corrected. These losses may be from vomiting (resulting in a hypokalemic, hypochloremic alkalosis) or from the diarrhea (resulting in a hypokalemic, hyperchloremic acidosis and moderate protein depletion). Oral correction of volume and electrolyte deficits may often be accomplished with glucose-rich electrolyte solutions, as glucose-facilitated sodium and water absorption by the gut is unaffected in Salmonella gastroenteritis. In many patients, however, intravenous replenishment, as directed by measurements of renal function, serum electrolyte pattern, and arterial pH, will correct deficits more rapidly. In patients with prolonged diarrhea, albumin supplementation is often necessary.

3. Symptomatic relief of nausea and vomiting may be accomplished with prochlorperazine (Compazine) or trimethobenzamide hydrochloride (Tigan). Suggested doses for adults are as follows: prochlorperazine, 5 to 10 mg. orally or intramuscularly every 4 to 6 hours, or a 25 mg. rectal suppository every 12 hours; trimethobenzamide

hydrochloride, 200 to 250 mg. intramuscularly, orally, or rectally every 6 to 8 hours. In children suggested doses are as follows: prochlorperazine, 2.5 mg. orally, rectally, or intramuscularly every 8 to 12 hours, or trimethobenzamide hydrochloride, 100 to 200 mg. orally or rectally every 6 to 8 hours.

4. *Severe* diarrhea may be alleviated with deodorized tincture of opium (DTO), 4 to 8 drops in water every 3 to 6 hours, or diphenoxylate dihydrochloride with atropine (Lomotil), 1 to 2 tablets every 6 hours, as needed. However, care must be taken not to suppress gut hypermotility too much, as this is an important host defense preventing salmonellal overgrowth and a higher rate of invasion and bacteremia. In practice, antidiarrheal medications are administered not to abolish diarrhea and cramps completely, but just to relieve major discomfort.

5. Enteric precautions are instituted while the patient is excreting salmonellae, with an emphasis on careful hand washing, disposal of fecally contaminated materials, and removal of the patient from contact with other patients or with foodhandling facilities. Three consecutive negative stool cultures, taken at weekly intervals, are a minimum requirement before a patient may be safely taken off these precautions.

6. Antibiotic therapy is *contraindicated* in the treatment of Salmonella gastroenteritis in the vast majority of patients, as all antibiotics tried thus far have failed to alter the rate of clinical recovery and have increased the incidence and duration of intestinal carriage of the organism. However, in a few selected patients this adverse effect is overbalance by the potential risks of bacteremia because of other medical problems simultaneously present. Antibiotic therapy to minimize the risks of bacteremia and metastatic infection should be considered for the following population groups: (1) neonates and the elderly; (2) those with lymphoproliferative disease; (3) those with abnormalities of the cardiovascular system such as prostheses, aneurysms or other vascular abnormalities, or rheumatic or congenital heart disease; (4) those with foreign bodies in their bones or joints; and (5) those with hemolytic anemias, particularly sickle cell disease. Antibiotic regimens similar to those used for bacteremia (see below) are used for periods of 10 to 14 days in these patient groups.

Bacteremia and Focal Infection

Although a transient bacteremia may occur as an insignificant concomitant of otherwise uncomplicated gastroenteritis, in patients with defects in host immunity—particularly lymphoproliferative disorders—and in patients who develop metastatic infection such bacteremias assume great importance. Sustained bacteremia, in which more than 50 per cent of multiple blood cultures are positive, usually connotes infection of the cardiovascular system, either at diseased endothelial surfaces of larger arteries or on damaged heart valves. As a result of either a sustained or a transient bacteremia, metastatic spread of infection to other sites may occur, particularly to the skeletal system, genitourinary system, the meninges, or any tissue in the body previously damaged by trauma or another disease process.

Management. 1. Supportive measures similar to those in patients with gastroenteritis are begun when indicated.

2. The level of bacteremia should be documented. In patients without defects in host defense in whom sustained bacteremia is demonstrated, careful evaluation of the cardiovascular system for evidence of focal disease by means of physical examination, ultrasonic, radionuclide, and phonocardiographic techniques is recommended. In patients over the age of 45 with sustained bacteremia, angiography is indicated to rule out the presence of an infected aneurysm, particularly of the aortoiliac system.

3. The definition of an aneurysm in a patient with sustained bacteremia mandates surgical replacement as well as prolonged antibiotic therapy. The demonstration of an infected heart valve will usually require surgical replacement as well as antibiotic treatment, although an initial trial of medical management alone is not unreasonable.

4. Antibiotic therapy of sustained bacteremia should always be parenteral and prolonged—4 to 6 weeks if no surgery is performed, and for at least 4 weeks following surgery. If the organism is susceptible, the bactericidal drug ampicillin in six divided doses of 10 to 12 grams per day (in children, doses of 200 to 400 mg. per kg. per day) should be employed, with close monitoring of the serum bactericidal level. The serum should be bactericidal at a dilution of $\geq$1:8 for the invading organism just before the next dose is due. In patients allergic to penicillins or with an ampicillin-resistant organism, intravenous therapy with chloramphenicol sodium succinate, 50 to 75 mg. per kg. per day in four divided doses, with close hematologic monitoring, should be employed. Oral therapy with trimethoprim-sulfamethoxazole, 4 to 8 tablets two to three times per day, should be used only as second-line therapy for this form of Salmonella infection; it is best suited for patients with resistant organisms or those who cannot tolerate ampicillin or chloramphenicol. (This use of trimethoprim-sulfamethoxazole is not listed in the manufacturer's official directive.)

5. The management of unsustained bacteremia and extraintestinal nonvascular infection includes 2 weeks of the antibiotics listed above and surgical drainage when indicated.

Enteric Fevers

The enteric fevers are characterized by prolonged fevers, a sustained Salmonella bacteremia without endothelial or endocardial involvement, hyperplasia and hypertrophy of the reticuloendothelial system, multiorgan dysfunction secondary to metastatic infection, the formation and deposition of immune complexes, and the effects of as yet undefined toxicity. Other than *S. typhi* (see pp. 73 to 76), the Salmonella serotypes most often responsible for enteric fever are *S. paratyphi, S. schottmülleri,* and *S. hirschfeldii*.

Management. 1. Supportive care, public health measures, and management of diarrhea (if present) are undertaken, as outlined under Gastroenteritis.

2. Antibiotic therapy should be continued for 10 to 15 days after the temperature has returned to normal. Intravenous therapy should be employed in the severely ill patient, with oral therapy being restricted to patients in geographic areas where intravenous therapy is not possible, to patients with mild disease, and to patients requiring trimethoprim-sulfamethoxazole* therapy because of resistant organisms or intolerance for the other drugs. Drug regimens recommended, in order of preference, are as follows: (a) Chloramphenicol, 50 mg. per kg. per day in divided doses every 6 hours, with close hematologic monitoring. (b) Ampicillin, 150 to 200 mg. per kg. per day in divided doses every 4 hours. (c) Trimethoprim-sulfamethoxazole,* 160 to 320 mg. and 800 to 1600 mg., respectively (2 to 4 tablets), two or three times per day.

3. The use of corticosteroids in this setting remains controversial, and is not recommended by the author.

Chronic Carrier State

The chronic carrier state may develop after symptomatic or asymptomatic infection of the gastrointestinal tract. Following symptomatic gastroenteritis, bacteria can be recovered from the stool in approximately 90 per cent of patients after 2, 40 per cent after 4, 15 per cent after 9, 10 per cent after 10, and 5 per cent after 20 weeks. No treatment is indicated other than the observation of strict enteric precautions until at least three negative stool cultures, taken at weekly intervals, are documented. Patients are considered "chronic Salmonella carriers" if they continue to excrete organisms more than 1 year after initial infection. This occurs in 0.2 to 0.6 per cent of patients infected with nontyphoidal salmonellae. The site of carriage is the biliary tract, with many of the patients having anatomic disease of the biliary tree, particularly stones, at least partially explaining their inability to clear these organisms.

*This use of trimethoprim-sulfamethoxazole is not listed in the manufacturer's official directive.

Management. 1. Noninvasive attempts to eliminate the chronic carrier state are probably indicated in all patients. The use of surgical as well as antibiotic therapy should be restricted to those with occupational needs (e.g., foodhandlers, medical personnel), those with poor personal hygiene, or those with other compelling public health reasons for undergoing such therapy.

2. In patients without biliary tract disease, and with ampicillin-sensitive organisms, treatment with ampicillin or amoxicillin in doses of 500 to 1000 mg. four times a day for 4 to 6 weeks will be successful 80 per cent of the time. In patients with penicillin allergy or ampicillin-resistant isolates, treatment with trimethoprim-sulfamethoxazole* in a dose of 2 tablets twice daily for a similar period of time may be tried.

3. In patients with chronic gallbladder disease, cholecystectomy under coverage with "bacteremic doses" of ampicillin or chloramphenicol (see above) for 10 to 14 days should be carried out.

4. In patients with chronic gallbladder disease in whom surgery is contraindicated, an attempt at a medical cure can be made with 4 to 6 grams of amoxicillin (this use of amoxicillin is not listed in the manufacturer's official directive), plus 2 grams of probenecid (Benemid), in four divided doses per day for 4 to 6 weeks, or intravenous ampicillin, 1 to 2 grams every 4 hours for 3 to 4 weeks.

*This use of trimethoprim-sulfamethoxazole is not listed in the manufacturer's official directive.

TETANUS

method of
WILLIAM R. SANDUSKY, M.D.
Charlottesville, Virginia

Tetanus is characterized by local or general spastic contractions of voluntary muscles resulting from the action of an exotoxin produced by the anaerobic spore-bearing gram-positive bacillus, *Clostridium tetani.* The disease can be prevented by the proper use of tetanus toxoid; specific antiserum will neutralize toxin; but after this extremely potent exotoxin, tetanospasmin, becomes fixed in the central nervous system, it cannot be neutralized by any presently available method.

Treatment

Once the clinical signs of tetanus become established, the opportunity for specific therapy is lost and one must rely upon supportive treatment until the effects of the toxin have worn off. Until this occurs, the management of an established case of tetanus requires (1) maintenance of adequate pulmonary ventilation; (2) control or prevention of muscle spasm; (3) neutralization of toxin which has not yet established an irreversible union with cells of the central nervous system; (4) elimination of the distributing focus of the exotoxin; (5) maintenance of fluid balance and nutrition; (6) prevention of secondary infections and other complications; and (7) active immunization.

Maintenance of Adequate Pulmonary Ventilation. Laryngeal spasm and respiratory compromise caused by spasm of the intercostal muscles or diaphragm or by involvement of the central respiratory center pose a threat to pulmonary ventilation throughout the course of the disease.

The patient must have the uninterrupted attention of an attendant competent to recognize the requirement for emergency artificial ventilation, as well as the need for urgent reinforcement of sedation. At the University of Virginia Medical Center, it is the practice to place patients with tetanus in a single room in an intensive care unit where there is ready for immediate use equipment for endotracheal intubation, tracheostomy, suction, oxygen administration, and artificial respiration, and where there are available, literally on a moment's notice, personnel capable of performing emergency artificial ventilation.

Removal of secretions from the respiratory passages by suction, preferably oropharyngeal suction, must be carried out with gentleness, using sterile-gloved hands and sterile catheters. Oxygen should be administered by mask when indicated, but it will not compensate for mechanically obstructed air passages caused by secretions or spasm. It must be remembered that its use may obscure the early signs and symptoms of mechanical obstruction and that precise measure of the adequacy of ventilation can be obtained only by the analysis of arterial blood gases and for pH. Facilities for these determinations should be available around the clock. There is no necessity to employ tracheostomy routinely; rather, its use should be reserved for patients selected because of laryngeal spasm, because copious or tenacious secretions cannot be removed easily by oropharyngeal suction, or because of therapeutic total paralysis.

Control or Prevention of Muscle Spasm. Measures must be taken to prevent or at least to minimize the painful and life-threatening muscular seizures which characterize tetanus. The patient should be kept in quiet surroundings, all external stimuli reduced to a minimum, and the necessary care and handling done with extreme gentleness.

Drugs for sedation and muscle relaxation have a very important place in the management of tetanus. The aim of therapy with these agents is to diminish the input of sensory stimuli and to prevent or diminish muscular spasm without making the patient unconscious and without abolishing his pharyngeal and cough reflexes.

Although a variety of drugs have been used for basal sedation, pentobarbital (Nembutal) is as effective, safe, and satisfactory as any. It may be used in doses ranging from 50 to 250 mg. for adults (proportionately less for children) given every 3 or 4 hours. The amount of this drug and the frequency of its administration must be regulated on the basis of individual response. Pentobarbital may be given by any of the usual routes of administration, with the choice being determined individually, depending upon whether the patient can swallow, upon the degree to which injections are disturbing, and upon the extent to which the patient is being maintained parenterally. When the need arises for temporary reinforcement of the basal sedation, an ultrashort-acting agent such as thiopental sodium (Pentothal) is employed intravenously, but it should be used as a very dilute solution (0.5 to 1.0 per cent). An indwelling intravenous catheter should be maintained throughout treatment for the purpose of administering the reinforcing agent. It should be connected to a three-way stopcock, which in turn is connected to a syringe containing the reinforcing drug. The common complications attending the use of an indwelling intravenous catheter—sepsis and thrombosis—can be minimized by aseptic and antiseptic technique during insertion and maintenance of intravenous equipment, change of all tubing and solutions proximal to the catheter needle hub every 24 hours, and change of the needle or catheter every 48 hours.

It is frequently necessary to employ one of the skeletal muscle relaxants to supplement sedation. Methocarbamol (Robaxin) selectively depresses the spinal cord internuncial neurons and produces relaxation of voluntary muscles without causing loss of consciousness, and is recommended for this purpose. It may be given by mouth or parenterally in an amount to be varied according to individual response, which is judged by the tonus of the neck or abdominal muscles. Intravenous increments of 1 to 3 grams every 6 hours or oral doses totaling 24 grams per day may be given with safety to adults; proportionately smaller doses should be used for children.

Diazepam (Valium), a drug having relaxant, anticonvulsant, and tranquilizing properties, has received favorable reception in the management of tetanus. It may be used as the sole agent of sedation and muscle relaxation, or it may be employed in combination with other drugs. The dosage depends upon the severity of symptoms and should be adjusted to the individual situation. It may be given orally, intramuscularly, or intravenously. The recommended adult dose ranges from 2 to 10 mg. two to four times daily, but quantities far in excess of this amount (e.g., 10 mg. per kg. per day) have been given without untoward results. When used intravenously, diazepam should be administered in small increments (e.g., 2 mg.) to titrate its effect. Moreover, it is irritating to veins, and when given by this route it is preferable to inject it into a freely running intravenous drip so as to dilute it.

When drugs such as those mentioned above do not control tetanic spasms and convulsions without causing deep coma, these muscular seizures may be prevented by total paralysis with curare, succinylcholine or other curare-like drugs, and artificial ventilation. This form of management is reserved, of course, for the severe cases, and theoretically it might be considered the ideal management, but its practical application requires specialized facilities and highly trained personnel and is not without considerable risk.

During the course of treatment it is frequently necessary to perform disturbing or even painful procedures which may precipitate spasms or convulsions; therefore such stimuli should be anticipated, and sedation should be reinforced prior to performance of the procedures.

Neutralization of Toxin Which Has Not Yet Established an Irreversible Union with Cells of the Central Nervous System. The signs and symptoms of tetanus do not become manifest until there is an interaction between the toxin and the cells of the central nervous system. Once this interaction has occurred, it cannot be reversed by antitoxin, a fact which dictates one of the aims of therapy—namely, neutralization of toxin by antitoxin from a human source before fixation occurs. Clinicians experienced in the treatment of tetanus do not agree on an appropriate therapeutic dose of tetanus immune globulin (human), TIG(H). Recommendations range from 3000 to 10,000 units, and a recent retrospective analysis from the Center for Disease Control suggests that 500 units may be as effective as a larger amount. In this perplexing setting in which authoritative opinion varies, and with recognition that antitoxin marketed in this country from human sources is relatively free from dose-related adverse reactions, it is prudent to err on the side of too much rather than too little. Therefore I recommend TIG(H) as a single dose in the amount of 5000 units. This must be given intramuscularly, as there is no preparation suitable for intravenous use. Intrathecal administration of antitoxin is not recommended. Sensitivity testing prior to administration of human globulin is not necessary. *Equine or bovine antitoxin should not be administered unless antitoxin from a human source is unavailable;* however, if its use becomes necessary, sensitivity testing is mandatory.

Elimination of the Distributing Focus of the Exotoxin. Once clinical tetanus is present, wound management should be directed at the elimination of the site where the microorganisms are multiplying and producing toxin. When a wound of entry can be identified, it should be incised widely, or, if compatible with anatomic considerations, it should be excised. It is obligatory that all foreign material and necrotic tissue be removed, that vascular integrity be restored, and that the wound be left open. Although antibacterial drugs do not neutralize tetanus toxin, there is evidence in the experimental animal that penicillin and oxytetracycline (Terramycin) may destroy or prevent multiplication of *Cl. tetani;* for this reason, one or the other of these antibiotics should be used as an adjunct to surgical wound management in the patient with established tetanus. It is recommended that wound surgery be performed after the administration of antitoxin.

Maintenance of Fluid Balance and Nutrition. It is essential that patients with tetanus be given an adequate intake of fluids, calories, proteins, and vitamins and be kept in proper electrolyte balance. Many patients can be managed so that they tolerate liquids or soft foods by mouth, but for others this is impossible owing to trismus, glottic spasm, or dysphagia. When such is the case, one has the alternatives of maintenance by vein, using total parenteral alimentation, or by gastrostomy.

Prevention of Secondary Infections and Other Complications. The measures pertaining to maintenance of pulmonary ventilation also are invaluable in the prevention of respiratory tract infection. Humidification to prevent inspissation of secretions, removal by coughing and oropharyngeal suction, and the use of patient-position to prevent their accumulation are of inestimable value. The patient must not be allowed to lie on his back but rather on one side or the other, and his position should be changed frequently. It is doubtful that antimicrobial agents offer additional help in the prevention of infection.

Spasm of the vesical sphincter, which occurs frequently, produces urinary retention and, in addition to discomfort, may lead to infection. If the patient is unable to void, intermittent catheterization or continuous bladder drainage by a closed system will be required. Anal sphincter spasm may abet fecal impaction, but this should pose no serious problem if the clinician is alert to the possibility. Also, one must be prepared to prevent or deal with injury which may arise during a convulsive seizure, such as a fracture or a bitten tongue. The latter is not infrequent and dictates the time-honored custom of having a padded tongue blade as part of the bedside equipment.

Isolation is not required from the standpoint of contagion, but protection of the patient against nosocomial infection is essential. The importance of avoiding the complications of the indwelling intravenous catheter, the necessity for a closed system of urinary bladder drainage, and the use of sterile-gloved hands and sterile catheters for respiratory tract suction are re-emphasized.

Active Immunization. It is not generally appreciated that tetanus does not confer immunity upon its victims. Therefore a program of active immunization must be made a part of the management of every patient who is being treated for established tetanus.

Prophylaxis

Any wound may be contaminated with either the spores or the vegetative forms of *Cl. tetani.* These organisms find an environment favorable for growth and toxin production in traumatized tissue. Prophylaxis of tetanus starts with prompt and adequate surgical care of the wound or trauma—i.e., the excision of dead tissue, the removal of foreign material, and thorough mechanical cleansing. The objective is to eliminate or reduce the number of microorganisms and the material on which they live and to ensure the vascular integrity of the part, so that the entire wound is in contact with well oxygenated arterial blood. In addition to careful wound surgery, the patient should receive specific protection against tetanus as indicated below.

There are several acceptable methods for active immunization against tetanus. In 1972, the Public Health Services Advisory Committee on Immunization Practices published the following immunization program:

For children 2 months through 6 years: the manufacturer's recommended dose of diphtheria and tetanus toxoids and pertussis vaccine (DTP) intramuscularly on four occasions—i.e., three doses at 4 to 6 week intervals, with a fourth dose approximately 1 year after the third injection.

For school children and adults: a series of three doses of tetanus and diphtheria toxoids, adult type (Td) given intramuscularly, with the second dose 4 to 6 weeks after the first, and the third dose 6 months to 1 year after the second dose.

Both preparations DTP and Td contain comparable amounts of tetanus toxoid, but the diphtheria component in Td is 15 to 20 per cent of that contained in the standard DTP preparation.

A person who has received active immunization with toxoid develops a measurable level of circulating tetanus antitoxin generally believed to be adequate for protection and keeps it for an indeterminate period, surely for at least 1 year, probably much longer. Beyond this period of active immunity, the person possesses the ability to recall a protective level of antitoxin when toxoid is administered again. Although it is not known how long he retains this ability, one report indicates that a protective titer may be recalled after a lapse of 25 years. The United States Public Health Service Advisory Committee on Immunization Practices recommends a booster every 10 years. This interval appears to be well within the limits of safety.

Temporary and passive immunologic protection can be obtained by administering preformed antitoxin from a human, equine, or bovine source. *Whenever human immune globulin is available, there is no excuse for subjecting the patient to the risks of foreign protein.* Two hundred and fifty (250) units of tetanus immune globulin (human), TIG(H), administered intramuscularly, gives an immediate level of antitoxin that is within the usual protective range and that lasts beyond the usual incubation period of *Cl. tetani.* Sensitivity testing is unnecessary when human immune globulin is used; but should it be necessary to administer antitoxin from a source other than human, sensitivity testing is mandatory. Whenever prophylactic antitoxin is given to an unimmunized person, it is highly desirable to start active immunization with toxoid at the same time; however, the two must not be given in the same syringe or into the same injection site.

Some of the antibacterial agents, notably penicillin and oxytetracycline (Terramycin), are effective in protecting against experimentally induced tetanus. Although their value in the prophylaxis of human tetanus has not been established, an antibiotic in addition to wound surgery should be used as an adjunct in the management of the "tetanus-prone" wound. It is important to remember that the mode of action of the antibiotic differs from that of antitoxin. The latter has no effect on the microorganism but neutralizes the exotoxin, whereas the antibiotic acts on the microorganism but has no effect on exotoxin.

Sometimes tetanus occurs after trivial or even unrecognized injury. Nonetheless, certain wounds provide a more favorable environment for the growth of anaerobic microorganisms than do others. Such wounds may be recognized by their extent, particularly their depth, by the amount of devascularization of tissue, by the presence of foreign material, or by the fact that adequate surgical care has been delayed. These criteria are not infallible, but they do provide useful guides for planning prophylaxis. When there is doubt, *even slight doubt,* the safe option is to assume that the wound in question is "tetanus prone."

A variety of schema for tetanus prophylaxis has been advanced by authoritative sources, including the American College of Surgeons Committee on Trauma and the United States Public Health Services Advisory Committee on Immunization Practices. Differences no doubt stem from doubt concerning the immune status of a person who has received only one or two injections of toxoid and from uncertainty as to how long a fully immunized person retains the ability to recall a protective titer. I follow a prophylactic schema more conservative than that recommended by the United States Public Health Services Advisory Committee on Immunization Practices, and one which adheres very closely to that of the Committee on Trauma, differing from the latter chiefly in the manner of presentation.

In addition to wound surgery, which is the sine qua non of tetanus prophylaxis, certain immunologic measures are recommended for specific situations, as follows:

Immunization completed previously; last booster within 1 year: No additional toxoid required.

Immunization completed within the previous 10 years; no subsequent booster: Give 0.5 ml. Td.*

Immunization completed more than 10 years previously; last booster within the previous 10 years: Give 0.5 ml. Td.*

Immunization completed more than 10 years previously; no booster within the previous 10 years; wound minor and relatively clean, treated promptly and adequately: Give 0.5 ml. Td.*

Immunization completed more than 10 years previously; no booster within the previous 5 years; wound other than minor and relatively clean and/or not treated promptly: Give 0.5 ml. Td* and 250 units TIG(H);† if wound is classified as "tetanus-prone," give 500 units.

No history or record of immunization; wound minor and very clean; wound surgery prompt and adequate: Begin immunization using 0.5 ml. Td;* give patient a written record of immunization and schedule appointments for completion of immunization.

No history or record of immunization; wound other than minor and very clean or not treated promptly or adequately: Give 250 units of TIG(H)† (if wound is classified as "tetanus-prone," give 500 units); begin immunization.

*Td=Tetanus and diphtheria toxoid, adult type.
†TIG(H)=Tetanus immune globulin (human).
When Td and TIG(H) are given concurrently, a separate syringe and needle and separate sites should be used.

TRICHINELLOSIS

(Trichinosis)

method of
THOMAS C. JONES, M.D.
New York, New York

Trichinellosis is a disease caused by migration through tissue of larvae released by the adult nematode *Trichinella spiralis*, which resides in the small intestine of the infected patient. During the migration and muscle encystment stages of the infection, the patient demonstrates a spectrum of signs and symptoms from mild muscle discomfort to severe myalgias, fever, and edema. A fatal outcome is unusual, but it may result from marked tissue damage to the myocardium, lung, and central nervous system during the period of larval migration.

Pathogenesis and Clinical Presentation

Encysted viable larvae of *T. spiralis* ingested in contaminated improperly cooked meats excyst by action of the gastric juices and mature in 48 to 72 hours into male and female adults in the upper small intestine; they copulate, the male dies, and the fertilized female burrows into mucosa and begins releasing larvae into vessels in the submucosa. This continues for several weeks before the adult worm is rejected from the intestine. The symptoms are determined by the amount of larval deposition during this period and the degree of the host's allergic reaction to them. Ultimately the larvae find appropriate skeletal muscle cells in which to enter and develop into infectious larvae capable of continuing the cycle when the muscle is ingested by another carnivore.

Epidemiology

During the past few years the incidence of trichinellosis in the United States has increased, associated with increased contamination of beef with pork products (recently said to be 10 per cent of ground beef), a decreased awareness of the danger of contaminated pork in improperly cooked (rare) sausage or meatballs, and sporadic epidemics after ingestion of bear and walrus meat. The disease occurs in the more industrialized societies because of increased potential for massive swine contamination by refeeding pork byproducts. It has been estimated that 0.13 per cent of swine going to market in the United States are infected, allowing a potential infection of 40 million humans. Cooking of pork products and prolonged freezing reduce the likely number of infections per year to 200,000. Only one in 1000 of these are reported. The rest either are misdiagnosed as other mild diseases or, in the case of light infections, are completely asymptomatic, detected only by antibody responses. Trichinella larvae are killed by thorough heating of meat to at least 58°C. or by freezing at −15°C. for 20 days.

Treatment

In mild cases symptomatic therapy with antipyretics, anti-inflammatory agents, and rest is adequate. The duration of symptoms may be several weeks even in these mild cases. If symptoms are more marked, the drug of choice is thiabendazole (Mintezol). This drug is of value because it has three actions of benefit in modifying the illness: (1) it is active against the adult worm in the intestinal tract, and thus it can potentially shorten the period of larval deposition; (2) it has some activity against the larvae in muscle; and (3) it has immunosuppressive actions which will contribute to reducing the fever and inflammatory response. The drug is given in a dose of 25 mg. per kg. twice daily until improvement is seen (usually several days). Then the dose can be reduced or given intermittently while the clinical response is observed. (The recommended maximal daily dosage in the manufacturer's official directive is 3 grams.) Thiabendazole may cause gastrointestinal symptoms (nausea, vomiting, and diarrhea), allergic reactions such as skin rash, and central nervous system effects such as restlessness. Rarely effects on liver and kidney function have been observed. An odor like that of asparagus occurs in the urine in patients receiving thiabendazole.

Corticosteroids can be used in those with severe involvement of the central nervous system or myocardium during the initial larval migratory stage. Thiabendazole should be given in addition to the corticosteroids, because adult worm persistence in the gastrointestinal tract may be prolonged in the presence of corticosteroids alone. A dose of 60 mg. of methylprednisolone per day or 12 mg. of dexamethasone per day should be used. Careful monitoring of myocardial and central nervous system function is important in severely ill patients, and appropriate supportive therapy should be provided as needed.

TULAREMIA

method of
CHARLES N. OSTER, M.D.
Frederick, Maryland

Tularemia, caused by *Francisella tularensis,* is primarily an enzootic disease which affects a wide variety of animals throughout North America, Europe, and Asia. Man usually becomes infected by contact with blood or tissues of diseased animals (most commonly, the cottontail rabbit), or via the bite of a blood-sucking vector (ticks, deer flies, or mosquitoes). In addition the disease may be acquired by eating undercooked, infected meat, drinking contaminated water, or inhaling infectious aerosols. The clinical presentation of tularemia in man is highly variable, ranging from subclinical through ulceroglandular or oculoglandular, glandular, gastrointestinal, pneumonic, and systemic illness. With the three last-named presentations, tularemia is difficult to identify, particularly when there are no local lesions. Such cases are often misdiagnosed and ineffectively treated. The case-fatality rate in untreated tularemia ranges from 6 to 7 per cent and decreases to less than 1 per cent with effective therapy. Therefore the attending physician must be alert to the possibility of tularemia and initiate therapy promptly in all suspected cases.

The drug of choice for the treatment of tularemia is streptomycin, 0.5 to 1.0 gram intramuscularly every 12 hours for 5 to 10 days. Patients so treated will respond dramatically with defervescence and symptomatic improvement within 24 to 48 hours. The dosage in children is 20 to 30 mg. per kg. per day and in newborns 10 to 20 mg. per kg. per day, given in two divided doses. The dosage of streptomycin must be reduced in patients with renal insufficiency; blood levels of the antibiotic must be monitored to guide therapy. Complications of streptomycin therapy include vestibular and auditory toxicity, nephrotoxicity, neuromuscular blockade, and rare hypersensitivity reactions. Other aminoglycoside antibiotics (such as gentamicin and kanamycin) are probably also effective treatment for tularemia, but they offer no advantage over streptomycin; experience with these drugs in the treatment of tularemia is limited.

Tetracycline is an effective alternative to streptomycin therapy for tularemia. It has the advantage of oral administration, but suffers the disadvantage that the disease may relapse after cessation of therapy, especially if treatment is initiated within the first week of illness or is not maintained for a full 14 days. Such a relapse is not due to acquired resistance of *F. tularensis,* and will respond promptly to retreatment with tetracycline. The recommended dosage of tetracycline is 1 to 2 grams per day in adults and 25 to 40 mg. per kg. per day in children, given in four divided doses. The use of tetracycline is contraindicated in pregnant females, children under 8 years of age, patients with known hypersensitivity to tetracyclines, patients with renal insufficiency or hepatic insufficiency, and patients taking tolbutamide, phenytoin sodium, oral anticoagulants, or phenformin. Complications of tetracycline therapy include gastrointestinal irritation, pseudomembranous and staphylococcal enterocolitis, superinfections with Candida or antibiotic-resistant gram-negative bacteria, photosensitivity, nephrotoxicity, and hepatotoxicity (particularly in patients who are pregnant or who have renal insufficiency and are receiving intravenous tetracycline).

Chloramphenicol, 50 mg. per kg. per day in four divided doses for 14 days, given orally or intravenously, may also be used for therapy of tularemia, but this drug offers no advantage over tetracycline. Dosage must be reduced in newborns (25 mg. per kg. per day), and in patients with liver disease; blood levels must be monitored in these patients to guide therapy. Dosage need not be altered in patients with renal insufficiency. Complications of chloramphenicol include dose-related marrow depression and, rarely, aplastic anemia.

Supportive care of the patient with tularemia will depend on the nature and the severity of the illness. The ulcer of the ulceroglandular form of the disease may heal slowly, even with effective antibiotic treatment, and requires only local care until healed. Involved lymph nodes usually require no special care; occasionally aspiration is necessary if rupture seems imminent. If a node ruptures and the patient develops a draining sinus, surgery may be required to remove the sinus tract and involved node.

Person-to-person spread of tularemia is not known to occur; therefore the infected patient presents no special hazard to attending personnel. However, tularemia may be acquired by accidental self-inoculation or by inhalation of aerosols of infectious material generated in the clinical laboratory. Therefore clinical and laboratory personnel must be alerted to the possibility of tularemia so that they may take proper precautions when handling specimens from the patient, and they must be reminded to immediately report any definite or suspected accidental exposure.

Postexposure prophylaxis of tularemia with streptomycin is effective in preventing disease. However, tetracycline and chloramphenicol are *not* effective prophylactic agents, as they only delay onset of the disease. An effective live attenuated vaccine is available for administration to persons at high risk; this vaccine is classified as an investigational new drug and is available only through the Biological Products Division, Immunobiologics Branch, Center for Disease Control, Atlanta, Ga. 30333. The older, inactivated vaccines offer little protection.

TYPHOID FEVER

method of
F. J. WRIGHT, M.A., M.D., F.R.C.P., F.R.C.P.E., D.T.M.&H.
Edinburgh, Scotland

Before the introduction, in 1948, of the antibiotic chloramphenicol, the treatment of typhoid fever was the supreme test of skilled nursing by supporting the patient until the body's defenses overcame the infection. The use of chloramphenicol, and, more recently, other antibiotics has greatly reduced the mortality rate, but it is still important to remember that it is the patient who is to be treated rather than the infection.

If the strain of *Salmonella typhi* affecting the patient is not of high virulence, or if the patient has some previously acquired immunity and the diagnosis is made early, the general condition of the patient is likely to be satisfactory and no special supportive treatment will be required other than bed rest and, to protect others, barrier nursing. In more severe infections and in later cases, correction of dehydration and electrolyte imbalance is necessary and skilled nursing desirable. The mouth should be kept clean; when it is available and the patient is cooperative, the chewing of pieces of pineapple, without swallowing the fiber, is for this purpose old fashioned but both effective and refreshing. The patient's skin needs constant attention. Headache may be temporarily relieved by paracetamol (acetaminophen) and the discomfort of fever by the gentle perspiration which follows sponging with hot water. For the fastidious, eau de cologne may be added to the water. If hyperpyrexia is present, tepid or cold sponging is indicated. No extravagant limitation of food intake is desirable. A nutritious diet acceptable to the patient should be maintained, avoiding those solids which are indigestible, especially those which tend to produce flatulence. It has been found in the Sudan (Abu-Asha et al., 1976) that patients with dimorphic, megaloblastic, and hemolytic anemia suffer severely. It may therefore be helpful to administer additional folate, particularly if the patient is malnourished. Aperients are best avoided; but if the patient is constipated, as is frequently the case in early stages, a simple soap and water enema gently administered on alternate days gives relief without tiring the patient. Ample fluids are required to counteract loss by perspiration and, at a later stage, perhaps by diarrhea also. Special measures to combat specific complications are indicated below.

Chemotherapy

As soon as the diagnosis is made, chemotherapy should accompany the general measures indicated above. Chloramphenicol and trimethoprim-sulfamethoxazole (co-trimoxazole) appear to be comparable in both efficacy and cost.

Chloramphenicol. Great experience has been gained with this drug, and a good response can be expected unless there is reason to believe that the infecting *S. typhi* may be resistant to chloramphenicol—as, for example, if *S. typhi* isolated from an earlier case in the same outbreak has been shown to be resistant. Outbreaks of typhoid fever are most common in developing countries with defective hygiene where economy in prescribing has to be exercised. The risk of aplastic anemia developing is very small; but if the patient's red cells are deficient in glucose-6-phosphate dehydrogenase, the danger of hemolysis from sensitivity to chloramphenicol makes the choice of an alternative antibiotic desirable.

If the patient is not vomiting, chloramphenicol is administered orally in a dose of 50 mg. per kg. of body weight daily in three or four divided doses. If oral treatment is not possible, chloramphenicol sodium succinate should be administered intravenously. If the parenteral preparation is not available, the drug may be administered through a nasogastric tube. The fever usually subsides in 3 to 5 days.

Corticosteroids. Only in the extremely toxic patient is the concomitant initial use of corticosteroids to be considered. Such a patient may benefit from hydrocortisone, 100 mg. (or an equivalent corticosteroid) intravenously every 8 hours for a few doses, gradually reduced as soon as there is improvement, over 3 days.

Duration of Chloramphenicol Therapy. If chloramphenicol is reduced in dosage or stopped prematurely, there is increased likelihood of a relapse. The optimal length of treatment is, in general, 14 to 21 days, but on economic grounds the dose may be reduced or the drug stopped after the patient has been afebrile for a week without much loss of efficiency. However, a few patients may relapse 1 or 2 weeks after stopping treatment prematurely and require a further course of treatment, the organisms usually still being susceptible to chloramphenicol. Unlike relapses which formerly sometimes followed spontaneous subsidence of fever, the relapses following inadequate chloramphenicol may be just as severe as the first attack and the patient still liable to suffer a serious complication. Chloramphenicol does not reduce the rate of subsequent permanent excretors of *S. typhi;* and as far more patients survive, the number of carriers tends to increase. However, if the locality was previously endemic for typhoid fever, this will make little difference to the community unless the carrier is employed in association with water supplies or the preparation of food (see below).

Co-trimoxazole (Bactrim, Septra). The standard tablet of trimethoprim-sulfamethoxazole (co-trimoxazole) contains 80 mg. of trimethoprim and 400 mg. of sulfamethoxazole; a double strength tablet is also available. Most or perhaps all strains of *S. typhi* so far isolated, including those showing sulfonamide resistance, are sensitive to co-trimoxazole. As it is probably as effective as chloramphenicol, although perhaps a little slower in action, some authorities now regard co-trimoxazole as the drug of choice. There are reports of its failure in individual patients followed by a satisfactory response on changing to chloramphenicol, and vice versa. It is contraindicated if the patient is allergic to sulfonamides. Three divided doses are given orally to a maximum of 480 mg. of trimethoprim and 2400 mg. of sulfamethoxazole daily and continued as recommended for chloramphenicol. (The use of trimethoprim-sulfamethoxazole for typhoid fever is investigational in the United States of America.) A parenteral preparation is now available for intravenous use (not available in the United States of America) if the patient is vomiting. The components of co-trimoxazole are excreted in adequate concentrations in the bile, and there is good evidence that the number of subsequent carriers is thereby reduced, although some relapses and some permanent excretors of *S. typhi* are recorded to have followed the use of co-trimoxazole.

Penicillin-Related Antibiotics. AMPICILLIN. This antibiotic was the first alternative drug to chloramphenicol, but it is less effective and more expensive than co-trimoxazole. It has been superseded by other antibiotics.

AMOXICILLIN. Amoxicillin is given orally in a dose of 100 mg. per kg. of body weight daily for 14 to 21 days; but for adults, 4 grams daily in four divided doses has proved to be satisfactory. (These doses may be higher than those recommended by the manufacturer.) Scragg (1976), in Durban, compared amoxicillin with chloramphenicol in the treatment of children and demonstrated the superiority of amoxicillin. With this antibiotic the clinical response was quicker, relapses were fewer, and there were no subsequent permanent carriers. However, strains of *S. typhi* resistant to ampicillin are equally resistant to amoxicillin, and no parenteral preparation of amoxicillin is available at the time of writing.

MECILLINAM. Mecillinam (not available in the United States of America) is closely related to the penicillins but has a different chemical structure and mode of action. It is very active against *S. typhi* and has been shown to be highly active also against ampicillin-resistant strains of *Escherichia coli*, except those which produce large quantities of β-lactamase. Mecillinam must be administered parenterally, either intravenously or intramuscularly. A derivative ester, pivmecillinam, is effective when given orally. Limited experience with this antibiotic (Clarke et al., 1976) indicated that it is effective in the majority of cases. As it is excreted in a satisfactory concentration in the bile, it is likely to prevent the occurrence of subsequent fecal excretors of *S. typhi*. Mecillinam is given in a dose of 30 to 40 mg. per kg. of body weight daily in four divided doses for 14 days. Initially the drug is administered parenterally, but after a clinical response is evident it is continued orally as pivmecillinam.

Complications

Meningitis. If the clinical signs suggest meningitis, lumbar puncture is indicated. The removal of cerebrospinal fluid will tend to relieve the symptoms, and examination of the fluid will indicate the nature of the meningeal reaction. No change in chemotherapy is necessary because of meningitis, other than the use of maximal doses of the antibiotic either parenterally or orally.

Intestinal Hemorrhage. A large hemorrhage into the lumen of the bowel from an eroded vessel in a Peyer patch leads to sudden collapse, with a fall of temperature, a rapid bounding pulse, perspiration, and air hunger. The essential of treatment is replacement of blood by a transfusion of compatible blood. If none is available, plasma or other intravenous fluids may be employed. Intramuscular morphine, 15 mg., together with 0.3 mg. of hyoscine, is indicated, particularly if the patient is restless.

Intestinal Perforation. Erosion of Peyer's patches in the ileum usually proceeds slowly with thrombosis of the small blood vessels in the wall of the intestine. When ulceration approaches the peritoneal covering, inflammatory lymph tends to seal a threatening hole and prevent escape of intestinal contents. When this process partly fails, an inflammatory mass develops adherent to neighboring intestine or mesentery. Exceptionally, gas and intestinal fluid contents escape abruptly into the peritoneal cavity, giving rise to the clinical signs of a perforation. Unless the patient is very toxic, severe pain is experienced and shock is evident, there being a sudden fall in temperature and a rapid thready pulse. Before the introduction of antibiotics, the results of surgery were bad, the best surgical results following the completion of the aforementioned process by minimal surgery after resuscitating the patient. Most surgeons who have the assistance of a skilled anesthetist or anesthesiologist now advocate surgery and correction of fluid and electrolyte deficiencies. Opinion is divided as to whether to delay operating for some hours until resuscitation has improved the patient's condition or to proceed without delay. It is salutary to recognize that some patients, deemed unfit for surgery, have survived under conservative medical treatment and that the mortality rate following surgery is still 15 to 30 per cent. Clear indications for surgery are evidence of an abrupt perforation in a patient who is not very toxic and the availability of a skilled surgeon and anesthetist. Contraindications include doubt as to the diagnosis or the ability of the patient to survive the operation. In all patients parenteral chemotherapy must be instituted, or continued, combined with general restorative measures. At laparotomy simple closure of the perforation (occasionally multiple) is generally preferable to more heroic measures, as the tissues are friable. Thorough peritoneal lavage is recommended. Postoperative correction of anemia is important.

Continued Fever. This may be due to the relative inaccessibility of the organisms in multiple small abscesses in the kidney or elsewhere, or to *S. typhi* having become resistant to the antibiotic being used. If *S. typhi* is being recovered from the patient, its sensitivity to antibiotics should be redetermined and, if indicated, a change of antibiotic made.

Periostitis and Osteomyelitis. When this complication occurs in early convalescence, a further course of antibiotic will usually lead to cure. In late cases the diagnosis is usually made after surgical drainage of a localized abscess, and the patient should be treated as if he were a carrier (see below).

Disseminated Intravascular Coagulation. This complication, reported particularly in children, is characterized clinically by shock, purpura, and hemorrhages. Urgent treatment is required, including the transfusion of blood or plasma, correction of electrolyte deficiencies, and administration of corticosteroids. There is no unanimity as to the use of heparin; if it is used, the prothrombin time must be closely monitored (Setiadhaima, 1973).

Carriers

Convalescent carriers may cease spontaneously to excrete *S. typhi*, but further doses of an antibiotic to which the organism is sensitive are indicated. Chronic carriers may be either fecal or urinary excretors of *S. typhi.* Fecal excretion is commonly associated with the presence of gallstones. In the past there was little hope of cure unless cholecystectomy was performed, and even then cure could not be guaranteed. If the gallstones have produced attacks of colic, cholecystectomy is clearly indicated; if not, the importance of ending the carrier state, having regard to the patient's intelligence, hygienic habits, and occupation, has to be weighed against the risks of an operation not clearly required for the patient's own well-being. In the Far East, the fluke *Clonorchis sinensis* is often found in large numbers in the biliary tract of carriers. Treatment of this fluke is not very satisfactory but consists of hexachloroparaxylol, 300 mg. per kg. of body weight daily for 3 days (investigational), or chloroquine, 600 mg. base daily (for an adult) for 14 days (investigational for this use). In countries where *Schistosoma haematobium* is endemic, this fluke is commonly found in urinary carriers and must be eliminated before there will be any prospect of success in eradicating *S. typhi*. *Schistosoma mansoni* is also suspected of maintaining the carrier state. A number of different treatments for schistosomiasis are in vogue; niridazole, 25 mg. per kg. of body weight orally daily for 7 days (available from CDC, Atlanta, Ga.), is usually effective but is contraindicated in disease of the liver.

In all patients an attempt should be made to eradicate *S. typhi* by the use of a modern antibiotic. A course of co-trimoxazole or pivmecillinam, as recommended for the initial illness, appears to hold out a good prospect of success. Subsequent repeated cultures of stools and urine are required. If the infection persists, the carrier must be barred from employment in the catering industry or in connection with water supplies and must be urged to practice meticulous hygiene, washing hands thoroughly after micturition and defecation.

Prophylaxis

Second attacks of typhoid fever rarely occur. Vaccines do not give perfect protection, but they reduce the likelihood of acquiring the infection. An intradermal dose of 0.1 ml. of the phenol-preserved heat-killed culture, followed by further doses after 4 to 6 weeks and again 6 to 12 months later, gives good protection. An acetone-killed vaccine administered subcutaneously is more potent but produces greater side effects.

The provision of safe water, clean food, and general good hygienic living, together with the control of carriers, are the main safeguards against typhoid fever.

Paratyphoid A and B

In general these infections may be treated in the same way as typhoid fever. Complications are rather less frequent. There is at present no vaccine of proved efficacy against *S. paratyphi B*; but in areas where *S. paratyphi A* occurs, notably the Balkans and India, the inclusion of this organism in the vaccine is indicated.

TYPHUS FEVER

method of
CHARLES L. WISSEMAN, Jr., M.D.
Baltimore, Maryland

Epidemic or louse-borne typhus *(Rickettsia prowazekii),* murine or flea-borne typhus *(R. mooseri),* and scrub or mite-borne typhus *(R. tsutsugamushi)* are distinct disease entities with independent geographic distributions and ecologies. Brill-Zinsser disease is recrudescence of epidemic typhus. *R. canada,* serologically related to *R. prowazekii* and *R. mooseri,* was originally isolated from ticks and may cause a spotted fever–like disease of man. Although precise information is not available about the pathophysiology of all these rickettsioses, all show similar basic lesions of the small blood vessels and display generally similar physiologic derangements, with some variation in severity and detail. Chloramphenicol and tetracycline drugs inhibit the growth of, but probably do not kill, all these obligate intracellular parasites. General principles of patient management rest upon (1) adequate antibiotic therapy to control the rickettsial agent until immunity develops, (2) such supportive measures as are required to prevent or correct physiologic abnormalities, and (3) prevention or treatment of secondary bacterial infections and other complications.

Therapy

Because louse-borne typhus tends to be the most severe of the diseases considered here, because epidemics usually occur where medical resources are primitive, and because recent experience in an epidemic under primitive conditions has led to important improvements and simplification of treatment, its management is described in detail. The other rickettsioses are managed according to the same principles which apply to comparable degrees of clinical severity, unless otherwise indicated.

Clinical Classification of Disease Severity. The patient is evaluated immediately on admission according to duration and general severity of disease, neurologic involvement (coma, delirium, lucid but unable to swallow), physiologic derangements (hypotension, shock, renal impairment, clotting derangement), state of nutrition and hydration, and presence or absence of complications. For practical management purposes, patients can then be classified as (1) mild or severe, (2) cooperative or uncooperative, and (3) uncomplicated or complicated. Even moderately severe but uncomplicated typhus in a cooperative patient is usually simple to manage with orally administered antibiotics, fluids, and nutriments. The uncooperative patient or the patient with complications requires added measures. Management is greatly simplified if the uncooperative patient can be brought quickly to the stage at which oral medications and fluids are possible (see below).

Antirickettsial Therapy. Prompt adequate antirickettsial therapy is the single most important factor in shortening the disease, reducing mortality, and speeding convalescence. In cooperative uncomplicated cases this may be the only medication required.

The tetracycline series of antibiotics and chloramphenicol are the drugs of choice. Penicillin, streptomycin, and sulfonamides are clinically ineffective. Practical concentrations of a wide range of aminoglycosides, semi-synthetic penicillins, and cephalosporins do not inhibit *R. prowazekii* growth in vitro in cell cultures. *Note: Except for chloramphenicol,* none of the drugs (ampicillin, amoxicillin, trimethoprim-sulfamethoxazole) used for the treatment of typhoid fever, a serious differential diagnostic problem in some areas, give clinical and/or in vitro evidence of effectiveness in typhus fever. Both chloramphenicol and tetracycline cause defervescence within 36 to 72 hours in uncomplicated epidemic or murine typhus and often sooner in scrub typhus. Presumed *R. canada* infections have responded to chloramphenicol and tetracycline. Oral medications containing aluminum hydroxide interfere with gastrointestinal absorption of tetracycline drugs. Because of rare instances of bone marrow depression or aplastic anemia following chloramphenicol, tetracyclines are usually given unless other factors strongly favor chloramphenicol. The usual precautions are observed in administering the antimicrobial, e.g., adjustment of dosage in patients with renal or hepatic dysfunction of rickettsial or independent origin, changes in microbial flora and superinfections, staining of developing teeth.

1. *Doxycycline,* a tetracycline derivative available for oral and intravenous use, is the treatment of choice for louse-borne typhus. This drug is rapidly and efficiently absorbed from the intestinal tract, even with food, and produces prolonged, effective blood and tissue levels with small doses. A *single* 100 mg. dose by mouth cures almost all adults with epidemic typhus without further antibiotic treatment. A *single* 200 mg. dose, even when given on the first day of disease, regularly cures this disease. A *single* 50 mg. dose regularly cures children up to the age of at least 10 or 12 years. We have had no experience in the treatment of infants with typhus with this drug. In the rare instance of "escape" from drug effect, 2 to 4 days after the first dose, another single 100 mg. dose suffices to effect a cure.

There is some suggestion that a single 200 mg. oral dose of doxycycline will cure *scrub typhus,* with occasional relapses. However, very limited experience with *murine typhus* suggests that a single dose is not adequate, and daily doses should be given as indicated below. *Note:* Rocky Mountain spotted fever is *not* cured by a *single* dose and requires daily administration of doxycycline.

2. *Tetracycline HCl* is given orally in a total daily dose of 25 to 50 mg. per kg. body weight. Two grams per day in divided doses at 4 to 6 or even 12 hour intervals usually suffices for adult patients.

3. *Chloramphenicol* is given orally in amounts of 50 to 75 mg. per. kg. body weight per day for adults and children, respectively, usually in divided doses at 4 to 6 or even 12 hour intervals. *Caution:* Doses larger than 25 mg. per kg. body weight may be severely toxic for *newborn infants.*

The uncooperative patient (delirious, comatose, unable to swallow) or the patient who is vomiting requires special management. When parenteral preparations are unavailable or intravenous drip therapy is impractical, oral preparations suspended in fluid may be administered by stomach tube. Intravenous tetracycline is given in doses of 0.5 to 1.0 gram every 6 to 12 hours to a maximum of 2 grams per day for adults. Though likely to cause pain or local reaction, up to 0.5 gram of the intramuscular tetracycline preparation may be given every 12 hours for a day or two until the patient can take the oral preparation. Chloramphenicol succinate, appropriately diluted, is given intravenously to adults in a dose of 1.0 gram every 8 to 12 hours. Parenteral therapy should be replaced with oral therapy as soon as the patient can swallow. At this point, a *single* 100 mg. dose of doxycycline usually completes the antibiotic requirement for louse-borne typhus.

Duration of Chemotherapy. With tetracycline HCl or chloramphenicol, optimal *duration* and *timing* of therapy are related to the rate of development of immunity and the rate of recovery of the particular organisms from the growth-inhibitory effects of the antibiotic employed. Since the drugs are primarily rickettsiostatic, ultimate "cure" depends upon development of an adequate immune response. Accordingly, treatment started very early in the course of disease usually must be maintained longer than treatment initiated later in the disease. If these drugs are discontinued too soon, the patient may experience a febrile relapse. With chloramphenicol, "relapse" may occur as soon as 12 to 24 hours after the last dose of drug in murine typhus or as long as 5 to 6 days in scrub typhus. A practical conservative guide to duration of chloramphenicol or tetracycline therapy is to give the drug at least until the patient has been afebrile for 48 hours and then for an additional period until the total time elapsed from *onset of disease* is 12 to 14 days—roughly the duration of untreated disease and the time required for an adequate immune response. Though not necessarily the *minimum* adequate regimen, it automatically compensates for the differing antibiotic requirements for treatment begun at any stage of the disease. Drug resistance, inducible in the laboratory, has not been encountered clinically. Relapse responds to retreatment with the same drug. Renal or hepatic impairment may permit toxic drug levels to develop with the usual doses of drug and may require reduction in daily dose.

Steroids. Though not rigorously controlled, studies have shown that corticosteroids given in conjunction with antibiotics may cause rapid defervescence, dramatic reversal of neurologic impairment (coma, difficulty in swallowing), and an apparent improvement in the general well-being of the patient without adversely affecting the infectious process. A comatose patient given steroid therapy in the evening may be sitting upon the side of the bed in the morning, conversing with his fellow patients and able to take medication and fluids by mouth. Similar effects may be seen in patients unable to swallow. One dispensary, although seeing an average of 200 to 300 epidemic typhus patients a month, did not need to give intravenous hydration after corticosteroids were incorporated into the initial therapy of uncooperative patients. This has been accomplished by giving 100 mg. of hydrocortisone intravenously and 200 to 300 mg. of cortisone acetate intramuscularly, in addition to 500 mg. of tetracycline intramuscularly, to a comatose typhus patient upon admission. *(Falciparum malaria must be excluded by blood smear in patients at risk to both diseases.)* Usually, within 24 hours the patient is able to swallow the final dose of antibiotic (100 mg. of doxycycline), to take oral fluids, to attend to elimination, and to move spontaneously to reduce the chances of developing pressure necroses or thrombophlebitis. Usually no more therapy of any kind, antimicrobial or steroid, is required and nutrition presents no problem. This therapy is reserved for seriously ill or "uncooperative" patients.

Supportive Therapy. Murine typhus and Brill-Zinsser disease, usually mild to moderately severe infections, do not ordinarily require intensive supportive measures and may be successfully managed in the home unless the patient is aged or debilitated. Epidemic typhus and scrub typhus may be much more severe. Even with these, the uncomplicated case responding rapidly to chemotherapy usually requires little special attention to hydration and nutrition. Bed rest, a diet liberal in protein and calories, adequate fluid intake, analgesia, and good nursing care are keystones of general supportive measures. However, severe rickettsial disease, regardless of type, may display marked physiologic disturbances (cardiovascular, central nervous system [CNS], renal, hepatic, hematologic) and may require special supportive or corrective measures. Barring other concomitant serious illness, mortality should be essentially zero in patients treated early. However, deaths still occur occasionally despite the most sophisticated therapy in severe disease when therapy is instituted late.

Nursing Care. Patients may be irrational or agitated and may injure themselves or even attempt self-destruction. Close observation and restraint may be required. Comatose patients should be turned frequently to prevent pressure necrosis, thrombophlebitis, and hypostatic pneumonia. Special skin care and protection of bony prominences may be desirable in view of the vascular damage associated with the disease. Good oral hygiene reduces the chances of suppurative parotitis.

Diet and Protein Balance. Negative nitrogen balance, hypoproteinemia, and loss of tissue proteins (weight loss, wasting) are common, even in moderately severe infections. A positive nitrogen balance, however, can be maintained by a diet high in calories and protein, given orally, by stomach tube, or parenterally as the situation demands. If oliguria or anuria is associated with significant azotemia, excessive protein supplements are avoided until renal function improves.

Fluid and Electrolyte Balance. Oral fluids

sufficient to ensure a daily urine output of at least 1500 ml. suffice for the conscious, cooperative patient. The comatose patient will require parenteral fluids to maintain an adequate urine output. Fluids should be given slowly so as not to tax the potentially labile cardiovascular system. Excess electrolytes contribute to the general edema and to cardiac load when the fluid re-enters the vascular compartment. Urine output, the presence of oliguria, and laboratory determinations will serve as guides to the proper volume and proportion of electrolytes, glucose, and water.

Hepatic and Renal Systems. The cause of the disturbed liver (abnormal tests, rarely jaundice) and kidney (azotemia, albuminuria, oliguria) functions remains controversial, but these abnormalities are usually transient and disappear with convalescence. Hence management, if required, is guided by identification of the specific abnormalities present through appropriate tests and by the presence of other complicating abnormalities.

Cardiovascular System, Including Blood. The most prominent manifestations of the typhus group of rickettsial diseases can be attributed to abnormalities of the cardiovascular system. Indeed, hypotension is common and "peripheral vascular collapse," frequently in the second week of disease, is a leading cause of death and has been difficult to manage. Its cause is only incompletely understood. However, the widespread focal lesions of the small vessels are assumed to be contributory to increased vascular permeability and collapse and may also account for some of the clotting abnormalities (thrombocytopenia, disseminated intravascular clotting as a result of endothelial damage and defective synthesis from liver impairment) which have recently been recognized in certain rickettsioses. This in turn would help explain certain complications—hemorrhage, arterial occlusion (gangrene, hemiplegia, others), and rarely thrombophlebitis—and would suggest more rational approaches to their prevention and management, especially when specifically identified by appropriate laboratory tests.

Accordingly, whole blood and plasma should be avoided. Albumin may be used to combat hypoproteinemia. Red cells are preferred to correct significant anemia. Heparin has been described in a single report as treatment for rickettsia-associated intravascular clotting.

The management of peripheral vascular collapse is empiric and of largely unproved benefit: (1) oxygen; (2) judicious use of salt-poor concentrated albumin as a plasma expander and to reduce edema; (3) vasopressor drugs, e.g., levarterenol bitartrate (Levophed); and (4) corticosteroids such as hydrocortisone.

Pulmonary edema and congestive heart failure, resulting from excessive intake of salt and water or from rapid resorption of edema fluid with vascular healing, are treated with digitalis. No guidelines are available for the use of diuretics, but if their use is contemplated, consideration should be given to the state of renal function.

Massive intravascular hemolysis, described in glucose-6-phosphate dehydrogenase deficient subjects with murine or scrub typhus, was managed successfully with peritoneal dialysis.

Other Complications. Secondary bacterial pneumonia, still frequent in epidemic typhus, or other bacterial infections are treated with appropriate antibiotics according to the causative organisms and their sensitivity patterns.

Gangrene, decubitus ulcers, and thrombophlebitis are treated by the usual surgical and medical methods. Unless caused by a large destructive process (hemorrhage or thrombosis of a large vessel), neurologic abnormalities usually resolve with convalescence, although personality changes and deafness have been known to persist in some patients for months.

Prevention and Control Measures

Special isolation or decontamination is required only of patients with epidemic typhus. Infected lice and louse feces present special hazards to all contacts, including physicians and attendants among whom infection is common. If proper decontamination is performed, nonimmune hospital personnel need take special precautions (gowns, masks, gloves) only from initial contact to final decontamination, provided that the wards are kept louse-free. Decontamination and disinsectization of the patient and his clothing (including blankets, hats, and the like) are performed immediately upon hospitalization of a typhus patient. Clothing is best decontaminated by heat, because this will kill the lice, their eggs, and the rickettsiae in the louse feces. The patient is bathed, deloused, and treated with appropriate lousicides at proper intervals. Since insecticide resistance among body lice all over the world is a growing problem, knowledge of the local resistance patterns will determine the choice of insecticide; 10 per cent DDT powder, 1 per cent malathion, 1 per cent lindane (gamma hexachlorohexane), and a new carbamate (Mobam) are the usual insecticides for use on human beings, but there is renewed interest in pyrethrins because of resistance to other compounds. Contacts should be deloused and observed for development of disease.

General control measures for epidemic typhus usually rely on isolation of patients and a louse control program for the population at risk, but this may not be adequate, depending upon local insecticide resistance patterns, "logistics," and many other practical considerations. Murine typhus is controlled by *first* eliminating the rat fleas in the area with appropriate insecticides and then instituting rat control measures. Control of scrub typhus is difficult. Area control of vector mites with persisting acaricides is possible but often impractical or undesirable because of environmental contamination problems. Personal preventive measures include avoidance of known endemic areas if possible or appropriate mite repellents applied to the skin or impregnated into the clothing (diethyltoluamide, M-1960) if such areas must be entered. Similar measures apply to ticks.

At present, commercial killed vaccines against epidemic typhus are variable in potency and unpredictable in antibody response. New specifications are being developed. An experimental living attenuated typhus vaccine gives strong protection under epidemic circumstances but is not yet generally available. No vaccines are commercially available for protection against murine typhus, scrub typhus, or *R. canada.*

WHOOPING COUGH
(Pertussis)

method of
HARRIS D. RILEY, Jr., M.D.
Oklahoma City, Oklahoma

Pertussis is an acute infection which affects children predominantly, but no age group is exempt. It is caused by *Bordetella pertussis,* a small gram-negative, nonmotile bacillus with rather fastidious growth requirements. *B. pertussis* shares certain antigenic components with *Bordetella parapertussis* and *Bordetella bronchiseptica*, both of which may cause respiratory disease resembling pertussis, but there is no evidence of cross-immunity with *B. pertussis.* It is highly contagious and more dangerous than is usually believed, especially for young infants. The young infant is not protected by transplacental antibodies. Pertussis is an important cause of morbidity and mortality among unimmunized infants and children and in those debilitated by underlying disease. Approximately 70 per cent of all deaths from pertussis occur in the first year of life. Pertussis is highly communicable, with secondary attack rates of 80 to 90 per cent in susceptible family members and 30 to 80 per cent in those with less intimate exposure. As a rule, one attack confers solid immunity, but the duration of immunity is likely not as long as it is generally thought to be. However, some of the reported secondary attacks may be due to infection with *B. parapertussis* or *B. bronchiseptica*. From 15 to 25 per cent of immunized children will contract the disease on exposure, but the disease is usually milder. The young infant is not protected by transplacental antibodies. Because of the presence of inclusion-bearing cells, certain other features (lymphocytosis, the interstitial character of the pneumonia and the encephalopathy), and the difficulty in recovering *B. pertussis*, the possibility that the disease is due to a viral agent, chiefly adenoviruses, has been repeatedly considered. Isolation of adenoviruses has occurred most frequently in unimmunized patients with the clinical picture of pertussis. However, serious questions remain as to the pathogenesis of the whooping cough syndrome associated with viral agents. Recent studies suggest that mixed bacterial and viral infections may be more common than suspected and confirm the continued importance of *B. pertussis* in the etiology of clinical disease.

Laboratory confirmation (by culture or the fluorescent antibody precipitin techniques) is particularly important in atypical cases.

Control of pertussis depends chiefly on immunization, although recently in Great Britain the efficacy of pertussis vaccine has been widely debated. A defect of presently available vaccines is the relatively short immunity which they invoke.

Recently, several outbreaks among adult hospital personnel have been described.

Treatment

General. The patient should be isolated during the first 4 weeks of illness, which is the usual accepted period of communicability, or from 3 weeks from onset of paroxysms, as this date usually can be set with more accuracy. Isolation serves not only as a protection for the patient from other infectious agents but also as a prophylactic measure for susceptible contacts. In particular, patients with active or potentially active cases of tuberculosis should be rigidly guarded against contact with pertussis. Nonimmunized children should be quarantined for 14 days following intimate exposure.

Hospitalization may be required to accomplish isolation when the home situation is not adequate or allows exposure to unimmunized infants or young children. It is usually indicated for children under the age of 2 years and always for patients with severe cases. Bed rest is indicated during the febrile period.

The importance of constant and resourceful nursing care cannot be overemphasized; in few other diseases is it as crucial, and it may spell the difference between life and death. Nursing attendants should be equipped to institute mechanical lifesaving procedures such as suctioning, insertion of an airway, and other measures. Choking attacks should be relieved by gently suctioning at frequent intervals.

Environmental temperature in a well-ventilated room should be constant to reduce the paroxysm of coughing produced by sudden fluctuations in temperature. Air conditioning is often helpful in controlling the paroxysms. Humidity should be maintained at a minimum of 40 to 50 per cent by either steam or other means of humidification. Oxygen is indicated for patients with respiratory complications or convulsions. Factors which provoke coughing, such as activity, excitement, and inhalant irritants, should be avoided. Cough suppressants should not be used.

It is important to maintain adequate nutrition and hydration. Small frequent feedings should be provided, and refeeding in the presence of vomiting associated with the paroxysms is important. Parenteral supplementation is necessary if hydration cannot be maintained by the oral route.

Specific. Pertussis immune globulin (human) has been widely recommended both for treatment of patients with active cases—particularly clinically severe cases occurring in infancy—and for prevention of pertussis in exposed susceptible individuals. In association with antimicrobials, it is prescribed by many experienced clinicians, especially for the treatment of young infants (1.25 ml. given daily for three to five doses, or 3.0 to 6.75 ml. as a single dose). However, its efficacy has not been scientifically established, and the results of controlled studies show little or no therapeutic benefit attributable to this form of therapy.

No antimicrobial agent has been established to be effective in modifying the severity or shortening the course of the pertussis, and the role of antimicrobial therapy is difficult to evaluate. *B. pertussis* is usually susceptible in vitro to sulfadiazine, the tetracyclines, chloramphenicol, erythromycin, streptomycin, colistin, ampicillin, and certain other agents. Erythromycin (40 to 50 mg. per kg. per day in four divided doses orally) or ampicillin (100 mg. per kg. per day in four divided oral doses) for 5 days has been used on the thesis that it produces bacteriologic conversion of cultures to negative and renders the child noncontagious. However, other studies have shown that tetracycline and ampicillin were not effective in eliminating *B. pertussis* from the respiratory tract. Antibiotics may be useful in the face of complicating bacterial infections, and the choice of drug should be guided by microbiologic test results. Chloramphenicol, because of its toxicity, should not be used. Infants with pertussis frequently are stimulated to a paroxysm and vomiting from resistance to administration of medication; if so, the same dose should be readministered immediately or ampicillin administered intramuscularly.

Because of the difficulty in diagnosis and the generally unsatisfactory therapy for the established disease, the control of pertussis lies in its prevention by means of active immunization. Vaccines are of no benefit, however, once clinical manifestations have begun.

Complications

Respiratory Tract. The most common and usually the most severe complication is pneumonia, which usually takes the form of an interstitial bronchopneumonia. It is usually caused by secondary invaders, most commonly *Hemophilus influenzae*, the pneumococcus and the Streptococcus. *B. pertussis* has been shown on occasion to be the predominating microorganism. Although every attempt should be made to identify the causative organism, this is only infrequently productive, and antibacterial therapy must be based on clinical grounds. Ampicillin or erythromycin may be used, because they are effective to varying degrees against the most common causative pathogens. If the causative organism is isolated, antimicrobial therapy may be guided by the results of in vitro susceptibility tests.

Atelectasis is a common complication, and it is often recognized only by radiographic examination. If it does not subside spontaneously, bronchoscopic aspiration may be necessary to prevent the development of bronchiectasis. No child with pertussis should be released from medical surveillance until the lungs have been shown to be clear roentgenographically.

Otitis media is a frequent complication, particularly in infants. Emphysema usually resolves spontaneously after the acute illness but may lead to interstitial emphysema or pneumothorax.

Central Nervous System. Convulsions are relatively common and represent a serious complication of pertussis. There are probably several different causes, including asphyxia from severe paroxysms, petechial hemorrhages, subarachnoid bleeding, or the development of a diffuse encephalopathy. Convulsions should be treated with sedatives, establishment of an adequate airway, oxygen, and lumbar puncture to relieve increased pressure. Phenobarbital (3 to 5 mg. per kg. per dose intramuscularly), because it does not ordinarily result in depression of the cough reflex, is recommended.

Other Complications. Hemorrhages, which are mechanical in origin, resulting from increased venous pressure and congestion associated with paroxysms, occur relatively frequently. Epistaxis and subconjunctival hemorrhages are particularly common; intracranial bleeding may also occur.

Other complications include hernia and prolapsed rectum associated with severe paroxysms and nutritional disturbances. Alkalotic tetany resulting from loss of acid gastric contents secondary to excessive vomiting should be treated with calcium gluconate intravenously. Digitalization should be done for the rare case of secondary cardiac failure.

Treatment of Contacts

Although inconsistent in its effectiveness, passive immunization is sometimes of value in protecting susceptible, exposed contacts. Its use should be limited to persons at high risk, such as subjects less than 2 years of age and children with serious underlying disorders such as decompensated heart disease or chronic pulmonary disease. In such situations, hyperimmune pertussis gamma globulin, 1.25 ml., should be given and this dose repeated in 5 days. If disease has not occurred by 14 days after contact, active immunization should be begun. Contacts not previously immunized should receive chemoprophylaxis in the form of erythromycin for 10 days after contact is broken or—if it is not possible to break the contact—for the duration of the cough in the infected contact. Immunized children less than 6 years of age exposed to pertussis should receive pertussis vaccine, 0.5 ml. (4 NIH units).

The prophylaxis or treatment of adult pertussis is based on use of erythromycin for 10 to 14 days, although there is some evidence that 5 days of oral therapy is adequate in adult as well as pediatric cases.

Acknowledgment

Appreciation is expressed to Toni Wood for typing the manuscript.

ACTIVE IMMUNIZATION FOR INFECTIOUS DISEASES

method of
H. BRUCE DULL, M.D.
Atlanta, Georgia

INTRODUCTION

Vaccines have become fundamental in the contemporary practice of preventive medicine. Dramatic evidence of their effectiveness is evident in the control of many infectious diseases by systematic vaccination programs.

The following review presents concepts of immunization in terms of current information, needs, and expectations. It is based largely on recommendations of the Public Health Service's Advisory Committee on Immunization Practices (ACIP) and disease status reports from the surveillance programs of the Center for Disease Control.

THE BASES OF IMMUNIZATION RECOMMENDATIONS

There are three basic questions to be answered in making vaccine recommendations:

1. What are the current risks from the disease for which vaccine is to be used—today's risks, not those when the vaccine was initially developed? How have epidemiologic characteristics of the disease influenced the timing and the manner in which vaccine can best be applied?

2. What are the characteristics of available vaccine(s), not only in terms of demonstrated effectiveness but also of inherent risk and ability to do the job which now exists? How much flexibility is there in scientific evidence to permit individual judgment in the vaccine's safe use when emergencies or medical preferences dictate?

3. How can the vaccine best practically be used within the general framework and patterns of good health care? How can unnecessary visits to physicians or clinics be avoided without jeopardizing an optimal response to vaccination or subjecting the patient to undue risks?

SOURCES OF IMMUNIZATION RECOMMENDATIONS

In the United States several medical and public health groups make immunization recommendations. This, at times, has led to confusion, especially when variations were detected. Differences were particularly disturbing to those who have chosen to interpret recommendations as pronouncements—the term "recommendation" being translated as "regulation."

Four major health agencies regularly publish on immunization practices:

The American Academy of Pediatrics' Committee on Infectious Diseases, the "Red Book" Committee, recommends primarily for the private practice of pediatrics, in which patients are brought with a certain predictable regularity to the physician's office.

The Public Health Service's Advisory Committee on Immunization Practices addresses its recommendations to organized public health. It is perhaps more conscious of the concerns in dealing broadly with community health while still expecting the same standard of preventive care.

The Armed Forces Epidemiology Board's Commission on Immunization orients its advice to military populations and their dependents who have, at times, clearly different needs and face different risks than either of the previous two groups.

The American Public Health Association includes vaccine recommendations among overall concepts of disease prevention in its manual, *Control of Communicable Diseases in Man* (12th edition, 1975). Immunization is only one part of a general review, which includes disease identification, reporting, quarantine and therapy as they are applied internationally.

In the past, minor differences have been found in immunization recommendations of these four sources. The differences were commonly inconsequential, often related to the date of revision or publication, interpretation of then available field and laboratory data, and specific needs of the particular audience to which the recommendations were addressed.

In recent years increasingly comparable recommendations have resulted from more formal liaison among groups actively considering immunization practices. But, even now, justifiable and logical differences in scheduling and general patterns of use can be expected.

GENERAL COMMENTS, CAUTIONS, AND CONTRAINDICATIONS

Several generalities underlie "applied immunology" and contemporary immunization practice.

Immunization Schedules

A schedule for immunizations is neither arbitrary nor rigid. The time for beginning is usually the earliest time that an antigen can be expected to be safe and effective, as well as the time when the disease to be prevented is either particularly prevalent or especially dangerous. Thus most of the live vaccines should be delayed until the second year of life, because maternal antibodies might interfere with adequate responses. However, it is best not to delay most primary immunizations beyond the second year, because the diseases to be prevented commonly occur in the susceptible preschool age groups; and furthermore, the risks of reactions from some of them may be greater at an older age. On the other hand, pertussis vaccine and other killed or inactivated antigens are given as early as possible in infancy, because the relevant diseases can be especially hazardous then.

The intervals between doses of vaccines which require more than one inoculation are selected both to complete the primary series expeditiously and to obtain an optimal antibody response. When evidence or extenuating circumstances indicate that the interval should be changed, either to accommodate new immunologic data or to combat increased disease risk, recommendations should be altered.

A common misconception in immunization practice, and another indication of "oversanctifying" the schedule, is that once a primary series is interrupted, it must be started over. This is incorrect both for inactivated and for live virus vaccines. When the initial antibody response has once been adequately stimulated, it appears that the immunologic "memory" may last for life.

Season for Immunization

At one time physicians were reluctant to vaccinate in certain seasons when naturally occurring illnesses might be prevalent and could theoretically add to the risk of immunization or interfere with suitable responses. Although a person should not be vaccinated when he has a severe febrile illness, there is no evidence in this country that season per se is a reason to postpone vaccination. Epidemic control of many diseases which occur seasonally is by widespread vaccination while the disease is prevalent.

Information to Parents and Patients

Parents and patients should be fully informed about the immunizations being given. They should know *what* is being administered and *why,* and what possibly or commonly associated reactions might be expected. A "threshold" should be established for when to notify the physician of a response which is severe or unusual and which may be related to the vaccine.

Immunization Records

Careful immunization data both in the physician's office record and in the patient's own health history are essential. The office record should completely identify vaccine by name, manufacturer, and lot number and indicate dose volume, route of administration, site of injection, and any untoward or associated events. A variety of cards and other personal health history systems have been developed by medical and public health groups. A suitable one should be used.

Inactivated vs. Live Virus Vaccines

In the United States both inactivated and live vaccines are widely used. Inactivated vaccines are generally given in multiple doses for primary immunization, plus regular boosters (e.g., DTP, rabies).

One live vaccine, oral poliovirus vaccine (trivalent), is given in multiple doses for primary immunization to achieve adequate response to all three types of poliovirus antigen combined in the vaccine. Most live vaccines, however, require only one dose (e.g., measles, rubella, mumps). Some need occasional reinforcing doses to maintain optimal levels of protection (e.g., smallpox, yellow fever).

In the United States live vaccines are generally preferred. The protection they stimulate is more like those that follow natural illness, persisting for longer periods of time than that generally produced by inactivated antigens.

Simultaneous Administration of Certain Vaccines

There are obvious practical advantages to giving more than one vaccine at the same time when this can be done safely and effectively. Experimental evidence and extensive field experience are strengthening the scientific basis for simultaneous administration of certain vaccines.

Generally, inactivated vaccine can be given on the same occasion at separate sites. When, however, vaccines known to be associated with local or systemic side effects are given simultaneously—vaccines such as those for cholera, typhoid, and plague—side effects could theoretically be accentuated. Persons known to experience such side effects should generally be given the vaccines on separate occasions.

An inactivated vaccine and a live, attenuated virus vaccine can generally be given at the same time at separate sites, observing the precautions that apply to the individual vaccines.

It has generally been recommended that administration of individual live virus vaccines should be separated by at least 1 month whenever possible. The rationale for this has been the theoretical concern that more frequent or severe side effects as well as diminished antibody responses might result. Field observations show, however, that with simultaneous administration of certain live virus vaccines, results of this type have been minimal or absent.

Antibody responses to trivalent oral polio vaccine (TOPV) given at the same time as the combination measles-mumps-rubella vaccine are comparable to those achieved when the same vaccines are given at different times. One might expect equivalent immunologic responses when other licensed combination live, attenuated virus vaccines or their component antigens are given at the same time as TOPV.

Smallpox and yellow fever vaccines have been given at the same time at separate sites and at varying intervals with the same effectiveness and safety as with individual vaccines. This is of special importance in vaccinating travelers to areas where both vaccines are needed.

Existing Acute Illnesses

Acute illnesses existing when vaccinations are scheduled may or may not require delay. Minor afebrile respiratory disease is not necessarily a contraindication to vaccination, but judgment is needed. Febrile illness usually does contraindicate vaccination—simply because it might be further accentuated by a vaccine which commonly induces a febrile response. Knowledge of what vaccine reactions might occur and when they would be expected should influence the ultimate decision to proceed or to delay immunization.

Altered Immune States

Protection afforded by vaccination depends on intact immunologic responsiveness. Persons with altered immune states, whether primary or induced by drugs or radiation, must be vaccinated with care and caution. Their responses to inactivated vaccines may or may not be completely adequate; only laboratory studies can demonstrate this. They should *not* be given live virus vaccines because of the risk of severe untoward reactions. Of particular concern should be patients with leukemia, lymphoma, or generalized malignancies and those with lowered resistance from therapy with steroids, alkylating drugs, antimetabolites, or radiation.

Pregnancy

Pregnancy per se does not call for primary or booster vaccination against any specific diseases. Pregnancy is a theoretical contraindication to live virus vaccine, because the attenuated viruses might infect the fetus with an unanticipated result. This risk must, of course, be weighed against need for protection when exposure to an important disease might occur.

In areas where neonatal tetanus continues to be prevalent, maternal prenatal care should include a review of the mother's tetanus immunity. If unprotected, the mother usually should be given tetanus toxoid for passive protection of the newborn.

Hypersensitivity to Vaccine Components

Vaccine antigens are produced in various substrates, some of them containing allergenic materials which can remain in small amounts in vaccines. These include antigens like those grown in eggs and used against such diseases as typhus, Rocky Mountain spotted fever, rabies, and yellow fever. Vaccines with such characteristics should not be given to persons known to be hypersensitive to components of the substrates.

Techniques of production and purification differ somewhat for each vaccine and can sometimes minimize any inherent risk of hypersensitivity reactions. For example, although prepared from viruses grown in embryonated eggs, influenza virus vaccine is highly purified during preparation and has only very rarely been reported to induce hypersensitivity responses. Screening persons by history of ability to eat eggs without adverse effects is a reasonable way to identify those possibly at risk from influenza vaccination.

Live virus vaccines prepared by growing viruses in cell culture are essentially devoid of potentially allergenic substances related to host tissues. There is no evidence that these vaccines cannot be given safely to all who need them.

Some vaccines contain preservatives or trace amounts of antibiotics to which patients may be hypersensitive. Label information should be reviewed carefully before deciding whether patients with known hypersensitivity to such preservatives or antibiotics can be vaccinated safely.

Untoward Reactions

All unexpected severe reactions to vaccines should be carefully documented and reported to local or state public health officials. The association of untoward reactions with vaccines must be clarified. Laboratory assistance may be required. (It is also the recommended common practice to notify the producer of the vaccine for his information and assistance.)

It is essential that there be nationally available data on the spectrum of associated reactions to vaccines to guide not only future vaccine development but also current patterns of use. Because severe responses fortunately are rare, they can be identified only from experience with very large numbers of vaccinations, usually millions.

Surveillance of Disease

To better understand the need for immunization and to evaluate its continuing effectiveness, it is important for all physicians and public health officials to diagnose and report infectious diseases conscientiously and consistently. The commitment to do so is an inherent part of relying on vaccines to prevent and control childhood diseases that were once common.

SPECIFIC DISEASES AND THEIR VACCINES

Diphtheria, Tetanus, and Pertussis

Routine immunization against diphtheria, tetanus, and pertussis during infancy and childhood has been widely advocated and generally practiced in the United States for more than 25 years. The effectiveness of this effort is evident in the resulting decline in incidence and mortality from these three diseases.

Diphtheria is now a rare disease in many parts of the country. In recent years only about 200 cases have been reported annually. Localized outbreaks do continue to occur in populations in which fully adequate immunization is not provided. Some increase in the proportion of cases in susceptible adults has been observed in recent years.

Tetanus remains an important public health problem, although its incidence in the United States has declined considerably in recent years. Universal active immunization is the only suitable method of protecting each individual from a disease originating in environmental exposure. Neonatal tetanus, still being reported from some parts of the country, can be prevented by adequate maternal tetanus immunization. In general, active tetanus immunization eliminates the need for passive therapy at the time of injury and is the basis for proper management of wounds which could result in tetanus infection.

Pertussis and its associated high infant mortality is the major rationale for DTP immunization in early infancy. Most pertussis deaths occur in infants, and almost half of the cases in infants occur in babies 3 months of age or younger.

Vaccines. The combination of diphtheria and tetanus toxoids and inactivated pertussis vaccine has become the traditional product for children. The adsorbed form is more widely used and is superior to the fluid preparation in inducing high titers of antibodies and more durable protection.

Older children and adults are immunized against tetanus and diphtheria with a preparation containing a standard dose of tetanus toxoid but only about 10 to 25 per cent of the diphtheria component. This "adult form," commonly known as Td, greatly reduces the likelihood of an unusually severe response to the diphtheria antigen in any person previously immunized. The pertussis vaccine component of DTP has not been felt to be needed by older children and adults, who also report a greater proportion of side effects from the vaccine.

Schedule. The primary immunization of infants and children through the time of entering school is three separate doses of DTP given intramuscularly at 4 to 8 week intervals beginning at approximately 8 to 12 weeks of age. A fourth or reinforcing dose is recommended 1 year after the third injection. This pattern produces not only the best initial responses but also durable protection. For children over approximately 6 years of age and adults, primary immunization is with Td given intramuscularly or subcutaneously on two occasions 4 to 6 weeks apart and a third or reinforcing dose approximately 6 months to 1 year after the second.

Booster immunization with DTP is recommended for children at the time of entering school, either kindergarten or elementary school, because the likelihood of their being exposed is accentuated. A single intramuscular dose is used. Thereafter, and for all older children and adults, a single intramuscular or subcutaneous dose of Td given at 10 year intervals will maintain high levels of antibody against tetanus and diphtheria.

At times of injury when tetanus exposure is clearly felt to be possible and the most recent Td booster was more than a year earlier, an additional booster of Td is usually recommended. The next regular booster is measured from that time. Td is used instead of tetanus toxoid alone to provide continuing diphtheria protection.

Poliomyelitis

Widespread use of poliovirus vaccines has resulted in the virtual elimination of paralytic poliomyelitis in the United States. In recent years, usually fewer than ten cases have been reported annually.

Vaccines. Oral polio vaccine (OPV), almost entirely the trivalent combination (TOPV), is much more widely used in this country than is inactivated poliovirus vaccine (IPV). It stimulates an immune response which appears to be more like that induced by natural poliovirus infection and involves both humoral and gastrointestinal tract immunity. Very rarely, however, cases of paralytic poliomyelitis occur among recipients of OPV in the 30 days after receiving vaccine or in their close contacts as a result of spread of vaccine virus. "Vaccine-associated" paralytic disease appears to occur at a rate of no more than one case for every 5 to 10 million cases of OPV administered.

A primary series of TOPV consisting of three adequately spaced doses will produce an immune response to all three poliovirus types in well over 90 per cent of recipients. A single dose of TOPV results in immunity to the three virus types in approximately 60 per cent of susceptible recipients.

Schedule. The primary immunization of infants with TOPV is commonly begun at the same time the first DTP inoculation is given, 8 to 12 weeks of age. The second dose preferably is administered approximately 8 weeks later at the time of the third DTP, and the third TOPV about 8 to 12 months later.

Older children and adolescents who have not had OPV should be given a comparable series of three doses of TOPV, the first two approximately 6 to 8 weeks apart, and the third 8 to 12 months after the second.

Routine immunization of adults in the United States is not necessary at present because of the extreme unlikelihood of exposure to polio. If risk of contracting polio is increased by virtue of contact with known cases or travel to areas where polio does exist, adults should receive TOPV according to the schedule outlined for older children and adults.

At the time of entering kindergarten or elementary school, all children who have completed primary immunization with OPV should receive a single follow-up dose of TOPV.

If inactivated poliovirus vaccine (IPV) is used, the primary series of four parenteral doses should be given, three at approximately monthly intervals, and the fourth, a reinforcing dose, 6 to 12 months after the third. Single booster doses of IPV have been recommended every few years thereafter if antibody titers are to be sustained. With the more potent IPV preparations now being prepared in many parts of the world, this schedule of relatively frequent booster doses may be more than necessary for adequate protection.

Measles (Rubeola)

The occurrence of measles in the United States has declined to less than 10 per cent of the level prior to widespread use of live measles virus vaccines. This dramatic change is the result of national efforts to eradicate measles by systematically vaccinating all susceptible children and incorporating measles vaccination into the regular immunization schedule for all children.

Vaccines. Live measles virus vaccine is highly effective and is produced in chick embryo cell culture from a vaccine virus strain attenuated to minimize the relatively common vaccine side effects, rash and fever. With the vaccine currently available in the United States, these short-lived and generally insignificant reactions, occurring in approximately 15 per cent of vaccinees, begin about the sixth day after vaccination and last up to 5 days.

Schedule. Live measles virus vaccine is indicated for all children who have not had measles. It should regularly be given at about 15 months of age when circulating maternal antibody will no longer interfere with optimal immune responses. When, however, there is the chance of exposure to natural measles at an earlier age, infants as young as 6 months old should be vaccinated. When this is done, recognizing that the rate of seroconversion declines with diminishing age, children vaccinated at 6 to 12 months of age may need to be revaccinated at an older age to assure continued protection.

Mumps

Mumps is most frequent in young school-age children. However, approximately 15 per cent of reported cases occur after the onset of puberty. All naturally acquired mumps infections, including the estimated 30 per cent which are subclinical, confer durable immunity.

Vaccine. Live mumps virus vaccine is prepared in cell culture of chick embryo and is highly effective and almost completely devoid of side effects.

Schedule. Live mumps vaccine should be given to children over age 12 months. When mumps vaccine is incorporated into licensed combination vaccines which also include the live measles antigen, the combination vaccine should not be given until about 15 months of age to assure optimal antibody response to the measles component.

Live mumps vaccine can be given to adults susceptible to mumps without any risk of side effects.

Rubella

Rubella is one of the common childhood exanthems. Most cases occur in school-age children, particularly during the winter and spring. By early adulthood approximately 80 to 90 per cent of residents of the United States have serologic evidence of immunity.

Rubella is generally a mild illness, but if the infection is acquired by a woman in the early months of pregnancy, it poses a considerable hazard to the fetus. This is a major consideration in controlling the disease.

Vaccine. Live rubella virus vaccines are highly effective and are prepared in duck embryo or rabbit kidney cell cultures. Approximately 95 per cent of susceptible vaccineees develop antibodies and long-lasting protection.

Rash and lymphadenopathy occur occasionally in children after vaccination, but transient arthralgia, usually of the small peripheral joints, has been the most common complaint. These side effects have varied in incidence from 2 to 9 per cent beginning 2 to 10 weeks after vaccination and generally persisting for 1 to 3 days. In adults, particularly women, arthralgia and generally transient arthritis following vaccination are more frequent and severe than in children.

Vaccinees may shed small amounts of virus in the pharynx briefly at some time between weeks 1 and 4 following vaccination. There is, however, no evidence of any resulting risk of transmitting vaccine virus to susceptible contacts.

It has been shown that rubella vaccine virus will infect the fetus in pregnancy; because of the theoretical risk that even attenuated virus might cause fetal anomaly, rubella vaccine should *not* be given in pregnancy.

Schedule. Live rubella virus vaccine is recommended for all children at any age after 12 months. In younger infants maternal antibody might interfere with optimal response. When rubella vaccine is incorporated into licensed combination vaccines, including the live measles antigen, the combination vaccine should not be given until about 15 months of age to assure optimal antibody response to the measles component.

Rubella immunization of susceptible adolescent girls and women of childbearing age is important in reducing the chance of rubella infection during pregnancy and consequent fetal anomaly. Vaccination in these instances should be on an individualized basis when susceptibility has been shown by serologic testing. In demonstrated susceptibles, vaccine should be given with the patient's assurance that she will avoid pregnancy for 2 to 3 months, being advised of the theoretical risk to the fetus from vaccine virus if pregnancy were to occur.

Rabies

Although rabies in humans is rare in the United States, about 30,000 persons receive post-exposure prophylaxis annually. The problem of whether or not to immunize those bitten or scratched by animals suspected of being rabid is perplexing for physicians.

Complete discussion of all relevant factors in rabies prophylaxis is beyond the scope of this review in that the approach to rabies prevention must be individualized. The reader is referred for additional information to the statement on rabies by the Public Health Service Advisory Committee on Immunization Practices and to consultation with local and state health authorities and the Center for Disease Control, Atlanta.

Rabies is minimal in the United States in domestic animals, although the majority of anti-rabies treatments follow bites by dogs and cats. Increasingly important, however, is rabies in wildlife—especially in skunks, foxes, raccoons, and bats—accounting for 70 per cent of all reported cases of animal rabies each year since 1968. Only Idaho, Vermont, Hawaii, and the District of Columbia report no wildlife rabies.

Vaccine. The only antirabies vaccine available in the United States is that produced in embryonated duck eggs from which fixed rabies virus is inactivated with beta-propiolactone. Duck embryo vaccine (DEV) is considerably less reactogenic than older vaccines and appears to be equally effective. A regular adjunct product to DEV is rabies immune globulin (human) (RIG). It is a standardized product containing neutralizing rabies antibody and is used now instead of antiserum of animal origin.

Local reactions to DEV are very common, although severe reactions such as anaphylaxis occur in less than 1 per cent of patients. Neuroparalytic reactions do occur with DEV, but only rarely.

Schedule. Postexposure rabies prophylaxis with RIG and DEV is undertaken only after careful evaluation of the species of biting animal, the circumstances of the biting incident, the type of exposure (e.g., bite, scratch), the vaccination status of the biting animal, and the presence of rabies in the area. In overall management of the bite wounds and scratches which could transmit rabies, local treatment is perhaps the most effective rabies preventive and should be prompt and thorough.

As indicated in Table 1, both RIG and DEV are given in postexposure rabies prophylaxis. The dose of RIG is based on body weight; a portion of it is infiltrated around the wound and the rest administered intramuscularly. Twenty-three doses of DEV should be given beginning on the day passive antibody is administered. There are options in the timing of doses, although in all instances two booster doses are included in the 23 recommended.

Persons at regular risk of exposure to rabies should be considered candidates for pre-exposure prophylaxis. These include veterinarians, animal handlers, certain laboratory workers, and persons living in places where rabies is a constant threat. Three injections of DEV are generally given, two doses 1 month apart, followed by a third 6 to 7 months after the second. All who receive pre-exposure vaccination should have rabies antibody determinations performed on serum collected 3 to 4 weeks after completing the vaccination series to document the response (Table 1).

TABLE 1. **Postexposure Antirabies Treatment Guide**

The following recommendations are only a guide. They should be applied in conjunction with knowledge of the animal species involved, circumstances of the bite or other exposure, vaccination status of the animal, and presence of rabies in the region.

SPECIES OF ANIMAL	CONDITION OF ANIMAL AT TIME OF ATTACK	TREATMENT OF EXPOSED HUMAN
Wild—skunk, fox, coyote, raccoon, bat	Regard as rabid	RIG + DEV*
Domestic—dog, cat	Healthy	None†
	Unknown (escaped)	RIG + DEV
	Rabid or suspected rabid	RIG + DEV*
Other	Consider individually	

*Discontinue vaccine if fluorescent antibody (FA) tests of animal killed at time of attack are negative.

†Begin RIG + DEV at first sign of rabies in biting dog or cat during holding period (10 days).

Influenza

Characteristically periodic epidemics of influenza and annual occurrence of the disease present special problems in influenza control. The biologic behavior of the virus makes forecasting epidemics and preparing suitably effective vaccine far from ideal.

The generally recommended policy for influenza vaccination in the United States is used to reduce severe illness and fatality and not to attempt to prevent disease in the general population. Those at risk of severe disease and fatality have regularly been demonstrated to be persons of all ages with chronic debilitating diseases, particularly those of the cardiovascular, bronchopulmonary, and metabolic systems. Also, it has been observed that persons in the older age groups generally, particularly above age 65, are at increased risk. For others in the civilian population, the risks from influenza are not great, and annual vaccination is not recommended.

Vaccine. Influenza vaccine is inactivated virus grown in embryonated chicken eggs. Vaccine formulation generally incorporates both type A and type B influenza viruses which are representative of prevalent strains. In the United States whole-virus and split-virus influenza vaccines are available. In general the split-virus vaccines are less frequently associated with side effects than whole-virus vaccines, although the latter vaccines may be more immunogenic. In adults, characteristic side effects of influenza vaccine include injection site soreness and erythema and transient systemic complaints with low-grade fever. These side effects are generally inconsequential, occurring in less than 2 to 5 per cent of vaccinees. In children, particularly those given whole-virus vaccines, 15 per cent or more may experience the same kind of, but often more pronounced, side effects.

As a result of the systematic surveillance of reactions to the influenza vaccines given during 1976 in preparation for a possible outbreak of A/New Jersey/76 virus (swine influenza virus), it was determined that the Guillain-Barré syndrome was associated with influenza vaccination at a rate of approximately 1 case per 100,000 or so vaccinations. Accurate risk data are difficult to collect because of regularly occurring cases of Guillain-Barré syndrome, presumably caused by various inciting factors.

Schedule. For persons receiving annual vaccination, except when an entirely new strain appears, a single dose of the current influenza vaccine formulation usually provides protection in about 70 to 80 per cent of recipients. Children, who might reasonably be given split-virus vaccine to minimize side effects, are probably better protected if they receive two doses of vaccine approximately 1 month or more apart. The dose volumes and more details on specific products are to be found in manufacturers' package labeling.

Being produced in eggs, influenza vaccine, although highly purified, can theoretically induce hypersensitivity reactions in persons highly allergic to eggs. Persons needing influenza protection who have history of such allergy should be vaccinated only after consultation with an allergist and hypersensitivity testing.

Meningococcal Disease

Meningococcal disease is endemic throughout the world. In the United States it caused serious epidemics approximately each decade from 1900 to 1945. An estimated 3000 to 6000 cases of meningococcal disease now occur in the United States each year. Since 1972, serogroup B meningococci have been the most common in this country. Serogroup C predominated from 1969 to 1971 but has been virtually eliminated in the military as the result of regular administration of group C meningococcal polysaccharide vaccine to all recruits since 1971.

Sulfa-sensitive serogroup B strains currently cause most cases of meningococcal disease in this country, with serogroup C strains causing about one third of them. Highest attack rates are in infants, although about 70 per cent of serogroup C cases appear in persons over 2 years old.

Meningococcal disease in civilians is primarily observed as single isolated cases and, infrequently, as small clusters of cases. Antibiotic prophylaxis has been the principal means of reducing the risk for immediate contacts of cases.

Vaccines. Three meningococcal polysaccharide vaccines, monovalent A, monovalent C, and bivalent A-C, are licensed for selective use in the United States. They are chemically defined antigens consisting of purified bacterial cell wall polysaccharides. They induce specific serogroup immunity following a single parenteral dose. Adverse reactions are infrequent and mild, consisting primarily of localized erythema lasting for a day or two. How long immunity lasts is not known.

Serogroup A vaccine appears to be effective in all age groups beyond the first year of life. Serogroup C vaccine is known to be effective in adults from experience in the military; it elicited antibody in all age groups, although older children and young adults reached the highest levels. This vaccine does not appear to be effective in children under 2 years of age.

Schedule. *Routine* vaccination of civilians with meningococcal polysaccharide vaccines is *not* recommended. Rather, serogroup specific monovalent vaccines should be reserved to control outbreaks of meningococcal disease. Vaccination may have some value for travelers to epidemic areas and might also be considered an adjunct to antibiotic chemoprophylaxis for household contacts of cases. This latter recommendation is based on the observation that half the secondary family cases occur more than 5 days after the primary case, a period long enough to yield potential benefits from vaccination.

Typhoid

The incidence of typhoid fever in the United States has declined steadily for many years. Cases are sporadic, primarily related to contact with carriers rather than to common source exposure. Routine typhoid immunization is therefore *not* recommended. Immunization is indicated *only* when there is known exposure to a typhoid carrier, as in a household, for example, or if there is likely to be exposure to typhoid where it is known to be prevalent.

Vaccine. Effectiveness of typhoid vaccine, an inactivated suspension of organisms, has varied with the degree of exposure to disease. Although not optimal, vaccine does provide some protection for incidental common source exposure.

Vaccination is commonly associated with transient local tenderness and perhaps induration. (For this reason, many elect to use the intradermal route for all booster doses.)

In the past, commonly available typhoid vaccine incorporated paratyphoid A and B antigens. These paratyphoid antigens have not proved to be effective; typhoid vaccine alone should be used.

Schedule. Adults and children over 10 years of age felt to be at risk to typhoid should receive primary immunization with 0.5 ml. vaccine given subcutaneously on two occasions, separated by 4 or more weeks. Children 6 months to 10 years are commonly given half this volume.

When conditions of continued or repeated exposure exist, booster doses should be given at least every 3 years. They can be administered either intradermally or subcutaneously with comparable results. If the subcutaneous route is elected, the volumes given in the primary series apply. If the intradermal route is used, all individuals can receive 0.1 ml.

SUGGESTED PATTERN FOR IMMUNIZATION

Figure 1 is a composite of many of the concepts already discussed: (1) range in suitable scheduling for immunization, (2) optimal period based on risks and responses, and (3) pattern which generally fits traditional health care practice.

The figure shows a *suggested pattern* of childhood immunization and the number of doses recommended within the first 24 months of life. The suggested pattern is superimposed on a continuing, *suitable period* for giving each vaccine. During the suitable period either primary or booster doses can be given at the recommended intervals.

The newer live virus vaccines, measles, rubella, and mumps, can be administered to children 12 to 15 months of age. As previously discussed, however, measles vaccine is best given at approximately 15 months to preclude any interference with antibody response from residual maternal antibody. When licensed combination vaccines, including the measles antigen and rubella and/or mumps, are to be used, the combination vaccine should not be given until about 15 months of age to assure optimal antibody response to measles.

The second segment of Figure 1 acknowledges the epidemiologic importance of entering kindergarten or elementary school when there is a heightened risk of exposure to the common childhood illnesses. This factor of risk, rather than age alone, justifies giving booster doses of the important antigens at the time of school entrance.

The third segment indicates the generally recommended pattern of booster immunization with diphtheria and tetanus toxoids in later school years and adult life. Trivalent OPV is suggested only at times of increased risk, such as with some foreign travel. None of the other "childhood vaccines" appear to require booster doses.

A tuberculin skin test is shown as optional at approximately 1 year of age. It is only under conditions of family contact with tuberculosis or exposure in a community where tuberculosis is common that one should expect to find a positive reactor. If the skin test is to be done either as part of routine health care or because of suspicion of an actual exposure, it should be carried out before measles vaccine is administered or about 2 to 3 months later. Otherwise, the attenuated measles virus infection could obscure the accuracy of the skin test.

Tuberculin skin testing of children entering school is generally of more value than when done earlier. Even at school entrance, however, the procedure is recommended not principally for case detection (the national average positive reactor

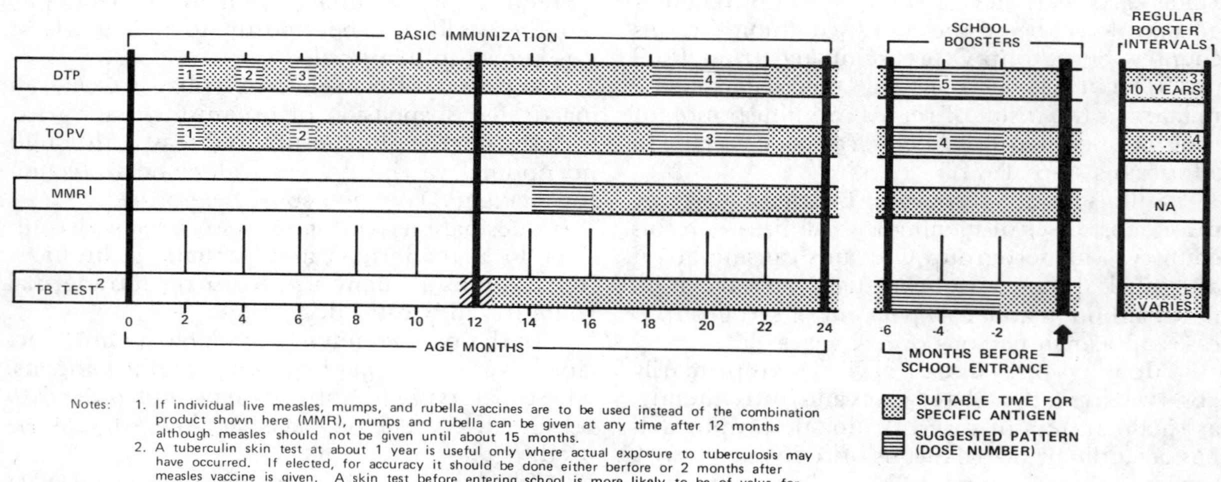

Notes:
1. If individual live measles, mumps, and rubella vaccines are to be used instead of the combination product shown here (MMR), mumps and rubella can be given at any time after 12 months although measles should not be given until about 15 months.
2. A tuberculin skin test at about 1 year is useful only where actual exposure to tuberculosis may have occurred. If elected, for accuracy it should be done either berfore or 2 months after measles vaccine is given. A skin test before entering school is more likely to be of value for documentation.
3. Td (adult type); basic to injury boosters.
4. Only for possible exposure, as with foreign travel to some areas.
5. Depends on local case-finding recommendations.

Figure 1. Childhood immunizations, booster doses, and tuberculin skin tests—suitable timing, suggested pattern, and number of doses.

rate is about 0.2 per cent at school entrance), but rather for documentation.

No regular schedule of tuberculin skin testing is shown thereafter, simply because the need varies from place to place and within particular segments of the population. Patterns and programs of tuberculosis case detection must be established by local medical and public health groups.

VACCINES FOR INTERNATIONAL TRAVEL

Some vaccines have particular application to international travel and therefore merit comment. Smallpox is, of course, one of them, but one which has become less important as we near the point of worldwide eradication of the disease. Others include cholera, plague, typhus, yellow fever, and sometimes rabies and typhoid. They are indicated only when itineraries could lead to exposure and when International Health Regulations dictate.

Many countries require travelers to present a validated International Certificate of Vaccination on arrival. Travelers are therefore advised to seek specific guidance when planning their trips. (Requirements are specified in the booklet entitled *Health Information for International Travel,* published as a supplement to the *Morbidity and Mortality Weekly Report* and available from the Center for Disease Control, Atlanta, Georgia 30333. Validation of International Certificates of Vaccination can be obtained at most city, county, and state health departments.

Smallpox

In the United States routine smallpox vaccination is no longer recommended. This is because of the near-worldwide eradication of smallpox. However, vaccination is still needed for travelers to countries requiring a validated International Certificate of Vaccination against smallpox. It is expected that the two countries in Africa where a few cases of smallpox still are occurring (1977) will soon have eliminated the disease.

Vaccine. Centuries of field observations on protective efficacy of smallpox vaccine well document its value. As with other medical procedures, however, smallpox vaccination carries a definite risk, particularly among primary vaccinees. The majority of reactions are eczema vaccinatum—avoidable in almost all cases if contraindications to smallpox vaccination are carefully observed. A smaller number of unusually severe reactions, including fatalities from postvaccinial encephalitis, can occur. Death resulted about once for each million primary vaccinations in the United States.

Schedule. Primary smallpox vaccination employing a potent vaccine is now indicated only for some foreign travel. Children under age 1 year are not generally vaccinated, because untoward reactions appear to be age related. For purposes of international travel, primary vaccination or revaccination within 3 years is needed for validating International Certificates. Evidence of smallpox vaccination is not required for entry or return to the United States from any part of the world.

Vaccination is generally by the multiple pressure method, using a standard or a "bifurcated" needle. Some prefer to use a puncture technique with the bifurcated needle. (Details of procedures are described in the vaccine labeling.) Vaccination is generally done on the skin over the insertion of the deltoid muscle in an area about one eighth inch in diameter. The remaining vaccine should be absorbed with dry, sterile gauze; no dressing should be applied.

The vaccination site should be inspected 6 to 8 days after vaccination and interpreted as follows: For primary vaccinations, a typical jennerian vesicle should appear. If none is observed, vaccination should be repeated with vaccine from other manufacturer lots until successful. For revaccination, only two responses are now accepted—a "major reaction," a vesicular or pustular lesion or an area of definite palpable induration or congestion surrounding a central lesion which may be an ulcer or crust; or an "equivocal reaction," any other response, none of which should be accepted as valid without revaccination using vaccine from another lot.

In addition to the general precautions on use of live virus vaccines specified earlier, *smallpox vaccine should not be given to patients with eczema or dermatitis or whose family or other close contacts have skin disorders.* Avoiding the risk of superinfection with vaccinia will markedly reduce the number of adverse reactions to smallpox vaccine.

Certain of the antiviral thiosemicarbazone derivatives can provide short-term protection against smallpox and some of the severe complications of vaccination. Information on thiosemicarbazones and on smallpox vaccination and management of complications should be sought from the Center for Disease Control, Atlanta, and from local or state public health agencies.

Cholera

Cholera generally occurs in endemic and epidemic form only in South and Southeast Asia. In recent years, however, it has also been epidemic in certain areas of the Middle East.

Infection is acquired principally from contaminated water or food.

Vaccine. Various inactivated cholera vaccines have been widely used, although it appears that the duration of vaccine-induced immunity is relatively brief. Protection seems to last no more than 6 months after the primary series or a booster.

Brief local reactions to cholera vaccine are relatively common and occasionally may be accompanied by fever, malaise, and headache. More severe reactions should preclude revaccination.

A primary vaccination or booster dose within the previous 6 months is generally required for persons traveling to or from countries with cholera. Individuals vaccinated against cholera must have a validated International Certificate of Vaccination for it to be acceptable by quarantine authorities.

Schedule. For travelers vaccinated in the United States, a single 0.5 ml. subcutaneous or intramuscular dose of cholera vaccines is considered adequate to satisfy the International Sanitary Regulations. The single dose for children is proportionately smaller (see Table 2). An intradermal dosage alternative is also shown for adults and children 5 years of age or more.

For adults traveling or working in areas where cholera is epidemic or known to be endemic and who live under conditions where sanitation is less than adequate, two doses of cholera vaccine, 0.5 ml., preferably given 1 month or more apart, are recommended. Boosters are recommended every 6 months as long as exposure persists.

Typhus

The last outbreak of louse-borne (epidemic) typhus occurred in the United States in 1922. The last reported case in 1950 did not result from an indigenous source.

Epidemic typhus was widespread in many foreign countries during World War II, but cases have generally declined steadily since 1945. A human reservoir of latent infections does, however, persist in some countries, and resurgence of disease could occur under conditions of war or disaster.

Vaccine. Typhus vaccine prepared from inactivated organisms grown in embryonated eggs has not been completely studied in field trials. Experience suggests, however, that the incidence and severity of cases are diminished among the vaccinated, especially if booster doses have been given.

Pain and tenderness at the injection site should be expected. Rarely, vaccinees have had exaggerated local reactions and fever, presumably as a manifestation of hypersensitivity.

Schedule. Vaccination may be indicated for travelers to rural or remote highland areas of Ethiopia, Rwanda, Burundi, Mexico, Ecuador, Bolivia, or Peru, and mountainous areas of Asia. It is principally useful for those whose work might bring them into close contact with indigenous populations where the disease actually occurs. It is not required under International Sanitary Regulations for entry into any country.

A primary vaccination consists of two subcutaneous injections of vaccine 4 or more weeks apart. The dose volume is indicated by the manufacturer. Booster injections of single doses of vaccine at intervals of 6 to 12 months should be continued as long as opportunity for exposure persists. Vaccine should not be administered to those with known hypersensitivity to eggs, in which the antigen is grown.

TABLE 2

	DOSE VOLUME (ML.)			
	INTRADERMAL*	SUBCUTANEOUS OR INTRAMUSCULAR		
	Age (Years)	*Age (Years)*		
DOSE NUMBER	*≥5*	*<5*	*5–10*	*>10*
1, 2, boosters	0.2	0.2	0.3	0.5

*Higher levels of protection (antibody) may be achieved in children less than 5 years old by the subcutaneous or intramuscular route.

Plague

Plague is a sylvatic infection of rodents and their ectoparasites in many parts of the world. In some countries of Asia, Africa, and South America, epidemics of plague result when domestic rats become infected. Currently the area of most intensive epidemic and epizootic infection is Vietnam.

Vaccine. Plague vaccine, although incompletely field tested, has been observed to reduce the incidence and severity of disease. It is prepared from organisms grown on artificial media and inactivated with formaldehyde.

Mild reactions of pain, redness, and swelling at the injection site are frequently seen. With repeated doses, systemic reactions of fever, headache, and malaise occur more frequently and become more pronounced. No fatal or disabling complications have been observed.

Schedule. Plague vaccine is recommended for persons whose vocations, field work, or travel bring them into frequent and regular contact with wild rodents in plague-enzootic areas of the western United States, Africa, or Asia. Mere travel in these areas is not sufficient justification for vaccination.

Adults and children over 10 years of age should receive three doses of vaccine in the primary series. The first two doses, 0.5 ml. each, should be administered intramuscularly 4 or more weeks apart, followed by the third dose, 0.2 ml., 4 to 12 more weeks after the second.

When less time is available, satisfactory, but less optimal, results can be obtained with two 0.5 ml. injections at least 3 weeks apart. For children less than 10 years old, the primary series is three smaller doses of vaccine (see Table 3).

Booster doses should be given every 6 months while individuals remain in an area where the risk of exposure persists, to a total of two boosters. Thereafter, booster doses at 1 to 2 year intervals should be adequate to sustain protection. Volumes are shown in Table 3.

TABLE 3

DOSE NUMBER	AGE (YEARS) UNDER 1	1–4	5–10	OVER 10
1 and 2	0.1 ml.	0.2 ml.	0.3 ml.	0.5 ml.
3 and boosters	0.04 ml.	0.08 ml.	0.12 ml.	0.2 ml.

Yellow Fever

At present, yellow fever cases are reported only from Africa and South America. Transmission is by the mosquito vector, *Aedes aegypti.* A principal part of disease prevention and control is eliminating the mosquito from urban areas where disease was previously epidemic.

Yellow fever virus persists as an enzootic disease in the jungles of certain countries in South America and Africa. Human cases of "jungle yellow fever" occur from exposure to the natural cycle of infection among nonhuman hosts spread by a variety of mosquito vectors. Immunization is the only feasible method of preventing disease acquired by exposure in this environment.

Vaccine. Yellow fever vaccine available in the United States is 17D strain of attenuated yellow fever virus. It is a highly effective live virus vaccine prepared from infected chick embryos and has essentially no untoward side effects. Protection is long lasting.

To be valid for purposes of international travel, yellow fever vaccine must be acceptable to the World Health Organization and administered at a Yellow Fever Center listed with WHO. Vaccinees should receive properly completed International Certificates of Vaccination bearing the validating stamp of the Center performing the vaccination. Individual country requirements are variable, and to avoid inconvenience and delay in South America and Africa it is advisable to have a valid International Certificate of Vaccination against yellow fever.

Schedule. Primary vaccination is recommended for all persons 6 months of age or older traveling or living in parts of Africa and South America where yellow fever occurs. A single subcutaneous injection of 0.5 ml. of reconstituted vaccine is used for both children and adults. Immunity has been shown to persist for more than 10 years, and revaccination need not be performed more frequently.

The vaccine should generally not be given to persons hypersensitive to eggs, but each case must be individualized on the basis of degree of hypersensitivity and need for protection. A waiver of yellow fever vaccination should be sought for travelers with clearly documented hypersensitivity.

SECTION 2

The Respiratory System

ACUTE RESPIRATORY FAILURE

method of
MORGAN DELANEY, M.D.,
and DONALD MASSARO, M.D.
Miami, Florida

The lung's major function is to eliminate CO_2 produced by the body's metabolic processes and to take up oxygen from the environment for subsequent delivery to the tissues. Lung failure (respiratory failure) may therefore be defined in terms of the arterial blood gases ($Paco_2$, Pao_2) and pH. Any elevation of $Paco_2$ above the normal value of 40 mm. Hg, which is not of a compensatory nature, i.e., due to metabolic alkalosis, represents a state of respiratory failure resulting from alveolar hypoventilation. This elevation of $Paco_2$ may be due to underlying lung disease or a chest wall abnormality (inadequate bellows function) or to the lack of adequate neural ventilatory drive—e.g., oversedation or head injury. A decrease in Pao_2, hypoxemia, invariably occurs when the $Paco_2$ is elevated. Hypoxemia can also occur without hypercapnia—indeed, in clinical practice, this type of respiratory failure is more frequently observed—and is usually due to ventilation-perfusion imbalance, i.e., a lung region having blood flow in excess of alveolar ventilation.

In general, acute respiratory failure, that is, a decrease in Pao_2 with or without an increase in $Paco_2$, usually occurs in one of two broad settings. On the one hand, it may represent an acute worsening of already abnormal arterial blood gases in a patient with some form of pre-existing obstructive airways disease such as chronic bronchitis, emphysema, or asthma. In patients with chronic bronchitis or emphysema (both conditions usually coexist in the same patient), acute bronchitis is the most common precipitating factor, but sedation, atmospheric pollution, hot weather, pneumonia, and pulmonary embolism are other predisposing factors. In patients with asthma there may be additional precipitating events such as allergic reactions and emotional upsets. In this category of acute respiratory failure, airways obstruction and excess bronchial secretions are the major problems. The second important setting for acute respiratory failure is in patients who, usually, have had preceding normal or relatively normal lungs; in this situation the major area of dysfunction is at the alveolar-capillary level rather than in the conducting airways.

ACUTE RESPIRATORY FAILURE IN THE PATIENT WITH UNDERLYING CHRONIC AIRWAYS OBSTRUCTION—CHRONIC BRONCHITIS AND EMPHYSEMA

The pathophysiologic events which lead to acute decompensation in a patient with chronic bronchitis or emphysema who has been functioning in a compensated state of chronic respiratory insufficiency are so similar that they will be discussed together. An acute insult, most commonly an episode of acute bronchitis, leads to secretion of bronchial mucus at a rate faster than it can be cleared from the lumina of the airways; increased bronchospasm is also frequently present. Airways obstruction is worsened, causing the distribution of ventilation within the lungs to become more nonuniform. The resultant alteration in the matching of ventilation to perfusion ($\dot{V}/\dot{Q}$ ratio) leads to alveolar hypoxia and hypoxemia—that is to say, many alveoli experience impaired delivery of atmospheric oxygen, and the blood flowing past those alveoli will be inadequately oxygenated.

To compensate for the inadequate oxygenation, the patient must increase ventilation of those lung units which are relatively free of obstruction. This increase in minute ventilation, although effective alveolar ventilation is low, increases the work of breathing because of the high airways resistance which exists. The oxygen cost of the extra work entailed can become quite high, so that many of these patients, both chronically and especially following an acute insult, cannot maintain a level of alveolar ventilation good enough to eliminate CO_2 at a normal rate. Alveolar hypoventilation with resultant hypercapnia, respiratory acidosis, and more profound hypoxemia ensues. These derangements of alveolar and arterial gas tensions and pH lead to an increase in pulmonary vascular resistance caused by the contraction of smooth muscle fibers within the walls of pulmonary arterioles. Pulmonary hypertension and possibly acute right ventricular failure may result.

If a patient manifests chronic alveolar hypoventilation with CO_2 retention, the normal drive to ventilation occasioned by the concentration of CO_2 in the blood is decreased. The coexistent hypoxemia becomes the more important stimulus for maintaining the level of alveolar ventilation. This is an important concept in the treatment of these patients, as elimination of hypoxia as a drive to ventilation by means of overaggressive use of supplemental oxygen therapy may fatally suppress alveolar ventilation.

Treatment of Acute Respiratory Failure in the Setting of Chronic Bronchitis or Emphysema

There are two basic principles involved in the treatment of acute respiratory failure in the patient with airways obstruction: (1) *Improve hypoxemia,* utilizing controlled low-flow oxygen. (2) *Clear the obstructed airways.*

Oxygen. Oxygen is a drug, and, like other drugs, it has therapeutic and toxic levels. Fortunately it is a drug whose blood levels may be rapidly determined. In administering oxygen certain conditions are fundamental and must be understood. First, it is the Fio_2 which is the major determinant of the toxicity of oxygen to the lungs, not the Pao_2. Oxygen toxicity increases rapidly as the Fio_2 rises above levels of about 60 per cent. Second, the body's oxygen stores are small, and hence decreases in the Fio_2 result in very rapid lowering of the Pao_2; intermittent oxygen therapy has no place in the management of acute respiratory failure. Third, the treatment of hypoxemia must be prompt, but, especially in patients with chronic lung disease, the Pao_2 should be brought toward but not to normal levels. In patients with chronic obstructive lung disease, especially those with chronic hypercapnia, complete correction of hypoxemia may result in severe alveolar hypoventilation and dangerous acidosis. Furthermore, there is almost never a reason to maintain arterial oxygen tensions above normal levels.

The goal of O_2 therapy should be to attain a Pao_2 in the range of 50 to 60 mm. Hg. This represents a hemoglobin O_2 saturation of 85 to 90 per cent. Above a Pao_2 of 60 mm. Hg, little further gain in additional O_2 content of the blood is achieved. In these patients, only small increments in Fio_2 (the fraction of O_2 in the inspired gas mixture) above ambient air are usually necessary to achieve this desired rise in Pao_2. This approach is rendered feasible because of the shape of the oxygen-hemoglobin dissociation curve, which, over the range of O_2 tensions that have been discussed, facilitates prompt loading of O_2 molecules onto the carriage molecule of hemoglobin, so that essentially full saturation of the blood is achieved at a Pao_2 of 55 to 60 mm. Hg.

There are several methods of delivering low concentrations of O_2. The most popular are by means of a soft rubber tube with small prongs which fit into the patient's nostrils (nasal cannulas), or by means of a commercially available mask which operates on the Venturi principle of high air flow with oxygen enrichment, mixing the O_2 in the final gas mixture which enters the mask surrounding the patient's nose and mouth; for example, to achieve an Fio_2 of 28 per cent, ten parts of room air are entrained and mixed with one part of 100 per cent oxygen.

We prefer to use nasal cannulas with a flow rate of 1 to 2 liters per minute as the initial O_2 delivery device in our patients, because they are more comfortable for the patient and allow him to cough and expectorate his secretions freely without the encumbrance of a mask about his face. It should be noted that when using nasal cannulas the flow rate is very important in determining the final Fio_2 delivered to the patient. In addition the Fio_2 delivered at any particular flow rate will vary, depending upon the patient's ventilatory rate and pattern. The adequacy and effect of oxygen administration must be monitored through repeated sampling of arterial blood gases.

The Venturi mask device allows much more precise control of the Fio_2, fairly independently of the flow rate set at the wall. Venturi masks are available to deliver O_2 concentrations of 24, 26, 28, 31, 35, and 40 per cent. Generally, the physician will choose a mask at 24 to 28 per cent when initiating O_2 therapy in a patient in acute respiratory failure superimposed upon chronic airways disease. The adequacy of oxygen therapy must then be assessed 20 to 30 minutes later by means of arterial blood gases. If the desired Pao_2 has not been achieved, a higher concentration of O_2 is delivered, with repeated monitoring of arterial blood gases.

Regardless of the device used to deliver controlled low-flow oxygen, it is usually feasible to achieve adequate tissue O_2 delivery without causing progressive ventilatory depression with worsening respiratory acidosis.

Measures to Clear the Airways. After O_2 therapy has been instituted, the physician must then direct his attention toward clearing the airway and/or treating other underlying causes of the acute decompensation.

1. *Chest physiotherapy:* Percussion and vibration of the chest, combined with encouragement to cough and to breathe deeply, aid the patient in raising his secretions. Sometimes the encouragement must be more than gentle. Continuous

badgering of the patient is necessary to produce an effective cough and to keep him awake. A physician, a nurse trained in respiratory care, or a competent respiratory therapist must be constantly in attendance to ensure that the patient remains awake, breathing, and coughing effectively.

2. *Nasotracheal suctioning* may be required to physically remove secretions and to further stimulate the patient to cough and to take deep breaths if these acts cannot be performed voluntarily.

3. *Bronchodilators* are usually given to decrease airways resistance. A continuous intravenous infusion of aminophylline (theophylline ethylenediamine) should be administered at a rate of 0.9 mg. per kg. per hour, after an initial loading dose of 6 mg. per kg. over 20 minutes. These dosage regimens should be decreased slightly in the presence of liver disease, congestive heart failure, or advanced age. A nomogram is available to guide initial therapy (Ann. Intern. Med., *86*:400, 1977). If signs of toxicity are witnessed (nausea, vomiting, arrhythmias, seizures, coma) or if lack of response is noted, theophylline serum levels should be obtained to guide further therapy (optimal therapeutic levels are 10 to 20 mg. per liter).

In addition, a bronchodilator of the adrenergic agonist class should be administered either topically or systemically. There seems to be a synergistic effect between the use of a theophylline salt and an adrenergic agonist in mediating maximal bronchodilatation. We prefer either isoproterenol (0.5 ml. of 1:200 aqueous solution in 2.5 to 5 ml. of isotonic saline) or isoetharine (0.5 ml. in 2.5 to 5 ml. of saline) aerosolized into the tracheobronchial tree via a side-arm nebulization device until the entire volume (3 to 5 ml.) has been delivered. There are few data to suggest an advantage to the use of intermittent positive pressure breathing (IPPB) in the delivery of topical bronchodilators in most patients, unless the patient is too feeble to take a deep breath.

Even if wheezing is not heard, bronchodilators should usually be given for the following reasons: (1) very slight changes in airway resistance can significantly improve flow rates; (2) the theophylline bronchodilators act as central respiratory stimulants; and (3) they enhance mucociliary clearance, thus aiding in the removal of bronchial secretions.

4. *Antibiotics* must be instituted if infection of the tracheobronchial tree is observed or suspected. The choice of antibiotic should be guided by the flora seen on Gram stain of the sputum. If no predominant organism is seen, ampicillin, 500 mg. orally every 6 hours, or tetracycline, 500 mg. orally every 6 hours, is a sensible choice for initial therapy because of the frequent implication of *Hemophilus influenzae* in the genesis of acute bronchitis in this setting. The sputum should be submitted for culture, with antibiotic therapy subsequently being tailored to the susceptibility pattern of the organisms that are grown.

5. *Adequate hydration* is essential for loosening and liquefaction of thick, tenacious secretions. We feel that it is necessary to deliver fluid either orally or parenterally to best achieve this goal. There is some question about the ability of nebulized water to penetrate mucus and alter its viscosity. The bronchitic should receive at least 2 to 3 liters of fluid each day after any fluid deficit has been corrected. Mucolytic agents such as acetylcysteine are of no proved value in the liquefaction of secretions when delivered as an aerosol; indeed, they may provoke bronchospasm.

6. *Corticosteroids* may be used if bronchospasm is a prominent feature of the disease; they always should be given to the asthmatic in acute respiratory failure. If indicated, they should be used early in the course. We usually give the equivalent of 40 to 60 mg. of prednisone each day.

Other Specific Measures. 1. *Diuretics* are indicated in the presence of left ventricular failure or if the patient is fluid overloaded. They should be administered cautiously, as there may be a risk of drying secretions if the patient is overdiuresed. It should be remembered that the right ventricle fails in this disease because of the profound rise in pulmonary vascular resistance caused by alveolar hypoxia and acidosis. Correction of the hypoxemia and acid-base balance is usually more effective in improving right ventricular function than are diuretics.

2. *Anticoagulants* are indicated if pulmonary emboli are strongly suspected or documented. Therapeutic anticoagulation with heparin should be employed under these circumstances. We frequently utilize "mini-dose" heparin (5000 units subcutaneously every 8 or 12 hours) if the patient has edema or will be confined to bed for any period of time, as prophylaxis against de novo pulmonary embolism.

3. The role of *digitalis* is controversial in the treatment of cor pulmonale. We administer digitalis in the setting of clear-cut left ventricular failure or for control of sensitive arrhythmias (e.g., atrial fibrillation, atrial flutter).

4. *Phlebotomy* should be performed if the hematocrit exceeds 55 per cent.

5. *Electrolyte disturbances,* especially potassium depletion, should be looked for and vigorously corrected. Potassium should be given as KCl.

6. *Sedation* is generally contraindicated in the

management of the chronic bronchitic in acute respiratory failure. Indeed, as indicated earlier, even very small dosages of sedatives or hypnotics may cause acute respiratory failure in these patients.

7. *Tube thoracostomy* should be utilized to evacuate a pneumothorax if one is documented.

Failure of Medical Management. The aforementioned measures, if conscientiously applied through a dedicated team effort, are of proved value in correcting acute respiratory failure in the setting of chronic bronchitis and emphysema. The object of therapy is to maintain oxygenation while clearing the airways and to avoid the necessity for endotracheal intubation and mechanical ventilatory support while accomplishing this objective. Nevertheless, despite impeccable care, an occasional patient will grow progressively more fatigued with worsening respiratory acidosis, requiring total mechanical ventilatory support.

Intubation. When mechanical ventilation is employed, a sealed connection between the ventilator and tracheobronchial tree must be established. This is accomplished by use of a flexible plastic tube with a balloon at one end which can be inflated to establish a seal against the tracheal wall. The endotracheal tube should be passed by a skilled person knowledgeable in the anatomy of the upper airway, larynx, and trachea. It can be inserted through either the nose or the mouth, through the pharynx and larynx into the trachea. The transnasal route is preferred in a conscious patient, because it is generally more comfortable. Once in proper position, the balloon or cuff is inflated with a volume of air great enough to prevent the leakage of any air around the tube when the lungs are inflated by the ventilator under positive pressure. Overinflation of the cuff can result in extraordinarily high pressures being exerted upon the tracheal mucosa, with possible impairment of capillary flow and resultant tracheal damage. Endotracheal tubes with high volume, low pressure soft cuffs should be used instead of the older, low compliance, stiff balloons.

The internal diameter of an endotracheal tube can be critically important, especially in terms of facilitating the weaning process (when the patient is removed from mechanical ventilatory support). One of the prime determinants of the resistance of tube is its radius. For example, reducing the radius of a tube by one half increases the resistance of the tube *16* times. Consequently one should always place the largest possible endotracheal tube that can be passed in a patient requiring intubation. Endotracheal tubes are generally numbered according to their internal diameter in millimeters. A size 7 or 8 mm. ID (internal diameter) endotracheal tube should usually be used. We will return to the issue of artificial airway resistance when we discuss weaning techniques.

The endotracheal tube allows direct access to the secretions within the airways; these are removed by periodic suctioning with a sterile soft rubber catheter.

An endotracheal tube bypasses the lung's normal humidification mechanisms in the nose. Consequently gas mixtures delivered through an endotracheal tube must be adequately humidified, as well as warmed to body temperature to prevent desiccation of the respiratory tract mucosa and its secretions.

Mechanical Ventilation. The cuffed endotracheal tube allows the delivery of gas mixtures into the lungs under positive pressure. A mechanical ventilator generates the positive pressure needed as a driving force to cause air to flow from the mouth down to the alveolus. Exhalation remains passive as the lungs' elastic recoil causes them to shrink back to their functional residual capacity (FRC) resting level.

A variety of mechanical ventilators are available at this time. They can be divided into two major groups: pressure-cycled machines and volume-cycled machines. On a pressure-cycled machine, the physician presets a pressure limit; respiratory flow continues after the timing mechanism turns the machine on until the pressure limit is achieved; the delivered tidal volume is variable, depending on the state of lung compliance and airways resistance (i.e., the pressure limit will be rapidly reached after delivery of a small tidal volume if the lungs are noncompliant or if airways resistance is high). All pressure-cycled machines have relatively low pressure capabilities; effective peak pressure is only 30 to 40 cm. H_2O. These machines cannot be used effectively in the patient with adult respiratory distress syndrome (ARDS). However, in most cases of acute respiratory failure in the setting of chronic airways obstruction, they can adequately ventilate the lungs, as the compliance is increased and the airways resistance, although greater than normal, is not extremely elevated. They also allow control of the inspiratory flow rate, which allows the operator to control the flow wave pattern, achieving great patient comfort and often better gas distribution within a pair of lungs whose individual units have varying degrees of obstruction within their conducting airways.

Volume-cycled ventilators will generate whatever pressure is necessary to deliver a preset volume, up to the maximum pressure-generating capabilities of the machine, which is generally on the order of 80 to 100 cm. H_2O. Considering that during normal spontaneous ventilation the airway pressures rarely rise above 5 cm. H_2O, levels of 80 to 100 cm. H_2O are more than adequate to achieve air flow even when the airways resistance is extremely high or lung compliance is severely decreased. Indeed, if pressures at this maximal level are required, the danger of alveolar rupture with resultant pneumothorax is great. Volume ventilators can be used in the management of the type of acute respiratory failure currently under discussion.

VENTILATING THE PATIENT WITH AIRWAYS OBSTRUCTION AND ACUTE RESPIRATORY FAILURE. Once placed on a mechanical ventilator, it is generally easy to oxygenate and ventilate these patients. The initial goals of ventilatory therapy will generally be as follows:

1. To ensure adequate oxygenation.
2. To clear the airways of secretions through frequent endotracheal suctioning.
3. To slowly lower the $Paco_2$.
4. To allow the exhausted patient, who has been working extremely hard to breathe for several days or weeks, to rest.

It is usually easy to establish the desired interface between machine and patient in this particular type of disease. The tidal volume should be on the low side, on the order of 8 ml. per kg. of body weight at a rate of 10 to 12 times per minute. The patient may be allowed to trigger the machine to initiate a respiratory cycle; indeed, this is often desirable, as it exercises the respiratory muscles and prevents the development of dyssynchronous respiratory movements which can make weaning from the ventilator difficult. The smaller minute volume allows for slow correction of the respiratory acidosis which has developed. Too rapid correction of this disturbance can result in a severe respiratory alkalosis with consequent seizures, coma, arrhythmias, and bronchospasm.

The patient with chronic CO_2 retention should never be ventilated rapidly to a normal $Paco_2$; he will definitely become alkalotic. The physician should aim for correction of pH, not $Paco_2$.

WEANING FROM MECHANICAL VENTILATION. After correction or improvement of the process which resulted in acute respiratory decompensation, the physician must institute weaning procedures to allow the patient to resume the work of breathing on his own, to break the interface with the machine, and to remove the artificial airway, so that the integrity of upper airway defense mechanisms may be restored. In the patient with altered respiratory mechanics, weaning can often be a prolonged and tedious process. In general, the longer the endotracheal tube is in place, the more difficult the weaning process is liable to be; therefore weaning should start as soon as possible. We practice a very aggressive approach to weaning. A trial at weaning the bronchitic from mechanical ventilation should be attempted as soon as he has had a rest for several hours, or overnight, and as soon as improvement is noted in his airways obstruction by diminished bronchospasm and thinning of secretions.

There are certain objective parameters which correlate with successful weaning and the ability to carry on spontaneous ventilation for a prolonged period of time. We recommend that the following parameters be measured and met by most patients prior to the onset of weaning: (1) A tidal volume of greater than 5 ml. per kg. (2) A vital capacity of 10 to 15 ml. per kg. (3) A maximum inspiratory force of at least -20 cm. H_2O.

Several additional parameters at a slightly more sophisticated level also convey information about the lungs' functional status: (1) Alveolar-arterial oxygen gradient breathing 100 per cent oxygen (P [A-aDo_2]) of less than 350 mm. Hg. (2) Dead space to tidal volume ratio (V_D/V_T) of less than 0.6. (3) Functional residual capacity of more than 50 per cent of predicted.

There are two general methods of weaning. One technique involves the use of a T-piece adaptor and the complete cessation of mechanical ventilator support. The procedural steps in the method are as follows:

1. The patient is first informed of the details of the process which is to take place.
2. He should be placed in a sitting position, either in bed or in a chair.
3. Vital signs and arterial blood gases should be measured and recorded prior to the onset of actual weaning.
4. The patient should be well suctioned.
5. A length of wide-bore tubing is connected to a high-flow humidified gas source, at the same or slightly higher Fio_2 than the patient has been receiving while on the machine. The tubing is connected to the endotracheal tube via a "T-piece" adaptor, and the ventilator is turned off. The patient is allowed to breathe spontaneously, drawing his inspired gas mixture from the high-flow system.
6. Vital signs (blood pressure, pulse, respiratory rate) should be monitored frequently. Measurement of arterial blood gases should be repeated after approximately 20 minutes and then at about hourly intervals.
7. If the patient seems to be tolerating the weaning procedure well without change in vital signs or arterial blood gases, the endotracheal tube should be removed at the end of a suitable period of time. One should remember that the artificial airway possesses a higher resistance than the normal upper airway. If the patient (who al-

ready has altered lung mechanics which demand greater work on his part to ventilate his diseased lungs) is asked to perform the work necessary to breathe against this added resistance for a prolonged period of time, he may grow fatigued. This would result in worsening CO_2 retention and progressive respiratory acidosis. Such events are often interpreted by the physician as a failure to wean. We feel that it is often beneficial to remove the endotracheal tube at an earlier point in the weaning process, before the patient evidences signs of fatigue. For example, if the arterial blood gases have remained stable after the first hour or hour and a half of weaning, the tube should be removed at that time.

8. If at any time during the weaning process the patient should evidence a change in his vital signs (hypertension, tachycardia, hypotension, tachypnea), complain of shortness of breath, become diaphoretic, or manifest a cardiac arrhythmia, he should immediately be placed back on the mechanical ventilator and a set of arterial blood gases should be drawn for subsequent documentation and correlation with the clinical situation which has been observed.

9. If the initial attempt at weaning is unsuccessful, the physician should attempt to identify those factors which may contribute to a failure to wean. Chief among these are inadequate resolution of the underlying acute pulmonary pathology; increased ventilatory requirements, such as might be occasioned by fever; or decreased muscle strength, often resulting from the patient's catabolic state. Problems occasioned by an increased work of breathing must also be considered; the issue of a small-bore endotracheal tube has already been mentioned. Remedial factors should be promptly corrected and attempts at weaning resumed.

10. Continued failure to wean demands the development of a coordinated plan of attack whereby the patient is allowed to gradually develop his physical and psychological independence of the machine. Several periods of weaning should be undertaken each day.

11. If the weaning process is prolonged beyond 7 to 10 days, the cuffed endotracheal tube, which has been inserted through either the nose or mouth, should be replaced by a tracheostomy. This not only contributes to greater patient comfort and lessens the total airway resistance; it also decreases the risk of damage to the tracheal mucosa. Bronchopulmonary toilet is facilitated through the shorter tracheostomy tube.

An alternative method of weaning, so-called intermittent mandatory ventilation (IMV), entails the gradual withdrawal of machine support, rather than the all-or-nothing, "sink or swim" approach demanded by the more traditional weaning procedures. Utilizing an IMV set-up, the ventilator is adapted to provide "mandatory" breaths to the patient at regular intervals (for example, at an IMV rate of 6, the machine would deliver the selected tidal volume every 10 seconds, or six times each minute). The patient is allowed to breathe spontaneously between IMV breaths, drawing his inspired gas mixture from a reservoir source (usually an anesthesia bag) set up in parallel with the machine. As the patient gains strength and displays his ability to function independently of the machine, the machine's component of the total minute ventilation is gradually reduced by decreasing the frequency of IMV breaths.

Unfortunately, although promising in theory, we have not found IMV to be particularly valuable in weaning many patients, especially those with chronic bronchitis and emphysema. The work of breathing against an artificial airway by a patient with abnormal lung mechanics generally proves to be too great; the bronchitic, in our experience, usually tires quickly in this setting. We have found it necessary to alternate between periods of rest and weaning during which the patient is performing essentially all the work of breathing.

ACUTE RESPIRATORY FAILURE IN THE PATIENT WITH PREVIOUSLY HEALTHY LUNGS

The patient who sustains an acute insult which damages the alveolar capillary membrane presents with a readily recognizable syndrome of clinical, physiologic, and pathologic features termed the adult respiratory distress syndrome (ARDS). The term is a nonspecific one, meant to encompass the many divergent causative events which give rise to the common clinical and pathologic features. The term is probably derived from the earlier-popularized "respiratory distress syndrome" of the newborn; however, it should be understood that the similarity in wording does not imply similar causes for these two disease entities.

In ARDS, damage occurs at the gas-exchange membrane, which results in two basic events: (1) altered permeability of the pulmonary capillaries, with movement of water, proteins, and cellular components of blood into the interstitial connective tissue of the lung as well as into the alveolar spaces themselves; and (2) loss of stability of alveoli and terminal airways so that they tend to collapse at low lung volumes (the role of surfactant deficiency in this alveolar instability is suspected but at present remains unsettled). If blood continues to flow through the lungs past fluid-filled and collapsed alveoli, it will not come into contact with oxygen, and consequently will not be oxygenated. This is known as shunting—i.e., the passage of blood from the right to the left side of the circulation without increase in oxygen content.

The clinical manifestations of this disease process stem from these underlying pathophysiologic disturbances. The fluid-filled and collapsed alveoli render the lungs stiff (noncompliant) and decrease the volume of air in the lungs (the functional residual capacity is decreased). These noncompliant lungs require greater pressures to inflate them, and consequently the work of breathing is markedly increased. O_2 uptake is usually markedly impaired, and the measurement of arterial blood gases will reveal profound hypoxemia and a compensatory respiratory alkalosis. If tissue oxygen delivery is below normal, a metabolic acidosis may be observed as anaerobic cellular metabolism ensues. The hypoxemia is resistant to the administration of supplemental oxygen; at even a very high Fio_2, oxygen simply never arrives at the gas exchange membrane where it can diffuse across into the pulmonary capillary blood.

Clinically, the patient complains of profound dyspnea and is noted to be markedly tachypneic and often cyanotic.

Clinical Situations Which Predispose to the Development of ARDS

A large and growing number of insults are associated with the development of ARDS:

1. Systemic hypotension ("shock lung")—hemorrhagic, traumatic, or septic.
2. Severe, diffuse pneumonia—viral, bacterial, or tuberculous.
3. Aspiration of gastric contents.
4. Local trauma to the lung.
5. Fat embolism.
6. Head injury or central nervous system (CNS) insult ("neurogenic pulmonary edema").
7. Breathing high concentrations of oxygen ("oxygen-toxicity lung").
8. Drug overdose, as in heroin abuse.
9. Infiltrative lung disease of diverse causes (e.g., miliary tuberculous, lymphangitic carcinomatosis).
10. Uremia.
11. Radiation pneumonitis.
12. Pancreatitis.
13. Prolonged cardiopulmonary bypass.
14. Disseminated intravascular coagulation.

Detection of ARDS

The measurement of arterial blood gases is necessary for the early detection of hypoxemia caused by developing ARDS. These should be measured *serially* in any patient with conditions predisposing to the ARDS and in any patient with tachypnea, restlessness, air hunger, confusion, or infiltration on the chest x-ray. In late stages of the syndrome cyanosis may be obvious, but arterial blood gases are still essential to guide therapy.

Having established the presence of diffuse pulmonary infiltration and hypoxemia, it is important to exclude those causes that may be remediable by specific therapy, particularly acute left ventricular failure. Unfortunately, clinical signs are often misleading and do not allow for conclusive exclusion of a diagnosis of left ventricular failure. For this purpose, all these patients should have their left atrial pressures estimated. The most reliable determination currently available clinically is the pulmonary capillary wedge pressure (PCWP), which is obtained by passing a Swan-Ganz catheter (balloon-tip flotation catheter) into a small pulmonary arterial branch. When the balloon at the catheter tip is subsequently inflated, one may measure the back pressure transmitted through the pulmonary veins and pulmonary capillary bed from the left atrium. PCWP thus reflects left atrial filling pressure. If the PCWP is elevated, some degree of left ventricular failure is present and should be treated with diuretics and inotropic agents. If PCWP is normal, the likelihood that the symptoms hypoxemia and pulmonary infiltration are due to ARDS is enhanced.

Therapy

The therapy of ARDS is primarily nonspecific, consisting of supportive measures. The goals are (1) to prevent the patient from dying of tissue anoxia and (2) to prevent further damage to the alveolar capillary membrane. One is in essence buying time for the lung to repair itself.

Oxygenation. The conventional methods of administering supplemental oxygen are generally not effective in improving the arterial oxygen content in this disease. In the face of a physiologic shunt of greater than 25 per cent of the total cardiac output, raising the Fio_2 to 100 per cent will achieve little improvement in the Pao_2. As explained earlier, the oxygen molecules do not physically reach the gas exchange membrane where they can diffuse across and into the capillary blood. In milder cases, however, when the percentage of shunting is low, increasing the Fio_2 may be sufficient to raise the Pao_2 to acceptable levels.

The use of oxygen is limited by the occurrence of oxygen toxicity at higher Fio_2. Oxygen toxicity causes cellular and subcellular changes which are perceived clinically as organ dysfunction. In the case of the lungs, there is damage to the alveolar-capillary membrane which is indistinguishable from the damage seen in ARDS—an obvious vicious cycle whereby the treatment becomes part of the disease itself. A major problem is thus to relieve hypoxemia without increasing the Fio_2 to levels at which oxygen toxicity occurs. In general, clinically significant O_2 toxicity rarely occurs below an Fio_2 of 40 per cent. Oxygen toxicity will occur rather frequently if the Fio_2 is above 60 to 80 per cent for more than 72 to 96 hours. The higher the Fio_2 and the longer the duration of exposure to O_2, the greater the risk of development of O_2 toxicity becomes. In practice when an Fio_2 of greater than 40 per cent is required to maintain a Pao_2 of 60 torr or greater, the patient should be placed on a ventilator, and positive end-expiratory pressure (PEEP) should be instituted in an attempt to improve the oxygenation.

Mechanical Ventilation of ARDS. 1. *Volume-cycled ventilators* are preferable because of the high distending pressures required to inflate lungs with decreased compliance.

2. *Large tidal volumes* on the order of 15 ml. per kg. should be employed in an attempt to reopen collapsed terminal lung units, and thus improve gas exchange.

3. *Establishing an interface* between the machine and the patient can often be quite difficult. A patient with stiff lungs tends to hyperventilate despite correction of hypoxemia. If he is allowed to trigger the respirator each time he takes a breath, he will develop respiratory alkalosis, sometimes of profound degrees. This can be corrected by sedating or paralyzing the patient, or by adding additional dead space to the ventilator circuitry so that the patient rebreathes CO_2, thus raising his $Fico_2$ and partially correcting the alkalosis. The problem of hyperventilation can also be solved by the use of IMV.

4. Intermittent mandatory ventilation (IMV) is a useful adjunct in ventilating patients with ARDS. It allows the patient who has stiff lungs to establish his own respiratory frequency. The mechanical ventilator is then adjusted to deliver only that additional amount of ventilation which is necessary to maintain a normal level of alveolar ventilation ($Paco_2$ of approximately 40 torr). This can generally be achieved at an IMV rate of 2 to 4. Such a procedure usually eliminates the need for heavy sedation or for muscular paralysis. Machine and patient are easily interfaced utilizing IMV.

Positive End-Expiratory Pressure (PEEP). Positive end-expiratory pressure refers to the maintenance of positive pressure within the airways at end-expiration. In other words, one is preventing the lungs from returning to atmospheric pressure; they remain partially inflated. The use of PEEP has been correlated with improvement in the Pao_2 when used in patients with ARDS. PEEP seems to exert this effect by (1) reinflating collapsed or closed alveoli and then maintaining them in a state of partial inflation, so that they will not collapse; (2) redistributing the fluid within a fluid-filled alveolus in a meniscus shape, so that the distance that O_2 must diffuse to reach the capillary blood is greatly reduced; and (3) conserving surfactant on the alveolar surface.

Blood flowing past re-expanded alveoli and alveoli in which the fluid has been redistributed now stands a good chance of coming into contact with O_2 and thereby increasing the total arterial O_2 content. Thus PEEP works by mechanical means to facilitate gas transport in the patient with ARDS.

PEEP, however, is not without adverse effects. Normally, venous return and hence cardiac output are enhanced during inspiration when a negative pressure exists within the thorax. When continuous *positive* pressure is maintained throughout the respiratory cycle, there may be serious impairment of cardiac filling, with resultant fall in cardiac output. One may thus have a situation in which the Pao_2 and the O_2 content of the blood are improved but the delivery of O_2 to the tissues is decreased by a fall in cardiac output. This potential decrease in O_2 transport to tissues (cardiac output × total arterial O_2 content) demands the measurements of parameters such as cardiac output and O_2 extraction as guides to the level of PEEP to use. The placement of a Swan-Ganz catheter allows such measurements to be made with minimal difficulty.

We generally will begin the patient on 5 to 10 cm. H_2O of PEEP, and then measure the resultant change in Pao_2 through arterial blood gases drawn 15 to 20 minutes after institution of PEEP. We will also at this time draw blood from the pulmonary artery for a mixed venous Pvo_2 and perform a cardiac output determination. If the desired improvement in gas exchange is not observed, further increments of PEEP are added until an optimal level of tissue O_2 delivery is achieved at an acceptable Fio_2 (less than 50 per cent).

Another potential complication related to the use of PEEP is barotrauma—i.e., pneumothorax, pneumomediastinum, and subcutaneous emphysema. The first of these must be treated with tube thoracostomy to evacuate the air. PEEP generally must be continued even in the face of such complications, as maintenance of acceptable oxygenation remains the paramount consideration.

Fluid Balance. In the face of altered pulmonary capillary permeability and an excess accumulation of water in the lung, fluid balance often can play a decisive role in determining the survival of the patient with ARDS.

1. *Dehydration:* In general, the physician should maintain these patients in a negative fluid balance. Lowering the hydrostatic pressure within the pulmonary capillary bed should potentially prevent the extravasation of further quantities of water into the interstitial compartment and into the alveolar spaces themselves. Patients on prolonged artificial ventilation tend to retain fluid unless their water balance is carefully monitored. We feel that all patients with severe ARDS, necessitating the use of PEEP for support of their oxygenation, require repeated monitoring of pulmonary capillary wedge pressures and cardiac outputs (using a Swan-Ganz catheter) to guide their fluid therapy. In general one is aiming for the lowest possible filling pressure which still maintains an adequate circulating blood volume and cardiac output. Daily weights should also be obtained. As a rule of thumb these patients, because they are in a catabolic state, should be expected to lose 300 to 500 grams of body weight daily.

2. *Diuretics* are frequently required to maintain an appropriate water balance. In some patients diuretics will mobilize a considerable amount of extravascular fluid from the lungs, and result in marked improvement in gas exchange. For this purpose, furosemide in appropriate dosages should be administered.

3. *Colloids:* Salt-poor albumin and other colloids may prove useful in selected patients by raising the oncotic pressure within pulmonary capillaries so that interstitial water re-enters the vessel. Unfortunately, one cannot reliably predict in which patients this effect can be expected to occur. Indeed, there is considerable risk that protein molecules will rapidly leave the pulmonary vessels with their altered permeability and enter the interstitial tissues and alveolar spaces, where they will serve to draw further water out of the vessels. There are no clear-cut guidelines for the use of colloids in this setting.

Other Therapeutic Modalities. *Corticosteroids* are of unproved value in the treatment of most conditions causing ARDS, despite the fact that many physicians routinely use them in all forms of ARDS. We generally administer corticosteroids in ARDS associated with chemical lung injury (e.g., aspiration pneumonia), in viral pneumonias, and if fat emboli are present. They should be given in high dosage (150 to 250 mg. of hydrocortisone equivalent every 4 to 6 hours) for 48 to 72 hours and then stopped if there is no improvement.

Antibiotics should be administered if one has documented a specific bacterial pathogen. Appropriate chemotherapy against tuberculosis would be indicated in the setting of miliary tuberculosis or overwhelming pulmonary tuberculosis.

Adequate nutrition should be maintained. The early use of enteral or parenteral alimentation to prevent protein catabolism may play a role in hastening tissue repair within the lung.

The patient should be assiduously monitored for the occurrence of *superinfection.* Gram stains should be made of the sputum every 2 to 3 days. If sheets of organisms are seen, appropriate antibiotic coverage should be instituted. Sepsis is a common cause of death in the patient with ARDS who has been successfully supported over the first few days of his illness.

Extracorporeal membrane oxygenation does not improve survival in this disease.

Course of ARDS

The course of the disease is often prolonged, demanding measures to support oxygenation for periods of several weeks. Early tracheostomy is frequently desirable to facilitate care of the artificial airway and for purposes of patient comfort.

When stabilization and improvement in gas exchange become apparent, the physician may cautiously begin to wean the patient from PEEP and mechanical ventilatory support. Often the mechanical support can be discontinued before weaning from PEEP. We generally begin to back off on PEEP by decrements of 5 cm. H_2O, following parameters of gas exchange and tissue oxygen delivery. It is generally desirable to attain a Pa_{O_2} of greater than 60 mm. Hg off PEEP with an Fi_{O_2} less than 40 to 50 per cent before removing the endotracheal tube. Weaning may be hampered by the patient's poor nutritional status with loss of muscular strength and an increased work of breathing resulting from residual scarring in the damaged lung.

RESPIRATORY FAILURE IN THE SETTING OF NEUROMUSCULAR DISEASE

Acute respiratory failure resulting from impairment of the normal bellows mechanism (e.g., drug overdose, neuromuscular disease) demands mechanical support of bellows function until the acute event has been reversed, if possible. Unfortunately, many of the neuromuscular diseases which affect the bellows are chronic in nature, and little or no improvement in ventilatory function can be expected. In such instances chronic mechanical ventilatory support is demanded. These patients are generally quite easy to ventilate, as their lungs are not diseased and possess normal compliance and normal resistance. One can utilize pressure-cycled, volume-cycled, or even negative pressure machines.

CHRONIC BRONCHITIS AND EMPHYSEMA

method of
STEVEN G. KELSEN, M.D.,
and NEIL S. CHERNIACK, M.D.
Cleveland, Ohio

Chronic bronchitis produces inflammation of the airways with excessive mucus production and can be diagnosed *clinically* by a history of cough and sputum production on most days for 3 consecutive months in 2 successive years. Emphysema, on the other hand, produces dilatation and destruction of air spaces distal to the terminal bronchiole and is diagnosed *pathologically*. In chronic bronchitis, the functional disturbances result from inflammatory narrowing and an increase in secretions within the airway lumen. In emphysema, they result from a disruption of the lungs' tissue elements which act to "tether" and maintain the patency of the intrapulmonary airways. Collectively, the two diseases make up the category of lung diseases described by the term chronic obstructive pulmonary disease (COPD). They are characterized functionally by (1) obstruction to airflow, (2) hyperinflation of the lungs with air trapping, (3) impaired efficiency of oxygen and carbon dioxide exchange, and (4) an increased work of breathing. The effects of emphysema and chronic bronchitis can be distinguished in the laboratory. Emphysema decreases lung elastic recoil and the D_LCO. This is, however, of little help clinically, because in the vast majority of subjects both processes are present simultaneously so that the therapeutic approach is the same.

Of great importance is recent evidence suggesting that the earliest lesions in COPD occur in the small (less than 2 mm. diameter) airways which produce no symptoms. Symptomatic, clinically evident disease develops only after many years when extensive involvement of the small airways has occurred. Detection of the disease in its subclinical form is now possible with readily available noninvasive techniques. These tests can be incorporated easily in the routine of the regular health check-up. Lesions detected at this stage of the disease may be completely reversible with elimination of the inciting factors such as cigarette smoke or industrial toxins.

Unfortunately, the majority of patients are first seen by the physician when the characteristic symptoms of shortness of breath and exercise limitation are already present. At this stage, normal lung function cannot be restored and the aims of medical management become (1) prevention of conditions which can accelerate pulmonary dysfunction, such as infection or exposure to bronchial irritants; (2) correction of reversible factors contributing to airflow obstruction (e.g., relief of bronchospasm and elimination of secretions); (3) treatment of secondary complications, such as congestive heart failure and acute respiratory failure; and (4) various supportive measures which improve the life style of the patient.

Overall Approaches

Minimizing the Progressive Loss of Pulmonary Function. The slow decrease in pulmonary function over time which occurs in most patients with chronic bronchitis and emphysema is greater than can be accounted for by an aging process alone. It is suspected that multiple factors contribute to the loss of lung function. One factor may be continued cigarette smoking. Although lung function deteriorates with age more rapidly in smokers than in nonsmokers, it is not clear if the rate of deterioration is affected by smoking in patients with *established* bronchitis and emphysema. It is known, however, that an acute increase in airway resistance may be produced by smoking only a single cigarette. Furthermore, most patients will report a reduction of the volume of sputum produced when cigarette smoking is discontinued, as well as a subjective improvement in the state of well-being. Therefore cessation of smoking is the first step in the therapeutic regimen for all patients.

A careful history is the key to pinpointing irritants in the work place and home environment which should be avoided. It is well known that the number of respiratory deaths increases during periods of severe atmospheric pollution. Patients living or working in areas with continuously high levels of air pollution which produce symptoms may benefit from a temporary or permanent change in their living or working location.

Inflammatory reactions introduce proteolytic enzymes which may digest lung tissue. This may explain why significant reductions in lung function may occur after acute respiratory infection. For example, a single acute bacterial pneumonia can produce respiratory failure in patients with borderline respiratory function. Furthermore, viral respiratory tract infections may account for as many as two thirds of all symptomatic episodes. Viral infections may interfere with lung clearance mechanisms and increase the susceptibility of the lung to bacterial colonization.

Given these considerations, patients with COPD should receive annual influenza vaccination against the prevalent strains. Studies have indicated that patients with chronic bronchitis given antibiotics prophylactically at the first sign of a respiratory tract infection (upper or lower) or simply when the sputum becomes purulent tend to have less morbidity in terms of hospitalizations and days lost from work. Furthermore, the duration of acute symptomatic exacerbations is reduced. This indicates that antibiotic therapy should be instituted early in all respiratory tract infections. Continuous administration of antibiotics over the winter months in some patients with repeated infections seems to be advisable.

Correction of Reversible Factors Which Contribute to Airflow Obstruction. In emphysema, airflow is reduced by airway collapse and by a decrease in the "driving" pressures (elastic recoil of the lung) which account for maximal flow. These factors cannot be reversed directly. However, the factors which produce airflow obstruction in chronic bronchitis are partly reversible and are present to some degree in all patients with COPD. Airflow obstruction in chronic bronchitis is produced by (1) increases in bronchomotor tone, (2) intraluminal mucus, and (3) mucosal edema.

Augmented parasympathetic nervous activity contributes to the heightened bronchomotor tone. A variety of α- and β-adrenergic agonists and anticholinergic blocking drugs are useful in relaxing bronchial smooth muscle.

Elimination of mucus may be achieved by physical measures which stimulate coughing and liquefaction of secretions and by the use of gravity or percussion to mechanically facilitate clearance. β-adrenergic drugs also increase the rate of mucociliary clearance.

Edema of the airways occurring in the acute stage of inflammation produced by exposure to noxious agents in the air or by antigen-antibody reactions is sometimes relieved by corticosteroids.

Treatment of Secondary Complications. RESPIRATORY FAILURE. Respiratory failure is usually considered to be present when the Po_2 is less than 50 mm. Hg or the Pco_2 is greater than 50 mm. Hg (at sea level in the absence of an accompanying metabolic alkalosis).

Subtle impairment of oxygen exchange, as indicated by increases in the alveolar-arterial oxygen tension gradient, is one of the earliest changes in COPD. However, because of the sigmoid shape of the oxyhemoglobin dissociation curve, the oxygen content of arterial blood is well maintained until the Po_2 falls below 60 mm. Hg. Hypoxemia results from poor distribution of inspired gas relative to pulmonary blood flow (ventilation-perfusion mismatch). However, reduction in the level of total ventilation (alveolar hypoventilation) may contribute to the development of hypoxemia when CO_2 retention is present. In most patients, increases in arterial CO_2 occur only when airway obstruction is severe and forced expiratory flow rates are less than 25 per cent of the predicted normal values (e.g., FEV_1 values of 1.0 to 1.5 liters or less). However, in some patients, impaired chemosensitivity with a failure of respiratory activity to increase appropriately in response to changes in blood gas tensions may also contribute to CO_2 retention.

COR PULMONALE AND CONGESTIVE HEART FAILURE. The prognosis of patients with COPD is poorer when there is pulmonary hypertension. The level of pulmonary artery pressure rises because hypoxia and hypercapnia produce vasoconstriction. Reduction in the volume of the pulmonary capillary bed caused by anatomic destruction of alveolar septa appears to be less important a cause of hypertension. In addition, severe hypoxia in patients with COPD may cause left ventricular dysfunction. Oxygen therapy and careful management of fluid and electrolyte balance are therefore important in the management of these patients.

Surgery. Resection of lung bullae rarely is of long-term benefit. A single bulla which is rapidly expanding and producing symptoms should be removed. Other surgical measures do not appear to be helpful in treating COPD. Intensive bronchodilator and antibiotic treatment to optimize lung function should precede elective surgical procedures in these patients.

Outpatient Management

Bronchodilators. In the past several years, significant advances have been made in understanding the physiology of bronchial smooth muscle constriction and in the development of improved bronchodilator drugs. These drugs can be given orally or in aerosol form and so are well suited for chronic outpatient care.

β-ADRENERGIC AGONISTS. β agonists relax bronchial smooth muscle by activating adenylcyclase and increasing the production of cyclic AMP. This bronchodilating action is mediated by a different set of β receptors (β_2) than those which produce cardiovascular (tachycardia and increased cardiac output) and central nervous system (CNS) effects (β_1). Newer preparations which have selective affinity for β_2 receptors are now available and provide potent bronchodilatation without the frequent adverse effects previously noted with isoproterenol, which has both β_1 and β_2 effects. Furthermore, the structure of the new drugs makes them less susceptible to the action of catechol-o-methyl transferases and monoamine oxidases, thereby prolonging their duration of action. Salbutamol, terbutaline, and metaproterenol are examples of these newer drugs that have been shown in clinical trials to be effective and safe in man. When given orally, these drugs have an earlier onset of action than ephedrine (a combined α- and β-adrenergic agonist) and greater degree and duration of bronchodilatation (4 to 6 hours). Because the onset of action of the oral β_2 preparations is sufficiently rapid for most outpatients, it is seldom necessary to prescribe aerosol preparations. We use terbutaline, 5 to 7.5 mg. orally every 6 hours, as the β stimulant in most outpatients.

Ephedrine is rarely used because of its relatively low potency and high incidence of side effects such as palpitations, insomnia, and urinary retention if prostatic enlargement is present. A frequent but short-lived side effect of terbutaline has been the development of hand tremor (a manifestation of β_2 stimulation on skeletal muscle). To date, there is no evidence of tachyphylaxis or paradoxical bronchospasm with terbutaline—either of which can occur when isoproterenol is used. In patients who cannot tolerate oral terbutaline because of idiosyncratic reactions, we use metaproterenol by Freon propellant aerosol (two to three inhalations [0.65 mg. metered dose each breath] every 6 hours).

XANTHINES. Xanthines such as theophylline increase the intracellular concentration of cyclic AMP, but do so by inhibiting the activity of diphosphoesterase which breaks down cyclic AMP. There is in vitro evidence for a synergistic interaction between adenylcyclase activators like the β agonists and diphosphoesterase inhibitors like theophylline. However, theophylline can be effective even when the sympathomimetics are not. Theophylline and its derivatives (methylated xanthines) are available in anhydrous form or in a variety of salts and solutions. About 90 per cent of uncoated aminophylline (theophylline ethylenediamine) and the choline salt of theophylline (oxtriphylline) are absorbed in the fasting state. They have a plasma half-life of 4 to 5 hours. The rates of excretion of the drug vary somewhat between individuals, but are sufficiently close enough to allow dosage to be based on body weight and the amount of anhydrous theophylline in each preparation. We generally use aminophylline tablets (80 per cent anhydrous theophylline by weight) in an initial dose of 3 mg. per kg. of anhydrous theophylline every 6 hours around the clock. This dose may be increased to a maximum of 6 mg. per kg. every 6 hours until the desired effect has been reached or toxicity develops. The blood level of the drug will plateau by 1 to 2 days. Thereafter, the dose of the drug can be increased every 2 to 3 days in an attempt to find an optimal level. Because rates of absorption are slower with oral administration, cardiovascular toxicity (hypotension, arrhythmias) and CNS toxicity (seizures) are rare, but anorexia, nausea, and vomiting can occur. Toxicity is usually associated with blood levels in excess of 20 micrograms per ml.

In Elixophyllin (a 20 per cent alcohol solution of anhydrous theophylline), the concentration of theophylline (80 mg. in 15 ml.) is relatively low. A substantial volume (45 to 60 ml.) must be ingested (9 to 12 ml. of alcohol) to deliver an adequate dose of theophylline.

ANTICHOLINERGICS. Recent evidence suggests that vagal reflexes contribute to the airway constriction that occurs in response to inhaled irritants or antigen-antibody reactions. The responses are diminished in animals by vagotomy and in man by blockade of efferent vagal fibers with an anticholinergic such as atropine. The role of these drugs in COPD is as yet unsettled. However, atropine, when given as an aerosol, increases the FEV_1 in patients with COPD. Concern about side effects of atropine (tachycardia and drying effects on tracheobronchial secretions) has led to the development of derivatives of atropine without these adverse actions. The most promising seems to be the methyl bromide of N-isopropyl nortropine known as Sch 1000. This is an inhaled bronchodilator with a potency equivalent to or greater than atropine and may be of particular value in patients with COPD and cardiovascular disease.

CORTICOSTEROIDS. The role of this class of drugs in COPD is controversial. Corticosteroids are available both as oral preparations and as aerosols containing derivatives with prominent pulmonary effects but little systemic effects because of poor absorption. Corticosteroids may help dilate bronchi and decrease inflammation. Their use is best limited to patients with (1) a substantial allergic component to their disease, (2) sputum or blood eosinophilia, (3) episodic bronchospasm, and (4) no evidence of pulmonary infection (e.g., inactive tuberculosis, suppurative bronchiectasis). Steroids are employed only when maximal doses of other bronchodilators have been given without sufficient improvement. We employ beclomethasone aerosol, two to four inhalations (50 micrograms metered dose per inhalation) four times a day. Candida pharyngitis is an occasionally reported complication.

Antibiotics. In contrast to normal subjects, in whom the lower respiratory tract is sterile, the lower respiratory tracts of patients with COPD appear to be colonized with gram-positive and gram-negative organisms (most commonly *Streptococcus pneumoniae* or *Hemophilus influenzae*). Continuous antibiotic treatment is helpful in some patients. In all patients, antibiotics should be used at the first sign of a respiratory infection or when the sputum becomes discolored. Either ampicillin, 500 mg. orally four times daily, or tetracycline, 250 mg. orally four times daily, for 7 days can be used. Amoxicillin, a derivative of ampicillin, is also reported to be well absorbed and to produce high levels in blood and sputum. Chloramphenicol is effective but should be used only as a last resort because of its hematologic toxicity. Clinical trials suggest that penicillin is relatively ineffective. Gram stain and culture of the sputum are of little help in most cases but should be obtained in patients with significant febrile illnesses or before antibiotics are changed.

Chronic Oxygen Therapy. Recent studies indicate that in severely hypoxemic subjects (Po_2 of less than 55 mm. Hg), chronic oxygen administration for at least 15 hours a day may be of value in (1) decreasing pulmonary artery pressure both at rest and during exercise, (2) minimizing polycythemia, (3) improving exercise tolerance, and (4) improving electroencephalographic (EEG) tracings and intellectual function. Furthermore, episodes of congestive heart failure seem to occur less frequently with oxygen administration. The effects of chronic oxygen therapy on long-term survival are less clear cut, however, but appear to be of benefit in patients living at high altitude.

Oxygen therapy may be particularly helpful during sleep. Arterial Po_2 may drop substantially during sleep in some patients with COPD because of an exaggeration of the normal hypoventilation of sleep and a worsening of ventilation-perfusion relationships. These changes are most marked during rapid eye movement (REM) sleep and should be sought in all patients who have a resting Po_2 of less than 60 mm. Hg while *awake*.

Several methods are now available to provide oxygen conveniently at home. A liquid oxygen system (Linde), consisting of a reservoir tank and portable (7 lb.) "walker," and a device which acts as a molecular "sieve" to concentrate oxygen by extracting nitrogen from room air are available. Regardless of the method chosen, domiciliary oxygen is expensive. Its use should be reserved for patients with (1) a Po_2 of less than 55 mm. Hg at rest, which declines still further with exercise or sleep, or (2) evidence of pulmonary hypertension. We give sufficient oxygen so as to maintain the arterial Po_2 above 60 mm. Hg.

Patients in whom chronic oxygen administration is considered should be hospitalized (1) to ascertain the effects of various oxygen flow rates on the Pao_2 and (2) to determine the increase in $Paco_2$ (generally slight) which results from the decrease in hypoxic chemical drive.

Diuretics and Digitalis. Intravascular volume is increased and peripheral edema is common even in the absence of heart failure in COPD. Diuretics are useful when extravascular salt and water are increased to prevent simultaneous accumulations in the lungs which can interfere with gas exchange.

The effectiveness of digitalis in improving right ventricular function even in the presence of heart failure is controversial. Also, patients with COPD develop serious arrhythmias with even small amounts of digitalis.

Improvement in Respiratory Drive. Reduced sensitivity of the respiratory "center" to chemical stimuli may aggravate hypoxemia and hypercapnia. In some patients with inherent disturbances in the function of the respiratory "center," respiratory failure may be produced by only slight degrees of airway obstruction. More common, however, are decreases in chemosensitivity "acquired" during the course of treatment. For example, metabolic alkalosis caused by intensive diuretic therapy may substantially blunt the response to CO_2. This should be prevented by administering adequate potassium and chloride. Also, sedatives and tranquilizers can diminish the responsiveness of the respiratory "center" to changes in Pco_2 or Po_2 and should be avoided. In *selected* patients agents to stimulate respiratory drive (e.g., medroxyprogesterone) are of benefit.

Physical Therapy. Patients with copious, thick secretions which are difficult to raise by coughing alone may be helped by postural drainage and chest percussion performed three to four times a day. These measures are generally more effective in mobilizing secretions than available expectorants and mucolytics. Incoordination of the breathing muscles has been implicated in some patients in causing poor gas exchange. In these patients breathing exercises are helpful, but in the majority of patients they are not. Patients with COPD are occasionally found to spontaneously employ pursed-lip breathing. This technique has been shown to be effective in some patients in relieving dyspnea and decreasing minute ventilation. The physiologic effect of pursed-lip breathing appears to be related to a reduction in expiratory flow and an increase in intra-airway pressure which minimizes airway collapse.

Left to themselves patients with obstructive pulmonary disease tend to become inactive, and deconditioning further limits exercise tolerance. A regular schedule of physical activity is beneficial in improving exercise performance. Physical training programs increase exercise tolerance and decrease oxygen consumption at any level of exertion. This improvement occurs without a measurable change in pulmonary function and appears to be the result of improved efficiency of both skeletal and cardiac muscle. Any attempt to increase the exercise tolerance of inactive patients should be attempted cautiously and only after physiologic studies of the effect of exercise on blood gas tensions and the cardiovascular system have been obtained.

Inhalation Therapy. NEBULIZATION-HUMIDIFICATION. A variety of devices have been employed to increase the water content of inspired air to help liquefy secretions and facilitate their removal. In normally hydrated patients breathing takes place through the nose and mouth, and the inspired air is 100 per cent saturated by the time it reaches the trachea. In addition, in nose- or mouth-breathing patients, very little of the water emitted by humidifiers and nebulizers reaches the lungs. Most is deposited in the upper airway or swallowed. Accordingly, we prefer to maintain hydration and sputum fluidity by having our patients drink 2 to 3 quarts of liquid daily.

IPPB. Intermittent positive pressure breathing (IPPB) per se does not improve pulmonary function and may even increase airway resistance and the work of breathing in subjects with reactive or easily collapsible airways. In patients with COPD, its use should be confined to the delivery of aerosol medication. Although IPPB is an effective means of delivering bronchodilator medication, several recent studies have shown that it is no better than hand-powered or propellant nebulizers. However, in subjects who cannot take or hold a deep breath, are weak, or lack coordination, IPPB "assist" may allow greater penetration of the drugs. Long-term use of IPPB as a means of delivering bronchodilators may produce overdistention of the lung, and it should not be used routinely in outpatient care.

Hospital Management

Acute respiratory failure, precipitated by acute infection, congestive heart failure, bronchospasm, or retention of secretions, is the most common cause of hospitalization in patients with COPD. Recognition of the precipitating factor(s) is the first step in hospital management. In general, however, the modalities used during hospitalization are the same as those used in the outpatient setting except for a greater intensity of application.

Oxygen Therapy. In most patients in acute respiratory failure, the most immediate threat to life is that of severe hypoxemia. Small, precise increases in oxygen concentration must be given so as to improve the arterial oxygen content without an excessive rise in P_{CO_2}. This can best be accomplished by any of a number of devices using the Venturi principle to deliver large volumes of gas with small (24 and 28 per cent) increases in oxygen concentration. Use of these Venturi devices (e.g., Ventimask) also prevents changes in either the level or pattern of breathing from affecting the inspired oxygen concentration in contrast to low flow systems.

Most patients in acute respiratory failure may be adequately treated without mechanical ventilation. Rather, intubation and mechanical ventilation should be reserved for the minority of patients in whom a progressive rise in P_{CO_2} occurs to the point at which either severe respiratory acidosis (pH < 7.25) or a CO_2-induced obtundation occurs. Rarely, the failure to obtain adequate oxygenation (P_{O_2} greater than 55 to 60 mm. Hg) using a facial mask may require mechanical ventilation. Patients on O_2 therapy with or without the aid of mechanical ventilation should be followed with measurements of arterial blood gases at regular intervals even when the clinical condition is apparently stable.

Bronchodilators. In the acute stage of the disease, aerosol and intravenous bronchodilators should be given because of their rapid onset and assured delivery.

We use aminophylline as a continuous infusion. This is always begun with a loading dose of 6.0 mg. per kg. given over 20 minutes, followed by a maintenance dose of 0.9 mg. per kg. per hour. In most patients, this dose will give a blood level of 10 to 15 micrograms per ml. Use of a loading dose produces a peak effect in 15 minutes, compared to 8 hours when the loading dose is not given. When a greater effect is desired, an additional dose of 3.0 mg. per kg. may be given over 20 minutes and the continuous dose increased to 1.35 mg. per kg. per hour. This larger dose will produce a blood level of 15 to 20 micrograms per ml. Patients with congestive heart failure or severe liver disease appear to have a decreased rate of clearance of the drug, and their maintenance dose should be decreased by one third and one half, respectively. The loading dose remains unchanged, however.

AEROSOL. There are at present no readily available β_2 aerosol *solutions*. We therefore make use of aerosolized isoproterenol, 0.5 ml. of 1:200 dilution given by IPPB machine over 15 minutes and repeated no more often than every 4 hours. In patients with cardiovascular disease, we use isoetharine in equivalent dose, because it may have less β_1 effect.

All bronchodilators may produce an initial decrease in P_{O_2}, because they dilate pulmonary blood vessels and may increase the perfusion more than the ventilation of some poorly ventilated regions. Consequently, bronchodilators in acute respiratory failure should be given only in conjunction with oxygen therapy.

ATELECTASIS

method of
JOE R. UTLEY, M.D.
San Diego, California

Localized Atelectasis

Atelectasis is the loss of volume of a part of the lung. Diminished volume may be secondary to bronchial obstruction, intrapulmonary or extrapulmonary compression, or fibrosis and contraction of the parenchyma. Atelectasis frequently occurs with patent bronchi and may be due to diminished ventilation or insufficient surfactant. Chronic atelectasis with infection may result in loss of lung architecture and parenchyma to a degree that expansion of the lung is not possible.

Ambulation and mobilization of the patient are encouraged to the degree permitted by associated conditions.

Inspired oxygen concentration (Fio_2) is increased to levels necessary to maintain arterial Po_2 between 75 and 100 mm. Hg. Prolonged Fio_2 above 40 per cent may produce lung damage. A high concentration of oxygen may reduce respiratory drive in hypercarbic patients.

Endotracheal suction is important in removing tracheobronchial secretions but is also useful in stimulating cough. Sterile, disposable nonreactive catheters and sterile gloves should be used.

Humidification of inspired gases is desirable if secretions are thick and difficult to remove by suction. Nebulization of fine water droplets may cause bronchial irritation and positive water balance. Humidification may be detrimental when secretions are copious and thin.

Positioning, postural drainage, percussion, breathing exercises, and training by conventional physiotherapy techniques are useful in hospitalized patients and may be taught to outpatients and their families. Blow bottles and incentive spirometry are useful in postoperative patients.

Relief of pain, particularly after thoracic or abdominal operations and trauma, is essential to achieve ventilation and expansion of collapsed lung. Morphine in small (up to 0.1 mg. per kg.), frequent (every 2 hours) doses is effective. Intercostal nerve blocks may be useful for chest wall pain. Binders, belts, and taping of ribs should be avoided.

Bronchodilators nebulized and inhaled are useful with asthma, bronchospasm, or wheezing. Isoproterenol, racemic epinephrine, or phenylephrine may be administered from an aerosol cartridge or nebulizer. These agents may also be useful in managing allergic or postintubation edema. Aminophylline (125 to 250 mg. every 15 to 60 minutes) may be used for more chronic forms of bronchospasm.

Thick tracheobronchial secretions may be difficult to remove by cough or suction. Antisialagogues such as atropine should be avoided in the presence of thick secretions. Thick secretions may be benefited by hydration, saturated solution of potassium iodide (SSKI, 15 drops in water or juice 4 times daily), or nebulized acetylcysteine (Mucomyst) or deoxyribonuclease (Dornavac).

Bronchial irritants, such as tobacco smoke, chemical fumes, spray agents, and hot steam, should be avoided.

Bronchoscopy is important in the diagnosis of broncho-occlusive lesions and may be essential for removal of thick secretions. Fiberoptic bronchoscopy at the bedside is useful in suctioning and lavaging subsegmental bronchi. Rigid bronchoscopy may be necessary to resect obstructing tumors, remove foreign bodies, and clear thick secretions.

Endotracheal intubation or tracheostomy may be necessary to remove large volumes of thick tracheobronchial secretions. Positive pressure ventilation, continuous positive airway pressure (CPAP), and positive end-expiratory pressure (PEEP) may be helpful in expanding collapsed lung.

Bronchial obstruction should be relieved by suction, lavage, and bronchoscopy. Tumors, external compression, stenoses, and foreign bodies should be removed by bronchoscopy or operatively. Unresectable tumors may be treated by radiation therapy. Chemotherapy is less likely to benefit localized obstructive lesions.

External compression caused by pleural effusion, pneumothorax, hemothorax, empyema, fibrothorax, and tumors should be relieved by surgical therapy.

Serial chest x-rays are important to determine resolution of atelectasis.

Diffuse Miliary Atelectasis (Adult Respiratory Distress Syndrome)

Diffuse miliary atelectasis may not be associated with radiographic signs of localized collapse. This syndrome is associated with a variety of clinical conditions, including trauma, cardiac surgery, multiple transfusions, fluid overload, left ventricular failure, and sepsis. Low arterial Po_2 with evidence of increased transpulmonary shunting of venous blood and increased alveolar-arterial oxygen gradient are characteristic of diffuse miliary atelectasis. Management includes maintenance of cardiac output, minimizing oxygen consumption, and improving oxygenation.

Fluids are restricted to diminish interstitial pulmonary edema. Sodium-containing fluids should be minimized and glucose and water limited to 1000 ml. per square meter of body surface per day. Expansion of blood volume should be accomplished with red cells, whole blood, albumin, or plasma protein fraction (Plasmanate), which remain mainly intravascular.

Diuresis to diminish interstitial pulmonary edema is important. Intravenous furosemide (Lasix), 0.5 to 1.0 mg. per kg. every 4 to 6 hours, increasing to 3 mg. per kg. if necessary, is preferred in acutely ill patients. Serum potassium should be monitored every 3 to 4 hours during brisk diuresis to avoid hypokalemia and arrhythmias.

Ventilator management: Patients should be intubated with sterile, nonreactive, disposable endotracheal tubes, which may be left in place for up to 7 days before tracheostomy is necessary. Tidal volume should be set at 8 to 10 ml. per kg. Inspired oxygen may be 100 per cent initially but should be diminished to 40 per cent or less as soon as possible, provided arterial Po_2 remains above 75 mm. Hg. Positive pressure ventilation increases the mean intra-alveolar pressure compared to spontaneous ventilation and aids the resorption of alveolar edema. Mean airway pressure may be increased further by adding positive end-expiratory pressure (PEEP). Airway pressure may be augmented by using continuous positive airway pressure (CPAP) during spontaneous breathing. CPAP is particularly useful in infants.

Adequate cardiac output is critical in the hypoxic patient to maintain oxygen delivery. Cardiac output may be maximized by producing an optimal heart rate, altering filling pressures (preload), arterial pressures (afterload), and contractility.

Oxygen consumption should be minimized when oxygen delivery is inadequate. The patient should be kept quiet and free of agitation. Diazepam (Valium), 0.1 mg. per kg. every 2 to 3 hours, or morphine sulfate, 0.1 mg. per kg. every 2 to 3 hours, is useful in sedating seriously ill patients. Controlled ventilation reduces the muscular work of breathing. In patients intubated and on a respirator, complete muscular paralysis further diminishes oxygen consumption. Pancuronium (Pavulon), 0.04 mg. per kg. every 2 to 3 hours or as indicated by the reappearance of muscular activity, is preferred. Patients should be allowed to return to spontaneous muscular activity once each day. The relative degree of paralysis may also be determined by nerve stimulation.

Body temperature should be controlled with antipyretics (acetylsalicylic acid [aspirin], 300 mg. every 4 hours) and hypothermia blankets. Body temperature should be maintained between 35 and 37°C. (95 and 99°F.).

Antibiotics should be used to treat specific infections as determined by repeated tracheal cultures.

MUCOPURULENT BRONCHITIS AND BRONCHIECTASIS

method of
JOSEPH L. POTTER, M.D.
Akron, Ohio

Mucopurulent bronchitis is an inflammation of the bronchial tree accompanied by a marked exudative process. The cause is infective, but may be secondary to injury from chemical or physical agents. The acute form is easily recognizable as a respiratory infection marked by cough and rather typical physical findings in the chest. The chronic form of the disease is generally a sequela of an acute process which may have remained subclinical for many years, and is characterized by mucosal edema, mucus hypersecretion, and some degree of obstructive disease. It may present simply with a mild, early-morning smoker's cough, and then progress over a variable period of time to pronounced signs of lung disease such as emphysema, pulmonary fibrosis, clubbing of the fingers, and bronchiectasis. This last term denotes a specific anatomic change involving widening of the bronchi.

General Principles of the Treatment Program

Mucopurulent bronchitis and bronchiectasis represent a spectrum of disease states, and thus the recommendations presented here must be tailored to the individual patient. It may be advantageous, particularly for patients with more advanced disease, to hospitalize the patient for baseline laboratory tests and for measurements of pulmonary function. At this time, any biochemical alterations should be corrected, and it must be assured that the patient is adequately hydrated. An extensive family history of disease should be taken. Agammaglobulinemia and other deficits of the various arms of the immune system, cystic fibrosis, Kartagener's syndrome, foreign bodies, and alpha–1–antitrypsin deficiency should be explored as possible causes of lung disease, and a thorough radiologic examination should be carried out. The therapeutic program can then be instituted under controlled conditions in an attempt to bring the disease into hand. It is extremely helpful at this time to educate the patient with respect to the nature of the disease and the prognosis, and to instruct him in such procedures as will become his own responsibility. A positive attitude should be instilled with respect to the program and unnecessary fears allayed. The patient should be advised to undertake appropriate physical activity and obtain required rest. He should take a nutritious diet, including vitamins, and reduction of weight should be achieved when indicated. When aggravating working conditions exist, it may be helpful for him to change his work environment; this may sometimes be accomplished within the framework of his present organization. Smoking in any form is to be prohibited, and it may be well to instigate an investigation of the home atmosphere, particularly with respect to possible allergic elements present in the home.

The core of the treatment program comprises appropriate antibiotic therapy to control the infectious component and postural drainage to remove excess or viscous secretions in an effort to promote pulmonary hygiene and function. Ancillary measures include nebulization therapy to add water to the secretions for the purpose of reducing their viscosity. Similarly, bronchodilators, mucolytic agents, antibiotics, and enzymes can be aerosolized into the pulmonary tree. It should be recognized that at least some of these agents are pulmonary irritants, and therefore they should be reserved for serious and refractory situations. The question of nebulization of water by mist tent or by intermittent aerosol therapy still remains controversial at this writing, with little objective evidence that it has a beneficial effect. It is still even questionable whether aerosolization is effective in reaching the desired site in the lung. It must further be recognized that many of these patients will have fixed anatomic changes which cannot be reversed by the program of therapy. However, the program may limit the extension of the disease, and a very positive psychologic benefit is often seen when a systematic program of therapy is instituted. Clinical improvement would certainly be a positive indication for continuation of aerosol treatment. However, long-term therapy with any of the ancillary agents should be based on objective measurements of improved pulmonary function.

The treatment program presented here is designed for patients with mild to moderately severe disease that can be managed on an ambulatory basis for the most part. For the critically ill patient in marked cardiorespiratory embarrassment, hypercapnic and hypoxic, admission to a specialized care unit is indicated until the disease can be stabilized at some reasonable level.

Treatment

Antimicrobial Drugs. The organism or organisms should be identified, preferably by culture of the sputum, and the sensitivities determined. If possible, a single drug should be used. The use of bactericidal drugs is usually preferable to bacteriostatic agents, but it is not always convenient to use certain bactericidal agents that must be administered parenterally. Prophylactic antibiotic therapy has been used in this disease, sometimes on a seasonal basis, but the possible emergence of drug-resistant organisms dictates against this policy. In general, because of the relative inaccessibility of the inflammatory site, one should treat with the maximal recommended dose of drug, and for the full period of time.

In a study of the sputum of patients with cystic fibrosis, bronchiectasis, and laryngectomy, a wide variety of bacterial flora was observed. There was no qualitative difference among the three groups of patients with respect to isolates. Most commonly observed in bronchiectasis were *Hemophilus influenzae*, *Diplococcus pneumoniae*, *Staphylococcus aureus*, Streptococcus (hemolytic and nonhemolytic), Proteus, Klebsiella, Aerobacter, *Escherichia coli*, and Pseudomonas. If the isolate is deemed to be part of the clinical picture of an active infection, it should be treated vigorously for a period of 1 to 2 weeks, and possibly longer if necessary.

Penicillin and tetracycline, because of their ease of administration and generally low host toxicity, are the mainstays of the treatment program. In children, ampicillin should be substituted for tetracycline whenever possible. For gram-positive infections sensitive to penicillin in adults, 2 grams per day in divided doses for 3 days, and then 1 gram per day for an additional week, should be used. Patients hypersensitive to penicillin should be given erythromycin at a dose of 500 mg. every 8 hours. For a staphylococcal infection resistant to penicillin, it is convenient to administer sodium oxacillin in a dosage of 4 grams per day. On the gram-negative side, tetracycline can be used at a dose of 2 grams per day for the first few days, and then be reduced to 1 gram per day for a period of a week. Doxycycline can be used at a dosage of 200 mg. for the first day and then reduced to 100 mg. a day. It has the advantage of requiring only 1 capsule each day. Ampicillin can be administered in a dosage of 2 grams per day initially, and then 1 gram per day if the organism is susceptible. Ampicillin is bactericidal, and less adverse effects have been observed with its use than with tetracycline. Pseudomonas infections remain a problem. Sodium colistimethate or gentamicin at a dosage of 2.5 to 5 mg. per kg. per day can be used. Carbenicillin can be used against susceptible Proteus or Pseudomonas, but very large doses are required. All three drugs have the advantage of a bactericidal mechanism but must be administered parenterally. Neomycin, kanamycin, polymyxin, and gentamicin are cationic compounds which tend to coprecipitate with anionic DNA in purulent secretions with consequent inactivation of the drug. Although effectiveness is thus diminished, their use is not contraindicated; they should be administered for sensitive gram-negative infections unless the organism also responds to ampicillin. However, the eighth nerve and/or kidney should be carefully monitored for toxic effects when any of this group of basic antimicrobial drugs is used. For very severe infections, higher doses and/or parenteral administration of antimicrobial agents may be indicated. In using large doses of drugs for extended periods, the physician should be on the alert for allergic and adverse host effects at all times, and it may be advisable to monitor blood levels of these agents. Direct aerosolization of antibiotics into the tracheobronchial tree may be a useful adjunct in some patients.

Postural Drainage. The introduction of the technique of postural drainage in the treatment of bronchiectasis, as well as in other pulmonary diseases, represents a significant advance in the management of these problems. The principle of the method is obvious and involves the positioning of an area of the pulmonary tree such that the infected secretions will drain by gravity into the larger bronchi, there to be coughed up. Since the flow of a viscous solution will necessarily be slow, clapping and vibration of the chest are helpful in loosening the secretions. The position that the patient adopts should be dictated from the bronchogram or, in its absence, clinical signs. Although a wide variety of methods have been advocated in different centers, there is little to recommend one over another. I have adopted the 1968 recommendations of the Committee on Therapy of the Medical Section of the National Tuberculosis Society. They are summarized briefly here. The patient is appropriately positioned and then he exhales slowly five to six times, during which time vibration is applied to the chest. Coughing and expectoration follow. This procedure is repeated several times during the treatment period. We have not been impressed with the use of hand vibrators, nor is their use entirely without hazard. The frequency of postural drainage is dictated by the severity of the disease. It may be advisable for the patient at home to drain the secretions at least on arising in the morning and at bedtime. Specialized equipment is not necessary for this treatment, and adaptation of beds and chairs will usually suffice.

The aforementioned measures will result in improved pulmonary hygiene. When there is an indication of spasm, or of edema of the bronchial mucous membranes, it will be helpful to administer isoproterenol and/or phenylephrine by aerosol prior to postural drainage. The aerosol treatment seems to be markedly superior to the systemic administration of similar reagents in terms of opening up the airways.

Ancillary Measures. Although antibiotic therapy and postural drainage remain the basis of the treatment program, there are a variety of other measures which can play a secondary role in the successful management of patients with bronchiectasis.

Humidification of the Airway. The addition of water to the secretion is, in theory, a simple and effective way of thinning it. The use of home humidifiers and air conditioners is to be recommended and will contribute to the comfort of the patient. The nightly use of a unit which generates cold mist has also been found to be of at least subjective value, but the particle size is such that only the upper airways are benefited. In severe cases, mist tent ultrasonic nebulization therapy can be used. It may be advisable to carry out the aerosol treatment in the hospital to drain the secretions frequently, and to obtain pulmonary function measurements.

Other Agents. Aerosolization of isoproterenol HCl and/or phenylephrine is quite useful in opening up the airway. Nine volumes of phenylephrine (0.125 per cent) and one volume of U.S.P. propylene glycol are mixed so that a final concentration of 10 per cent propylene glycol is attained. Two ml. is aerosolized three or four times a day. If desired, a solution containing 1.6 ml. of the phenylephrine–propylene glycol mixture and 0.4 ml. of isoproterenol HCl 1:200 can be aerosolized. Parenteral aminophylline and steroids should probably be reserved for hospitalized patients who have severe disease and require close supervision. The administration of expectorant agents such as potassium iodide and ammonium chloride has not been found to be particularly helpful. Detergents, enzymes, and other mucolytic agents such as N-acetylcysteine have been used in this disease with rather variable results. This may, in part, be due to the spectrum of severity in this disease, and in part to the method of administration. Objective measurements of the efficiency of these agents and their possible adverse side effects are still needed. A trial of oral bronchodilators containing theophylline will sometimes bring relief to certain patients, but it is important to be aware of the side effects of these preparations.

General Measures. Instruction of the patient in breathing exercises and in the development of an effective cough to expel secretions is a valuable adjunct to the treatment program. The removal of the patient from contact with noxious fumes and other pulmonary irritants is helpful, as is the avoidance of exposure to situations in which respiratory infections are epidemic. Prophylactic treatment against infectious disease, such as immunization with influenza vaccine, is desirable, because viral infection undoubtedly can lead to a bacterial proliferation in the lung. Allergies and sinusitis should be treated intensively, and the patient is advised to seek regular dental care.

Surgery. Patients with bronchiectasis can be classified into two general categories, although each category again represents a spectrum of diseases. In the first group, there will be found extensive and severe bronchial disease, possibly associated with other pulmonary pathology. In this group, surgical intervention is not advisable. The second group will have more localized disease, and it is among these patients that the most favorable response to medical management is observed. In the past, surgery has been recommended for those patients with rather localized disease, such as in a single lobe or segment, and when there is no evidence of pulmonary disease elsewhere. It is obviously not always possible to establish these criteria with certainty. The response to surgery appears to be more favorable in younger patients. In patients whose normal activities are hampered by their disease and in whom the criteria for surgery seem to be present, good results after resection may be seen. Before recommending surgery, the physician should make an intensive effort to bring the disease under control by medical management.

PRIMARY LUNG CANCER

method of
ROBERT J. GINSBERG, M.D.
Toronto, Ontario, Canada

Introduction

Carcinoma of the lung continues to be the most common cause of cancer death in males in North America. Its incidence has reached almost epidemic proportions. Lung cancer in females shows a similar alarming increase.

Despite vigorous attempts to improve early diagnosis and methods of therapy, little has been done to improve survival figures. About 90 per cent of patients will be dead from their disease within 5 years.

Surgical therapy still offers the best hope of cure in lung cancer. If complete resection can be performed, approximately 25 per cent of those resected will survive 5 years. Unfortunately, in less than one third of the patients suffering from this disease can the tumor be completely resected.

Palliative resections, leaving residual tumor behind, rarely are indicated. These resections do not improve survival rates and offer no better palliation than other forms of therapy.

Preoperative Assessment

We try to avoid unnecessary thoracotomies, resulting in failure to resect for cure as well as avoidable morbidity and mortality. Therefore preoperative assessment must identify (1) tumors that can be totally excised (tumor assessment) and (2) patients who can tolerate the operative procedure and loss of functioning pulmonary tissue (patient assessment).

Tumor Assessment. It is important in assessing the tumor to stage the disease according to the size of tumor and spread to lymph nodes or distant areas. We adhere fairly well to the clinical staging system proposed by the American Joint Committee of Cancer Staging and End Results Reporting, but differentiate those tumors with extrathoracic disease (Table 1). As well, tumors behave differently according to histologic type. The classification we use is as follows: (1) squamous cell, (2) adenocarcinoma, (3) undifferentiated large cell carcinoma, (4) undifferentiated small cell (oat cell) carcinoma (Table 2). It is known that squamous cell carcinoma has the best prognosis, no matter what stage of the disease. Adenocarcinoma and undifferentiated large cell carcinoma have less optimistic results but are similar. Undifferentiated small cell carcinoma is a lethal disease no matter what the stage.

TABLE 1. **Staging**

Occult carcinoma	Positive cytology only
Stage I	A tumor 3 cm. or less with only adjacent nodes involved
Stage II	Large tumor or any tumor with ipsilateral hilar nodes involved
Stage III	Tumor with mediastinal nodes involved
Stage IV	Extrathoracic disease

The diagnosis of carcinoma of the lung usually presents no problem. Proximal lesions can be easily biopsied and/or cytologic material obtained from bronchoscopy. Peripheral lesions are now amenable to cytologic diagnosis by fine needle aspiration biopsy or transbronchial brushings with radiologic control.

Once the diagnosis has been proved histologically, all efforts must be made to stage the tumor. Characteristically, lung tumors spread by both lymphatic and hematogenous routes.

Extensive mediastinal spread or distant metastases are contraindications to surgical excision for cure.

On physical examination, scalene node involvement, superior vena cava obstruction, and, in most cases, recurrent laryngeal nerve palsies indicate extensive tumor spread in the mediastinum, beyond hope for cure. Less obvious mediastinal node involvement is best assessed by a mediastinoscopy or anterior mediastinotomy with lymph node biopsy. In our experience, mediastinal tomograms, to assess mediastinal involvement, have been shown to be inaccurate in approximately one

TABLE 2. **Histologic Classification**

Squamous cell
Adenocarcinoma, including alveolar cell
Undifferentiated large cell
Undifferentiated small cell (oat cell)

third of cases. Both false negative and false positive results can occur. We have not assessed the accuracy of gallium scanning.

Hematogenous spread most frequently involves bone, liver, and brain. A detailed history and physical examination is indicated with special attention to these areas of possible involvement. An elevated alkaline phosphatase indicates the necessity for a further search for bony or liver involvement. We have found that routine skeletal surveys or radioisotope studies of bone and liver have not proved valuable in identifying unsuspected metastases without an elevated alkaline phosphatase. Similarly, brain scans without neurologic signs or symptoms have not proved useful in our hands. We limit these isotopic investigations to those patients exhibiting signs or symptoms suggestive of organ involvement or having an elevated alkaline phosphatase.

A pleural effusion associated with carcinoma of the lung, especially if bloody or containing malignant cells, is an ominous sign; however, occasionally, obstructive atelectasis and pneumonia are associated with a nonmalignant effusion. Pleural biopsy or thoracoscopy is indicated to identify diffuse parietal pleural spread. This type of spread is a contraindication to surgical treatment.

Although local tumor extension to neighboring organs (pericardium, atrium, chest wall, diaphragm, trachea) is a poor prognostic sign, it is not an absolute contraindication to excisional curative therapy.

Similarly, paraneoplastic syndromes in themselves are not contraindications to surgical treatment of the disease.

Patient Assessment. One must consider whether the patient can tolerate the rigors of anesthesia and thoracotomy. Added to this, one has to gauge whether the patient has the pulmonary reserve to withstand resection of functioning pulmonary tissue.

Pneumonectomy can be performed only on those patients with sufficient pulmonary reserve. Chronic hypercarbia, or fixed pulmonary hypertension, is a contraindication to this form of resection. Other guidelines that seem valuable include a maximum voluntary ventilation (MVV) of less than 50 liters per minute and hypoxemia on exercise testing. The classic "two-flight stair walking" (i.e., walking up two flights of stairs without significant dyspnea or tachycardia) is a good rough guide of cardiopulmonary reserve with exercise.

Generally speaking, lobectomy or lesser resections of pulmonary tissue will be tolerated by most patients who are fit enough for general anesthesia and thoracotomy. In these patients, mild chronic respiratory failure is not an absolute contraindication to surgery.

In the case of hilar lesions, pulmonary angiography with right heart catheterization can give important preoperative information with respect to whether lobectomy or pneumonectomy is required and can be tolerated.

Surgical Therapy

Surgical treatment aims at complete excision of the tumor, preserving as much functioning pulmonary tissue as possible.

Pneumonectomy. Historically, pneumonectomy was considered the only effective operation for resectable lung cancer. This offered complete excision of the tumor and as much lymphatic drainage excision as was technically feasible. Currently, most tumors involving the proximal main stem bronchi, crossing the major fissure, involving the left or right main pulmonary arteries, or involving the proximal perihilar lymph nodes (i.e., Stage II) will require pneumonectomy. As mentioned, limited pulmonary reserve or pulmonary hypertension contraindicates this operation. Previously age was considered a major factor. However, cardiopulmonary function is much more important.

Lobectomy. In those fortunate patients with peripheral tumors or with tumors limited to one lobe, lobectomy is the treatment of choice. This has become the most common operation performed for curative bronchogenic carcinoma. Segmental and lobar lymph nodes are removed with the specimen.

By adding a sleeve resection of main stem bronchi, lobectomy can be performed on patients with tumors minimally involving main stem bronchi. Occasionally, a concomitant sleeve resection of the right or left pulmonary artery can also be done in order to preserve pulmonary tissue.

Smaller Resections. Although not considered to be adequate "cancer operations" by some, segmental resection and wedge excision of tumors may be considered in those patients with very limited pulmonary reserve who have peripherally placed small tumors. Survival figures indicate that this type of resection can offer up to 35 per cent 5 year survival rate in selected patients.

Locally Extensive Procedures. Direct tumor extension into the pericardium, phrenic nerve, chest wall, diaphragm, or low trachea does not necessarily obviate complete surgical excision for cure. Resection of the tumor-bearing lung may be carried out "en bloc" with the affected structure. Left recurrent laryngeal nerve palsies usually indicate extensive mediastinal node involvement. However, local involvement of the descending vagus or recurrent nerve within the thoracic cavity occasionally occurs and may allow total surgical excision.

If low mediastinal lymph nodes on the same side as the tumor are involved by lymphatic spread, these can be removed "en bloc" with the upper lobe or entire lung.

All these locally extensive lesions have a more ominous prognosis. Of these lesions, squamous cell tumors are much more favorable. Adenocarcinoma or large cell carcinoma yields very poor results with locally extensive disease.

Small Cell Anaplastic Carcinoma

Small cell anaplastic carcinoma has to be considered as a separate entity. This is a highly malignant disease with a very unfavorable prognosis. Most of these patients cannot be cured by surgical therapy. Recent British experience demonstrates that radiotherapy alone or radiotherapy in combination with chemotherapy yields higher survival rates than surgical therapy alone. Only in the very favorable, peripherally placed small tumor would a surgical excision be considered.

Alveolar Cell Carcinoma

In its diffuse form, alveolar cell carcinoma, a form of adenocarcinoma, is not a curable disease. However, many of these tumors are single peripheral nodules and can be considered in the same manner as other lung cancer.

Surgical Adjuvant Therapy

Because of the generally poor results in the treatment of carcinoma of the lung, intensive study has been made of several modalities of adjuvant therapy added before or after surgery in the hope of improving cure rates.

Radiotherapy. Despite attempts at pre- and postoperative radiotherapy in conjunction with surgery, no controlled trial has shown any significant improvement in survival rates. Selected uncontrolled studies suggest some improvement with tumors involving the chest wall or mediastinum. Significantly, Pancoast's tumors, preoperatively irradiated, seem to do better after surgical resection.

Chemotherapy. Adjuvant chemotherapy has not been shown to improve the results of surgical therapy in controlled studies.

Immunotherapy. Immunotherapy is being extensively studied as an adjunct to surgery in the treatment of carcinoma of the lung. It is known that patients with carcinoma of the lung have a suppressed immune response. Attempts to increase host immunity have been made using nonspecific immunotherapeutic agents (bacille Calmette Guérin [BCG], Levamisol, *C. parvum*) and/or specific immunotherapy with lung cancer antigens. Early results using both forms of therapy show some promise. The most optimistic results are obtained in those patients who have had total excision of their tumor prior to immunotherapy (i.e., Stage I disease).

Palliative Resections

Occasionally, incomplete resection may improve the quality of life. Patients suffering from carcinomatous abscess or severe forms of paraneoplastic syndromes (e.g., hypercalcemia, pulmonary osteoarthropathy) which do not respond to symptomatic therapy may have improvement in their quality of life if the tumor is resected.

Prognosis

The lung cancer with the most favorable prognosis (Stage I), when resected, will recur in about 50 per cent of cases. Worse survival figures occur in Stages II and III. Local extension to adjacent organs or spread to low mediastinal glands is a grave prognostic sign. Less than 15 per cent of those resected survive 5 years. As mentioned, squamous cell carcinoma has a much more favorable prognosis than large cell or adenocarcinoma in other than Stage I disease.

Once the tumor has spread beyond the confines of total surgical excision, less than 1 per cent of patients will live 5 years.

Since the surgical mortality for resection is about 5 per cent, we must be careful in the selection of those patients to whom surgical therapy is offered. We must always be cognizant of the fact that there is a significant mortality associated with the operation. If the risk of operation is higher than the rate of cure, other forms of therapy should be offered.

Radiotherapy

In Stage I carcinoma of the lung, radiotherapy can offer cure in some instances. If cancericidal doses (5000 to 6000 rads) can be administered to the tumor, one can expect up to a 5 to 10 per cent 5 year survival rate. This treatment can be offered those patients who cannot tolerate surgery.

Radiotherapy is an extremely useful modality in the treatment of inoperable carcinoma for palliation of symptoms. It is especially effective in squamous cell and small cell anaplastic carcinoma. Painful metastases, cough resulting from endobronchial lesions, superior vena cava obstruction, and pathologic fractures will all benefit by radiotherapy. It is possible that reduction of the tumor mass will improve symptomatic well-being.

In our center, radiotherapy is the treatment of choice for inoperable carcinoma of the lung localized to the chest but beyond the limits of curative resection.

Chemotherapy

Currently, chemotherapy offers only short-term regression of symptoms in a small number of patients with metastatic disease. However, in small cell anaplastic carcinoma, it is as effective as radiotherapy. Combination chemotherapy and radiotherapy may be the optimal choice in this disease.

Other histologic types respond less well to chemotherapy. However, in a patient with extrathoracic metastases at the time of diagnosis, this form of therapy, with alkylating agents, may offer a slim chance of regression of disease. Benefit usually only lasts 3 to 6 months.

In patients with superior vena cava obstruction, the combination of radiotherapy and alkylating agents is often the best form of therapy.

We had found that, in patients with dyspnea associated with alveolar cell carcinoma or diffuse lymphangitic spread of carcinoma, high dose steroids (e.g., prednisone, 100 mg. daily) followed by chemotherapy may promote a useful regression of symptoms.

There is continuing study of various combinations of chemotherapy. At the moment, no single drug or combination of drugs seems to have a much more beneficial effect than the standard for therapy—cyclophosphamide.

COCCIDIOIDOMYCOSIS

method of
HANS E. EINSTEIN, M.D.
Bakersfield, California

Introduction

Coccidioidomycosis is a major health problem in the southwestern United States, particularly southern California, southern Arizona, southern Nevada, southern New Mexico, and west Texas. This area continues to be a heavily traveled part of the country by tourists and continues its postwar population growth, thereby bringing nonimmune people into the area continuously, some of whom acquire the disease and then are seen outside the endemic area with puzzling pulmonary infections. In addition, the increasing use of immunosuppression and organ transplantations has resulted in old infections reappearing in areas far removed from the endemic area. Although less than one third of the total number of infections are severe enough to require a physician's attention, the remainder do occasionally produce problems in management.

Therapy for Primary Infections

The primary coccidioidal infections are pulmonary, and do not require amphotericin treatment. Recovery is usually rapid and complete, with only anatomic residuals such as cavities or granulomas remaining. These require excision or biopsy upon occasion, usually without chemotherapeutic coverage.

Amphotericin B Therapy

Chemotherapy with amphotericin B is indicated in the following circumstances:

Primary Pulmonary Disease. 1. Infants.

2. Debilitated elderly patients.

3. Progressive primary pneumonia, persistence of hilar adenopathy with a rapidly rising antibody titer, particularly in non-Caucasian patients, diabetics, pregnant women, patients receiving immunosuppressive therapy, or those with underlying immunosuppressive illnesses.

4. Occasionally for surgical coverage, particularly when disease is extensive or recent, or antibodies are high; for postoperative complications; or for repeat surgery.

Disseminated Disease. All disseminated lesions are treated with amphotericin.

1. Meninges: systemic and local therapy (injection into the cisterna magna, lumbar area with hyperbaric glucose, occasionally into the ventricles) (Ommaya reservoir).

2. Bone lesions: these are treated systemically and locally by debridement and perfusion with amphotericin.

3. Skin lesions: systemic treatment and local treatment if drainage is present.

4. Viscera: systemic treatment only, unless accessible locally. The mortality of nonmeningeal dissemination has been reduced to less than 10 per cent in nonmeningeal cases and to 40 per cent in meningeal cases. Treatment must be persistent and vigorous. New antifungal agents are under investigation currently, with miconazole the most extensively studied. Immunotherapy with transfer factor is also undergoing investigational trial.

Amphotericin is administered intravenously and locally, as mentioned above. For the former purpose, it is dissolved in 5 per cent dextrose and water in concentration of 0.10 mg. per ml. A small needle in a peripheral vein is used, starting with 5 to 10 mg. the first day and increasing by 10 mg. increments to the usual maximal daily infusion of 50 mg. This can be built up to the level of 1.0 mg. per kg. The infusion is usually given over the course of approximately 1 hour; it has been found that this is much better tolerated by the patient than the usually recommended 3 to 4 hour course. The total dosage of amphotericin depends on the clinical situation: but generally for progressive primary disease, meningitis without other systemic involvement, bone lesions amenable to local therapy, empyema, and surgical coverage, 2 grams or less is sufficient, with 1 gram frequently adequate. This important limitation tends to decrease renal damage, which is dose related, and therefore allows subsequent retreatment. In view of the prolonged half-life of amphotericin, every-other-day administration is adequate and works out well, particularly in outpatient situations.

Chills, fever, anorexia, vomiting, and hypokalemia are almost invariable accompaniments of amphotericin treatment. These can be ameliorated somewhat with antiemetic, antipyretic, and antihistamine medications. Potassium supplementation is routinely given. Moderate azotemia is inevitable but is usually self-limited. This is best detected and followed by serum creatinine or creatinine clearances. Most follow-up studies show return of renal function to pretreatment levels, even when rather large doses have been given. Anemia, probably on a hemolytic basis, is invariably present but is usually self-limited.

As mentioned above, intravenous dosage should be supplemented whenever possible by local therapy. In bone, joint, and skin lesions, this is usually done by a daily drip of between 50 and 150 mg. of amphotericin (this use is not listed in the manufacturer's official directive). The intrathecal dosage is started with 0.10 mg. and is then built up by thrice weekly injections to the best tolerated dose, usually around 0.5 mg. This therapy is then continued for an indefinite period until all parameters in the spinal fluid have been negative for at least a year. I have found the cisterna magna to be the safest and most useful site of injection, although the lumbar and ventricular routes have also been used as secondary alternatives. The intrathecal use of amphotericin continues to be considered experimental by the Food and Drug Administration.

Corticosteroids are used both locally and systemically to suppress the severe inflammatory effects of the disease and to ameliorate the toxic effects of amphotericin B in critically ill patients. This occasionally allows the continuation of therapy when it would otherwise have to be interrupted. Corticosteroids are also used locally in intrathecal or intra-articular injections.

Surgery

In addition to the orthopedic procedures, residual pulmonary lesions require surgical attention. It is our practice to resect cavities that have been present for more than a year, particularly those which have bled or are threatening to rupture. This is usually done by lobectomy. Routine amphotericin coverage has not been necessary. It is used in patients with high serologic titers, in empyema, or in those of susceptible races. Diabetics do poorly with cavity resection, having a high recurrence rate; consequently resection is not done in such patients unless it is absolutely necessary. Solid granulomas, so-called coccidioidomas, need not be removed unless they present a diagnostic problem as to their cause. In that case, frequently biopsy procedures are successful in identifying the benign nature of the lesion.

Summary

The treatment of pulmonary and disseminating coccidioidomycosis involves the intelligent use or nonuse of amphotericin B, with the risk of the disease being carefully weighed against that of the drug in each case. Early use of amphotericin usually allows less total dosage and thus less permanent renal damage. It is hoped that secondary agents, immunotherapy, and an effective vaccine will soon become available to the profession for the benefit of the continuing large number of patients.

HISTOPLASMOSIS

method of
FRANCIS F. FOUNTAIN, Jr., M.D.,
and WHEELAN D. SUTLIFF, M.D.
Memphis, Tennessee

Histoplasmosis is a very common worldwide granulomatous infection. It is caused by the thermophilic dimorphic fungus, *Histoplasma capsulatum*. In the past, this has been classified as an imperfect fungus, but since the identification of the perfect form, *Emmonsiella capsulata,* a heterothallic ascomycete, this has not been appropriate. It is found in soil containing increased nitrogen, especially associated with the guano of birds and bats. However, when injected into birds it will be found only in the feathers. It has been found almost everywhere it has been sought, but is less common in Europe than the climatic conditions would suggest. In the United States it is endemic in wide areas of the Ohio-Mississippi valley. But even in endemic areas there are scattered areas of high concentration, and it will occasionally be found outside the endemic area in restricted environmental conditions such as caves. A humidity of 67 to 87 per cent with temperatures of 68 to 90°F. (20 to 32.2°C.) is associated with the largest incidence of exposure demonstrated by positive skin tests in man.

When the spores are inhaled, they are transformed into a tubular form and then into a single budding, small (2 to 5 microns in diameter) yeast with a narrow neck, frequently found in the reticuloendothelial system. Mycelial growth is not seen in vivo, but will occur in appropriate culture media at ambient temperature. The presence of tuberculate chlamydospores at ambient temperature aids in specific diagnosis.

A firm diagnosis should be made prior to treatment if at all possible, because of the toxicity of the primary drug, amphotericin B. If treatment is started without a firm diagnosis, there is a temptation to interrupt therapy sooner than would otherwise be the case when toxicity occurs. Except if the diagnostic procedure is too dangerous or the clinical situation is worsening too rapidly, a firmly established etiologic diagnosis should be sought. The diagnosis is definitively established by culture as described above. The yeast resembles other yeast forms, especially small forms of Candida, in the sputum when stained with silver methenamine, periodic acid–Schiff (PAS), or Giemsa. An immunofluorescent stain method for specific identification has been developed and, it is hoped, will be useful when it is more widely available.

Primary Pulmonary Histoplasmosis

Asymptomatic Primary Histoplasmosis. Ninety-five per cent of the patients are asymptomatic, with only single or multiple calcifications in the lungs and a positive skin test as evidence of previous infection. This form of the disease does not require treatment.

Symptomatic Primary Histoplasmosis. Symptomatic patients may have the gradual development of a dry cough, hoarseness, dyspnea, pleuritic pain, and, in more severe cases, night sweats, fever, and weight loss. Radiographically, multiple pulmonary infiltrates or nodules with unilateral or bilateral hilar lymphadenopathy are frequently seen. The pulmonary lesions resolve slowly with calcification. Occasionally a miliary pattern will be noted, which resolves. During this phase of the illness, occasional dissemination to lymph nodes, liver, and spleen will occur. The organism is occasionally found in both the sputum and bone marrow. Infrequently the disease will be severe enough to require treatment with amphotericin B.

Acute Reinfection Pulmonary Histoplasmosis

The patient who was previously infected is relatively immune from reinfection. However, if such a patient has been exposed to a high concentration of spores, exogenous reinfection may occur with onset 7 to 10 days after exposure to infected areas such as chicken yards or caves. This can be associated with a mild or a severe acute febrile illness resembling hypersensitivity pneumonitis, and may benefit from a short course of corticosteroids as well as amphotericin B. Except for such unusual circumstances, steroids and amphotericin B are to be avoided.

Sequelae. Several special situations are recognized as early or late sequelae to acute primary disease: mediastinitis, subacute endocarditis, traction diverticula of the esophagus, and bronchial obstruction resulting from lymphadenopathy with secondary infection. Occasionally mechanical complications of healing acute pulmonary histoplasmosis, such as broncholithiasis, bronchial obstruction, or fibrosing mediastinitis, are observed.

Chronic Pulmonary Histoplasmosis

Chronic pulmonary histoplasmosis is the most frequent clinical form of the disease. It is most common in males and is indistinguishable clinically from tuberculosis, frequently causing upper lung field fibronodular or cavitary lesions. It may proceed directly from a primary pulmonary infection or as an endogenous reinfection. Symptoms include weight loss, fever, hemoptysis, and dyspnea. Untreated, the disease follows a slow, progressive course, with periodic exacerbations and spreading pulmonary lesions. Pulmonary tuberculosis may complicate chronic pulmonary histoplasmosis, and may occur before, during, or after histoplasmosis is recognized in up to 20 per cent of the patients.

The excellent studies of the Veterans Administration Armed Forces Study Group are the only large-scale prospective randomized studies available on the treatment of histoplasmosis. They clearly show the need for treatment with amphotericin B for chronic pulmonary histoplasmosis. The optimal dose was also determined. Although a low total dose over the course of the illness, 500 mg. in adults, is helpful for some, larger doses are needed. A high total dose, 2500 mg. in adults, was uniformly effective but was also more toxic. An optimal dose is probably in the range of 20 to 35 mg. per kg. or from 1 to 1.5 grams in adults intravenously in divided doses of not over 1.5 mg. per kg. per day. There are no prospective controlled studies showing the need for surgery. If surgery is used, amphotericin B should seriously be considered to avoid relapses. Histoplasmomas, granulomatous solitary nodules usually less than 4 cm. in diameter, are a form of chronic pulmonary histoplasmosis that may occur without bacteriologic or serologic confirmation, usually with some calcification and rarely slowly enlarging. They may require excision for differentiation from neoplasia.

Disseminated Histoplasmosis

Benign dissemination frequently occurs early in the disease but is rarely diagnosed at that stage. It is noted retrospectively by calcifications outside the lungs. Treatment is not usually needed. Occasionally at this stage of the disease, organisms may be recovered from the sputum or bone marrow.

Clinically apparent disseminated histoplasmosis has a mortality rate, if untreated, of from 85 to nearly 100 per cent. Such patients deserve treatment with amphotericin B. It is realized that the disease in an occasional patient will clear without treatment.

Dissemination in childhood is associated with lymphadenopathy, hepatosplenomegaly, and bone marrow involvement. Amphotericin B in uncontrolled series has shown a dramatic improvement in fatality rates and should regularly be used.

Dissemination in adults was the first type described by Darling, and was similar symptomatically to leishmaniasis. Pulmonary symptoms are not usually prominent, but hepatosplenomegaly, anemia, and weight loss are seen. There may be occasional massive involvement of the lungs. Mucocutaneous involvement of the mouth, pharynx and larynx, and small intestines is noted, as well as occasional involvement of the skin and rheumatic involvement. There is frequent adrenal involvement, leading to adrenal insufficiency with disseminated histoplasmosis, and adrenal function should be evaluated in all patients. Meningitis occurs and may require intrathecal treatment with amphotericin B, although the intrathecal use is not listed in the manufacturer's official directive. The intrathecal therapy may be given by repeated lumbar punctures, cisternal punctures, or intraventricularly by a subcutaneous reservoir, the Ommaya reservoir. Because of the high mortality rate of disseminated histoplasmosis in adults, treatment should be instituted with amphotericin B if at all possible.

Treatment

Amphotericin B is the treatment of choice. Amphotericin B is a polyene antibiotic which is not absorbable from the gastrointestinal tract and must be administered intravenously. It combines with cholesterol in the cell membrane, thereby altering its permeability. It also damages host cells. It is available as a bile salt complex. When mixed with 5 per cent glucose in water, it forms a colloidal suspension. It should not be mixed with saline or with excessive acid, as this destroys the micelle suspension, producing a cloudy solution. It is quite stable in 5 per cent dextrose and water for 24 hours even in the presence of light. After intravenous injection, serum concentrations reach 0.5 to 2.0 micrograms per ml. Ten per cent of the dose remains in the plasma bound firmly to plasma protein. The urine concentration parallels the plasma concentration, and it is so low that reduced urinary function has no effect on serum concentration. Its affinity for cholesterol is such as to suggest that the antibiotic is chiefly bound to sterol-containing cell membranes throughout the body. Details of distribution and catabolism are unknown.

The method that we use for administration is similar to that of the Veterans Administration Armed Forces Study Group. The dry powder is mixed with 10 ml. of sterile preservative-free water or 5 per cent dextrose in water until completely clear. This is then added to 5 per cent dextrose in water so that the solution is no more dilute than 1 mg. per 10 ml. Some advise giving 1 mg. intravenously as a test dose for idiosyncratic reactions; but since reactions may still occur, and we have not seen this difficulty if mixed as described above, we do not routinely perform this test. We normally give 10, 20, 30, 40, and 50 mg. on consecutive days, or a maximum dose of 1 mg. per kg. in patients weighing less than 50 kg., and then give that dose on Mondays, Wednesdays, and Fridays. Techniques for measuring the amount of amphotericin B required to inhibit a recent fungal isolate, and the correlated value, the optimal therapeutic blood amphotericin B concentration, are not well established. In practice we have not found it necessary to routinely measure the minimal inhibitory concentration of the infecting organism or blood levels, or to give amphotericin B daily, although others have found these measures helpful.

Amphotericin B is given via scalp vein needle in alternating arms and veins, avoiding any bandage pressure, positional venous obstruction, or general sedation or muscular tension contributing to diminished blood flow in the veins. Until a volume greater than 300 ml. is given, we allow it to run in as fast as it will flow through the small needle. Larger volumes are given over a 2 hour period because of the fluid entailed. In patients with cardiac impairment, smaller volumes may be used. We have not found a slow infusion needed, and patients given a choice of slow or rapid infusion will almost invariably choose a rapid infusion. It should be noted, however, that there is a report of one cardiorespiratory death when 50 mg. was given rapidly as the initial dose.

Amphotericin B is toxic, regularly causing chills, fever, and nausea, for which we routinely use premedication. As treatment continues, these symptoms are usually less severe. It regularly causes increases in blood urea nitrogen (BUN) and decreases in creatinine clearance as well as renal acidosis and renal tubular damage leading to calcifications. Most renal function abnormalities are reversible; some are not, and renal function should be closely monitored. The place of intravenous mannitol and alkali is under investigation in the hope of modifying renal toxicity. It will be necessary also to investigate any effect on the efficacy of amphotericin B or enhanced toxicity of these combinations.

An anemia is regularly found, caused by bone marrow depression and changes in the red blood cell wall. Hypokalemia is frequent, and monitoring should be performed in order to replace potassium. Liver toxicity currently is uncommon. Numerous other toxicities are described in the manufacturer's package insert. Phlebitis is seen, and some advocate the use of heparin. We have not found this needed. Steroids also have been used to modify the phlebitis, but because of the possibility of increased cardiotoxicity and decreased host resistance they should be used with caution. Toxicity, or pre-existing renal damage, may require modification of the doses listed above.

Experimental Drugs

Miconazole, a broad-spectrum antifungal agent, is under investigational use for histoplasmosis. There is currently a problem of hyperlipidemia, possibly associated with the vehicle, which remains to be resolved. The methyl ester of amphotericin B is less toxic, but possibly less effective, and is unstable for storage and transport. Combinations of amphotericin B and other drugs are under consideration. Rifampin in particular has been found useful in animal infection. Rifampin, however, has been shown to depress cellular immunity, and may have a different toxicity when combined with amphotericin B. It therefore awaits further studies. Other drugs may be found helpful in combination with amphotericin B which would alter the permeability of the cell wall to these drugs, even though they are not themselves helpful when used alone. Transfer factor, a dialysable extract of leukocytes, has been used by us and others to convert positive skin tests on anergic patients. Clinical improvement has not been noted to regularly follow the prompt conversion of the skin test in patients with histoplasmosis. This method of treatment awaits prospective control studies.

Histoplasmosis Duboisii

A clinically distinct form of histoplasmosis is found primarily in moist equatorial Africa. It is caused by an organism called *Histoplasma duboisii* or *Histoplasma capsulatum* variety *duboisii*. This organism is antigenically indistinguishable from two strains of typical *Histoplasma capsulatum*. The *duboisii* strain is a single budding yeast 12 to 15 microns in diameter, resembling *Blastomyces dermatitidis* but lacking the broad-based bud. Clinical types of disease include (1) localized cutaneous, lymphatic, subcutaneous, or bone lesions and (2) multifocal disseminated types with many organs involved. Skeletal lesions are seen in as many as two thirds of disseminated cases. The yeast is found in giant cells rather than in histiocytes. It is suspected that the infection is acquired through the lungs, but pulmonary involvement is uncommon. Amphotericin B is the treatment of choice. Doses used have been 0.25 to 1.0 mg. per kg. One to 3 grams is necessary for a full course of treatment. Alternate day therapy may be used.

NORTH AMERICAN BLASTOMYCOSIS

method of
GUY D. CAMPBELL, M.D.
Jackson, Mississippi

North American blastomycosis is caused by the fungus *Blastomyces dermatitidis*. In the United States cases are most commonly found along the Ohio-Mississippi River valleys and the middle Atlantic states. Patients with blastomycosis diagnosed in other areas usually have been residents of the endemic regions. The disease has also been reported from Africa, Canada, and Latin America.

As with most deep systemic mycoses, infection follows inhalation of the mycelial spore of this dimorphic fungus. Within the lungs at body temperature the spore phase becomes a yeast form which spreads to various other organs, principally the skin, bone, and genitourinary system. Although documentation of the source of *B. dermatitidis* is far less secure than in histoplasmosis and coccidioidomycosis, *B. dermatitidis* is also thought to be indigenous to the soil despite few isolations from this source.

A smear from sputum or exudate revealing a typical budding yeast with double refractile walls and a wide pore between the mother and daughter cells is sufficient evidence to begin therapy when viewed by an experienced observer. Using special stains, particularly Gomori's methenamine silver technique or the periodic acid–Schiff method, biopsy specimens, when positive, are diagnostic of blastomycosis, but both the smear and tissue section should have cultural confirmation. Occasionally the diagnosis is first made when the organism is seen in sputum collected for cytology studies for malignancy.

Treatment

With rare exception a diagnosis of blastomycosis makes treatment mandatory. Isolation of the patient is not required, as human-to-human transmission does not occur.

Amphotericin B. This antibiotic is the most effective agent for treatment of blastomycosis. It has many side effects, most of which are unpleasant, but rarely some are more serious. Amphotericin B is indicated in patients with dense pulmonary disease with or without cavitation, multiple system disease, or miliary or central nervous system involvement, and in patients who fail to respond or who relapse after adequate treatment with 2-hydroxystilbamidine.

Amphotericin is a polyene antibiotic derived from the soil actinomycete, *Streptomyces nodosus.* The mechanism of action is not completely elucidated but probably is related to antibiotic binding to a sterol moiety present in the membrane of susceptible fungi, allowing leakage of intracellular components. Following cessation of therapy, the drug may be excreted in the urine for weeks.

Because of annoying side effects and the need for long duration of intravenous therapy, many physicians are reluctant to use amphotericin B. In over 200 patients treated, we have never seen a serious or life-threatening reaction, nor has any patient been left with significant compromised organ insufficiency despite a total dose up to 16 grams. Nevertheless, there are bothersome side effects which cause patient discomfort and require a physician's attention with careful monitoring.

Amphotericin B is packaged as a lyophilized powder in vials containing 50 mg. of the antibiotic, buffers, and sodium deoxycholate to effect a colloidal dispersion. The powder is reconstituted by adding 10 ml. of sterile water for injection U.S.P. *without a preservative* and mixing thoroughly to form a solution of 5 mg. per ml. The antibiotic is then added to 5 per cent dextrose injection U.S.P. (*never* saline solution), so that there is 100 ml. of 5 per cent dextrose injection U.S.P. for every 10 mg. of amphotericin B. This should be made fresh for each infusion and given immediately. If any precipitate or foreign matter is present on reconstitution or after adding to the infusion, the solution should be discarded. Amphotericin B should not be given through an infusion set with a membrane filter, because the drug is in colloidal form and will be removed by the filter.

Many schemes are recommended for administering amphotericin B, and the convenience and cost to patient (hospitalization) may influence the method chosen. Administration of the drug should be initiated while the patient is hospitalized. After the patient's condition has stabilized, he may receive the antibiotic on an outpatient basis with proper monitoring. When symptoms subside, the patient is able to return to his occupation while continuing amphotericin B on an outpatient basis.

ADMINISTRATION. 1. The initial dose is 5 or 10 mg. of amphotericin B in 100 ml. of 5 per cent dextrose injection U.S.P. This intravenous infusion is given in about 1 hour. Subsequent doses are administered in 30 to 60 minutes with 45 minutes for an average infusion. Fewer and less severe side reactions occur with this rapid administration than when the 6 hour infusion recommended in the package insert is followed.

2. The dosage is increased stepwise by 10 mg. of amphotericin B in each infusion until 30 to 35 mg. is being given, and then 5 mg. increases are employed until a maximal dose of 50 mg. is reached. As the amount of amphotericin B is increased, it is necessary to increase the 5 per cent dextrose injection U.S.P. being used as the vehicle. A good rule of thumb to remember is to add 50 ml. for each 5 mg. of amphotericin B.

3. In severely ill patients the initial dose should be 15 to 20 mg., increasing the dose by 10 to 15 mg. *daily* until a daily dose of 50 mg. is achieved.

4. Do not exceed a daily dose of 50 mg. of amphotericin B. Often patients cannot tolerate a dose this large even on a Monday-Wednesday-Friday regimen because of severe side effects and/or significant anemia or urea retention. Good results have been obtained with lesser doses, even as low as 15 to 20 mg.

5. As the dose increases, the patient may go from essentially no complaint to severe side reactions, primarily chills, fever, headache, nausea, vomiting, anorexia, or malaise. These side reactions may occur with the first or early dosages. By holding the dosage at the same level for several infusions, most patients develop a "tolerance" and can then accept a 5 mg. increase in dose. This approach may require repetition with each increase in dose.

6. As the blood urea nitrogen rises, patients usually become anemic, but this is not always so. An effort should be made to keep the hematocrit above 29 per cent and the blood urea nitrogen below 51 mg. per cent. Rather than discontinue therapy to achieve these goals, it is best to reduce the individual dose sufficiently until improvement occurs, after which the dose can again be slowly increased. In rare patients packed red cells may be required to keep the hematocrit within a safe range. After therapy is completed, the blood urea nitrogen returns to normal (or near normal) and the hemoglobin and hematocrit correct themselves.

7. The antibiotic is usually given daily for 7 to 10 days in order to relieve symptoms and to shorten hospitalization. As the patient improves,

most clinicians choose a Monday-Wednesday-Friday regimen unless the patient is critically ill or has widely disseminated disease.

8. A large majority of patients have some difficulty with amphotericin B. The most common complaints are chills, fever, anorexia, nausea, vomiting, headaches, and malaise. The most common findings are thrombophlebitis at the site of infusion, anemia, urea and creatinine retention, and hypokalemia. Hepatitis is unusual but may occur. Each infusion should contain approximately 2500 units of heparin to lessen thrombophlebitis, and the infusion should be given at different sites, beginning with the distal veins. Diphenhydramine (Benadryl), 50 mg. orally, is beneficial in ameliorating allergic reactions and is given routinely 30 minutes before the infusion. Aspirin is helpful in treating chills, fever, malaise, and headaches. Prochlorperazine (Compazine), 5 or 10 mg. orally, helps control nausea, vomiting, and anorexia. When indicated, both aspirin and prochlorperazine should be given 30 minutes before the infusion. Peripheral neuropathy is a rare manifestation of amphotericin B therapy and occurs almost exclusively in patients who have received a large total dose.

9. Steroids are often recommended to ameliorate or control troublesome side effects. We have been able to avoid steroids by adjusting individual doses, using rapid infusion, allowing the patient to develop "tolerance" to the individual dose before proceeding with the next higher dose, and using the medications mentioned above.

10. Before therapy, baseline serum glutamic oxaloacetic transaminase, potassium, blood urea nitrogen, creatinine, creatinine clearance, hemoglobin, hematocrit, and urinalysis determinations should be obtained. While the patient is receiving daily therapy, he should be monitored two or three times weekly by all the aforementioned tests except creatinine clearance. When he is converted to a three-times-weekly treatment, the same tests once a week usually suffice. Hypokalemia develops infrequently in the latter regimen, but supplementary potassium may be required if the patient is on daily therapy.

The minimal effective daily dose as well as the total dose is yet to be defined and varies from patient to patient, probably relating not only to the number of organs but also to specific organ involvement. It has been proposed that an adequate daily dose should give serum levels of amphotericin B that are twice the minimal inhibitory concentration. However, few laboratories are prepared to supply these results.

Most clinicians feel that a total dose of 2 grams of amphotericin B in a patient who becomes culture negative is adequate therapy. A minimal dose should not be less than 1.5 grams. Rarely, patients remain active despite large doses. If amphotericin B is reasonably well tolerated, it would seem logical in such a patient to continue amphotericin B three times weekly while adding daily 2-hydroxystilbamidine.

Miliary blastomycosis carries a serious prognosis and a 50 per cent mortality. If the patient requires a ventilator because of inadequate oxygen transfer, daily amphotericin B and 2-hydroxystilbamidine appear justified, although no studies are available documenting two-drug treatment as being more effective than amphotericin B alone. Those patients developing an acute respiratory distress syndrome probably benefit from intravenous steroids during the acute episode. Such acutely ill patients may require a larger total dose of amphotericin B.

2-Hydroxystilbamidine. 2-Hydroxystilbamidine (hydroxystilbamidine isethionate) is an aromatic diamidine which is less toxic but also less effective than amphotericin B for the treatment of blastomycosis. Patients with cutaneous lesions only or those with cutaneous and minimal noncavitary pulmonary blastomycosis usually have a very satisfactory response to 2-hydroxystilbamidine. The antibiotic is also indicated when patients are unable to tolerate or fail to respond to amphotericin B.

2-Hydroxystilbamidine is supplied in a 20 ml. ampule containing 225 mg. of sterile powder. The powder is dissolved immediately prior to use in 200 ml. of either 5 per cent dextrose injection U.S.P. or sodium chloride injection U.S.P. If the solution is turbid, it should be discarded. Both the ampule and the prepared solution must be protected from light and heat. A black covering should be slipped over the bottle until the infusion is completed.

The recommended daily dose is 225 mg. administered over a 45 to 60 minute period (a 2 or 3 hour infusion is recommended in the package insert). Although most patients have no difficulty, minor reactions may be noted, consisting of formication, weakness, headache, myalgia, anorexia, nausea, vomiting, diarrhea, chills, and fever. If the solution is given too quickly, patients may develop weakness, dizziness, pleuritis, tachycardia, or circulatory collapse. Hepatitis is an uncommon but potentially serious toxicity. Patients receiving 2-hydroxystilbamidine should be monitored prior to therapy and weekly during therapy with serum glutamic oxaloacetic transaminase, blood urea nitrogen, and urinalysis determinations.

The minimal effective dose is yet to be determined but should not be less than 8 grams. Because of individual response to therapy, some patients may require as much as 12 to 16 grams.

Lesions usually show continued improvement after the drug is discontinued, probably related to the continued presence of 2-hydroxystilbamidine for weeks after cessation of therapy. After the patient is stabilized and no significant toxicities are associated with the infusion, the medication may be continued on a daily outpatient basis while the patient returns to his normal activities. After discharge some physicians omit the Sunday dose for the convenience of the patient.

Surgery. Except for diagnosis, there is rarely any indication for surgery in blastomycosis. Surgery has been mistakenly employed to excise what was thought to be a malignancy. Antifungal therapy should be administered even when it appears that the lesion has been completely removed and when the roentgenographic appearance seems to confirm this impression. Unless antifungal therapy is administered, there is distinct possibility that the lesion may recur in the lungs or disseminate to other areas, including the spine.

EMPYEMA THORACIS

method of
HUGH E. STEPHENSON, JR., M.D.
Columbia, Missouri

Most suppurative pleural disease is effectively treated with a combination of antibiotic medication and properly selected and adequate drainage techniques. Since Evarts A. Graham in 1918 established the basic principles for managing a collection of pus in the pleural space, the goals have continued to be those of adequate drainage and obliteration and sterilization of the empyema cavity.

Although the incidence of tuberculous empyema has been markedly reduced, one continues to encounter empyema as a sequela of pneumonia, lung abscess, pulmonary neoplasm, bronchopleural fistula, and retained foreign body in the pleural space, as well as in association with a variety of postoperative complications in addition to post-thoracotomy such as subphrenic abscess. A post-traumatic, infected, clotted hemopneumothorax may develop subsequent to thoracentesis or even intercostal tube drainage for hemothorax. Failure to employ proper preventive measures or to institute prompt isolation of the offending bacteriologic agent and begin early therapy still results in much morbidity and prolonged hospital stay. Most deaths are encountered in the infant under 2 years or in the older patient with associated debilitating disease.

Treatment

Timing is a key consideration, not only in the early identification of the causative organism but also in removal of the fluid and re-expansion of the lung. Chronicity adds much to the challenge of proper therapy because of thickening of the pleura, loculation of the fluid, entrapment of the lung with reduced pulmonary function, and general inanition. Therefore early acute pleural empyema requires the measures listed.

Microbiology of Empyema. Early identification of the offending organism should be made. Smears, cultures (aerobic and anaerobic), and sensitivity studies should be done on pus obtained by thoracentesis. In our institution the microorganisms most frequently isolated include *Staphylococcus aureus* (coagulase positive), *Pseudomonas aeruginosa,* pneumococcus, hemolytic Streptococcus, *Escherichia coli,* and *Aerobacter aerogenes. Streptococcus pyogenes, Streptococcus pneumoniae,* Bacteroides, and Klebsiella may be involved. The Citrobacter species need to be separated from *Escherichia coli. Citrobacter diversus* is a potential pathogen, especially in patients with compromised host defenses. All culture sites in addition to pleural fluid should be utilized, when applicable, including sputum, bronchial washing, blood culture, and wound culture. Resistant organisms and mixed cultures are to be expected. Repeat cultures should be obtained throughout treatment, especially if progress appears delayed. Since amebiasis may occasionally provoke an empyemic infection, fluid obtained should be examined for *Entamoeba histolytica,* especially if of an anchovy-sauce consistency.

What Is the Etiology? Accurate categorization of the causes of the empyema is necessary, because empyema is always secondary to disease originating elsewhere. For example, pleural suppuration after rupture of the esophagus usually requires immediate drainage. If radiologic study demonstrates the multiple translucent zones of staphylococcal pneumonia in infancy, one must consider the possibility of a tension pyopneumothorax. Tuberculous empyema requires special consideration, because one wishes to prevent open drainage of a cutaneous fistula. Secondary contamination of the tuberculous empyema cavity will further seriously complicate management. Although empyema after a pneumonic process is still the most common causative factor, many other possibilities exist. Direct contamination of the pleural space during traumatic injury may be the obvious cause. Fortunately, postoperative empyema has decreased in frequency. Patients on immunosuppressive therapy and steroids appear more susceptible to empyema, owing often to their associated debilitating disease.

Nevertheless postoperative empyema still occurs with annoying frequency. Antimicrobial prophylaxis is not generally a routine for patients requiring thoracic procedures. At least one institution, however, uses systemic cephalosporins in what they believe to be an effective measure:

1. Cephalexin, 0.5 gram by mouth the evening before operation, and cephalothin, 1.0 gram intramuscularly or intravenously on call to the operating room.

2. Cephalothin, 1 gram intramuscularly or intravenously every 6 hours for 2 days, followed by cephalexin, 0.25 gram by mouth four times daily for 3 days.

Irrigations of the pleural cavity with a solution of 1 gram of kanamycin or 1 gram of cephalothin in a liter of isotonic saline solution is often included in the regimen.

A pulmonary abscess caused by neoplastic obstruction may rupture into the pleural space. Bronchiectasis, foreign bodies, or a subphrenic abscess may be the source of infection.

Drainage. A decision must be made as to which method will ensure the most effective drainage and obliteration of the pleural space. With acute empyema one should elect a method of drainage based on the following criteria:

THORACENTESIS. Generally speaking, thoracentesis is primarily a diagnostic procedure aimed at determining the bacteriology of the pleural empyema. In an occasional instance thoracentesis along with systemic antibiotic therapy will suffice. Needle thoracentesis may not always accomplish the goal of complete cavity aspiration. It is difficult to position the needle in the most satisfactory fashion. For this reason I prefer to thread a polythene catheter through the bore of the needle (as described by Gray, 1959), remove the needle, and allow the catheter to seek the most dependent position in the cavity. The catheter technique lessens the possibility of producing a pneumothorax and obviates the need for a critically ill patient to be maintained in an upright position during thoracentesis. A much greater amount of fluid can be removed in this fashion.

Antibiotics suitable for intrathoracic instillation may be added at the conclusion of aspiration. Appropriate antibiotics are also administered systemically. Bacteriologic studies are repeated upon each aspiration.

TUBE THORACOSTOMY. Although thoracentesis is a diagnostic measure and may serve as a primary means of therapy in selected patients, early closed thoracostomy is more often the best means of achieving adequate drainage and obliteration of the empyema cavity through complete and continued removal of the infected fluid.

The intercostal tube insertion is done with strict aseptic precautions, with adequate local anesthesia, and with the patient in a sitting position. The decision whether to drain anteriorly, laterally, or posteriorly will be determined by the biplane radiographic studies and auscultation and percussion of the chest. The tube is inserted after a small incision is made over the rib edge superiorly and extended down to the pleural space. One may pass the tube, usually a plastic chest catheter, into the pleural space through a chest trocar or simply by following behind the dissection with a blunt hemostat. It is obviously important to place the tube in the most dependent portion of the infected area.

After fixation of the tube to the skin with suture and tape, it is connected to an underwater seal and suction. X-rays are then taken to check the position of the tube. The tube should not be removed until all drainage has ceased and lung expansion is evident. Irrigation with saline solution may be helpful from time to time. Clagett's solution of 250 mg. of neomycin per 100 ml. may be instilled, if indicated. (This use of neomycin may not be listed in the manufacturer's official directive.) Bacitracin, 25,000 units per 100 ml., sodium colistimethate (Coly-Mycin), 150 mg. per 100 ml., or both are often used, because frequently both Staphylococcus and Pseudomonas are cultured from the cavity. (See manufacturer's official directive before using bacitracin and sodium colistimethate as recommended.)

Tube drainage will usually be required for at least 8 to 14 days. Patency of the drainage tube should be monitored constantly. Simply shortening the tube over a period of time without removal will help to completely obliterate the empyema cavity.

Closed drainage of empyema with a large tube is particularly effective in patients with large empyemas, in the acutely ill and toxic patient, and in the infant with acute empyema secondary to staphylococcal pneumonia.

Supportive Therapy. Bed rest is recommended in the early acute febrile phase, with ambulation permitted as soon as the toxic state is corrected. Bronchoscopy may be done early to rule out the presence of an obstructing lesion and to obtain material for bacteriology and cytologic studies. Bronchoscopy may also be helpful in enhancing drainage by the removal of any inspissated material, necrotic slough, retained secretion, or foreign body that might be present.

Other supportive nonspecific measures include a high caloric diet rich in vitamins and abundant fluid intake to help thin the secretions. Occasionally blood transfusions may be indicated.

This course of therapy should be continued as long as there is clinical or radiologic improvement or until the disappearance of all symptoms.

Open Drainage. Some pleural empyemas will be seen late in the course of the process or will not respond to closed-tube thoracostomy. In such instances rib resection and open drainage will be required for adequate management, including continuous removal of the purulent exudate and encouragement of lung re-expansion with obliteration of the empyema cavity. If all debris is to be removed from the empyema cavity, the opening must be of sufficient size and in a dependent position. A small encapsulated empyema may not yield to easy drainage with a tube thoracostomy.

Decortication. Chronic, thick-walled cavities and major pulmonary collapse will usually require a decortication procedure. Seldom is this necessary before 4 to 5 weeks after the initial therapy.

Despite antibiotics and tube drainage, pleural infection may complicate chest trauma. Earlier pleural decortication is often indicated in posttraumatic empyema and may even be carried out before the organization of the pleural exudate. Especially is early decortication to be considered if a residual air-fluid level persists despite chest-tube drainage or if ventilatory function is markedly compromised by pleural restriction. Decortication may be attempted as early as 2 to 3 weeks after bacterial empyema formation. Early and adequate treatment of acute empyema will lessen the need for lung decortication.

Complications. Complications secondary to an empyemic infection include a variety of possibilities such as extension of the infection to the ribs, cartilage, or sternum. Although rare, the infection may rupture into the esophagus or pericardial sac. Empyema necessitatis (spread of pus through the tissue planes of the chest wall) is seldom encountered today. More commonly, however, a bronchopleural fistula is encountered with empyema and requires early drainage of the infection to avoid persistent contamination of bronchi with purulent material.

PRIMARY LUNG ABSCESS

method of
NICHOLAS D'ESOPO, M.D.
West Haven, Connecticut

Primary lung abscess is the result of a necrotizing pneumonia caused by bacteria aspirated from the oropharynx following states of clouded consciousness, especially alcoholism. A few are caused by staphylococci or Klebsiella, which along with *Mycobacterium tuberculosis* should be looked for in the sputum in each patient.

Studies of the bacteriology of simple lung abscess have shown that the causative organisms are anaerobic bacteria, either alone or together with aerobic bacteria. The majority of these are susceptible to penicillin. The role of *Bacteroides fragilis*, which is resistant to penicillin, is not clear. However, patients in whom *B. fragilis* are found respond satisfactorily to penicillin.

The demonstration that a simple lung abscess is due to anaerobic bacteria requires culture of material from tracheal lavage or of pus obtained directly from the abscess by lung puncture. These procedures are not required in the management of simple lung abscess. If smear and culture of the sputum do not suggest that staphylococci or gram-negatives are the cause of the abscess, the clinician may confidently assume that the abscess is due to anaerobic bacteria.

The treatment of anaerobic lung abscess is penicillin. The dose is 2 million units a day intramuscularly. In very ill patients doses as high as 10 million units are sometimes used, although without evidence that these large doses are necessary. Their disadvantage is their potential for superinfection.

Patients who are allergic to penicillin may be treated with parenteral clindamycin in doses of 1.8 grams daily. Cephalosporins and the semisynthetic penicillins are not recommended.

Lung abscesses will not heal unless they drain adequately. In most cases drainage promptly follows the institution of antibiotic therapy. In others, however, methods to promote drainage must be vigorously pursued: postural drainage, chest physiotherapy, hydration, and ultrasonic nebulization. Such measures are essential in a patient whose abscess continues to show a fluid level, especially when such a patient is raising only a small amount of sputum. Bronchoscopy, bronchial brushing, and small arterial catheters directed into the cavity under fluoroscopic control may also be used to promote drainage.

Whether or not bronchoscopy should be done in every patient is an open question. Some physicians employ bronchoscopy in every patient to rule out the presence of a foreign body, neoplasm, or other bronchial obstruction. Others withhold it so long as the patient's clinical and roentgenographic course is favorable.

Supportive therapy is required as in any patient with a febrile illness; but in addition it should be remembered that many patients with primary lung abscess are alcoholics whose pulmonary infection has been preceded by a period of poor nutrition and neglect. Many patients have carious teeth to which attention should be given at an appropriate time.

The duration of chemotherapy cannot be precisely determined. Penicillin should be continued until serial x-rays (viz., 1 to 2 weeks apart) are more or less stable, as evidenced by the resolution of the pneumonic component surrounding the abscess, the size of the abscess cavity, and the thickness of the cavity wall. By this time the sputum is no longer purulent and sputum volume has approached the patient's baseline amount. Most patients with primary lung abscess are chronic bronchitics who have daily sputum. This will continue even after successful treatment of the abscess. The persistence of the abscess cavity as a thin-walled, cyst-like structure is not in itself an indication for continued therapy.

The average duration of chemotherapy is approximately 6 weeks, but some patients, especially those with large cavities of some duration prior to chemotherapy, may require longer treatment. When patients are over the acute phase, oral chemotherapy may be used: usually phenoxymethyl penicillin, 500 mg. four times daily.

Medical treatment results in cure of the abscess in almost 100 per cent of the patients. A few patients die of overwhelming sepsis within the first few days of treatment, and exsanguinating hemorrhage accounts for a few additional deaths. Surgery is now rarely necessary. Some cavities take months to disappear, and a few remain permanently as thin-walled structures. Surgical removal of such residual cavities is not warranted. A few may become reinfected or hemorrhage. These complications can be managed when they occur. An important indication for surgery is life-threatening hemorrhage. What is considered a life-threatening hemorrhage is a matter of judgment in each patient; however, experience indicates that hemorrhage of more than 400 ml. over a 24 hour period carries a bad prognosis on medical treatment alone, and is considered by many an indication for surgery. Another important though rarely needed indication for surgery is failure of an abscess to drain. Occasionally, a severe inflammatory bronchial stenosis proximal to the abscess prevents adequate drainage even by some of the maneuvers cited above. Surgery may be considered when the patient remains septic with minimal sputum production or when air-fluid levels persist after 7 to 10 days of antibiotic therapy. Such patients may require external tube drainage (after ensuring symphysis of the pleural membranes) or resection. Patients occasionally present with an abscess already complicated by empyema and bronchopleural fistula. The empyema should be drained.

It should be remembered that because of alcoholism, epilepsy, and other predisposing conditions associated with loss of gag reflex, patients with primary lung abscess are subject to repeated pulmonary infections. Removal of functioning lung should not be done unless absolutely necessary. Surgery should be employed only after a long trial of chemotherapy and efforts at cavity drainage have been unsuccessful.

OTITIS MEDIA

method of
PAUL A. SHURIN, M.D.
Cleveland, Ohio

Otitis media is most frequent in the first years of life but occurs at all ages. The condition is defined clinically by the presence of middle ear effusion. Both bacterial and nonbacterial effusions are common and cannot be differentiated without examination and culture of the middle ear fluid. Infections of the middle ear are usually treated without complication, but may be important foci for such serious infections as mastoiditis, meningitis, labyrinthitis, and cerebral or parameningeal abscess. Chronic otitis media may be complicated by cholesteatoma formation.

Tympanocentesis or aspiration of the middle ear is not generally required for assessment of cases of otitis media, but should be performed when identification of the causative organism would confer significant clinical benefit. Suitable indications include (1) otitis media in patients who are seriously ill or appear toxic, (2) an unsatisfactory response to initial antimicrobial therapy, (3) the onset of otitis media in a patient who is receiving antimicrobial agents, (4) the presence of suppurative complications of otitis, or (5) otitis in the newborn or in patients with immune deficiency, in whom infection with unusual organisms is more likely. Prior to aspiration, the ear canal should be cultured with a swab and cleansed with 70 per cent alcohol. The ear canal culture is often helpful in determining whether organisms recovered in the middle ear fluid are contaminants from the ear canal or pathogens from the middle ear itself. Tympanocentesis is performed through the inferior portion of the tympanic membrane, using an 18 gauge spinal needle attached to a syringe or suction apparatus.

Etiology of Middle Ear Infections

The major causative agents are as follows:

1. *Streptococcus pneumoniae* accounts for approximately 40 per cent of cases. These infec-

tions are likely to be of sudden onset and associated with severe pain and high fever, although otitis of any type may be subclinical in presentation.

2. *Hemophilus influenza* causes 20 per cent of cases and is an agent of otitis at all ages. Bilateral involvement and an insidious onset are common. Strains resistant to ampicillin have recently appeared and may present an increasing problem.

3. *Neisseria catarrhalis* has been isolated in pure culture from 5 to 10 per cent of patients.

4. Group A beta-hemolytic Streptococcus has been isolated from approximately 5 per cent of cases of otitis.

5. Twenty-five to 50 per cent of effusions from acute otitis media are bacteriologically sterile.

Therapy of Otitis Media

The antimicrobial drugs selected should be those active against both *S. pneumoniae* and *H. influenzae* unless the specific causative agent is known. The following regimens are of proved effectiveness in sterilizing middle ear effusions:

1. Ampicillin, 50 to 100 mg. per kg. per day given orally in four divided doses for 10 days (250 mg. four times daily for adults), or amoxicillin, 25 to 40 mg. per kg. per day orally in three doses.

2. Penicillin V or penicillin G, 25,000 to 50,000 units per kg. per day, plus triple sulfonamides or sulfisoxazole, 125 mg. per kg. per day given orally in four divided doses for 10 days.

3. Erythromycin, 40 to 50 mg. per kg. per day, plus triple sulfonamides or sulfisoxazole, 125 mg. per kg. per day given orally in four doses. This is the most useful regimen for patients who are allergic to penicillin, or for those in whom infection with ampicillin-resistant *H. influenzae* is suspected.

Parenteral therapy may be required initially for patients with severe otitis or for patients who cannot tolerate oral medication. Antibiotics other than those mentioned are not at present of well-established efficacy and should, in general, be considered only when the sensitivity of the infecting organism is known.

Decongestants and antihistamines may be used for symptomatic relief but are not of established efficacy in treatment of middle ear effusion. Analgesics may be used, but for severe earache needle aspiration or myringotomy is most effective.

It is important for the physician to establish that symptoms have begun to resolve within several days and that complete resolution of the ear effusion has occurred within 2 to 6 weeks. Patients who have persisting effusions may be given a trial of prophylactic antimicrobial therapy with either (1) ampicillin, 125 to 250 mg. given once daily, or (2) sulfisoxazole, 40 mg. per kg. twice daily.

In patients in whom antimicrobial prophylaxis is unsuccessful after a 1 to 3 month trial, or when there is significant hearing loss, myringotomy and placement of tympanostomy tubes will afford relief of the effusions and improvement in hearing.

Recurrent Acute Otitis Media and Persistent Middle Ear Effusion

These conditions are very common in children and are thought to cause deficits in language acquisition in some patients. Hearing loss may be subtle and episodic. Consequently persistent middle ear effusion is better diagnosed with otoscopic examination or tympanometry than with pure-tone audiometry. However, effective therapy and good follow-up are crucial when conductive hearing loss is present, and hearing should be tested in patients who are at risk and who are old enough to cooperate with the test. The therapeutic options for patients with persistent or recurrent otitis media are as follows:

1. Antimicrobial therapy of acute symptomatic episodes, as outlined above.

2. Prolonged (1 to 3 months) administration of either ampicillin or sulfisoxazole (as above) in an attempt to suppress infection and permit healing of the middle ear mucosa.

3. Myringotomy, aspiration of effusion, and insertion of ventilating tubes. A myringotomy incision alone will generally heal rapidly without lasting benefit. Ventilating tubes remain in place for 2 to 6 months and provide a marked improvement in hearing. Otitis media developing while tubes are in place is manifested by otorrhea and should be treated with systemic antibiotics. Ear drops such as those containing hydrocortisone, neomycin, and polymyxin B may be used for this condition in addition to oral antibiotics. Ventilating tubes may also be helpful for patients with atelectasis of the middle ear if hearing loss is significant, or if deep retraction is present in the posterosuperior portion of the tympanic membrane. Chronic otitis media with perforation requires surgical management when healing has not followed adequate antimicrobial therapy, when the perforation is posterosuperior or marginal, or when cholesteatoma is suspected.

BACTERIAL PNEUMONIA

method of
JAMES R. BONNER, M.D.
Mobile, Alabama

Effective treatment of patients with bacterial pneumonia requires both general supportive measures and specific antimicrobial agents directed against the causative microorganisms.

General Measures

Most patients need hospitalization, at least initially, in order to assure adequate rest, good diet, and prompt treatment of any complications which may arise. Dehydration is a frequent concomitant of pneumonia, and proper fluid balance should be assured either orally or by the administration of appropriate intravenous fluids. Mobilization of purulent material should be promoted, if necessary, by humidified air, vibropercussion, and postural drainage. Airway obstruction can result from inflammatory edema, secretions, or bronchospasm. When wheezing is heard, bronchodilators such as aminophylline, 100 or 200 mg. every 6 hours (adult dose), may be helpful. Therapeutic bronchoscopy is sometimes indicated to remove inspissated secretions. Supplemental oxygen may be required for hypoxia, and arterial blood gases should be measured in all patients with cyanosis or respiratory distress. Patients with chronic obstructive lung disease may need a hypoxic stimulus for respiration, and oxygen therapy may result in respiratory depression and carbon dioxide retention. Limited amounts of oxygen with careful monitoring of arterial blood gases is necessary in these patients. Ventilatory support may be needed in seriously ill patients and is discussed in the article on Acute Respiratory Failure. The use of aspirin or other antipyretics is of doubtful value, as it may negate the usefulness of the temperature response in following the patient's course and sometimes causes wide swings in temperature, resulting in uncomfortable chills and sweats. Fever should be treated in patients with heart disease, in whom the accompanying tachycardia could be dangerous, and in patients with temperatures above 105°F. (40.5°C.). Pleuritic pain leads to shallow respirations and should be relieved by analgesics such as indomethacin, 25 mg. three times daily (with meals) (this use of indomethacin is not listed in the manufacturer's official directive), or codeine, 15 to 30 mg. intramuscularly or 30 to 60 mg. orally every 4 hours. Codeine is a cough suppressant but has the advantage of not affecting temperature

Identification of Pathogen

Attempts to identify the specific pathogen should precede initiation of antimicrobial therapy. Careful examination of a Gram stain of a good sputum specimen remains the best test in determining initial therapy. The presence of numerous polymorphonuclear leukocytes is evidence that an adequate specimen has been obtained. Transtracheal aspiration is recommended by some in order to avoid contamination of sputum by upper respiratory bacteria. This procedure is particularly useful if precise anaerobic cultures are desired but carries some risk and should not be performed routinely. Specimens obtained by bronchoscopy offer little advantage over expectorated sputum except in patients who are unable to produce a proper specimen. Sputum can sometimes be obtained by nasotracheal or orotracheal suctioning. Before initiating treatment, sputum and blood cultures should be obtained.

The drugs of choice for specific bacterial infections, along with alternative drugs, and the usual doses are listed in Table 1.

Specific Treatment

Pneumococcal Pneumonia. *Streptococcus pneumoniae* is still the most common cause of bacterial pneumonia, especially in previously healthy young adults. It characteristically produces an acute illness with fever, a single chill, pleuritic chest pain, and expectoration of rusty brown sputum. Patients sometimes develop a sterile pleural effusion, but empyema and abscess formation are unusual. Demonstrable bacteremia occurs in about 30 per cent of patients with pneumococcal pneumonia, and these patients have a poorer prognosis than patients whose blood cultures are negative. Arthritis, endocarditis, and meningitis are infrequent complications of pneumococcal bacteremia. Confusion and lethargy should not be attributed to "toxicity" or hypoxia without first examining the cerebrospinal fluid.

The drug of choice for pneumococcal pneumonia is penicillin G. For patients allergic to penicillin, erythromycin may be substituted. Antibiotics should be continued for 1 week or until the patient has been afebrile for 2 to 3 days, whichever is longer. Patients usually show marked clinical improvement with defervescence within 24 to 48 hours, but occasionally 3 to 4 days elapse before improvement is noted. It is important to remember that radiographic clearance often does not accompany clinical improvement. Signs of consolidation may persist for up to 10 weeks, and volume loss and streaking may persist for over 4 months. Clinical improvement and radiographic clearance are most often delayed in patients with

TABLE 1. **Antibiotic Treatment for Adult Bacterial Pneumonia**

MICROORGANISM	DRUG OF CHOICE*	ALTERNATIVE DRUGS‡
Streptococcus pneumoniae	Procaine penicillin G, 600,000 U. I.M. q. 12 h.	Erythromycin, 500 mg. P.O. q. 6 h.
Staphylococcus aureus	Nafcillin, 1–2 grams I.V. q. 4 h. *or* Aqueous penicillin G, 20 million U. I.V.q.d. in divided doses (when bacteria susceptible)	Cephalothin, 1–2 grams I.V. q. 4 h. Cephalothin, 1–2 grams I.V. q. 4 h. Vancomycin, 1 gram I.V. over 30–40 min. q. 12 h.
Hemophilus influenzae	Ampicillin, 1–2 grams I.V. q. 6 h. *or* Amoxicillin, 500 mg. P.O. q. 8 h.	Chloramphenicol, 0.5–1 gram I.V. q. 6 h.
Streptococcus pyogenes	Same as for *S. pneumoniae*	Same as for *S. pneumoniae*
Klebsiella	Gentamicin, 1–1.5 mg./kg. I.V. or I.M. q. 8 h. *plus* Cephalothin, 1–2 grams/kg. I.V. q. 4 h.	Chloramphenicol, 0.5 gram I.V. q. 6 h.
Enterobacter	Gentamicin, 1–1.5 mg./kg.I.V. or I.M.q.8h. *plus* Carbenicillin, 5 grams I.V. q. 4 h.	Chloramphenicol, 0.5–1 gram I.V. q. 6 h.
Escherichia coli	Ampicillin, 1–2 grams q. 6 h. I.V. (when bacteria susceptible) *or* Gentamicin, 1–1.5 mg./kg. I.V. or I.M. q. 8 h.	Cephalothin, 1–2 grams I.V. q. 4 h. Chloramphenicol, 0.5–1 gram I.V. q. 6 h.
Proteus mirabilis	Ampicillin, 1–2 grams q. 6 h. I.V. (when bacteria susceptible) *or* Gentamicin, 1–1.5 mg./kg. I.V. or I.M. q. 8 h.	Cephalothin, 1–2 grams I.V. q. 4 h. Chloramphenicol, 0.5–1 gram I.V. q. 6 h.
Other Proteus species	Gentamicin, 1–1.5 mg./kg. I.V. or I.M. q. 8 h. *plus* Carbenicillin, 5 grams I.V. q. 4 h.	Chloramphenicol, 0.5–1 gram I.V. q. 6 h.
Serratia marcescens	Gentamicin, 1–1.5 mg./kg. I.V. or I.M. q. 8 h. *plus* Carbenicillin, 5 grams I.V. q. 4 h.	Chloramphenicol, 0.5–1 gram I.V. q. 8 h.
Pseudomonas aeruginosa	Tobramycin, 1–1.5 mg./kg. I.V. or I.M. q. 6 h. *plus* Carbenicillin, 5 grams I.V. q. 4 h.	
Aspiration pneumonia	Penicillin, 20 million U.I.V. q.d.† (in divided doses)	Clindamycin, 300 mg. I.V. q. 6 h. Chloramphenicol, 0.5–1 gram I.V. q. 6 h.

*Dosages are for adult patients with normal renal function. Except for *Streptococcus pyogenes* and pneumococcal pneumonia, the final choice for antibiotics is dependent upon laboratory sensitivity studies.

†For aspiration pneumonia, high dose penicillin is recommended when the patient is first seen and is severely ill. Once there is clinical improvement with defervescence, low dose penicillin such as that used for pneumococcal pneumonias can be given.

‡Cephalosporins should not be used in patients with penicillin allergy if the allergy is of the anaphylactic type.

chronic obstructive lung disease, elderly patients, and those with extensive disease. Patients with persistent radiographic changes should have chest x-rays repeated every 4 to 6 weeks to rule out other pulmonary disorders.

Staphylococcal Pneumonia. *Staphylococcus aureus* is responsible for 1 to 2 per cent of adult bacterial pneumonia. The pneumonia may be "primary" or may result from hematogenous spread from staphylococcal disease elsewhere. Primary staphylococcal pneumonia occurs most commonly in patients with chronic debilitating disease, as a nosocomial infection, or following an episode of influenza. Hematogenous staphylococcal pneumonia can complicate staphylococcal bacteremia from any cause such as skin infection, drug addiction, acute bacterial endocarditis, or contaminated intravenous sites. Staphylococcal pneumonia is characterized by early empyema, pneumatocele, and pyopneumothorax.

Except in those rare instances in which the organism is susceptible to penicillin G, a penicillinase-resistant semisynthetic penicillin such as nafcillin is the drug of choice. Alternative drugs are vancomycin and the cephalosporins. Cephalosporins should probably be avoided in patients with a history of immediate anaphylactic reactions to penicillin.

Drainage of empyema is an important part of therapy; this usually requires surgical placement of a chest tube. Recovery is characterized by gradual clinical improvement, with complete defervescence only after a 1 to 2 week period. Treatment should be continued for a total of 3 to 4 weeks in patients with primary pneumonia and for 4 to 6 weeks in pneumonia of hematogenous origin. In either case antibiotics should be continued until the patient is clinically better and the x-ray changes have cleared or become stable (this is a necrotizing pneumonia, and residual scarring is not uncommon).

Hemophilus Pneumonia. *Hemophilus influenzae* causes pneumonia in children under 4 years old and rarely in adults (usually patients with chronic obstructive lung disease). Ampicillin is the drug of choice. *H. influenzae* is occasionally resistant to ampicillin, and in these instances, as well as in patients allergic to penicillin, chloramphenicol should be used. This is not a necrotizing pneumonia, and clinical improvement is usually rapid.

Streptococcal Pneumonia. *Streptococcus pyogenes* (group A beta-hemolytic Streptococcus) is presently a rare cause of pneumonia. The disease is associated with streptococcal outbreaks in the community and sometimes follows influenza or measles. Characteristically there is abrupt onset of chills, fever, cough productive of thin pink sputum, and early empyema formation. Antibiotic therapy is the same as for pneumococcal pneumonia.

Aerobic Gram-Negative Rod Pneumonia. Klebsiella is a cause of acute lobar pneumonia in debilitated patients, especially alcoholics. It may have a predilection for the right upper lobe and is characterized by acute illness with fever, chills, and production of tenacious brown sputum. Klebsiella and other gram-negative bacilli also cause nosocomial infections, often in severely ill patients who are already receiving antibiotics and those requiring respiratory support. Microorganisms involved include *Escherichia coli,* Proteus species, *Serratia marcescens,* Enterobacter, and *Pseudomonas aeruginosa*. These bacteria produce necrotizing pneumonias sometimes complicated by abscess or empyema. Antibiotic sensitivities may vary in these species, and therapy must be based on susceptibility data. Pending sensitivity data a cephalosporin and an aminoglycoside such as gentamicin or tobramycin should be started (tobramycin is recommended as the initial drug in suspected or proved Pseudomonas pneumonia, and in this situation carbenicillin is included, as it may be synergistic with the aminoglycosides against Pseudomonas). Treatment should be continued for 2 to 3 weeks or until there is clinical improvement and x-rays show complete clearing or stabilization of the infiltrates (gram-negative pneumonia often leaves a residua of scar tissue apparent roentgenographically).

Aspiration Pneumonia. Aspiration of oropharyngeal or gastric contents can cause severe necrotizing pneumonia and lead to formation of chronic lung abscess. Aspiration can occur secondary to swallowing disorders or unconsciousness (e.g., alcoholism, seizures, general anesthesia). Antibiotic coverage is directed against upper respiratory flora, e.g., alpha-hemolytic streptococci and anaerobic bacteria such as Fusobacterium and Bacteroides species. Most of these microorganisms are susceptible to penicillin, and this drug has been proved effective even when resistant anaerobes such as *Bacteroides fragilis* are involved. If the patient does not respond to penicillin or has a history of penicillin allergy, chloramphenicol or clindamycin should be substituted. If the patient was seriously ill before the aspiration event or was receiving antibiotics, prior colonization of the upper respiratory tract by penicillin-resistant organisms may be assumed. In such situations staphylococci or enteric gram-negative bacilli may predominate, and treatment should be based on the results of Gram stain and culture. If gastric contents are involved and if the patient is seen within a few hours of aspiration, corticosteroids such as methylprednisolone, 250 mg. intravenously, may be given to reduce inflammation, and bronchoscopy with suctioning may be necessary.

Patients severely ill with bacterial pneumonia of any cause in whom the specific pathogen is uncertain should initially receive therapy for *Staphylococcus aureus* and gram-negative enteric bacilli. The combination of tobramycin and cephalothin is recommended in these situations. When results of sputum and blood cultures are available, therapy may be modified.

NONBACTERIAL PNEUMONIA

method of
GREGORY H. SZEYKO, M.D.
El Paso, Texas

Acute nonbacterial pneumonias are caused by both infectious and noninfectious agents. Infectious agents include viruses, Mycoplasma, Bedsonia, fungi, protozoa, Rickettsia and metazoa. Noninfectious causes that can mimic the presentation of viral pneumonia include a variety of physical and chemical irritants inducing hypersensitivity reactions or pulmonary edema, and those associated with uremia, irradiation, collagen vascular disease, trauma, pulmonary emboli, and malignancy. Specific therapy depends upon differentiation of these pneumonias from bacterial pneumonia, as well as upon establishing a precise diagnosis. Such a diagnosis is based upon clinical presentation, consideration of predisposing factors and epidemiology, and interpretation of chest x-rays and Gram stained smears of sputum and pleural fluid, as well as cultures of blood and pleural fluid. Sputum cultures should not be used to establish or exclude a diagnosis of bacterial pneumonia, as cultures alone can be misleading. Rather, the sputum culture should confirm what is seen on the Gram stained sputum smear.

Viral Pneumonia

Acute viral pneumonias are usually uncomplicated, self-limited infections of mild to moderate severity requiring only supportive therapy. Occasionally they are severe and complicated by respiratory failure and/or bacterial superinfection and require more intensive therapy.

A number of respiratory viruses are responsible for primary viral pneumonia in otherwise healthy infants and children; these include respiratory syncytial virus (RSV), parainfluenza virus, influenza A and B, adenovirus, variola and varicella, rubeola, and occasionally the enteroviruses (coxsackievirus and echovirus). Influenza virus is an important cause of viral pneumonia in adults, especially the elderly, those with underlying cardiopulmonary disease (particularly mitral stenosis), and pregnant women in the third trimester. Immunosuppressed patients are particularly susceptible to infection with cytomegalovirus (CMV), varicella-zoster virus, and herpes simplex virus (type 1).

General Principles of Therapy. Uncomplicated viral pneumonia in an otherwise healthy person can usually be treated symptomatically at home. General supportive therapy includes bed rest, hydration, and antipyretics. Analgesics may be necessary for systemic manifestations. Aspirin, 300 to 600 mg. (5 to 10 grains) every 4 to 6 hours, is very effective for systemic manifestations; it should be given continuously with meals or buffered to avoid gastrointestinal upset. Aspirin substitutes such as acetaminophen (Tylenol, Datril), 325 to 650 mg. orally every 4 to 6 hours, or propoxyphene (Darvon), 65 mg. every 4 to 6 hours, may also be used. Cough suppressants may be necessary for the distressing nonproductive cough commonly associated with viral (and mycoplasmal) pneumonias. Codeine, 15 to 30 mg. every 4 to 6 hours, seems to be more effective than hydrocodone (Hycodan) or dextromethorphan. Cough suppressants should be avoided in patients with productive cough.

Complications. Patients with serious underlying diseases, immunosuppressed patients, and those with complicated illness (e.g., dyspnea, dehydration, myocarditis, or meningoencephalitis) must be hospitalized, as additional therapy may be required. Once the diagnosis is established, the most important aspects of therapy are early recognition and management of complications. Therapy includes the following measures:

1. *Blood gas analysis:* Hypoxemia can at times be profound with interstitial pneumonia. Clinical evaluation of hypoxemia (cyanosis, restlessness, agitation, tachycardia, and arrhythmias) is helpful but at times may be misleading. Frequent assessment of arterial blood gases during therapy is essential for proper management.

2. *Oxygen* is initially administered by Venturi mask (24 to 28 per cent) to maintain a Po_2 of at least 60 mm. Hg (at sea level). Patients with underlying chronic pulmonary disease may tolerate a lower Po_2. When Pco_2 is not known initially, it is wise to begin therapy with 24 per cent Fio_2. High concentrations of oxygen (Fio_2 of 60 per cent for more than 48 hours) should be avoided because of the increased risk of oxygen toxicity. Inspired oxygen should be humidified.

3. *Endotracheal intubation* and *ventilatory assistance* may be required in more serious cases and are indicated if adequate oxygenation (Po_2 at least 60 mm. Hg) cannot be achieved by mask with high Fio_2 concentrations, if exhaustion or a decreasing level of consciousness is present, or if the arterial Pco_2 is 45 to 50 mm. Hg or higher. A volume-cycled respirator (Bennett MA-1, Emerson, Engstrom, Ohio 560) should be used. A chest x-ray should be obtained after intubation to assess location of the tube. Endotracheal intubation may be continued for several days without significant complications if proper care is given, but if prolonged ventilatory assistance is anticipated, consideration must be given to elective tracheostomy. Some patients may tolerate assisted ventilation, but severe cases usually require controlled synchronized ventilation with suppression of respiratory drive.

4. *Sedation* should be administered cautiously. The most useful drugs are morphine, 5 to 15 mg. intravenously every 6 hours, or diazepam (Valium), 5 to 15 mg. intravenously every 3 to 4 hours, but both may precipitate or aggravate existing hypotension. If synchronization cannot be achieved with these drugs, neuromuscular blockers such as pancuronium bromide (Pavulon), which has five times the potency of d-tubocurarine, can be used effectively. Pavulon has little effect on the cardiovascular system other than to increase the pulse rate. Pavulon is administered intravenously at an initial dose of 0.1 mg. per kg., with supplemental doses being administered at 0.01 mg. per kg. until control is achieved. Except for neonates, dosage for children is the same as for adults. (See manufacturer's official directive before using in children under the age of 10 years.) The drug should be used cautiously in patients with underlying renal disease, because a

major portion is excreted unchanged in the urine. Sedatives should not be given to hypoxemic patients whose respirations are not being controlled with mechanical ventilation.

5. *Positive end-expiratory pressure (PEEP)* should be used when oxygen concentrations greater than 60 per cent are required to maintain a Po_2 of 60 mm. Hg or if a patient has been on at least 60 per cent Fio_2 for more than 48 hours. The use of PEEP at 5 to 15 cm. H_2O can increase Pao_2 while allowing one to decrease Fio_2 to safe levels. PEEP is not without risk, and one must be aware of the possibility of hypotension, pneumothorax, and/or pneumomediastinum.

6. *Steroids* may be beneficial in overwhelming viral pneumonia when there has been a progressive downhill course in spite of appropriate therapy. Steroids are not indicated for routine cases.

7. *Antimicrobial agents* have no proved therapuetic or prophylactic value in the treatment of viral pneumonia and may actually predispose to lethal secondary bacterial infections. They should not be given unless bacterial suprainfection has occurred. Patients should be examined daily, and Gram stained sputum specimens should be monitored on a daily basis to facilitate early diagnosis of bacterial complications. Influenza, varicella, variola, and rubeola pneumonias tend to be associated with a high incidence of bacterial suprainfection, whereas parainfluenza and herpes simplex virus are associated with a moderate incidence. Others have a relatively low incidence of secondary bacterial infection. Most cases of bacterial pneumonia associated with influenza are caused by pneumococci or staphylococci, but *Hemophilus influenzae* and other gram-negative organisms may be the causative agents, especially in compromised hosts. It is imperative that one institute early appropriate antibiotic therapy based on a presumptive diagnosis made from the Gram stained sputum smear. Attention must then be paid to (1) airway maintenance, (2) adequate oxygenation, (3) removal of secretions, (4) administration of appropriate intravenous fluids, (5) maintenance of electrolyte and acid-base balance, and (6) frequent monitoring of vital signs. Patients should also be monitored for arrhythmias, which may occur as a result of myocarditis or hypoxemia. It is also helpful to obtain periodic chest x-rays and Gram stained sputum smears in addition to following other clinical parameters to assess clinical response.

Specific antiviral chemotherapy is not available at present. Several agents are under investigation and may prove efficacious in the future.

Postviral asthenia, for which there is no specific therapy, is a not uncommon occurrence and may be prolonged. Postinfluenzal patients especially should be cautioned that resuming full activity too quickly may precipitate relapse.

Prevention. Avoidance of contact with infected persons is the principal means of prevention. Isolation of other patients and visitors is wise, especially infants, pregnant females, the elderly, and the immunosuppressed. Prophylactic vaccines are presently available for influenza and measles. The effectiveness of amantadine hydrochloride for prophylaxis and early treatment of influenza A_2 is controversial. The drug should be used cautiously in the elderly and in patients with a history of a convulsive disorder because of an increased risk of central nervous system dysfunction—e.g., depression, lethargy, and ataxia. Prophylactic dosage is 200 mg. once daily or 100 mg. two times daily.

Mycoplasma Pneumonia (Primary Atypical Pneumonia, Cold Agglutinin Pneumonia, Eaton Agent Pneumonia)

Mycoplasma pneumonia is usually a benign self-limited infection, and many patients recover spontaneously without specific treatment. General supportive therapy is indicated for the usual patient. Patients with dyspnea or extrapulmonary complications should be hospitalized. Pleural effusions are common but are rarely detected. Massive effusions may occur, requiring thoracentesis for diagnosis and occasionally for relief of dyspnea. Specific antimicrobial therapy is indicated when systemic manifestations such as fever, malaise, and myalgias are prominent. Antimicrobial therapy does not significantly affect respiratory symptoms and does not hasten disappearance of the organism from the respiratory tract. *M. pneumoniae* is sensitive to several antimicrobial agents in vitro. Erythromycin, 500 mg. every 6 hours, is the therapy of choice. Effective alternatives are tetracycline, 250 mg. every 6 hours, or doxycyline, 100 mg. every 12 hours. Tetracyclines should not be used in pregnant females or in children under 8 years of age. The penicillins and cephalosporins are not effective against Mycoplasma, because the organism lacks a cell wall. Antimicrobial therapy should be continued for 5 to 7 days. Clinical response may take 2 to 5 days. Some advocate continuing therapy for 2 to 3 weeks for severe pneumonia because of continued shedding of the organism and occasional relapse after shorter courses of therapy.

Complications. Rarely the pneumonia is fulminating, with severe hypoxemia and respiratory alkalosis. Oxygen therapy and assisted ventilation may be necessary as previously described.

Administration of corticosteroids (e.g., methylprednisolone sodium succinate [Solu-Medrol], 40 mg. every 6 hours) may be beneficial if the patient's condition continues to deteriorate in spite of appropriate antibiotic and supportive therapy. Steroids should be discontinued as soon as possible. Their use is clearly not indicated in the routine case because of the usual benign nature of the illness. Mixed infection or bacterial superinfection is uncommon. A self-limited Coombs-positive hemolytic anemia usually associated with high titers of cold agglutinins $\geq$ 1:512) occurs occasionally. It is rarely serious enough to warrant transfusion and does not require steroid therapy. Chilling should be avoided, and antipyretics should not be used if possible.

Generalized malaise and a dry, hacking, nonproductive cough may persist for several weeks. The latter is best controlled with an antitussive such as codeine. Pulmonary infiltrates tend to persist after clinical improvement and are no cause for concern unless symptoms persist or recur.

Pulmonary Aspiration

Proper therapy of pulmonary aspiration depends upon establishing the nature of the aspirated material, which can be bacterial, chemical, mechanical, or thermal. Differentiation of the material aspirated is readily accomplished by investigation of the clinical circumstances associated with the aspiration as well as careful interpretation of a Gram stained sputum specimen.

Aspiration of infected oropharyngeal secretions containing predominantly anaerobic flora may result in anaerobic pneumonia, empyema, and/or lung abscess. Effective antimicrobial therapy is required, the details of which are presented elsewhere in this text.

The pathophysiology of gastric aspiration is entirely different, resulting in an acute inflammatory chemical or obstructive pneumonitis, depending upon whether nonparticulate gastric juice with a pH of 1.5 to 2.4 (fasting state) or food particles are aspirated. The severity of pneumonitis produced by gastric aspiration depends on the pH and volume aspirated. Mild aspiration does not require specific therapy other than supportive measures and careful observation for secondary bacterial complications. Extensive aspiration of acid gastric juice may result in severe hypoxemia, generalized bronchospasm, pulmonary edema, and shock. Therapy should begin with arterial blood gas analysis to assess oxygenation and with oxygen administration if indicated. Depending then upon the clinical status of the patient, therapy may require endotracheal intubation, mechanical ventilation with a volume ventilator and high Fio_2 with humidification, positive end-expiratory pressure (PEEP), sterile tracheal suction and/or bronchoscopy to facilitate removal of secretions, central venous pressure (CVP) monitoring, electrolyte solutions and/or vasopressors as required, daily sputum Gram stains to monitor the possibility of secondary bacterial infection, and bronchodilators if bronchospasm is prominent. Fever is *not* an indication for broad-spectrum antimicrobials, because it is nonspecific and secondary to the chemical pneumonitis. A useful procedure if done immediately after aspiration is to measure the pH of tracheobronchial secretions. A markedly acid pH is suggestive of gastric aspiration.

Aspiration of large foreign bodies may result in laryngeal obstruction, the so-called "café coronary." Smaller objects or food particles result in atelectasis or obstructive emphysema. Bronchoscopy should be performed to remove foreign bodies. Large volume bronchial lavage with saline, sodium bicarbonate, or steroid preparations is futile; it may enhance dissemination and introduce bacterial contamination. The use of systemic steroids is unnecessary in mild cases. Proof of the efficacy of systemic steroids in overwhelming gastric aspiration is lacking, but many advocate their use if they are administered early. There is no evidence that infection plays an early role in aspiration of chemicals or solid particles. The only exceptions to this may be achlorhydric patients or those who aspirate feculent material. However, late complications frequently involve bacterial superinfection. Antimicrobial therapy is not indicated unless there is evidence of bacterial invasion. This is best accomplished by evaluation of Gram stained sputum smears in addition to clinical evaluation.

Prevention of recurrent aspiration is an important part of therapy. Attention must be paid to risk factors such as general anesthesia, unconsciousness, seizure disorders, neuromuscular disease, cardiac resuscitation, tube feedings, gastrointestinal obstruction, esophageal disease, and patients with endotracheal tubes and tracheostomies. Unconscious or semiconscious patients should not be placed in the supine position, which favors aspiration; they should be placed in a lateral or semiprone position. Preoperative patients should be fasted for at least 8 hours prior to surgery.

Smoke inhalation and thermal burns of the respiratory tract require treatment of airway obstruction. All patients with smoke inhalation must be hospitalized for observation, because the extent of injury may not be apparent for 12 to 24 hours after exposure. Except in mild cases, bacterial superinfection will eventually occur. Strict isolation as a means of prevention is essential.

Lipoid pneumonia is rarely seen nowadays. An organizing fibrosis may develop which in some patients may require surgical therapy.

PULMONARY EMBOLISM

method of
KENNETH M. MOSER, M.D.
San Diego, California

Pulmonary embolism continues to be a major cause of morbidity and mortality in patient populations around the world. In the United States alone, it is estimated that at least 50,000 deaths per year are due to embolism. If one makes the legitimate assumption that embolism leads to death in fewer than 10 per cent of patients, this translates into an annual incidence exceeding 500,000 embolic episodes. Further, if one assumes that fewer than 10 per cent of venous thrombi lead to embolism, then some 5,000,000 patients—at a minimum—are having episodes of deep venous thrombosis each year in this country. These minimum figures indicate that the problem of venous thromboembolism is, indeed, a major one.

In the past, the therapy of venous thromboembolism has focused primarily upon its most dramatic event—namely, massive pulmonary embolism. However, it has become clear that this therapeutic emphasis has been misplaced. Pulmonary embolism is not a disease per se; rather, it is a preventable *complication* of the real problem: deep venous thrombosis. Therefore the highest therapeutic priority should be placed upon prevention of venous thrombosis. If venous thrombosis is prevented, pulmonary embolism is automatically avoided. The second highest priority should be prompt detection and treatment of venous thrombosis. If these goals are achieved, embolism should become an uncommon event.

Prevention of Deep Venous Thrombosis

Although effective prophylactic regimens for deep venous thrombosis have long been sought, a major deficiency inhibited their development—namely, the lack of sensitive, reliable and noninjurious techniques for early detection of deep venous thrombosis and for following its course. Without such techniques, valid studies of the efficacy of various prophylactic measures were not possible. Such techniques have now emerged, and their impact has been substantial. Three noninvasive techniques—the ^{125}I-fibrinogen leg scanning method, impedance phlebography, and Doppler ultrasound—standardized against and supplemented by contrast venography, have provided the essential diagnostic tools. Studies with these approaches have firmly established several facts critical to prophylaxis: (1) The clinical diagnosis of acute deep venous thrombosis (DVT) of the lower extremities is highly unreliable. (2) In the patient over 40 years of age undergoing major abdominal, thoracic, or gynecologic surgery, the incidence of deep venous thrombosis is high (20 to 40 per cent or more), and such thrombi most often develop *during* or immediately following surgery. (3) A high frequency of DVT also is associated with other forms of major surgery and with immobilizing medical illnesses such as myocardial infarction.

These diagnostic advances have led to prophylactic trials with several agents and maneuvers. The most effective of these approaches has been the use of low dose ("mini-dose") heparin.

Mini-dose heparin is simple to apply. It consists of administering 5000 units of heparin subcutaneously every 12 hours. Although some trials have employed an every-8-hour regimen, the every-12-hour regimen has proved as effective in the prevention of deep venous thrombosis. No laboratory control is necessary.

Studies to date have indicated that this regimen should be applied to all patients above the age of 40 who are to undergo major abdominal-thoracic or abdominal surgery, provided that preoperative screening (platelet count, prothrombin time, partial thromboplastin time) discloses no hemostatic defect. Heparin should be commenced 2 to 4 hours prior to surgery and continued until the patient is ambulatory.

The risk of hemorrhage in these surgical patients cannot be used as a rationale for withholding prophylaxis, because investigations have shown that heparin-treated patients are *not* subject to significant hemorrhagic risk, aside from a modest increase in wound hematomas. Furthermore, the available evidence indicates that prophylaxis achieves a reduction not only in the incidence of deep venous thrombosis but also in the frequency of pulmonary embolism and lethal pulmonary embolism.

The value of mini-dose heparin in other high risk situations is less clear. Its efficacy in hip replacement, for example, has not been demonstrated, even though such patients do have a high incidence of venous thromboembolism. In prostatic surgery, the risk of hemorrhage appears to balance out the benefits to be gained. In myocardial infarction, the regimen decreases the frequency of venous thrombosis but has not been shown to reduce the frequency of lethal and nonlethal *embolism*.

Therefore, until further data are available, the application of mini-dose heparin to other medical and surgical patients is a judgmental matter. Our own policy is to apply it to all such patients in whom a combination of risk factors is present. For example, we use mini-dose heparin in patients with myocardial infarction who also have left ventricular failure or a prior history of venous thromboembolism or obesity. Similarly, in the third trimester of pregnancy (and in the postpartum state), a prior history of venous thrombosis would lead us to recommend low dose heparin. Until further studies in additional patient subgroups become available, the physician must weigh the very small hemorrhagic risk of this new regimen against the risk of thrombosis and embolism (extrapolated from other patient groups).

How can such small doses of heparin be so effective in preventing deep venous thrombosis and its complications? The efficacy of low dose heparin is based upon its enhancement of the inhibition of activated factor X. By potentiating the naturally occurring inhibitor (antithrombin III), these small doses halt the progress of the coagulation cascade early, *before* the elaboration of thrombin occurs. Such early action amplifies the antithrombotic effect of these small doses.

Other prophylactic regimens have, of course, been applied to high risk groups. Thus far, it has been shown that mechanical approaches to prevention of stasis in the postoperative patient (such as early ambulation, elastic stockings, and pneumocompression devices) do reduce the frequency of deep venous thrombosis, but are *not* as effective as mini-dose heparin. Other pharmacologic agents also have been studied extensively. Dextran infusions have not been shown to be of value in most studies. Aspirin prophylaxis also has had no consistent beneficial effect, although occasional studies have suggested its value. Currently, further prophylactic trials are underway employing aspirin and other "antiplatelet" agents. The results of these trials may alter present views of optimal prophylactic regimens.

Prothrombinopenic drugs were, of course, the original agents used in prophylaxis of venous thromboembolism (dicumarol, warfarin). At this time, they are still the agents of choice in the prophylaxis of patients with orthopedic trauma to the lower extremities, patients in whom their efficacy has been well established for more than a decade. Such patients should be placed on prophylaxis as soon as their condition has stabilized and any hemorrhagic risk from other injuries has been evaluated. Although they will not be in therapeutic range for 24 to 48 hours, prior studies have indicated the value of prothrombinopenic agents applied in this manner. The patient should be maintained in therapeutic range (prothrombin time 1.5 to 2.5 times control) until fully ambulatory. The hemorrhagic risks of prothrombinopenic therapy are well recognized. However, until a better regimen is established, it remains the approach of choice in this patient group.

Treatment of Deep Venous Thrombosis

Obviously, despite the introduction of effective prophylactic regimens, deep venous thrombosis will continue to occur. Prompt and adequate therapy of deep venous thrombosis has three goals: (1) halting the propagation of the venous thrombosis; (2) limiting venous thrombotic residuals by hastening the resolution of the thrombus; and (3) preventing pulmonary embolism.

Effective anticoagulant therapy should accomplish the first objective by preventing the layering of additional platelets and fibrinogen onto the surface of the thrombus. The second objective, acceleration of thrombus removal, is accomplished indirectly by anticoagulant therapy. No anticoagulant regimen is known to be capable of enhancing fibrinolytic activity. However, by halting the formation of *additional* thrombus, anticoagulant drugs allow fibrinolysis to proceed unopposed by the simultaneous build-up of additional thrombotic material.

The last objective, prevention of embolism, is less secure, even with an optimal anticoagulant regimen. Effective anticoagulation cannot prevent the detachment or fragmentation of the thrombus leading to embolization, except indirectly by inhibiting thrombus growth and permitting dissolution and/or organization to occur.

Therapy of venous thrombosis should be started as soon as the diagnosis is entertained. However, since the clinical diagnosis of deep venous thrombosis often is uncertain, diagnostic confirmation by one of the previously mentioned techniques is often warranted after the initiation of treatment. The ^{125}I-fibrinogen method will not detect thrombi in the presence of heparin therapy, which, ideally, prevents fibrinogen accumulation at the thrombotic site; but impedance, Doppler, and contrast venography remain suitable. ^{125}I-fibrinogen should be used in this context only when sufficient diagnostic uncertainty exists to warrant a delay in therapy, because this method cannot detect venous thrombosis with assurance until at least 24 hours after injection. Furthermore, ^{125}I-fibrinogen will not be incorporated into old thrombi—i.e., thrombi which are no longer actively growing.

There is no debate about the drug of choice for the initial treatment of acute deep venous thrombosis. That drug is heparin. This choice is based on the following factors: (1) The antithrombotic effects of heparin are exerted immediately. (2) Heparin achieves its antithrombotic action by interfering with the coagulation system in several ways—e.g., at the level of inhibiting activated factor X, thereby halting thrombin generation, and by inhibiting thrombin itself. Thus an immediate, widespread antithrombotic effect is what is needed in venous thrombosis, and heparin satisfies this need.

There is, however, substantial debate about the optimal heparin regimen, in terms of both dosage and route of administration. There is no controversy about what would constitute an "ideal" regimen. Such an ideal would combine 100 per cent efficacy (antithrombotic effect) with 100 per cent safety (no hemorrhagic risk); or, at the least, the best possible toxic:therapeutic ratio attainable in the variable-laden world of clinical medicine.

Unfortunately, there have not yet been definitive studies to identify the characteristics of this "ideal" regimen. Until such studies emerge, it is best to recognize the lack of finite guidelines and allow the physician to exercise options based on those data which are available.

Four basic regimens have been widely used in the United States for some years: (1) continuous intravenous administration of approximately 1000 units of heparin per hour; (2) intermittent intravenous administration of approximately 5000 units every 4 hours; (3) subcutaneous administration of 5000 units every 4 hours; and (4) subcutaneous administration of 10,000 units every 8 hours. All these regimens approximate a dose of 30,000 units per 24 hours, a total which is substantially below those long employed empirically in the Scandinavian countries.

In selecting one of these regimens, the physician faces three questions: (1) Which is the most effective? (2) Which is associated with least hemorrhagic risk? (3) Which is the most convenient and reliable in a given hospital setting? The question of convenience and reliability obviously is the least important if one regimen is clearly superior.

Unfortunately, no one regimen can lay claim to that designation. The corollary to that statement is the fact that no laboratory test yet described provides the physician with a "therapeutic range" in which confidence can be placed. If such a laboratory derived therapeutic range *did* exist, selection of a regimen would be simple; one would provide that number of units (continuously or intermittently) that maintained all patients in that "range."

Such ranges have, of course, been suggested. The tests recommended have been the whole blood clotting time (WBCT) and the partial thromboplastin time (PTT). In most institutions, the PTT has replaced the WBCT because of its greater reproducibility. The therapeutic ranges commonly stipulated have been as follows: (1) for continuous infusion, maintenance of the PTT at 1.5 to 2.5 times the control value; and (2) for intermittent schedules, to assure that the PTT just prior to the next scheduled dose is at least 1.5 times the control value.

Whether or not such ranges are superior to the empirically selected doses mentioned above rests on the demonstration that such ranges either are (1) associated with less bleeding risk or (2) capable of providing better therapeutic effects such as prevention of thrombotic extension, reduction in the extent of thrombotic residual, or a decrease in the incidence of embolism. None of these criteria has been consistently satisfied by investigations performed to date. From the available literature, one can marshal data to support or refute the value of such ranges as guides to heparin regimens. Badly needed are studies employing the diagnostic and follow-up techniques now available and *relating* these results to heparin doses and the PTT (or other tests), while carefully monitoring bleeding incidence and degree.

Until such data become available, the physician can choose between empiric dosage and "PTT monitored" regimens. We currently do not use monitoring in patient management but rely upon empiric doses, although we are continuing investigations of certain potentially valuable monitoring techniques. Until it can be shown clearly that the "tests" correlate with the "events" at issue (bleeding, thrombosis extension, embolism), we prefer not to rely upon tests which may provide us with a false sense of security with respect to both safety and efficacy.

In terms of selection of route, therefore, convenience and reliability remain valid concerns. Continuous intravenous therapy is certainly the most popular regimen, but it requires expensive and reliable infusion pumps. If such pumps are not available or if experience indicates that intravenous bottles are not promptly hung or infusion rates oscillate widely, this route of administration should be abandoned in favor of intermittent intravenous injections. Furthermore, if regulations or practices in a given hospital make it unlikely that intravenous heparin will be administered on schedule (e.g., if nurses are not allowed to give intravenous injections under any circumstances), subcutaneous administration is advisable.

In addition to heparin therapy, other supportive measures may be employed. With substantial edema and pain, leg elevation may make the patient more comfortable. Application of dry or wet heat to the involved extremity also may be helpful, but care should be taken to avoid methods capable of burning or macerating the skin, and heat should *not* be applied if significant arterial disease coexists. Elastic stockings should be applied to encourage venous return so long as they do not cause discomfort or induce venous stasis by compressing the popliteal space. Mild analgesia may be required, but aspirin and other agents with effects on the coagulation system should be avoided, as should all intramuscular injections.

Once initial therapy is instituted, three related therapeutic decisions remain: (1) When should the patient be ambulated? (2) How long should heparin therapy be continued? (3) Should anticoagulant therapy be continued beyond discharge?

On a theoretical basis, these questions are easy to answer. The patient should be ambulated when ambulation does not cause discomfort and does not enhance the risk of embolization. Heparin therapy should be continued until the thrombotic process has fully resolved. Anticoagulant therapy need be continued beyond discharge only when there is significant risk of recurrence of venous thrombosis.

Unfortunately, again, data to translate these theoretical answers into practical terms do not presently exist, although they are slowly being accumulated. What is at issue here is the natural history of treated (and untreated) venous thrombosis in man. If we knew this course in large patient groups—or could follow it in the individual patient—we could make these decisions easily. Studies are in progress in which the "activity" of the thrombus (by ^{125}I-fibrinogen) and the extent of the residual (by impedance, Doppler, and venography) are being assessed. These should clarify the validity of our current approach.

Our present knowledge indicates that venous thrombi resolve (by either dissolution or organization) within 7 to 10 days. Therefore, within this time period, the venous thrombi have been either removed (by fibrinolysis) or organized into the venous wall and endothelialized. Thus the hazards of thrombotic extension and embolization are over.

Based on this sequence, we begin ambulation of the patient on the eighth day of heparin therapy (provided that this does not cause pain). However, we allow the patient use of a bedside commode from the start, because struggling with bedpans, we feel, places the patient at greater hazard of potential embolism.

If a decision has been made not to continue anticoagulant therapy after discharge, we maintain full heparin dose for 7 days, institute minidose heparin on days 8 and 9, and discontinue heparin on the tenth day. After 24 hours off heparin and ambulating, the patient is discharged.

This brings us to the final question: Who merits "long-term protection" and how is this provided? It is our view that long-term anticoagulation is required only in patients who are at risk of recurrence. We feel that such patients represent a minority of those with deep venous thrombosis. Who, then, are those "at risk?" Some are easy to identify. For example, the patient with an extremity fracture remains at risk until fully ambulatory and should receive anticoagulant protection until that state is achieved. The patient with postoperative thrombosis also should be protected until fully ambulatory. Patients with congestive heart failure should continue treatment until their failure is fully controlled. Persons with prior episodes of deep venous thrombosis merit long-term protection, as do markedly obese persons.

How long should those meriting continued protection be maintained? The theoretical answer is simple: until the inciting factor(s) associated with the initial venous thrombosis have subsided (leg fracture healed, congestive failure treated). In others, the answer is more difficult. For example, how long should the patient with recurrent venous thrombosis be treated? How about the patient with persistent congestive failure or cancer or obesity? Clearly, in the absence of definitive data about recurrence, one must be arbitrary. The usual recommendation (and one to which we adhere) is to maintain prophylaxis for 3 to 6 months and then observe the patient. However, it would not be incorrect (or subject to challenge) if shorter or longer periods were elected.

If patients do not fall into clear categories of increased risk, we do not elect to offer them protection beyond the hospital stay, and our experience with negligible recurrence rates over the years has led us to maintain this policy. However, no one can challenge the physician who, until further data are available, wishes to provide an arbitrary period of post-discharge protection to all his patients.

When it has been decided that a patient should receive long-term anticoagulant therapy, how is this best done? There are currently two options: prothrombinopenic agents and minidose heparin. Prothrombinopenic agents remain the most widely used. The decision to employ them should be made early during the hospitalization, because it is likely that the antithrombotic action of these agents is not fully achieved until the patient has been "in range" for at least 3 days and preferably 5 days. The therapeutic "range" for prothrombinopenic agents is defined by the prothrombin time. The optimal range is between 2.0 and 3.0 times the control level. Above this range, bleeding risk is exaggerated; below it, efficacy is less certain. However, the particular thromboplastin used to determine the prothrombin time may condition the proper "range" so that, in some laboratories, that range is 1.5 to 2.5 times control. Physicians are advised to check the situation in the particular laboratory they use. It should also be noted that the prothrombin time can be influenced by heparin therapy. This is a special hazard if the blood sample is taken at the "peak effect time" of an intermittent heparin schedule. Taken at the "trough" or during continuous intravenous administration, the effect is modest.

Mini-dose heparin is a well established prophylactic regimen in patients at risk of thrombosis. It has not yet been widely used in prophylaxis following venous thrombosis. However, we have been using it in a progressively larger number of such patients, because (1) it may be associated with less hemorrhagic risk, (2) it requires no laboratory control, and (3) it is likely to be at least as effective as coumarin-type drugs. The disadvantage is that the patient (or someone in the home) must learn to give the twice-a-day injection. This is not possible in some instances. If, however, this can be accomplished, transition to mini-dose heparin is simple. It can be started at the conclusion of full dose heparin and continued beyond discharge.

There is one major contraindication to long-term anticoagulant therapy—namely, the patient's ability to cooperate. If the patient is "unreliable" for either organic or psychologic reasons, hemorrhagic complications and/or lack of efficacy are likely, as wide experience has shown. In these circumstances, it is in the patient's best interest not to attempt long-term maintenance. Lack of patient understanding of the problems of such therapy is, to us, an almost absolute contraindication.

Pulmonary Embolism

As in the case of venous thrombosis, the therapy of pulmonary embolism has been clarified by the availability of improved methods for diagnosis and follow-up. These methods, chiefly ventilation and perfusion pulmonary scintiphotography and pulmonary angiography, have demonstrated that (1) the clinical diagnosis of pulmonary embolism is uncertain, with a substantial number of both "false positive" and "false negative" diagnoses; (2) most pulmonary emboli resolve over days to weeks with restoration of blood flow to the involved region(s); (3) infarction is an uncommon (<15 per cent) complication of pulmonary embolism; and (4) in the patient with massive embolism who survives long enough to achieve diagnosis and initiation of anticoagulant therapy, survival rates are extremely high.

Taken together, these observations indicate that prompt and adequate medical therapy of embolism is associated with very low mortality and an excellent functional result in terms of restoration of vascular patency. The *promptness* of anticoagulant therapy depends upon a high index of suspicion plus confirmation by appropriate diagnostic tests. The *adequacy* of therapy depends upon the use of heparin. As in venous thrombosis, heparin is the drug of choice; and, as in venous thrombosis, the optimal regimen is unsettled.

There is agreement that the initial dose of heparin in pulmonary embolism should be given intravenously to achieve an antithrombotic effect promptly. However, the size of this initial dose depends upon one's view of data regarding the role of platelets in the initial pulmonary and hemodynamic events following embolism. There is convincing evidence from experiments in animals that platelets coat fresh emboli, and, further, that aggregation and disintegration of these platelets result in the release of pulmonary vasoconstrictive and bronchoconstrictive mediators (e.g., serotonin). This release can significantly increase the rise in pulmonary vascular resistance, as well as the pulmonary mechanical abnormalities, which are associated with embolic obstruction per se. It has been further shown that doses of heparin large enough to prevent thrombin-induced platelet aggregation can prevent this sequence. To block this sequence in man requires an initial intravenous bolus of 15,000 to 20,000 units.

Whether or not this sequence occurs in man is unknown. However, our position has been that the evidence that it *may* occur in man is sufficiently impressive to warrant use of an initial large bolus, and our initial dose is 15,000 to 20,000 units intravenously. Others, who do not find the evidence as persuasive, use smaller initial doses.

After this initial dose, we then use one of the maintenance regimens described under "deep venous thrombosis." If continuous intravenous heparin is chosen, it is begun within an hour after the first large bolus. If one of the intermittent intravenous or subcutaneous regimens is selected, it is begun 4 hours after the first bolus. The criteria for selection and monitoring (or not monitoring) these regimens have been discussed previously. Our own preference is for either of the intravenous regimens, without monitoring.

Some physicians prefer to administer larger heparin doses during the first 24 to 36 hours after an embolus. This position is based on sequential studies of the behavior of the partial thromboplastin time and a concern that larger doses are needed to assure complete thrombin inhibition over this period. Therefore an every-4-hour schedule of 7500 to 10,000 units intravenously or 1500 to 2000 units per hour by continuous infusion is often given. We do not administer these larger doses, but there are no data regarding patient outcome to favor one choice over the other.

In addition to prompt initiation of one of these regimens, various supportive measures may be indicated in a given patient. If hypoxemia is present, supplementary oxygen should be given. Chest pain should be relieved by appropriate analgesics. The presence of hypotension presents another therapeutic choice. Intravenous isoproterenol has often been recommended because of its pulmonary vasodilator and cardiac inotropic qualities. However, this agent also lowers systemic resistance, potentially exaggerating hypotension, and may promote cardiac arrhythmias. Dopamine infusion therefore is now generally preferred.

Once the patient has been stabilized, we encounter the same sequence of decisions as in the patient with deep venous thrombosis: ambulation and duration of therapy. Our recommendations in these regards are the same as those for deep venous thrombosis, because the sequence of resolution of emboli parallels that described for venous thrombi. Assuming that the clinical course is the usual one of progressive improvement, we reduce the patient to mini-dose heparin on the eighth day, stop therapy on day 10 and ambulate the patient, with discharge on day 11. There is one difference: we follow the patient with perfusion lung scans at 3 to 5 day intervals. If there is a residual abnormality on the initial follow-up (day 3 to 5), we place this patient in our increased-risk and therefore long-term treatment category. Aside from this, our indications and methods for long-term anticoagulation are the same as for deep venous thrombosis.

Thrombolytic Therapy

For some years, the concept of using intravenous urokinase and streptokinase to enhance fibrinolytic activity and hasten thrombus dissolution has been under investigation. Neither agent is yet available for clinical use. However, even if they were, the available evidence does not indicate that they are of benefit to patients with venous thrombosis or pulmonary embolism. It has been shown that urokinase will hasten resolution of emboli in man. However, no improvement in morbidity or mortality has been demonstrated. Perhaps future studies will demonstrate such effects; until that time, thrombolytic therapy cannot be recommended.

Surgical Management

Two surgical procedures merit consideration in the management of patients with venous thromboembolism: venous interruption and pulmonary embolectomy.

In the past, ligation of various lower extremity veins distal to the inferior vena cava has been practiced to prevent embolization. However, such procedures have largely been abandoned because of equivocal results and because deep venous thrombosis often is bilateral. Therefore interruptive procedures now are almost exclusively directed toward the inferior vena cava. In the past, decision for caval interruption most often has been based on two assumptions: (1) that recurrent emboli would lead to permanent obstruction of pulmonary arteries, and (2) that interruption would prevent recurrence. Neither assumption is correct, because (1) most emboli resolve, and (2) all interruptive procedures can be followed by embolic recurrence. Recurrence may occur through large collaterals (after ligation), through any interruptive device, or from the right cardiac chambers above the interruption. We regard interruption as a procedure which will prevent the *early* recurrence of *large* emboli. Therefore we employ it almost exclusively in patients with substantial emboli (leading to significant cardiopulmonary compromise) in whom early recurrence (which cannot be securely prevented by heparin) could be life threatening. Choice of the interruptive procedure (ligation, plication, clip, umbrella) often depends on the local expertise available. Our preference is for insertion of the umbrella filter, which does not require surgery.

Other indications for caval interruption are substantially more controversial. In the patient who has a proved embolic event and an absolute contraindication (active bleeding) to anticoagulation, the procedure is indicated. With relative contraindications to anticoagulant therapy (recent bleeding, other factors which enhance bleeding risk), the choice is more difficult. We often choose low dose heparin in such patients rather than inferior vena cava (IVC) interruption as our first choice. In patients who have "recurrent embolization on anticoagulant therapy," we require assurance (1) that recurrence has indeed occurred, and (2) that adequate anticoagulant therapy was in place. If these requirements are met (and they rarely are), we may recommend caval interruption, particularly when the patient is a poor resolver or nonresolver of emboli.

Emergency embolectomy is rarely indicated. Several investigations have disclosed that, even in the hypotensive patient with extensive embolization, medical therapy is associated with a lower mortality than embolectomy. Therefore our option is to treat all patients medically unless there is a set of quite special circumstances (e.g., proved massive embolism in a patient with an absolute contraindication to anticoagulation). A surgical team experienced in cardiopulmonary bypass is a requisite for this procedure.

Surgical removal of nonresolved emboli which are of sufficient extent to cause pulmonary hypertension is an indication for embolectomy. Actually, this is a thromboendarterectomy, because such occlusions are no longer thromboemboli but are masses of organized tissue. If the thrombi are in proximal vessels (lobar or more central), the procedure should be considered, as it is the only means of dealing with this potentially reversible form of pulmonary hypertension. In our experience, emboli that have remained unchanged for 6 to 8 weeks (by scan or angiography) will not resolve thereafter.

Final Comments

The difficult therapeutic decisions faced in patients with suspected venous thromboembolism cannot be minimized. Many patients present special features which must be "factored in." Furthermore, new therapeutic options are under investigation which may change present recommendations. However, the keys to decision making regarding therapy will remain unchanged: (1) documentation that thrombosis and/or embolism has occurred, and (2) rigorous attention to present knowledge of the risk: benefit ratio of the available options. Until a number of current uncertainties regarding risk vs. benefit are resolved, the details of therapy (e.g., heparin regimens) will continue to require decisions by individual physicians treating individual patients within the guidelines described here.

SARCOIDOSIS

method of
LOUIS E. SILTZBACH, M.D.
New York, New York

Sarcoidosis is a multisystem granulomatous disorder of unknown cause most commonly affecting young adults and presenting most frequently with bilateral hilar lymphadenopathy, pulmonary infiltration, and skin or eye lesions. The diagnosis is established most securely when clinicoradiographic findings are supported by histologic evidence of widespread noncaseating epithelioid cell granulomas in more than one organ or a positive Kveim-Siltzbach skin test. Immunologic features are depression of delayed-type hypersensitivity suggesting impaired cell-mediated immunity and raised or abnormal immunoglobulins. There may also be hypercalciuria with or without hypercalcemia. The course and prognosis may correlate with the mode of onset; an acute onset with erythema nodosum heralds a self-limiting course and spontaneous resolution, whereas an insidious onset may be followed by relentless progressive fibrosis. Corticosteroids relieve symptoms and suppress inflammation and granuloma formation.

Therapy

Because of the frequency of asymptomatic sarcoidosis and the high level of spontaneous remission, only about one third of all patients ever require treatment. The most effective agents are the corticosteroids. Chloroquine and its derivatives and phenylbutazone are also useful under certain circumstances (this use of these agents is not listed in the manufacturer's official directive). These agents are suppressive in their action, not curative. Other anti-inflammatory and immunosuppressive drugs are less useful, and bed rest, radiotherapy, and physical therapy have no place in management. Special diets are not indicated, aside from a low calcium diet sometimes prescribed for patients with persistent hypercalcemia and hypercalciuria.

Corticosteroid Therapy. Corticosteroids act by halting the deposit of new granulomas in the various organs which are affected. The hormones have no effect on lesions which have already undergone fibrosis and hyalinization. Hence, propitious timing of therapy may prove crucial to recovery with a minimum of organ dysfunction. The anti-inflammatory effects of the corticosteroids can manifest themselves within a few days with recession of edema, hyperemia, and nonspecific inflammation around or at some distance from the granulomas. The epithelioid granulomas themselves begin to undergo involution and resorption within 2 weeks of the start of therapy. Abatement and damping down of the granulomatous process and the resorption of many granulomas leave smaller areas of residual scarring of the organs than might ensue if the process were allowed to proceed untreated.

INDICATIONS FOR CORTICOSTEROID THERAPY. Indications for treatment mainly concern lesions in which further involvement portends dire consequences if they are allowed to progress without therapy. Prompt therapy is required for the following manifestations:

1. Ocular lesions.
2. Diffuse pulmonary lesions with significant respiratory symptoms and with deterioration of lung function.

3. Central nervous system lesions with involvement of brain, spinal cord, and meninges.

4. Intrinsic myocardial lesions.

5. Splenic involvement with associated hypersplenism (leukopenia, anemia, thrombocytopenia, and hemorrhagic tendency).

6. Hypercalcemia or persistent hypercalciuria with renal damage.

Only about 10 per cent of the patients fall into the aforementioned group with indications for urgent therapy.

Corticosteroids are also required, but not so urgently, by patients whose course is less predictable and who can be observed for 2 to 6 months to discern the trend toward resolution or progression before a decision to treat need be made. This category of treated patients includes about 20 per cent of the roster:

7. Slowly worsening pulmonary status.

8. Persistent and debilitating constitutional symptoms.

9. Disfiguring lesions of skin, salivary glands, and superficial lymph nodes.

10. Vexing symptoms from nasal, pharyngeal, and bronchial mucosal lesions.

11. Persistent facial palsy.

12. Prolonged muscle and joint pains.

Treatment is regarded as unnecessary for those with isolated hilar node or mediastinal node enlargement or with localized pulmonary involvement, unless cough or dyspnea becomes troubling. Erythema nodosum, which is self-limiting, can be managed with an interim course of indomethacin. (This use of indomethacin is not listed in the manufacturer's official directive.) Nor are minor superficial lymph node enlargement, asymptomatic hepatosplenomegaly, and bone cysts of themselves indications for therapy. Many patients with asymptomatic miliary nodulation of the lung fields of recent onset show spontaneous clearing and one may temporize with therapy, but frequent radiographic monitoring will detect those with persistence and progression of the lesions which eventually do require intercession. Patients with widespread flocculent pulmonary lesions, however, almost always require therapy, particularly if significant restrictive and diffusion defects in lung function are demonstrated.

Dosage. Prednisone and prednisolone are most widely used. Daily doses, once or twice a day, totaling 20 to 30 mg. initially, are maintained for 1 month or 6 weeks, after which the dose may be reduced gradually to a maintenance level of 10 to 15 mg. Alternate day therapy of equivalent doses is borne well by many patients with reduction of some of the drug's side effects.

Duration of Therapy. Treatment generally extends over a year or longer, because shorter courses of therapy are frequently followed by relapse. For patients with advanced pulmonary fibrosis whose cough and dyspnea may reach disabling intensity, maintenance therapy may have to be continued indefinitely. When to end the course of therapy is determined empirically and is governed by an assessment of whether maximal enduring benefit has been achieved. At that point, tapering of dosage is carried out over a period of 6 weeks to 3 months.

Relapse

Approximately half of the treated group suffer a recurrence of activity of intrathoracic lesions after discontinuation of therapy, but most relapses are mild and retreatment courses need be undertaken in only a minority of them. Recovery of the patient's adrenocortical function, suppressed in varying degrees during exogenous intake, often results in secondary clearing of lesions some weeks or months after halting therapy. Although cutaneous sarcoids respond regularly, most chronic skin lesions tend to recur with reduction of dosage or cessation of therapy. When the lesions involve exposed areas, patients prefer the mild risk associated with therapy to bearing the sometimes abhorrent disfigurement.

Complications of Therapy

Side effects on low dosage schedules are not troublesome. In a minority, there are cushingoid facies, hirsutism, the uncovering of latent diabetes, and, occasionally, retention of fluid. Complicating pulmonary tuberculosis in corticosteroid-treated patients has been growing rarer. Prophylactic doses of isoniazid during the course of therapy are prescribed only for patients with positive tuberculin reactions. Fungal colonization of bullae is no more frequent among corticosteroid-treated patients than in the untreated. Hemoptysis from a mycetoma may be severe enough to require excisional surgery if the patient's pulmonary reserve permits.

Effects on Various Organs

Lung and Mediastinal Nodes. Fresh granulomatous lesions respond to therapy more rapidly and regularly than older ones. Two thirds of these patients show either clearing of pulmonary densities or substantial improvement. Coarse nodular lesions are slower to respond than patchy or fine miliary densities. Enlarged hilar and mediastinal nodes regress at an uneven pace; but once they dwindle, recurrence of enlargement is infrequent. Cough, dyspnea, fever, weight loss, and easy fatigability usually are promptly controlled, but ebbing of symptoms may be slower in patients with extensive pulmonary densities of long duration.

Ocular Lesions. Iridocyclitis involving the anterior uveal tracts is treated topically with eyedrops containing 1 per cent prednisolone or 0.1 per cent dexamethasone administered four to six times daily, combined with 1.0 per cent atropine drops or 0.25 per cent scopolamine drops twice a day. If the response is unsatisfactory after 10 days, a subconjunctival deposit of 0.25 or 0.50 ml. (10 to 20 mg.) of methylprednisolone is sometimes helpful in refractory cases. For posterior uveitis, the usual course of oral therapy, beginning with 20 to 30 mg. of prednisone daily, is prescribed, and later the dose is tapered to maintenance levels of 10 to 15 mg. Frequent monitoring of ocular tension is mandatory to detect the insidious onset of glaucoma. Repeated determination of ocular tension and observation for incipient cataract formation are a necessary routine for all patients receiving prolonged corticosteroid therapy.

Cutaneous Lesions. For chronic skin sarcoids of the nodular and plaque-like variety, including lupus pernio, chloroquine, 250 mg. a day, or hydroxychloroquine, 200 mg. daily, is often useful. (This use of these agents is not listed in the manufacturer's official directive.) Close surveillance is required for possible toxicity manifested by corneal opacities which are reversible and retinal damage which may be irreversible. Nine month courses alternating with 6 month free intervals are recommended. Alternatively, corticosteroids at the accepted oral dosage or local intralesional injection of triamcinolone acetonide (Kenalog-10), 10 mg. per ml., diluted with equal parts of lidocaine (Xylocaine) using a 22 to 27 gauge needle, may prove of aid in stubborn individual lesions.

Hypercalcemia and Hypercalciuria. Persistence of hypercalcemia and hypercalciuria eventually can result in grave renal damage. Corticosteroids effectively and promptly lower the enhanced level of calcium absorption from the gut, restoring normal fecal excretion of calcium and lessening its urinary excretion. A low calcium diet and avoidance of increased vitamin D intake, even in pregnancy, may also prove beneficial.

Other Organ Involvement. In myocardial sarcoidosis, antiarrhythmic drugs, such as procainamide (Pronestyl), quinidine, or propranolol, may help control arrhythmias. In some instances of heart block, a pacemaker may become advisable. Corticosteroid therapy for neurosarcoidosis has usually proved to be disappointing, although in patients with acute lesions involving meninges, central nervous system, or cranial and peripheral nerves, a gratifying result is sometimes encountered. Splenomegaly, which may attain giant proportions and be associated with significant hypersplenism, may require splenectomy, which often proves to be hematologically curative. Milder hypersplenism may be treated with corticosteroids.

SILICOSIS

method of
WILLIAM C. BAILEY, M.D.
Birmingham, Alabama

Silicosis is caused by inhalation of respirable particles of free crystalline silica, and exposure is a hazard in certain occupations. The most common occupations producing respirable particles of silicon dioxide (SiO_2) and thereby associated with silicosis are hard rock mining (e.g., gold mining), rock drilling, quarrying, and sandblasting. Silicosis is also a hazard to ceramic clay workers, foundry workers, and those exposed to diatomaceous earth in the manufacturing of paints and varnishes.

Particle sizes most likely to produce the disease are those in the range of 0.5 to 5 microns. The percentage of free silica, however, tends to be less in the smaller particles. The exact mechanism of injury by silicon dioxide is not fully understood, and several pathogenic mechanisms have been proposed. The one with the most supporting evidence is the theory that absorption of protein on the silica particles enables the protein to act as a nonspecific antigen to which an antibody is formed.

This has been proposed as a type III immunologic lung reaction in which there is a reaction between an antigen and a 7-S precipitating antibody. Serum levels of gamma globulin have been shown to be increased in patients with silicosis. At the histologic level, the antigen-antibody complex is thought to be deposited in the collagen fibril of the silicotic nodule. The proponents of this theory feel that this mechanism would explain why the disease progresses for such long periods after the patient has been removed from exposure to silica. It is felt that the antigen-antibody complexes activate several fractions of complement and attract polymorphonuclear cells, causing them to release lysosomes. The lysosomes released in turn produce inflammation or tissue necrosis with the formation of an Arthus reaction.

An alternative theory, or at least another mechanism that should be considered, is the fact that the particles may cause lysosomal instability when phagocytosed. Cellular breakdown with the re-release of the particles can occur together with hydrolic enzymes producing tissue necrosis. Also, removal from further accumulation of new particles does not dispose of those already in the interstitium.

Silica content of the lung is an age-related factor but rarely ever exceeds 0.2 per cent of the dry weight of normal lungs as compared to 15 to 20 grams in silicotic lungs.

The disease varies from minimal nodular deposition of silica with almost no fibrosis to severe airways disease and destruction of lung parenchyma from fibrosis and conglomerate masses. Obstructive and restrictive functional impairment varies in severity and does not necessarily correlate with radiologic abnormalities. Acute intense exposure may result in an accelerated form of the disease, the most acute variety resembling alveolar proteinosis. Complications are many and varied but primarily relate to increased susceptibility to infection, particularly those seen when cell-mediated hypersensitivity is impaired; destructive lung changes; and associated autoimmune disease.

Prevention

There is no specific treatment for silicosis demonstrated to be effective, so prevention is the mainstay of management. Increasing the understanding of both labor and management to the circumstances under which silicosis may be expected to occur and the serious consequences thereof is very important. Effort should of course be made to reduce the dust concentrations of respirable particles and, when possible, to use processes in which such particles are not generated. If these conditions cannot be obtained, then protective devices, including hoods, even with outside sources of air, must be worn. Sandblasting in enclosed spaces is one of the most dangerous and difficult-to-control occupations. The only real solution to this problem is the substitution of abrasive materials containing very little free silica. This has become standard in Great Britain.

Once a person develops clinical silicosis, he should be removed from further silica exposure; even then, the disease may progress.

Treatment

Acute Silicosis. Lung lavage has been tried on occasion with silicosis and makes the most sense in the acute variety resembling alveolar proteinosis. No good documentation of its efficacy is available, but it should be considered, particularly in acute silicosis. Acute steroid therapy has also been recommended in acute silicosis, and since this is such a severe life-threatening disease, even though no data are available to support it, our clinical impression is that some benefit may be derived. If it is tried, a high dose, 40 to 60 mg. of prednisone per day or its equivalent, should be initiated. After a period of 4 to 6 weeks if there has been evidence of clinical improvement, the dose may be tapered to a maintenance dose of 10 to 15 mg. per day. This then could be continued for varying periods of time, ranging from 6 months to a year, depending on the clinical circumstances, and then gradually reduced until discontinued. If there has been no evidence of clinical response after 4 to 6 weeks, gradual tapering until discontinued should be done at that time.

Obstructive Airways Disease. If airways disease develops, the resulting obstruction can be treated in the following manner:

1. Bronchodilation therapy is employed, using aminophylline as a base of therapy and aiming for a blood level of 15 micrograms per ml. Dose requirement is quite variable because of the individual variation in metabolic degradation, but 200 mg. every 6 hours is a good place to start. Blood levels should be done to determine the exact dose. If after adequate therapeutic levels of aminophylline the patient still continues to have evidence of bronchospasm, sympathomimetic amines may be used as an additional drug. Terbutaline, 5 mg. orally three times daily, or metaproterenol (Alupent), 10 mg. orally three times a day, are drugs we have used with some success. They are reported to produce a bit less cardiovascular toxicity than some of the other sympathomimetic drugs. Metaproterenol (Alupent) may also be used by the inhaled route with proper supervision. Under such circumstances no more than two puffs of a commercially available metered dose should be given every 4 to 6 hours.

2. If secretions are a problem, vibropercussion with postural drainage, plus proper humidification, is a very important and effective means of producing improvement in obstructive airways disease. This treatment is so basic that it is often neglected, but it is vital in the therapy of any obstructive airways disease and must be pursued with vigor even in patients with very severe disease.

3. Continued purulent sputum or frequent attacks of acute bronchitis often occur in patients with chronic obstructive airways disease. Since *Hemophilus influenzae* and the *pneumococcus* are the two most frequent offending agents, tetracycline or ampicillin is often indicated. These can be used in a variety of ways, depending on the frequency of infection. For patients with only occasional problems with purulent sputum, one of these antibiotics instituted at the first sign of purulent sputum, usually in a dose of 250 to 500 mg. every 6 hours for a course of 10 days, often is sufficient. In patients who continually have purulent sputum, one may use antibiotics quite frequently. We most commonly alternate tetracycline with ampicillin, giving it the first week of each month. On rare occasions these patients must be on almost continuous antibiotic therapy, but almost always periodic alternation of the antibiotic is required. When the infection does not respond immediately

to the antibiotic chosen, a Gram stain, sputum culture, and sensitivity should be done to determine the appropriate antibiotic therapy.

Respiratory Failure. If the airways or parenchymal disease progresses to the point of respiratory failure, supplemental oxygen may be required. This is particularly beneficial in patients who have pulmonary arteries unduly responsive to hypoxemia. It may prevent or delay the progression of cor pulmonale. Because of the frequent association of airways disease leading to hypercapnia, it is desirable to use the lowest possible concentration of oxygen to elevate the Po_2 a little above 60. An Fio_2 of 0.24 or 2 liters of nasal oxygen is a good place to start, but continued administration must be monitored by arterial blood gases.

Mechanical ventilatory support is at times necessary, and it is most helpful when a specific correctable abnormality is identified. Pneumothorax is a not uncommon mode of exodus for patients with end-stage silicosis, and chest tube drainage is of course the treatment of choice. The complication of bronchopleural fistula may ensue, and under such circumstances surgical intervention may be considered.

Infections. Because of the interference with macrophage function and perhaps other alterations to the immune mechanism, specific infectious complications occur. Infection with *Mycobacterium tuberculosis,* as reflected by positive skin test to intermediate purified protein derivative (PPD), definitely deserves isoniazid (INH), 300 mg. daily for 1 year. Continuation beyond the traditional 1 year of therapy is considered appropriate by many, and some people recommend continuation of INH therapy for life in silicotics with positive skin tests. There are no data to support treatment beyond a year, although the severity of the insult to cellular hypersensitivity causes us to treat patients with positive skin tests often for periods ranging from1 to 2 years and sometimes longer if significant parenchymal disease is noted. Acute active pulmonary disease with either *Mycobacterium tuberculosis* or other mycobacteria requires multiple drug therapy. Until several negative sputa have been returned, it may be difficult to rule out active pulmonary disease in patients with extensive radiologic changes from silicosis associated with a positive skin test. Therefore it is often wise to begin multiple drug therapy until the bacteriologic status is definitely established. We usually begin with INH, 300 mg. a day, and rifampin, 600 mg. a day, in either proved or suspected active disease. An alternative regimen is INH, 300 mg. a day, ethambutol, 15 mg. per kg., and streptomycin, 1 gram per day, for varying periods of time, depending upon the estimation of the bacterial population. Patients with minimal disease may not require streptomycin at all, but patients with many organisms require streptomycin for as long as a month to 6 weeks—rarely beyond this, in my experience. Proper drug therapy usually results in sputum conversion. The use of combination therapy beyond the standard 18 months to 2 years is controversial but often done. The length of time varies with the extent of residual disease; but again, no data are available to support therapy beyond the standard 2 years.

Autoimmune Disease. Autoimmune disease has been noted to occur in association with silicosis, and under such circumstances the appropriate immunosuppressive therapy for that disease may be considered. Acute steroid therapy as indicated for acute silicosis is occasionally given such patients, and of course treatment with other agents such as salicylates for joint disease may also be considered.

In an attempt to prevent the effects of inhaled silica a number of agents have been tried, but so far no evidence has been gathered to support their effectiveness. Most agree that inhalation of aluminum powder, which has been tried in the past, is not effective, and the theoretical positive effect of D-penicillamine is probably outweighed by its definite toxic side effects. Polyvinylpyridine-N-oxide is a polymer which may inhibit the bonding of silicic acid with membranes; it is presently being investigated as a possible means of treating silicosis, but no data have yet been gathered to document its efficacy.

SINUSITIS

method of
PHILIP M. SPRINKLE, M.D.,
and FREDERICK T. SPORCK, M.D.
Morgantown, West Virginia

Sinusitis in our era of mass media advertising has become a very popular complaint among the general public. It is many things to many people and so needs to be defined. At present headaches and most nasal problems, including normal postnasal discharge, allergic rhinitis, vasomotor rhinitis, and nasopharyngitis, all are attributed to sinusitis.

Sinusitis by definition is an inflammatory change in the mucosal lining of one or more of the paranasal sinuses. There are four pairs of paranasal sinuses in the human: the maxillary, frontal, ethmoid, and sphenoid. The ethmoid and maxillary are the most commonly involved with sinusitis, followed by the frontal and sphenoid in that order. Involvement may be unilateral or bilateral or both, and may involve one group or all. Involvement of the sphenoid alone is very rare and, in older age groups, should call to mind a malignancy. We will deal mainly with maxillary sinusitis and touch briefly on frontal sinusitis.

Etiology

Most cases of sinusitis probably follow a viral insult to the upper respiratory tract such as the common cold. If the disease remains viral, no treatment other than symptomatic management is necessary. Frequently, however, there is a secondary bacterial involvement. Because the sinus is a closed cavity, it is difficult to isolate a pure culture. Cultures taken from the nose may be contaminated by local flora. In most series in which pure cultures were obtained by antral aspiration, the predominant organisms have been *Diplococcus pneumoniae*, *Hemophilus influenzae, Staphylococcus aureus,* and *Strepotococcus pyogenes.*

Contributing factors may be changes in pressure from forcible nose blowing, swimming and diving in contaminated water, facial trauma, and dental disease. Nasal allergy with or without nasal polyps can certainly be implicated. As we learn more about immunology, it appears that some cases of chronic sinusitis may be a type III immune-complex disease.

Treatment

The aim of treatment of sinusitis is to establish drainage of the involved sinus and eradication of the infecting organism by appropriate antibiotic therapy.

Acute Maxillary Sinusitis. 1. Topical decongestants are useful during the acute phase of sinusitis (2 per cent ephedrine, 0.25 per cent phenylephrine (Neo-Synephrine), and oxymetazoline). These must be used judiciously, however, because of their ability to produce a rebound phenomenon and rhinitis medicamentosa. They probably should not be used more than 5 to 7 days in succession.

2. Systemic decongestants or antihistamines alone or in combination play an important part in the management of acute sinusitis. There continues to be controversy regarding the use of these two types of drugs in combination. Some studies have suggested that alpha-adrenergic drugs may have the effect of increasing histamine release. Other studies indicate that adrenergic agents may act synergistically with antihistamines.

Decongestants should of course be used with caution in patients with glaucoma, hypertension, and diabetes and in those taking monoamine oxidase inhibitors and tricyclic antidepressants. If decongestants alone are used, ephedrine and the pseudoephedrines are probably the most effective.

Antihistamines are divided into five classes, and some patients may respond better to one class than another. Generally speaking, the propylamine class is the most commonly used (chlorpheniramine, brompheniramine, pyrrobutamine, and triprolidine).

In our practice we generally use a combination drug in those patients in whom there is no contraindication to the decongestant component. We like to use these for 3 to 4 weeks after the symptoms have resolved so that the ostia will remain patent and obstruction does not recur.

3. As the predominant organisms in most series are *H. influenzae* and *D. pneumoniae,* we prefer to use a broad-spectrum antibiotic such as ampicillin. The dosage varies from 250 to 500 mg., depending on the patient and the severity of the disease. In penicillin-sensitive patients, erythromycin is a good choice. For chronic infections tetracycline is usually our choice. We normally use a 10 to 14 day course of antibiotics in most instances and longer if symptoms do not resolve in that period of time.

4. In many cases aspirin or acetaminophen will provide sufficient analgesia. If not, we generally use a combination of one of these with codeine or propoxyphene.

5. The place of antral puncture and irrigation is currently somewhat controversial, with many recommending that it not be done until the patient has had several days of antibiotic therapy to reduce the danger of producing an osteomyelitis. In our practice we find that a certain number of patients who are particularly symptomatic experience a good deal of relief with acute antral puncture and irrigation. There is little question that in patients in whom there has been little resolution of symptoms or findings after a week to 10 days of appropriate medical therapy, antral puncture and irrigation is in order.

6. The application of moist heat over the involved sinus is also recommended for symptomatic relief and to help resolve the inflammation. Humidification of the environment is also thought to be helpful, and adequate fluid intake is a necessity.

Acute Frontal Sinusitis. Involvement of the frontal sinus with an air fluid level and pain and tenderness over the involved frontal sinus is a serious problem, as this indicates that the nasofrontal duct is occluded. If allowed to go unchecked, the infection may spread through the posterior table via the veins of Breschet to the epidural space with the danger of intracranial complications.

Immediate treatment consists of large doses of antibiotics, preferably intravenously, infracturing of the middle turbinate, and spot suctioning in an attempt to open the ostium. The other steps outlined for acute maxillary sinusitis also hold true here. If symptoms fail to resolve within 24 to 48 hours, trephination through the floor of the frontal sinus is done with insertion of a drainage and irrigation catheter. This is irrigated two to three times a day with an antibiotic solution until spontaneous drainage begins via the nasofrontal duct.

Acute Ethmoiditis. In uncomplicated ethmoiditis the management is similar to that for acute maxillary sinusitis. When ethmoiditis becomes complicated with extension into the orbit, periorbital abscess, and ensuing ocular complications, it becomes an acute surgical emergency, and an external ethmoidectomy must be done.

Chronic Sinusitis. Chronic sinusitis is a more difficult problem. Many of these patients will have a strong allergic component to their disease and should be skin tested and desensitized. They should also be evaluated for food allergies with rotational diets. Those with nasal polyps usually require polypectomy, although we have found that the use of dexamethasone sodium phosphate (Decadron Turbinaire) two to three times daily results in marked improvement and sometimes resolution of polyps in many of our patients.

In those patients in whom long-term medical management with antihistamines, decongestants, antibiotics, and allergic management fails to produce a response, surgical management becomes a necessity. The aims of such management are to restore a functioning nasal airway, restore more normal drainage for the sinus, eradicate diseased tissue, and prevent complications of sinus disease.

The surgery usually done for chronic maxillary disease is a nasoantral window either alone or in combination with a Caldwell-Luc procedure.

For chronic frontal sinusitis an osteoplastic frontal flap is done through either a spectacle or coronal incision. The mucosal lining is removed, the nasofrontal duct is plugged with fascia, and the cavity is filled with a free abdominal fat graft.

In chronic ethmoiditis the ethmoidectomy may be done either through an external approach or intranasally, with the external approach probably being more popular today.

STREPTOCOCCAL PHARYNGITIS

method of
FRANK A. DISNEY, M.D.
Rochester, New York

The method of treatment of streptococcal pharyngitis should be individualized, based upon the clinical picture and the bacteriology.

Acute Illness

The findings of an acute febrile illness with erythematous tonsillopharyngitis (occasionally with petechiae), yellow or gray follicular exudate, enlarged tender anterior cervical lymph nodes, a white blood count elevated above 12,000 per cu. mm. with a left shift, and a culture positive for Group A beta-hemolytic streptococci comprise a classic picture indicating therapy. This, however, occurs in only 6 per cent of streptococcal throat infections, and, although some of those symptoms and signs may be present in the other 94 per cent, the decision of when to start treatment in this latter group requires more critical clinical judgment. In the classic strep throat, specific therapy can justifiably be started on clinical signs alone; but when there is some question of the diagnosis, it is advisable to await the confirming bacteriologic report.

Carriers

Some patients are asymptomatic carriers of streptococci, and thus pose problems in diagnosis. With unrelated illnesses their throat cultures will be positive (sometimes strongly) and yet the organisms are not responsible for their present clinical condition, and they are not necessarily in need of therapy. Actually there is some evidence that persistence of the carrier state (even for months) may confer a degree of immunity upon these persons, and there are studies showing that they are not necessarily an epidemiologic threat to those around them. However, the existence of the carrier state as a potential source of secondary complication of the basic illness must be equated in the therapy decision in such patients. Additionally, it is always advisable to be certain that the patient has a Group A organism, especially in carriers, as non–Group A streptococci do not require therapy in throat infections.

Specific Therapy

Specific therapy includes many antibiotics effective against the Streptococcus; to minimize the chance of development of nonsuppurative complications and of clinical or bacteriologic recurrence of the infection, any treatment program must be continued for a 10 day period.

Penicillin. Penicillin is still the preferred drug for treatment of streptococcal infections, and it may be administered intramuscularly or orally.

1. Intramuscular benzathine penicillin G may be given in doses of 600,000 units in children under 12 years of age, or 1,200,000 units in those over 12 years of age; a recently reported combination of 900,000 units of benzathine penicillin G and 300,000 units of procaine penicillin G appears to give the best results.

2. Oral phenoxymethyl penicillin may be given in the following weight-related doses: less than 40 lbs. (18 kg.), 125 mg. three times a day; 40 to 60 lbs. (18 to 27 kg.), 125 mg. four times a day; 60 to 120 lbs. (27 to 54 kg.), 250 mg. three times a day; more than 120 lbs. (54 kg.), 250 mg. four times a day.

Erythromycin. Erythromycin is an effective drug for use in those allergic to penicillin. It is given to children in the total daily dose of 25 mg. per kg. of body weight divided into three doses. The total daily dose may be divided into two doses a day, but it must be realized that if one dose is forgotten, the desired level of the drug will not be maintained throughout the 24 hour period.

Cephalexin. This is also an effective drug. It is given to children in a total daily dose of 25 mg. per kg. of body weight divided into three doses. The adult dose is 250 mg. four times a day.

Other Drugs. Many other antibiotics may also be used; but some, such as ampicillin, might better be reserved for infections in which a broader coverage is indicated. Two drugs not recommended are tetracycline and sulfonamides. Tetracycline-resistant streptococci have been isolated in as many as 40 per cent of patients in some studies. Sulfonamides may improve the patient's clinical condition but do not eliminate the organisms from the throat.

General Measures. In addition to specific therapy, the patient should be given antipyretics, sedatives, and lukewarm sponges to help alleviate his symptoms during the acute phase of his infection.

Family Contacts and Infection

Prophylactic treatment of other members of the family is not effective and hence is not recommended. Routine throat cultures of all other members of the family after identification of the primary case can be difficult logistically and are frequently unrewarding. However, throat cultures may be indicated when two or more family members have simultaneous streptococcal illnesses (not necessarily of the throat), or when many members are having repeated recurrences, with each infection responding to treatment but recurring soon after cessation of therapy. In such situations we recommend treatment of the ill members in the usual manner for 10 days, followed by treatment with phenoxymethyl penicillin, 125 mg. daily to each child and 250 mg. daily to each adult for 1 month. This usually eliminates the organism from the household.

Rheumatic Fever Prophylaxis

Prophylaxis against beta-hemolytic infection is recommended for all patients who have an attack of acute rheumatic fever. This can be accomplished by any one of the following methods: (1) benzathine penicillin G, 1,200,000 units intramuscularly once a month; (2) oral phenoxymethyl penicillin, 125 mg. twice daily to children under 50 lbs. and 250 mg. twice daily to children over 50 lbs. and to adults; or (3) sulfadiazine, 0.5 gram daily to children weighing less than 50 lbs. and 1.0 gram daily to those patients weighing more than 50 lbs.

TUBERCULOSIS AND OTHER MYCOBACTERIAL DISEASES

method of
WHITNEY W. ADDINGTON, M.D.
Chicago, Illinois

The recently revised classification* of tuberculosis simplifies the categorization of patients with mycobacterial exposure, infection, and disease. This new classification enables the physician to prescribe an effective and safe course of chemotherapy. The principles of antituberculous chemotherapy are discussed in the text. The doses and side effects of the individual drugs are listed in Tables 1 and 2.

Adequate chemotherapeutic regimens produce uniformly excellent results. Prognosis is not determined by factors other than chemotherapy; for example, rest, the amount of fresh air or sunshine, diet, smoking habits, length of hospitalization, and alcohol use or abuse by themselves do not influence outcome. All that matters is that the patient receive the medication!

*Diagnostic Standards and Classification of Tuberculosis and Other Mycobacterial Diseases. New York, American Lung Association/American Thoracic Society, 1974.

TABLE 1. **Treatment of Mycobacterial Disease—First-Line Drugs**

FIRST-LINE DRUGS	DAILY DOSAGE	MOST COMMON SIDE EFFECTS	TESTS FOR SIDE EFFECTS	REMARKS
Isoniazid	5–10 mg./kg. up to 300 mg. P.O. or I.M.	Peripheral neuritis, hepatitis, hypersensitivity	SGOT/SGPT (not as a routine)	Bactericidal; pyridoxine, 10 mg. as prophylaxis for neuritis; 50–100 mg. as treatment
Ethambutol	15–25 mg./kg. P.O.	Optic neuritis (reversible with discontinuation of drug; very rare at 15 mg./kg.), skin rash	Red-green color discrimination and visual acuity	Use with caution with renal disease or when eye testing is not feasible
Rifampin	10–20 mg./kg. up to 600 mg. P.O.	Hepatitis, febrile reaction, purpura (rare)	SGOT/SGPT (not as a routine)	Bactericidal; orange urine color; negates effect of birth control pills
Streptomycin	15–20 mg./kg. up to 1 gram I.M.	Eighth nerve damage, nephrotoxicity	Vestibular function audiograms; BUN and creatinine	Use with caution in older patients or those with renal disease

TABLE 2. **Treatment of Mycobacterial Disease—Second-Line Drugs**

SECOND-LINE DRUGS	DAILY DOSAGE	MOST COMMON SIDE EFFECTS	TESTS FOR SIDE EFFECTS	REMARKS
Viomycin	15–30 mg./kg. up to 1 gram I.M.	Auditory toxicity, nephrotoxicity, vestibular toxicity (rare)	Vestibular function audiograms; BUN and creatinine	Used with caution in older patients; rarely used with renal disease
Capreomycin	15–30 mg./kg. up to 1 gram I.M.	Eighth nerve damage, nephrotoxicity	Vestibular function audiograms; BUN and creatinine	Used with caution in older patients; rarely used with renal disease
Kanamycin	15–20 mg./kg. up to 1 gram I.M.	Auditory toxicity, nephrotoxicity, vestibular toxicity (rare)	Vestibular function audiograms; BUN and creatinine	Used with caution in older patients; rarely used with renal disease
Ethionamide	15–30 mg./kg. up to 1 gram P.O.	Gastrointestinal disturbance, hepatotoxicity, hypersensitivity	SGOT/SGPT	Divided dose may help gastrointestinal side effects
Pyrazinamide	15–30 mg./kg. up to 2 grams P.O.	Hyperuricemia, hepatotoxicity	Uric acid, SGOT/SGPT	Combination with an aminoglycoside is bactericidal
Para-aminosalicylic acid (aminosalicylic acid)	150 mg./kg. up to 12 grams P.O.	Gastrointestinal disturbance, hypersensitivity, hepatotoxicity, sodium load	SGOT/SGPT	Gastrointestinal side effects very frequent, making cooperation difficult
Cycloserine	10–20 mg./kg. up to 1 gram P.O.	Psychosis, personality changes, convulsions, rash	Psychologic testing	Very difficult drug to use; side effects may be blocked by pyridoxine, ataractic agents, or anticonvulsant drugs

Categorization and Treatment

Category 0—No tuberculosis exposure, not infected: No therapy is necessary.

Category I—Tuberculosis exposure, no evidence of infection:

Some contacts not yet proved to be infected (P.P.D. negative) are candidates for "primary prophylaxis" because the tuberculin skin test may be in the process of conversion. All household contacts should be considered for such treatment. Primary prophylaxis is standard for children, being especially important for those less than 5 years of age and essential for neonates. Isoniazid is the only drug with demonstrated effectiveness. The usual duration of treatment is until approximately 3 months after the contact has been broken, unless the patient changes to Category II.

Category II—Tuberculous infection without disease:

The treatment of persons who are infected but do not have disease (P.P.D. positive; chest roentgenogram and bacteriology negative) is based on the concept that the lifetime risk of developing tuberculosis for an untreated infected person exceeds the risk of therapy with 1 year of isoniazid. Positive reactors who are less than 35 years of age are candidates for therapy. Persons older than 35 who have an additional risk factor, such as corticosteroid therapy, immunosuppressive therapy, or a disease state that impairs the immune response, should also be treated. (For additional details concerning treatment of infection, see Preventive therapy of tuberculous infection, American Thoracic Society. Amer. Rev. Respir. Dis., *110*:371, 1974.)

Category III—Tuberculous infection with disease:

Past tuberculosis previously untreated: Persons who have had tuberculosis but who have not previously received adequate chemotherapy or persons who are tuberculin skin test reactors with roentgenographic findings consistent with tuberculous scarring but with negative bacteriology should receive isoniazid preventive therapy for 1 year.

Current tuberculosis (bacteriology positive): Isoniazid, ethambutol, rifampin, and streptomycin are considered to be first-line or primary drugs. The most frequently used regimen is isoniazid and ethambutol for 18 months. When the bacterial population is thought to be particularly large (extensive cavitary lesions) or the patient is from an area where drug-resistant tuberculosis is prevalent, daily streptomycin may be included in the regimen, usually not longer than 3 months, until the bacterial population is reduced.

Rifampin combined with isoniazid is as effective as any three drug regimen in the treatment of extensive cavitary disease. After the sputum bacteriology becomes negative, ethambutol may be substituted for the rifampin, with the total duration of therapy lasting 18 to 24 months.

Patient acceptance, drug toxicity, and cost must be as important considerations in selecting therapy as is the efficacy of the drug. An orally administered regimen (isoniazid-rifampin; isoniazid-ethambutol) lends itself to an outpatient program much more than one with streptomycin, which is delivered by painful injections administered by a medical professional. Total cost is the sum of expenditures to the patient by loss of time from work and transportation, as well as program personnel and drug expenses. The actual duration of therapy necessary is under study, but a course of two drugs for 18 to 24 months is almost always successful.

Isoniazid and ethambutol are the preferred combination when treatment during pregnancy is necessary.

Since the advent of effective antituberculous chemotherapy, surgery is only rarely indicated in patients with tuberculosis. The concept of surgically removing a "target" of pulmonary tuberculosis has been proved to be unnecessary if appropriate chemotherapy is received by the patient and ineffective if the patient does not receive an adequate course of chemotherapy.

Disease Caused by Drug-Resistant Bacilli

Second-line drugs are used only to treat disease caused by *Mycobacterium tuberculosis* resistant to first-line drugs or to replace first-line drugs in patients for whom they are contraindicated. These are listed in Table 2. Viomycin, capreomycin, kanamycin, and streptomycin should generally not be used together because of possible eighth nerve damage and nephrotoxicity. Second-line drugs are definitely more toxic and in some cases less effective than the primary drugs and usually should be prescribed only by physicians familiar with their use.

Regimens that include second-line drugs should be based on the susceptibility pattern of bacteria and on the potential for toxicity in any given patient. The patient with drug-resistant organisms should always be receiving at least two and preferably three drugs to which the organisms are known to be susceptible. More than 18 months of therapy may be required in some of these patients.

Tuberculosis in Children

Treatment of tuberculosis in children follows the same guidelines as for adults. When large numbers of bacilli are harbored, two or more drugs are indicated. Rifampin is not approved for use in children, although it has been used in this group without a risk any greater than for adults. Ethambutol cannot be used in children too young to report signs of visual toxicity. Thus para-aminosalicylic acid (PAS), a relatively weak drug, is a common companion drug with isoniazid and streptomycin in this age group. After the patient is bacteriologically negative, the streptomycin is discontinued and PAS and isoniazid are continued for 12 months, followed by isoniazid alone for a total period of 18 months. In many instances of initial infection in children, the diagnosis of pulmonary tuberculosis is based upon the epidemiologic situation, a positive skin test, and a pulmonary infiltrate without cavitation. Cultures of sputum or other material are frequently not positive in these instances, and treatment is initiated with two drugs such as isoniazid and PAS. Cultures during treatment are not ordinarily obtained from these children, and progress is measured by serial chest roentgenograms and clinical assessment. When the roentgenogram is stable, the PAS can be discontinued and isoniazid given alone for a total of 18 months.

Extrapulmonary Tuberculosis

The chemotherapeutic guidelines for the management of extrapulmonary tuberculosis are the same as for pulmonary tuberculosis. It was once believed that surgical treatment was necessary more often in extrapulmonary lesions, but potent chemotherapy has virtually abolished the need for nephrectomy in genitourinary infections and has greatly reduced the indications for fusions, drainage, and other surgical procedures in skeletal tuberculosis.

Treatment of Atypical Tuberculosis

Mycobacteria other than *Mycobacterium tuberculosis* account for about 10 per cent of all pulmonary disease caused by organisms in this species. Two organisms account for most of these—*Mycobacterium kansasii* and *Myobacterium intracellulare*. In children cervical lymphadenitis may be due to *Mycobacterium scrofulaceum*.

Treatment of *M. kansasii* is usually successful, even though drug susceptibility studies may show that the organism is resistant to one or all of the drugs the patient received. The explanation for such a favorable result is not known. Initial treatment with isoniazid, rifampin in the usual doses, and ethambutol in a dose of 25 mg. per kg. will give excellent results in almost all cases. The ethambutol dose may be reduced from 25 to 15 mg. per kg. after the first 3 months of treatment.

Treatment of *M. intracellulare* infection is difficult because the organisms are usually resistant to all drugs tested, and the patients involved are mostly older and may be debilitated with other medical problems such as emphysema, diabetes mellitus, or rheumatoid arthritis. The therapy is sometimes worse than the disease. Patients suffering from *M. intracellulare* infection should be under the care of a physician experienced in the treatment of drug-resistant tuberculosis.

Discharge of Tuberculosis Patients from Medical Surveillance

The most critical determinant of the course that will be followed by the patient with tuberculosis is the adequacy of the chemotherapy. Experience with drug therapy convincingly indicates that if adequate antituberculous chemotherapy is received by the patient, tubercle bacilli are rapidly eradicated from the sputum, and after completion of chemotherapy relapse is uncommon. Therefore the long-term surveillance policies designed and utilized in the prechemotherapy era are no longer appropriate for tuberculosis patients who have completed adequate drug therapy. Indeed, several reviews of the productivity of long-term follow-up indicate that the majority of relapses are not detected by routine surveillance procedures.

Before discharge from the tuberculosis treatment program, the patient should be instructed as to what symptoms might be associated with reactivity of the tuberculous process and of the importance of the prompt evaluation of these symptoms. The patient should be referred for continuing general health care, making sure that a history of successfully treated pulmonary tuberculosis is noted on the medical record.

Patient Compliance

Organizing an effective ambulatory care facility is the most important and often most challenging problem that must be solved in caring for patients with tuberculosis. Whether one is involved in a large urban program or in a rural setting with a few patients, the basic issue is patient compliance. The only meaningful measure of success is the percentage of patients who complete therapy.

An approach must be fashioned around the specific needs of the patient population. For example, a skid-row population will require the availability of social services and a clinic staff that can relate humanely to patients who are alcoholics. Working and family people may need more assistance in advocacy and in educating their employers and community to accept them. The staff must be able and willing to diplomatically accomplish these tasks.

Because of the difficulty in determining which patient will be noncompliant, it is necessary to approach every patient as potentially noncompliant. A punitive or parental approach has been proved ineffective. Rather, the approach should be to work with the patient in removing as many barriers to compliance as possible. The patient should be clear about his role in curing the disease. In patients with multiple medical problems, each problem and its therapy should be distinct. Too often the medical mandate is combined: "Stop drinking, stop smoking, and take your pills." The result is noncompliance with them all.

VIRAL RESPIRATORY INFECTIONS

method of
MAURICE A. MUFSON, M.D.
Huntington, West Virginia

More than 200 antigenically different viruses can infect the human upper respiratory tract and cause acute respiratory tract disease. These viruses belong to several major groups, including the myxoviruses, paramyxoviruses, adenoviruses, picornaviruses, and coronaviruses. Their frequency of occurrence and the severity of illnesses they produce vary, depending upon the virus group involved; they can cause a spectrum of respiratory tract illnesses, including the common cold, exudative and nonexudative pharyngitis, afebrile and febrile respiratory disease, and influenza and influenza-like illnesses. Morbidity from viral respiratory tract infections accounts for cumulatively more days lost in school and work by affected persons than any other type of illness.

Among infants, acute viral infections of the respiratory tract frequently involve the lower respiratory tract and tend to be more severe. Older children and adults infected with the same agents usually experience much milder upper respiratory tract illnesses. Except for influenza virus infections, the clinical manifestations of most viral respiratory tract infections are brief, usually lasting several days to 1 week. Influenza virus infection characteristically causes more severe illness, including high fever, cough, malaise, and involvement of the lower respiratory tract. It can be an especially serious infection in the elderly and in persons with intercurrent diseases.

Etiologic differentiation of viral respiratory tract infections cannot be accomplished on the basis of clinical findings alone. Establishing a specific etiologic diagnosis requires virus recovery from secretions of the respiratory tract, the detection of viral antigen in smears of nasal and pharyngeal epithelium by immunofluorescence, or the detection of a diagnostic four-fold rise in antibody between serum collected at the onset of illness and that collected during convalescence. These tests are available on a limited basis and usually only in a specialized laboratory. The results from the immunofluorescent procedure can be obtained within hours, but the other tests require 2 to 3 weeks until the results are reported. Treatment must be instituted without access to the definitive diagnostic laboratory examinations.

Treatment of viral respiratory tract infections should provide maximum symptomatic relief from the distress of the illness while the disease abates naturally. Therapy is directed at suppressing or eliminating the distressing symptoms of the disease—fever, headache, rhinorrhea, nasal obstruction, sore throat, cough, anorexia, and malaise. Strict isolation of affected persons is not required; however, ill persons should avoid close and direct contact with their associates, dispose of nasal secretions hygienically, and wash their hands after touching the face and wiping the nose.

Since the intracellular events accompanying virus replication are not inhibited by antibiotics, these drugs are not indicated in the treatment of uncomplicated viral respiratory tract diseases. Secondary bacterial invasion seldom occurs during most viral respiratory tract infections, and the routine use of antibiotics during the course of viral respiratory tract infections should be avoided. Occasionally, secondary bacterial infections such as otitis media, sinusitis, and pneumonia complicate an acute viral respiratory tract illness. These complications usually become manifest 5 to 10 days after the onset of the acute illness, and appropriate antibiotic therapy is indicated for these conditions.

As general measures, bed rest, adequate diet, and abundant liquid—water, juices, carbonated drinks—are advisable, especially for the person with marked malaise, fatigue, fever, and sweats. Except for providing fluid replacement, citrus fruits and juices and vitamin C per se have no therapeutic effect in the treatment of viral respiratory tract infections.

The control of fever encourages a feeling of well being, decreases fluid loss from sweating, and lessens the metabolic demand in adults, which is especially important in patients with diminished cardiac reserve. In children, prompt reversal of fever diminishes the chance of febrile convulsions; in this regard, tepid water sponge or tub baths and, if necessary, alcohol sponges are a useful adjunct in the control of high fevers. For fever up to 101°F. (38.3°C.) in the young child, no special measures need be taken except when a history of convulsions exists.

Acetylsalicylic acid (aspirin, U.S.P.) should be given to children in doses of 60 mg. per year of age every 4 to 6 hours, not to exceed four doses in a 24 hour period. A fruit-flavored chewable aspirin is more palatable for children. The adult dose of aspirin is 0.6 gram every 3 to 4 hours. If the aspirin causes gastric distress, it can be taken with a small amount of milk. Aspirin suppositories are effective for the relief of fever in the patient experiencing retching or emesis; a dose comparable to the indicated oral dose should be used.

Alternatively, acetaminophen (Tylenol elixir or Liquiprin), a nonsalicylate analgesic-antipyretic, can be employed for infants and younger children. The dosage of Tylenol elixir for children under 1 year of age is ½ teaspoonful; for 1 to 3 years, ½ to 1 teaspoonful; for 3 to 6 years, 1 teaspoonful; and, over 6 years, 2 teaspoonfuls three or four times daily. As chewable tablets, the dose of acetaminophen (Tylenol tablets) for children 3 to 6 years is 1 tablet three or four times daily, and for children over 6 years it is 2 tablets at these times. The dosage of Liquiprin for children under 1 year of age is 1.25 ml.; for 1 to 3 years, 1.25 to 2.5 ml.; and, 3 to 6 years, 2.5 ml.

Treatment of rhinitis and obstruction in infants includes intranasal instillation of a 0.05 per cent solution of xylometazoline (Otrivin) drops in each nostril; in adults 0.1 per cent solution of xylometazoline (Otrivin) or 0.05 per cent oxymetazoline (Afrin) is used as a nasal spray. Two squeezes are instilled into each nostril three or four times daily. Humidification of the room air by a portable cold air humidifier also decreases nasal congestion.

A number of antihistamines can provide diminution in rhinorrhea. Recommended are chlorpheniramine (Chlor-Trimeton), 4 mg. every 6 hours for adults or 1 to 2 mg. tablet every 6 hours for children; or chlorpheniramine elixir (Novahistine elixir), ½ to 1 teaspoonful four times a day for children 1 to 6 years of age and 2 teaspoonfuls four times a day for older children. In adults, sustained acting capsules of chlorpheniramine maleate (Ornade Spansule) provide effective relief of rhinorrhea; the dosage of this medication is 1 capsule every 12 hours.

When cough is persistent, nonproductive, and distressing, any one of a number of antitussive medications can be prescribed. Depending upon the clinical situation, cough suppressants or expectorants are administered. Physiologically, expectorants are preferred to clear secretions and maintain the cough reflex intact. Recommended are expectorants containing antihistamines (Novahistine elixir or diphenhydramine [Benylin expectorant]). The dosage of Novahistine elixir is 1 tablespoonful four times a day for adults, and for Benylin expectorant it is 1 to 2 teaspoonfuls four times a day. For severe and persistent nonproductive cough, an antitussive such as codeine should be used in combination with antihistamines (Novahistine DH). The dose of Novahistine DH for adults is 2 teaspoonfuls four times a day. For children 1 to 6 years of age, the dosage of Novahistine DH is ¼ to ¾ teaspoonful, and for children 6 to 12 years, it is 1 teaspoonful four times a day.

Sore throat can be relieved by frequent gargling with warm saline solution (¼ teaspoonful of sodium chloride in ½ glass of warm water). Aspirin and acetaminophen in the usual doses can relieve sore throat. Room humidification with a cold water mist is helpful also.

Immunoprophylaxis

Inactivated influenza virus vaccines are the only commercially available vaccines for immunization against any of the many viruses which infect the human respiratory tract. Influenza virus vaccines effectively prevent infection with the prevalent types of influenza. These vaccines are reformulated annually, based on predictions concerning the specific influenza strains which can be expected to appear in the ensuing winter. Usually the vaccines are bivalent, containing the most recent individual influenza virus A and B strains. However, depending upon the pattern of occurrence or anticipated occurrence of influenza virus strains in the nation, monovalent A or B strain vaccines or bivalent vaccines containing differing A strains may be available also. In these instances, the recommendations for use and dosage of the vaccines issued by the Center for Disease Control should be followed.

The vaccine virus is grown in embryonated eggs and is purified to remove most egg protein and pyrogenic materials. Some preparations may be treated further with either ether or tri-n-butyl phosphate to disrupt the whole virus (virion) particle; these specially treated vaccines are designated split product vaccines. Split product influenza virus vaccines have been recommended for use in children, as they produce fewer side reactions in this age group. Persons sensitive to egg protein should not receive influenza virus vaccines.

Influenza virus vaccine is recommended for individuals suffering from chronic debilitating diseases, including congenital and rheumatic heart disease, hypertensive and arteriosclerotic heart disease, chronic respiratory diseases, and diabetes mellitus and other chronic metabolic disorders, as well as aged persons and persons essential to community services. To be effective, immunization with influenza virus vaccines must be repeated annually in the fall, and with the current formulated vaccine.

Chemoprophylactic Drugs

Except for amantadine, no chemotherapeutic drugs are available for the treatment of viral respiratory tract infections. Amantadine (Symmetrel) is an effective chemoprophylactic drug for influenza virus type A2 infections. Since it prevents viral attachment to uninfected cells, it must be administered before infection occurs. Amantadine is ineffective for the treatment of established influenza virus or other respiratory virus infections, and it is not recommended for these purposes.

Because of its limited antiviral spectrum, the drug should be given to high risk patients only when outbreaks of influenza virus A2 strains have been identified in the community. The dose for adults is 200 mg. daily. Higher daily doses produce central nervous system side effects, including nervousness, dizziness, inability to concentrate, and depression. Patients in the high risk group can be given influenza virus vaccine and amantadine and the drug stopped soon after an antibody response to vaccine can be expected to develop. Amantadine is contraindicated in pregnant women.

SECTION 3

The Cardiovascular System

ACQUIRED DISEASES OF THE AORTA

method of
JOHN J. COLLINS, Jr., M.D.
Boston, Massachusetts

Acquired diseases become clinically significant when they result in obstruction, expansion, or rupture of the aorta. The most common acquired aortic disease is arteriosclerosis, which may cause any or all of these problems. The cause of arteriosclerosis is uncertain despite much experimental and clinical research. The pathogenesis is also not clearly understood, although various forms of the disease have been experimentally produced and certain clinical factors are known to promote progression of the disease.

Management of Arteriosclerotic Aortic Disease

Medical Measures. Patients with clinically significant arteriosclerotic lesions of the aorta should have their blood pressure carefully controlled by medication or surgery in appropriate instances. They should not use tobacco in any form. Diabetes, when present, should be carefully controlled, although such control is not certain to impede the progression of the process. Patients with hyperlipidemias are wise to pursue a dietary program to control levels of cholesterol and lipoproteins, although dietary management has not been proved to arrest or reverse the disease in human beings. There is evidence from some laboratory animal models that lipid deposition in arterial walls may be controlled or even reversed by diet changes. Consideration of the physical condition of concentration camp survivors gave rise to some speculation following World War II that severe dietary restriction might possibly even reverse lesions in human beings, although no firm evidence has yet been produced.

Whether any benefit may result from the chronic use of aspirin or other drugs to reduce platelet adhesiveness is entirely speculative. Similarly, no advantage has been described for hormone manipulation, although there may be emerging some suggestion that certain contraceptive medications may render susceptible women more prone to premature atherosclerosis.

The metabolic impact of small bowel exclusion operations or redirection of portal blood flow has been studied in some patients with hyperlipidemic syndromes. Results to date are controversial and no striking benefit has been reliably documented, although lipid levels may be dramatically lowered in some patients.

The potential benefit of exercise programs and measures to diminish stress has been widely described without convincing documentation.

Surgical Management. Rupture of the aorta is an always clear-cut indication for operation if the patient is to survive for long. Obstruction of the aorta is nearly always best treated by operation. Transverse expansion of the aorta beyond one and one half times its usual diameter in a local segment is an indication for surgery in patients otherwise healthy, but longitudinal expansion of the aorta is well tolerated and does not require operation in most instances even though the roentgenographic appearance of the tortuous contrast-filled artery may be alarming.

The decision to operate on a patient for an aortic lesion must be based upon the surgeon's conviction that life expectancy, comfort, or limb viability is more threatened by the disease than by the contemplated operation. The indications thus depend upon the risk of surgical correction as well as the realistic assessment of the hope for rehabilitation. A highly skilled surgeon is justified in taking a more aggressive approach in an early or asymptomatic lesion than a less skilled one. Skill and experience are more important as the difficulty and complexity of operation increase.

Several techniques are available for correction of aortic lesions. The aorta may be directly repaired, replaced with an artificial conduit, bypassed, or disimpacted of obstruction. The selection of operation depends upon the nature of the lesion, the condition of the adjacent arterial walls, the general health of the patient, and the experience of the surgeon.

Aortic rupture, as a complication of arteriosclerotic aortic disease, most commonly occurs as a complication in the natural history of aortic aneurysm. On occasion, however, transmural aortic rupture may occur with a very small aneurysm or through an area of ruptured plaque with no appreciable aneurysm whatsoever. Arteriosclerotic aortic rupture is more common in the abdominal than in the thoracic aorta. The diagnosis is most frequently suspected in the emergency room. It has become our practice under these circumstances to perform minimal resuscitative measures in the emergency room. Usually, one or two large bore intravenous routes are established and blood is drawn for crossmatch. The patient is transferred forthwith to the operating room where the remainder of necessary manipulations are completed. An arterial monitoring line is placed, usually in the radial artery, and a Foley catheter is placed in the bladder. Additional large bore intravenous access is obtained to a total of three reliable conduits. An antistaphylococcal antibiotic is given intravenously. We prefer a cephalosporin or lincomycin. The entire chest, abdomen, and groin are rapidly prepared with benzalkonium chloride (Zephiran) and alcohol and draped in a sterile manner. A midline incision is made and the state of the abdominal aorta assessed. If there is a relatively small retroperitoneal hematoma and if the neck of the aneurysm is obviously approachable below the renal arteries, the retroperitoneum is dissected minimally and an occluding clamp placed from a vertical direction just above the beginning of the aneurysm and below the renal arteries. No attempt is made to pass a tape around the aorta. Following this, control can easily be obtained around the common iliac arteries. If the aneurysm involves the origin of the common iliac arteries, it is necessary to use a bifurcation graft replacement. If the aneurysm involves only the distal aorta, it has been the practice at the Peter Bent Brigham Hospital to utilize a straight graft. Following isolation, the aneurysm can be incised anteriorly and the clot evacuated. Bleeding lumbar vessels should be controlled with a few sutures. If desired, 5000 or 7500 units of heparin may be administered at this point. We do not use heparin in patients with a ruptured aneurysm except to instill a small amount in saline into the iliacs after clamping. It is unwise to administer heparin before controlling the neck of the aneurysm in any case. A suitable graft of Teflon or Dacron is then sutured in place with continuous suture. If the aneurysm is not septic, the graft is placed entirely within the aorta without transecting the posterior aortic wall. Deep, closely spaced posterior bites ensure absence of posterior bleeding following completion of the anastomoses. With a straight graft, the entire prosthesis lies within the aneurysm. The redundant aneurysm wall may then be trimmed following completion of the proximal and distal anastomoses and closed over the graft. If the aneurysm shows evidence of infection or is known to be septic, the entire aneurysm should be resected. This is a more formidable undertaking and carries with it a considerable increase in the hazards of bleeding from the aneurysm bed and injury to the inferior vena cava. If there is aneurysmal involvement of the iliac bifurcation, a bifurcated graft must be used with individual anastomoses to the iliac arteries on either side. This may be accomplished by proximal ligation of the common iliac arteries, and end-to-side anastomosis of the distal limbs of the bifurcation prosthesis to the common or external iliac vessels, or the iliac anastomoses may be performed inside the aneurysms in a manner similar to that used for the proximal aortic anastomosis. Protamine is administered following completion of the anastomoses and removal of the aortic clamp (if heparin has been used).

Under ordinary circumstances, no more than 30 to 45 minutes of aortic crossclamping is necessary. Under these circumstances, severe hypotension with removal of the clamp is unusual. However, the anesthesiologist should be prepared at the time of unclamping of the aorta to transfuse vigorously should the need arise. Under these circumstances, it is wise to consider the possible deleterious effect of infusion of cold potassium-rich blood on the myocardial action. Rewarming the blood prior to transfusion and the judicious utilization of intravenous calcium may have a place at this point. Although we have not routinely utilized mannitol during aortic aneurysm resection, the possibility of compromise of the renal circulation should always be borne in mind, and if there is any threat of this, 6.0 to 10.0 grams of mannitol should be given intravenously at an early moment. The presence of mannitol in the circulation may prolong the tolerable renal ischemia time in the event that clamping the aorta above the renal arteries becomes necessary for control of bleeding. In addition, the production of a large urine volume may be protective against the effects of hypotension and multiple transfusion and the tendency to acute tubular necrosis under these circumstances.

When, upon examination of the retroperitoneal hematoma, the neck of the aneurysm is not immediately evident, it may become necessary to place an aortic crossclamp above the renal arteries or occasionally immediately beneath the diaphragm. Under these circumstances, minimal dissection should be used and a large atraumatic clamp should be applied from the anterior aspect of the aorta. As soon as the hemorrhage is controlled and the aneurysm is anatomically identified, the clamp should be moved to a position below the renal arteries with re-establishment of renal blood flow. In the event that it appears such a repositioning of the clamp may not be possible for a period of time beyond 30 minutes, it is probably wise to establish local renal hypothermia and even to consider perfusion of the kidney with a membrane stabilizing solution.

Surgical treatment of intact arteriosclerotic aneurysms of the abdominal aorta is advised when the diameter of the involved segment exceeds 5 cm. Suspected areas of aortic ectasia smaller than that should be examined at frequent intervals and operation advised if enlargement occurs or if the onset of pain and tenderness suggests expansion even though measurable dimensions have not changed. If other vital systems are diseased, the surgeon should be cautious in suggesting surgery for asymptomatic small lesions. The most troublesome illnesses commonly associated with abdominal aortic aneurysm are chronic obstructive pulmonary disease, arteriosclerotic heart disease, and arteriosclerotic cerebrovascular disease.

An antibiotic with staphylococcidal capability is given on the evening before operation, intravenously during the procedure, and for several days after surgery. In many patients pulmonary artery pressure is monitored using a flow-directed balloon-tip catheter, and albumin may be administered sufficient to maintain wedge pressures of 6 to 10 mm. Hg. Hypotension upon release of the aortic clamp is thereby minimized.

A midline incision is most often used. Evisceration is useful in obese patients with large aneurysms. In most patients the abdominal contents may simply be packed away with moist gauze. Careful exploration is important. Malignant tumors of the pancreas or stomach take precedence unless there is threatened rupture of the aneurysm. A small tumor of the colon probably is best left for a later procedure. If the aneurysm resection goes smoothly and quickly, a stone-filled gallbladder should be removed if this can be readily accomplished. Postoperative cholecystitis and jaundice can be a bother or worse. Operations involving entry into the stomach or duodenum are best avoided because of the potentially high cost of prosthetic graft contamination.

The duodenum is carefully dissected from in front of the aneurysm and packed away with a suitable retractor. The left renal vein should be identified and kept from harm. One must be wary of a possible retroaortic course of this structure or of the presence of a left-sided vena cava. The inferior mesenteric vein is ligated and divided. Aberrant arteries of the lower poles of the kidneys may require division.

The iliac arteries should be freed over several centimeters length beyond any area of adherence to the iliac veins. The ureters must be kept in mind, but it is not necessary to search them out specifically.

It is not necessary to dissect behind the aorta in most instances. Usually the fingers of the right hand can squeeze the aorta forward sufficiently to allow placement of a clamp by the left hand in an anteroposterior attitude on the aorta just beneath the renal arteries. Encircling the iliac arteries is also unnecessary, prolongs dissection, and increases the hazard of iliac vein injury. After the lesion is isolated by application of clamps, it is opened longitudinally on the anterior aspect. Lumbar vessels are ligated with sutures. The posterior aortic wall is preserved. A straight or bifurcation graft is implanted as with ruptured lesions. Following closure of the aortic wall over the graft, the peritoneum is repositioned with absorbable sutures and the abdominal contents replaced.

Rupture of arteriosclerotic aneurysms above the diaphragm is distinctly less common, although such a complication can be devastating. In addition to pain, such rupture of an intrathoracic aneurysm may be manifested by hemoptysis. Unless the patient is moribund, it is wise to obtain a thoracic aortogram before operating on patients with suspected rupture of the thoracic aorta. Often it may be possible, utilizing this technique, to localize the site of aortic injury and to plan the operative approach to provide adequate exposure of the involved area. Most arteriosclerotic aneurysms will occur in the descending aorta distal to the left subclavian artery. In such a case, it should be possible to obtain access to the aorta above the aneurysm and below the aneurysm without undue difficulty. The area immediately overlying the site of rupture may be densely adherent to the lung from previous inflammatory change, and the planes of desired dissection may be obscured by hematoma. Control may be obtained above and below and the aorta clamped using an external shunt from the transverse arch of the aorta to the descending aorta below the distal clamp or utilizing partial cardiopulmonary bypass to decompress the central circulation and perfuse the distal aorta.

Some surgeons simply clamp the aorta above and below the lesion, utilizing intravenous trimethaphan or nitroprusside to control the proximal aortic pressure while performing the necessary graft interposition. If it is possible to complete the operation in 40 minutes or less, this approach has provided excellent results. It has been our usual practice to utilize a silicone-rubber tubular shunt from the transverse arch of the aorta to the descending aorta. Heparinization is not absolutely necessary, but 5000 units may be administered. Polyvinylchloride tubing coated with TDMAC (tridodecylmethylammonium chloride) is commercially available in suitable configurations, and heparin need not be used. An attempt should be made to dissect the lung away from the involved segment of aorta. If this appears to threaten the involved segment of lung, the aorta may be incised and sufficient of the aneurysm excised to free the lung, leaving a portion of the wall of the aneurysm on the lung, or, using a stapling device, a portion of the lung may be left on the aortic wall and later resected. In any event, it is advisable to isolate the involved segment of aorta with as little dissection as possible, open it, and control bleeding from the intercostal arteries with suture ligation, damaging as few as possible. A prosthetic cloth graft is then sutured entirely within the aortic lumen above and below. Care should be taken to employ a prosthesis of at least 1 inch diameter. The collapsed aorta may appear to have a smaller internal diameter than 1 inch, but in virtually all instances the aortic wall should be stretched to accommodate the graft so that an artificial coarctation will not be produced by introduction of too small a prosthesis. Continuous suture of plastic material is used above and below. The redundant aorta is then trimmed and the aorta closed over the graft.

We have preferred the use of woven grafts as opposed to weave-knit or knitted grafts. It is essential to use woven material if the graft is to be placed while the patient is on cardiopulmonary bypass with full heparinization. Otherwise, the extent of hemorrhage will be quite astonishing and possibly even fatal through the interstices of the graft. Even the woven grafts at times show a troublesome amount of ooze from the pores between the fibers.

If under any circumstances weave knits or knitted grafts are to be used for aortic conduits, such grafts should be carefully preclotted.

Rupture of arteriosclerotic aneurysms involving the arch of the aorta constitute one of surgery's most formidable problems. Arteriosclerotic aneurysms of the ascending aorta are uncommon. When a ruptured aneurysm involves the arch of the aorta, a left thoracotomy incision through the fourth intercostal space traversing the sternum into the third or fourth intercostal space on the right side is usually necessary for adequate visualization. It may be necessary to sacrifice a portion of the upper lobe of the lung in order to obtain adequate visualization of the aortic arch. It will then be necessary to isolate the ascending aorta proximal to the takeoff of the innominate artery and to isolate the descending aorta at a suitable point as high as possible. Before crossclamping the aorta, the patient is totally heparinized and cardiopulmonary bypass established using the left common femoral vein and left common femoral artery. It may be necessary to place a second venous cannula either into the pulmonary outflow tract or into the right atrium if that is accessible in order to obtain adequate flow. When this has been accomplished, the patient should be cooled to about 24°C. During the process of cooling, the descending aorta may be transected and a straight cloth graft of suitably redundant length anastomosed end-to-end with the distal descending aortic segment.

The head should now be inclined downward and the branches of the aortic arch individually clamped or secured with tourniquets. A proximal aortic clamp is now applied and the aortic arch isolated. The aortic arch is then opened and the distally attached cloth graft placed within the arch of the aorta. A button of aorta containing the orifices of the great vessels is resected from the surrounding aorta and sutured to an appropriately devised aperture on the cloth graft, or such an aperture on the cloth graft may be sewn to the otherwise intact aortic wall around the orifice of the great vessels. The proximal portion of the cloth graft may then be clamped and, with the great vessels still occluded, blood flow introduced from below into the cloth aortic arch replacement. When all air has been removed, the head vessels may be released to allow them to be perfused from the cardiopulmonary bypass apparatus in a retrograde fashion. The proximal anastomosis may now be completed and continuity of the aortic arch re-established. More than 15 minutes of cerebral ischemia may be damaging.

Some surgeons prefer to utilize perfusion of the innominate and left common carotid arteries from the heart-lung machine during completion of the anastomoses. This may be done using coronary perfusion pumps or by a Y-connection from the arterial perfusion line.

The principal problems in surgical operations on the aortic arch are (1) obtaining adequate exposure, (2) providing adequate cerebral blood flow while avoiding air embolism or atheromatous embolism to the brain, and (3) avoiding hemorrhage from the suture lines. In addition, many patients with aneurysms involving the aorta may be elderly and generally debilitated. Often such patients may be unable to withstand the enormous surgical trauma attendant upon resection of the aortic arch. Such operations should be attempted only in those centers where adequate experience with the use of cardiopulmonary bypass, hypothermia, and aortic resection offers some reasonable hope for survival. In instances in which direct resection of the aortic arch is deemed impossible or inadvisable, it may occasionally be possible to construct a prosthetic aortic arch from the ascending aorta around the hilum of the right lung through the diaphragm and through the retroperitoneal space connecting to the abdominal aorta. Grafts may then be constructed from the arch of the prosthetic conduit to the head vessels in the base of the neck. Following this, the head vessels can be ligated and the arch of the aorta excluded from the circulation by oversewing. This is still a formidable operation, although the advantage of not interrupting the cerebral circulation may be considerable.

Obstruction of the Aorta

Aortic obstruction most commonly occurs as the result of embolization to the distal aorta at or just proximal to the iliac bifurcation. Partial obstruction, particularly of the distal aorta, may result from severe proliferation of atherosclerotic plaque with superimposition of thrombosis. In instances of aortic obstruction caused by embolization of blood clot, it is usually possible to remove the clot by the Fogarty embolectomy technique, utilizing bilateral femoral arteriotomies with retrograde catheterization to clear the clot. This procedure may be done under local anesthesia if the condition of the patient dictates.

Chronic distal aortic obstruction resulting from atherosclerotic plaque with or without thrombosis requires a more direct surgical approach. When the obstruction is localized and the iliac vessels or aorta distally have walls of good quality, endarterectomy may be possible. Following longitudinal incision of the aortic adventitia, a plane is established in the media where relatively easy dissection will shell out the atheromatous core. The proximal extent of dissection may be variable. When the dissection has been carried to an area where the lumen is no longer compromised, the intima may be trimmed in a suitable circumferential fashion. A few tacking sutures may be necessary, but often these are not needed. Distally, the dissection should be carried to a point where the intima is as normal as possible. The intima should then be carefully trimmed, and tacking sutures are often necessary to assure that the intima remains in close and intimate contact with the adventitia. If this is not carefully attended to, a dissection may result in the area with consequent obstruction. Closure of the aorta may be accomplished by direct suture or using a woven cloth patch graft if needed.

In the many circumstances under which endarterectomy is inappropriate, it is possible to transect the distal aorta, performing an end-to-end anastomosis to a prosthetic graft and leading the bifurcated distal graft into anastomoses end-to-side with the external iliac or common femoral vessels or performing an end-to-side anastomosis both above and below. Aortofemoral grafts are preferable to endarterectomy when aortic disease extends above the inferior mesenteric artery origin or when obstruction extends beyond the iliac bifurcations.

Arteriosclerotic obstruction of the major arterial branches of the aorta may be surgically treated by end-to-side suture of the appropriate grafts to the side of the aorta and subsequent end-to-side graft to recipient artery anastomosis beyond the areas of obstruction. This technique is suitable for obstructions to the brachiocephalic vessels or to major intra-abdominal vessels. Saphenous vein conduits are preferable to cloth grafts for most reconstructions of the abdominal arteries. A major consideration in such operations is obtaining adequate exposure. A lateral oblique extraperitoneal approach may be used for exposure of the common iliac artery of one side and the distal-most portion of the aorta. For any other purpose a generous midline transperitoneal approach is preferable. Some surgeons utilize paramedian incision.

Management of Dissecting Aneurysms

In most patients the occurrence of aortic dissection is a recognizable acute event accompanied by chest, back, or neck pain which may be quite severe. Some patients may be encountered in whom the acute episode was either unnoticed or not investigated. These persons may present with syndromes of peripheral ischemia, aortic valve malfunction, or enlarging saccular aneurysms.

Patients with acute aortic dissections most commonly present with pain, shock, cardiac failure, or neurologic deficits. The syndrome depends upon the site of origin of the lesion, the extent of progression of intramural hematoma, and the peripheral distribution of aortic branches which may have become obstructed. The objects of therapy are to prevent aortic rupture, to control progression of the hematoma, and, if necessary, to re-establish aortic valve function and satisfactory peripheral organ perfusion. In some patients the location of the hematoma rapidly produces life-threatening disability such as acute aortic insufficiency, coronary artery compression, or cerebral ischemia from brachiocephalic arterial compression. Paralytic syndromes may result from spinal artery compression. Aortic rupture may occur early in the course of illness into the pericardium, mediastinum, or pleural space. Retroperitoneal rupture is uncommon.

A precise diagnosis, including localization of the site of origin of the hematoma, is necessary for selection of appropriate therapy. Transfemoral or transaxillary percutaneous aortic angiography provides high quality contrast safely in skilled hands. Intravenous angiography generally does not provide as satisfactory a study. If the patient's condition is precarious, angiography may be delayed or abandoned. Surgery without angiography should be undertaken only when cardiac tamponade is not controlled by aspiration or when heart failure, hypotension, or hemorrhage is otherwise likely to be rapidly fatal.

Initial management includes blood pressure control, establishment of intravenous access routes and an arterial pressure monitoring line, and provision for measurement of urinary output. If hypotension is persistent or if continuous intravenous antihypertensive medication is indicated, a urinary catheter should be inserted.

Our experience, supported by reports from other centers, indicates that immediate operation yields better results for patients with lesions originating in the ascending aorta (DeBakey Types I and II). Medical management is reasonable for patients in whom the dissection begins distal to the left subclavian artery unless the hematoma continues to progress, saccular aneurysm or rupture develops, or peripheral vital organ ischemia develops. Proximal extension of hematoma from a descending aortic origin to rupture into the pericardium or produce aortic valve incompetence is rare. We have seen only one such case.

Medical Therapy. 1. Patients are admitted to an intensive care unit. The electrocardiogram is monitored as well as arterial blood pressure and urinary output.

2. Systolic blood pressure is maintained at 90 to 100 mm. Hg, presuming no evidence of cerebral, renal, or myocardial ischemia develops. We prefer intravenous nitroprusside for control of hypertension. A solution of 50 mg. nitroprusside in 1000 ml. 5 per cent dextrose in water is prepared and shielded from light by metal foil. Intravenous infusion of 0.5 ml. per minute is begun and increased at intervals of 3 to 5 minutes by 0.5 ml. per minute until adequate control is obtained. Serum thiocyanate level is obtained each day in patients in whom infusion is continued for more than 24 hours. Thiocyanate of 10 mg. or more per 100 ml. is potentially toxic and may necessitate stopping the infusion. Trimethaphan in a solution of 1 or 2 mg. per ml. may be substituted with proper regard for the side effects of ganglionic blockade which may result.

3. A program of long-term antihypertensive medication should be started soon after admission. Propranolol, 1 mg. intravenously by infusion over 20 minutes or 20 mg. orally, is administered every 6 hours unless the heart rate is slowed below 60 per minute or other side effects dictate cessation. Alpha-methyldopa is begun with 250 mg. intramuscularly or by mouth at 4 to 6 hour intervals. If alpha-methyldopa is contraindicated or not well tolerated, reserpine, 0.25 mg. every 12 hours, or guanethidine, 25 to 50 mg. every 12 hours, may be used. A thiazide diuretic is also employed in most cases.

4. Portable chest roentgenograms are obtained at appropriate intervals. In early acute cases a film is obtained on admission and again in 4 to 6 hours. If progression has not occurred, further examinations are performed in 12 to 24 hours and daily during the intensive care stay.

5. When adequate control of hypertension has been maintained for 24 hours, intravenous medication is tapered and gradually discontinued. Bed rest and sedation programs are relaxed over several days after 3 to 4 days of recumbency. Care to avoid postural hypotension is needed, as well as observation of blood pressure to ensure adequate hypertension control during this phase of rehabilitation. Most patients are ready to leave the intensive care area in 5 to 7 days for another 7 to 10 days of graduated ambulation on the general wards.

6. If medical therapy fails as indicated by continuance or recurrence of pain, enlargement of the dissecting hematoma, development of ischemia of vital organs, or impending aortic rupture, operation should be undertaken without delay.

Surgical Therapy. Patients with acute or chronic manifestations of aortic dissection may require operation. For most patients with chronic aortic insufficiency secondary to dissecting aneurysm, replacement of the aortic valve as well as of the ascending aorta will be necessary. The proximal aorta may be hugely dilated in some patients, and the aortic annulus may be stretched or deformed to such an extent that adequate repair is impossible. In such instances a prosthetic or bioprosthetic aortic valve may be sutured in place and a woven plastic cloth conduit directly sutured to the fixation ring of the valve. The coronary ostia are sutured to appropriately fashioned apertures in the cloth graft. This may be done without trimming the aorta around the ostia, lessening the chance for bleeding from these suture lines. The cloth graft may then be fixed to the aortic wall from within just proximal to the origin of the innominate takeoff. The aneurysm is trimmed and the remaining aortic wall closed snugly around the prosthetic conduit, leaving little or no exposed aorto-prosthetic suture line. Bleeding from the thinned fragile aorta is thereby minimized and the operation made simpler and safer than when resection of the entire aortic circumference is attempted. Often in proximal aortic dilatation with dissection the posterior aortic wall (along the interior curve of the aortic arch) may be intact and the dilatation may be entirely anteriorly and laterally directed. In such instances it may be possible to resect the aneurysm anteriorly and laterally, leaving the posterior wall intact and restoring continuity by use of a wedge-shaped patch of woven graft material. This may be rather quickly performed, with or without aortic valve replacement, and avoids a troublesome posterior suture line from which bleeding may be difficult to control.

Acute dissections originating in the ascending aorta may be treated more conservatively in most instances, as the intima may not be particularly dilated and the aortic valve may be anatomically normal save for dehiscence of its moorings.

Surgical management of acute dissecting aneurysm of the ascending aorta is accomplished as follows. With the usual intravenous conduits and arterial monitoring necessary for open-heart surgery, the patient is appropriately prepared and draped in a sterile manner. The heart and aorta are exposed through a median sternotomy incision. Only a single venous cannula is used through a purse-string in the right atrium. If the dissection extends into the arch of the aorta, it may be necessary to utilize retrograde femoral arterial cannulation and perfusion for cardiopulmonary bypass. In some instances it may be possible to cannulate the arch of the aorta along the inner aspect of the lesser curve of the arch. In this area, dissection rarely splits the intima away from the adventitia.

After establishment of cardiopulmonary bypass, an atraumatic clamp should be applied to the ascending aorta immediately proximal to the origin of the innominate artery. It is usually possible to visualize the dissecting hematoma and to recognize some extravasation of blood into the adventitia, particularly over the pulmonary outflow tract and proximal pulmonary artery. There may have occurred some leaking of blood, particularly in this area, and free blood may be found in the pericardial cavity.

The aorta should be opened anteriorly to expose the interior of the false lumen of the aorta. In most instances, the intima would be found to be of normal size and the blood in the false lumen will still be liquid. The blood can be aspirated. If the hematoma has dissected far enough proximally to unhinge the attachments of the aortic valve, it is possible at this point to reposition the aortic valve and to line the cavity of the false lumen with either prosthetic cloth graft material or prosthetic felt material in a carefully tailored manner so as to resuspend the native aortic valve in a competent fashion. The commissures of the aortic valve are buttressed in a through-and-through fashion with pledget reinforced sutures passed through the aortic intima, through the cloth or felt, and through the adventitial aortic layers. When these sutures are tied, the valve should be quite competent. The aortic adventitia should be trimmed so that the entire extent of the false lumen may be oversewn incorporating the new prosthetic media. The distal segment of the ascending aorta may then be either resected or lined with cloth in a fashion similar to that of the proximal segment. In either event, the distalmost retained aortic portion should be cloth-lined and oversewn. If the aorta is then to be primarily reanastomosed, this can be accomplished using large bites of simple suture in an over-and-over fashion. Since there is prosthetic material now in the media of the aorta, the utilization of externally applied pledget material is unnecessary. If a prosthetic graft has been chosen to replace the ascending aorta, such a graft can be easily inserted. Even in these instances, it may be wise to retain the posterior aortic wall to avoid the possibility of bleeding from a hidden suture line. Our experience with over a dozen patients in whom severe aortic insufficiency occurred with acute dissection, and in whom resuspension of the aortic valve had been carried out, indicates that the mortality for surgical repair is low (under 10 per cent), and the follow-up period up to 7 years has shown no significant progression of aortic incompetence or proximal aortic dilatation. Aortic valve replacement in acute aortic insufficiency caused by dissecting aneurysm may be necessary if the leaflets themselves have been damaged by previous disease or if they are congenitally abnormal, or if the proximal aorta is sufficiently dilated that apposition of the edges of the aortic valve leaflets can only be obtained by narrowing the annulus. In general, operations in which the annulus of the aorta is shortened have met with only mediocre success and have frequently been complicated in time by dilatation.

If aortic valve replacement is chosen, it may be carried out in a fashion similar to that described for aortic valve replacement and ascending aortic replacement for chronic dissecting aneurysm. A central flow orifice valve should be chosen rather than a ball valve. Turbulence around the ball valve outflow area may cause late ascending aorta dilatation with rupture.

Following completion of the anastomoses, cardiopulmonary bypass is discontinued in the usual manner, utilizing left atrial monitoring as well as constant measurement of intra-arterial blood pressure to determine the need for cardiotonic drugs. We have not utilized coronary arterial perfusion for the past 5 or 6 years. We prefer systemic hypothermia on cardiopulmonary bypass to about 28 to 30°C. and topical cardiac hypothermia induced by infusion of lactate Ringer's solution (4°C.) into the pericardium in a constant stream using intravenous tubing. In addition, the interior of the heart is copiously irrigated three to five times during the course of operation with cold lactate Ringer's solution. This technique provides adequate myocardial protection for up to 2 hours of ischemia. Cannulation of the coronary arteries for perfusion in patients with acute dissecting aneurysms involving the ascending aorta poses a greater than usual hazard of coronary arterial injury. We have had no significant experience with the use of membrane stabilizing solutions in these patients, although some additional benefit may possibly be derived from this technique.

Following the conclusion of cardiopulmonary bypass, it is important to avoid hypertension. Appropriate anesthetic agents may be administered to maintain the systolic blood pressure at 100 to 110 mm. Hg while the patient remains in the operating room during closure of the chest. Following return to the intensive care unit, any inordinate rise in systolic blood pressure may be controlled by appropriate manipulation of the blood volume as dictated by the left atrial pressure. If the left atrial pressure is below 8 mm. Hg, it is unwise to deplete the blood volume further. Under these circumstances a constant infusion of nitroprusside is a safer technique for obtaining blood pressure control. A solution of 50 mg. nitroprusside in 1000 ml. 5 per cent dextrose in water is utilized in a fashion similar to that described for medical management of acute dissecting aneurysm. Longer acting antihypertensive agents may then be added as indicated.

Chronic dissecting aneurysms involving the descending aorta may attain a very large size. Their very bulk may make it difficult to approach them surgically. A left thoracotomy incision through the bed of the fourth rib or through the fourth intercostal space generally provides adequate exposure. It may occasionally be necessary to transect the sternum for additional exposure. The lung must be carefully dissected away from the mass of the aneurysm. Limited pulmonary resection may sometimes be necessary to provide adequate exposure. The aorta should be encircled with a tape above and below the aneurysm. If there is sufficient room, it may be possible to utilize a bypass conduit for maintenance of aortic flow during the period when the aneurysm is clamped. Often, however, it may be difficult or impossible to obtain a proper spot on the proximal aorta for establishment of a bypass conduit. Under these circumstances it may be elected to simply cross-clamp the aorta and proceed with the operation, having the anesthetist control the proximal aortic blood pressure with medication; or, as we more frequently do, it may be necessary to utilize femorofemoral bypass to control proximal aortic pressure and provide distal aortic perfusion. If bypass is to be used, proximal and distal control should be obtained if possible prior to heparinization.

When the aorta has been clamped, the dissecting hematoma is entered and the condition of the aortic lumen assessed. It is necessary to find the origin of the dissection. When this has been done, a conservative amount of aorta is resected. In some instances, no aortic resection at all is necessary and a prosthetic conduit may simply be sutured inside the lumen of the descending aorta from a point above the origin of the dissection to a point well below. If this technique is chosen, great care must be taken to obliterate the false lumen both above and below. This is readily accomplished by interposition of Teflon felt and oversewing the cut edges. The remaining aortic wall may be closed over the prosthetic graft. The fragile consistency of the aortic wall and particularly of the intima in these patients cannot be overemphasized. Enormous care must be taken to damage these walls as little as possible, and, wherever necessary, reinforcing pledgets should be used to prevent the sutures tearing through. Even so, the most common major complication of this sort of operation is continued hemorrhage from the suture lines, with a sometimes fatal outcome.

The management of acute dissecting aneurysms originating in the descending aorta is similar to that for chronic dissecting aneurysm originating in this area except that reconstruction of the aorta may more frequently be possible. The essential maneuver in the surgical management of these aneurysms is localization and elimination of the intimal tear of origin and obliteration of the false lumen above and below this area. We have utilized the cloth lining of the false lumen technique with oversewing of the proximal and distal margins to accomplish this objective. In some instances, primary anastomosis of the cut ends of the aorta may be possible, although often a short graft interposition is necessary. Care should be taken to preserve as many intercostal arteries as is possible. The question of utilization of cardiopulmonary bypass or a shunt, or of simply crossclamping the aorta, depends upon the age of the patient and the ease with which the operation is to be performed, based upon the appearance of the pathologic anatomy. If the patient is young and the operation appears to be straightforward, it is probably quite safe simply to crossclamp the aorta with pharmacologic blood pressure control for periods up to a half hour. If the operation is going to take longer than this, some provision should be made for distal aortic perfusion during the period of clamping. A shunt is excellent for this purpose if there is sufficient room above and below the aneurysm.

Aortic Injuries

Severe deceleration trauma of the chest is common in automobile and motorcycle accidents. Disruption of the aorta occurs most commonly just beyond the origin of the left subclavian artery. Avulsion of major branches may also occur. Widening of the mediastinum on chest roentgenogram is enough to justify prompt aortography. Only life-threatening injuries elsewhere should delay investigation and operation. Even total aortic disruption may be contained for days or longer within the mediastinum in some instances, but the false aneurysm involved should be considered an urgent problem when discovered.

Surgical management is like that for aneurysms in similar locations. We have tended to use a short cloth graft for reconstruction in nearly all cases so that suture lines have no tension.

Penetrating injuries may involve the aorta in any location. Such wounds may allow prolonged survival with opportunity for definitive repair.

Nonspecific Aortitis ("Pulseless Disease")

The aorta may occasionally be involved with a proliferative inflammatory process possibly of hypersensitivity origin. Therapy with antituberculosis medication has been of little benefit. Some improvement has been noted in some patients with corticosteroid therapy. Surgical excision or bypass grafting may be necessary in many patients, particularly when hypertension (coarctation syndrome) or vital organ ischemia results. Long-term benefit is uncertain, and such operations are often more difficult than expected because of the inflammatory process.

ANGINA PECTORIS

method of
KENNETH A. POPIO, M.D.
Rochester, New York

Pathophysiology

Angina pectoris is the consequence of inadequate regional myocardial perfusion relative to the metabolically generated need for energy sources supplied by blood flow. This imbalance of supply and demand is characteristically transient in angina. It is created by situations which increase the demand for oxygen and nutrients beyond the capacity for their supply, and it is rapidly alleviated by any changes that diminish the need. This simple supply-demand relationship is the basis for the pathophysiology of angina. A thorough understanding of the various factors in the pathophysiology is important to the practical management of patients with angina pectoris. As will be shown, the physician who can identify contributing elements to both supply and demand can modify them and thereby effectively treat the patient with chest pain. The various forms of current therapy may be understood as active interventions designed to rebalance inadequate supply-demand states.

The factors most prominent in determining myocardial oxygen need are heart rate, contractility, systolic intraventricular pressure, ventricular size, and ventricular wall thickness. Increases in any of these parameters can promote oxygen demands and, where supply is limited, the clinical syndrome of angina pectoris. On the other hand, the ability to supply needed oxygen is dependent upon the patency of the coronary arteries, the oxygen-carrying ability of the blood, and the ability to provide oxygen to be carried by the blood. Although the "simple" supply-demand relationship has become more complicated when its subunits are considered, several important and clinically accessible parameters emerge as helpful in the management of this syndrome. A less obvious one is obtained by simply multiplying heart rate by systolic pressure. This product provides a good approximation of myocardial oxygen needs and may be very useful in monitoring the effectiveness of clinical treatment. Since patients with angina experience pain only episodically, the relevant measurement must be made during pain.

Initial Approach to Treatment

Once the diagnosis of angina is secure, treatment should begin by searching for factors other than the state of the coronary arteries that might affect the supply-demand relationship. This permits the identification of conditions which may exacerbate the clinical syndrome in patients with otherwise adequate supply-demand ratios. The removal and/or specific treatment of such extracoronary factors may greatly reduce or even eliminate the need for further treatment directed at angina per se.

Certain clinical syndromes, such as thyrotoxicosis, obesity, and hypertension, require increased myocardial oxygen. Cardiac diseases other than coronary artery obstructions may also be associated with increased oxygen need and angina. Any obstruction to left ventricular outflow (e.g., aortic stenosis and idiopathic hypertrophic subaortic stenosis), pulmonary hypertension, "billowing mitral leaflet" syndrome, and many kinds of tachyarrhythmias are examples. Treatment for these is often very different from that required for coronary obstructive disease.

Excessive use of caffeine (coffee, tea, cola drinks) can lead to tachycardia and angina. Certain medications can promote increased oxygen needs. For example, nasal decongestants, bronchodilators, and some "diet aids" (containing thyroid and/or amphetamines) are capable of increasing heart rate and blood pressure. Steroids with fluid-retaining side effects can worsen angina by increasing heart size. Even though resting heart rate or blood pressure may seem unaffected, remarkable increases may occur with stresses of exercise or emotion. All such medications should be stopped if possible. Many of these offending agents are sold without a physician's prescription, and the search for their presence must be careful and specific.

The ability to supply sufficient oxygen to the myocardium can be affected by anemia, any cardiorespiratory disorder that causes arterial unsaturation, and/or any abnormality of hemoglobin-oxygen affinity. Examples of the last include methemoglobinemia, carboxyhemoglobinemia, or inherited structural defects of hemoglobin that impair oxygen release to the tissues. Some disorders can affect both supply and demand. Examples include aortic insufficiency and arteriovenous fistulas, which increase heart rate and ventricular size and thickness while decreasing coronary perfusion pressure in diastole.

Preliminary Efforts to Increase Supply

Having looked for and eliminated (as far as possible) all these extracoronary elements, one must now attempt to rebalance the supply-demand equation in more direct ways. One is relatively restricted in approaches that potentially increase supply. As noted above, anemia may be corrected and attempts made at increasing arterial saturation when appropriate. The most important and commonly applicable way to improve supply, however, is to advise against all smoking. Cigarette smoking is by far the worst offender, but all forms of smoking are associated with increases in heart rate, blood pressure, and blood carbon monoxide levels. Thus an increased need for oxygen is created while the ability to supply it is diminished. Vigorous education and encouragement are needed to overcome the strong resistance of most smokers. The frequency of chest pains is often much improved by this single change in life-style. Furthermore, although the risk of future myocardial infarction is eight times higher in those smoking one pack of cigarettes per day than in similar nonsmokers, it is substantially lowered within 3 months of stopping smoking.

Another major therapeutic approach is designed to increase blood supply: surgery. However, there is an obvious risk to operation, and results are still not completely established. Most physicians reserve its use until simpler measures have been exhausted. It seems appropriate, then, to discuss it after forms of therapy designed to diminish myocardial oxygen requirements.

Efforts to Decrease Oxygen Demand

Life-Style Manipulations. An effective plan of treatment must be based upon a thorough understanding of the circumstances that precipitate angina for each individual patient. Angina often occurs repeatedly in association with the same activity. Such activities are usually associated with some stress, either emotional or physical. All such stresses produce increases in heart rate, blood pressure, and contractility. In addition, at least some forms of exercise increase ventricular volume. The stress associated with a given activity may be further increased by certain superimposed factors such as performance after meals or in the presence of hot or cold ambient temperatures. Modification or elimination of these stresses can decrease oxygen needs and thus improve the frequency of anginal attacks.

It is much easier for patients to follow advice aimed at modifying physical activity than that aimed at emotional stress. Physical exercise can be restricted or performed more slowly, only before meals, or only in moderate temperatures. It is much harder for patients not to "worry." It is best to advise patients to entirely avoid emotional situations likely to promote angina when this is possible. A restriction should also be placed upon air travel for some patients. Patients who develop angina upon climbing a flight or less of stairs should travel by air only with supplemental oxygen, because alveolar air content is decreased at increasing altitudes.

Although it may be possible to almost totally eliminate angina by the restriction of activities, the resulting life-style may not be acceptable as the patient contemplates his future. Depression is common no matter how slight the restriction. Patients should be encouraged to be optimistic and informed that angina may persist for years without worsening. During this time many patients can lead fairly normal lives. One must be careful to encourage whatever degree of activity is possible as long as symptoms are not produced. However, if the degree of restriction necessary to provide a comfortable existence is unacceptable, drug therapy may be able to produce the desired decrease in myocardial oxygen need in the presence of greater levels of activity than would otherwise be possible.

Drug Therapy. NITROGLYCERIN. Nitroglycerin is still the most powerful agent for the treatment of an acute anginal attack. Employed in dosages from 0.15 to 0.60 mg. sublingually, it can produce dramatic relief of pain within 1½ to 3 minutes. Treatment should begin with 0.3 mg. tablets, and patients should be instructed to use one whenever and as soon as an anginal attack occurs. They should be warned that burning of the tongue, headache, and dizziness may be experienced. The first trial should be made while the patient is seated so that he can judge the magnitude of these effects in a safe position. The patient should also be informed that the upright position potentiates the effect of the drug. However, if extreme light-headedness should occur, the patient should be instructed to sit down with his head between his knees or lie down. If the headaches are intolerable, reducing the dosage of nitroglycerin may still relieve angina without causing headache.

If pain is not relieved within 5 minutes, another dose may be taken; if there is still no relief after an additional 5 minutes, another may be used. Pain still unrelieved should prompt an immediate visit to a hospital emergency room for evaluation of the possibility of myocardial infarction. These tablets should be carried at all times, and patients should be strongly urged to use the tablets whenever angina first strikes. They should be reassured that many doses can be used daily without development of dependence or tolerance. Nitroglycerin is also very effective when used prophylactically in circumstances in which the patient can reliably predict that angina will develop. A nitroglycerin tablet used within 5 to 10 minutes before an activity will protect for about ½ to 1 hour. This use is often neglected but is very important. All patients should be warned that this medication may lose its potency after about 6 months. The burning sensation under the tongue associated with its use is a good marker for clinical potency. Only small, frequently replenished quantities in tightly stoppered glass vials should be carried by patients.

Nitroglycerin acts through a potent effect on smooth muscle relaxation. By this means it produces both arterial hypotension and venous pooling. Both these actions tend to decrease myocardial oxygen demand—the former via reduction in intraventricular systolic pressure, and the latter by decreasing venous return and thus ventricular volume. Some evidence suggests that nitroglycerin may also produce some dilation of coronary arterial vessels and collaterals. A reflex increase in heart rate seems to be outweighed by the substantial decrease in cardiac work mediated by the aforementioned factors.

LONG-ACTING NITRATES. The use of these preparations continues to be controversial. Results of studies comparing the efficacy and duration of action of these preparations with ordinary nitroglycerin are inconclusive. Still, there is no doubt that certain patients seem to enjoy great benefit from these agents. A trial is always indicated in patients using more than a few nitroglycerin tablets per day. There are many preparations but only the sublingual ones are useful, because hepatic metabolism inactivates most of the absorbed orally administered agents. Therapy may be begun with 5 to 10 mg. of sublingual isosorbide dinitrate (Isordil) three to four times per day, including bedtime. This dose may be administered more frequently (as often as every 2 hours) in patients with truly unrelenting pain.

One of the oldest attempts at prolonged nitroglycerin effectiveness has recently received rekindled interest. Two per cent nitroglycerin ointment (Nitrol) takes advantage of absorption through the skin to provide its benefit. Several recent studies have shown hemodynamic benefit and symptomatic relief for 2 to 3 hours, with onset occurring within 15 to 20 minutes. The magnitude of its effect on both arteriolar and venous vessels is similar to the faster-acting sublingual nitroglycerin. It is quite useful as bedtime treatment in patients with nocturnal angina and as intensive treatment for those with incapacitating pain. It is administered as 1 to 5 inch strips covered by an occlusive dressing.

BETA-BLOCKADE. The other major pharmacotherapeutic tool in the treatment of angina is beta-blockade. The use of these competitive antagonists of epinephrine and isoproterenol lowers heart rate and contractility. In higher doses, there is also a decrease in blood pressure. These effects diminish left ventricular work and oxygen consumption, leading to an amelioration of angina. Many studies have shown that the use of beta-blockade in effective doses can lead to a reduction in the frequency of anginal episodes and in the consumption of nitroglycerin for 80 to 100 per cent of the patients examined. Furthermore, many studies employing repeated exercise testing have shown that patients can perform more work before the onset of angina or typical electrocardiographic changes. There can be no question that beta-blockade is an important part of the modern treatment of angina. Its use should be attempted in most patients requiring more than 2 to 3 nitroglycerin tablets per day (exceptions as below).

In the United States, the single approved beta-blocking drug is propranolol (Inderal). There is a wide range in the usual effective oral dose (160 to 400 mg. per day) because of widely variable differences in individual hepatic metabolism. It is therefore important to tailor propranolol therapy to each patient. Many physicians have used reduction in resting heart rate to about 60 beats per minute as a parameter of effective dosage. This has, however, been shown to be relatively insensitive and has led to many patients being erroneously considered "medical failures." The marked reduction or abolition of heart rate response to exercise is a much better criterion for adequate beta-blockade. In the absence of need for caution (see below), propranolol may be started in doses of 20 to 40 mg. four times daily and increased weekly until an effective dosage is reached. If symptomatic benefit is not seen at daily doses of 320 to 640 mg., higher doses will also probably be ineffective. (The manufacturer's official directive states that the value and safety of dosages exceeding 320 mg. per day have not been established.)

The modes of action of nitroglycerin and propranolol are complementary. We have found that the regular use of sublingual isosorbide dinitrate (Isordil) added to effective beta-blockade often provides even greater relief.

Propranolol is capable of affecting beta receptors in other tissues, most notably pulmonary airways. This can lead to one of its major limitations, the production of bronchoconstriction. Bronchoconstriction is clearly shown to occur only in asthmatics, in whom the drug should be avoided. In patients with other forms of obstructive airway disease, caution should be exercised. It is best to begin treatment with small doses (5 to 10 mg. four times daily) and close observation for 2 to 3 days. If wheezing and/or dyspnea do not worsen, one may double the dosage every 2 to 3 days until an effective dose is reached. Forced expiratory volume in 1 second is a simple, easily obtained, and sensitive measurement for monitoring.

Caution is likewise needed when treating patients who have been in congestive heart failure. Propranolol can seriously worsen heart failure by its hemodynamic effects and by promoting sodium and water retention. No patient should be given propranolol in the presence of acute failure, but should first be treated for that. Any patient suspected of previous myocardial damage or failure should be begun on low doses (5 to 10 mg. two to four times daily) of propranolol and followed closely for about 5 days before increasing the dose. One can monitor daily weights, vital capacity, and symptoms. Although the onset of heart failure is insidious in these circumstances, it should be apparent after 5 days. If all goes well, one can proceed to increase dosages as above. Ordinarily, failure or bronchoconstriction will occur early if either is to occur. Patients who have been treated for heart failure and continue to have pain may be given propranolol in the presence of digitalis preparations. Propranolol should not be used in patients with second or third degree atrioventricular block and used only cautiously in those with intraventricular conduction defects. One should proceed cautiously when using propranolol in insulin-dependent diabetics, especially those prone to hypoglycemic episodes. In this circumstance recovery from hypoglycemia may be prolonged and the important sign of hypoglycemia—tachycardia—masked. Any of these complications can be treated by using isoproterenol to overcome propranolol's competitive inhibition.

A final word of caution is needed concerning the cessation of propranolol treatment. Worsening of angina and myocardial infarction have been reported when propranolol was suddenly withdrawn after large doses had been taken for long periods of time. This has not been noted in hospitalized patients. Current recommendations are thus for gradual tapering and/or activity restriction in this situation.

OTHER DRUGS. Heart failure can lead to worsening of angina through increased myocardial oxygen demands mediated by enlarged volume and diminished net perfusion pressure. The treatment of congestive failure with digoxin and diuretics can greatly ameliorate or even eliminate angina. Nocturnal angina sometimes reflects borderline cardiac compensation in that the increased venous return associated with recumbency initiates the cycle of enlarged heart. A trial of diuretics in those with nocturnal attacks may be effective. However, nocturnal angina may rather be the result of disturbing dreams. The distinction between these two causes of nocturnal attack is important, because in the first case it suggests advanced disease with left ventricular enlargement which should be treated as heart failure. The latter circumstance is much less ominous and usually responds to treatment with beta-blockade, whereas such treatment worsens the former. It is usually best to begin with a trial of diuretics when one is unsure as to which cause is at work.

Premature beats as well as tachyarrhythmias

may have a deleterious effect upon angina. Increased exercise capacity has been noted in angina patients whose exercise-induced ventricular premature beats have been controlled by treatment of the rhythm abnormality. Bradycardias have also been associated with typical angina, and some patients improve just by increasing heart rate with a pacemaker.

Combined systolic and diastolic hypertension, when associated with angina, should always be treated to lower oxygen needs. Such treatment often contributes to good total therapeutic response. There is, however, much controversy regarding the treatment of systolic hypertension. Although elevation of systolic pressure could conceivably lead to increased oxygen needs, most authorities do not currently treat it. Thought should be given to its therapy in patients for whom all else has been done without success. Hydralazine (Apresoline) should be avoided, as it produces an increase in heart rate.

Since most angina patients either have had longstanding anxiety preceding diagnosis or have developed it after diagnosis, relatively small doses of mild sedatives and tranquilizers (e.g., 5 mg. of diazepam [Valium] every 6 hours as needed) are often useful. This is especially so if emotional stress has been a major provocative component. On the other hand, certain antidepressant drugs can worsen angina by increasing heart rate and/or blood pressure. These include nortriptyline hydrochloride (Aventyl), thioridazine (Mellaril), and amitriptyline hydrochloride (Elavil). The vogue for the use of anticoagulants in the treatment of angina has passed, and they cannot be recommended. There is much current interest in the use of antiplatelet drugs (aspirin and dipyridamole) to prevent myocardial infarction. This trend derives from preliminary epidemiologic data, but as yet the issue is not proved. These agents are thus not currently routinely recommended except as part of investigative efforts.

Physical Conditioning. Appropriate degrees of exercise should form an integral part of the medical treatment of angina. Before conditioning, patients who undergo supervised stress testing will develop angina reproducibly at an individually constant blood pressure–heart rate product. After physical conditioning, the blood pressure–heart rate product at which pain appears may remain the same, but more work is done before achieving it. Additionally, about half of the conditioned patients will not develop angina until they reach a higher "double product." An important goal of drug therapy is also the augmentation of exercise capacity. Patients can and should be helped to use this benefit to improve their level of physical conditioning so that a mutually dependent system is developed in which drug therapy and physical conditioning are used together to extend a patient's physical capability and thus his adaptation to his disease.

A program of regular exercise should be encouraged quite early in the course of medical treatment of angina. Ideally, an exercise prescription can be formulated using the results of multistage exercise testing on a treadmill. Once a level of exercise is determined that is just below the level that produces pain, regular training can be done. This is best done under the careful supervision of a staff trained in the goals and special needs of such patients. As conditioning occurs, the amount of exercise done may be gradually increased so that the amount of work prescribed is always just below the anginal threshold.

If no such exercise facility exists, similar goals can be reached by a careful practicing physician. The patient can be advised to begin by walking at a slow pace which he can gradually increase. The initial distance may also be small when angina supervenes. The patient should be instructed to stop and rest and take nitroglycerin when pain intervenes. Gradually a patient may be able to extend his exercise ability with the help of pharmacotherapy and conditioning itself. When the patient can walk 1 mile in 15 to 20 minutes, other forms of exercise may be attempted. Recommended exercises are those in which steady exercise can maintain graded increases in heart rate for 20 to 30 minute periods of time. Examples are jogging, bicycling, and swimming. Forms of exercise with bursts of activity (doubles tennis) or isometric stress (weight lifting) should be avoided. All exercise periods should begin and end with 3 to 4 minute warm-up and cool-down periods of milder exercise. Careful supervision by the physician is recommended during the period of increasing physical conditioning, ideally with repeated exercise treadmill testing to document current levels and direct future efforts.

Exercise not only has measurable cardiovascular effects; it is also very important in psychologic terms. Exercise can demonstrate to the patient that he is not necessarily crippled by his disease and can also show him that he can improve himself to some degree independent of drugs.

Final Approach to Increasing Supply: Surgery

Essentially every cardiologist will agree that when all efforts to modify myocardial oxygen supply-demand balances have failed, one must attempt to increase supply by coronary artery bypass surgery. However, before this can be undertaken, such patients must have selective coronary angiography and ventriculography. These techniques not only define operability but also guide the surgeon in the operative design by showing which vessels are operable and defining the possible coexistence of ventricular dysfunction. Skilled performance and interpretation are essential to meaningful and safe preoperative assessment. Risks of catheterization should be relatively small —major morbidity (myocardial infarction, cerebral embolus) equals about 0.1 per cent in the best series and mortality about 0.2 per cent. Operability is largely dependent upon the presence of patent vessels distal to localized obstructions and preserved left ventricular function.

About 75 to 90 per cent of patients who are good operative candidates and survive surgery will have either disappearance or marked reduction of angina. There is, however, still controversy as to whether surgery prolongs life. It is generally agreed that life expectancy is probably increased in those with the worst projected natural history without operation, left main and/or three vessel disease. The results and risks of operation are obviously heavily dependent upon the skill of the surgeon. The risk of death should not exceed 4 per cent for good operative candidates. About 10 to 25 per cent of patients undergoing bypass surgery will develop perioperative myocardial infarctions. Risk of mortality increases markedly in those with ventricular damage without a well defined aneurysm. On the other hand, a ventricular aneurysm may, of itself, account for angina by increasing left ventricular volume and tachycardia. Thus aneurysmectomy alone may be beneficial as treatment for angina as well as heart failure. Furthermore, the risk of aneurysmectomy when added to bypass surgery is not as great as bypass alone in patients with generalized left ventricular dysfunction.

The results of catheterization are not always as the clinician predicts. Although about 90 per cent of patients presenting with typical clinical angina pectoris will have obstructive coronary artery disease, the other 10 per cent do not. These may have one of the situations already alluded to under Initial Approach to Treatment (p. 163) or a peculiar syndrome in which arteries seem normal and yet none of these factors are present. The prognosis for these last patients is excellent, and treatment is a continued vigorous medical regimen.

In similar fashion, some patients with suggestive but atypical histories will elude all attempts at clinical diagnosis. For these patients exact diagnosis is essential to proper treatment. Coronary angiography is essential to diagnosis *and* treatment. Some will be found to have obstructive coronary disease and be treated as described in this article; others will not and will require more noncardiac investigation.

Special Clinical Variations of Angina

Unstable Angina. There have been many definitions of this term, but all have implied "impending infarction" and therefore urgency. A currently accepted definition is "worsening (increased frequency or severity) of chest pain in a patient with previously stable angina supported by electrocardiographic evidence of ischemia during pain." Such patients have been thought to have a very serious prognosis with high risk of myocardial infarction and death. Recent studies challenge this view. Nevertheless, such patients should be admitted to hospital bed rest and closely observed for the possible development of an infarction. While being observed, there should be a thorough search for mitigating factors as listed under Initial Approach to Treatment. Any such factor found should be eliminated as far as possible. Pharmacologic therapy should be intensive and should include sedation, beta-blockade, and frequent nitrate administration. Many centers advise coronary angiography once infarction is eliminated and the anginal frequency is controlled. Operation is then advised for those with left main obstruction or severe three vessel coronary artery disease.

The new onset of angina was formerly considered a form of "unstable angina" and therefore dangerous. Current data suggest that this is not so, and it is simply treated as the beginning of the whole spectrum of angina pectoris (see above).

Prinzmetal's Variant Angina and Arterial Spasm. In 1959, Prinzmetal described an unusual form of cardiac pain occurring almost invariably at rest rather than with physical exertion or emotional stress. A cardinal sign of this syndrome was the development of electrocardiographic ST elevation rather than depression. Ventricular arrhythmias and conduction blocks complicate the syndrome, as does sudden death. Patients have had varying degrees of coronary atherosclerotic occlusions, varying from no obstructions to all grades. It has clearly been shown that at least some such patients have arterial spasm during painful episodes. This spasm has produced almost total acute lack of blood flow and is presumed responsible for the dramatic electrocardiographic changes. Nitroglycerin is usually effective in relieving both the spasm and the pain. Frequent doses have been prophylactic in some patients. Beta-blockade has likewise been useful in some. Bypass surgery has been attempted occasionally but has been ineffective.

CARDIAC ARREST

method of
CHARLES H. DART, JR., M.D.
Ventura, California

Introduction

Standards for cardiopulmonary resuscitation and emergency cardiac care have been outlined by the National Conference on Standards for Cardiopulmonary Resuscitation. These standards have been improved upon when dictated by newer research methods and experience. The method presented incorporates these principles.

Since irreversible brain damage occurs after 3 to 5 minutes of circulatory arrest, until proved otherwise, an unconscious person with absent pulses and respiration should be considered to have respiratory and/or cardiac arrest. Cardiopulmonary failure is the definition of this state and should be suspected in all persons who appear to be unconscious. An unconscious patient can be confused with one sleeping or recovering from the effects of a stroke or epileptic seizure. If an unconscious patient fails to respond to stimuli, he should be considered to have signs of cardiopulmonary failure.

The treatment of cardiopulmonary failure is divided into (1) basic life support, with the use of the ABC steps of cardiopulmonary resuscitation—airway, breathing, and circulation; and (2) advanced life support, which includes electrocardiogram monitoring, defibrillation, endotracheal intubation, intravenous infusion, drug therapy, and other sophisticated life support systems. The aim of both of these life support or cardiopulmonary resuscitation procedures (CPR) is to establish body circulation and respiration which will provide adequate oxygen to the heart, brain, and other organs.

Basic Life Support

Basic life support is emergency institution of cardiopulmonary resuscitation sufficient to maintain life until the patient recovers sufficiently to be transported or until advanced life support is available. This phase includes the ABC steps of cardiopulmonary resuscitation (see bottom of this page).

Rapidly, an airway must be established; if adequate ventilation is not present, artificial ventilation should be instituted, and if adequate circulation does not exist, external cardiac compression must be provided. Except in extraordinary circumstances, time must not be wasted in transport or in moving a patient to a more convenient location for the institution of further treatment. Since seconds and minutes can count, transportation must await stabilization.

Airway. Immediate unobstructed airway is essential for successful resuscitation. The placement of a patient on his back on a flat hard surface is necessary for artificial ventilation and cardiac compression. Unfortunately, this position in an unconscious patient can produce obstruction of the airway, because the normal curvature of the cervical area becomes flattened, flexing the head, thus producing acute pharyngeal angulation and airway obstruction at the level of the epiglottis. The flaccid epiglottis and tongue fall posteriorly, compounding the obstruction.

Obstruction can be removed in one of two ways. In the head tilt maneuver, a patent airway is established by the resuscitator, placing one hand under the patient's neck and another on the forehead. Simultaneously, the resuscitator lifts the neck with one hand and tilts the head backward by forehead pressure with the other hand. Acute pharnygeal angulation is relieved as the maneuver overcorrects the obstructing flexure of the head on the cervical region. The second maneuver can be used when the head tilt procedure fails to produce an obstructed airway. This procedure, called the jaw thrust (or mandible thrust) maneuver, overcorrects the obstructing flexion by triple airway manipulation. (1) The resuscitator places his fingers behind the angle of the patient's jaw and forcefully displaces the mandible forward. (2) Using a hand behind the neck or forehead pressure, the head is tilted backward. (3) The mandible-holding hand then retracts the patient's lip, using thumb pressure, thus allowing breathing to occur through the mouth as well as the nose.

Breathing. After establishment of an airway, artificial ventilation should be started if the patient fails to resume adequate spontaneous breathing as evidenced by rhythmic chest movement. Mouth-to-mouth ventilation should be instituted immediately if adequate respiration is questioned. This is performed while maintaining upward pressure on the patient's neck with one hand and backward pressure on the forehead with the

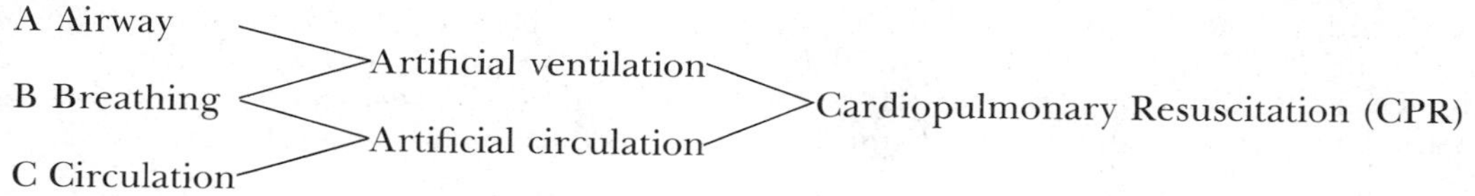

other. The resuscitator grasps the patient's nose between thumb and forefinger, sealing the nostril. The resuscitator takes a deep breath, seals the patient's mouth with his, and blows directly into the patient's mouth. The respiration cycle is completed by the resuscitator's removing his mouth and allowing the patient to exhale passively. With the institution of the first breath, the resuscitator can determine if ventilation is adequate or if the airway is patent. Should the chest not rise sufficiently, a larger breath volume should be used. If airway resistance is encountered, repositioning of the head, using the described manuevers, may relieve obstructions. Should a foreign body such as dentures be encountered, it can be removed by rolling the patient to one side, forcing the mouth open, and probing into the oral pharynx with the index and middle fimger in a sweeping motion toward the base of the tongue and out the oral cavity.

Immediately after establishing artificial ventilation, four full breaths are given.

Circulation. Cardiac arrest is recognized by lack of pulsation in large arteries in an unconscious patient requiring ventilation. While the head tilt is maintained with one hand on the patient's forehead, the carotid artery can be palpated just lateral to the trachea between the thyroid cartilage and the sternomastoid muscles in the anterior neck area.

If carotid pulsation is absent, external cardiac compression should be instituted immediately. In an adult, the sternum can easily be depressed posteriorly for about 5 to 6 cm. Such posterior displacement compresses the heart and mediastinum, because equal intrathoracic pressures prevent lateral displacement. With each sternal compression, the heart is thus compressed, ejecting blood from the ventricles into the ascending aorta and aortic arch. As the descending aorta is also somewhat compressed, the majority of the blood volume is directed to the coronary arteries and arch vessels.

Cardiac compression is performed by the resuscitator's placing himself beside the patient with the heel of one hand parallel to and over the lower half of the sternum. The xiphoid area is avoided. Palpating the xiphoid process, the heel of the hand is placed 6 to 7 cm. cephalad to the tip of the xiphoid. The other hand is placed on top of the first, bringing the resuscitator's shoulders directly over the patient's sternum. Keeping his shoulders straight, the resuscitator depresses the patient's sternum 5 to 7 cm. Pressure on the sternum should be completely released and relaxed immediately following compression. The compressions are regular, smooth, and uninterrupted. The heel of the hand should remain on the patient's chest during the entire cycle.

External cardiac compression rate for two resuscitators is 60 compressions per minute. The artificial ventilation rate is 12 ventilations per minute, timed so that the ventilation coincides with the relaxation phase of the cardiac compression cycle. The ventilation-compression ratio is 1 to 5. A single resuscitator must perform 2 lung ventilations for each 15 chest compressions. Since a pause in compression occurs, a rate of 80 compressions per minute is necessary to achieve an effective heart rate compression of 60 per minute.

Infants and Children. Airway relief is achieved with less hyperextension of the head than in adult patients. Ventilation usually is performed through both nose and mouth with less volume and more rapidity than in adults (20 to 25 per minute). The rate of compression approximates that with adults. The cardiac compression is performed higher on the chest in the midsternal area, using the heel of the hand for children and the tips of the index and middle fingers for infants. Infants require a 1.5 to 2.0 cm. depression of the sternum; young children, 2.0 to 3.5 cm. Compression rates between 80 to 100 per minute are achieved with ventilation after each 5 compressions.

Foreign Bodies. Airway obstruction not relieved by finger extraction may be difficult to dislodge without laryngeal instruments. Aspirations of a bolus of food may be dislodged by an upward thrust of the heel of the hand in the upper abdomen below the rib cage. Gastric dilatation may be relieved by exerting moderate abdominal pressure in the left upper quadrant, with the patient's head and shoulders turned to the side to avoid aspiration of gastric contents.

Witnessed Cardiac Arrest. Occasionally, when cardiac arrest is of short duration and myocardial ischemia has been brief, a quick thump of the closed fist from a point 25 cm. above the midpoint of the sternum may restore circulation. This situation occurs when a patient is seen to undergo cardiovascular collapse or has been seen to experience cardiac arrest while attached to an electrocardiographic monitor. Resuscitation efforts should not be delayed by repeated attempts with this maneuver.

Advanced Life Support

Advanced cardiopulmonary resuscitation combines basic life support with specialized equipment and personnel as it becomes available in a clinical situation. It should be stressed that basic cardiopulmonary resuscitation procedures should not be delayed while awaiting these supportive measures, as sophisticated equipment is not essential for most cases of cardiopulmonary resuscitation.

Airway and Ventilation Assistance. Oropharyngeal or nasopharyngeal airways may be quite helpful in relieving pharyngeal obstruction. Care is required in the placement of both, as incorrect placement can further displace the tongue, thus producing more obstruction.

A well fitting ventilation mask combined with bag ventilation can be used effectively to improve oxygenation when administered by trained and experienced personnel. Supplemental oxygen to reduce hypoxemia is also required.

Endotracheal intubation is indicated when trained personnel are available and ventilation is not satisfactory by other means, when the patient is not able to maintain a satisfactory airway, or when prolonged ventilation is anticipated. Resuscitation attempts should not be delayed while intubation is attempted or performed. Rarely is tracheostomy justified except in mechanical oropharyngeal problems.

Cardiac Compression Assists. Manual or automatic piston chest compressors assist in eliminating operator fatigue, thus providing a more regular and uninterrupted cardiopulmonary resuscitation. When combined with artificial ventilation cycling, a smoother resuscitation is achieved if resuscitation is prolonged. Unfortunately, most assisting devices are limited to adult use.

Internal cardiac compression is occasionally indicated when external compression would be ineffective. Such cases would be traumatic or penetrating wounds of the heart, tension pneumothorax, and chest or spinal deformities. Left thoracotomy through the fifth intercostal space should be performed only by knowledgeable personnel with special equipment and facilities.

Cardiac Monitoring and Defibrillation. Electrocardiographic monitoring should be established as soon as possible on all patients undergoing cardiopulmonary resuscitation. Electrocardiac dysrhythmias are identified and treated. If ventricular fibrillation is present, defibrillation should be immediate, using direct current depolarization of the heart. Ventricular tachycardia without a peripheral pulse is also an indication for electrical countershock. Drug therapy as indicated below is combined with defibrillation. Patients with other dysrhythmias, such as cardiac asystole or bradycardia, should receive appropriate drug therapy. If electrocardiographic monitoring is not immediately available, an initial attempt at defibrillation may be justified.

Arterial blood pressure monitoring, using a No. 18 to 20 Teflon cannula in the radial or femoral artery, is useful for measuring the effect of resuscitation procedures as well as delineating arterial hypoxemia and acidosis.

Defibrillation Procedure. The output regulator should be set at 400 watt-seconds (joules) for adults, and at 10 to 60 watt-seconds for infants and children. One paddle is placed to the right of the sternum at the level of the third rib and another near the midaxillary lines, fifth interspace. Electrode jelly should be applied to both paddles. Defibrillation may not be accomplished if the myocardium is not adequately oxygenated.

Definitive Drug Therapy. Concomitant with basic life support procedures, No. 16 or 18 plastic cannulas are inserted in internal jugular, subclavian, or femoral veins. Adequate fluid is given to maintain circulation and to administer drugs.

Following the introduction of the intravenous cannula, sodium bicarbonate, 1 mEq. per kg., should be given by bolus or metriset. Further administration should be regulated by arterial pH measurement. In the presence of ventricular fibrillation, lidocaine may prevent recurrence, repeated ventricular premature contractions, or ventricular tachycardia. An initial dose of 50 to 100 mg. slowly, intravenously, followed by a continuous infusion of 2 to 4 mg. per minute, may be maintained. In the event of asystole, epinephrine, 0.5 ml. of 1:1000 solution, should be given intravenously and repeated as necessary every 5 minutes to improve myocardial contractility. Defibrillation attempts may also be enhanced with this drug. Sinus bradycardia may respond to atropine sulfate, 0.5 mg. intravenously. In the absence of atrial activity, atropine is ineffective. Calcium chloride, 0.5 to 1.0 gram intravenously, may also improve myocardial contractility and tone. These drugs are considered essential for resuscitation and are listed with their dosages in Table 1.

TABLE 1. **Essential Drugs**

	INITIAL DOSE	REPEATED DOSE
Sodium bicarbonate	1 mEq./kg. I.V.	Repeated as indicated by arterial blood gas
Lidocaine	1 mg./kg. I.V.	2–4 mg./minute Solution—2 grams/ 500 ml. 5% D/W (4 mg./1 ml.)
Epinephrine	0.5 ml. of 1:1000 solution I.V. (1 mg./ml.)	Repeated every 5 minutes PRN
Atropine sulfate	0.5 mg. I.V.	Repeated every 5 minutes PRN
Calcium chloride	0.5–1.0 gram I.V.	Repeated every 10 minutes PRN

Should low blood pressure continue despite adequate basic life support, levarterenol, 4.0 mg. per 4 ml. (1 ampule) in 500 ml. of 5 per cent dextrose in water run at a rate of 0.5 to 1.0 ml. per minute, may be indicated if peripheral vasoconstriction is absent. Dopamine, 200 mg. in 250 ml. of 5 per cent dextrose in water, may also be used.

Isoproterenol, 1.0 mg. in 250 ml. of 5 per cent dextrose in water at a rate up to 1 ml. per minute, may be useful in treating patients with profound bradycardia. Methylprednisolone, 30 mg. per kg. intravenously, has been helpful in the treatment of cardiogenic shock and shock lung. Postresuscitation cerebral edema has also responded to dosage of 60 to 100 mg. every 6 hours. Furosemide, 40 mg. intravenously, can be given for decreasing urinary output. These drugs are considered support drugs and are listed in Table 2.

Termination of Cardiopulmonary Resuscitation

Termination of cardiopulmonary resuscitation depends upon medical evaluation of cerebral and cardiac death. Absence of spontaneous ventilation, fixed and dilated pupils for longer than 15 to 30 minutes, and deep unconsciousness are indicative of cerebral death. Absence of ventricular activity for 10 minutes during adequate cardiopulmonary support and appropriate drug therapy usually indicates cardiac death.

Postresuscitation

Following a successful resuscitation effort, continued monitoring of central venous pressure, arterial pressure, electrocardiogram, and ventilation should be carried out to prevent possible recurrence of arrest conditions. Complications of basic life support procedures include rib fractures, costochondral separations, and liver lacerations. Less frequently, perforations of the stomach and fat embolism have occurred. Renal failure and cerebral ischemia from compromised circulation are not uncommon. These complications should be anticipated and treated appropriately in the postresuscitation period.

TABLE 2. **Support Drugs**

	SOLUTION	DOSAGE
Levarterenol	4 mg. in 500 ml. 5% D/W	Titrate I.V. (8 micrograms/ ml.)
Dopamine	200 mg. in 250 ml. 5% D/W	Titrate I.V. (800 micrograms/ ml.)
Isoproterenol	1 mg. in 250 ml. 5% D/W	Titrate I.V. (16 micrograms/ ml.)
Methylprednisolone	—	30 mg./kg. I.V.
Furosemide	—	40 mg. I.V.; repeat PRN

ATRIAL FIBRILLATION

method of
ROBERT N. SCHNITZLER, M.D.,
and ROBERT A. O'ROURKE, M.D.
San Antonio, Texas

The appropriate therapy of atrial fibrillation is best initiated by identifying and correcting, when possible, the underlying cause or precipitating factors. Atrial fibrillation is a common finding in patients with rheumatic mitral valve disease or coronary atherosclerosis and occurs frequently in association with congestive or restrictive cardiomyopathies, pulmonary diseases resulting in hypoxemia (e.g., pulmonary emboli, chronic obstructive lung disease), and degenerative myocardial disease affecting elderly patients. Other causes include hypertensive cardiovascular disease, pericarditis of any cause, the "bradycardia-tachycardia" syndrome, and thyrotoxicosis. Additionally, atrial fibrillation occurs in some patients with the "click-murmur" syndrome and in certain persons with ventricular pre-excitation. Atrial fibrillation may be precipitated by the use of caffeinated beverages, marijuana, certain narcotics, alcohol, antihistamines, and over-the-counter preparations including cold tablets and decongestants which contain sympathomimetic agents.

Approach to Therapy

Atrial fibrillation occurs in either of two clinical situations: the patient is hemodynamically compromised (urgent), or the patient is stable and, if symptomatic, has only a fluttering sensation in his chest or other nonspecific complaints (elective).

Urgent Therapy

Electrical Reversion. The patient with atrial fibrillation who is hemodynamically compromised requires urgent treatment. Our approach is to determine immediately whether the patient has been receiving digitalis preparations prior to the onset of the current problem. If not, a synchronized DC precordial shock is used to revert the patient's atrial fibrillation to sinus rhythm. This is our treatment of choice in the patient who exhibits hypotension or pulmonary edema whether or not the ventricular response to atrial fibrillation is rapid (>120 beats per minute). If the patient has been receiving digitalis, lidocaine (100 mg. intravenously) is administered prior to the attempt at electrical reversion in order to avoid the occurrence of ventricular irritability which so often results from DC cardioversion in the presence of digitalis therapy.

Pharmacologic Control. Pharmacologic therapy is used when the situation is somewhat less serious. Short-acting intravenous digitalis preparations (digoxin, lanatoside C [cedilanid]) and/or beta-blocking agents are employed in this circumstance. Usually we administer digoxin, 0.5 mg. intravenously immediately and 0.25 mg. intravenously every 2 hours until the ventricular rate is controlled between 90 and 110 beats per minute. The beta-blocking agent propranolol is not used if hypotension is present, but is otherwise used as described below.

Possible complications, although small in number and uncommon in occurrence, include systemic embolization following reversion, hypotension associated with the use of anesthesia, and failure to establish a stable sinus rhythm. Hypotension may occur as a complication of beta-blocking drugs when a significant negative inotropic effect results before the ventricular response is controlled.

Elective Therapy

Electrical Reversion. Elective synchronized DC cardioversion is our preferred form of therapy for (1) any patient with a stable arrhythmia which has not been present for more than 6 months and (2) any patient with the new onset of atrial fibrillation which does not revert to sinus rhythm with appropriate treatment of the underlying disease. Under the aforementioned conditions, we believe that every patient deserves an attempt at reversion to sinus rhythm, because our experience indicates that atrial fibrillation per se is often responsible for the subsequent clinical deterioration of certain patients.

It must be emphasized that DC cardioversion with subsequent maintenance of sinus rhythm is destined to fail unless the underlying cause and/or precipitating factors have been corrected. In our experience, atrial fibrillation is likely to recur when (1) the arrhythmia has been present for longer than 6 months; (2) there is uncontrolled thyrotoxicosis; (3) there is persistent hypoxemia from chronic pulmonary disease or recurrent emboli; (4) sick sinus syndrome or the "bradycardia-tachycardia" variant is present; (5) there is severe myocardial dysfunction; (6) there is continued drug abuse (e.g., alcohol); (7) severe rheumatic mitral disease or atrial disease (e.g., atrial septal defect) is present; or (8) there is acute or chronic pericardial disease resulting from systemic disorders, such as lupus erythematosus.

After carefully selecting the patient, we prefer to attempt elective reversion with the assistance of an anesthesiologist, using either the recovery room or the intensive care unit to ensure the maximum in available facilities should the need arise. We prepare the patient as for any procedure requiring anesthesia—i.e., we withhold food on the night prior to the reversion. If the patient is receiving a digitalis preparation, we withhold it for at least a period of one half-life (36 hours for digoxin and 5 days for digitoxin). We do not routinely employ anticoagulation prior to cardioversion unless there has been a previous embolic episode or the patient has a prosthetic mitral valve. Two hundred mg. of quinidine sulfate is administered orally 2 hours prior to the reversion, although some physicians prescribe 300 mg. every 6 hours for four doses prior to the reversion attempt. A small percentage of patients will return to sinus rhythm prior to the scheduled cardioversion with the latter approach. The monitoring equipment should include an oscilloscope and electrocardiographic recorder and should be grounded to the same ground source as the defibrillator. The monitor is then attached to the patient, and sedation to somnolence is accomplished with either diazepam (10 to 20 mg. intravenously) or a short-acting barbiturate. When the patient is definitely asleep, a synchronized DC countershock is delivered to the precordium. Our starting point is 80 joules (watt-seconds) *delivered* energy (new defibrillators indicate "stored" and/or "delivered" energy on their energy control settings), which is discharged through two well-lubricated paddles placed over the second right intercostal space and apex, respectively. If the 80 joule energy level fails to revert the patient's rhythm, 160 and 320 joules are subsequently utilized. If reversion does not occur with 320 joules, we abandon further attempts.

If cardioversion is successful, the patient is allowed to awaken, started on quinidine sulfate (200 to 300 mg. every 6 hours), and monitored for the remainder of the day. Although unusual in our experience, systemic embolization has been reported to occur for up to 6 days following elective countershock.

Pharmacologic Reversion. Although it is our opinion that synchronous cardioversion is a safer approach to the problem, pharmacologic reversion has been used by others with success. When utilized, various dose schedules are employed—from 200 mg. of oral quinidine sulfate every 6 hours to as much as 400 mg. every 3 hours—until either side effects or toxicity occur or the atrial fibrillation reverts to sinus rhythm.

Control of the Ventricular Response. Except in emergency circumstances, the initial therapy of atrial fibrillation is always aimed at controlling the ventricular response. The goal of successful therapy is to slow the transmission of the electrical impulses through the AV node, thus reducing the ventricular rate. The two classes of agents used to accomplish this end are digitalis and the beta-blocking drugs. Any digitalis preparation may be utilized, and each has its own method of use. We prefer digoxin because it is a drug with a rapid onset of action and can be used both intravenously and orally.

Intravenous digoxin is used when a rapid response to therapy is necessary, such as in the patient who is in severe congestive heart failure; the oral form is given to less ill patients. The end-point of appropriate digitalis therapy, regardless of the preparation used, is a ventricular rate appropriate for the clinical setting and which does not increase excessively during mild to moderate exercise. For example, a short walk down the hall should not increase the ventricular rate above 100 to 110 beats per minute when the resting rate is 80 to 90 beats per minute.

Various formulas are available for determining the dose of digoxin and digitoxin necessary to produce adequate blood concentrations. These formulas are often difficult to use and inaccurate in individual patients. It is far more important to be cognizant of the patient's renal function, because digoxin is excreted mainly by the kidneys. In general, however, the ventricular rate is a far more accurate way of judging the amount of maintenance digoxin for patients with atrial fibrillation. In many patients, the ventricular response is best controlled by oral digoxin taken every 12 hours. The maintenance dose of digoxin necessary may vary from 0.125 mg. every other day in a patient with severe renal disease to 0.5 mg. every 12 hours in a difficult-to-control patient.

It recently has been shown that high serum concentrations of digoxin often are recorded in patients with chronic atrial fibrillation, and many physicians reduce the dose of digoxin needed by adding a beta-blocking agent to achieve sufficient slowing of the ventricular response.

Propranolol is a beta-adrenergic blocking agent that affects the ventricular response in atrial fibrillation by its ability to delay conduction through the AV node. However, it should be remembered that this drug also is a negative inotropic agent and therefore depresses myocardial contractility. Its action on smooth muscle in arteries and bronchi also makes it relatively contraindicated in patients with asthma or chronic lung disease. We use propranolol in the treatment of atrial fibrillation when (1) rapid slowing of the ventricular response is necessary in patients without moderate or severe heart failure and (2) the dose of digoxin is apparently entering a potentially toxic range.

We found propranolol most useful when atrial fibrillation results from thyrotoxicosis, alcohol ingestion, marijuana use, or excessive use of sympathetic amines (such as nose drops). We utilize it in combination with digitalis if the risk of toxicity is increased by the need to use large doses of digoxin to control the ventricular rate. Propranolol may be given intravenously or orally. When used intravenously, 1 mg. is administered every 5 minutes with close monitoring of the blood pressure. Adequate control of the ventricular response usually occurs between 3 and 5 mg. (total dose). Oral therapy is occasionally used, and adequate results are achieved with doses between 40 to 120 mg. daily given in divided doses every 6 hours.

We treat patients in whom atrial fibrillation has been successfully reverted to sinus rhythm with oral quinidine sulfate, 200 to 400 mg. every 6 hours, dependent on serum concentration, and digoxin, 0.25 mg. daily. Our only exception to this policy is in those patients who have experienced a paroxysm of atrial fibrillation but have no apparent underlying cardiac disorder. If the attacks continue without an apparent cause, propranolol, 40 to 120 mg. daily, or digoxin, 0.25 mg. daily, is prescribed.

We do not routinely use anticoagulants for patients with the recent onset of atrial fibrillation. For elective conversions, we use sodium warfarin (Coumadin), 5 to 10 mg. daily with appropriate therapeutic levels (prothrombin time 2 to 2.5 times normal or a 20 per cent activity) maintained for at least 14 days prior to DC cardioversion. The drug is continued postreversion for a similar 14 day period and is then stopped.

If the rare complication of cerebral embolism were to occur, we would promptly reverse the anticoagulant effect with vitamin K and reinstitute the anticoagulant after 48 hours. We do not routinely anticoagulate a patient who is in chronic atrial fibrillation without significant congestive heart failure.

PREMATURE BEATS

method of

J. THOMAS BIGGER, JR., M.D.

New York, New York

Introduction

"Premature beats," i.e., premature cardiac depolarization, may arise in the atria, atrioventricular (AV) junction, or ventricles, and are very common. They may result from heart disease, from abnormal physiologic states caused by diseases of other organ systems, or from therapy gone awry, or they may occur in apparently normal persons. Whether these arrhythmias occur in normal persons or those with disease, they may be triggered or aggravated by stimuli commonly encountered in daily life—e.g., caffeine, nicotine, or psychological stresses; many of these influences are apparently mediated via the autonomic nervous system. Supraventricular or ventricular premature depolarizations may be harmless, may cause serious hemodynamic abnormalities, or may augur sudden arrhythmic death. The wide variety of possible consequences of premature depolarizations should be given due consideration when contemplating the management of an arrhythmia. A certain electrocardiographic diagnosis is an important cornerstone of effective antiarrhythmic management. Diagnosis always requires skill in electrocardiography and often requires that special procedures be done. However, it should be emphasized that type and extent of heart disease and other physiologic aberrations are at least as important in determining the patient's outcome and the strategy of therapy as the characteristics of the arrhythmia itself.

It is unfortunate that most of the treatment modalities available for use in managing premature depolarizations have serious undesirable effects or are, at the very least, inconvenient. There is much more to the management of these rhythm disturbances than the application of drugs, electronic devices, or surgery. Whether or not any of these specific treatment modalities are instituted, the physician has much to offer in the management of the patient and his arrhythmia.

Atrial Premature Depolarizations

Normal Persons. When frequent atrial premature depolarizations (APD's) are found in normal patients, they can often be ascribed to drugs the patient is using—e.g., caffeine, nicotine, amphetamines, sympathomimetic drugs. Often, reducing the exposure to the culprit drug will reduce or abolish the arrhythmia. Also, some patients will develop APD's when fatigued or anxious. Again, advice about prudence in life style usually suffices to control the arrhythmia. It is important *not to treat* such arrhythmias with antiarrhythmic drugs.

Ischemic Heart Disease. ACUTE MYOCARDIAL INFARCTION. In acute myocardial infarction, APD's most often indicate left ventricular dysfunction, although they may signal atrial infarction or pericarditis. Because of their association with left ventricular dysfunction, APD's are associated with increased hospital mortality (about two-fold), but specific treatment of the APD's does not reduce mortality. APD's usually require no specific treatment in acute infarction and often decrease in frequency when left ventricular function improves (as with vasodilator therapy). If APD's repeatedly trigger atrial fibrillation, they should be treated with digitalis. A 0.5 mg. oral or intravenous dose of digoxin can be given immediately and the dose repeated orally once or twice at 4 to 6 hour intervals. A maintenance dose of 0.125 to 0.25 mg. should be chosen on the basis of judgments about absorption, renal function, and cardiac response. It should be recalled that ischemic myocardium can show increased sensitivity to digitalis. Serum digoxin concentrations can be useful in monitoring therapy. If APD's persist after digitalization and require treatment, quinidine or procainamide should be used. Quinidine sulfate, 400 mg. orally every 6 hours, or procainamide, 500 to 1500 mg. orally every 4 to 6 hours, is usually effective.

In chronic ischemic heart disease, treatment of APD's is guided by the same principles as treatment in other chronic diseases of the heart (see below).

Chronic Heart Disease. APD's are often seen in chronic ischemic, valvular, or myopathic heart diseases. In this circumstance, APD's may be caused either by the kinds of factors responsible for their occurrence in normal patients or by left ventricular failure. In rheumatic mitral valve disease, cardiomyopathies, or pericardial diseases, the atrium may be the site of intrinsic injury quite apart from stretch caused by increased LV filling pressure. Particularly when APD's occur in the presence of increased left atrial size (established by radiography or echocardiography) and a widened P wave, APD's should be considered for treatment because atrial fibrillation is likely to occur. Digitalis therapy alone often suffices. If not, then quinidine or procainamide should also be used. Dosage is similar to that given under Acute Myocardial Infarction, above.

Other Conditions. APD's may occur in a variety of other conditions, e.g., severe electrolyte imbalance (hypokalemia) or chronic obstructive pulmonary disease with abnormal blood gases. In such circumstances, the main thrust of therapy is to correct or remove the problem generating the arrhythmia and to avoid causing drug toxicity with therapy; for example, digitalis is likely to cause severe arrhythmias.

APD's which otherwise would not be treated should be considered for treatment if the patient has known AV nodal re-entrant supraventricular tachycardia or the Wolff-Parkinson-White syndrome. In such patients the APD's are likely to trigger more serious or symptomatic supraventricular tachyarrhythmias. The objective of therapy may be to remove the triggering APD, in which case digitalis, quinidine, or digitalis and quinidine are useful. On the other hand, the objective of therapy may be to prevent APD's from triggering supraventricular tachyarrhythmias; for this purpose, propranolol may be helpful alone or in combination with quinidine.

Ventricular Premature Depolarizations

Normal Persons. Often, ventricular premature depolarizations (VPD's) are encountered in "normal" persons. Unless VPD's are a signal of occult coronary disease or myopathy, they do not exert a significant mortality force. Selection of therapy is usually based on symptoms or character of the VPD's. In either case, an effort should be made to find an association between the VPD's and factors in the patient's life—e.g., excess caffeine, excess smoking, fatigue, or certain psychological situations. If such a factor is identified, therapy centers on removing the factor or altering the patient's response to it. Asymptomatic patients are usually not treated with antiarrhythmic drugs unless ventricular tachycardia (VT) is detected on electrocardiographic (ECG) recordings. Symptomatic patients are treated much as patients with heart disease (see Ischemic Heart Disease, above), except that the physician may use drugs which alleviate symptoms rather than effectively eradicating the arrhythmia. For example, propranolol in very small doses (20 to 40 mg. four times per day orally) may have no effect on the frequency or character of VPD's but may reduce or abolish the patient's perception of them.

There is a group of patients who, although apparently normal, have manifestly malignant ventricular arrhythmias—i.e., symptomatic VT or bouts of ventricular fibrillation (VFIB). These patients must be treated aggressively with the objective of preventing VT or VFIB. Because of the life-threatening nature of this problem, therapy should be initiated and adjusted under strict surveillance in the hospital. Often the arrhythmia is aggravated or precipitated by strenuous exercise. This association is helpful in arriving at effective therapy. Propranolol is a reasonable therapy to try first. Graded doses of 160 mg. up to 1000 mg. can be administered and exercise repeated until exercise can no longer precipitate the arrhythmia. If propranolol is not effective, quinidine sulfate or a combination of quinidine and propranolol can be tried. After effective drug therapy is found in this test circumstance, continuous ECG recordings should be made while the patient engages in any activity previously known to be associated with severe arrhythmias. At times recurrent VT or VFIB which is very resistant to drug therapy will respond to combined pacemaker and drug therapy.

Acute Myocardial Infarction (AMI). PREHOSPITAL PHASE. A large percentage of deaths in AMI occur within the first hour or two and usually before the patient enters the health care system. At present the treatment of this phase of AMI is experimental and involves three major approaches: (1) community-based resuscitation programs, (2) self-administration of drugs such as lidocaine or atropine, or (3) antiarrhythmic prophylaxis. The latter two strategies depend heavily on identifying patients who are at high risk to AMI or sudden death.

CORONARY CARE UNIT PHASE. There has been a steady evolution in the management of patients in the coronary care unit phase of AMI from prompt resuscitation to treatment of "warning arrhythmias" (frequent VPD's, the R on T phenomenon, bigeminy, multiformed VPD's, or VPD's occurring in runs). Recent studies show that almost half of the patients with AMI who develop primary VFIB in the coronary care unit have no warning arrhythmia. This finding led to the proposal that antiarrhythmic prophylaxis be given all patients with AMI in the first 24 to 48 hours. Lidocaine prophylaxis does not reduce primary VFIB unless high doses are used. The following regimen was successful in reducing primary VFIB in a small, well controlled study: (1) 100 mg. lidocaine intravenously on admission, and (2) a 3 mg. per minute lidocaine infusion for 48 hours. This regimen also will produce a significant incidence of undesirable effects (about 20 per cent), most commonly in older patients. Even though primary VFIB is reduced by prophylaxis, there is no significant improvement in mortality rate over that achieved by treatment of "warning arrhythmias" and prompt resuscitation of primary VFIB when controlled trials are done. However, prophylaxis seems an attractive approach for many coronary care units, particularly if patients over 70 years of age are not treated. The older patient (over 70) has a low incidence of primary VFIB and a high incidence of adverse effects to lidocaine. Very careful control of infusion rate *must* be maintained. After 48 hours, the lidocaine infusion can be abruptly stopped and the patient observed for 6 to 12 hours. If lidocaine is ineffective, or if the physician prefers, procainamide prophylaxis can be utilized: (1) a loading dose of 750 mg. can be infused intravenously over 35 minutes, and (2) 2 to 4 mg. per minute infused over 48 hours. The procainamide infusion can be discontinued abruptly at 48 hours.

THE POSTHOSPITAL PHASE. The death rate is higher in the first year following AMI than after this critical period; the death rate in the first 6 months is particularly impressive. At present there can be no general recommendation for antiarrhythmic treatment of this group, but this is a group that is being enrolled into clinical trials. By testing patients before hospital discharge, it is possible to select patients who are at low risk and who therefore should be spared the inconvenience and risk of therapy. Patients are at low risk of dying in the first year after AMI if they (1) show no evidence of significant left ventricular failure during their hospital course, (2) have a normal-sized heart by 6 foot chest x-ray 2 weeks after AMI, and (3) have less than 1 VPD per hour and lack ventricular tachycardia on a 24 hour ECG recording 2 weeks after AMI. Patients who have left ventricular dysfunction and ventricular arrhythmias are at very high risk and should be considered for treatment.

DRUG THERAPY. Although it is not known that control of VPD's in the first 6 to 12 months after acute infarction will prevent sudden death from VFIB, this is the assumption underlying antiarrhythmic drug therapy during this period. If therapy is elected, a dose of antiarrhythmic drug which has significant effect (50 to 75 per cent or more decrease) on VPD's should be used. Quinidine, procainamide, propranolol, and phenytoin are available for long-term oral therapy. Drug dosage should be adjusted based on *the response of VPD's* to treatment; this is best judged by analysis of prolonged ECG recordings. Also, it is good practice to measure the plasma concentration of the drug found to be effective in suppressing the VPD's. Care should be taken to note the precise time that blood concentrations are measured in relationship to the dose. The most valuable time to obtain a level is just prior to a dose in the steady state of dosing. Samples drawn during the first 3 hours after an oral dose are difficult to interpret. This initial drug blood level often proves helpful in dealing with problems encountered in follow-up. The excess mortality force in ischemic heart disease which is imparted by acute infarction dissipates by the sixth postinfarction month and is most intense in the first 3 months. Therefore it is rational to discontinue therapy about 3 to 6 months after infarction.

SPECIFIC AGENTS. *Quinidine* sulfate, 300 to 600 mg. every 6 hours, is usually effective for VPD's in ischemic heart disease; effective plasma concentrations are usually in the range of 2 to 5 micrograms per ml. Doses given after meals or snacks are less likely to cause gastrointestinal upset. Quinidine gluconate seems less likely to cause gastrointestinal symptoms than the sulfate salt, but absorption of the gluconate is more erratic and incomplete. The most serious undesirable effect during prolonged quinidine therapy is thrombocytopenia. Several important cardiovascular drug interactions may occur during long-term therapy with quinidine. Quinidine may increase the likelihood of bleeding on warfarin therapy. Nitroglycerin may cause profound hypotension in patients on quinidine; phenytoin usually causes a decrease in quinidine blood level; and quinidine treatment may cause an increase in the serum digoxin concentration.

Procainamide is usually effective in doses of 750 to 2000 mg. given every 6 hours. The package insert for procainamide suggests that doses be given every 3 to 4 hours; this is not practical for long-term oral therapy; neither is it usually necessary, because the half-life for procainamide elimination is increased after infarction. Effective plasma concentrations are 3 to 10 micrograms per ml. It is worth remembering that N-acetylprocainamide, an active metabolite, may be in the plasma in high concentration but is not measured by spectrophotometric or fluorometric methods. The most frequent and important undesirable effects of procainamide therapy are fever (at the outset of therapy), a lupus erythematosus–like syndrome, or agranulocytosis.

Propranolol is not well studied for its antiarrhythmic effect in the posthospital phase of acute infarction. Some arrhythmias will respond to low (40 mg. four times daily) or conventional doses (60 to 80 mg. four times daily). However, some patients require much larger doses to control VPD's (1000 mg. or more per day). Effective levels range from 30 to 1000 nanograms per ml. If patients tolerate propranolol at the outset of therapy, it is relatively free of late undesirable effects.

Phenytoin can be effective in treating VPD's in doses of 300 to 800 mg. per day and can be given once or twice a day (e.g., 200 mg. twice daily); effective plasma concentrations are 8 to 18 micrograms per ml. (This use of phenytoin is not listed in the manufacturer's official directive.) Among antiarrhythmics, phenytoin is unique for its dose-dependent metabolism. As plasma concentrations reach a critical value, elimination switches from first order to zero order kinetics, resulting in an unexpectedly large increase in plasma concentration. This property can cause puzzling effects during dose adjustment to eradicate arrhythmias. During short-term (months) therapy, phenytoin is relatively free of undesirable effects. Phenytoin is known to interact with many other drugs by altering their metabolism.

Drug combinations have not been formally studied in the postinfarction period. Propranolol and quinidine can be effective when neither is alone. Procainamide and phenytoin can be effective together. We try to avoid the quinidine-phenytoin combination.

Other Conditions. VALVULAR HEART DISEASE AND CARDIOMYOPATHY. VPD's occur frequently in aortic valve disease, in mitral regurgitation, and in cardiomyopathy. Lacking good natural history data, it is difficult to establish criteria for treating these arrhythmias. Currently, we treat these arrhythmias if they are symptomatic or if they contribute to hemodynamic abnormalities. Chronic oral therapy is conducted, using the guidelines discussed under Ischemic Heart Disease. When left ventricular failure is present, greater caution must attend the use of propranolol.

Sudden death is presently considered a risk in patients with click-murmur syndrome (Barlow's syndrome, floppy mitral valve) and frequent VPD's. These patients are usually treated with propranolol in a dose which will decrease the frequency of VPD's significantly.

VPD's may be lethal in patients who have congenitally prolonged QT intervals. These patients have been successfully treated with propranolol, phenytoin, and surgical sympathectomy of the cervicothoracic chain. The utility of sympathectomy can be evaluated using sympathetic blockade so that surgery is offered only to patients who stand to benefit.

DRUG TOXICITY. A number of drugs can cause ventricular arrhythmias when their concentration is excessive. *Digitalis toxicity* is the most important in this category. In many cases, observation and discontinuance of digitalis are sufficient therapy; but if the arrhythmias are complex, suppressive therapy is indicated. When hypokalemia is present or the patient is depleted of potassium, potassium therapy is indicated. Intravenous infusion permits finely controlled therapy; a solution of 100 mEq. K^+ per liter of 5 per cent glucose can be infused at the rate of 15 mEq. per hour. Often ventricular arrhythmias improve strikingly after only a few mEq. of K^+ has been administered. Phenytoin is very effective against digitalis-induced ventricular arrhythmias. Doses of 100 mg. are given by intravenous injection every 5 minutes. (This use of phenytoin is not listed in the manufacturer's official directive.) The arrhythmias usually respond after 200 to 400 mg. Lidocaine has been used less than phenytoin in digitalis toxicity, but should be effective. A 100 mg. injection should be followed by constant rate infusion of 1 to 4 mg. per minute.

Quinidine and procainamide toxicity can be manifest by severe and bizarre ventricular arrhythmias. Recently, imipramine hydrochloride has been shown to have antiarrhythmic effects similar to those of quinidine and to produce similar arrhythmias when toxic plasma concentrations are present. Therapy with antiarrhythmic drugs or potassium will *worsen* the arrhythmias caused by these drugs. They should be treated with molar sodium lactate (40 to 50 mEq. intravenously), isoproterenol, or dopamine infusion and cardiac pacemaker.

HEART BLOCK

method of
KENNETH B. LEWIS, M.D.
Baltimore, Maryland

Approach to the Patient

Heart block is defined as a delay or interruption of impulse transmission in any portion of the cardiac conducting system. The abnormality may occur at the level of the sinus node, at the atrioventricular node (AV) when it is designated intranodal, or in the bundle branches distal to the His bundle (infranodal block). It may be partial or complete and may occur transiently, occur intermittently, or persist permanently.

The conduction abnormality may be due to sclerodegenerative changes in the conducting system, usually related to aging; to chronic ischemic changes in the myocardium; or to metabolic abnormalities such as hyperkalemia or hypoxia. Heart block is not infrequently the result of drug therapy with digitalis, quinidine, procainamide, propranolol, diphenylhydantoin, and antihypertensive agents such as reserpine and alphamethyldopa. Acute myocardial infarction can produce heart block, but this is usually transient. Infiltrative diseases such as rheumatoid arthritis, sarcoidosis, and metastatic tumor can also produce varying degrees of heart block.

It is the reduction in cardiac rate secondary to the heart block which is responsible for symptoms. The presence of heart block or reduced cardiac rate is not in itself an indication for therapy. A few patients tolerate rates of 40 per minute without symptoms. Treatment is indicated when the slow cardiac rate is associated with symptoms such as (1) sudden loss of consciousness (Stokes-Adams attack), (2) congestive heart failure, (3) progressive mental deterioration, (4) azotemia secondary to decreased renal blood flow, (5) ischemic cardiac pain, or (6) bradycardia-triggered ventricular arrhythmias.

Frequently, and particularly in older patients, it may be difficult to ascertain whether symptoms of lightheadedness, brief mental lapses, or unsteadiness of gait are due to the conduction disturbance or to other factors such as transient cerebral ischemia. In this circumstance a temporary pacemaker may be tried to determine whether control of the rate abolishes the symptoms. Intermittent heart block may be difficult to confirm, because by the time the patient is seen by the physician, the conduction disturbance causing syncope or other symptoms may have reverted to normal. These intermittent symptoms may recur for some time before the cause is determined. Patients with episodic symptoms suggestive of intermittent heart block should be studied with a 24 hour Holter electrocardiographic tape recorder to detect intermittent heart block. A patient's family may be taught to take the pulse and to record this observation at the time the patient is symptomatic. If symptomatic heart block is documented, appropriate therapy may be instituted. Treatment may also be necessary in asymptomatic patients who require drugs such as digitalis or propranolol but in whom these drugs cannot be given to full therapeutic levels because of excessive slowing of the heart rate.

Pharmacologic Therapy

The increasing reliability and sophistication of electronic pacemakers has reduced the need for pharmacologic therapy in the management of heart block in most clinical situations. Drug therapy may be required temporarily until pacemaker implantation can be accomplished. On rare occasion a patient with symptomatic heart block may refuse permanent pacemaker implantation, and chronic drug therapy may be all that can be offered.

Vagolytic Therapy. Vagolytic drugs are useful only when the conduction disturbance affects the sinus or AV node, as there is little vagal influence in the ventricle. Atropine should be given intravenously, beginning with 0.5 mg. An effect is expected in 2 minutes. If there is no response, repeat 0.5 mg. doses may be given up to a total dose of 2.0 mg. over 10 to 15 minutes. Doses of atropine less than 0.5 mg. should not be given, for they may produce paradoxical slowing of the sinus node and AV conduction owing to a central vagotonic effect. If a clinical response is not obtained with 2.0 mg. of atropine, it is futile to give more; alternative therapy with a temporary pacemaker may have to be considered. If effective, the drug may be given every 3 to 4 hours intravenously. If this regimen is used for more than a short time, there is a high incidence of complications, including urinary and gastric retention, agitation or frank psychosis, and increased intraocular pressure. This is especially true in older patients. Long-term therapy of sinus or AV node dysfunction with oral atropine, 0.6 mg. four to six times daily, or propantheline bromide (Pro-Banthine), 15 mg. four to six times daily, is generally not satisfactory because of variable absorption and high incidence of side effects. If the patient is symptomatic with sinus or AV node dysfunction, implantation of a permanent pacemaker is more reliable.

Sympathomimetic Drugs. Drugs in this category enhance rhythmicity of both upper and lower (ventricular) pacemakers, thereby increasing the effective cardiac rate even when heart block occurs below the His bundle. In addition they may improve conduction through the AV node to increase the ventricular rate. Isoproterenol is the most effective and may be administered intravenously in doses of from 1 to 5 micrograms per minute. This can most easily be accomplished by diluting 1 mg. of isoproterenol in 500 ml. of 5 per cent dextrose and water, which gives a concentration of 2.0 micrograms per ml. This should be administered carefully with a microdrip infusion set or an infusion pump, beginning at 0.5 microgram per minute and increasing the infusion rate in increments of 0.5 microgram per minute. Isoproterenol increases ventricular irritability so that ventricular arrhythmias may limit the amount which can be administered. It also increases myocardial oxygen consumption, making the use of this drug inadvisable in the setting of myocardial infarction or ischemia. Long-term therapy of heart block with sublingual preparations of isoproterenol, 10 or 20 mg. every 4 hours, or ephedrine is unreliable and rarely effective, and should only be used in patients who refuse permanent pacemaker therapy.

Pacemakers

Since the introduction of permanent implanted cardiac pacemakers in 1958, these devices have made the greatest contribution to medical care of any of the products of biomedical engineering. These units have become smaller, more reliable, and longer lived and are the treatment of choice in symptomatic heart block. Cardiac pacing systems consist of electrodes which may be positioned within the heart through a vein or sewn onto the external surface of the heart and the pulse generator, which consists of the electrical circuitry and batteries. In 95 per cent of the permanent pacemaker implantations in the United States today, the electrode is inserted into the apex of the right ventricle under fluoroscopic control through the cephalic or external jugular vein. The electrode is then connected to the pulse generator, which is placed in a subcutaneous pocket usually on the anterior chest wall but on occasion in the anterior abdominal wall. This procedure is usually done under local anesthesia using lidocaine and thereby avoiding the potential morbidity of general anesthesia. The use of local anesthesia has been of particular value in pacemaker insertions in very elderly patients. In 5 per cent of patients satisfactory pacing cannot be established using the transvenous approach, usually because the electrode catheter repeatedly moves within the right ventricle. In those circumstances it may be necessary to suture electrodes into the epicardium. The leads are then brought out through the chest wall and connected to a subcutaneously implanted pulse generator.

Most pacemakers utilized today are of the demand type. These devices through the catheter electrodes sense the intrinsic activity of the heart and are inhibited if the heart is beating at a rate faster than that of the pacemaker. If the intrinsic cardiac rate falls below the pacemaker rate, the pacemaker begins functioning at its set rate. This type of device permits the heart's intrinsic rhythm to function if it is capable of doing so and provides a backup during intermittent malfunction. It also prevents competition between an intrinsic cardiac rate and the pacemaker beats, as occurred in fixed rate pacemakers. Fixed rate pacemakers were set to function at a given rate and were unresponsive to intrinsic activity. Pacemakers manufactured today are shielded from outside electromagnetic interference such as microwave ovens and engine spark coils, although this type of interference was a problem some years ago.

The most common problem with transvenous pacing systems is malposition of the electrode, which requires repositioning. Electrode breakage, perforation of the heart, infection, and thrombophlebitis at the site of catheter insertion occur but are not common problems. Battery exhaustion and the necessity for replacement of the pulse generator have been the main limitations of pacing systems. Initially mercury zinc batteries were used in pacemakers, and their average length of life was 18 months. Although newer mercury cells and improved efficiency of circuitry have increased the life span to 3 to 4 years, mercury cell pacemakers are now obsolete with the development of newer types of batteries. Lithium iodide batteries are now powering pacemakers with an anticipated life of 3 to 7 years. Rechargeable nickel cadmium batteries and nuclear batteries are powering long-term pacemakers with anticipated functional life spans of 20 years.

In addition to patients with symptomatic heart block, some patients require a combination of pacemaker and pharmacologic therapy to control their problem. Some patients who require digitalis to control their cardiac failure and yet develop marked bradycardia on the drug are well managed on this combination therapy. The pacemaker controls their rate so that adequate digitalis can be administered for its inotropic effect. Combined pacemaker and drug therapy may also be necessary in controlling certain arrhythmias.

Management of Specific Forms of Heart Block

Sinus Node Disease. 1. Sinus bradycardia may occur in well conditioned people. It may also occur as a consequence of metabolic disease such as hypothyroidism or hyperkalemia; in drug therapy with digitalis, propranolol, or antihypertensive agents; or as a manifestation of aging. If the rate is above 40 and there are no symptoms, no specific therapy is indicated. When specific causative factors can be implicated, treatment of the metabolic disease or withdrawal of drugs is obviously necessary. In some persons sinus bradycardia is an indication of disease of the sinus node and has been termed the "sick sinus syndrome." This may be responsible for symptomatic bradycardia or failure of a sinus impulse to develop after SA block or sinus node suppression. When symptoms related to inadequate cardiac output are produced by sinus node disease, pacemaker therapy is indicated as drug therapy is not consistent or reliable.

2. The bradycardia-tachycardia syndrome is a manifestation of sinus node disease in which chronic sinus bradycardia permits the development of tachyarrhythmias such as atrial tachycardia, atrial flutter, or fibrillation. Therapy of the tachyarrhythmias with digitalis, propranolol, or quinidine may cause further slowing of the sinus rate so that patients without symptoms from the initial bradycardia may require pacemaker therapy to permit adequate suppressive doses of antiarrhythmic drugs.

3. Various forms of sinoatrial block or sinus node suppression are generally well tolerated and do not require therapy unless inadequate cardiac output results.

4. In rare instances the sinus node may be suppressed so that after the spontaneous termination of a tachyarrhythmia such as paroxysmal atrial tachycardia, cardiac asystole, and syncope result. When this is documented, a demand pacemaker is necessary for management.

Intranodal Block. Heart block arising within the atrioventricular node usually produces a QRS complex of normal duration. When block is complete, the usual idioventricular rate is maintained at about 40 per minute. Drugs such as digitalis, acute inflammatory processes such as rheumatic fever, vagotonic influences, and acute ischemia during inferior myocardial infarction are particularly likely to produce an intranodal block that is reversible.

1. First degree heart block requires no specific therapy but may represent digitalis intoxication and can be a harbinger of more advanced heart block.

2. Second degree heart block has been classically divided into Mobitz type I (Wenckebach) or Mobitz type II block. In most instances the Wenckebach type reflects dysfunction within the AV node. It is often due to digitalis excess and may be corrected by withdrawal of the drug. It is a relatively stable form of heart block and rarely requires pacemaker therapy. In acute situations intravenous atropine may be effective in improving conduction.

3. Congenital complete heart block is due to the interruption of the conducting pathways within the AV node. It may occur in persons without other evidence of congenital heart disease and may be well tolerated for many years. It does not necessarily require pacemaker therapy unless syncope occurs. It may, however, be associated with congenital malformations of the heart such as ventricular septal defect, endocardial cushion defect, or corrected transposition of the great vessels.

4. Rarely complete intranodal block may result from digitalis intoxication, acute myocarditis, or infiltrative diseases of the heart such as sarcoidosis, hemochromatosis, or metastatic tumor. Temporary or sometimes permanent pacing may be required in these settings.

Infranodal Block. Most chronic heart block in adults is due to disease of the distal conducting pathways in the ventricles below the AV node and the bundle of His. Coronary artery disease may be responsible for some of these cases, but the majority are due to an idiopathic sclerosing process not necessarily associated with arterial disease. In this form of heart block the QRS complexes are widened, and when the complete block occurs the ventricular rate is below 45 per minute. It is convenient to consider the distal conducting pathways as a trifascicular system consisting of the right bundle branch and the anterior and posterior branches of the left bundle. Complete heart block, permanent or intermittent, is commonly preceded by evidence of block in one or two of the fascicles.

1. Isolated right and left bundle branch block are common electrocardiographic abnormalities which do not require treatment unless the patient presents with syncope documented as being due to intermittent heart block. In this setting the presence of intermittent block may be difficult to establish, and the 24 hour tape recorder may be valuable in its assessment. Other causes of syncope must be excluded.

2. Mobitz type II block usually indicates the presence of distal conducting disease even when the QRS complex is of normal duration. Patients with this disorder are prone to syncope or progression to complete heart block. Permanent pacing is indicated in the majority of these patients.

3. The presence of bifascicular block is suspected when the electrocardiogram demonstrates left anterior or posterior hemiblock with right bundle branch block, left bundle branch block with first degree heart block, or alternating right bundle branch block with left hemifascicular block. If the patient is asymptomatic, no therapy is indicated. When syncope occurs in a patient with any of these electrocardiographic abnormalities, intermittent complete heart block should be assumed even if it cannot be documented on sporadic ambulatory monitoring. A pacemaker should be implanted in these patients. Digitalis can usually be given in these patients without fear of aggravating the block.

4. Partial block in one fascicle with complete block in the other two, i.e., prolonged PR interval with right bundle branch block and left anterior or posterior hemiblock or alternating right and left bundle branch block, indicates trifascicular block. As in other forms of heart block, symptoms should dictate therapy and asymptomatic patients should not be treated routinely with pacemakers. Patients with trifascicular block should have temporary demand pacemakers in place during major surgery.

5. The presence of complete heart block is not in and of itself an indication for pacemaker therapy. Some patients tolerate this arrhythmia for long periods without symptoms. The first occurrence of symptoms related to inadequate cerebral profusion is an urgent indication for a pacemaker.

Heart Block Complicating Myocardial Infarction. The aggressive use of temporary pacemakers in the management of acute myocardial infarction, which was recommended in the early 1960s, is no longer considered necessary. Observations over the years have indicated that most patients with inferior infarction and AV block do well with or without pacemaker therapy. In inferior infarction dysfunction of the sinus or AV nodes is reversible and may be related to excessive vagal stimulation. It does not necessarily correlate with infarct size. In anterior infarction the development of heart block is indicative of disease of the distal conducting system and is evidence of extensive myocardial damage. The myocardial damage is a more important determinant of prognosis than the rhythm disturbance. Many of these patients die of ventricular failure despite adequate management of their heart block with a pacemaker.

INFERIOR INFARCTION. First degree AV block does not require specific therapy. Wenckebach second degree AV block or sinus dysfunction will usually respond to intravenous atropine, and pacing is not required. With third degree block, a ventricular rate of 40, and no symptoms, a temporary pacemaker is not always required. The presence of heart failure, shock, ventricular arrhythmias, or altered cerebral profusion indicates the need for inserting a temporary pacing catheter. The pacing unit should be left in place for a minimum of 72 hours after normal conduction has returned. There is no need to consider permanent pacing in these patients.

ANTERIOR INFARCTION. Temporary pacing is mandatory when second degree (Mobitz type II) or third degree block complicates anterior infarction. In addition the development of trifascicular block or prolongation of the PR interval with left or right bundle branch block or left posterior fascicular block should prompt pacemaker insertion as a standby precaution. Bifascicular block in this setting must be carefully observed; if evidence of further conduction abnormality is found, a temporary pacemaker is inserted. The pacing electrode should be left in place at least 96 hours after stabilization of the rhythm disturbance. As noted above, despite the control of the conduction abnormality with a pacemaker, the extensive myocardial damage which caused the problem may still result in the patient's death.

Recent studies have suggested that patients who develop advanced conduction system disease during the course of anterior infarction are at high risk for sudden death after hospital discharge. It has been suggested that inserting a permanent demand pacemaker can reduce the late mortality. Although the evidence to support this is limited, I would recommend that strong consideration be given to permanent pacing in the patient with an anterior infarct who has had established transient heart block or persistent evidence of trifascicular disease.

TACHYCARDIA

method of
C. GLENN SAWYER, M.D.,
and FREDERIC ROSS KAHL, M.D.
Winston-Salem, North Carolina

Tachycardia exists when the heart rate or a heart chamber rate is greater than 100 beats per minute. In some instances of tachycardia, however, the heart rate may be less than 100 beats per minute because an ordinarily dormant subsidiary pacemaker discharges at an accelerated rate, as in nonparoxysmal atrioventricular (AV) junctional tachycardia with a rate of 60 to 100 beats per minute.

Appropriate and effective treatment of tachycardia requires precise identification of the abnormal heart rhythm, and this is usually accomplished by careful analysis of the scalar electrocardiogram. In some instances, however, intracardiac electrograms (atrial electrogram or His bundle electrogram) are needed to define the tachycardia. Tachycardia should not be viewed as an isolated electrocardiographic finding; rather, the entire clinical status of the patient with tachycardia should be assessed so that optimally appropriate and effective treatment can be applied. A number of secondary causes may either precipitate or aggravate tachycardia, and correction of these problems may be sufficient to control the tachycardia. Examples include tachycardias induced or aggravated by hypokalemia, hypoxia, acidosis, and drug intoxication. The decision to specifically treat a tachycardia and how to treat it is definitely related to the clinical status of the patient and an appreciation of the natural history of the tachycardia under consideration. Catastrophic tachycardias such as ventricular fibrillation demand immediate defibrillation by DC countershock; sinus tachycardia often requires no treatment whatsoever. Finally the decision to treat a tachycardia is predicated on the fact that the treatment is properly applied for optimal results and that the hazards of treatment are not greater than the underlying tachycardia itself. This is especially true for each form of drug therapy for tachycardia as well as for cardioversion and pacemakers, all of which may produce significant adverse reactions which outweigh clinical benefits.

Sinus Tachycardia

Sinus tachycardia is characterized by sinus P waves of a constant contour firing at a rate of usually 100 to 160 per minute, although higher rates may be seen in healthy young adults during strenuous exercise. Ordinarily the P-R interval is normal (0.12 to 0.20 second), and the QRS complexes are identical to ones present in normal sinus rhythm. Sinus tachycardia may be seen in a wide variety of situations. Physiologic sinus tachycardia is often noted in healthy persons, especially during strenuous activity or states of high emotional tension and also in infants. Sinus tachycardia can be produced by a variety of pharmacologic agents such as atropine and over-the-counter drug preparations which contain antihistamines and sympathomimetic amines. Coffee, tea, alcohol, and cigarettes may also elicit sinus tachycardia. A diverse group of pathologic states may produce sinus tachycardia, including fever, chronic infection, anemia, lung disease, hyperthyroidism, hypoglycemia, pulmonary embolism, myocardial infarction, congestive heart failure, and shock. Consequently, the clinical significance of sinus tachycardia is related to its underlying cause, and treatment of sinus tachycardia is aimed at correcting the underlying disorder. Rarely, no apparent explanation for sinus tachycardia can be found, and in these instances simple reassurance about the benignity of sinus tachycardia usually is sufficient. Mild sedatives may also be helpful, and only very rarely is it necessary to treat sinus tachycardia primarily with specific drugs. If such treatment is necessary, propranolol (Inderal), 10 to 40 mg. orally four times daily, is effective.

Atrial Tachycardia

Atrial tachycardia is characterized by six or more consecutive premature atrial beats, and the rate of sustained atrial tachycardia is usually 160 to 200 beats per minute, although occasionally faster rates are present. The P wave contour usually differs from the sinus P wave but is still upright in lead II and inverted in lead aVR. Sometimes identification of the P waves in atrial tachycardia is difficult, because they are superimposed on the ST segment or T wave of the preceding QRS complex. The rate of atrial tachycardia is usually precisely regular, and the QRS complex typically is identical to that of normal sinus beats, although aberration and functional bundle branch block may develop with the tachycardia. AV conduction in paroxysmal atrial tachycardia is usually preserved with a 1:1 response; in atrial tachycardia caused by digitalis intoxication, AV block may be present with 2:1 AV block. It is useful to determine whether the atrial tachycardia is due to re-entrant (circus movement) tachycardia, which is the common mechanism of paroxysmal atrial tachycardia, or due to an accelerated ectopic atrial focus, which occurs with digitalis intoxication. Paroxysmal atrial tachycardia caused by re-entry is often seen in patients without underlying heart disease and also in patients with rheumatic heart disease, acute myocardial infarction, mitral valve prolapse, congenital heart disease, pulmonary disease, thyrotoxicosis, and the Wolff-Parkinson-White syndrome. Atrial tachycardia caused by an accelerated ectopic atrial focus is almost invariably associated with underlying heart disease or digitalis intoxication.

Many instances of paroxysmal atrial tachycardia are brief with spontaneous conversion to normal sinus rhythm. In patients without organic heart disease, who have only infrequent episodes of paroxysmal atrial tachycardia which do not produce significant symptoms, specific antiarrhythmic treatment is not indicated. These patients should attempt to modify habits, such as heavy smoking or tea, coffee, or alcohol ingestion, which may precipitate the paroxysm of atrial tachycardia. If periods of emotional stress precipitate the atrial tachycardia, mild sedatives such as diazepam (Valium), 5 mg. orally three or four times daily, are useful. Patients with mild and infrequent episodes of paroxysmal atrial tachycardia should be instructed about the use of the Valsalva maneuver and mild carotid sinus pressure to break the paroxysm. If the paroxysm persists or is associated with significant cardiovascular symptoms, the patient should be instructed to seek prompt medical attention.

There are a variety of methods to terminate the acute episode of paroxysmal tachycardia. Vagal stimulation is often effective, and the simplest vagal maneuvers are the Valsalva maneuver and carotid sinus pressure. Prior to applying carotid sinus pressure, the carotid arteries must be examined by palpation and auscultation to be certain that occlusive vascular disease of the carotid arteries is not present. Carotid artery compression should be applied to either the right or left carotid and never to both simultaneously. Continuous monitoring of the electrocardiogram during carotid sinus compression is mandatory, and the pressure should be released when the paroxysm is converted or ventricular ectopic beats are elicited. Carotid sinus compression should not be applied for more than 5 seconds and should not be used if digitalis intoxication is suspected. If the paroxysm is not responsive to compression of one carotid, then it can be repeated on the other side, often with good results. Rapidly acting cholinergic drugs may also terminate acute paroxysmal atrial tachycardia, and the preparation of choice is edrophonium. A test dose of 1 mg. is given intravenously; if no untoward reactions occur, the remainder of the 10 mg. is administered intravenously.* Pressor agents may also break an acute paroxysm of atrial tachycardia associated with arterial hypotension, particularly when vagal maneuvers are applied after the blood pressure has been restored to normal. One hundred mg. of metaraminol* is dissolved in 500 ml. of 5 per cent dextrose solution and infused slowly intravenously to return the blood pressure to normal. It is not necessary to produce even moderate arterial hypertension for metaraminol to be effective in paroxysmal atrial tachycardia.

Should the paroxysmal atrial tachycardia persist, digoxin (Lanoxin), 0.5 mg. intravenously, is administered in the undigitalized patient. Again, vagal maneuvers, particularly carotid sinus pressure, may be employed after intravenous digoxin to terminate the atrial tachycardia. Alternatively, propranolol (Inderal) administered intravenously can terminate paroxysmal atrial tachycardia, provided there are no contraindications to the use of this agent such as heart failure, rhinitis (allergic), or bronchial asthma. Propranolol is given as 0.5 to 1.0 mg. boluses intravenously every 1 to 5 minutes, and the total dose should not exceed 3 mg.

In instances of paroxysmal atrial tachycardia resistant to vagal maneuvers and intravenous drug therapy, cardioversion or atrial pacing is effective. Of the two, cardioversion is considered the standard intervention; after the patient has been anesthetized with either intravenous diazepam or a short-acting barbiturate, low energy (50 to 150 joules) synchronized DC countershock is applied. Atrial pacing is employed as either isolated atrial stimuli or rapid atrial pacing at rates 25 to 50 beats per minute faster than the tachycardia rate and may restore normal sinus rhythm. Atrial pacing has the advantage of also treating sinus bradyrhythmia or cardiac standstill which may develop when the atrial tachycardia is terminated and is particularly useful in patients with the sick sinus syndrome.

Chronic treatment of paroxysmal atrial tachycardia aims at abolishing or reducing the frequency of episodes of tachycardia. The drug of choice for suppressive therapy is oral digoxin (Lanoxin), 0.25 mg. daily. Digoxin usually is quite effective as suppressant therapy in paroxysmal atrial tachycardia and has the advantage, in terms of patient compliance, of a single daily dose. Propranolol (Inderal), 10 to 40 mg. orally four times daily, is also effective for suppression of paroxysmal atrial tachycardia either alone or in combination with digoxin. In some instances, quinidine may be required as an additional antiarrhythmic agent; quinidine gluconate (Quinaglute), 324 mg. two to four times daily, is used because of a lower incidence of gastrointestinal reactions compared to quinidine sulfate. In patients refractory to drug therapy with frequent and symptomatic recurrences of paroxysmal atrial tachycardia, permanent atrial pacemakers have been used with a radiofrequency device to activate a short burst of rapid atrial pacing during the paroxysm of atrial tachycardia and convert it to sinus rhythm.

The treatment of atrial tachycardia resulting from an accelerated ectopic atrial focus is quite different from the treatment of paroxysmal atrial tachycardia produced by re-entry. Atrial tachycardia caused by an accelerated ectopic atrial focus is usually not paroxysmal and may be a chronic stable arrhythmia in patients with advanced organic heart disease, or it may be due to digitalis intoxication. In instances of digitalis-induced atrial tachycardia, the first action is to discontinue administration of the digitalis preparation. If the patient is clinically stable, no further therapy is needed unless the serum potassium level is low (<3.5 mEq. per liter), in which case oral potassium supplementation, 15 to 20 mEq. four times daily, is used. In instances of atrial tachycardia resulting from digitalis intoxication with serious clinical symptoms or excessive tachycardia (>150 per minute), more aggressive treatment is indicated. Low serum potassium levels (<3.5 mEq. per liter) should be corrected with parenteral potassium, 60 to 160 mEq. in 24 hours. Intravenous phenytoin is also a very effective agent for this arrhythmia. (This use of phenytoin is not listed in the manufacturer's official directive.) It is given at rates of 25 to 50 mg. per minute and no more than 100 mg. every 5 minutes until the atrial tachycardia is abolished or a total of 1000 mg. phenytoin is used. In cases resistant to these therapies, propranolol (Inderal) administered intravenously may be effective; 0.5 to 1.0 mg. per minute is given every 1 to 5 minutes to a total dose of 3 mg. Cardioversion is not indicated in cases of atrial tachycardia caused by digitalis intoxication, because more severe grades of toxic arrhythmias, such as ventricular tachycardia or fibrillation, may be unleashed. Atrial pacing ordinarily is not effective in atrial tachycardia caused by digitalis intoxication.

Chronic atrial tachycardia resulting from organic heart disease and not digitalis toxicity is rare and difficult to treat. Suppressive therapy with

*This use of this agent is not listed in the manufacturer's official directive.

quinidine, in the form of quinidine gluconate (Quinaglute), 324 mg. two to four times daily, or phenytoin,* 300 to 400 mg. daily, may be tried but often is not effective. Frequently the therapeutic goal in this form of atrial tachycardia is to produce AV block to slow the ventricular rate to normal range. Oral digoxin (Lanoxin), 0.25 mg. daily, is the drug of choice to achieve this aim; occasionally, low doses of propranolol (Inderal), 5 to 20 mg. four times daily, are required to supplement the action of digoxin and to slow AV conduction.

Multifocal Atrial Tachycardia

The characteristic electrocardiographic findings in multifocal atrial tachycardia are two or more ectopic P waves of different configurations and two or more different interectopic intervals. Thus the rhythm is not regular, and atrial rates vary from 100 to 250 per minute. Often the P-R intervals vary and some atrial impulses are not conducted to the ventricles, resulting in slower ventricular rates (100 to 150 per minute). Multifocal atrial tachycardia usually occurs in seriously ill, elderly patients. Chronic lung disease and cor pulmonale account for many instances of this tachycardia. The arrhythmia may also be caused by digitalis intoxication and occurs rarely in patients with hypertensive cardiovascular disease, valvular heart disease, pulmonary embolism, and septicemia. The treatment of multifocal atrial tachycardia is directed at correcting the underlying clinical disorder responsible for the arrhythmia. Most important is improving ventilatory performance and correcting blood gas abnormalities in patients with chronic lung disease. Digitalis should be used prudently in multifocal atrial tachycardia and discontinued if digitalis intoxication is suspected. Acute interventive drug therapy for multifocal atrial tachycardia has not been clearly defined. Propranolol (Inderal) may be effective, but its use is limited by the frequently associated condition of lung disease with cor pulmonale. Phenytoin* and quinidine may also be effective for suppressive therapy of multifocal atrial tachycardia.

Atrial Flutter

Atrial flutter is diagnosed when atrial activity consists of flutter waves which are discrete oscillations, usually with a sawtooth configuration, best seen in leads II, III, aVF, V_1 and V_2. The atrial rate in atrial flutter is usually 250 to 350 per minute and is ordinarily precisely regular. Quinidine and procainamide may slow the flutter rate, whereas digitalis may accelerate the flutter rate. A 2:1 AV block is usually present in atrial flutter with a resultant ventricular rate of 150 per minute, although occasionally 1:1 AV conduction is present with ventricular rates of 250 to 300 per minute. More advanced AV block with periods of alternating 2:1, 4:1, and even 6:1 AV conduction can result in an irregular ventricular rate. The configuration of the QRS complex is usually normal in atrial flutter, although aberration and functional bundle branch block may occur during rapid ventricular responses. Atrial flutter almost always indicates some form of heart disease such as rheumatic heart disease, coronary artery disease, or hypertensive cardiovascular disease. It also occurs occasionally in patients with the Wolff-Parkinson-White syndrome, sick sinus syndrome, thyrotoxicosis, pulmonary embolism, cardiomyopathy, or congenital heart disease. Rarely atrial flutter can be produced by digitalis intoxication. Atrial flutter may be either a paroxysmal or chronic tachyrhythmia.

Treatment of atrial flutter depends on the clinical status of the patient. In instances in which serious cardiovascular symptoms are produced by atrial flutter or when there is 1:1 AV conduction with a rapid ventricular response, immediate cardioversion is indicated unless digitalis intoxication is suspected. The patient is lightly anesthetized with intravenous diazepam (Valium) or a short-acting barbiturate, and synchronized DC countershock is applied with low energy settings (25 to 150 joules). Alternatively, rapid atrial pacing may be used to terminate atrial flutter. Pacing rates of 400 to 800 impulses per minute may be necessary and will either convert the atrial flutter to sinus rhythm or to atrial fibrillation, which frequently reverts to sinus rhythm spontaneously.

For less urgent episodes of atrial flutter, the first approach is to increase AV block and slow the ventricular response. This can be accomplished with digoxin (Lanoxin) either intravenously or orally. Initially 0.5 mg. is used, and subsequently 0.25 mg. every 4 to 6 hours is given until adequate AV block is achieved. Often, however, atrial flutter is resistant to digoxin alone, and adequate rate control requires large doses of digoxin with consequent elevations of the serum digoxin level into the toxic range. Propranolol (Inderal) is a useful adjunct to digoxin for rate control in atrial flutter. For a rapid response, intravenous propranolol, 0.5 to 1 mg. every 5 minutes to a total dose of 3 mg., is effective; orally, propranolol is given as 5 to 20 mg. four times daily and is ordinarily effective.

Occasionally, the paroxysm of atrial flutter will be terminated by the use of digoxin and propranolol alone. Often, however, quinidine in the form of quinidine gluconate (Quinaglute), 324 mg. three times daily, is added to digitalis and

*This use of phenytoin is not listed in the manufacturer's official directive.

propranolol to terminate atrial flutter. Quinidine should not be used as the sole agent in the treatment of atrial flutter, as it may elicit 1:1 AV conduction and an unacceptable acceleration of the ventricular rate. If the atrial flutter is not abolished by the addition of quinidine given for 2 to 3 days, cardioversion or rapid atrial pacing may produce reversion to normal sinus rhythm. If cardioversion is contemplated, digoxin is discontinued 24 hours earlier and quinidine and propranolol are continued. The digoxin is stopped because cardioversion may elicit significant arrhythmias resulting from digitalis excess. Usually low energy synchronized cardioversion (25 to 150 joules) reverts atrial flutter to sinus rhythm. Rapid atrial pacing at rates of 400 to 800 per minute is also effective in abolishing atrial flutter and restoring sinus rhythm either directly or after a brief period of transient atrial fibrillation.

Suppressive therapy of atrial flutter consists of oral digoxin, 0.25 mg. daily, quinidine (as Quinaglute), 324 mg. twice to four times daily, and, if necessary, propranolol (Inderal), 10 to 40 mg. four times daily.

Atrial Fibrillation

On the electrocardiogram atrial fibrillation is characterized by the absence of coordinated atrial activity; rather uncoordinated atrial oscillations at a rate of 400 to 650 per minute are present and are best seen in leads II and V_1. The ventricular response to atrial fibrillation is ordinarily irregular, and in the undigitalized patient it is rapid with rates of 120 to 200 beats per minute. The configuration of the QRS complex may be identical to that of normal sinus rhythm or aberrant, simulating premature ventricular contractions or even ventricular tachycardia.

Atrial fibrillation is a common tachycardia and may be chronic or may occur paroxysmally. It is observed in a variety of cardiac disorders such as rheumatic heart disease, coronary artery disease, hypertensive cardiovascular disease, thyrotoxicosis, the Wolff-Parkinson-White syndrome, and the sick sinus syndrome. Occasionally atrial fibrillation is present in patients with cardiomyopathy, myocarditis, and congenital heart disease. Rarely atrial fibrillation is a manifestation of digitalis intoxication. In a very small group of patients with paroxysmal atrial fibrillation, no underlying cardiac disorder is present, and these patients are considered to have "lone" or idiopathic atrial fibrillation.

As with atrial flutter, the treatment of atrial fibrillation depends on the clinical circumstances. In patients with extremely rapid ventricular rates or serious cardiac symptoms attributed to the tachycardia, cardioversion is indicated. After light anesthesia with intravenous diazepam (Valium) or short-acting barbiturates, synchronized DC countershock is performed with moderate energy settings (100 to 200 joules). In instances of atrial fibrillation with only modest cardiac distress and only a moderately rapid ventricular response (140 to 160 beats per minute), treatment with drugs can be employed. Digoxin (Lanoxin) is the drug of choice and may be used either orally or intravenously. In the undigitalized patient, digoxin, 0.5 mg., is given, followed by 0.25 mg. digoxin given each 4 to 6 hours until adequate rate control is achieved or a total of 1.5 to 2.0 mg. digoxin is reached. Propranolol (Inderal) is a useful adjunctive drug to slow the ventricular response to atrial fibrillation. In situations in which rapid rate control is necessary, 0.5 to 1.0 mg. propranolol is administered intravenously every 5 minutes until the ventricular response is slowed or a total dose of 3 mg. is given. In patients who persist with a moderately rapid ventricular response to atrial fibrillation despite adequate digitalis therapy, oral propranolol, 10 to 30 mg. four times daily, usually reduces the ventricular rate to satisfactory levels.

Digitalization alone may terminate a paroxysm of atrial fibrillation, but in many patients additional antiarrhythmic therapy is required. After the ventricular response has been slowed with drugs (digoxin and/or propranolol), quinidine in the form of quinidine gluconate (Quinaglute), 324 mg., is given two to four times daily; after several days, restoration of normal sinus rhythm may occur. A high rate of success of drug conversion of atrial fibrillation has been achieved with a combination of digoxin, quinidine, and propranolol, all given in the usual doses. Patients who do not revert to sinus rhythm with drug therapy may be considered for DC conversion if restoration of sinus rhythm is hemodynamically important and can be accomplished with a reasonable expectation that sinus rhythm will persist. Patients with longstanding atrial fibrillation (greater than 5 years), cardiomegaly, or significant left atrial enlargement are poor candidates for cardioversion, as they frequently revert to atrial fibrillation soon after cardioversion. Ordinarily such patients should be allowed to remain in atrial fibrillation with adequate control of ventricular rates. In patients who are judged good candidates for cardioversion, synchronized DC countershock under light anesthesia is performed with 100 to 250 joule energy settings. Quinidine is continued without interruption, but digoxin is discontinued 24 hours prior to the DC cardioversion and then renewed the day after the cardioversion. The use of anticoagulants prior to elective cardioversion of atrial fibrillation is prudent in patients with known rheumatic mitral stenosis or a prior history of arterial embolism.

Prevention of recurrent episodes of atrial fibrillation is often successful with maintenance oral digoxin (Lanoxin), 0.25 mg. daily, and oral quinidine gluconate (Quinaglute), 324 mg. two to four times daily. Occasional patients may require in addition propranolol (Inderal), 10 to 40 mg. four times daily.

Atrioventricular (AV) Junctional Tachycardia

There are two varieties of AV junctional tachycardia, paroxysmal and nonparoxysmal. Paroxysmal AV junctional tachycardia often occurs in healthy persons and is manifest as a regular supraventricular tachycardia with usual rates between 160 and 200 beats per minute. The QRS complexes are ordinarily similar to and often identical to those of normal sinus rhythm. The P wave configuration is variable; but, often, retrograde P waves inverted in lead II are seen just before or after the QRS complex. The treatment of paroxysmal AV junctional tachycardia is similar to that used in the treatment of paroxysmal atrial tachycardia (see above). Nonparoxysmal AV junctional tachycardia, nearly always associated with organic heart disease or digitalis intoxication, is characterized by a regular supraventricular rhythm with rates usually of 70 to 130 beats per minute. The QRS configuration is similar or identical to sinus conducted beats, and the P wave configuration, if seen, is characterized by retrograde P waves preceding or following the QRS complex. The treatment of nonparoxysmal AV junctional tachycardia, especially if it is due to digitalis intoxication, is similar to the treatment of ectopic atrial tachycardia (see above).

Ventricular Tachycardia

Ventricular tachycardia is defined as the presence of three or more consecutive ventricular ectopic impulses. The rate of this arrhythmia is quite variable but usually constant; ordinarily the rate of ventricular tachycardia is 180 to 250 beats per minute. Rates of as low as 70 beats per minute can occur; these are referred to as accelerated idioventricular rhythms or "slow ventricular tachycardia" and may not require specific treatment. The QRS complexes in ventricular tachycardia are wide and bizarre, and often, but not invariably, the QRS configuration is constant. Usually the ventricular tachycardia is regular. When gross irregularities appear associated with alterations in the QRS configuration, the disorder is designated as multiform ventricular tachycardia. Usually there is complete AV dissociation so that normal sinus P waves are present but are unrelated to the QRS complexes; occasionally retrograde capture of the atrium by the ventricular tachycardia occurs with retrograde P waves following each QRS complex. Ventricular tachycardia is usually seen in patients with heart disease and particularly in the setting of acute myocardial infarction. Ventricular tachycardia may be present in patients with chronic coronary heart disease, especially when associated with ventricular aneurysms, and also in patients with valvular heart disease, hypertensive cardiovascular disease, cardiomyopathies, and the prolonged Q-T syndrome. It may be associated with myxedema coma or intracranial hemorrhage or trauma. Other important causes of ventricular tachycardia include intoxication with a variety of drugs, including digitalis, quinidine, procainamide, phenothiazines, and the tricyclic antidepressants.

The treatment of ventricular tachycardia depends on the clinical setting. If there is an exceedingly rapid ventricular rate or severe cardiac distress resulting from the arrhythmia, emergency cardioversion is indicated and may be lifesaving. Synchronized DC countershock is used with high energy settings (200 to 400 joules). Immediately after successful cardioversion, suppressive antiarrhythmic therapy should be instituted.

Suppressive therapy of ventricular tachycardia involves initially administration of intravenous lidocaine (Xylocaine). An initial bolus of 100 mg. is administered, followed by continuous infusion of 2 to 4 mg. per minute. The total dose should not exceed 300 mg. per hour. If the ventricular tachycardia is not abolished by a low infusion rate of lidocaine, an additional 25 mg. bolus of lidocaine should be given, and the infusion rate should be increased to a higher level but not to exceed 4 mg. per minute. In ventricular tachycardia not responsive to intravenous lidocaine, intravenous procainamide (Pronestyl) is the next drug of choice. Procainamide may be administered at a rate of 50 mg. per minute but no more than 100 mg. in 5 minutes until the ventricular tachycardia is abolished or a total of 1000 mg. of procainamide has been given. To sustain the blood levels of procainamide, a continuous intravenous infusion of 1.5 to 5.0 mg. per minute is administered. Should these agents fail to control recurrent severe acute ventricular tachycardia, intravenous phenytoin* is used at a rate of 50 mg. per minute, and 100 mg. can be given every 5 minutes until the ventricular tachycardia is abolished or a total dose of 1000 mg. has been given. Alternatively, intravenous propranolol (Inderal) may be used, with 0.5 to 1.0 mg. given every 5 minutes to a total of 3

*This use of phenytoin is not listed in the manufacturer's official directive.

mg. If these combinations of agents are not successful in preventing recurrent acute ventricular tachycardia, rapid atrial or ventricular pacing, 100 to 140 beats per minute, may be employed to produce overdrive suppression of ventricular tachycardia. Occasionally faster-paced rates for brief periods may be necessary. In patients with severe refractory ventricular arrhythmias not responsive to these approaches and in whom a ventricular aneurysm is suspected, cardiac catheterization is performed; if a discrete ventricular aneurysm is present, emergency open heart surgery is performed to resect the aneurysm.

In patients with less catastrophic but clinically significant episodes of ventricular tachycardia in whom chronic suppressive therapy is indicated, a variety of antiarrhythmic agents may be employed on a trial and error basis under close medical supervision. Initially single agents are used, and the dose is adjusted to achieve therapeutic plasma levels. If one agent is not successful, another is tried, again with doses adjusted to establish effective plasma levels. If no single agent is effective, then multiple antiarrhythmic drug regimens are employed. The initial drug to use is quinidine in the form of quinidine gluconate (Quinaglute), 324 mg. two to four times daily to reach the therapeutic plasma level of 1 to 6 micrograms per ml. Next, oral procainamide (Pronestyl) is tried, 250 to 500 mg. every 3 to 6 hours, adjusting the dose until a plasma level of 4 to 8 micrograms per ml. is reached. Phenytoin* may also be used; a loading dose of 700 to 1000 mg. is given on the first day, and thereafter the maintenance dose is 300 to 400 mg. once daily, adjusted to establish plasma levels of 10 to 18 micrograms per ml. Another agent is propranolol (Inderal), 10 to 40 mg. four times daily. If these agents either alone or in combination are not effective, adjunctive therapy with rapid atrial or ventricular pacing for overdrive suppression is considered next. Initially a temporary pacemaker is used to establish the effectiveness of this therapy and the optimal rate and site of pacing for overdrive suppression. If this approach is effective, a permanent pacemaker is then implanted. Cardiac catheterization and coronary arteriography also should be performed in patients with refractory ventricular tachycardia to search for abnormalities which may be corrected by open heart surgery such as ventricular aneurysm, obstructive coronary artery disease, or intracardiac tumor. Recent experience suggests that a certain proportion of patients with serious refractory ventricular tachycardia may respond to oral digitalis therapy.

*This use of phenytoin is not listed in the manufacturer's official directive.

In asymptomatic patients with brief salvos of ventricular tachycardia (three beat ventricular tachycardia), specific antiarrhythmic therapy may not be indicated. It is important to assess the clinical benefits expected of antiarrhythmic therapy in these patients in relation to the hazards posed by the use of these potent drugs.

Ventricular Flutter and Fibrillation

Ventricular flutter and ventricular fibrillation are catastrophic and lethal arrhythmias. Ventricular flutter is characterized by a rapid ventricular rate 180 to 250 beats per minute, and the configuration of the QRST complex is rounded so that the distinction between its discrete elements—the QRS complex, ST segment, and T wave—is lost. Ventricular fibrillation is manifest by rapid, chaotic oscillation of varying contour. These lethal ventricular tachyrhythmias are seen in the same clinical settings as ventricular tachycardia. The immediate treatment of ventricular flutter and fibrillation is emergency DC defibrillation with 400 joules. Suppressive antiarrhythmic treatment for recurrent ventricular flutter or fibrillation is the same as for ventricular tachycardia (see above).

Tachycardia Due to Digitalis Intoxication

The common tachycardias produced by digitalis intoxication are nonparoxysmal AV junctional tachycardia, atrial tachycardia, and ventricular tachycardia. Very rarely, atrial flutter and atrial fibrillation may be produced by digitalis excess. Frequently, multiple digitalis-induced arrhythmias coexist, such as atrial tachycardia with AV block and simultaneous atrial and nonparoxysmal AV junctional tachycardia (double tachycardia). Whenever these arrhythmias are noted in patients receiving digitalis, drug intoxication should be suspected and blood samples should be drawn for digitalis glycoside assays to confirm the diagnosis. Digitalis intoxication is seen most often in elderly patients, patients with poor renal function, and patients who are receiving excessive doses of digitalis.

The initial therapeutic action is to discontinue further administration of digitalis. Further therapy depends on the type of tachycardia and the clinical consequences of the arrhythmia, and occasionally no further specific therapy is indicated. However, in patients who are symptomatic because of excessively rapid rates of the tachycardia, therapy is required. If the serum potassium is less than 3.5 mEq., potassium supplementation is indicated. Elixir of KCl, 10 per cent, may be administered orally, 15 to 30 ml. four times daily (60 to 120 mEq. KCl), depending on the degree of potassium deficiency. Intravenous KCl is used in more urgent situations of digitalis-induced tachycardia associated with hypokalemia; 60 to 160 mEq. in 24 hours may be required and should be infused no faster than 15 mEq. per hour. Intravenous phenytoin* is effective for all digitalis-induced tachycardias; it is administered at a rate of 50 mg. per minute, and 100 mg. can be infused every 5 minutes until the arrhythmia is abolished or a total dose of 1000 mg. is given. In instances of digitalis-induced ventricular tachycardia, lidocaine (Xylocaine) may be effective intravenously; a 100 mg. bolus is given, followed by a continuous infusion at a rate of 2 to 4 mg. per minute.

Cardioversion ordinarily should not be attempted to correct the tachycardias of digitalis intoxication, as it may unleash more advanced and catastrophic arrhythmias. Only under very exceptional circumstances is cardioversion indicated—i.e., only in instances of ventricular tachycardia resistant to potassium, phenytoin,* and lidocaine. If the ventricular tachycardia is life threatening, cardioversion should be performed with the lowest energy settings expected to revert the tachycardia. Prophylactic administration of intravenous phenytoin* just prior to cardioversion in these situations may prevent the occurrence of more serious digitalis-induced arrhythmias.

Tachycardias Associated with the Wolff-Parkinson-White Syndrome

A variety of supraventricular tachycardias, including paroxysmal atrial tachycardia, atrial flutter, and atrial fibrillation, are encountered in patients with the Wolff-Parkinson-White syndrome and its variants. These patients have ventricular pre-excitation caused by an accessory AV bypass tract which is manifest on the electrocardiogram by a short P-R interval and a delta wave on the upstroke of the QRS complex. The existence of the accessory AV bypass tract and the normal AV node permits re-entrant (circus movement) supraventricular tachycardias to occur. Also, since the refractory period of the accessory AV bypass tract may be very short, exceedingly rapid ventricular responses to atrial flutter (1:1 AV conduction) and atrial fibrillation may occur, with ventricular rates of 250 to 300 per minute. The most common supraventricular tachycardia in patients with Wolff-Parkinson-White syndrome is paroxysmal atrial tachycardia; atrial flutter and atrial fibrillation are encountered less often in these patients.

The treatment of the tachycardias associated with the Wolff-Parkinson-White syndrome differs from the treatment of supraventricular tachycardias in patients without pre-excitation. Since patients with the Wolff-Parkinson-White syndrome may sustain rapid ventricular rates, cardioversion often is indicated as the initial treatment. This is particularly so in instances of atrial flutter with 1:1 AV conduction and atrial fibrillation with ventricular rates in excess of 200 beats per minute. Light anesthesia with diazepam (Valium) or short-acting barbiturates is achieved, and low-energy synchronized DC cardioversion is employed with energy settings of 50 to 150 joules. If countershock is not indicated by the clinical status of the patient, the first agents of choice are quinidine or procainamide (Pronestyl) in the usual therapeutic doses. These agents depress conductivity through the accessory AV bypass tract. Should these agents not be successful, digoxin or propranolol (Inderal) in the standard doses may be added to terminate the supraventricular tachycardia. Digoxin and propranolol should not be used alone, as they may produce block in the normal AV node and facilitate the rapid conduction of impulses through the accessory AV bypass tract leading to a paradoxical increase in the heart rate. If drug therapy does not abolish the supraventricular tachycardia, cardioversion is then indicated.

To suppress recurrent episodes of supraventricular tachycardia in patients with the Wolff-Parkinson-White syndrome, quinidine or procainamide should be used initially. Adjunctive digoxin or propranolol may be effective if these agents fail, but digoxin or propranolol should not be administered as the sole agents, as they may accelerate the ventricular response during the tachycardia. In patients with severe recurrent supraventricular tachycardias resistant to drug therapy, surgical interruption of the accessory AV bypass tract should be considered.

Tachycardias Associated with the Sick Sinus Syndrome

The sick sinus syndrome is characterized by disordered sinus node impulse formation and sinoatrial conduction disturbances resulting in atrial bradycardias such as sinus bradycardia, sinus arrest, and sinoatrial block. Paradoxically a certain proportion of patients with the sick sinus syndrome have episodes of paroxysmal supraventricular arrhythmias such as atrial tachycardia, atrial flutter, and atrial fibrillation. During these atrial tachyrhythmias, the heart rate is usually rapid, and these patients consequently are plagued by periods of bradycardia alternating with periods of tachycardia and may be severely symptomatic.

The treatment of the supraventricular tachycardias in the sick sinus syndrome must be

*This use of phenytoin is not listed in the manufacturer's official directive.

modified, because many of the drugs used—digoxin, quinidine, and propranolol—may aggravate the sinus node dysfunction, producing serious bradyrhythmias. In these patients, effective treatment is often accomplished by implanting a permanent pacemaker, either atrial or ventricular, to prevent episodes of bradycardia. Occasionally this will suffice alone and the episodes of supraventricular tachycardia will no longer occur because the basic heart rate is normal. If recurrent supraventricular tachycardias persist after pacemaker implantation, conventional therapy with digoxin, quinidine, and propranolol may be employed without fear of producing pathologic bradycardia.

CONGENITAL HEART DISEASE

method of
JAMES E. GIBBONS, M.D.,
and GEORGE F. COLLINS, M.B.
Montreal, Quebec, Canada

Anatomic malformations caused by defective cardiac embryogenesis in intrauterine life are present at birth (congenital malformations of the heart) and may result in significant disability in the neonatal period or at some later time in infancy or childhood. Surgical repair is the definitive treatment of congenital heart disease, but many children with simple anomalies can lead normal, unrestricted lives without surgical intervention. The decision to operate is based on an understanding of the natural history of the lesion and the results of surgery.

Congenital malformations of the heart occur in approximately 8 per 1000 live births. The mortality rate is still significant in the first year of life, particularly in the newborn period. Fortunately, recent technical advances have made it possible to successfully treat ill newborns and infants, and the emphasis today is on early investigation and aggressive treatment of these young patients.

Emergency Management of the Sick Newborn

Heart disease may not be easily detected in the newborn baby. Yet prompt recognition is essential. Subtle early clinical signs may precede by hours a dramatic deterioration and fatal termination. The signs are those of respiratory distress, lethargy, heart failure, and/or cyanosis. However, it must be emphasized that critical hypoxemia (arterial oxygen tension less than 35 mm. Hg with progressive metabolic acidosis) can occur in the newborn without recognizable cyanosis. Tachypnea, particularly rapid, shallow respirations, may be the only early sign of serious heart disease. At this age a heart murmur is more often absent than present, and the initial chest x-ray and electrocardiogram may be normal. Nurses, residents, and physicians who work in newborn nurseries have considerable responsibility to appreciate the significance of subtle early signs of heart disease and to arrange for their prompt investigation. It is no longer appropriate to observe overnight with oxygen and digitalis. Proper management includes early consultation and the arrangement for prompt transfer to a regional neonatal intensive care unit, where facilities exist for complete cardiac investigation and emergency surgical management.

In preparing for transfer, capillary blood gas analysis may identify metabolic acidosis or CO_2 retention and lead to preliminary treatment with sodium bicarbonate, digoxin, and diuretics. During transportation and with subsequent examinations and investigations, careful attention must be given to temperature regulation and oxygen requirement. Echocardiography in experienced hands can be extremely valuable, both to exclude the possibility of a cardiac lesion (e.g., persistent fetal circulation) and to pinpoint such common problems as the hypoplastic left heart syndrome or complete transposition of the great vessels. Most infants, however, require a prompt anatomic and physiologic diagnosis by cardiac catheterization and selective angiography. During this investigation, specific treatment, in the form of an atrial balloon septostomy (transposition) or the infusion of prostaglandins (pulmonary atresia) can lead to dramatic improvement. The investigation is not complete until the anatomic findings have been reviewed with the surgeons and decisions made as to further surgical management.

Congestive Heart Failure in Infancy

Congestive heart failure complicating congenital heart disease usually occurs in the first year of life. It rarely occurs for the first time later in childhood unless there is an associated bacterial endocarditis. In infancy heart failure is most commonly due to an increase in pulmonary blood flow, as a result of a large intracardiac left-to-right shunt (volume overload). It can also occur with obstructive heart lesions (pressure overload), either alone or in association with increased flow. Pump failure, however, is rare, as most children have normal myocardial contractility. As a result, medical management, although often producing an amelioration in symptoms, is seldom curative. Advantage should be taken of the initial clinical improvement to carry out the necessary investigations to determine the underlying anatomic abnormality in preparation for possible future surgery.

General Supportive Measures. REST AND SEDATION. The presenting clinical picture varies from the infant with mild respiratory distress, feeding poorly, and slow to gain weight, to the acutely distressed child, apprehensive, fighting for breath, and in severe pulmonary edema. The management varies accordingly. Most infants are apprehensive and benefit initially from mild oral sedation (diazepam, 0.2 mg. per kg.). Morphine sulfate (0.1 mg. per kg.), subcutaneously or intramuscularly, is required by those in pulmonary edema. Such a child requires careful monitoring, including blood gas analysis. In all children breathing is facilitated by maintaining the semisitting position. This is comfortably achieved in older infants by using an infant seat.

NUTRITIONAL REQUIREMENTS. Most infants in heart failure feed poorly and gain weight slowly. Caloric requirements are increased in the presence of heart failure, yet oral feeding is rapidly exhausting and may be impossible in the acutely distressed child. Such children require nasogastric tube feedings, and occasionally intravenous alimentation is indicated to prepare a severely malnourished child for heart surgery. Rest is facilitated in those who are less ill by feeding small amounts of high calorie milk preparations more frequently (2-hourly) or by alternating oral and nasogastric tube feedings. Growth is severely retarded in children in chronic heart failure, and unless an oral intake of at least 100 calories per kg. per day can be maintained after the institution of medications to control the failure, it may be appropriate to consider early surgical repair. Low salt milk preparations are available, but these preparations are relatively unpalatable, making it difficult to maintain adequate nutrition during long-term use. Rather than restrict salt or fluid intake in infants, the current practice is to feed liberally with high calorie milk formulas and utilize diuretics to control excessive fluid accumulation. As a general rule the higher caloric value of milk products over cereal is justification for delaying the introduction of solid foods, but in this practice care must be exercised to supplement the diet with vitamins and oral iron when necessary.

OXYGEN THERAPY. When cyanosis results from an intracardiac right-to-left shunt, oxygen administration has no effect on arterial oxygen saturation. However, an oxygen-rich environment is most beneficial to the child in pulmonary edema. It is inappropriate, even dangerous, to give oxygen by mask because of the risk of vomiting and aspiration in infants. A well sealed Isolette or Croupette will provide ambient oxygen concentrations of 40 to 50 per cent. High oxygen tensions are dangerous for premature infants, and in such patients both environmental oxygen and arterial oxygen tensions should be monitored. Occasionally endotracheal intubation and assisted ventilation are necessary in the presence of carbon dioxide retention.

INTERCURRENT INFECTIONS. Sepsis in the newborn period and pneumonia later in infancy may complicate congenital heart disease and can precipitate heart failure. Antibiotic therapy appropriate for the age of the child and type of infection is an important part of therapy. If antibiotics are given by the intravenous route, the type and volume of fluid given should be controlled to prevent aggravating the already existent fluid overload.

ANEMIA AND/OR ELECTROLYTE DISTURBANCES. Mild to moderate degrees of anemia are common in chronically ill and malnourished infants. Such anemia can respond to oral iron supplements, but occasionally blood transfusions are important in the management of seriously ill infants in heart failure. Given as packed cells, such transfusions are usually well tolerated.

When diuretics are used regularly, serum electrolytes should be measured weekly. Occasionally potassium supplements are needed. It should also be noted that either hypoglycemia and/or hypocalcemia can accompany heart failure in the newborn period. Specific correction of the metabolic disturbance may alleviate the signs of heart failure.

Specific Medical Management. DIGOXIN. Cardiac glycosides remain the cornerstone of drug therapy for children, just as they are for adults, in heart failure. With children, however, special care is needed because of the small dosage, calculated on the basis of age and body weight. Errors in both prescription and administration are easily made. As with adults, there is an individual patient variation in tolerance, and the optimal therapeutic dose is closely related to the toxic levels. Digoxin is usually given orally, as a green liquid preparation, elixir digoxin (Lanoxin)—a stable medication, with a concentration of 0.05 mg. per ml., which is easily measured using a graduated dropper pipette. There is also a pediatric parenteral preparation containing 0.1 mg. per ml.

In those in mild distress, effective digitalization can be achieved in 4 or 5 days by beginning with the daily maintenance dose of digoxin orally in divided doses every 12 hours (Table 1). Those who are critically ill are digitalized more rapidly over a 24 to 36 hour period, giving one half of the digitalizing dose immediately, then one fourth

TABLE 1. **Digoxin Dosage in Pediatric Practice**

AGE	TOTAL DIGITALIZING DOSE (TDD), ORAL* (OVER 24 TO 48 HOURS)	DAILY MAINTENANCE†
Premature infants	0.04 mg./kg.	0.01 mg./kg.
Newborn–6 months	0.06 mg./kg.	One third to one forth of TDD
6 months–2 years	0.05 mg./kg.	One third to one forth of TDD
2–5 years	0.04 mg./kg.	One fourth to one fifth of TDD
>5 years	0.04 mg./kg. (1.0 mg. maximum)	One fifth (maximum, 0.25 mg. daily)

*If given intravenously, use 75 per cent of oral dose.
†Give as divided doses every 12 hours.

and one fourth at 12- to 18-hourly intervals (Table 1). It is best to administer these doses parenterally to avoid problems with emesis and gastrointestinal absorption. The patient should be carefully assessed and an electrocardiogram rhythm strip recorded before the third dose. Again it should be stressed that calculations of the digitalizing dose should be carefully checked; it is too easy to misplace the decimal point!

Certain patients—e.g., premature infants, patients with myocarditis, those with impaired renal function and/or electrolyte disturbances—may be unusually sensitive to cardiac glycosides, so it is best to use only half the calculated dose, given cautiously with electrocardiographic monitoring. In older patients, 5 to 10 years of age, toxicity may result if the total digitalizing dose is based only on body weight. In this age group total digitalization should not exceed 1.0 mg. in 24 hours. As there is considerable variation in individual tolerance, the observation of any of the following signs should result in withholding the next dose and a reconsideration of further requirements: (1) marked slowing of the heart rate; (2) obvious sinus arrhythmia in the young infant; (3) premature ventricular contractions; or (4) anorexia or vomiting.

DIURETICS. Oral diuretics are usually added to the therapeutic regimen in moderately severe heart failure. The most common drugs are the thiazide derivatives (hydrochlorothiazide) given with or without aldosterone antagonists (spironolactone [Aldactone]). The dosage is empirical, 2 to 4 mg. per kg. daily for 5 days each week, or, in patients with less severe failure, on alternate days. On such a regimen potassium depletion is uncommon (although with persistent long-term use,serum potassium should be checked periodically). Supplemental potassium is rarely necessary, apart from daily ingestion of citrus fruit juice.

In the acutely ill child, parenteral diuretics, such as furosemide or ethacrynic acid, are administered as necessary (dosage, 1 mg. per kg. intravenously, intramuscularly, or orally). These medications may cause significant electrolyte disturbance when used frequently or on a long-term basis. They should not be used as a replacement for thiazide derivatives in the management of chronic heart failure; but when added 1 to 2 times per week to a thiazide-Aldactone regimen, additional beneficial diuresis can often be achieved.

All infants who present with heart failure will require complete investigation, including echocardiography and cardiac catheterization, to determine the underlying pathology. The latter investigation may become a matter of some urgency, but can usually wait a day or two for the initial clinical improvement.

Cyanotic Heart Disease

Cyanosis in the newborn period may be a medical emergency; its occurrence later in infancy and childhood requires prompt and careful cardiac evaluation to determine the nature of the underlying lesion. Children with cyanotic congenital heart disease will require surgical intervention. The type and timing of surgery depends on the severity of the clinical picture, the complexity of the lesion, and the surgical experience. For those who are relatively asymptomatic, such surgery is usually planned just prior to starting school; however, progressive cyanosis and secondary polycythemia will require earlier intervention, either with a palliative procedure or an open-heart operation.

Children who are cyanosed may be handicapped with fatigue and irritability. They may be slow to gain weight and retarded in the achievement of their "milestones." Such a child needs extra attention and can cause stress in family relationships. These patients require regular clinical evaluations while awaiting surgery; the parents need considerable support.

Hemoglobin and hematocrit levels, repeated at intervals of 3 to 6 months, are valuable in assessing progress of the cyanotic infant. Hemoglobin estimates alone can be misleading in infancy when iron intake is poor. Even when the hemoglobin is "normal for age," additional iron may be beneficial to maintain the mean corpuscular hemoglobin concentration (MCHC) above 30 per cent, optimizing the oxygen-carrying capacity of the blood. An unduly high hemoglobin and hematocrit are cause for concern. A hemoglobin over 20 grams per 100 ml. or a hematocrit greater than 60 per cent is associated with increased blood viscosity and the risk of a cerebrovascular accident. Common childhood illnesses associated with dehydration—i.e., febrile illnesses, diarrhea, and vomiting—can cause an acute rise in hematocrit. Special precautions are needed in these children to prevent dehydration, including early hospitalization and institution of intravenous fluid replacement.

Hypoxic Spells. Intermittent hypoxic or cyanotic spells in cyanotic heart disease are unique to tetralogy of Fallot. Such a history in infancy must be taken seriously and investigated thoroughly. In these children, the right ventricular outflow obstruction is muscular and reactive. The infundibular "spasm" which results from increased sympathetic tone aggravates the right-to-left intracardiac shunt, causing progressive cyanosis, hypoxemia, and metabolic acidosis. The child may die in either the first or any subsequent "spell" or may be left with permanent brain damage. Thus early surgical intervention is mandatory.

Emergency management of the hypoxic spell includes the following measures:

1. Placing the child in the knee-chest position.
2. Oxygen administration.
3. Morphine sulfate, 0.1 mg. per kg. subcutaneously.
4. Propranolol, 0.1 mg. per kg. intravenously, to relieve infundibular spasm by beta-adrenergic blockage. A *slow* infusion (over a 5 minute period) is important; monitor heart rate and avoid undue bradycardia.
5. Correction of metabolic acidosis with intravenous sodium bicarbonate (2 mEq. per kg.).
6. Phenylephrine HCl, 2 to 5 micrograms per kg. per minute by constant intravenous infusion. Prepare a 10 microgram per ml. solution by diluting 1 ml. of 0.2 per cent phenylephrine HCl in 200 ml. saline. Use constant infusion pump and infuse at the lower dose, 2 micrograms per kg. per minute, with increments at 5 minute intervals to the maximum dose of 5 micrograms per kg. per minute to achieve an increase of 30 to 40 mm. Hg in systemic blood pressure and a 10 per cent reduction in heart rate.

The Child with a Heart Murmur

Innocent or functional heart murmurs are common in childhood, occurring at some time or other in approximately 40 per cent of all children. Unfortunately many people, including some physicians, equate heart murmurs with heart disease. A great deal of anxiety may result from finding a heart murmur in a child. All too often, this anxiety causes unnecessary restrictions at school and in play. Such an attitude can be most unfortunate, predisposing to the development of a cardiac neurosis in later life.

It is important to appreciate that only 1 in 40 children with a murmur will have heart disease, and that most of these children can be identified by a good history and physical examination, with perhaps the support of an electrocardiogram, chest x-ray, and echocardiogram. In an asymptomatic child who is growing and developing normally, a careful cardiac examination that detects palpable femoral pulses, a normally located apex beat, a quiet precordium, and normal (variable) splitting of the second heart sound will exclude the important congenital heart lesions and facilitate reassurance.

Even if the child has a congenital heart lesion, there is rarely an indication to limit normal physical activity. Most patients who are hypoxemic or have chronic heart failure establish their own level of activity. Those who have critical aortic stenosis or significant pulmonary hypertension (Eisenmenger syndrome) should avoid the sudden stress of competitive sports or track and field, but even they can usually play, swim, or ride their bicycles for pleasure. However, all other children should be encouraged to lead active lives, participating in physical activities to the limit of their tolerance.

Infective Endocarditis

Bacterial endocarditis is a relatively uncommon complication of congenital heart disease, but when it occurs it is a potentially life-threatening illness. The occurrence of bacteremia in children with an anatomic abnormality of the heart may result in an infective endocardial focus. The risk is highest when the congenital heart lesion causes turbulent blood flow—i.e., small ventricular septal defect, aortic stenosis, patent ductus arteriosus (PDA), coarctation, and mitral insufficiency. The problem is of increasing importance for those patients with artificial heart valves. All such children at risk should have regular twice yearly dental supervision beginning at age 3 years. There is a significant incidence of bacteremia during dental extractions, bronchoscopic and cystoscopic manipulations, and tonsillectomy. For such procedures the risk of endocarditis is minimized if appropriate antibiotics are given in therapeutic doses—e. g., oral penicillin G, 400,000 units three times each day for 3 days, starting on the day of the procedure. Alternatively a single intramuscular dose of procaine penicillin G (400,000 units) can be given 1 to 2 hours prior to the procedure, repeating the same dose on the next 2 days, or using oral penicillin as described. Patients sensitive to penicillin may be given erythromycin; when gram-negative organisms are anticipated, ampicillin may be used.

Prostaglandins and Prostaglandin Antagonists

Prostaglandins are potent vasoactive agents present in most human tissues. They do not seem to act as circulating hormones in adults, because biologically neutralizing enzymes in the lung remove about 95 per cent of any prostaglandin which finds its way into the venous system. However, in the fetal circulation such substances bypass the pulmonary circulation and act as circulating vasoactive hormones on large arterial vessels, including the ductus arteriosus.

Recently prostaglandin E has been used experimentally and in newborn infants with cyanotic congenital heart disease in whom imminent closure of the ductus threatened to cut off the blood supply to the lungs (i.e., pulmonary atresia). There is convincing evidence that this treatment will dilate the ductus and increase the arterial Po_2, allowing a less hurried approach to surgery in ductus-dependent severe cyanotic congenital heart disease in the newborn period. As an extension of this work, prostaglandin inhibitors have been used experimentally to promote closure of a persistent ductus arteriosus in premature infants with heart failure. As yet, not enough is known about the effects of these inhibitors to justify general use. Until more is known about possible side effects, their use should be restricted to life-threatening illness in which conventional treatment is unlikely to succeed.

Management of Specific Congenital Heart Lesions

Ventricular Septal Defect. Within a few weeks of birth, the size of the shunt at ventricular level is a reflection of the size of the septal defect. Subsequent management depends on the child's symptoms and an understanding of the natural history of the lesion. Small defects are well tolerated, and many will close spontaneously later in childhood.

When the defect is large and causing symptoms in infancy, cardiac catheterization is necessary to evaluate the size of the shunt, the pulmonary artery pressure, and the pulmonary vascular resistance. These large defects also tend to decrease in size and may also close spontaneously. However, approximately 15 per cent of these children are at risk of developing progressive pulmonary arteriolar disease, and such vascular changes can occur by the end of the first year of life. Such patients, and those in whom severe heart failure cannot be controlled by medical therapy, require early surgical intervention. In experienced centers, direct closure of the defect seems more appropriate than a palliative pulmonary artery band.

Atrial Septal Defect. Atrial septal defects rarely produce cardiac failure in infancy. If there is a significant left-to-right shunt, with a pulmonary–to–systemic flow ratio greater than 1.8:1, surgical closure of the defect should be carried out, preferably between the ages of 5 and 7 years.

Patent Ductus Arteriosus. Infants with cardiac failure resulting from a large patent ductus arteriosus should initially be treated medically, after which the diagnosis should be confirmed by cardiac catheterization. Since there is a significant risk of developing pulmonary vascular disease later in life and little chance of "spontaneous" closure, early surgery is advised. The tiny premature infant, critically ill with a large patent ductus, poses special challenging problems. Spontaneous closure occurs frequently. Medical therapy for this special group should be aggressive, reserving surgical intervention for those infants in whom cardiac failure cannot be controlled or for instances in which it is felt that the increased pulmonary blood flow is interfering with the mechanics of ventilation. The older infant or child relatively asymptomatic with a smaller patent ductus should have elective surgery prior to age 18 months or after 4 years.

Aortic Valve Stenosis. The majority of children with this lesion remain asymptomatic for many years. Occasionally infants with "critical" aortic stenosis present with congestive heart failure and signs of low cardiac output. Intensive medical treatment and emergency surgery are indicated. Older infants and children with "critical" aortic stenosis may have symptoms such as dyspnea, angina, or syncope, and surgical intervention is also indicated. However, since the majority of patients are asymptomatic, the decision for surgery is usually based on specific data obtained at the time of cardiac catheterization. A resting peak systolic gradient between the left ventricular and aorta exceeding 60 to 70 mm. Hg is usually an indication for operation. Recently echocardiography has been found helpful to identify patients with significant obstruction. Long-term follow-up is mandatory, because aortic stenosis may be progressive.

Pulmonic Valve Stenosis. "Critical" isolated pulmonic stenosis in early infancy requires emergency pulmonary valvotomy. This condition is characterized by cardiomegaly, evidence of severe right ventricular hypertrophy and strain on the electrocardiogram, and, at times, cyanosis. Less critical obstruction in older infants and children is well tolerated. Elective operation is indicated when the resting right ventricular pressure is at or above 60 to 70 per cent of the systemic pressure.

Transposition of the Great Vessels. Complete d-transposition of the great vessels, with intact ventricular septum, usually presents as an emergency in the newborn period. Lack of intracardiac mixing results in critical hypoxemia and metabolic acidosis. An atrial balloon septostomy carried out during the diagnostic study can be a most dramatic lifesaving procedure. Occasionally when there is an excessive pulmonary blood flow in association with a large patent ductus arteriosus, the septostomy is followed by surgical ligation of the ductus. After a successful atrial septostomy, an open operation with an intra-atrial pericardial "baffle" is carried out between 9 and 15 months of age. Frequently, with persistent critical cyanosis, an earlier surgical approach is required.

With transposition of the great arteries and a large ventricular septal defect, pulmonary blood flow is excessive and the early presentation is congestive heart failure, with the risk of developing early progressive pulmonary arteriolar damage (Eisenmenger reaction). An atrial septostomy is performed. It is usually also necessary to band the pulmonary artery, or proceed with early definitive surgical repair, particularly if the lungs are not protected.

When transposition with a ventricular septal defect is associated with pulmonary stenosis, the clinical presentation resembles tetralogy of Fallot with diminished pulmonary blood flow. The pulmonary obstruction is often subvalvar and difficult to repair as it may involve the mitral valve apparatus. If surgery is necessary in early life, a palliative systemic-pulmonary shunt is preferred. Definitive correction can then be postponed until later in childhood.

Tetralogy of Fallot. The severity of symptoms in these children depends on the severity of the pulmonary obstruction. Surgical repair, involving relief of the pulmonary valve and infundibular stenosis and patch closure of the ventricular defect, is ideally carried out between the ages of 2 and 5 years, although primary repair can be performed in the first year of life in those with troublesome cyanosis or cyanotic spells. The risk of primary repair in infancy is increased when the pulmonary valve ring and artery are extremely hypoplastic, and such children may benefit from a preliminary systemic-to-pulmonary artery shunt. Such selected patients may later require tubular conduits to connect the right ventricle to the pulmonary artery.

Tricuspid Atresia. When pulmonary blood flow is markedly reduced, a surgical shunt will be necessary in infancy (Blalock or Glenn shunt). If critical cyanosis recurs, further improvement can be expected from a second palliative shunt. For older children, the recent experience with a more complete hemodynamic correction, closing the atrial septal defect and connecting the right atrial appendage via a conduit to the pulmonary artery, is very encouraging.

Total Anomalous Pulmonary Venous Return. In the obstructed infradiaphragmatic form of total anomalous pulmonary venous return, death in early infancy is the rule unless a corrective surgical operation can be carried out.

With "obstructed" supradiaphragmatic total anomalous pulmonary venous return, medical management is usually ineffective, and an early open surgical approach is preferred. There may be some infants who can be improved with atrial balloon septostomy and heart failure therapy and for whom a later operation is more appropriate. However, the selection of those infants for whom surgery can be deferred may be quite difficult.

CONGESTIVE HEART FAILURE

method of
DEAN T. MASON, M.D.
Davis, California

Congestive heart failure (CHF) is the pathologic condition in which severely impaired cardiac performance is responsible for the inability of the heart to deliver blood at a rate commensurate with the basal metabolic requirements of the organs throughout the body. Recent findings obtained from experimental and clinical studies on the control of force and velocity of ventricular contraction have clarified that the function of the intact heart is governed by intimate integration of four principal determinants that regulate stroke volume and cardiac output: (1) *preload* (ventricular end-diastolic volume), (2) *contractility* (variable force of ventricular contraction independent of loading), (3) *afterload* (intraventricular systolic tension during ejection), and (4) *heart rate*. The first two determinants are fundamental, intrinsic mechanisms inherent in the contractile machinery of the myocardium, whereas the last two are largely under extrinsic autonomic modulation. When considering cardiac function in coronary heart disease, it is important to add a fifth determinant, one that adversely affects ventricular performance: (5) *dyssynergy* or abnormal temporal sequence of segmental ventricular contraction. The terms cardiac function and ventricular performance are used in the general sense to refer to the combined action of these determinants of cardiac output and not necessarily to the single determinant, contractility (inotropism), itself. The disturbed mechanisms operative in all types of clinical heart disease can be evaluated and accurately characterized within the framework of isolated or composite disorders of these five major determinants of cardiac performance. The recent development of improved techniques and concepts for the assessment of cardiac function in patients by both hemodynamic methods and myocardial mechanics has provided the means for differential analyses of the nature and degree of importance of the roles of each of these fundamental determinants and their interrelations with cardiac compensatory mechanisms governing stroke output in heart disease.

Pathophysiologic Mechanisms of Heart Failure

Clinical heart disease can be broadly classified on a pathophysiologic basis according to three general types of cardiac functional abnormalities: (1) *primary contractility disturbance,* as in idiopathic or ischemic myocardial disease; (2) *diastolic mechanical inhibition* of cardiac performance (ventricular underloading) in which ventricular hypertrophy does not develop, as in restricted ventricular filling in mitral stenosis or pericardial tamponade; and (3) *systolic mechanical ventricular overloading,* characterized by excessive pressure loading, as in aortic stenosis or essential hypertension, or increased volume loading, as in mitral or aortic regurgitation. CHF in systolic ventricular overloading and in primary inotropic disorders occurs when there is substantial depression of contractility; decompensation ensues when the impairment of contractile state becomes particularly severe.

General Approach to Therapy

At the outset, it is important to emphasize that cardiac dysfunction should not be allowed to reach refractoriness to medical therapy in congenital heart disease or acquired valvular disorders. Indeed, definitive evaluation by cardiac catheterization and surgery, if appropriate, generally are carried out electively prior to symptoms in congenital heart disease and when cardiac symptoms occur with ordinary activity (greater than stable Class II symptoms by the New York Heart Association criteria) in chronic rheumatic valvular heart disease. In severe valvular malfunction, valve replacement should not be delayed to the stage of refractory CHF, as the secondary abnormalities in ventricular contractility remain after operation corrects the mechanical burden on the ventricle in patients with chronic cardiac symptoms occurring with mild activity (Class III) or at rest (Class IV) prior to heart surgery.

In patients with chronic CHF, even if idiopathic cardiomyopathy is the suspected diagnosis, it is our policy to carry out detailed right and left heart catheterization to establish positively the type of heart disease involved and to quantify the extent of cardiac and myocardial dysfunction. In patients with unsuspected congenital or acquired heart disease, corrective or palliative surgery may be possible. In some patients with cardiomyopathies and marked secondary mitral regurgitation, mitral replacement has been helpful, despite the increased operative risk, prolonged convalescence, and incomplete benefit. In chronic coronary artery disease, elective saphenous vein bypass by itself has not consistently produced improvement in chronic ventricular dysfunction, except in occasional patients with frequent angina in whom satisfactory anastomosis substantially improves blood flow to the ischemic regions of the ventricle. Patients with CHF caused by chronic coronary artery disease, however, usually do not have prominent anginal symptoms, as they often do not have substantial ischemic, potentially normal functioning myocardium; their heart failure is more on the basis of muscle fibrosis with generalized abnormalities of wall motion. On the other hand, in chronic coronary CHF, surgical resection of a ventricular aneurysm may be performed successfully in patients in whom the area of segmental dyssynergy is not too extensive and is well demarcated from a considerable quantity of normally functioning remaining left ventricle.

In many instances of chronic refractory CHF, careful re-evaluation of history, physical examination, laboratory tests, and results of cardiac catheterization does not reveal previously unrecognized diseases or conditions to which special medical or surgical therapy can be applied. Chronic refractory CHF in such patients is caused by myocardial heart disease (the specific, idiopathic, and ischemic cardiomyopathies), with severe reduction in contractility without chronic hemodynamic overload. Ventricular dysfunction may be largely irreversible in these situations. The remainder of this article on management of refractory heart failure deals with the difficult and relatively incomplete therapeutic modalities that can be used in chronic pump dysfunction resulting entirely from markedly depressed inotropic state.

Medical therapy is somewhat limited and nonspecific in chronic CHF caused by primary ventricular muscle dysfunction. Nevertheless, salutary effects can be achieved in most instances. The physiologic approach to treatment is based on improving the aforementioned principal determinants of cardiac function. Thus the four major factors regulating cardiac performance (preload, contractility, afterload, and heart rate) are therapeutically adjusted to provide optimal circumstances for the depressed contractile force of the failing pump to deliver a normal cardiac output. Treatment is often best initiated in the hospital, with diminution of physical activity and the use of bed rest. Management usually centers on improving two principal aspects of the congestive failure state: (1) impaired contractility and (2) body salt and water retention. In addition, certain electrical measures sometimes may be applied to optimize heart rate and improve ventricular filling. Furthermore, reduction of the impedance to left ventricular ejection by the use of peripheral vasodilator agents constitutes a new therapeutic approach to raising low stroke output.

Bed Rest

Bed rest must be individualized in CHF. Bed rest reduces preload (by decreasing augmented venous return) accompanying muscular activity, diminishes afterload (by reducing arterial blood pressure), and declines heart rate. Mild to moderate CHF is adequately controlled by medication. Strict bed rest may even be deleterious and may promote venostasis with pulmonary emboli. Normal activity should be attained as soon as possible to prevent the various complications that might ensue. Effective management of CHF also requires the exclusion of precipitating and aggravating factors.

Digitalis

Since the basic abnormality of the failing myocardium leading to refractory circulatory congestion is marked disturbance of contractile state, the first principle of management is to consider positive inotropic agents for enhancing cardiac performance. Improvement of depressed contractility elevates the entire ventricular function curve toward normal, thereby raising the lowered cardiac output and reducing the excessive left ventricular end-diastolic pressure. Rational treatment generally begins with the digitalis glycosides. Since the beneficial effects of these agents stem from their direct stimulatory action on the force of contraction of the myocardium, using these drugs produces some improvement in the depressed contractile state and rise in low cardiac output. Furthermore, the glycosides exert an overall indirect effect of vasodilation in congestive heart failure; elevated peripheral vascular resistance is reduced by the elevation of the diminished cardiac output, thereby allowing withdrawal of sympathetically mediated vasoconstriction, which overrides the mild direct vasoconstrictor action of digitalis. In regard to myocardial oxygen requirements of the failing heart and digitalis, it is important to point out that, despite the increased oxygen cost of increasing contractile state per se, the overall glycoside effect is to improve cardiac efficiency and reduce myocardial oxygen consumption, because the predominant indirect action of the agent is to diminish heart size, thereby decreasing intramyocardial systolic tension.

Oral and Parenteral Administration. Pharmacodynamic studies of tritiated digoxin have shown that oral digoxin is absorbed considerably better than had been previously appreciated. Eighty per cent of an oral dose is absorbed, and therefore the total oral digitalizing dose should now be only 2 mg. In contrast to digitoxin, digoxin is little bound to serum proteins, and therefore, after absorption, digoxin is rapidly bound to the myocardium and other tissues, resulting in a myocardial-to-serum ratio of approximately 30:1. Digitalis slowly accumulates within the body after institution of a daily maintenance regimen, without an initial loading dose. The body retains daily a certain constant percentage of the quantity of systemic glycoside—30 per cent in the case of digoxin. In normal persons taking 0.5 mg. oral tritiated digoxin daily, the plateau concentration of radioactive digoxin in the blood is the same after 6 days, whether or not an initial loading dose is given. Consequently, only maintenance doses of digoxin (average, 0.25 mg.) are required to achieve therapeutic concentrations in a few days in nonurgent conditions of CHF. In situations when rapid digitalization is required, the agent may be given intravenously or intramuscularly. Since parenteral digoxin is completely absorbed, the full digitalizing dose is only 1.50 mg. In such instances, parenteral digoxin is usually given as an initial 0.50 mg. dose, with subsequent 0.25 mg. doses every 6 hours as necessary.

The traditional concept of the relation between the dose and the positive contractile action of digitalis has been that little contractile benefit is achieved until a certain digitalizing dose is reached, and that the positive contractile action of the glycoside then diminishes as higher doses are administered and toxicity is approached. Recent evidence indicates, however, that there is a linear therapeutic dose–to–contractile response relation. This linear dose-response relation has been shown in isolated, cat ventricular papillary muscles—for digitoxin, digoxin, ouabain, and acetyl strophanthidin. Thus small or large quantities of the glycosides have the same qualitative contractile action, the extent of which is proportional to the dose employed, and a patient need not receive a maximally tolerated dose of digitalis to achieve some salutary effect. Even small amounts of the glycoside provide some therapeutic action, a point to be kept in mind if the agent is used in patients who may be prone to toxicity.

Potassium and Digitalis. The serum potassium concentration importantly influences the actions of digitalis. Both the toxic and contractile actions of digitalis are increased when the glycoside is given in the presence of hypokalemia, and these actions are reduced when the glycoside is administered during hyperkalemia. The relation between potassium and the digitalis contractile action was recently examined in isolated, supported cat papillary muscles. The linear dose-to-contractile response curve for acetyl strophanthidin added to the muscle bath with an extracellular potassium concentration of 3.5 mM. was markedly depressed when the drug was added to an extracellular bath of 7.0 mM. potassium concentration, showing that digitalis inotropic stimulation is attenuated by pretreatment with potassium. In contrast, increasing the extracellular potassium concentration in the muscle bath, from 3.5 to 7.0 mM., after pretreatment with digitalis did not alter the force of cardiac muscle contraction. From these and related observations, potassium and digitalis seem to compete for myocardial binding sites. But potassium is bound to the myocardium relatively loosely, and it delays subsequent digitalis binding. In contrast, digitalis is firmly bound to myocardial receptors, and thus potassium has little effect on glycoside already attached to the heart before potassium is administered. Translated into the clinical setting, alterations in serum potassium effected before treatment with digitalis have marked influences on the toxic and contractile actions of the glycoside. But potassium has relatively little influence on the toxic and contractile effects of digitalis when it is given after the glycoside has been taken up by the heart.

Radioimmunoassay. One of the most important advances in clinical digitalis pharmacology has been the recent development of the radioimmunoassy method for measuring glycoside concentrations. Since the original development of the immunologic methods for measuring digoxin concentration, the radioimmunoassay has become available for routine clinical use in many medical centers. The digoxin assay is based on competition between serum nonradioactive digoxin and a constant amount of tritiated digoxin for a constant number of digoxin-antibody binding sites. Since nonradioactive digoxin interferes with tritiated digoxin binding, radioactive digoxin-bound antibody is reduced with higher concentrations of serum digoxin, measured by a liquid scintillation counter. The precise concentration of serum digoxin is then determined from a standard curve.

Patients on from 0.25 mg. to 0.50 mg. oral maintenance digoxin daily, without toxicity, usually have therapeutic concentrations of from 1 to 2 nanograms per ml. serum, whereas approximately 90 per cent of patients with electrical toxicity have levels above 2 nanograms per ml. Although the range of overlap between nontoxicity and toxicity is 1.5 to 3.0 nanograms per ml., it is generally prudent to discontinue digoxin therapy in patients with levels above 2 nanograms per ml. until the serum level falls below this concentration. But patients with atrial fibrillation, who require more than 0.50 mg. digoxin daily for rate control, seem to be relatively insensitive to development of toxicity, and they may have levels of more than 2 nanograms per ml. Other conditions in which digitalis dosage may be increased include hyperthyroidism, impaired intestinal absorption in malabsorption syndromes, infancy, altered digitoxin metabolism, and rare instances of digitalis antibodies. On the other hand, there is increased sensitivity to toxicity in ischemic and primary myocardial disease, hypothyroidism, hypoxia, hypokalemia, hypomagnesemia, hypercalcemia, and alkalosis. There is considerable variation in the biologic availability of oral digoxin tablets produced by different manufacturers. Digoxin serum concentrations varied widely after ingestion of different brands containing the same digoxin content, which indicated nonequivalent absorption because of differing product formulation, leading to unequal disintegration and dissolution rates. Lanoxin is now recognized to be the digoxin brand providing uniform and optimal potency.

Electrophysiologic Effects. The influences of digitalis on the electrophysiologic properties of heart muscle are complex. These effects vary considerably with dose, type of cardiac tissue involved, and autonomic activity. In diastole during intracellular negativity, excitability is raised by the reduced resting potential. Also in diastole, digitalis stimulates automaticity, thereby enhancing subsidiary ectopic pacemakers. In the process of depolarization, the rate of rise of the action potential determining conduction velocity is diminished by digitalis, particularly in the atrioventricular node, thereby leading to various degrees of heart block. Since the speed of depolarization is directly related to the level of resting membrane potential, digitalis depresses membrane responsiveness. The reduction of conduction velocity in the atrioventricular node by digitalis is of major therapeutic significance for slowing the rapid ventricular rate in atrial fibrillation and, thereby, furthering decremental conduction and increasing the functional refractory period of the atrioventricular node. The repolarization process is altered by digitalis, and thus the duration of the action potential in cardiac tissues is shortened, leading to decrease in refractoriness in myocardial conductive fibers which, in the ventricles, is seen in the narrowing of the QT interval on the surface electrocardiogram. The effects of digitalis on conduction velocity and the refractory period underlie the drug's provocation of re-entrant tachyarrhythmias.

Treatment of Digitalis Toxicity. Although

glycoside toxicity can be reversed with digitalis antibodies clinically, no practical specific antidote is currently available for the too common problem of digitalis intoxication in patients. But special advantages pertain to the use of potassium, phenytoin, lidocaine, propranolol, bretylium, and cardiac pacing. Although, in experimental animals, the administration of potassium or antiarrhythmic drugs after the onset of electrical toxicity can suppress digitalis-induced tachyarrhythmias, the accumulated dose of digitalis at which these arrhythmias become refractory and fatal is not increased by this treatment. Similarly, in dogs, ventricular overdrive pacing, begun at the onset of ouabain-provoked tachyarrhythmias, can transiently overcome these rhythm disorders, but the maximum tolerated dose of ouabain before death was not altered in comparison with that in control animals receiving digitalis in the same manner. In clinical practice, however, digitalis is discontinued at the onset of toxicity, and antiarrhythmic measures are employed to suppress ectopic activity until the glycoside is excreted or metabolized.

A clinical problem in the use of countershock to electively convert supraventricular arrhythmias has been that life-threatening ventricular arrhythmias attributable to digitalis may be provoked by electrical discharge, even without prior digitalis toxicity. In this case, the amount of discharge energy required to produce ventricular tachycardia is reduced in the digitalized heart. Thus some clinicians have reduced or withdrawn maintenance digitalis before the use of electroconversion. In contrast, our approach is to continue the drug therapy because of the risk of exacerbating heart failure and developing a rapid ventricular rate before cardioversion and to use small amounts of electrical energy at the time of electroshock. The frequency of ventricular tachyarrhythmias after electroconversion of supraventricular arrhythmias in the presence of digitalis can be reduced, if the shock energy is at the lowest level necessary to achieve conversion. This is done by using initially small, incrementally increasing energy levels of countershock for restoring sinus rhythm and using lidocaine to suppress any premature ventricular contractions occurring with direct current shock.

Isoproterenol

The powerful sympathomimetic isoproterenol sometimes is useful in refractory heart failure. Stimulation of contractility and heart rate by the agent is produced by its direct action on beta-adrenergic receptors in the heart. The maximal inotropic effect of isoproterenol usually exceeds that of digitalis prior to the onset of toxicity. Furthermore, the elevation of cardiac output at comparable levels of enhanced contractility is greater with isoproterenol than with digitalis, as the catecholamine produces direct vasodilation by its stimulation of beta receptors in the peripheral arteriolar beds. The influence of isoproterenol on blood pressures varies. When the diseased ventricle is relatively unable to improve its depressed contractile state, the drug produces only a small rise in cardiac output relative to a greater decline in peripheral vascular resistance; therefore there may be a tendency for blood pressure to decrease. Since isoproterenol reduces systemic resistance to left ventricular ejection, it may be of special benefit when mitral regurgitation complicates severe cardiomyopathies. Isoproterenol has been more useful in chronic refractory heart failure from causes other than coronary artery disease. The agent is given by slow intravenous drip for several hours at an initial rate of 1 to 3 micrograms per minute. Isoproterenol must be administered cautiously because of the rapid heart rate, ventricular tachyarrhythmias, and hypotension that the agent may provoke. In our experience, it has been a valuable agent in the recovery of patients with the low cardiac output syndrome after cardiac surgery. In addition, for patients with aortic stenosis who have delayed corrective surgery too long, isoproterenol has been useful in causing sufficient reduction of considerably elevated blood urea nitrogen resulting from markedly lowered cardiac output, to allow for safer performance of cardiac catheterization and valve replacement. Isoproterenol may also provide temporary improvement of impaired organ perfusion in chronic cardiomyopathies.

Dopamine

The biologic precursor of norepinephrine, dopamine, possesses certain advantages compared to isoproterenol; therefore our current choice is dopamine over isoproterenol. The beta receptor–stimulating property of dopamine exerts a positive inotropic effect, and there is mild reduction of total peripheral vascular resistance. Dopamine acts somewhat similarly to epinephrine, with elevation of cardiac output and a directional change of arteriolar resistance intermediate between that of the vasodilation of isoproterenol and the vasoconstriction induced by norepinephrine. In addition, dopamine possesses the beneficial effect of direct, non-beta receptor–mediated renal vasodilation. Dopamine is administered slowly by intravenous drip at an initial rate of 2 to 5 micrograms per kg. per minute. Epinephrine can be given in the same manner at an initial rate of 1 to 2 micrograms per minute. To obtain the desired effects on cardiac output and blood pressure, the simultaneous use of dopamine with isoproterenol, or of phentolamine with dopamine or norepinephrine, may be more effective than any single agent.

Other Cardiotonic Agents

The recently synthesized sympathomimetic agent dobutamine possesses the advantage of relatively selective myocardial beta receptor stimulation, which produces substantial positive inotropic effect with little influence on peripheral vascular resistance and heart rate. In our experience, glucagon has not been useful in patients with chronic refractory congestive heart failure. Aminophylline exerts a positive inotropic action by its influence on the intracellular beta-sympathomimetic pathway; the agent inhibits the enzyme phosphodiesterase that deactivates cyclic AMP, thereby prolonging the action of cyclic AMP within the myocardial cell. Aminophylline sometimes is useful clinically to augment the positive inotropic effects of sympathomimetic agents.

A unique, although still investigational, approach in the therapy of ventricular dysfunction has been provided by a new class of positive inotropic compounds, termed ionophores, which alter the permeability of cardiac cell membranes. These agents augment cardiac contractility through enhanced calcium delivery to the contractile proteins by increasing transport of calcium ions into the cell and by releasing calcium intracellularly. The ionophores are microbial metabolites that concentrate in the lipid of cell membranes, where they form ionophore-cation complexes, thereby serving as mobile cation carriers across the membrane surface. In experimental studies, the intravenous administration of the calcium ionophore RO 2-2985 (X537A), an antibiotic produced from a Streptomyces strain, has been shown to result in a sustained, marked increase in myocardial contractility and cardiac output, accompanied by a rise in systemic arterial pressure with little or no change in systemic vascular resistance and heart rate. Considerable attention presently is focused on the therapeutic potential of calcium ionophores in the therapy of heart failure and cardiogenic shock.

Electrical Modalities

Electrical methods to improve cardiac pump function include cardioversion of tachyarrhythmias and pacemaker catheters in sinus bradycardia and complete heart block. Restoration of atrial transport after electroconversion of atrial fibrillation may substantially improve ventricular preload and cardiac output, particularly in hypertrophic cardiomyopathies, coronary artery disease, and systolic ventricular pressure overloading. Although it is difficult to maintain normal sinus rhythm with pressure or volume increase in the left atrium, elective atrial fibrillation electroconversion should be attempted in chronic CHF. Occasionally, even short periods of sinus rhythm are associated with reduction in heart failure, even if atrial fibrillation recurs. Elective defibrillation can be carried out safely without inducing digitalis toxicity when the patient is receiving therapeutic doses of glycoside by using initially small incremental levels of countershock.

Systemic Vasodilators

In the clinical management of acute and chronic CHF, systemic vasodilators constitute a new approach through their reduction of elevated left ventricular wall tension during systole (ventricular afterload) by decreasing aortic impedance and/or by diminishing venous return to the heart. Thus the agents may result in elevation of lowered cardiac output by reducing peripheral vascular resistance and/or in decline of increased ventricular end-diastolic volume (ventricular preload) by lowering venous tone. In addition, these agents cause concomitant reduction in myocardial oxygen requirements, of special importance in ischemic heart disease.

Nitroglycerin, Nitroprusside, and Phentolamine. The vasodilators used most commonly—nitroglycerin (sublingual, 0.4 mg.), nitroprusside (intravenous, 75 micrograms per minute; range, 25 to 125 micrograms), and phentolamine (intravenous, 1.3 mg. per minute; range, 0.75 to 2.0 mg.)—produce disparate modifications of cardiac function by their differing alterations of preload versus impedance, which are dependent upon their relative effects on systemic resistance and capacitance vessels characteristic of each agent. (This use of nitroprusside and phentolamine is not listed in the manufacturer's official directive.) In this regard, nitroglycerin principally acts on veins and phentolamine on arterioles, whereas nitroprusside has a balanced vasodilator effect on the venous and arteriolar beds. Translated to cardiac function, nitroglycerin lowers elevated ventricular end-diastolic pressure (relieves pulmonary congestion) without raising cardiac output, whereas nitroprusside reduces end-diastolic pressure while increasing depressed cardiac output, and phentolamine raises lowered cardiac output to a greater degree than elevated end-diastolic pressure is reduced, provided that left ventricular end-diastolic pressure is not diminished below the upper limits of normal (12 mm. Hg). In addition, it should be pointed out that nitroprusside is of special advantage in mitral regurgitation and in aortic regurgitation, because the agent not only improves forward cardiac output while lowering elevated end-diastolic pressure, but also reduces the regurgitant fraction. The same is the case with ventricular septal defect in which the agent reduces the magnitude of left-to-right shunt, while concomitantly raising cardiac output and lowering end-diastolic pressure.

Nitroprusside and Dopamine. The use of certain positive inotropic agents in conjunction with the systemic vasodilator drugs is of special value in the treatment of acute and chronic congestive heart failure. Thus vasodilator drugs and inotropic agents are capable of augmenting cardiac function by unrelated but complementary actions. In this regard we have found the combined intravenous application of nitroprusside (70 micrograms per minute) and dopamine (6 micrograms per kg. per minute) to be especially beneficial clinically in a variety of types of cardiac disease with congestive heart failure. Thereby a synergistic effect is achieved in which low cardiac output is considerably raised while elevated left ventricular end-diastolic pressure is markedly reduced, more so than with either agent administered separately.

Nitroprusside and Counterpulsation. In left ventricular pump failure caused by acute coronary heart disease, a potential hazard of systemic vasodilation is reduction in coronary perfusion pressure consequent to decline in aortic diastolic pressure. Thus further reduction of coronary blood flow may extend the area of myocardial ischemia and necrosis with resultant additional left ventricular pump dysfunction. Aortic diastolic pressure augmentation provided by intra-aortic balloon pumping or external counterpulsation, coupled with the system vasodilator action of nitroprusside, allows improvement of coronary diastolic perfusion concomitant with reduction in ventricular outflow impedance. This combination of therapeutic modalities offers decided hemodynamic and cardiac metabolic advantages in the particularly difficult condition of left ventricular failure in acute myocardial infarction with normal, or even reduced, systolic blood pressure.

Long-Acting Nitrates. The sublingual and oral long-acting nitrates are also useful in the management of acute coronary patients with unstable angina, and in the therapy of left ventricular dysfunction resulting from myocardial infarction or from several types of chronic congestive heart failure. Impressive hemodynamic benefit results for approximately 4 to 5 hours following the sublingual or oral administration of isosorbide dinitrate, similar to but more prolonged than the 15 to 30 minute action of sublingual nitroglycerin. In addition, cutaneous nitroglycerin ointment provides sustained actions similar to those of the oral long-acting nitrates. Thus the long-acting nitrates reduce myocardial oxygen needs with decline in anginal symptoms, as well as relieving pulmonary congestion by diminishing elevated left ventricular end-diastolic pressure, usually without affecting cardiac output.

Consistent with these observations is that peripheral venodilation occurs following oral sustained-release nitroglycerin, and abolition of pulmonary edema in consort with prolonged lowering of increased ventricular preload is induced by oral controlled-release nitroglycerin (Nitro-Bid, 6.5 mg. nitroglycerin capsules). In addition, we have observed sublingual nitroglycerin, 0.4 mg., to reduce myocardial ischemia in patients with acute myocardial infarction as estimated by the multiple 35-electrocardiographic lead precordial blanket and in patients with coronary stenoses as judged by measurements of coronary blood flow, myocardial oxygen extraction, and consumption indices, provided that coronary perfusion pressure is maintained within the normal range. It should be emphasized that the short- and long-acting nitrates do not consistently decrease peripheral vascular resistance, and in this respect they are not useful in improving low cardiac output. However, the nitrates are efficacious as antianginal agents and in the relief of pulmonary congestion, thereby providing a unique means for extending in-hospital vasodilator therapy to chronic outpatient management.

Hydralazine and Prazosin. Most recently, the ability to utilize impedance reduction therapy in the chronic outpatient management of congestive heart failure has been provided by the demonstration that orally administered hydralazine* (50 to 75 mg. four times daily) or prazosin (Minipress)* (2 to 6 mg. four times daily) causes long-lasting systemic arteriolar dilation, thereby raising lowered cardiac output. In our experience the two agents have different actions on the peripheral circulation. Thus hydralazine produces only systemic arteriolar dilation, whereas prazosin causes systemic vasodilation of both the arteriolar and venous systems. Thereby ingested prazosin alone acts like intravenous nitroprusside but with the duration of effect of the former being considerably more sustained, whereas the combination of ingested hydralazine with a long-lasting nitrate would be required to achieve a persistent nitroprusside-like effect.

---

*This use of this agent is not listed in the manufacturer's official directive.

Sodium Restriction

Salt restriction is usually not required in early or mild heart failure, as diuretic agents with digitalis suffice. More advanced CHF, however, does require sodium restriction in the range of 2 grams of sodium (5 grams of salt) per day. In severe CHF, it is necessary to restrict sodium to 1 gram per day, often limiting daily water intake to below 1 liter, with the use of maximum diuretic therapy. Under these circumstances, salt restriction reduces preload by decreasing circulating blood volume and may also diminish afterload by decreasing blood pressure.

Diuretics

Although it may be difficult to correct the basic defect in refractory heart failure by improving depressed contractile state, usually it is possible to mobilize excessive body salt and fluid accumulation by rational selection of diuretic agents. The development of the potent oral diuretic drugs (chlorothiazide, ethacrynic acid, furosemide, and spironolactone) in the past decade has greatly enhanced the ease and success of relieving relatively intractable circulatory congestion.

Thiazides. Modern diuretic therapy begins with oral thiazides. These agents interfere with dilution of urine (inhibiting free water formation) in the ascending loop of Henle and distal tubule by preventing reabsorption of sodium, chloride, and potassium, with resultant excretion of these ions with water. Hydrochlorothiazide (50 mg.) or chlorothiazide (500 mg.) is administered once or twice daily.

Aldosterone Antagonists. If the thiazides prove inadequate, an oral aldosterone antagonist should be added. Either spironolactone (Aldactone, 25 mg. four times daily) or triamterene (100 mg. daily) is the agent used. The aldosterone antagonists inhibit the exchange of potassium for sodium in the distal tubules that is produced by aldosterone, excreting sodium while potassium is retained. The aldosterone inhibitors are less powerful than the thiazides, ethacrynic acid, and furosemide, but they promote considerable natriuresis when administered daily for several weeks. An aldosterone antagonist combined with a thiazide makes potassium supplementation hazardous.

Loop Diuretics. If the combination of chlorothiazide with spironolactone or triamterene is unsuccessful, one of the most potent oral diuretics, ethacrynic acid (Edecrin), 50 to 100 mg. once or twice daily, or furosemide (Lasix), 20 to 80 mg. once or twice daily, is substituted for the thiazide. These newer agents, ethacrynic acid and furosemide, block sodium transport from the ascending loop of Henle, thereby interfering with urinary concentrating ability by rendering the renal medullary interstitium less hypertonic for water reabsorption in the collecting ducts. These loop diuretics also possess the thiazide action of inhibiting the dilution of urine in the ascending loop of Henle and the distal tubules. In some refractory conditions, initiation of diuresis appears to be aided by beginning ethacrynic acid (50 mg.) or furosemide (40 mg.) therapy by the intravenous route.

Organomercurials. Although the organomercurials remain useful and powerful diuretics that inhibit isosmotic reabsorption of salt and water in the proximal and distal tubules, they must be given intramuscularly to be effective. For potent diuresis in resistant congestion there no longer is need for the complex combined regimen of acidifying chlorides, carbonic anhydrase inhibitors (to prevent proximal tubular urine acidification, thereby inhibiting exchange of hydrogen for sodium and reducing sodium reabsorption), mercurials, and aminophylline (to increase renal blood flow).

Cardiac Homotransplantation and the Artificial Heart

In patients with ischemic or primary cardiomyopathies who develop chronic end-stage congestive heart failure that is truly refractory to the judicious use of all medical measures, and in whom a palliative operation is not applicable, it is not imprudent to consider the possibility of cardiac homotransplantation in carefully selected patients at medical centers highly experienced with this procedure. However, cardiac homotransplantation is quite restricted in availability and also limited in success. Mechanical cardiac assist devices have not been useful in the management of chronic heart failure, although such devices have provided at least temporary benefit in the treatment of severe cardiac dysfunction caused by acute myocardial infarction. The major inroads in the management of absolutely intractable myocardial failure incompatible with life in chronic coronary heart disease and the cardiomyopathies must await the development of a successful permanently implantable artificial heart.

Acknowledgments

This work was supported in part by Research Program Project Grant HL 14780 from the National Heart, Lung and Blood Institute, NIH, Bethesda, Maryland, and by Research Grants from California Chapters of the American Heart Association, Dallas, Texas. The author gratefully acknowledges the technical assistance of Leslie J. Silvernail.

INFECTIVE ENDOCARDITIS

method of
W. MICHAEL SCHELD, M.D.,
and MERLE A. SANDE, M.D.
Charlottesville, Virginia

The clinical spectrum of infective endocarditis has witnessed a gradual evolution since the advent of antibiotic therapy. The older classification of "acute" (a fulminant illness usually caused by staphylococci, pneumococci, gonococci, or group A beta-hemolytic streptococci) and "subacute" (a more protracted illness usually caused by the "viridans" streptococci) endocarditis has been gradually supplanted by a classification based on the causative organism, with its implications of appropriate antimicrobial therapy. The clinical syndrome has changed with an increase in elderly patients, and the special problems of endocarditis in heroin addicts and prosthetic valve endocarditis have emerged.

Infective endocarditis is an uncommon infectious disease, accounting for 0.3 to 3.0 cases per 1000 hospital admissions, but morbidity and mortality remain high. Fifty-four to 69 per cent of patients are males, and approximately half of all patients are over 50 years old. Rheumatic heart disease is present in 40 to 60 per cent of the patients (with involvement of the mitral valve in greater than 85 per cent), and congenital heart disease in 7 to 16 per cent; no diagnosable cause of heart disease can be determined in 20 to 40 per cent of the patients, although most are probably degenerative in origin. A slight increase in aortic and tricuspid involvement, with a corresponding decrease in mitral involvement, has been noted. Fever is almost invariably present and is remittent; murmurs are present in more than 85 per cent of cases, but the classic "changing" murmur is rare; major embolic phenomena occur in about one third; and neurologic and renal manifestations are frequent.

Streptococci and staphylococci cause 90 to 95 per cent of cases of infective endocarditis; the most common organisms are the "viridans" group of streptococci (30 to 40 per cent), enterococci (10 per cent), "other" streptococci (20 to 30 per cent), *Staphylococcus aureus* (9 to 27 per cent), *Staphylococcus epidermidis* (1 to 3 per cent), and gram-negative aerobic bacilli (1 to 5 per cent). Fungal and diphtheroid endocarditis are rare but require special therapy.

An animal model of endocarditis, utilizing rabbits, has been developed and has contributed to our understanding of the pathogenesis, therapy, and regimens of prophylaxis for this disease.

Principles of Therapy

Since the metabolic state of the organisms within the vegetation is low and a leukocytic response is minimal, infective endocarditis represents an example of an infection in an area of impaired host resistance. Therefore the cardinal rule of therapy is to use bactericidal antibiotics by the parenteral route for prolonged periods of time. Failure to do so may result in uncontrolled infection, increased complications, relapse, and/or death.

Four to five blood cultures obtained over a period of several hours, each 10 ml. and incubated aerobically and anaerobically for 3 weeks, should be obtained prior to the institution of antimicrobial therapy in "subacute" cases. In more emergent circumstances, three blood cultures taken over an hour prior to therapy should suffice. It is essential to isolate the infecting organism, because specific treatment is based on the sensitivity of the bacteria to antimicrobial agents. Tube dilution sensitivities of the isolate and minimum bactericidal concentrations (MBC's) should be obtained, as the Kirby-Bauer disc sensitivity may be misleading. The serum bactericidal test is an excellent gauge of the antibacterial activity obtained with the antimicrobial agent. Levels of 1:8 or greater have correlated well with successful treatment. It is wise to monitor antibiotic levels in patients with renal insufficiency, especially if aminoglycosides are used. Anticoagulants are contraindicated, and corrections for the large cation loads administered with high dose penicillin therapy (approximately 130 mEq. Na for 30 grams carbenicillin, for example) may be necessary.

Specific Infections (All Dosages Are for Adults)

Penicillin-Sensitive Streptococcal Endocarditis (e.g., minimum inhibitory concentration (MIC) 0.1 microgram or less). Our recommendation is based on the New York Hospital–Cornell Medical Center experience, in which 100 cases of penicillin-sensitive streptococcal endocarditis were treated without a relapse. The regimen is as follows: aqueous penicillin G, 10 to 20 million units intravenously daily, *or* procaine penicillin G, 1.2 million units intramuscularly every 6 hours for 4 weeks, combined with streptomycin, 0.5 gram intramuscularly every 12 hours for the first 2 weeks. In the penicillin-allergic patient, cephalothin, 2 grams intravenously every 4 hours, *or* cefazolin, 1 to 2 grams intramuscularly every 6 hours, combined with streptomycin 0.5 gram intramuscularly every 12 hours for the first 2 weeks *or* vancomycin, 0.5 gram intravenously every 6 hours for 4 weeks, is appropriate therapy. High doses of penicillin alone for 4 weeks is standard therapy in many medical centers and may be nearly as effective as the combination. Therefore in elderly patients with a high risk to develop streptomycin ototoxicity, the streptomycin can be dropped.

Penicillin-Resistant Streptococcal Endocarditis (e.g., penicillin MIC greater than 0.1 microgram per ml.). Enterococci are the third most common cause of bacterial endocarditis and demonstrate variable sensitivity to penicillin (MIC range, 1.6 to 6.2 micrograms per ml.). Synergy between penicillin and streptomycin is demonstrable for approximately 60 per cent of strains in vitro. Most consultants recommend a total treatment regimen encompassing 6 weeks. Our recommendation is aqueous penicillin G, 20 million units intravenously daily for 6 weeks, combined with streptomycin, 1 gram intramuscularly every 12 hours for the first 2 weeks, followed by 0.5 gram intramuscularly every 12 hours for the final 4 weeks. Although 40 per cent of enterococci are highly resistant to streptomycin (MIC >2000 micrograms per ml.) and are sensitive to gentamicin in vitro, the aforementioned regimen will cure over 80 per cent of all patients. In vitro and in animal models a combination of penicillin plus gentamicin is superior to penicillin and streptomycin against these highly resistant strains. However, greater efficacy of the penicillin-gentamicin combination over the standard penicillin-streptomycin regimen remains unproved in patients. In penicillin-allergic patients, vancomycin, 0.5 gram intravenously every 6 hours for 6 weeks, is appropriate therapy; many authorities would combine this with an aminoglycoside, but renal toxicity may be additive.

Staphylococcal Endocarditis. The mortality in this disease still approaches 50 per cent. The preferred regimen incorporates a penicillinase-resistant penicillin (nafcillin, methicillin, or oxacillin, 2 grams intravenously every 4 hours) or a cephalosporin (cephalothin, 2 grams intravenously every 4 hours, or cefazolin, 1 to 2 grams intramuscularly every 6 hours) given for 6 weeks. The addition of gentamicin has been demonstrated to be synergistic in the animal model, and a multicenter cooperative study in patients is in progress. If the organism is sensitive to penicillin (MIC <0.1 microgram per ml.), penicillin G, 20 million units intravenously daily, may be substituted. In penicillin-allergic patients, vancomycin, 0.5 gram intravenously every 6 hours for 6 weeks, is alternative therapy. With methicillin-resistant strains (especially *Staphylococcus epidermidis*), a cephalosporin or vancomycin may be used.

Unusual Bacterial Causes. In pneumococcal, meningococcal, or gonococcal endocarditis, aqueous penicillin G, 20 million units intravenously per day, should be administered for 4 weeks. If endocarditis is caused by an aerobic gram-negative bacillus, full in vitro testing is necessary, and full doses of a penicillin or cephalosporin (as above) combined with gentamicin, 1.0 to 1.7 mg. per kg. intramuscularly every 8 hours, is necessary for 4 weeks. In Pseudomonas endocarditis, carbenicillin, 500 mg. per kg. intravenously every 4 hours, plus gentamicin is suggested. Anaerobic endocarditis is rare, but the mortality rate is high; the mainstay of therapy is penicillin G, 20 million units intravenously per day for 4 weeks. This may be combined with clindamycin, 450 mg. intravenously every 6 hours, or chloramphenicol sodium succinate, 1 gram intravenously every 6 hours.

Fungal Endocarditis. The most common causes of fungal endocarditis are Candida, Aspergillus, and Histoplasma. Although blood cultures are usually positive in Candida endocarditis, they are usually negative with the latter two agents. Large, friable vegetations often lead to large systemic emboli, and the diagnosis may be made by culture and histologic study of resected emboli. Surgery is often required in these patients. Antimicrobial therapy consists of amphotericin B, 0.5 mg. per kg. intravenously per day for at least 6 weeks. Amphotericin B may be associated with fever, chills, nausea, vomiting, phlebitis, bone marrow depression, nephrotoxicity, renal tubular acidosis, hypokalemia, and anorexia. The addition of 5-fluorocytosine, 150 mg. per kg. orally per day, may be advisable in these difficult cases, but surgery is usually required for cure.

Prosthetic Valve Endocarditis. This is a devastating complication of prosthetic valve replacement and occurs in 2 to 4 per cent of such patients. The most common organisms are staphylococci (especially *S. epidermidis*), diphtheroids, streptococci, micrococci, gram-negative aerobic bacilli, and fungi (chiefly Candida and Aspergillus spp.). The mortality rate remains high, approximately 60 per cent, and is highest for "early" (less than 2 months postoperatively) endocarditis. The aortic valve is most frequently involved, and newer tests (echocardiography, cinefluoroscopy, and phonocardiography) may aid in diagnosis and management. It is of note that gram-negative bacteremia in the "early" postoperative period may not reflect endocarditis, and a vigorous search should be undertaken for a source of infection. We recommend a minimum of 6 weeks of parenteral bactericidal antimicrobial therapy, usually consisting initially of cephalothin, 2 grams intravenously every 4 hours, plus aqueous penicillin G, 20 million units intravenously per day, plus streptomycin, 0.5 gram intramuscularly every 12 hours, until results of in vitro susceptibility are available. Vancomycin, 0.5 gram intravenously every 6 hours, may be substituted in the penicillin-allergic patient, in combination with streptomycin, 0.5 gram intramuscularly every 12 hours, or gentamicin, 1.7 mg. per kg. intramuscularly every 8 hours. The value of prolonged oral therapy after completion of parenteral therapy remains unproved, and we do not recommend its use. If absolutely necessary, anticoagulants can be continued, but the prothrombin time should be monitored carefully. In selected patients with poor prognostic features (nonstreptococcal cause, new regurgitant murmur, or significant heart failure), early valve replacement is mandatory. Some authorities recommend prompt valve replacement for all patients except those with favorable prognostic signs ("late" streptococcal "viridans" endocarditis, highly sensitive to penicillin, and with no complications).

Endocarditis in Addicts Who Use Narcotics Intravenously. The most common causative organisms in this group are *Staphylococcus aureus,* gram-negative aerobic bacilli, and Candida. Right-sided involvement is common, with frequent embolic manifestations (infarct, septic pneumonia, abscesses) in the pulmonary tree. Treatment should include the regimen specific for the causative organism.

Culture-Negative Endocarditis. Although reported as high as 7 to 28 per cent in some series, our experience is that culture-negative cases represent less than 5 per cent of all cases of endocarditis. We recommend therapy as outlined for enterococcal endocarditis, above.

Surgical Management

The indications for surgical replacement of the infected valve are as follows: refractory heart failure, more than one serious systemic embolic episode, valve dysfunction, uncontrolled infection, recurrent relapses, or no available effective regimen (i.e., fungal endocarditis). The indications for surgery in prosthetic valve endocarditis are somewhat broader, and prompt valve replacement may be necessary in up to 70 per cent of these patients (see above).

Prophylaxis of Infective Endocarditis

Although the optimal approach to prophylaxis is the correction of the underlying cardiac defect that predisposes to infection, this is seldom accomplished; therefore measures to reduce the bacteremia burden after invasive procedures are employed. General principles include maintenance of good oral hygiene, avoidance of intravascular catheters, and vigorous therapy of other infections. The 1972 recommendations on prophylaxis by the American Heart Association have been called into question by recent work in the experimental model of endocarditis which demonstrates that high blood levels of an effective antimicrobial agent must be maintained for at least 6 hours after the initiation of the bacteremic episode.

Although minor modifications are possible before publication in the fall of 1977, the following summarizes the new recommendations of the American Heart Association for prevention of bacterial endocarditis. Prophylaxis is recommended for patients with most types of congenital heart disease (with the exception of uncomplicated secundum atrial septal defect), rheumatic or other acquired valvular heart disease, idiopathic hypertrophic subaortic stenosis, mitral valve prolapse syndrome if clinical evidence of mitral insufficiency is present, and prosthetic heart valves. The dosages assume normal renal function, and the timing of doses for children is the same as for adults.

The recommendations are as follows:

1. For all dental procedures which are likely to result in gingival bleeding (including surgery or instrumentation of the upper respiratory tract): For adults, use *either* aqueous penicillin G, 1,000,000 units intramuscularly, mixed with procaine penicillin G, 600,000 units intramuscularly, alone *or* with the addition of streptomycin, 1.0 gram intramuscularly (the addition of streptomycin is particularly recommended for patients with prosthetic cardiac valves), *or* phenoxymethyl penicillin, 2 grams orally, given 30 to 60 minutes prior to the procedure. Each of the three possible regimens is followed by phenoxymethyl penicillin, 500 mg. orally every 6 hours for eight doses. In penicillin-allergic patients, use vancomycin, 1.0 gram intravenously 30 to 60 minutes prior to the procedure, *or* erythromycin, 1.0 gram orally 90 to 120 minutes prior to the procedure; both are followed by erythromycin, 500 mg. orally every 6 hours for eight doses. For children, *either* aqueous penicillin G, 30,000 units per kg. intramuscularly, mixed with procaine penicillin G, 600,000 units intramuscularly, alone *or* with the addition of streptomycin, 20 mg. per kg. intramuscularly, *or* phenoxymethyl penicillin, 2.0 grams orally. Again, each is followed by phenoxymethyl penicillin orally (in children under 60 lbs., use 250 mg. orally every 6 hours for eight doses). In the penicillin-allergic patient, use erythromycin, 20 mg. per kg. orally, followed by 10 mg. per kg. orally every 6 hours for eight doses.

2. For genitourinary tract and gastrointestinal tract surgery or instrumentation: For adults, aqueous penicillin G, 2,000,000 units intramuscularly or intravenously, *or* ampicillin, 1.0 gram intramuscularly or intravenously, *with* the addition of either streptomycin, 1.0 gram intramuscularly, *or* gentamicin, 1.5 mg. per kg. (not to exceed 80 mg.) intramuscularly or intra-

venously, given 30 to 60 minutes prior to the procedure, followed by the same regimen every 8 hours (if gentamicin is used) or every 12 hours (if streptomycin is used) for two additional doses. In penicillin-allergic patients, use vancomycin, 1.0 gram intravenously, *plus* streptomycin, 1.0 gram intramuscularly, 30 to 60 minutes prior to the procedure and repeat in 12 hours. For children, use aqueous penicillin G, 30,000 units intramuscularly or intravenously, *or* ampicillin, 50 mg. per kg. intramuscularly or intravenously, with the addition of either streptomycin, 20 mg. per kg. intramuscularly, *or* gentamicin, 2.0 mg. per kg. intramuscularly or intravenously. In the penicillin-allergic patient, use vancomycin, 20 mg. per kg. intravenously, *plus* streptomycin, 20 mg. per kg. intramuscularly. Timing of doses for children is the same as for adults.

3. For cardiac surgery: Use a penicillinase-resistant penicillin (e.g., nafcillin, methicillin, or oxacillin) *or* cephalothin, 2 grams intravenously, 30 to 60 minutes prior to surgery and repeated at 4 hour intervals for up to 3 days.

Prophylaxis directed primarily against *S. aureus* (a penicillinase-resistant penicillin) is also indicated for patients undergoing surgery on any infected or contaminated tissue. Patients who have had a documented previous episode of endocarditis, even in the absence of clinically detectable heart disease, should receive the appropriate prophylactic regimen when undergoing any of the procedures outlined above. Prophylaxis is not routinely suggested for cardiac catheterization or angiography, uncomplicated vaginal delivery, barium enema, or sigmoidoscopy.

HYPERTENSION

method of
MICHAEL A. WEBER, M.D.,
and JOHN H. LARAGH, M.D.
New York, New York

Our approach to the treatment of hypertension has changed markedly in the last 10 to 15 years. Perhaps the main spur to our now more aggressive intervention in hypertensive disease has been the realization that this condition not only is exceptionally common but also is probably the major factor in the genesis of most forms of cardiovascular disease. It is now clearly documented that hypertensive patients are far more likely than their normotensive counterparts to suffer from strokes, ischemic heart disease, or heart failure, and to be more susceptible to peripheral vascular disease and renal impairment. These findings help explain what has long been known to life insurance actuaries: that patients with untreated hypertension have substantially reduced life expectancies.

The magnitude of the challenge in treating this condition on a wide basis is emphasized by epidemiologic surveys which, depending on the criteria used, have estimated that between 12 and 25 per cent of the adult population have elevated levels of blood pressure. In the practice of the average physician concerned with primary care medicine, approximately a quarter of all patients seen have hypertension as a primary problem or at least in association with some other condition.

An important breakthrough in our attitudes toward the treatment of hypertension has been stimulated by the growing evidence that treatment of hypertension clearly lowers the incidence of cardiovascular diseases. Until fairly recently, many physicians were loath to treat their asymptomatic hypertensive patients, because the relatively severe side effects of the then available antihypertensive medications made it difficult to justify a treatment program with as yet unproved benefits. But the advent of a large array of effective and more palatable medications during the last decade, together with the realization that the treatment of patients with established hypertension is clearly mandated, has provided the physician with the tools and the incentive to tackle this important task.

When to Treat

In the past, it was customary to withhold antihypertensive treatment until patients developed definite stigmata of hypertension or presented with a major cardiovascular complication. But now, the treatment of hypertension has become a constructive exercise in preventive medicine. We know that young hypertensive patients, even with only mild elevations of blood pressure and without any objective signs of cardiovascular damage, are at increased risk of heart disease, stroke, and renal failure, and may anticipate a reduced life span. Potentially, therefore, it is the young, mildly hypertensive patient who has not yet been affected by cardiovascular complications who has most to gain from the physician's early intervention.

We do not yet have available to us the data that would allow us to stipulate a specific blood pressure level at which treatment should be started. The Veterans Administration Cooperative Study showed that treatment of patients with diastolic blood pressures of over 104 mm. Hg conferred clear benefits in reducing the incidence of stroke and heart failure. But at the same time, we also know that diastolic pressures of as low as 90 mm. Hg in younger patients are associated with reduced longevity, even though we do not yet have proof that treating this level of blood pressure will reduce the likelihood of cardiovascular disease. Thus decisions as to whether or not to start treatment in the large number of patients whose diastolic pressures are in the range of 90 to 104 mm. Hg still must be made judgmentally and on an individual basis.

Variations in an individual patient's blood pressure readings can also confuse the picture. For instance, in some patients allowed to rest in either the seated or lying position for 20 or 30 minutes, an initially high blood pressure reading will fall to a lower level. However, in such patients it is generally wisest to base treatment decisions on the first and higher reading, as most of the data used to guide these decisions are derived from studies based on single casual blood pressure readings. But some patients have truly labile hypertension. On some occasions their blood pressure will be clearly elevated, yet at other times it will be appreciably lower and perhaps even normal. The assessment of such patients can be difficult, for long-term follow-ups have shown that some of them will develop true sustained hypertension, whereas others will retain a labile pattern.

In making a judgment whether to start treatment, factors other than the level of blood pressure can be helpful in making a decision. As a rule, men appear to be more at risk of hypertensive complications than women and should be treated at an earlier stage. Similarly, black people appear to be more susceptible than whites to hypertensive vascular disease, especially in younger age groups, and deserve more aggressive treatment. In general, the decision to start treatment should be based on more than one baseline reading unless the blood pressure is very high or there are overt vascular complications.

The existence of objective signs of vascular damage provides a strong incentive to start treatment even when blood pressure levels are only moderately elevated. Electrocardiographic evidence of left ventricular hypertrophy or ischemia, or an enlarged heart on chest x-ray, is a useful pointer. Similarly, biochemical evidence of reduced renal function can alert the physician to early hypertensive damage. Careful examination of the optic fundi also will provide a useful index of hypertensive vascular disease; the finding of early changes in a young patient is a strong indication to bring blood pressure under control as quickly as possible.

Since our aim in treating hypertension is to try to protect the patient from premature cardiovascular disease, the finding of other concurrent risk factors should also serve as an incentive to initiate therapy or at least observe the blood pressure state very closely. Certain of these risk factors, including diabetes, hyperlipidemia, and hyperuricemia, appear to occur more commonly in hypertensive persons than in those with normal blood pressure. Thus these factors should always be looked for and taken into account when deciding whether to begin treatment. In this context, a strong family history of hypertensive or cardiovascular disease would act as another signal for the early initiation of antihypertensive therapy.

There is now good and growing evidence that the measurement of plasma renin activity can provide a valuable prognostic insight in evaluating hypertensive patients. By using a renin-sodium nomogram (discussed later in this article), it is possible to divide patients with essential or other forms of hypertension into three renin subgroups: low, normal, or high. It has been found that patients in the high renin subgroup, comprising approximately 15 to 18 per cent of the hypertensive population, are particularly at risk of premature heart disease, malignant hypertension, stroke, and kidney failure. We believe that an aggressive approach to the diagnosis and treatment of these highly susceptible patients is imperative. At the other end of the spectrum, patients with low renin forms of hypertension appear to be in a relatively protected state as far as vascular complications are concerned. However, the classification of a hypertensive patient into the low renin subgroup should not be used as an indication to withhold treatment. Until the natural history and long-term prognosis of low renin hypertension are more fully clarified, the decision whether or not to start treatment should be based on the criteria and considerations discussed previously.

There has been some recent controversy concerning the treatment of elderly patients, especially those aged 70 years and above. In particular, elderly patients do not tolerate the side effects of antihypertensive medications as well as younger patients. It is probably reasonable not to treat, or to treat only with great caution, those elderly patients who do not have a history or gross signs of cardiovascular disease, unless the blood pressure readings are remarkably high. On the other hand, cautious treatment should be started in those instances in which an elderly patient is hypertensive and appears to be at risk of a major cardiovascular event.

Sometimes physicians are hesitant about starting treatment in patients who have already incurred major vascular damage. In patients who have suffered a recent stroke or have signs of encephalopathy, apprehension is sometimes expressed that starting antihypertensive treatment will exacerbate cerebral ischemia. In such cases, it should be remembered that the hypertension is far more of a risk to the patient than the theoretical problems that may be created by treatment. Indeed, with effective treatment, the cerebral vasculature may become less vasoconstricted and the supply of oxygenated blood to brain tissue may actually increase. However, when treatment is started under these circumstances, especially in older patients, dramatic or sudden reductions in blood pressure should be avoided. Similarly, it is sometimes felt that lowering blood pressure will reduce renal function in patients with already impaired kidneys. More often than not the reverse is true, and effective treatment of the hypertension will often improve basic renal function or at least keep it at a steady level. It is likely that during treatment, particularly if diuretics are employed, there will be an increase in blood concentrations of urea and creatinine. However, these changes may reflect dehydration with renal vasoconstriction and do not as a rule denote a true deterioration in renal function.

Nonspecific Approaches to Treatment

In general, patients with established hypertension depend on a well planned and systematic regimen of treatment employing appropriate antihypertensive medications. However, a number of other treatment modalities may sometimes be considered as part of the overall program. These include methods for dealing with stressful or anxiety-producing situations, changes in dietary, drinking, and smoking habits, and the role of exercise. Although the value of these various maneuvers in contributing to hypertension control is somewhat debatable, these issues are often raised by patients themselves. It is possible that some discussion of these matters at an early stage of treatment may help promote a greater degree of patient compliance with the more specific therapies.

It has been commonly believed that hypertension may result from stress or anxiety. Because of this, anxiolytic agents have sometimes been prescribed routinely as the first mode of treatment. There is, in fact, no objective evidence to support the idea that hypertensive patients are more subject to these problems than the population as a whole; moreover, there is little or no evidence to suggest that treatment with anxiety-relieving agents confers any sustained benefits as far as blood pressure control is concerned. Indeed, the prescribing of such agents as a routine may be positively harmful, as a false sense of security can result.

More recently, there has been great interest in nonpharmacologic techniques such as transcendental meditation, self-hypnosis, and biofeedback. There is no question that many patients who practice these techniques feel an improved sense of well-being. But once again, evidence that these approaches produce any meaningful or long-term reductions in blood pressure is still lacking; these practices should at most be considered a complement to conventional antihypertensive treatment and not a substitute.

Diets designed to help obese patients lose weight may sometimes be helpful in producing a degree of blood pressure reduction. Moreover, obesity is of itself a cardiac risk factor, and the achievement of weight reduction in appropriate patients can be an important part of an overall program designed to minimize the chances of serious cardiovascular disease.

Because of the likelihood that sodium retention plays a part in sustaining increased blood pressure levels in a proportion of hypertensive patients, diets restricted in salt frequently have been advocated as part of the treatment of hypertension. Unfortunately, to produce a degree of volume depletion equivalent to that produced by even a mild diuretic agent requires an exceptionally stringent diet, and very few patients are able to adhere to this over a prolonged period of time. Even then, there is no convincing evidence as yet concerning the ideal sodium intake for individual patients. In fact, in only about a third of hypertensive patients can blood pressure be significantly improved or normalized by even the most stringent sodium depletion, as exemplified by the experience with the rice diet. In the remainder, other (vasoconstrictor) mechanisms may be far more important, so that in some of these sodium depletion might even have an adverse effect. It is probably reasonable therefore to advise patients to adopt a compromise in the matter of salt ingestion, a sodium intake in the range of 50 to 200 mEq. daily (3 to 12 grams of salt) being consistent with the effective working of diuretic and other antihypertensive agents.

Although a moderate intake of alcohol probably has no deleterious effect on hypertension or its treatment, recent studies have shown that the regular intake of excessive amounts may induce or amplify hypertension. Thus patients should be advised to be prudent in their consumption of alcohol. There is little evidence that cigarette smoking has any sustained effects on blood pressure or its treatment. But this habit is of itself a cardiac risk factor, and cessation is an advisable part of overall treatment.

The role of exercise in the management of hypertension and in promoting cardiovascular integrity is not yet defined. By producing a general sense of well-being and improving morale, a moderate degree of exercise is probably beneficial. However, highly vigorous activities, especially those involving isometric exercises of the upper limbs, should be avoided, as dramatic upward swings in blood pressure may occur.

Principles of Treatment

The treatment of hypertension has undergone an evolution during the last two decades. During this period, we have passed from the purely empiricial to a much more rational approach based on our rapidly expanding knowledge of the pathophysiologic mechanisms that sustain high blood pressure. Intermediary to this process have been various schemes, some of which are still in use and designated as "stepped-care" programs, that employ the panoply of antihypertensive agents now available in a fixed sequence. Although the "stepped-care" approaches represent an improvement over the earlier empiricism by virtue of combining drugs having complementary mechanisms of action on blood pressure regulation, they still assume homogeneity of the hypertensive population and fail to discriminate between differing underlying mechanisms in hypertension.

Since our current protocols in the diagnosis and therapy of hypertension represent a departure from the methods still used in many clinical settings, it may be important to comment first on the tradition and second on the research and rationale supporting the new direction. In fairness, the newer protocols we will describe have their empirical aspects, too, but we believe them to be given clearer direction by a recently attained ability to analyze causes of hypertension and to predict the effects of drugs.

Most traditional approaches to hypertension rest on the assumption that the common denominator in all forms of hypertension is the blood pressure itself, so that its reduction, by whatever means, is the critical issue. Diuretic therapy has been the first step and cornerstone in almost every treatment program. The protocol generally begins with diuretics, and then goes on when necessary to add sympatholytic agents, vasodilators, and ganglionic blockers. This "stepped-care" process continues until normal blood pressure has been obtained or when, despite the simultaneous deployment of as many as four or five different drugs, the physician accepts whatever level of blood pressure control has been achieved. This not uncommon predicament underscores another weakness in the "stepped-care" approach: its total reliance on drug addition, rather than on a balance between addition and subtraction designed to define and then tackle the underlying hypertensive mechanisms. Quite clearly, when a combination of three or more drugs fails to control blood pressure, it can be presumed and even shown that some or all of these agents are noncontributory or, worse, counterproductive.

Even when a diuretic-based treatment system appears to work, its appropriateness can sometimes be questioned. Doubts begin to appear when we entertain the notion that high blood pressure, like high temperature, is symptom and not disease. It is possible to relieve a symptom; but if that relief is not addressed to the basic lesion, the price of the relief may be a masking and even an exacerbation of the lesion. When hypertension results from salt and water retention, reduction of blood pressure by diuresis is indeed a relevant and specific therapeutic retort. However, if the problem is elsewhere, forced blood pressure reduction by diuresis may not be relevant and, in fact, may in the long term do harm by its reactive stimulation of the real abnormality.

The preceding considerations and doubts are given substance by recent research establishing that essential hypertension, far from being a uniform disease, is a manifestation of several different disorders that are clearly different in etiology, in biochemistry, and in their response to different treatments. Practical means of identifying which of several mechanisms sustains hypertension in individual patients have emerged and allow designation of relevant and specific therapy.

A New Approach

The basis for this new approach is the exposure of the renin-angiotensin-aldosterone axis as the central control system for the maintenance of electrolyte balance and blood pressure homeostasis. Although not the sole regulator of these functions, the system participates in all blood pressure events of any duration, and by its adjustments of vasoconstriction and volume factors it accommodates and counterbalances pressor or depressor influences elsewhere. Potential abnormalities of this system are reflected by the concentrations of its plasma constituents, providing a biochemical profile (the renin-sodium profile) that can be diagnostic when correctly interpreted. An abnormality so revealed may indicate either a derangement in the regulatory system itself or a reaction to influences elsewhere; in either case it helps dissect mechanisms that may be involved in sustaining hypertension.

It will become apparent that chronic hypertension is sustained, if not triggered, by either of two polar mechanisms or an inappropriate combination of them. At the more familiar end of the spectrum, hypertension is entirely dependent on volume accumulation produced by excessive salt and water retention. But at the other end of the spectrum, hypertension may be entirely dependent on an abnormality of renin production that inappropriately induces vasoconstriction as well as aldosterone-mediated volume retention. In the area between, the two forces overlap and summate their effects.

It will be further seen that the two forces—renin influence and volume retention—have a complementary relationship and that the balancing of their interplay is the means by which a physiologic level of blood pressure is maintained. A significant implication of this is that these two mechanisms react to each other so that the inhibition or stimulation of one results in an opposite effect on the other. That implication can become critical in therapy, especially if treatment is applied to the wrong end of the spectrum.

From these concepts emerges the new system of analysis and treatment we will describe. We will set forth the steps by which the contributions of renin and volume may be assessed, either with or without an advanced laboratory back-up, and by which specific therapy may be applied and effectively titrated. In this therapy system a new first-line role is assigned to beta-adrenergic blocking drugs such as propranolol.

The Renin System. The renin-angiotensin-aldosterone system is a cascade of hormones activated by renal secretion of renin and exercising a pressor influence composed of both vasoconstrictor and volume components. Stimulated by low perfusion pressure in the renal arterioles and inhibited by high pressure, the system thereby incorporates a negative feedback loop in its cybernetic regulation of blood pressure.

Figure 1 represents a scheme of this system, to provide a convenient frame of reference for the description that follows.

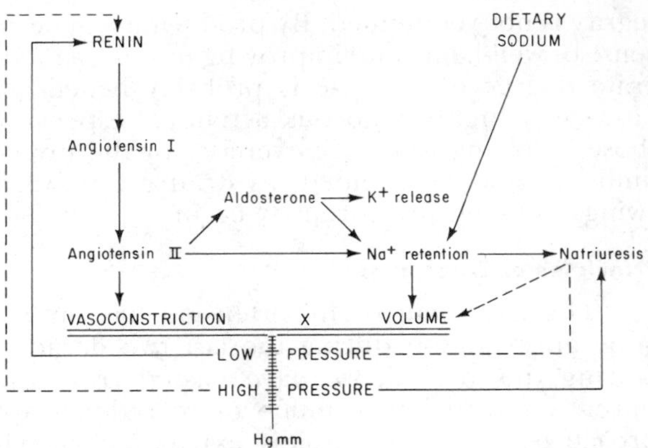

Figure 1. Schema of the renin-angiotensin-aldosterone axis and its regulation of the vasoconstriction and volume components of blood pressure. Dotted lines indicate negative feedback.

The first hormone, renin, is an enzyme secreted by the juxtaglomerular cells. It has no direct physiologic effect of its own. When released into the bloodstream under the stimulus of lowered perfusion pressure, it reacts with a circulating alpha$_2$-globulin substrate of hepatic origin to produce the decapeptide angiotensin I. Neither does angiotensin I have a direct physiologic action, but during passage through the pulmonary circulation it encounters converting enzymes that hydrolyze it into the octapeptide angiotensin II, which is the first active component of this system.

The biologic activity of angiotensin II is formidable. By weight it is the most potent pressure known, its vasoconstrictive action being about ten times more powerful than that of norepinephrine. It has a direct and immediate myotropic effect on smooth muscle cells, but also indirectly activates hormones of the autonomic nervous system and may even summon some central nervous system effects.

At the same time, angiotensin II musters increased fluid volume to reinforce the more directly elevated pressure. It increases fluid volume by two mechanisms. One of these is a direct sodium-retaining effect on the kidney seen at lower concentrations, but which tends to be reversed with higher concentrations. The tubular reabsorption may be associated with renal vasoconstriction and reduced glomerular filtration.

But by far the more important component of fluid retention is secondary to angiotensin's stimulation of adrenal cortical secretion of aldosterone, the second effector hormone of the system. Aldosterone induces a slow but cumulatively potent sodium retention and increased fluid volume. An important mechanism in this action is the establishment of an electrochemical gradient favoring sodium reabsorption in exchange for potassium at the distal tubular site; thus a price of this sodium retention is potassium excretion. This accounts for the potassium wastage observed in primary aldosteronism.

The combined effects of the brisk vasoconstriction produced by angiotensin II and the more slowly developing volume expansion raise blood pressure. The elevated pressure then exerts a negative feedback stimulus that acts on both the vasoconstrictive and the volume sides of the equation. Pressure natriuresis, releasing pressure by fluid escape, acts as a safety valve against excessive blood pressure surges, while the raised pressure also shuts off the renin production that began the cycle.

In this way the renin-angiotensin-aldosterone system provides hour-to-hour and day-to-day regulation, maintaining blood pressure at physiologic levels in response to other circumstances that can alter it. Although the renin system can be shown to respond appropriately to short-term blood pressure events induced by such factors as posture and exercise, the chief antagonist against which it plays its counterbalancing role is the volume of the blood pool itself. In essence, renin's counterpart in this relationship is the state of sodium balance, which in turn is determined by salt intake and the integrity of sodium retaining and releasing mechanisms.

The level of renin system activity, then, can be considered normal or abnormal only in relation to the state of salt balance and the level of blood pressure being maintained. This is the subject we will next explore.

The Renin-Sodium Index. Now that plasma renin activity may be assayed (by methods to be discussed later), it is fruitful to examine to what extent the renin level may be correlated with the various hypertensive states, and thereby to see what diagnostic aid and therapeutic guidance such a measurement can provide, especially in the matter of essential hypertension. A number of investigators have studied this question, but until recently no consistent relationship has been uncovered except for the general agreement that renin activity is almost always markedly high in malignant hypertension.

One of the reasons for the inconclusive results of earlier renin studies may be that investigators often failed to take into account the renin-sodium relationship in their study of patients or of normal controls. As noted above, body fluid volume varies widely with fluctuations in dietary salt intake, and it is body fluid volume that determines the appropriateness of a given level of renin production. Some investigators recognized this, but they related renin measurements to bracketed ranges of normal renin activity for controlled levels of salt balance. A problem with bracketed ranges of normal relationships is that they overlap and often fail to discriminate important but subtle abnormalities.

A few methodologic changes help bring greater consistency to the study of renin and make this technique more feasible for broad clinical application. For one, instead of indexing renin values against salt balance as determined under tedious balance ward conditions, the index is made against the 24 hour sodium excretion. It has been established that the 24 hour urine collection, except in those very few patients who cannot maintain salt balance, accurately reflects the state of sodium balance. It probably provides a more reliable insight into a patient's appetite for salt than does interrogation. But most importantly, its simplicity allows for the evaluation of large numbers of subjects on an outpatient basis and so offers a richer statistical base for plotting the normal relationships between renin and sodium.

Another methodologic change involves the method of plotting the normal relationships. Instead of employing bracketed ranges at stepped and overlapped levels, the normal values are plotted graphically so as to provide a nomogram of the type illustrated in Figure 2. It can be seen that the normal range in such a nomogram is continuous and easily defined through all levels of sodium excretion and renin activity.

Besides providing a sharp reference for determining the appropriateness of a patient's renin-sodium index, the nomogram dramatically illustrates the interdependence of renin and sodium. When the 24 hour sodium is low, reflecting low salt intake and minimized body fluid volume accretion, plasma renin is correspondingly high as it meets the challenge of maintaining effective blood pressure. When salt excretion and salt intake are high, the associated high volume sustains an effective level of blood pressure and renin is not required.

Measuring Plasma Renin Activity. Since antihypertensive drugs affect the renin axis, it is good practice to withdraw all such medications for at least 3 weeks before obtaining a diagnostic baseline renin-sodium profile. The blood is collected with the patient in the seated position after having been ambulatory for a few hours. In our laboratory we usually perform the measurements

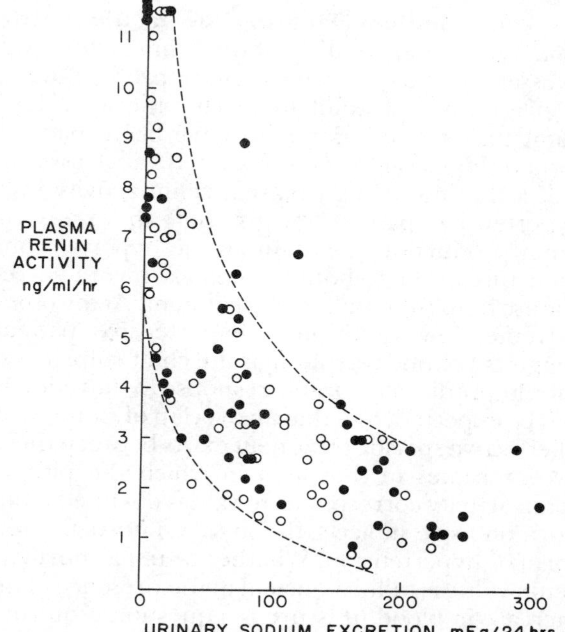

Figure 2. Renin-sodium nomogram. Individual points represent values obtained in normotensive control subjects. Dotted lines define "normal" range.

after a 5 to 7 day period of mild sodium deprivation, a protocol that lightly stimulates renin secretion into a range at which deviations from normal may be easier to perceive. The 24 hour urine collection is made on the day preceding the clinic visit. We normally provide a plastic container for the urine, together with written instructions for the proper collection of a 24 hour sample.

The laboratory methodology for measurement of plasma renin activity has been described elsewhere. But it should be emphasized here that in order to discriminate renin values below the normal range, it may be necessary to prolong the plasma incubation step for as long as 18 hours. With such long incubations the laboratory method must include steps for complete inhibition of plasma angiotensinases; this can be done by using ethylenediamine tetra-acetic acid (EDTA) and a bacteriostatic agent plus diisopropylfluorophosphate (DFP) or paramethyl sulfonyl fluoride (PMSF) at the optimal acid pH for renin (5.5 to 6.0). It is a mistake to drop the pH below 4 in order to destroy substrate and angiotensinases; it is now clear that this maneuver produces artifactually high renin values by activating an inactive form of renin, possibly prorenin. Chilling of the blood sample immediately after withdrawal from the patient produces a similar result, and this, too, should be avoided in the collection period. Undoubtedly, the failure to observe these refinements of method accounts for much of the inconsistency in renin findings reported in the literature.

Renin-Sodium Profiling as a Diagnostic Tool. An understanding of the renin system and its assessment by the renin-sodium profile can aid in diagnosis and point to specific therapy. This point may be considered to have been made if certain things can be demonstrated. If we assume that a finding of high plasma renin activity in a hypertensive patient means that an excess of renin production is sustaining the hypertension, then this finding should predict a favorable response to specific antirenin treatment. At the other extreme, low renin in a hypertensive patient suggests volume retention as the chief culprit and should predict a favorable response to diuretics. It can be expected, too, that an overlap of causes and of effective specific treatment exists between these two extremes in that area in which the plasma renin activity corresponds to values obtained from normotensive subjects, the so-called normal renin form of hypertension. Whether or not a "normal" renin value is indeed normal in the presence of an increase in blood pressure is a question requiring further study and clarification.

Renin, Aldosterone, and Sodium in Specific Forms of Hypertension. Although we are chiefly concerned here with the treatment of essential hypertension, a class comprising the vast majority of hypertensive patients, it may be illustrative to review briefly the findings that showed renin profiling to be useful in characterizing and treating other forms of hypertensive disease.

MALIGNANT HYPERTENSION. The renin-angiotensin-aldosterone axis was first discovered in studies of patients with malignant hypertension in whom we demonstrated, quite unlike essential hypertension, massive oversecretion of aldosterone. We suspected that this was a consequence of renal damage with inappropriate secretion of excessive renin loading to marked excesses of angiotensin. This link was established when we showed that angiotensin II selectively stimulates the adrenal cortical secretion of aldosterone in normal subjects. Thus angiotensin II emerged as the major physiologic stimulus for aldosterone, excesses of which explain the aldosterone oversecretion of malignant hypertension. Moreover, inappropriate levels of angiotensin and aldosterone in this disorder appeared as the cause not only of the hypertension but also of the attendant diffuse vascular damage.

PRIMARY ALDOSTERONISM. Specific derangements in the renin axis cause at least two different forms of hypertension—not only malignant hypertension but also primary aldosteronism. These two diseases then represent the polar extremes of oversecretion of the two limbs of the hormonal system—i.e., either primary renin (i.e., angiotensin II) excess (malignant hypertension) or primary aldosterone excess (primary aldosteronism). It is noteworthy that the latter is in contrast a benign disease and is associated with suppressed levels of plasma renin activity, whereas malignant hypertension is instead a virulent condition associated with diffuse necrotizing arteriolitis, uremia, and often an early death. Malignant hypertension differs in that it is accompanied by excesses of *both* angiotensin and aldosterone, because the primary hyperreninemia also induces secondary hyperaldosteronism. Thus when the hypertensive process involves both limbs of the hormonal system, the hypertensive state is much more severe.

RENOVASCULAR HYPERTENSION. A third type of hypertension associated with and caused by specific abnormalities in the renin axis is unilateral renovascular hypertension, commonly called Goldblatt hypertension. Goldblatt showed in 1934 that clamping of one renal artery could cause hypertension. But for a long time thereafter it was unclear whether abnormal plasma renin levels contributed to this disorder. However, with appreciation of its link to sodium balance, with improved methodology and the development of the renin profile, and with an understanding that patients with bilateral renal hypertension usually have normal or low renin values, renin measurements have become clinically meaningful in dealing with the problem. Most patients with curable unilateral renovascular hypertension have abnormally high circulating plasma renin activity in relation to their sodium balance so that hypersecretion of renin actually maintains the elevated blood pressure and is an important diagnostic indicator for predicting surgical curability. Renal vein renin measurements are especially useful to determine which kidney is secreting excessive renin, the degree of its ischemia, and whether renin secretion from the contralateral kidney is appropriately suppressed, all requirements for surgical curability.

Renin Profiling in Essential Hypertension. When the improved methods of renin-sodium profiling described earlier were brought to bear in the classification of patients with essential hypertension, three subgroups were identified: high renin, 15 per cent; normal or medium renin, 55 per cent; and low renin, 30 per cent. A study of the clinical and epidemiologic features of these groups revealed significant differences among them. All groups had a fairly similar incidence of left ventricular hypertrophy and similar levels of such indicators as plasma uric acid, cholesterol, and fasting blood sugar. However, the high renin group had perceptibly higher diastolic blood pressure and blood urea, a greater incidence of retinopathy and proteinuria, and tended—expectedly, in view of a more active aldosterone level—to hypokalemia. The suggestion that high renin patients were at greater risk was strengthened by finding that these patients tended to be younger and with shorter duration of disease.

The most striking observation was the difference in the incidence of heart attack and stroke. The high renin patients suffered an incidence of 14 per cent, and the normal, 10 per cent; but the low renin patients had not one case of either of these complications. Since that original study our series has grown to over 600, and among the more than 100 of them with low renin there has been only one myocardial infarction.

The inference is irresistible that excess renin production is associated with greater hazard of cardiovascular sequelae, possibly in consequence of angiotensin's vasculotoxic pressor effect. This suggests the importance in therapy of addressing the renin factor directly and to do nothing that would inadvertently stimulate it—this concept is one of the foundation stones in the program of therapy we will discuss. Low renin patients, whose hypertension is chiefly sustained by factors of sodium retention, appear to be better protected against cardiovascular damage despite their hypertension. This may well explain the longstanding clinical enigma of that small subgroup of patients who ignore treatment and yet appear immune to the complications of hypertension.

It can be further inferred that essential hypertension is not a uniform disease but a group of disorders different in cause and biochemistry, each requiring its own specific treatment. If the role of the renin system is indeed what has been described so far, and if the renin-sodium profile is an accurate indicator of renin involvement, high renin patients should respond to antirenin therapy alone and low renin patients to diuretics alone, whereas "normal" or medium renin patients may require an appropriate balance of conjoint antirenin and antivolume therapy.

At any rate, the diagnostic and therapeutic validity of these inferences can be proved if the response to specific antirenin and antivolume therapy corresponds to the predictions made possible by renin profiling. We need not search very far for specific antivolume therapy; a wide assortment of diuretics has been part of the therapeutic armamentarium for some time. Specific antirenin therapy, however, is another matter, and it bears some discussion before we outline our program of therapy.

Antirenin Therapy. A number of drugs now available for treating hypertension can be shown to depress renin production. However, the beta-adrenergic blocker propranolol, probably through a direct action on the renal juxtaglomerular cell, exhibits the greatest potency and specificity in this respect. Propranolol has been known to be antihypertensive since 1964. It has been speculated that its antihypertensive effect comes from its reduction of cardiac output, the anti-inotropic purpose for which it is chiefly prescribed in cardiology. However, this suggestion does not stand up very well before the demonstration that the drug reduces cardiac output *but not blood pressure* in low renin patients or in most normotensive subjects.

We have already mentioned the experience with beta blockade in treating malignant hypertension emergencies. In many of these, propranolol completely normalized blood pressure, with parallel reduction of renin levels, without any other therapy being needed. In some the pressure reduction was not complete despite the normalization of renin levels; in these, blood pressure was normalized by the addition of diuretics, testifying to and quantifying the separate but additive participation of renin and volume factors in these patients. Of equal importance in understanding the antihypertensive action of propranolol, we have found that in patients with renal hypertension the identification of surgical curability in those with high renin was matched by a positive response to propranolol in both the reduction of blood pressure and plasma renin activity. Hence, the clinical response to propranolol has a diagnostic utility that appears to parallel renin profiling and might be used as a screening modality in circumstances in which it is not possible to assay renin directly.

But most importantly, the specificity of propranolol has been confirmed in patients with essential hypertension. In average doses (about 160 mg. daily), propranolol reduces blood pressure, together with renin levels, often all the way to normal, in most high renin patients. Normal renin patients also show a definite but somewhat lesser response, and their residual hypertension generally is treatable with conjoint diuretics. But for the most part, the drug has virtually no effect in patients with low renin values. These patients normally respond well to volume depletion alone—and here it should be mentioned that in our experience it makes little difference which type of diuretic is used.

It is of interest that nearly a third of low renin patients, together with an even higher proportion of normal and high renin patients, exhibit only a small or a transitory response to diuretics. This apparent failure of treatment appears to be related to the especially potent reactive renin and aldosterone stimulation that is evoked in some patients by diuretic-induced volume depletion. In the management of this important group of patients, an understanding of renin mechanisms during treatment, and ideally the ability to obtain direct measurements of renin and aldosterone, can be of considerable help in determining the next appropriate step in therapy.

Whereas the specificity of propranolol in treating various forms of hypertension has been inferred from broad clinical and experimental experience, the confirmation of renin's role in essential hypertension has derived from studies using the experimental drugs saralasin and SQ20881. The effects of these agents are confined to ablating the renin-angiotensin system, saralasin by competitively blocking the action of angiotensin II upon its receptors and SQ20881 by inhibiting the enzymatic conversion of angiotensin I to angiotensin II. It is not the role of this article to discuss the interesting but complex pharmacology of these exciting new diagnostic probes. However, the message from studies already performed in man is clear. The blood pressure reductions achieved when either of these agents is used to block the renin-angiotensin system are proportional to the pretreatment renin measurements, confirming the direct relationship between the level of renin in the plasma and its participation in sustaining hypertension. As a corollary of this, these agents dramatically lower and often normalize blood pressure in high renin patients, have little or no effect in low renin patients, and elicit an intermediate response in normal renin patients. If patients are pretreated with diuretics, saralasin or SQ20881 produces even greater falls in blood pressure, documenting the role of reactively stimulated renin in sustaining blood pressure in conditions of volume depletion.

Based on our understanding of the participation of renin and volume factors in hypertension, both before and during treatment, let us now consider the strategies available to us for the rational therapy of hypertension.

Rationale for a Modern System of Therapy. We can now propose a system of analysis and treatment based on the evaluation of the renin component in hypertension and its specific monotherapy when it can be identified as the major factor, or, conversely, the specific monotherapy of the volume component when the renin factor is absent, and to appropriately titrated conjoint therapy when both factors operate. The virtues of using only one drug instead of two, or two instead of three or more, scarcely need justification; such simplicity and specificity minimize the incidence of side effects and maximize the patient's compliance while conserving money and time.

In contrast to traditional protocols, which generally start with a trial of diuretics, the system we will describe prefers to first employ antirenin therapy except in those patients in whom the clinical circumstances contraindicate the use of a particular antirenin drug, or in whom a low renin profile suggests that such therapy will prove ineffective. Part of the thinking behind such a change in sequence is strongly influenced by the evidence that excessive renin production appears to enhance the likelihood of cardiovascular complications. Thus it is advisable to identify the renin involvement and treat it first. Inappropriate treatment with volume depletion may reactively increase renin production and place the patient in an undesirable physiologic state despite the sphygmomanometer's optimistic readings. In fact, even when antivolume therapy is appropriate, as in the case of a purely volume-dependent patient, it may be found that conjoint light doses of renin blockade may help dampen reactive renin swings.

Our preference for the first step in antirenin therapy is propranolol. The close parallel in its action to that of specific pharmacologic probes and the ability of the renin-sodium profile to predict that action make a strong case for the drug's specificity and usefulness. It is well tolerated, with a minimum of side effects, and those patients who can be normalized on propranolol alone will find that the drug generally does not affect mentation, produces no postural or postexercise hypotension, and only rarely interferes with sexual potency. Until a better antirenin agent comes along, which may well happen when some European beta-adrenergic blockers become approved here, propranolol must serve as a basic or primary agent in the modern therapy of hypertension.

Analysis by Renin Profile and Pharmacologic Probes. Figure 3 is a schematic concept of the spectrum of patients in terms of the dependency of their hypertension upon renin production at one end, volume retention at the other, and both factors in the middle. It is at the same time a representation of the therapy program—propranolol against renin and diuretics against volume, with an appropriate blend of the two when both factors are present.

The initial step is to analyze where a specific patient stands in the scheme. The renin-sodium profile, if it is obtained by the methods described earlier, will suggest those patients most likely to benefit from propranolol (i.e., those with high or normal renin) and those most likely to respond to volume depletion (low renin patients).

After having made such an identification, the clinician can proceed to trial and titration of the therapy suggested by the profile, according to the protocol described below. A more elaborate approach, when other agents become available for broad use, might be to go on to the employment of pharmacologic probes such as the converting enzyme inhibitors or angiotensin II antagonists. Such testing can also serve in periodic re-evaluation of the patient's changing hormonal pattern and will materially cut down the time and expense of an empirical search for the appropriate therapeutic formula.

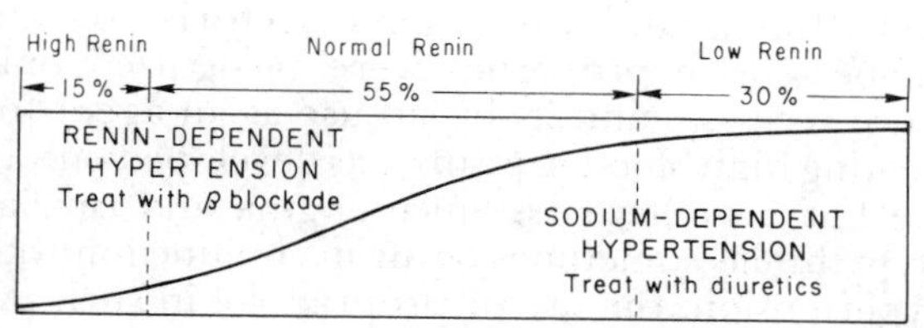

Figure 3.

It would be useful and convenient to be able to call for a renin assay as readily as for a hematocrit or serum cholesterol; we have not yet reached that point in the laboratory facilities available to most practitioners, although it may not be too long before we do.

However, it is quite possible to achieve much the same sort of analysis, quantification, and titration by exploiting the known properties of propranolol and interpreting the results achieved with this agent on the basis of our knowledge and understanding of the renin-angiotensin system. That is, we can consider the response to propranolol to be the clinical equivalent of renin profiling and pharmacologic probing. Whereas the renin profile, if it is available, will separate those to be tried first on propranolol from those on diuretics, the treatment-titration method begins all patients on propranolol except when clinically contraindicated.

The Treatment-Titration Plan. Figure 4 represents a decision tree and outlines the steps—and the de-stepping—in our system of therapy. The group to be started on propranolol alone will comprise most patients: those found by renin profiling to have high or normal renin, or, in the absence of renin profiling, all patients except those in whom the use of this drug is clinically contraindicated. When the use of propranolol is not feasible, other agents having renin-lowering properties, such as clonidine, can be substituted.

It will be found that most patients can safely be started on propranolol. Our average dose is 40 mg. four times daily or 80 mg. twice daily—less if the patient's clinical circumstances suggest caution or a mild degree of renin involvement. The response is then observed for a period that may range from 1 to 3 weeks, depending on the progress of the illness, the pace of the response, and the convenience of outpatient visits. If the starting dose succeeds in normalizing the blood pressure, the dose is then reduced to test for the minimum dosage for maintenance. We have found some patients showing complete correction on as little as 20 mg. of propranolol twice daily. If the starting dose brings about an incomplete response, the dose may be increased to see if further correction can be made, although we have not usually gone beyond a daily total of 320 mg. When these trials produce complete correction, therapy with propranolol alone can be continued, with periodic reevaluation and subtraction of the dose to test for

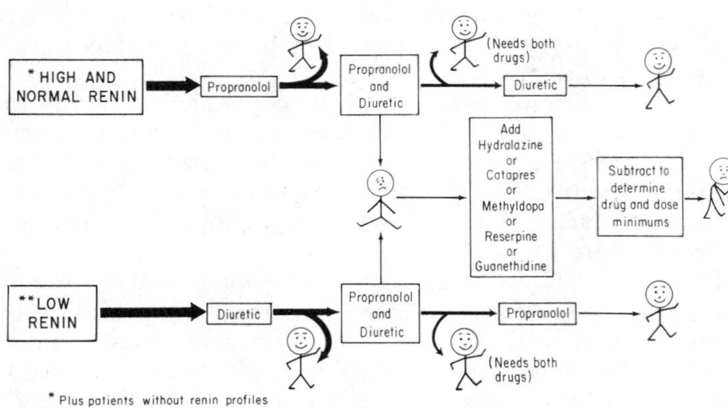

Figure 4. Treatment strategies in hypertensive patients either classified according to their renin status or unclassified. Full explanation is given in the text.

any changes in the hormonal picture and to adjust for the minimal maintenance dose.

If complete correction is not achieved or if it is apparent that there is no response at all, a diuretic is added to the propranolol to test for volume factors. In our experience this combined regimen achieves normalization in up to 85 per cent of patients. The procedure is the same as with propranolol: a starting dose to see if there is a response and then an increase in dosage until full correction is achieved or until it is evident that full correction will not be attained. The selection of the diuretic, considering the large numbers available, is largely a matter of the physician's prejudice. We generally start with chlorthalidone, because it is long acting and needs to be given only once a day. We begin with 50 mg. and, if necessary, then double the dose. An acceptable alternative is hydrochlorothiazide, starting at 25 mg. twice daily and increasing to 50 to 100 mg. twice daily. Spironolactone, in a range from 25 to 100 mg. twice daily, is a useful backup diuretic in the presence of potassium depletion. Needless to say, should the starting dose of diuretic achieve full correction, it is reduced to test for the minimum needed.

After a patient has been normalized on such a combined regimen, the propranolol is *subtracted* to see if the patient can be maintained on diuretic alone. If so, or if the propranolol needs to be restored, he is put on maintenance with periodic re-evaluation and trial de-stepping.

In the comparatively rare event that the combined regimen does not normalize the blood pressure, the physician will then have to revert to what is essentially the classic empirical approach and test serially other drugs such as hydralazine, prazosin, clonidine, methyldopa, reserpine, or guanethidine, until complete control is achieved. At that point, an active process of subtraction must be undertaken to test for the least number of drugs and their minimum doses.

Those patients to be begun first on diuretic will follow a parallel course. Diuretic is tried first, and propranolol is added if the diuretic fails. If combined therapy succeeds, the diuretic is subtracted to see if the patient truly needs both drugs or can be sustained on propranolol alone. If combined therapy fails, a trial of the third-line drugs may begin. As with those begun on propranolol, the subtraction trial for minimum dose and drug is a key feature of the strategy.

Antihypertensive Agents

A list of the antihypertensive agents discussed in this article is given in Table 1. Although we have already explained how these various agents may best be deployed in the treatment scheme for hypertension, a few further remarks concerning the characteristics of some of these drugs may be helpful.

Propranolol. This beta-adrenoreceptor blocking agent was first introduced into this country in the early 1960s as a treatment for cardiac arrhythmias and for angina pectoris. Its antihypertensive properties were recognized only more recently, and its broad use as an agent for treating high blood pressure has developed only in the last 2 or 3 years. Since angina and cardiac arrhythmias sometimes occur in conjunction with hypertension, the use of propranolol in such pa-

TABLE 1. **Major Oral Antihypertensive Agents**

	ADULT DOSE RANGE (PER DAY)	ROLE
Propranolol (Inderal)	20–320 mg.	First drug of choice in most patients; second line in low renin patients
Diuretics:		
Chlorthalidone (Hygroton)	25–100 mg.	First drug of choice in low-renin patients; otherwise, second-line drug
Hydrochlorothiazide (Hydrodiuril, Esidrix)	25–100 mg.	
Spironolactone (Aldactone)	25–200 mg.	
Triamterene (Dyrenium)	50–200 mg.	
Clonidine (Catapres)	0.2–1.2 mg.	Third-line drugs; can substitute as first-line if propranolol contraindicated
Methyldopa (Aldomet)	500–2000 mg.	
Reserpine (Serpasil)	0.1–0.5 mg.	
Hydralazine (Apresoline)	20–200 mg.	Third-line drugs
Prazosin (Minipres)	3–15 mg.	
Guanethidine (Ismelin)	10–150 mg.	Alternative to earlier drugs if they fail to work

tients is particularly attractive, as it allows the treatment of two diseases with only one drug.

Different authorities have advocated a wide range of doses of propranolol for treating hypertension. Some physicians start treatment with as little as 20 to 40 mg. daily; others are willing to push as high as 1 to 2 grams per day. We believe that in the vast majority of cases effective beta blockade and renin suppression can be achieved with doses of 160 or at most 320 mg. per day. The patient's pulse rate provides the physician with an inbuilt monitor of the drug's beta-blocking effectiveness. Thus pulse rates above 70 beats per minute suggest that further dose increases can be justified, whereas rates in the low 60s suggest that an adequate degree of beta blockade has been achieved. Although additive blood pressure–lowering effects can be seen with very large doses of propranolol, it is possible that the drug is then working by mechanisms other than beta blockade. It is probably more realistic to add a second type of medication to the propranolol at this stage rather than to build the dose to inordinately high levels. Propranolol seems to have a comparatively long biologic half-life, and normally can be administered on a twice-daily basis.

Because of its inhibitory action on the heart, propranolol should not be given to patients in heart failure except with great caution. This drug also has an inhibitory effect on bronchodilator mechanisms, and should not be used in patients with asthma. In this context, it is generally wise to withhold propranolol in patients with hay fever or other seasonal allergies in whom there is a danger of bronchoconstriction. Patients with chronic obstructive lung disease may also be embarrassed by the use of propranolol. Because it may mask the important warning symptoms of hypoglycemia, propranolol should be used with extreme care in patients receiving insulin for diabetes mellitus. Peripheral vascular disease or Raynaud-like phenomena are also relative contraindications to the use of propranolol.

In the large majority of patients, propranolol is well tolerated. Occasionally it may produce changes in sleep patterns and in the frequency and nature of dreams. Some patients may complain of mild drowsiness. Rarely, reversible impotence may occur in men taking this agent.

Clonidine. This imidazoline compound is a comparatively new and powerful antihypertensive agent. Like propranolol, it has renin-lowering properties, but additionally has a sympathoinhibitory effect mediated by its alpha-agonist action in the central nervous system. In patients in whom propranolol is contraindicated, clonidine can be substituted as the first line drug. In some patients, a dose as small as 0.1 mg. twice daily is sufficient to produce a powerful antihypertensive effect; if necessary, the dose can be increased to 0.4 mg. three times per day.

The most common side effects of clonidine are dryness of the mouth and drowsiness. In most instances when these side effects occur, they will tend to disappear after a few days or, at the most, 2 or 3 weeks of treatment. Occasionally these side effects prove intolerable to the patient and may necessitate a switch to another agent. Rarely, rebound hypertension may be seen in patients who precipitously discontinue taking clonidine. As a general rule, this is seen only in those patients in whom a dramatic reduction in blood pressure occurred when clonidine treatment was first begun. It is important to advise patients not to stop their medication abruptly but to slowly taper their dosage over a period of days. If rebound does occur, restarting the drug will generally solve the problem. In those very rare instances in which a pressor rebound reaches alarming proportions, treatment with phentolamine or other alpha-adrenergic blocking agents will act specifically to lower the blood pressure.

α-Methyldopa. As with clonidine, methyldopa exerts at least some of its antihypertensive effects through an action in the central nervous system that results in a reduction of sympathetic outflow. In addition, methyldopa has some renin-lowering properties, and this too may result from substituting its methyl-norepinephrine metabolite for norepinephrine in central or peripheral alpha-receptor terminals. The range of dosage of this agent is from 500 to 2000 mg. daily. In general, it is effective if given as a twice daily regimen.

Until the more recent appreciation of newer agents such as propranolol or clonidine, the relative palatability and effectiveness of methyldopa had made it a mainstay of antihypertensive treatment throughout the world. Like clonidine, methyldopa can produce a degree of sedation and dryness of the mouth in a proportion of patients. Perhaps of greater importance, methyldopa produces reversible interference with sexual function, ranging from changes in libido to failure of erection or ejaculation, in a considerable proportion of male patients. Approximately 10 to 15 per cent of patients receiving this drug will develop a positive direct Coombs reaction. Changes in liver function and hemolytic anemia are uncommon side effects, but are troublesome when they occur. Rebound hypertension can occur in some patients if the drug is stopped abruptly; the management of this problem is the same as for clonidine.

Reserpine. This agent is one of the rauwolfia compounds that have enjoyed wide use in the treatment of hypertension for several years. Reserpine has both central and peripheral inhibitory actions on the sympathetic nervous system, and also exhibits a degree of renin suppression. Reserpine is usually effective when taken as a single daily dose of 0.2 to 0.5 mg.

The chief factor in the falling popularity of this drug is the high incidence of depression that it produces. This can vary from subtle changes in personality to profound melancholia and even suicide. Unwanted sedation, dry mouth, and nasal stuffiness can also pose problems during treatment. After discontinuing the drug, reversal of side effects, especially depression, can take several weeks or even months.

Guanethidine. This agent is a specific antagonist of the sympathetic nervous system. It appears to have little or no action in the central nervous system, but seems to work almost entirely in peripheral nerve terminals. The dose range of this drug is between 25 and 150 mg. per day. The drug is most commonly administered on a twice daily basis, but the major proportion of the total daily dose is often given in the evening so as to minimize side effects. Recently, some studies have indicated that guanethidine may be effective in a number of patients if given as a single daily dose.

The effectiveness of guanethidine can be blocked by agents such as the tricyclic antidepressants, including imipramine, desipramine, and amitriptyline, which prevent its uptake at nerve endings. Some phenothiazines and amphetamine can also impair its action. Although guanethidine is a powerful agent, its antihypertensive effects are chiefly postural. Apart from producing symptoms, questions have been raised concerning its efficacy in producing a constant lowering of blood pressure. Monitoring of blood pressure over 24 hour periods during administration of this drug has revealed that blood pressure is low when patients are in the erect posture, but that it can rise to high levels when patients are seated and especially when they are recumbent. Hence, guanethidine's status as a second-line drug is open to some question; its use may best be reserved for the occasional patient resistant to other agents. Because it does not enter the central nervous system in appreciable concentrations, guanethidine does not produce the sedation and other central side effects that can complicate the use of other agents. Apart from symptoms related to changes in posture, the most common complaint of patients receiving this drug is diarrhea. Additionally, a proportion of men taking this drug suffer from a reversible interference with sexual function, the classic manifestation being retrograde ejaculation.

Hydralazine. This agent remains the most commonly used oral vasodilator for the treatment of hypertension. Hydralazine appears to work through lowering peripheral vascular resistance by directly relaxing smooth muscle in small arteries and arterioles. The dosage range of this agent is from 20 to 200 mg. daily, and can be given in two equally divided doses.

In most cases, hydralazine must be used as part of a three drug regimen. This arises because of two compensatory reactions that occur during hydralazine administration: first, a substantial degree of fluid retention; and second, accompanying increases adrenergically mediated in plasma renin activity and in heart rate and cardiac output. For these reasons, hydralazine is usually only effective if given in company with a diuretic and with agents such as propranolol that can reduce renin secretion and lower pulse rate and cardiac output. Hence, in approaching the treatment of hypertension, hydralazine is best regarded as a third-line drug.

Apart from headaches early in the course of treatment and occasional episodes of orthostatic symptoms, hydralazine produces relatively few side effects. However, in susceptible patients in whom hepatic metabolism of the drug is not sufficiently rapid, concentrations can build to a point of producing a form of systemic lupus erythematosus. Although this problem is reversible upon discontinuation of the drug, it is generally wisest to restrict total daily dosage to 200 mg. and thereby avoid this potential difficulty.

Prazosin. This newly available agent was first thought to be a vasodilator similar to hydralazine. However, more recent research has indicated that it is probably an alpha-adrenergic blocking agent more related to substances such as phentolamine. The normal dose range is from 3 to 15 mg. per day given in three equally divided doses. Although fairly well tolerated, severe postural symptoms can occur during the first few hours of treatment, and it is advised that the very first dose be given shortly before the patient retires to bed. It can be expected that prazosin will prove to be a good third-line drug choice, working well in combination with propranolol and with diuretics.

Diuretics. The most commonly used diuretics in the treatment of hypertension are the sulfonamide agents. There are a large number of equally effective products available to the physician. Hydrochlorothiazide is probably the most commonly used of the shorter-acting agents, whereas chlorthalidone is the most frequently used longer-acting agent. Although there has been controversy concerning the mechanism of action of these agents, it is now widely accepted that they lower blood pressure as a result of reducing extracellular fluid volume. If diuretics are being used as the sole form of treatment, as in patients with low renin hypertension, hydrochlorothiazide should be used in a total daily dosage of 100 to 200 mg. divided into two equal doses, and chlorthalidone should be given as a single daily dose of 50 to 100 mg. However, when used in conjunction with other types of antihypertensive agents, lower doses are usually adequate.

Diuretics are fairly well tolerated; impotence, depression, and decreased exercise tolerance are sometimes reported. Most of the side effects and problems associated with diuretic treatment relate to the physiologic changes that are produced by these agents. Hypokalemia is an almost invariable accompaniment of the use of diuretics in their full effective doses. Apart from the dangers of cardiac dysrhythmias and possible myocardial damage caused by sustained hypokalemia, patients may complain of weakness and muscle discomfort, especially in hot weather. Serum potassium concentrations can be kept at acceptable levels in most patients by increasing their intake of orange juice, bananas, and other potassium-rich foods. Because of the wide swings in serum potassium concentrations that they produce and the possibility that small bowel ulceration may sometimes occur, pharmacologic potassium supplements should be used with caution.

Through their action to retard insulin secretion, sulfonamide diuretics will often increase blood glucose concentrations. Although this is not a problem in most patients, it will sometimes push a borderline diabetic into the range at which specific treatment becomes necessary, or it may create temporary difficulties in controlling blood glucose levels in patients already receiving diabetic therapy. Increases in serum uric acid concentrations produced by diuretics can also present problems in a fairly large number of patients. Because of the risk of clinical gout or of urate-induced renal damage, it is sometimes necessary to add agents such as allopurinol or probenecid. Increases in blood concentrations of cholesterol and triglycerides also commonly occur during diuretic treatment; the implications of these increases in plasma lipid concentrations have not yet been fully evaluated. Other concomitants of diuretic therapy, inevitable in the induced state of dehydration, are hemoconcentration and increased blood viscosity and coagulability, in more severe and unusual circumstances expressed by azotemia, weakness, and postural hypotension.

Because of the various cardiovascular risk factors that they seem to invoke, it would seem unwise to regard diuretics as totally benign agents that can be used indiscriminately. In low renin patients in whom excessive volume factors are implicated directly in sustaining the hypertension, the use of diuretics in full effective doses is a specific approach to therapy and appears to be justified. But in the majority of patients who comprise the high and normal renin subgroups, and in whom volume plays a lesser part in sustaining hypertension, propranolol or the sympatholytic agents should comprise the cornerstone of therapy. Although some fluid retention may occur in these patients secondary to the hypotensive actions of these agents, this can generally be dealt with by comparatively low diuretic doses.

Furosemide and ethacrynic acid, more powerful diuretics that act in the loop of Henle, have also been advocated as a treatment for hypertension. However, these agents produce biochemical changes similar to those of the diuretics discussed previously, and they have another possible disadvantage in that more frequent administration, up to three to four times a day, may be needed. However, furosemide is the ideal diuretic for treating hypertension in patients with renal impairment, because it retains its diuretic potency better than other diuretic agents in the face of reduced kidney function.

Spironolactone, an agent that produces its diuretic effect by specifically antagonizing the action of aldosterone in the kidney, is also effective in treating hypertension. It has the advantage of not producing the hypokalemia and the hyperglycemia that can complicate treatment with the sulfonamide diuretics. In doses over 100 mg. daily, spironolactone may cause breast swelling and tenderness, especially in male patients, and can produce reversible sexual dysfunction. Triamterene, another potassium-sparing diuretic that works in the distal renal tubule, can also be used in the treatment of hypertension. However, it has a fairly weak diuretic action and is generally used in combination with thiazide diuretics so as to exploit its mild potassium-conserving properties.

Setting Treatment Goals

It is well established that lowering blood pressure in hypertensive patients reduces the likelihood of major cardiovascular events and will almost certainly prolong life. In the treatment of young or middle-aged patients it would obviously be desirable to maintain blood pressure at "normal" levels such as 120/80 or even 110/70 mm. Hg. In a number of patients this goal can be achieved using only one or two antihypertensive agents in modest doses, particularly if a rational approach to treatment such as we described earlier is employed. However, blood pressure in a proportion of patients can be normalized only by the use of multidrug regimens and at the expense of excessively troublesome side effects. In such patients, the physician must use judgment and balance the negative aspects of treatment against the likely benefits. There is also the risk that overly aggressive treatment that impairs the patient's ability to enjoy an acceptable quality of life may result in disillusionment and the complete abandonment of the treatment program. Although firm data are not yet available, previous studies would indicate that any reasonable reduction in blood pressure, even if it does not fall to normal levels, should provide at least some improvement in the patient's cardiovascular prognosis.

Although blood pressure levels provide the most practical monitor of treatment effectiveness on a week-to-week or month-to-month basis, it should not be forgotten that the success of treatment can be gauged only on the basis of the patient's vascular status. Thus it is imperative that regular checks of the optic fundi, the electrocardiogram, and electrolyte metabolism and renal function be made during the long-term phase of treatment. These tests, equally important as the blood pressure measurements themselves, will tell the physician whether the treatment program is effective or whether more complete control of the blood pressure should be striven for.

Apparent Treatment Failure. Despite the use of a systematic approach to the treatment of hypertension, including the use of appropriate drugs and drug combinations in suitable doses, a small proportion of patients fail to respond adequately to treatment. Although there may be a very small residuum of patients who, for reasons not yet fully understood, appear completely refractory to treatment, possible explanations for treatment failure should be carefully explored in each case. These possibilities are listed in Table 2.

The most common and important cause of apparent resistance to treatment is a lack of compliance by the patient with the prescribed therapeutic regimen. There may be a number of reasons for poor compliance. Three principal causes stand out: inadequate instruction and insufficient awareness on the part of the patient of the importance of careful and continuing adherence to the treatment program; troublesome side effects of treatment that may lead a patient to decide that accepting the risks of discontinuation or reduction of his medications is preferable to the discomforts of treatment; and states of depression that commonly are associated with chronic illness and which may leave the patient uninterested in the quality of his own care. All these problems are potentially solvable by the physician. Good patient education, including discussion of the risks and nature of hypertension and of the problems and probable need for a lifelong duration of treatment, is an essential part of good management. Careful questioning of the patient, therefore, is a

TABLE 2. **Inadequate Treatment Response**

Poor patient compliance with treatment: inadequate instruction, excessive side effects of treatment, mental depression
Unsatisfactory medication program: inappropriate drug selection, inadequate dose schedule
Conflicting medications: e.g., sympathomimetic agents, tricyclic antidepressants, certain antihistamines, oral contraceptives
Unsuspected forms of secondary hypertension: e.g., occult renal disease, renal artery stenosis, pheochromocytoma

vital first step in evaluating an apparently unsuccessful treatment program.

Poor treatment response resulting from inappropriate drug selection can occur when medications are prescribed without sufficient thought being given to their mechanisms of action. As we have discussed earlier, antihypertensive medications should be added to and subtracted from the regimen according to a logical pattern that takes into account the basic mechanisms of the hypertensive process and the changes likely to be induced by the drug. For example, agents such as propranolol or clonidine, which work by inhibiting renin or sympathetic mechanisms, may require the addition of small doses of diuretics in order to deal with the fluid accumulation that can occur during their use. Similarly, if a diuretic is being used, it is likely that the renin-angiotensin system will be strongly stimulated and will produce marked vasoconstriction; in such patients the addition of an agent having renin-lowering properties is clearly indicated to improve blood pressure control. The addition of an inappropriate drug will not only be unhelpful in these instances, but may actually be counterproductive and produce further increases in blood pressure. In this context, it is worth re-emphasizing that when patients are responding poorly to multidrug regimens, it is often more advantageous to undergo a subtraction process than to consider the addition of yet further agents.

Occasionally, apparent treatment failure may be caused by using inadequate amounts of a particular drug. For instance, with the use of diuretics, agents such as chlorthalidone or metolazone need be given only once daily, but agents such as chlorothiazide or benzthiazide should normally be given twice daily. Furosemide must be given three or four times daily to be effective for blood pressure control. Although it has become conventional to use agents such as propranolol, clonidine, methyldopa, and hydralazine in twice daily dosages, some patients will require more frequent administrations for a full 24 hour control of blood pressure. It can sometimes be helpful to measure blood pressure at different times of the day so as to evaluate the overall effectiveness of treatment, and on the basis of this to make any necessary adjustments to the spacing and size of the doses.

The concurrent use of medications that mutually antagonize each other's mechanisms of action is sometimes responsible for a poor treatment result. For example, in patients receiving sympathetic inhibitors for their hypertension, the use of sympathomimetic amines, such as mental stimulants or nasal decongestants, may produce exaggerated and potentially dangerous upward swings in blood pressure. It should also be noted that amphetamines, some antihistamines, and the commonly used tricyclic antidepressants can interfere with the actions of antihypertensive agents, particularly ganglionic blockers such as guanethidine. In female patients whose blood pressure responses are inadequate, it is worth checking as to whether they still may be taking oral contraceptives. Even when these agents are not directly responsible for causing the hypertension, they may prevent an appropriate response to treatment with antihypertensive medications.

If one of the aforementioned causes cannot be shown to be responsible for a poor result, it is important to consider once again the possibility of an underlying secondary cause for the hypertension. An intravenous pyelogram may well be justified in such patients to look for a previously unsuspected renal artery stenosis or for some occult renal or urinary tract condition. Similarly, pheochromocytoma is often very poorly responsive to conventional antihypertensive medications, and it may be useful to discontinue all medications and reassess this possible diagnosis in patients resistant to treatment.

Emergency Treatment of Hypertension. Sometimes in the course of poorly controlled or undiagnosed hypertension, blood pressure acutely can reach levels that may place the patient in immediate jeopardy of a major cardiovascular catastrophe. This may occur in previously uncomplicated essential hypertension, but is commonly seen when the hypertension is associated with renal damage, or it may be entirely secondary to established renal disease.

The major hypertensive emergencies are (1) malignant hypertension, (2) hypertensive encephalopathy, (3) hypertension with transient ischemic attacks or impending stroke, (4) severe hypertension with left ventricular failure, (5) hypertension with dissecting or bleeding aneurysms, and (6) toxemias of pregnancy.

Diastolic blood pressures of 140 mm. Hg or above are cause for concern and will generally warrant the immediate admission of the patient to hospital. When these high blood pressures are associated with strong evidence of vascular disease, including advanced retinopathy and either hematuria or proteinuria, a state of malignant hypertension is diagnosed. As with other forms of hypertension, malignant hypertension can be classified according to renin status. However, in contrast to essential hypertension, high renin forms constitute the large majority of malignant hypertension cases, whereas normal or low renin forms are less commonly seen.

In the ideal situation, patients with malignant hypertension should be immediately tested with a powerful antirenin agent such as SQ20881. This would enable immediate classification of the condition to be made, and would enable the physician to commence treatment with the most appropriate therapeutic agent. However, until the rapidly acting agents for evaluating renin status become a standard part of the emergency room or office armamentarium, the majority of physicians will be dependent upon their own clinical judgment in choosing a drug with which to initiate treatment.

The best approach to patients with acutely elevated blood pressures is to divide them into three groups: those whose blood pressures are high but in whom there is no clinical evidence for encephalopathy or other hyperacute clinical problems; those in whom the high blood pressure is associated with symptoms or signs of an impending vascular disaster; and those in whom there is evidence of fluid overload—e.g., signs of pulmonary edema or severe heart failure, recent history of weight gain.

In patients with high levels of blood pressure but in whom there is no evidence of an imminent clinical event, the best approach is to assume a high renin state and to immediately commence treatment with comparatively high oral doses of propranolol (e.g., 40 mg. four times daily). In most patients, this will reduce blood pressure to more acceptable levels within 24 to 48 hours. If there is no response within this time period, or if the response is deemed to be inadequate, a diuretic can be added to the regimen. If at any time anxiety is felt concerning the patient's well-being, it may be necessary to respond quickly with a rapidly acting parenteral agent (see below). However, it should be recognized that in the majority of cases dramatic intervention is not required. Nor should the benefits of hospitalization and bed rest per se be overlooked.

In patients with the full syndrome of malignant hypertension and in whom an imminent vascular event is feared, treatment should be started immediately with a parenteral drug. Although intravenous administration of agents such as hydralazine or diazoxide will generally reduce blood pressure rapidly in these situations, they are fairly long-acting and do not allow the physician to modulate blood pressure to a desired level; there is always the risk of a prolonged period of absolute or relative hypotension. Probably the best available agent for use in these patients is sodium nitroprusside. The nitroprusside is prepared by making up 50 mg. in 500 ml. of 5 per cent dextrose in water. Because this agent decays rapidly in the presence of light, the entire intravenous giving-system must be carefully enveloped in aluminum foil to ensure its continued potency. Owing to its exceptionally rapid action in lowering blood pressure, there is no established infusion rate. The physician or a trained nurse must be in attendance at all times, making frequent and careful adjustments to the flow rate so as to ensure that the blood pressure is reduced to a reasonable level, and then maintained without excessive upward or downward fluctuations. Ideally, this treatment should be carried out in an intensive care unit. When it is not possible to use nitroprusside, diazoxide can be administered as a single intravenous bolus of 100 to 300 mg. This agent is also rapidly acting and has a short duration of action. Sometimes repeated dosages have to be administered in order to keep blood pressure down to an acceptable level. Because of its powerful and rapid action, the use of diazoxide can sometimes be associated with a marked hypotensive period, and the physician must carefully observe the patient for several minutes after the drug has been given. In the very rare instances in which nitroprusside and diazoxide fail to adequately lower blood pressure, an intravenous infusion of phentolamine, given at approximately 0.5 to 1.0 mg. per minute, can be given. Regardless of the intravenous agent used, treatment with conventional oral medications, administered according to the principles described earlier, should be started as soon as possible.

In the final group of patients, those in whom volume factors are presumed to be the chief cause of the rapid increase in blood pressure, immediate treatment should be started with a single intravenous bolus of furosemide, 40 mg. If this maneuver is successful, the patient can be continued on chronic diuretic treatment, together with any other antihypertensive medications found necessary. However, if there is no response to the furosemide, nitroprusside or the other rapidly acting agents discussed earlier must be employed.

Summary

A system of therapy in hypertension is presented that represents a conceptual change from traditional practice. In this new approach beta-adrenergic therapy is the cornerstone of treatment, whereas diuretic therapy, up to now the basic treatment approach, moves into a secondary but still essential role. The major current issue becomes whether long-term beta blockade of the renin secretory mechanism and the autonomic nervous system, which acts more directly to reduce peripheral resistance, is preferable to chronic volume depletion for reducing peripheral resistance.

We believe that the greater specificity of this newer approach allows effective blood pressure control to be achieved in the individual patient with fewer drugs, lower dosages, and less side effects. By constructively using a systematic process of drug subtraction as well as addition, rather than being confined by a rigid unidirectional protocol, the physician is able to define and then treat the principal mechanisms underlying the hypertension. The proof for these new and attractive possibilities rests with more clinical research and experience, both of which are gaining steadily.

ACUTE MYOCARDIAL INFARCTION

method of
LEWIS C. BECKER, M.D.
Baltimore, Maryland

Prehospital Emergency Treatment

When a patient with suspected acute myocardial infarction is seen outside the hospital, the most important consideration is immediate transport to an emergency room where constant observation and resuscitation equipment are available. This is because the risk of ventricular fibrillation is markedly increased in the first few hours of an infarct. It is estimated that 50 per cent of the deaths from infarction occur suddenly and unexpectedly before the patient reaches medical attention. It is likely that most of these deaths could be prevented by emergency defibrillation.

Therapy may sometimes be required before the patient arrives at the hospital. Severe chest pain is treated with morphine sulfate, 5 to 10 mg. intravenously or subcutaneously. Atropine, 0.5 to 1 mg., is given intravenously or subcutaneously for bradycardia accompanied by hypotension, cold clammy skin, or frequent premature ventricular beats. The dose of atropine may be repeated in a few minutes if the response is inadequate. Bradycardia which is uncomplicated does not require treatment. Lidocaine (Xylocaine), 50 to 100 mg., is given intravenously for frequent premature ventricular beats or runs of ventricular tachycardia, unless bradycardia is present, in which case atropine is used first. Recent evidence suggests that lidocaine should be considered for routine use in all patients with acute infarction, as it provides protection against ventricular fibrillation whether or not premature ventricular beats are present. For prevention of ventricular fibrillation, 50 to 100 mg. may be used intravenously or 300 mg. intramuscularly in the deltoid muscle. The intramuscular route gives more sustained blood levels of lidocaine, but this is balanced against a longer time for peak effect and a possible increase in serum enzyme levels.

Initial Hospital Evaluation

Electrocardiographic monitoring should begin as soon as the patient arrives at the hospital. An intravenous catheter should be inserted and "kept open" with a dextrose/water solution. The patient should then be accompanied from the emergency room to the coronary care area by a physician or trained nurse.

After the patient is admitted to the coronary care unit, a detailed history and physical examination should be performed. Particular attention should be paid to the adequacy of peripheral circulation, as well as to the presence or absence of pulmonary rales, abnormal precordial impulse (indicating a ventricular aneurysm), gallop sounds, pericardial friction rub, or cardiac murmurs. A systolic murmur may indicate mitral regurgitation caused by papillary muscle infarction or ventricular septal defect from a ruptured septum. A portable x-ray film of the chest should be obtained in each patient to assess the degree of pulmonary congestion. A noncardiac cause for the patient's chest pain may sometimes be revealed, such as a lung tumor, pericardial effusion, mediastinal emphysema, or dissecting aortic aneurysm.

Treatment in Coronary Care Unit

Relief of Pain. Narcotics are most commonly used for relief of pain in acute myocardial infarction. Morphine, 10 mg., and meperidine (Demerol), 75 mg., are approximately equivalent. These agents are best given intravenously in graded doses to titrate the patient's discomfort, but the subcutaneous route may be used when the circulation is not impaired. Too much narcotic may cause hypotension, respiratory depression, and nausea and vomiting, mimicking cardiogenic shock. Some patients are sensitive to the gastrointestinal side effects and may require antiemetics or atropine. Nitroglycerin does not relieve pain of acute infarction, and because of the risk of hypotension it should not be used except for specific indications, including unstable angina, acute pulmonary edema, or low output syndrome (see below). Narcotics are usually needed only for the first day of an acute infarction. Pain continuing after the first day generally represents pericarditis, although impending rupture of the heart, extension of the infarct, or undiagnosed aortic dissection must also be considered. When pain is due to pericarditis, aspirin, 600 mg. every 4 hours, or indomethacin, 25 mg. every 6 hours (this use of indomethacin is not listed in the manufacturer's official directive), is much more effective than narcotics.

Oxygen. Oxygen should be given routinely by face mask or nasal cannula at 4 liters per minute. Recent studies have shown a reduction in ST segment elevation when 40 per cent oxygen is given compared to room air. Patients in pulmonary edema or shock may require higher inspired oxygen concentrations or assisted ventilation to maintain adequate arterial Po_2 levels.

Activity. Patients with uncomplicated infarction are allowed up in a chair for short periods on the day after infarction. Progressive ambulation is begun 7 days after an infarction; if there are no complications, patients are discharged at 2 weeks. Patients with significant arrhythmias or congestive heart failure are ambulated more slowly and kept in the hospital longer. Earlier ambulation in general has reduced the problems of pulmonary embolism and deep venous thrombosis. After 4 to 6 weeks of home convalescence, patients return to light work, and by 3 months they are usually back to work fulltime.

Bowel Movements. Patients generally use a bedside commode rather than a bedpan to move their bowels. Use of a commode involves less energy expenditure and more effectively prevents constipation. Stool softeners such as dioctyl sodium sulfosuccinate (Colace) or mild laxatives are used routinely.

Diet. A light diet is usually given for the first few days. Very hot or cold foods are avoided, and salt is restricted if congestive heart failure is present. Subsequently the patient is given a diet low in saturated fat and cholesterol. If he is obese, weight reduction is recommended.

Sedation. Moderate doses of sedatives are used to allay patient fear and prevent anxiety-induced arrhythmias. Sedation may also be useful as an adjunct in the patient with severe chest pain resistant to large doses of morphine. Around-the-clock sedative administration to keep the patient "snowed under" has obvious dangers and has not been proved to be of benefit. If the patient is being treated with one of the coumarin drugs, it must be remembered that certain sedatives, notably barbiturates, chloral hydrate, glutethimide (Doriden), meprobamate, and ethchlorvynol (Placidyl), stimulate microsomal enzymes, which metabolize the coumarin drugs and lead to decreased anticoagulant levels. Drugs such as hydroxyzine (Vistaril), diazepam (Valium), chlordiazepoxide (Librium), and promethazine (Phenergan) may be preferable, as they do not seem to interfere.

Anticoagulation. Despite many clinical trials, the question of anticoagulation remains controversial. Anticoagulants have been shown in retrospective but not prospective trials to reduce mortality. Prospective studies have, however, indicated a reduction in pulmonary and systemic emboli with anticoagulants, suggesting a reduction in deep venous and left ventricular mural thrombosis. For this reason, most patients with acute infarction are given anticoagulants. A constant intravenous infusion of heparin is used in doses sufficient to prolong the clotting time to about 20 minutes; 30,000 to 40,000 units every 24 hours is usually required. With this technique, bleeding complications are very uncommon. "Minidose" heparin, 5000 units every 12 hours subcutaneously or intravenously, protects against deep venous thrombosis without prolonging the clotting time, but it is unknown whether pulmonary emboli and particularly systemic emboli are prevented. Warfarin sodium (Coumadin) may be used instead of heparin, but the dose is more difficult to control precisely. All patients with congestive heart failure, shock, or recurrent arrhythmias are anticoagulated unless they are actively bleeding, as the risk of thromboembolism is high. Anticoagulants are not usually stopped because of pericarditis unless postinfarction (Dressler's) syndrome is thought to be present. They are usually discontinued after the patient is ambulatory.

Treatment of Complications

Arrhythmias. Arrhythmias are particularly frequent in patients with infarction. The presence of ischemic areas of myocardium produces an uneven spread of excitation and recovery over the ventricles, leading to "re-entry" of excitation waves from slowly recovering areas into more quickly recovering ones, and causing ectopic ventricular contractions. Heart block and bradycardias may result from infarction or edema of the sinus or atrioventricular nodes, or from involvement of the more distal portions of the conduction system. Atrial arrhythmias may occur from pericarditis, from infarction of the atria, or as a result of left ventricular failure with rising left atrial pressure and left atrial dilatation. Finally, drugs used in the treatment of myocardial infarction, such as morphine or digitalis glycosides, may produce arrhythmias on their own account.

TACHYRHYTHMIAS. Sinus tachycardia occurs in as many as one third of patients with acute infarction and is most often due to anxiety, fever, pericarditis, or increased levels of circulating catecholamines. When sustained, it may be a manifestation of cardiac failure and indicate a poor prognosis. Ordinarily sinus tachycardia is not treated except to deal with underlying causes. Occasionally the beta-adrenergic blocking agent propranolol (Inderal) is given if the tachycardia is excessive (over 120 beats per minute) and heart failure is not present. This is done to reduce myocardial oxygen demands and thereby limit myocardial ischemia. Propranolol should be started in low doses and increased stepwise as needed. Orally 10 mg. every 6 hours is used, but intravenously the dose is much lower, 1 mg. every 4 hours.

Atrial and junctional (nodal) tachyrhythmias are managed in patients with infarction much as they are in other settings. Basically, the choice of therapy is dictated by the clinical state of the patient. If the arrhythmia has produced serious clinical deterioration, DC countershock should be used. However, electrical conversion of a patient with digitalis toxicity should be avoided, as dangerous postconversion ventricular arrhythmias may result. If the situation is less critical, drug therapy may be employed as in patients without infarction.

Because atrial arrhythmias are frequently recurrent in the first week of an infarction, procainamide (Pronestyl), 250 to 500 mg. orally every 3 to 4 hours, or quinidine, 0.8 to 1.2 grams daily in divided doses, may be required. In all cases of atrial tachyrhythmias, left ventricular failure and pulmonary emboli should be considered as precipitating factors.

Ventricular arrhythmias are generally a greater problem than atrial arrhythmias in acute myocardial infarction. Ventricular premature beats (VPB's), particularly when frequent or multifocal, are potentially lethal. A VPB occurring during the vulnerable period of repolarization, on the ascending portion and peak of the T wave, may directly induce ventricular tachycardia or fibrillation. VPB's are therefore aggressively suppressed with drugs during the early period of infarction. Intravenous lidocaine (Xylocaine) is the drug of choice for suppressing ventricular irritability. Because its onset of action is very rapid and its duration of action short, danger of overdosage is minimized. However, it is rapidly metabolized by the liver, and a blood level must be established by bolus injection and maintained by continuous intravenous infusion. An initial dose of 1 mg. per kg. is given and repeated in 5 minutes if necessary. If this is successful, an infusion of 20 micrograms per kg. per minute (1 to 2 mg. per minute) is started. If ectopic beats return, an additional small bolus is given and the infusion rate increased. Rates in excess of 50 micrograms per kg. per minute (roughly 3.5 mg. per minute) frequently produce neurotoxic side effects: tinnitus, visual scintillations, acute agitation, obtundation, or seizures. Patients with low cardiac output or liver disease should generally receive only half the usual rate because of reduced drug clearance and increased risk of toxicity. Recent studies showing that ventricular fibrillation can occur without any premonitory VPB's have led to the suggestion that lidocaine should be used routinely in all patients for prophylaxis against fibrillation. Protection can be achieved at a dose of 3 mg. per minute, but the incidence of side effects is high. Other studies using 2 mg. per minute do not show protection. Prophylactic lidocaine should be considered most strongly for patients presenting early in their infarction, when the risk of fibrillation is highest.

Procainamide is usually given when lidocaine is unsuccessful in managing ventricular ectopic activity. A dose of 100 mg. is administered intravenously every 5 minutes until ectopic beats are suppressed or 1 gram is reached. A 1 gram loading dose can also be given orally. This initial dose is followed by 250 to 500 mg. orally every 3 to 4 hours or a constant infusion of 20 to 50 micrograms per kg. per minute. In the event of toxic side effects, such as hypotension, diminished cardiac output, or QRS prolongation (greater than 25 per cent), the dose must be reduced or the drug discontinued. Dose levels should also be reduced in the presence of hepatic or renal dysfunction.

Less frequently used drugs for suppressing ventricular premature beats include quinidine, phenytoin sodium (Dilantin), and propranolol (Inderal). Quinidine is given in a dose of 200 to 300 mg. every 4 to 6 hours; however, in some instances, the Q-T interval prolongation caused by the drug may increase rather than decrease the tendency to ventricular fibrillation. Phenytoin is given intravenously in loading doses similar to those of procainamide and may be particularly useful in digitalis-induced arrhythmias. (This use of phenytoin is not listed in the manufacturer's official directive.) Propranolol, given in 1 mg. increments intravenously, may be useful in the absence of heart failure.

When ventricular premature beats are refractory to drug therapy, a difficult management problem arises. If dosage levels of suppressant drugs are "pushed," toxic myocardial side effects and circulatory failure may result. There is a real risk of doing more harm than good in this situation, and careful clinical judgment must be exercised.

Ventricular tachycardia is the most dangerous arrhythmia short of ventricular fibrillation. It usually results in a prompt and severe fall in cardiac output and degenerates into ventricular fibrillation. It is usually terminated immediately by DC countershock, but a hard thump on the sternum with the fist may occasionally suffice. If the rhythm is tolerated and the patient remains conscious, an intravenous bolus of lidocaine, 50 to 100 mg., may also stop it.

Recurrent ventricular tachycardia or frequent ventricular premature beats refractory to drug therapy may be treated by cardiac pacing. A transvenous ventricular pacemaker is inserted, and the heart is paced at a rate of 90 beats per minute or greater to prevent recurrences of ventricular tachycardia. Brief periods of pacing may also be used to convert ventricular tachycardia to sinus rhythm.

Ventricular fibrillation is treated by immediate DC shock. While the defibrillator is being brought to the patient's bedside, a sharp blow to the precordium should be given and external cardiac compression instituted. There must be no delay in administering DC shock, because the longer ventricular fibrillation continues, the harder it is to resuscitate the patient. If initial resuscitation efforts are unsuccessful, endotracheal intubation should be performed, sodium bicarbonate and epinephrine administered, and resuscitation continued as in other cardiac arrest situations.

BRADYRHYTHMIAS. Sinus bradycardia is seen in as many as 40 per cent of patients monitored very early in the infarction and is more common in inferior than in anterior infarctions. Sinus bradycardia is now treated with atropine only if it is associated with hypotension, signs of low cardiac output, or ventricular irritability. Uncomplicated bradycardia is no longer treated because of evidence that atropine may induce sustained sinus tachycardia, ventricular ectopic beats, or ventricular fibrillation. Other side effects include urinary retention, precipitation of glaucoma, and mental aberration. Side effects may be minimized by using an initial dose of 0.5 mg. of atropine intravenously and giving more only if needed.

The most serious bradyrhythmia is complete heart block, although the prognosis, as well as incidence and presentation, differs for inferior and anterior infarctions. In inferior infarctions, heart block is more common and is produced by ischemia of the atrioventricular node. There is usually a transition through first- and second-degree atrioventricular block. Complete block is usually associated with an escape focus of normal QRS duration and rate over 45 beats per minute. On the other hand, in anterior infarctions, heart block, although less common, carries a far worse prognosis. This is because the infarction is larger and is frequently associated with heart failure or shock. Block is produced by injury to the bundle branches distal to the His bundle, and often occurs suddenly without going through lesser degrees of block. Frequently, the presence of an interventricular conduction defect, particularly a bundle branch block pattern with abnormal electrical axis, is the only clue of imminent heart block. The escape focus tends to be slower and more unstable than in inferior infarctions, and the QRS complex tends to be wide and bizarre. Asystole may occur without warning.

In inferior infarctions with heart block, a temporary transvenous pacemaker should be inserted in the following situations: (1) if the heart rate is less than 40 beats per minute; (2) if there is hypotension or loss of consciousness; (3) if ventricular irritability is present; or (4) if there is associated bundle branch block, especially of acute onset. If the heart rate is above 40 beats per minute, the QRS complexes are narrow, and the rhythm is well tolerated, it is not necessary to insert a pacemaker. In anterior infarctions with heart block, however, the situation is different. Because of the danger of sudden asystole, all patients with second-degree or complete atrioventricular block in the setting of acute anterior infarction should have a pacemaker placed immediately, even if the rhythm is well tolerated. Patients with bundle branch block should probably also have a pacemaker, particularly if the bundle branch block is acute.

The risks of transvenous pacing are real and must be borne in mind. Pacing catheters may perforate the right ventricle, become infected, or mechanically induce ventricular arrhythmias. Pacing should not be attempted if experienced personnel and appropriate facilities are unavailable.

Drug treatment of complete heart block has little place in acute infarction except as a temporary emergency measure. Atropine, 0.5 to 2.0 mg. intravenously, or isoproterenol, 1 to 5 micrograms per minute infusion, may be administered while arrangements are being made to insert a pacing catheter. If asystole suddenly develops, it is better to insert an emergency pacing wire. A semi-floating wire can be passed percutaneously from a peripheral vein or a transthoracic wire can be passed through the chest wall into the right ventricular cavity.

Unstable Angina. An unstable anginal syndrome may develop in the early postinfarction period characterized by repeated episodes of transient myocardial ischemia occurring at rest. This syndrome is more common in patients with a small infarct in which ischemic viable myocardium remains in the region of infarction. Frequently there are changes in heart rate and blood pressure and transient changes in ST segments or T waves in the electrocardiogram during the ischemic episodes. These findings may allow differentiation from pericardial or chest wall pain. Treatment includes sublingual nitroglycerin for the acute attack, and long-acting nitrates, propranolol, and anticoagulants for prevention of repeated attacks. Isosorbide dinitrate (Isordil) is given sublingually,

5 to 10 mg. every 2 to 3 hours, or orally, 10 to 40 mg. every 4 to 6 hours. The oral preparation gives a longer-lasting effect, but requires higher doses to compensate for "first pass" inactivation by the liver via the portal circulation. Nitroglycerin may also be given cutaneously (Nitrol ointment, 2 per cent nitroglycerin) ½ to 2 inches every 4 to 6 hours, spread thinly over a 6 inch square area under plastic wrap. Propranolol is begun in low dose, 10 mg. every 6 hours, and increased until symptoms abate, side effects occur, or full beta-adrenergic blockade is achieved. "Full" blockade is judged by a resting pulse under 60 beats per minute and the lack of increase with activity. Doses as high as 100 mg. every 6 hours may be required, but the drug must be used with caution in the presence of heart failure. If the unstable anginal syndrome cannot be controlled medically, an intra-aortic balloon is generally used to provide relief. Coronary angiography is then performed and the patient sent for coronary artery bypass graft surgery if he proves to be a suitable candidate.

Hypertension. Hypertension is common in patients with acute infarction because of catecholamine excess. Usually no specific therapy is necessary beyond bed rest, sedation, and relief of chest pain. If hypertension persists for several hours, a rapidly acting diuretic such as furosemide (Lasix) or an antihypertensive agent such as alphamethyldopa (Aldomet) is given. If blood pressure is markedly elevated (more than 190/130), an intravenous infusion of sodium nitroprusside (Nipride) may be used, particularly if there is associated heart failure or persistent chest pain. To avoid a precipitous fall in blood pressure, very close blood pressure monitoring is required, usually through a radial artery catheter.

Congestive Heart Failure. A mild degree of left ventricular failure is common in patients with acute infarction and is not necessarily a bad prognostic sign. Severe left ventricular failure with pulmonary edema, however, carries a very grave prognosis. Signs of right-sided heart failure, such as edema, congested liver, and elevated venous pressure, are not present unless there is a history of chronic heart failure or unless the patient has infarcted the right ventricle.

Diuretics are used first to treat congestive failure. Furosemide, 20 to 40 mg., or ethacrynic acid, 25 to 50 mg., is commonly chosen because of rapid action. If diuretics are unsuccessful, digitalis glycosides may be added, but they must be used with caution because of their potential for causing arrhythmias, and the possibility that they may increase the extent of injury by increasing myocardial oxygen demands. Digitalis should generally be continued in patients with acute infarction who have been taking it chronically. Congestive heart failure refractory to diuretics and digitalis may respond to vasodilator treatment. Nitrates may be used sublingually, orally, or cutaneously, or nitroprusside may be given intravenously. Therapy is best monitored using systemic arterial and pulmonary arterial catheters. Acute pulmonary edema is treated as in other situations with upright posture, rotating tourniquets, oxygen (with positive pressure if necessary), morphine, rapidly acting diuretics, bronchodilators, and phlebotomy as a last resort.

Shock. Cardiogenic shock accounts for about 40 per cent of the hospital deaths from acute myocardial infarction and has an 80 to 90 per cent mortality. The shock syndrome is characterized by mental confusion, low urinary output, poor peripheral perfusion, and central hypoxia. There are severe reductions in cardiac output and systemic blood pressure. Left ventricular filling pressure and pulmonary artery pressure are elevated, and because peripheral circulation is inadequate, acidosis and tissue injury result. The inadequacy of present therapy is clearly indicated by the high mortality. It is therefore most important to distinguish certain conditions that may mimic cardiogenic shock. These include morphine overdose, hemorrhage from an occult gastrointestinal lesion (especially in a patient on anticoagulants), and dehydration.

In managing cardiogenic shock, precipitating causes, such as arrhythmias or myocardial depression from antiarrhythmic drugs, should first be ruled out. Oxygen and digitalis are given, and adrenergic stimulants such as dopamine (Intropin) or norepinephrine (Levophed) may be used. The aim of therapy with adrenergic stimulants is to improve cardiac output and coronary perfusion pressure (aortic blood pressure) without disproportionately increasing myocardial oxygen demand or peripheral vasoconstriction. If blood pressure is reasonably well maintained (over 90/60), vasodilators such as nitroprusside are given cautiously in preference to adrenergic agents in an effort to reduce systemic resistance, improve cardiac output, and increase organ blood flow. Beneficial effects can often be achieved without further reduction in blood pressure. Acidosis is corrected and artificial ventilation initiated if spontaneous respirations become inadequate.

Management is aided by catheters to measure urinary output, systemic arterial pressure, and pulmonary artery pressure. The pulmonary artery diastolic pressure correlates well with left ventricular filling pressure in the absence of mitral valve or chronic pulmonary disease; if filling pressure is low, volume expansion may improve cardiac output. Central venous pressure has been found to be very misleading for this purpose.

Circulatory-assist devices are currently being used for management of cardiogenic shock refractory to medical therapy. Of the various techniques, intra-aortic balloon counterpulsation is the most widely used. The aim is to improve cardiac output without increasing myocardial oxygen consumption and to limit infarct size by improving diastolic coronary perfusion. Some patients who improve temporarily on circulatory assist but relapse into shock when it is discontinued have had emergency coronary arteriography and coronary saphenous vein bypass grafts or infarctectomy. The patients most likely to survive are those with their first infarct who have a correctible process contributing to the depth of shock, such as arrhythmia, sepsis, myocardial ischemia adjacent to the infarct region, mitral regurgitation, or a new ventricular septal defect (see below). Considering the enormous effort required, the overall results of this aggressive approach have been disappointing.

Surgical Complications of Acute Myocardial Infarction

Occasional patients develop rupture of a papillary muscle, resulting in severe mitral regurgitation, or rupture of the interventricular septum with formation of a large left to right shunt. Both these complications are heralded by the presence of a new systolic murmur. Although they may be difficult to distinguish clinically, a ruptured septum generally presents a more medially located murmur accompanied by a left parasternal thrill and signs of right ventricular failure. Diagnosis can usually be made by right heart catheterization. With a ruptured septum, blood taken from the pulmonary artery and right ventricle will be more fully saturated with oxygen than blood from the right atrium. With a ruptured papillary muscle, large "V" waves may be seen in the pressure tracing recorded from a catheter wedged in a distal branch of the pulmonary artery, but a left ventricular angiogram may be necessary to confirm the diagnosis.

If the patient's clinical condition permits, these defects are repaired 6 to 12 weeks after the acute infarction, when the scar has become firm and sutures are more likely to hold. However, if the patient deteriorates in the early stages of infarction, surgical repair must be attempted under nonideal circumstances; in this setting the risks of surgery are very high but are justified in view of the 90 to 100 per cent mortality with conservative management.

CARE AND REHABILITATION AFTER MYOCARDIAL INFARCTION

method of
ROBERT J. CORLISS, M.D.
Madison, Wisconsin

Care and rehabilitation after a myocardial infarction must be individually adjusted, because coronary atherosclerosis is so multifaceted in its clinical presentation. Following the acute phase of a myocardial infarction, the aims should be as follows:

1. To minimize the potential complications of depression, physical deconditioning, negative nitrogen balance, and pulmonary emboli that are often associated with a myocardial infarction and prolonged bed rest.
2. To minimize the period of hospitalization and convalescence and return the patients to a normal life as soon as possible.
3. To minimize (ideally) the chance of recurrent myocardial infarction or progression of the atherosclerotic process by modifying the associated risk factors.
4. To inform and educate patients and their families about the disease.

Ambulation

A program of progressive ambulation should be started as soon as efforts to reduce myocardial oxygen consumption are stabilized; pain, congestive heart failure, and arrhythmias are controlled; and the acute enzyme (CPK) has peaked or begun to decrease. This is generally on the second or third day of infarction. Up until that time, passive range of motion and voluntary extremity movements should be encouraged.

The use of changes in the heart rate for monitoring exercise and ambulation is recommended and has the following advantages:

1. Physical work and myocardial oxygen consumption are linearly related to the heart rate, but the heart rate per unit of workload is an individual characteristic determined by age, physical conditioning, and the cardiac status. Consequently, exercise prescribed by heart rate (based on age) compensates for individual differences in physical conditioning and varying myocardial oxygen requirements for the same activity in different persons.
2. Precise instructions may be given to the hospital staff and the patient and written as a prescription or physican order.

3. The heart rate can continue to be used as a guide for physical activity and conditioning programs after discharge.

To initiate the program of ambulation:

1. Patients should be instructed in taking their own heart (pulse) rate.

2. A target heart rate is assigned the patients based on their age.

3. Ambulation prescriptions are calculated daily and modified as indicated by the clinical course and then written as a specific instruction to the hospital staff.

The following formula:

$$[(\text{Target heart rate} - \text{resting rate}) \times (\%\ \text{increment increase})] + (\text{resting heart rate}) = \text{exercising heart rate for that given day}$$

is used to provide a guide for activity (Table 1). The "target heart rate" is age related and can be adjusted up or down, depending on the philosophy of the attending physician. The per cent increment increase in heart rate per day will determine the time of hospitalization—a 10 per cent increment increase will provide about 12 days of hospitalization; a 5 per cent increase, about 3 weeks. The trend is toward more rapid ambulation and shorter hospitalization.

TABLE 1. **Example of Ambulation Program Following Myocardial Infarction**

DAY POSTINFARCT	% INCREASE	TIME (MINUTES)	SETS PER DAY
1	0	Passive range of motion and voluntary extremity movements	
2	0		
3	10	3	2
4	20	3	3
5	30	4	3
6	40	4	3
7	50	5	4
8	60	5	4
9	70	6	4
10	80	7	4
11	90	8	4
12	100	8	1

AGE	TARGET HEART RATE
70	105
60–69	110
50–59	115
40–49	120
Under 40	125

Example: 52-year-old male; resting heart rate, 84; day 7.

$$[(115 - 84) \times 50\%] + 84 = 99$$

Patient exercised with heart rate of 99 to 100 5 minutes four times.

The patient should be exercised up to the predetermined heart rate, and this level of exertion should be maintained during the exercise period. The activity should be dynamic as opposed to isometric; always limited to within the production of chest pain, arrhythmias, or undue fatigue; and performed at least 1 hour after meals. Initial exercise periods to generate the estimated heart rate will have great patient-to-patient variability and can be performed in the patient's room or at the bedside. During the latter stages of the program, the exercise will consist primarily of bench stepping and walking in the halls. The length of the exercise period can range from 3 to 10 minutes per session, with two to four sessions per day. The shorter and less frequent sessions are recommended early in ambulation.

A single lead electrocardiogram and the blood pressure should be monitored during the first few days and the last day of the exercise program. When not formally exercising, patients may be fully ambulatory but should always limit their activity to within the production of approximately 75 per cent of that day's prescribed exercising heart rate. Patients should not be allowed to exercise unsupervised.

Activity and Discharge

By the time of discharge, patients should be able to accurately check their own heart rate and adjust their activity accordingly. The patients are assigned a maximum heart rate, which should be approximately 90 per cent of their "target heart rate." They may then engage in any activity at home (physical, emotional, or sexual), as long as they do not exceed this maximum heart rate. They also should be given a "training heart rate," more arbitrarily determined, but approximately 75 to 80 per cent of their hospital "target heart rate." They should be instructed to exercise to this level several times daily but not immediately after meals. As their convalescence progresses, the training rate can be increased.

Four to 8 weeks after the infarction, a progressive exercise tolerance test should be done to determine the safe maximum work capacity. Based on the exercise tolerance test, a further training program can be started. Generally patients can exercise at 70 per cent of their individually determined maximum workload. Since the heart rate and workloads are linearly related, the heart rate may still be used as a guide. If the initial phase of the training cannot be done under some form of supervision, a lower percentage (50 to 60 per cent) of the maximum work capacity should initially be used. The exercising periods are gradually increased up to 30 to 45 minutes per day, 3 to 5 days per week, with a warm-up and cool-down period. The total work capacity determined by the exercise tolerance test can be compared to the estimated energy requirements of the patient's occupation and used as a guide for returning the patient to work.

It must be emphasized that patient motivation, coordination, interest, and previous experience vary, and any exercise rehabilitation program will have to be individually adjusted.

Risk Factors

Even though changes in the progression or possibly regression of coronary atherosclerosis have not been documented when the risk factors are limited, common sense dictates their modification when possible. Patients should adjust their eating habits by limiting both the saturated fat content and the caloric intake of their diet in an effort to reduce their total body fat to under 10 per cent (weight of most individuals in their early 20's). Cigarette smoking should be discontinued. The patient should engage in a physical conditioning program as previously outlined. Personality should be modified as much as possible by fostering "Type B" characteristics and eliminating "Type A." Hypertension should be vigorously treated. Hyperlipidemia, diabetes, and hyperuricemia can be modified by diet and treated if necessary. Admittedly, these idealistic objectives are rarely obtained, but they should nevertheless be sought.

Drugs

The use of drugs in asymptomatic patients in the convalescence phase of myocardial infarction cannot be routinely recommended until adequate clinical studies are completed. Anticoagulants are suggested only if there are special conditions predisposing to thromboembolism. The platelet antiaggregate, aspirin, because of the required low dose, minimal side effects, low cost, and effects in experimental models may prove useful. Beta-blockers also have been proved effective in certain experimental models. Because of their potential benefits, they should be considered primary drugs for the treatment of certain arrhythmias and hypertension when associated with coronary atherosclerosis.

Complications

Patients who have limiting or progressive angina in spite of adequate therapy, those with poor exercise tolerance tests, those with atypical or unusual manifestations of their infarct or convalescence, and those employed in certain occupations should be considered for coronary arteriography or myocardial imaging. Persistent or exercise-induced arrhythmias should be evaluated by continuous ambulatory monitoring to determine their significance. Complications such as ventricular aneurysm, papillary muscle dysfunction, or pericarditis may not become evident until weeks or months after the infarct and require special evaluation.

PERICARDITIS

method of
WILLIAM H. GAASCH, M.D.
Boston, Massachusetts

Optimal management of pericarditis includes (1) specific treatment of the underlying cause; (2) treatment of pain; (3) treatment of arrhythmias; (4) management of pericardial effusion, including pericardiocentesis for tamponade; and (5) pericardiectomy when the diagnosis of constrictive pericarditis is made.

Etiology

Acute benign (idiopathic) pericarditis is probably the most common form of pericarditis seen in clinical practice, and no specific treatment is available. Management consists of pain control (e.g., aspirin, indomethacin; see below) and observation to detect the presence or development of pericardial effusion.

Purulent pericarditis is treated with systemic antibiotics and surgical drainage of the pericardial space. As soon as the diagnosis is made, treatment (appropriate for most likely organisms) is begun; the combination of methicillin, 12 grams per day intravenously or intramuscularly (this dose may be greater than that listed in the manufacturer's official directive), and gentamicin, 2 to 4 mg. per kg. per day in divided intramuscular doses, may be used until the results of culture are available. Cultures of the pericardial fluid, sputum, pleural fluid, and blood should be obtained; a simple Gram stain may allow a more specific approach while awaiting the culture and sensitivity results.

Tuberculous pericarditis requires prolonged treatment with antituberculous chemotherapy, and thus all possible diagnostic approaches should be utilized before committing the patient to 2 or more years of combined drug therapy. Initial therapy consists of streptomycin, 1 gram intramuscularly daily; isoniazid, 400 to 600 mg. per day; and ethambutol, 15 mg. per kg. per day. After the acute stage, generally 2 to 3 months, streptomycin is discontinued; isoniazid and ethambutol are continued for a period of 2 years. Other agents (rifampin, para-aminosalicylic acid) may be substituted, and pyridoxine should be used during isoniazid therapy to prevent neurotoxicity. Prednisone, 80 mg. daily in divided doses, is indicated in patients with a significant pericardial effusion; the rationale for this includes a more rapid resolution of the effusion and a reduced incidence of late pericardial constriction. Corticosteroids are generally tapered and discontinued within 1 to 2 months; a recurrence of pain or effusion is not rare during the period of steroid dose reduction.

Acute pericarditis may also be due to a host of other causes, including trauma, neoplasm, radiation, uremia, immunologic disease (including drug hypersensitivity), and others. *Traumatic pericarditis,* such as that produced by blunt chest trauma or myocardial perforation by a pacemaker wire, is treated conservatively with careful observation for bleeding and tamponade. Tamponade is an urgent indication for pericardiocentesis, and recurrent tamponade requires surgical drainage of the pericardium. *Neoplastic pericarditis* is treated with local and systemic chemotherapy, mediastinal irradiation, and open drainage for recurrent effusion with tamponade. *Uremic pericarditis* generally occurs with markedly elevated blood urea nitrogen; however, pericarditis may also develop during dialysis when the blood urea nitrogen has been lowered. Therapy consists of indomethacin,* 25 to 50 mg. every 6 hours; steroids are occasionally used. Anticoagulants should not be used if there is evidence of pericardial bleeding and generally should be avoided in patients with pericarditis.

Pericardial Pain

Aspirin, 600 mg. every 4 hours, or indomethacin,* 25 to 50 mg. every 6 hours, is an effective analgesic and anti-inflammatory agent. Prednisone, 60 to 80 mg. per day, is sometimes employed during the early phase of pericarditis to attenuate the inflammatory response and to reduce the effusion. During the reduction in steroid dosage, the patient should be treated with aspirin or indomethacin* in an attempt to reduce the rebound inflammatory response and pain that may occur. If pain is severe, meperidine hydrochloride or morphine may be used. Pericardiectomy may be necessary for refractory pain.

*This use of indomethacin is not listed in the manufacturer's official directive.

Arrhythmias

Supraventricular tachyrhythmias (e.g., atrial fibrillation, atrial flutter, paroxysmal atrial tachycardia) are common in patients with acute pericarditis, and they are managed just as they would be in patients without pericarditis. Digitalization is generally effective, although some refractory cases may require additional antiarrhythmic agents.

Pericardial Effusion

Pericardial effusion in acute idiopathic pericarditis, in tuberculous pericarditis, and in most other forms of pericarditis generally resolves when anti-inflammatory therapy is initiated. The simple presence of a pericardial effusion, even a large effusion, is not an indication for pericardiocentesis. Although the echocardiogram has been found to be a very sensitive tool in the diagnosis of pericardial effusion, cardiac tamponade is not an echocardiographic diagnosis; the echocardiogram should be used only to confirm the presence and to estimate the volume of the fluid. In some cases, an acute seroconstrictive process may result in cardiac compression within weeks and, because of the thickened pericardium, tamponade may occur in the presence of only modest effusion.

Pericardiocentesis is indicated as a therapeutic maneuver when tamponade is present and as a diagnostic maneuver (1) when purulent pericarditis is suspected, (2) when tumor cells are likely to be found in the pericardial fluid, (3) when tuberculous pericarditis is under consideration, and (4) under certain other conditions when the diagnosis remains in doubt. However, the yield of a diagnostic pericardiocentesis is often disappointingly low; for instance, if tuberculous pericarditis is under consideration, a pericardial biopsy (in addition to fluid examination and culture) is much more likely to be useful than is a simple pericardiocentesis.

Except under the most urgent conditions, pericardiocentesis should be carried out in an intensive care unit or laboratory where monitoring and resuscitation equipment is readily available. Continuous electrocardiographic monitoring is essential, and it is useful to follow the central venous pressure during the procedure. The patient may be premedicated with diazepam; atropine, 0.6 to 1.0 mg. subcutaneously, is employed to prevent vagal reactions.

The costoxiphoid area is cleansed and draped using standard techniques, and the patient is positioned on his back in a steep (60 degrees) head-up posture. The skin and subcutaneous tissue to the left of the xiphoid are anesthetized.

An 18 gauge needle (8 cm. long) is connected to a 30 to 50 ml. syringe via a three-way stopcock; sterile tubing is connected to the stopcock to allow fluid collection. The needle may be connected to the V-lead of the electrocardiogram for monitoring purposes. However, care must be taken to ensure proper grounding of the electronic equipment, as current leaks may induce ventricular fibrillation. This potential problem is especially prominent when a metal needle is surrounded by a plastic sheath or cannula; in this situation the needle is insulated except at its tip, and a current leak may be delivered directly to the heart.

The needle is advanced in a posterosuperior direction, with the needle at an approximately 30 to 40 degree angle to the skin; the needle is directed toward the midline or slightly toward the right shoulder; it is advanced, and a distinct "give" or "pop" is commonly felt when the needle pierces the pericardium. If the needle touches the epicardium, ST elevation is seen on the exploring (V-lead) electrode and extrasystoles may develop. Once the needle is in the pericardium, a clamp may be attached to the needle at the skin surface to stabilize the needle. Fluid is aspirated and, in general, removal of only a small amount of pericardial fluid will result in a prompt reduction in the central venous pressure and dramatic symptomatic improvement. If the fluid is bloody, its hematocrit is measured and compared to a venous sample. Although pericardial fluid generally fails to clot, a recent pericardial bleed might produce an aspirate which clots. Samples are withdrawn for appropriate bacteriologic, histologic, or other tests.

Pericardial aspiration may be carried out with the needle or through a catheter which may be placed in the pericardial space; a guidewire can be advanced through the needle into the pericardium, the needle is withdrawn, and a catheter (with multiple side holes) is advanced over the guidewire. This catheter may be secured and left in place for 24 to 48 hours to allow continued pericardial drainage, or it may be used for instillation of cytotoxic agents in patients with malignant disease of the pericardium. The instillation of CO_2 or air into the pericardium has been suggested to evaluate the pericardial thickness or tumor mass following pericardiocentesis; the volume should not exceed 20 to 30 per cent of the amount of fluid aspirated. A chest x-ray should be obtained following pericardiocentesis in all patients.

Cardiac tamponade is manifest by increased jugular venous pressure, pulsus paradoxus, and hypotension, and it is by definition due to markedly elevated pericardial pressure. The life-saving treatment is immediate removal of the pericardial fluid. Very temporary support may be produced by rapid intravenous infusion of volume and by the administration of 2 to 4 micrograms of isoproterenol per minute. These temporizing measures should be used only briefly while one is preparing for pericardiocentesis.

Constrictive Pericarditis

Although it is said that constrictive pericarditis does not occur following acute rheumatic fever, it is probably safe to assume that pericarditis may progress to constriction in any of the other different etiologic classifications; tuberculous or radiation pericarditis is more likely to produce constriction than acute (benign) idiopathic pericarditis. Once the characteristic findings of constriction are present, the diagnosis should be confirmed by cardiac catheterization, severe congestion should be treated medically, and a pericardiectomy should be performed. Postponing surgery can only result in progression of the constricting process to a point at which the surgical procedure becomes more difficult and the risk increases.

Preoperatively, the patient should be treated with salt restriction, diuretics, and digitalis. However, the overuse of diuretics should be avoided as some degree of elevation of the central venous pressure is important in maintaining cardiac output. Medical therapy is generally continued for a time postoperatively, as it may take several months for the maximum benefit of pericardiectomy to become apparent.

DEGENERATIVE ARTERIAL DISEASE

method of
WILSON V. GARRETT, M.D.,
and ROBERT W. BARNES, M.D.
Iowa City, Iowa

Acute Ischemia

Manifestations of acute limb ischemia include severe pain, pallor, coolness, and eventual neurologic dysfunction in the extremity manifested by either sensory or later motor deficits. The cause of acute ischemia, excluding obvious traumatic causes, includes embolism of thrombotic material from a more proximal point in the vascular tree and thrombosis locally in the area of pre-existing arteriosclerotic stenosis. More and more frequently, iatrogenic causes of acute ischemia following cardiac catheterization, radiologic procedures, and the insertion of monitoring catheters into the arterial system have been identified.

The differentiation of embolus versus thrombosis is important, because the type of surgery required, the immediate therapy instituted, and the planning for operative intervention are considerably different. Patients suffering from acute embolization of thrombotic material usually have no history of pre-existing claudication or other symptoms of chronic ischemia. Most of these patients have associated cardiac disease with a history of recent myocardial infarction, ventricular aneurysm, cardiac arrhythmias (particularly atrial flutter and atrial fibrillation), or rheumatic valvular disease. More recently, other disease processes in the more proximal vasculature have been incriminated as sources of embolic material. These processes include ulcerated plaques and aneurysmal disease of the aorta. Patients suffering an acute thrombosis because of local arteriosclerotic occlusive disease will give a history of past claudication or other evidence of chronic ischemia. If the stenosing process has been gradual, an acute thrombosis of the vessel may produce an increase in ischemic symptoms distally, but the viability of the distal extremity may not be threatened. In such patients, acute intervention utilizing embolectomy catheters may be unwise because of the lack of satisfactory preoperative planning and may cause unnecessary trauma to severely diseased vessels.

Given the patient with no pre-existing history of peripheral occlusive arterial disease who suddenly develops symptoms of acute ischemia in an appropriate setting of pre-existing cardiac arrhythmias or myocardial infarction, diagnosis of arterial embolization can be made with a high degree of certainty. Our treatment regimen for *acute embolus* includes the following steps.

1. Immediate heparinization is carried out with 5000 to 10,000 units of heparin given intravenously.

2. Analgesics are administered to patients suffering severe pain.

3. Prompt arterial embolectomy is performed, utilizing Fogarty embolectomy catheters. (a) In the unusual case of arterial embolization to the upper extremity, exploration is carried out at the antecubital fossa so that embolectomy catheters can be passed proximally and distally via the brachial artery. (b) When a lower extremity is affected, exploration is carried out at the groin, utilizing the common femoral artery as the site for passage of embolectomy catheters. Utilizing this approach, even saddle emboli to the aortic bifurcation can be treated successfully without laparotomy. Adequate inflow is assured by the passage of the embolectomy catheter proximally.

4. Adequate outflow is assured by the passage of the catheters distally and then either arteriography to assess the patency of the distal circulation or the utilization of noninvasive measures such as Doppler assessment of ankle pressure. In considering the patient with emboli to the lower extremity, one must carefully evaluate the opposite extremity because of the frequency with which both sides are affected. One leg may be more symptomatic than the opposite leg, but preoperative assessment of flow in the lower extremities by careful physical examination as well as Doppler evaluation of ankle pressures may suggest the presence of clot in the less affected extremity. In such instances, both groins should be explored.

5. If adequate inflow cannot be achieved via the groin, one may assume safely that either aortic or iliac thrombosis is the cause of the patient's acute ischemia. One must be prepared to perform indicated bypass procedures in such patients, including aortofemoral, femorofemoral, or axillofemoral bypass.

6. Both the profunda femoris and the superficial femoral artery must be cleared of thrombus prior to closure of the arteriotomy.

7. Because of the infrequent situation in which thrombosis is the cause of the acute ischemia, cephalothin sodium (Keflin), 1 to 2 grams intravenously, is administered prior to the exploration because of the potential for placement of a prosthetic graft.

8. Exploration of the groin as well as the antecubital fossa can be carried out under local anesthesia, and the patient can be given a general anesthetic should bypass grafting be required.

9. Following successful embolectomy, an extensive workup should be performed to determine the origin of the embolic material. (a) Complete cardiac evaluation may be required to rule out ventricular aneurysm, valvular heart disease, or episodic arrhythmias. (b) If such a cardiac evaluation fails to reveal the source of embolic material, complete thoracic and abdominal aortography is indicated to look for ulcerations of arteriosclerotic plaques or aneurysmal disease which cannot be confirmed by physical examination.

10. Our routine has been to keep such patients on anticoagulation for a period of 7 to 10 days following the embolectomy.

11. Patients are also carefully observed for the occurrence of subsequent emboli, particularly emboli to the superior mesenteric artery. Any such patient who develops abdominal pain should receive prompt aortography with views of the superior mesenteric artery. This vessel is frequently affected because of the obliquity of its takeoff from the abdominal aorta.

The diagnosis of *acute thrombosis* of a vessel can be determined preoperatively in most instances. If the viability of the extremity is threatened, prompt surgical intervention is required.

Heparinization is performed prior to any surgical intervention, and, if time permits, angiography should be carried out so that proper planning of the required bypass procedure can be done. More frequently, however, the viability of the extremity is not immediately threatened and the patient has suffered the acute onset of rest pain in a setting of pre-existing peripheral occlusive disease. Arteriographic evaluation is performed without the necessity of heparinization in these patients, and planning of the operative intervention required can be performed at a more leisurely pace. Patients whose severely diseased peripheral arteries thrombose acutely have usually had time to develop sufficient collateral circulation so that the viability of the extremity is not immediately threatened. Some patients will improve during a period of observation.

Some patients present with irreversible changes of the extremity, and only amputation can be offered. When irreversible changes in an extremity are present, we have been careful in our approach because of our observation that revascularization of an extremity containing necrotic muscle will not prevent the necessity for amputation and may lead to acute renal failure secondary to myoglobinuria. Patients who have reinstitution of peripheral flow to an extremely ischemic extremity may experience tremendous muscle swelling and should be observed closely postoperatively. Should the patient begin to complain of numbness between the great and second toes of the affected extremity accompanied by tenderness over the anterior compartment, fasciotomy is indicated. Successful fasciotomy of all compartments of the lower extremity is best carried out utilizing a lateral approach with resection of the fibula, allowing decompression of all the anterior compartment and the deep and superficial compartments posteriorly. The clinical examination is adequate to determine the need for fasciotomy in most instances. Pressures can be obtained by introducing a needle into the anterior compartment. When the pressure within the compartment approaches diastolic pressure, fasciotomy is indicated. The muscles in the anterior compartment are particularly at risk because of their end-arterial blood supply and the confining fascial boundaries present.

Chronic Ischemia

Patients suffering from obstructive vascular lesions experience symptoms because of the reduction of blood flow either at rest or, more commonly, with exercise distal to an area of arterial narrowing. Decreased flow which is insufficient to maintain adequate oxygenation of distal muscle groups expresses itself as *claudication* (pain accompanying exercise) of the affected muscles. Stenotic arterial disease affecting the aortoiliac areas characteristically produces buttock or thigh claudication and may be accompanied by calf claudication with prolonged exercise. Calf claudication results from femoropopliteal occlusive disease. Claudication appears at a reproducible distance and is relieved by a period of 3 to 5 minutes of inactivity. With progression of the occlusive disease with serial resistances in the arterial circuit, *rest pain* may result. The pain, described as a numb ache, begins in the forefoot across the heads of the metatarsals. The pain is brought on by recumbency, interrupts sleep characteristically, and is relieved by a position of dependency of the lower extremity. Some patients obtain relief by a short period of ambulation. The gravitational improvement in capillary filling of the foot is sufficient to relieve the ischemic pain. Although ischemic neuritis may play a role in the cause of the patient's discomfort, the pain in the forefoot is felt to result primarily from insufficient perfusion pressure at the ankle to overcome the gradient of the upright foot in the recumbent position. Some patients with severe disease may have pain in the heel as well, but characteristically their original rest pain began in the forefoot. With further diminution of flow or acute thrombosis of small vessels in the foot, *gangrenous changes* or unrelenting rest pain may occur. In patients with severe circulatory compromise of the foot, small areas of trauma may lead to *nonhealing ulcers.*

Recently a group of patients has been identified exhibiting chronic ischemia specifically of the toes. Such patients present with painful toes with a cyanotic discoloration but may have normal pulses at the ankle. This collection of findings has been termed the "blue toes syndrome" and results from the embolization of atheromatous material or platelet-fibrin particles to the distal circulation. The proximal ulcerated plaques are most frequently located in the femoropopliteal area. Arteriography, utilizing oblique views if necessary, is indicated to determine the source of the emboli. Symptoms of the blue toes syndrome can be relieved by endarterectomy of the area containing the ulcerated plaque or by vein bypass procedures excluding the area.

Many patients with chronic ischemia, particularly those with claudication, can be managed medically. We have become considerably more conservative in the management of patients with combined aortoiliac and femoropopliteal disease with symptoms of claudication. Such patients require aortoiliac bypass procedures to improve inflow, and approximately one third of such patients will continue to be symptomatic, some requiring secondary distal operations for relief of persisting claudication. Because of the magnitude of surgery required to relieve some patients of their claudication, medical management of such patients is indicated if possible. Several studies in the past have demonstrated the benign nature of claudication. Very few patients progress to the point of necessitating surgical intervention because of rest pain or impending gangrene, and the attrition rate because of accompanying cardiopulmonary disease is great. The program of medical management utilized at our institution includes the following measures:

1. Patients are advised to walk to the point of claudication five consecutive times daily. The exposure of the extremity to repeated episodes of ischemia is felt to improve collateral flow, and we have observed rather dramatic improvement in some patients placed on an exercise program.

2. Patients are admonished to cease smoking cigarettes. The cessation of smoking can be accompanied by dramatic improvement. Unfortunately, very few patients can discontinue or limit their cigarette smoking.

3. Patients exhibiting trophic changes of the feet with a loss of subcutaneous tissues, dependent rubor, and hypertrophic nail changes are advised to keep the feet cleansed and dry. Lanolin or baby oil may be used to prevent fissures in dry scaly skin. Trichophytosis is aggressively treated, and the patients are warned about the importance of avoiding foot trauma. Podiatric consultation is obtained if necessary so that shoes are well fitting and that callous lesions or plantar warts can be managed carefully.

4. If other risk factors are present, particularly hyperlipidemia, dietary and, if necessary, drug therapy is instituted.

5. We do not use vasodilators as a part of the medical management or postoperative management of patients with peripheral arterial occlusive disease. Our feeling is that such agents probably decrease flow beyond areas of arterial obstruction by dilating the normal arterial beds, with a resultant decrease in perfusion pressure to the involved limbs.

When claudication is disabling, in that the patient cannot fulfill employment responsibilities or is severely incapacitated by his symptoms, surgery is indicated but only after a trial of approximately 6 months of medical management. Patients with rest pain or gangrenous or pregangrenous changes of the feet require earlier operative intervention if reconstruction is possible. Our preoperative approach includes the following steps:

1. If medical management is to no avail, an arteriogram is ordered to outline the extent and location of the disease, even though the location of the offending lesions has been previously identified by a thorough history and physical examination.

2. In patients who have aortoiliac occlusive disease and absent pulses in an extremity, segmental pressure measurements utilizing Doppler ultrasound have been of value in determining the physiologic extent of the lesions seen on arteriography. During the medical management of such patients, periodic determinations of ankle pressure at rest or after exercise or reactive hyperemia give an objective assessment of the circulatory status.

3. If the patient's disease is confined to the aortoiliac area, aortofemoral bypass grafting can be expected to provide complete relief of symptoms. If the patient's disease is confined to the femoropopliteal area, one may expect complete relief of symptoms after femoropopliteal bypass. In patients with femoropopliteal disease, however, medical management is usually effective, and femoropopliteal bypass grafting is infrequently required for the claudicant.

4. Patients with mild rest pain in the presence of additional cardiac or pulmonary risks are given a trial of medical management. A few of these patients who adhere to an exercise program and discontinue smoking may experience a dramatic relief of their symptoms. A few patients have mild rest pain which they can tolerate, but most patients come to surgery. The aim of operative intervention is limb salvage in these patients and not total symptomatic relief. The surgeon is not faced with the dilemma of persistent symptoms as in the claudicating patients with multilevel disease. If aortoiliac disease is present, relief of the inflow obstruction is generally sufficient to relieve the patient of rest pain and preserve the extremity.

If multiple resistances are present distally in the limb, additional femoropopliteal or more distal grafting may be required.

For correction of aortoiliac occlusive disease, aortofemoral bypass using a Dacron prosthesis is indicated in patients who do not represent a prohibitive risk for an intra-abdominal operation. Femorofemoral bypass grafting may be utilized in patients who have unilateral iliac occlusion; axillofemoral grafting is used for bilateral aortoiliac disease in high risk cardiac and pulmonary patients. As experience with the seondary operations of femorofemoral bypass and axillofemoral bypass has increased, the results have been surprisingly good. However, in our hands, aortofemoral bypass grafting has provided the most satisfactory results in patients who can tolerate this procedure. The bypass material of choice in femoropopliteal or femorotibial bypass is a reversed saphenous vein. When the saphenous vein is unsatisfactory because of varicosities, previous vein stripping, or inadequate diameter (less than 4 mm.), alternative materials have to be utilized. When the bypass can be performed in the femoropopliteal location above the knee, knitted Dacron materials have been satisfactory. When the bypass has to extend across the knee joint, however, a composite Dacron and saphenous or cephalic vein can be constructed. We have had little experience with the use of expanded polytetrafluoroethylene (Gore-Tex). When the bypass extends to the lower third of the leg, we have been reluctant to perform such procedures if an intraoperative arteriogram does not reveal a satisfactory plantar arch and therefore satisfactory runoff. The success rate of bypass grafting to a distal artery with such poor runoff is low.

Rarely one may perform endarterectomy of localized lesions in the femoropopliteal area or in the aortoiliac area. Those with aortoiliac occlusive disease appropriate for aortoiliac endarterectomy are young patients exhibiting claudication with aortoiliac occlusions confined to the aorta and common iliac arteries. Most of the endarterectomy procedures performed in the femoropopliteal area have been performed for the "blue toes syndrome."

Following revascularization procedures, postoperative medical management is of great importance. Hyperlipidemia must be controlled, and the patients should be on a regular exercise program. If obesity or hypertension or both are present, they should be controlled. The cessation of smoking is strongly advocated, although our success rate in controlling this particular risk factor is low. Patients are warned of the presence of an acute change and are advised to return promptly should such a complication occur. Patients who have prosthetic materials placed for the bypass are given prophylactic antibiotics preoperatively, intraoperatively, and postoperatively until all invasive devices such as intravenous lines and bladder catheters are removed. Care is taken to avoid postoperative wound hematomas or seromas by careful technique. Meticulous preparation of the skin is carried out prior to the operation, and generous use of antibiotic irrigating solutions intraoperatively has been our routine. Patients who have plastic prostheses should be warned that before any invasive procedures in the future which could result in an episode of bacteremia or in the event of overt bacterial infection, antibiotic prophylaxis should be given to prevent potential infection of the implanted graft. Utilizing these precautions, the incidence of graft infection should be low.

Sympathectomy at the time of arterial reconstruction has not been our routine. We have not been able to demonstrate an increased long-term patency of grafts in patients who receive sympathectomy. Sympathectomy will reduce the foot arterial resistance, however, and we have occasionally utilized it in the presence of extensive distal disease with skin involvement.

Diabetic patients exhibit a particular pattern of calcific arteriosclerotic occlusive disease with more severe involvement in the lower leg. The distal disease combined with the problems of diabetic neuropathy, decreased resistance to infection, and the propensity toward podiatric problems make the diabetic patient especially likely to develop necrotizing infection in the foot, necessitating amputation. Because of the diabetic involvement of small arteries, some patients will present with gangrenous toes with ankle pulses. Calcified vessels make ankle pressure determinations as well as other segmental leg pressure determinations somewhat suspect in the diabetic; hence, the importance of angiography in diabetic patients with threatened gangrenous changes of the foot and decreased pulses. A great many diabetic patients have nonhealing ulcers of the feet which will heal with adequate revascularization. An aggressive approach toward correcting occlusive lesions in such patients can produce gratifying results, with preservation of feet or lowering of the levels of amputation. Very careful foot care in the diabetic is of extreme importance.

Buerger's disease or thromboangiitis obliterans is seen in young men who smoke. The inflammatory arterial lesion present tends to affect medium-sized arteries such as the posterior tibial, anterior tibial, peroneal, radial, and ulnar vessels. These patients experience episodes of severe distal pain and ulceration. These episodes generally respond to the discontinuation of smoking, the administration of antibiotics, and local wound care. The cessation of smoking will prevent the progression of the disease. However, the discontinuation of smoking for such patients is peculiarly difficult, and the medical treatment of the condition is generally unsuccessful because of this fact.

When confronted with the patient with peripheral arterial occlusive disease who has irreversible changes causing gangrene or who has unreconstructable disease and rest pain, amputation will be required. Formerly, most amputations for vascular disease were performed at the above-knee level. There has been a progressive change recently to an increased number of below-knee amputations. The decision to proceed to an above-knee amputation must be tempered by the fact that rehabilitation in such patients is much more difficult than in patients who have healed a below-knee amputation. We have found that patients who have a popliteal signal by Doppler ultrasound and a below-knee pressure of 70 mm. Hg should heal a below-knee amputation. Seventy-five per cent of patients who have a popliteal Doppler signal present and a below-knee pressure of less than 70 mm. Hg will heal below-knee amputations. Should the Doppler signal be absent, one should consider initial above-knee amputation, because all patients with such findings have failed to heal a below-knee amputation. We have found that patients requiring foot amputations who have ankle pressures greater than 60 mm. Hg should heal such amputations. In diabetic patients, the ankle pressure predictive of healing is 80 mm. Hg. If reconstructive surgery can be performed to improve the inflow to the foot so that a foot amputation rather than a higher amputation can be carried out, such an operation should be considered.

We have utilized equal anterior and posterior flaps for above-knee amputations and a long posterior flap for below-knee amputations. The technique of below-knee amputations is important, and great care is taken to prevent an anterior flap which rides over the tibial prominence. Drains are generally not used in such amputations except in the presence of persistent oozing from the wound. When drains are used, they are removed shortly after surgery and the opening through which the drain exits is closed promptly. Soft dressings have been utilized at this institution, because a study in this laboratory comparing soft dressings to immediate post-operative prosthetic fittings showed no difference in the length of time required for healing between the two groups. Rehabilitation time is shortened by immediate postoperative prosthesis fitting, but the increased personnel and time required to satisfactorily perform this technique have led us to prefer soft dressings. Upon healing of the wound, prosthetic application is performed.

In patients suffering iatrogenic arterial occlusion following cardiac catheterization or the placement of monitoring catheters, an aggressive approach to avoid chronic arterial insufficiency of the limb is indicated. Most of the complications occur in the upper extremity. If a question of arterial obstruction results after cardiac catheterization via the brachial artery, exploration of the brachial artery is performed. Generally, satisfactory thrombectomy of the vessels can be performed with reconstitution of normal flow to the hand. We have seen several patients in whom such an aggressive approach was not utilized who later complained vigorously of hand claudication and discomfort. In the arterial reconstruction of neglected cases, long vein bypass procedures are necessary from the axillary artery to the distal radial or ulnar arteries. Similarly, when common femoral thromboses occur as a result of transfemoral radiologic procedures or cardiac catheterization, an aggressive approach is utilized to reinstitute normal flow to the lower extremity. In pediatric patients, a similarly aggressive approach is warranted because of the fear of later limb growth disturbances.

Vasospastic Arterial Disease

Vasospastic arterial disease can affect both the upper and lower extremities. Most frequently, involvement is confined to the upper extremities and the vasospastic phenomena are limited to the distal circulation. Most patients who exhibit vasospastic changes have Raynaud's *phenomenon;* i.e., they have vasospastic arterial disease secondary to a basic underlying cause, most frequently collagen-vascular disease. Most of the patients who manifest collagen-vascular disease have scleroderma. Patients who have Raynaud's *disease* have no apparent underlying cause. Most of these patients are young females who experience the onset of their symptoms with exposure to cold or anxiety.

Patients with arterial vasospastic conditions are usually quite sensitive to cold and will experience pain and a bluish discoloration of the digits upon cold exposure. Their symptoms may progress to the point of fingertip ulceration with very exquisitely tender lesions in the subungual area of the fingertip. One form of arterial vasospasm which can affect large and small arteries is seen in patients exceeding the accepted dosage of ergotamine in the management of migraine headaches. Such patients present as diagnostic dilemmas. Once the diagnosis of ergotism is made and the drug discontinued, relief is shortly forthcoming. Vasodilators and sympathectomy have been utilized in the management of patients intoxicated by ergot. Vasodilators may be beneficial, but no therapeutic effect of sympathectomy has as yet been demonstrated objectively.

Patients who demonstrate the more usual form of peripheral arterial vasospasm with painful digits may be treated nonoperatively, especially if the involvement affects all four extremities. Therapy for vasospastic conditions includes the following measures:

1. Oral agents can be tried, including reserpine, alpha-methyldopa, and low doses of guanethidine. We have only a limited experience with the use of these oral agents and they are investigational for this use. Most of the patients we see have Raynaud's phenomenon and have not been substantially benefited by oral preparations.

2. Intra-arterial injections of reserpine have been utilized; however, the benefit of such an

approach with short periods of relief must be balanced against the risk of intra-arterial injections. (This use of reserpine is not listed in the manufacturer's official directive.)

3. Patients are advised to dress warmly and protect their extremities during the cold months of the year, and such an approach is normally sufficient for preventing digital complications.

4. In an occasional patient, however, the presence of apparent impending gangrenous changes, severe pain, or ulceration necessitates surgical intervention. (a) We have been able to obtain some prediction of the benefit of lumbar or cervical sympathectomy in such patients by performing either strain gauge or photoelectric digital plethysmography at the time of lumbar sympathetic or cervical sympathetic block. If an improvement of blood flow in the extremity can be objectively demonstrated by plethysmographic techniques and the patient experiences relief of his symptoms accompanied by warming of the extremity, benefit from sympathectomy can be expected. (b) A cervical sympathectomy can be performed by either a supraclavicular or transaxillary approach, removing the Tl through T5 sympathetic ganglia. Obtaining the distal exposure is difficult through the cervical incision, and the likelihood of phrenic nerve or thoracic duct injury is less with a transaxillary approach. Patients almost universally prefer the supraclavicular approach, however, when bilateral cervical sympathectomies have been done, one via a transaxillary and one through a supraclavicular approach. There is dispute over how often an adequate cervical sympathectomy can be achieved without removal of the entire stellate ganglion. Removal of the stellate ganglion will result in ipsilateral Horner's syndrome. In patients who genuinely need a cervical sympathectomy, the presence of Horner's syndrome postoperatively is not bothersome. We have usually removed the entire stellate ganglion to achieve satisfactory sympathetic effect, warning the patients preoperatively of the presence of postoperative Horner's syndrome. (c) A few patients require lumbar sympathectomy for relief of lower extremity vasospastic disease. Removal of the L2 through L5 lumbar sympathetic ganglia is sufficient to obtain a satisfactory result.

Peripheral Arterial Aneurysms

The most important aspect of the evaluation of a patient manifesting peripheral arterial aneurysms is complete and thorough angiography because of the frequent association of aortic, iliac, femoral, and popliteal aneurysms. Some patients have a widespread arteriomegaly affecting virtually all the arterial tree.

Popliteal aneurysms are most frequently seen and are treacherous because of their propensity to clot suddenly, resulting in acute ischemia of the lower leg. Rarely popliteal aneurysms can enlarge sufficiently to produce local symptoms of pain and venous or nerve compression. With acute thrombosis of a popliteal aneurysm, prompt surgical intervention is necessary to save the limb. When such a catastrophe has not occurred, a popliteal aneurysm can be suspected by the presence of a prominent popliteal pulse and in some cases by the presence of a palpable aneurysm. Popliteal aneurysms are frequently bilateral, and one should strongly suspect the presence of an accompanying aneurysm in the contralateral extremity. It should be ruled out with arteriography. Most frequently the aneurysms are fusiform but can be saccular. They very rarely progress to rupture. The treatment is surgical excision or exclusion from the arterial system with proximal and distal ligation and saphenous vein interposition or bypass. A significant number of popliteal aneurysms are associated with proximal aneurysmal disease; hence, the importance of thorough angiography.

Femoral aneurysms are also frequently associated with aneurysmal disease in more proximal locations. These aneurysms do not as frequently thrombose but more commonly rupture. Upon their discovery they should be excised, and either saphenous vein or prosthetic material should be utilized as an interposition graft. We have chosen to follow small femoral aneurysms less than 2 to 2.5 cm. in size because of their availability for frequent inspection. We have applied this approach as well to the presence of false aneurysms at the distal anastomosis of aortofemoral bypass grafts. When, however, these aneurysms exceed 2 cm. in size, consideration should be given to their excision.

MASSIVE THROMBOPHLEBITIS OF THE LOWER EXTREMITIES

method of
MICHAEL HUME, M.D.
Jamaica Plain, Massachusetts

Heparin given intravenously and followed by warfarin will prevent extension of venous thrombosis and pulmonary embolism. A standard plan of management for major (including massive) venous thrombosis is presented here, along with alternatives that may be required in special circumstances.

Proof of Diagnosis

Treatment with anticoagulant drugs is prolonged, complex, and potentially hazardous. Proof of the diagnosis confirmed by phlebogram should be required in order to avoid complications in patients unnecessarily treated. Treatment should begin forthwith; any unavoidable delay in obtaining a phlebogram should be covered by commencing heparin treatment provisionally. After a few hours of elevation of the legs, edema will lessen and it may be technically easier to obtain a phlebogram the following day.

Heparin Dosage

Flexible dosage is appropriate, because early in treatment more heparin is required, and later, less. Response to the initial dose, reflected in prolongation of the partial thromboplastin time (PTT), guides changes in subsequent dosage. Depending on body weight, 5000 to 10,000 units is initially given intravenously. The interval between the dose and the time at which blood is collected for determination of partial thromboplastin time must be noted carefully. At 3½ hours, the test should be prolonged from 1½ to 2 times the control value. Sometimes this interval is difficult to keep standard, or poor communication delays the decision regarding altered dosage. These variables do not affect continuous infusion of heparin after the first dose, and the daily dosage will be easier to relate to the patient's response with this technique. Continuous infusion of heparin is adjusted to keep the partial thromboplastin time between 50 and 80 seconds. To reflect the effect of hourly dosage, blood should be drawn for this test at least 4 to 6 hours after the priming dose. Daily testing is required, but additional determinations during the first 24 hours are generally needed. At least 1000 units hourly will be required during the first day, and this amount should be ordered to follow the priming dose; after the first PTT, an increase is often needed. Intermittent heparin doses given intravenously every 4 hours are equally effective; with due care in laboratory control, either may be successfully used. Heparin is given for 7 to 10 days; additional days of treatment follow if symptoms respond slowly or the expected response in the prothrombin time from warfarin given concurrently is delayed.

Continuous Infusion Pumps

Continuous infusion pumps for heparin should be battery powered to allow progressive ambulation. Between the pump and the reservoir bottle which contains the 24 hour dose there should be a calibrated burette chamber. This allows the nurse to monitor the rate of infusion and limits the volume of heparin which might run in if the tubing becomes misplaced off the pump head. The pump should be out of reach of confused patients.

Failure of heparin to control thromboembolism is unusual if the partial thromboplastin time is kept in the range of 50 to 80 seconds, or approximately twice the control. Bleeding complications can occur during heparin therapy even though this test is maintained in the desired range. Serious hemorrhage is reported to be significantly less frequent if heparin is given by continuously pumped infusion than if injected intermittently. It is necessary to consider the risk of bleeding for any patient given heparin, noting the following points.

Risk of Bleeding

Drug interaction is the most common cause of bleeding, and aspirin—or compound drugs that contain aspirin—is the worst offender. A complete drug history is essential. Elderly patients, particularly postmenopausal women, incur more bleeding complications from heparin than other subjects. The platelet concentration should be estimated by blood smear or platelet count, and/or the template bleeding time should be measured. After specific surgical operations, the risk of bleeding during anticoagulant therapy varies from a relative to an absolute contraindication for heparin, even several weeks after surgery. Taking into account the interval between surgery and the need for heparin, an absolute contraindication exists after surgery of the retina, central nervous system, or retroperitoneal area, and a relative contraindication after prostatectomy and major joint replacement. When all these factors have been reviewed, the risk of bleeding may be regarded as sufficiently high to require an alternative to heparin.

Warfarin Treatment

After the proper response to initial heparin therapy, warfarin is begun. A large initial dose is not appropriate, for the risk of bleeding is thereby increased without achieving early antithrombotic effect. Warfarin therapy requires at least 5 to 7 days to be effective. Ten mg. of warfarin is given daily until the prothrombin time is twice that of control. Occasionally, larger doses are necessary. Continuous infusion of heparin does not spuriously prolong the prothrombin time, but if intermittent heparin is used, it is necessary to be certain that at least 3½ hours have elapsed between the last dose of heparin and blood collection for determining the prothrombin time. Warfarin is continued for several weeks after heparin has been stopped. This interval may have to be extended if factors are still present which may contribute to rethrombosis, such as failure of the patient to resume full regular activity. Recurrence of thrombosis is less frequent if warfarin is used for 12 to 14 weeks after heparin therapy than if it is not used for this period. Afterward, the occurrence of rethrombosis is approximately the same whether or not warfarin is used. Because some risk of bleeding complication attends very long-term use of warfarin, it is prudent to discontinue treatment at about 12 to 14 weeks. Prothrombin time is determined at 1 to 3 week intervals after discharge from the hospital, depending on how radically the dose has to be adjusted; weekly blood testing is needed if there is much variation, less frequent testing if the response is stable.

Intrafat Heparin, Alternative to Warfarin

Pregnancy is a special circumstance, because warfarin treatment may affect the prothrombin time of the fetus. Nearly all complications of warfarin treatment during pregnancy occur at the period about term. Low doses of heparin, 5000 units twice a day, are an alternative for patients who can be taught this method. This technique, which is most appropriate in pregnant patients to prevent rethrombosis, may be applied to other subjects who are competent to administer their own heparin and whose circumstances indicate that laboratory control with the prothrombin time is not going to be easy to arrange.

Physical Measures

Physical measures contribute much to the management of venous thrombosis. Progressive ambulation is required as soon as leg symptoms allow. Bathroom privileges and hourly periods of walking are begun. The period of out-of-bed activity every hour is increased daily in 5 minute increments. Chair sitting is limited during the first period to the time required to eat a meal at table. Control of edema is essential and assured by elevating the foot of the bed on 8 inch (20 cm.) blocks. The patient should recline on the bed for the balance of the hour after the walking activity is performed. Pressure gradient elastic stockings are fitted as soon as any edema is brought under control by bed rest, with or without compression bandaging of the legs with Ace bandages. Knee-length stockings are sufficient unless serious symptoms in the thigh persist, but full-length stockings for this reason are rarely needed. Elevation of the bed and pressure gradient stockings are employed consistently until edema is no longer demonstrable. Any compromise of this precaution risks serious chronic venous insufficiency in later years.

Thrombolytic Therapy

Thrombolytic therapy should be used before heparin is begun in very extensive venous thrombosis. This is a matter of judgment and is best described as follows: thrombolytic agents, either streptokinase or urokinase, should be considered if venous thrombosis is so extensive that it can reasonably be predicted that serious venous insufficiency will persist if only heparin is given. It is important to estimate the age of the thrombotic process, because old thrombi respond less well to thrombolytic therapy than do fresh thrombi. The following evidence should be considered: the patient's symptoms are a crude indicator, but the appearance of the thrombus in the phlebogram is more helpful. Most useful is a finding of "split products" in the blood; fibrin monomer and fibrin degradation products will certainly be demonstrable in such extensive fresh thrombosis as to lead to a consideration of thrombolytic agents. As indicated, the diagnosis must be established by a phlebogram. Special laboratory tests are required: thrombin time for regulating the sustaining dose, and the streptokinase resistance test to reveal whether unusual resistance to streptokinase can be expected. A syringe pump is required with close observation, such as in an intensive care unit. Febrile reaction is common, and pretreatment with steroids is routine; a standard loading dose of streptokinase is given (250,000 units), followed by an hourly maintenance dose—initially, 100,000 units per hour. Adjustment of the hourly dose may be required in the second 12 hour period, depending on the result of the thrombin time. Any circumstance which would preclude the use of anticoagulant drugs represents a distinct contraindication to thrombolytic therapy; neither should they be used during the first 2 weeks after surgical operation or deep needle biopsy.

Alternative Medical Therapy

Alternative medical therapy for established venous thrombosis may be justified if certain relative contraindications to anticoagulant drugs exist. Only dextran can be considered as effective for the control of thrombosis (and prevention of embolism) but at somewhat lower risk of bleeding than heparin therapy entails. Cardiac compensation and renal function require attention, but if they are not impaired, 500 ml. of Dextran 70 is given daily for 3 days and every third day thereafter until warfarin dosage has been regulated. External pneumatic compression of the calf, which is said to be effective for the prevention of venous thrombosis under some circumstances, should not be considered an alternative to anticoagulant therapy in established venous thrombosis. So applied, it may be hazardous. Among all the treatments for venous thrombosis there are degrees of effectiveness, and certain drug programs for the prevention of venous thrombosis cannot be considered as appropriate for the treatment of established thrombosis.

Surgery

When anticoagulant drug therapy is absolutely contraindicated or has been properly used and has failed to prevent extension of the process as shown by a repeat phlebogram, surgery must be considered. The primary purpose of surgical intervention is to prevent major pulmonary embolism, principally by interruption of the inferior vena cava. Surgical removal of thrombus must be mentioned additionally.

Interruption of the vena cava can be effected by direct surgical approach—ligation, plication, or use of a clip externally applied—or by the insertion of the "umbrella" filter mounted on a catheter and passed into proper position under fluoroscopic control through a limited dissection at the base of the neck by way of the internal jugular vein. The occurrence of distal propagation of venous thrombosis and recurrent embolism differ little among these several techniques. Partial interruption of the vena cava spares the acute hemodynamic consequences of total ligation. The umbrella filter technique avoids general anesthesia and offers the additional advantage that it can be carried out during heparin therapy if that is not precluded by the circumstances which required surgical intervention. Personal experience with the technique as described by Mobin-Uddin, routine cavography, and the use of the 28 mm. filter have presented no complications and few difficulties with the procedure; indeed, it is extremely well tolerated by the patient. Caval ligation is reserved for septic pelvic thrombophlebitis and is now seldom needed. The gonadal veins are ligated also for this indication, and this requires a transperitoneal approach.

Thrombectomy is likely to be used little hereafter. Those severe forms of venous thrombosis for which it was once considered to be the only alternative to heparin treatment may now be the very ones most appropriate for thrombolytic therapy. Will there remain any circumstance for which thrombectomy is the one best plan? At once, one needs to consider phlegmasia cerulea dolens, especially with venous gangrene or other signs of poor tissue perfusion. Under such conditions, it would be hard to withhold thrombectomy while waiting 12 or more hours for thrombolytic therapy to reverse the process.

Minor Venous Thrombosis

Minimal venous thrombosis and thrombosis in superficial veins, including varicose veins, need mention. Warfarin can be given to outpatients; in my experience, minor venous thrombosis and superficial phlebitis resolve more rapidly during warfarin therapy than on other symptomatic treatment, including anti-inflammatory drugs. It is, of course, necessary not to overlook the possibility that deep venous thrombosis accompanies apparently minor or superficial phlebitis. Impedance (IPG) testing seems to be a convenient, noninvasive method of determining whether occult deep vein thrombosis accompanies these superficial manifestations.

Dermatitis and Leg Ulcers

Dermatitis and leg ulcers caused by chronic venous insufficiency constitute a special problem which deserves attention and demands persistence and skill beyond that often given to this stubborn and painful condition. Ligation of incompetent perforating veins, excision of ulcers and skin grafting, and the management of dermatitis are complex problems beyond the scope of the present discussion.

PRIMARY VARICOSE VEINS

method of
KARL A. LOFGREN, M.D.
Rochester, Minnesota

Primary varicose veins develop spontaneously as abnormally dilated superficial veins of the lower extremities during early life. From the standpoint of treatment and prognosis, this condition should be differentiated from secondary varicose veins, which develop as a sequela to deep venous insufficiency and associated venous hypertension, often in later life. Primary varicose veins respond well to surgical treatment; secondary varicose veins are less amenable to surgical improvement unless they are definitely incompetent, and even then the underlying deep venous insufficiency remains as a permanent, often major impairment to the patient.

Heredity undoubtedly plays a primary role in the development of varicose veins. Extreme dilatation produces incompetency of the venous valves, and abnormal elevation of venous pressure results. In severe venous insufficiency, chronic venous stasis causes pigmentation, dermatitis, cellulitis, and superficial ulceration in the ankle and lower leg area. With primary varicose veins, the stasis changes in the skin and subcutaneous tissues are reversible if an adequate surgical procedure is done to eliminate the malfunctioning veins and thus restore normal venous physiology.

Treatment is governed by the nature of the varicose problem and by the general health status of the patient. Surgical and nonsurgical methods can be used, either alone or in combination. For primary varicose veins that have been judged to be incompetent by clinical test results, surgical elimination is the treatment of choice. A malfunctioning varix that is removed surgically ceases to be a problem for the patient. If the health status of the patient prohibits the risks of an operation, nonsurgical methods—such as elastic support, periodic elevation of the legs, exercises, and sclerotherapy in selected conditions—are substituted. Sclerotherapy is not used as primary treatment of incompetent varicosities because of its unpredictable, often short duration and the risk of complications; nonetheless, it is useful in obliterating spiderbursts and minor cutaneous venules that sometimes develop in the long-term postoperative follow-up period.

Surgical Treatment

Our present-day operation for varicose veins consists of thorough stripping and excision of incompetent saphenous veins, all tributaries, and incompetent perforating veins. For this procedure, which was developed gradually at the Mayo Clinic 30 years ago, a flexible intraluminal stripper is used. To date, we have done this type of operation in more than 12,000 patients.

Indications. 1. Symptomatic varicosities—aching, heaviness, swelling, cramps, itching.

2. Complicated varicosities—pigmentation, dermatitis, cellulitis, superficial thrombophlebitis, bleeding, or ulceration (the last usually posttraumatic).

3. Asymptomatic varicosities—incompetent and large, becoming progressively worse.

4. Cosmetic varicosities—incompetent, unsightly, and distressful to the patient.

Contraindications. 1. Occlusive arterial disease of the lower extremities.

2. Significant cardiovascular, metabolic, neuromuscular, or orthopedic disorders.

3. Recent malignancy with uncertain prognosis.

4. Deep thrombophlebitis of recent origin.

5. Pregnancy (surgical treatment is postponed until the postpartum period, when venous physiology has normalized).

Technique. 1. Preoperatively, incompetency of the saphenous system must be confirmed by clinical tests (Brodie-Trendelenburg tourniquet test and manual compression test). Competent or normal saphenous veins should not be destroyed. All visible and palpable varicosities are marked meticulously with indelible marking solution—a key step for an efficient, successful operation.

2. General anesthesia is necessary, with sodium thiopental induction. A split-leg operating table permits easy access to both legs for all assistants during the operation. The foot of the operating table is elevated 10 degrees during the operation to lessen bleeding; blood loss is generally minimal.

3. With the *greater saphenous vein,* high ligation at the saphenofemoral juncture is done first before strippers are introduced. Simple and transfixion ligatures with chromic catgut (1–0) are used. The important principle is to ligate flush with the femoral vein without trauma from clamps. Low ligation is a common cause of recurrence of varicosities postoperatively.

4. A long, flexible, intraluminal stripper (100 cm.) with a small acorn (¼-inch diameter) of the Myers type is introduced into the greater saphenous vein on the dorsomedial aspect of the foot and threaded upward to the groin while the progressing tip is palpated. Trauma to the saphenous nerve must be avoided by using the smallest acorn. Distally, the saphenous vein is tied around the stripper with heavy fishline. The stripper remains as a landmark until the tributaries have been removed.

5. All marked tributaries are stripped or dissected out, as marked. For this procedure, a short intraluminal stripper (36 cm. long) with a small tip is most useful. Unstrippable, tortuous varicosities or plexuses are dissected out from the subcutaneous layer with a curved Carmalt forceps, which is used to extract the veins between incisions.

6. Incompetent perforating veins, usually marked preoperatively with an "X," are exposed through separate incisions and ligated where they emerge through the deep fascial layer, and the attached superficial tributaries are removed by excision or stripping.

7. The main channel stripper is finally pulled out in a cephalad direction, from foot to groin. Other unmarked tributaries or parallel channels are sought and removed through additional incisions. The saphenous vein is telescoped upon the stripper and removed through the groin incision. (In an alternative method, the saphenous vein is

stripped upward from foot to knee level and downward from the groin to the knee with a separate stripper.)

8. Generally, longitudinal skin incisions are used because they cause less trauma to lymphatic vessels and sensory nerves. Except for the groin and foot incisions, few ligatures (Dexon 3–0) are required. For closing the skin, interrupted mattress sutures of 4–0 silk on an atraumatic needle are preferable to clips, Steritapes, or intracutaneous sutures. Surgical dressings, cotton pads, and elastic rubber-reinforced bandages are applied from the foot to the groin.

9. With the *lesser saphenous vein,* the ligation close to the saphenopopliteal juncture may be done with the patient in either the supine or the prone position. The latter provides the easiest exposure of the popliteal fossa. After incising the popliteal fascia longitudinally, the lesser saphenous vein is ligated under slight tension with the knee slightly flexed. The short intraluminal stripper is threaded upward into the saphenous vein from the incision on the lateral aspect of the ankle. Great care must be taken to avoid injury to the sural nerve. Adequate exposure and use of a stripper with the smallest acorn help to prevent nerve trauma. Tributaries and perforating veins are removed as already described for the greater saphenous vein.

Postoperative Course. 1. The foot of the bed is elevated about 10 degrees. Elastic bandages are reapplied daily for comfort. The surgical dressing is changed in 3 days and the skin sutures are removed in 7 days.

2. Bathroom privileges and gradually increased ambulation begin on the first postoperative day. No sitting or prolonged standing is allowed. Elastic bandages are used for 6 weeks, or longer if needed.

3. Antibiotics or anticoagulants are not used unless a specific indication arises. Blood loss is generally minimal, and transfusions are not necessary.

Complications. The morbidity is low. Suspected minor pulmonary emboli occurred in 0.39 per cent of 4080 patients during a 10 year period. Hematomas are minor problems, usually prevented by careful hemostasis and by expulsion of pooled blood from incisions and stripped-out channels with bimanual pressure before application of surgical dressings and elastic bandages. Saphenous or sural nerve injury is largely preventable by careful exposure of structures and by use of a stripper with the smallest acorn. Stripping in the cephalad direction (upward) produces less wadding in the lower leg area and less trauma to the adjacent nerves.

Long-Term Results. A carefully executed operation that removes all incompetent varicosities will prevent early recurrences. Late recurrences, although infrequent, are not always preventable in the particularly susceptible patient or in those whose normal venous hemodynamics have been disrupted by deep thrombophlebitis or pregnancy. A regular follow-up program is therefore essential for the best long-term care of the patient, for it provides the opportunity to control any minor recurrences and also to assess the effectiveness of the surgical technique.

In a long-term follow-up review of our surgical patients, strict criteria of evaluation were used. If any recurrent varicosity was more than 3 mm. in diameter, the results were classified as fair rather than excellent or good. By these criteria, approximately 85 per cent of patients examined by us were in either excellent or good condition with reference to the previous vein surgery, 10 or more years before. The condition of the remaining 15 per cent of patients was fair, most of whom felt fine and declined any further treatment at follow-up examination.

Nonsurgical Treatment

1. *Sclerotherapy* is used as cosmetic treatment of spiderbursts and smaller venules, as follow-up treatment for minor recurrences postoperatively, and as direct treatment of eroding or bleeding cutaneous varicosities. It is not used as primary treatment of incompetent varicosities. Thus it is useful but has a limited role in our therapeutic program. Presently available sclerosants in the United States include 5 per cent sodium morrhuate and 1 per cent or 3 per cent Sotradecol (sodium tetradecyl sulfate). Sotradecol is used in most clinics, but we are still using Monolate (monoethanolamine oleate) for sclerosing purposes at our institution.

Sclerotherapy has an unpredictable duration of effect and sometimes causes residual pigmentation of the skin. In sensitive persons, occasional allergic reactions are seen. Excessive injections may also damage deep major veins.

For larger venules, the empty-vein technique (elevation of the leg before injecting) produces a better sclerosing effect when it is used in combination with compression bandages for several days. For spiderbursts, a foamy sclerosing solution produced by shaking the half-empty syringe is less irritating and allows better visualization of the injected sclerosant.

2. *Elastic support* alleviates symptoms of chronic venous insufficiency by compressing incompetent superficial veins, preventing edema, and supporting the musculovenous pump mechanism of the calf. This can be used effectively as

substitute therapy for patients who cannot tolerate a surgical procedure for incompetent varicose veins and is also indicated for varicose veins in the pregnant patient and for those associated with postphlebitic conditions and severe deep venous insufficiency. Elastic support is the primary treatment in the management of the postphlebitic leg.

Type and weight of elastic support are determined by the severity of the venous insufficiency. Elastic rubber-reinforced bandages, heavy- or medium-weight elastic stockings, leotards, pantyhose, and support hose all serve useful purposes. Custom-made elastic stockings generally are indicated for legs of unusual configuration when ready-made ones would not fit satisfactorily. Elastic support is needed primarily around the ankle and lower leg and rarely above knee level, except during pregnancy when waist-high support often provides more comfort.

3. *Elevation of the legs* relieves symptoms of varicosities by emptying out the venous blood and lowering the venous pressure. It also reduces edema fluid in the subcutaneous tissues. This technique is not effective unless the feet are elevated about 10 inches above heart level; sitting with the legs elevated lowers the venous pressure to a much lesser degree and is therefore not adequate.

4. *Exercise*—walking, running, bicycling, swimming, or forceful movement of the ankles—produces better venous flow by activating the musculovenous pump of the calf musculature. Exercise lowers the venous pressure and helps to relieve symptoms of venous insufficiency, whether superficial or deep.

Summary

Primary varicose veins that are judged to be incompetent by clinical test results are best treated by complete surgical removal. This operation involves thorough stripping and excision of all visible and palpable varicosities of the greater or lesser saphenous systems and of all incompetent perforating veins. Normal or competent saphenous veins should not be destroyed, particularly in patients who might have potential future needs for autogenous vein grafts.

Sclerotherapy and other nonsurgical methods serve useful, supportive roles in the management of primary varicose veins in those patients whose varicosities are minor or whose health status prohibits surgery.

SECTION 4

The Blood and Spleen

APLASTIC ANEMIA

method of
S. M. LEWIS, M.D., F.R.C.PATH.
London, England

Aplastic anemia may be caused by ionizing irradiation, by cytotoxic drugs which have a dose-related effect on the bone marrow, and by a number of drugs and chemicals (and possible infections) which appear to be harmful only to susceptible subjects. There is also a chronic acquired type which occurs at all ages and in which no causal agent is identified. Other variants of aplastic anemia differ from the chronic acquired type in course and prognosis; these include a hereditary type (Fanconi's syndrome), and transient marrow depression, which may occur as a secondary event in patients suffering from severe infections, uremia, or hemolytic anemias. Aplastic anemia results in granulocytopenia and thrombocytopenia as well as anemia. Hypoplasia of the marrow affecting only the erythroid cell occurs as a congenital disorder (Diamond-Blackfan syndrome) or an acquired type, usually termed "pure red cell aplasia."

Management of aplastic anemia depends, to an extent, on the type. There is no specific therapy, but the treatment is directed to several aspects of the disease and its direct complications.

Identification and Removal of the Cause

In only one third of all cases of acquired aplastic anemia is there a history of some drug or toxin which may be considered as a possible cause. Even when there is such a history, it may be impossible to be sure of its significance. Thus, while the American Medical Association Register of drugs causing blood dyscrasias listed (in 1967) approximately 350 substances which had been reported over a period of 11 years, they ranged from those which have an undoubted aplastogenic action, such as chloramphenicol, to aspirin and other presumably innocuous drugs. In the majority of cases removal of the cause or presumed cause does not seem to influence the ultimate prognosis, which depends on the extent of the initial damage to the bone marrow. There is no means of identifying susceptible subjects in advance, and great care must be taken in using drugs that are especially liable to cause aplastic anemia in susceptible subjects. On the other hand, as cytotoxic drugs affect the bone marrow in all subjects, administration of such drugs must be carefully controlled by regular blood counts, especially platelet counts. If aplastic anemia follows administration of gold or arsenical compounds, the patient should be treated with dimercaprol (BAL), 800 mg. per day intramuscularly in divided doses for 2 to 3 days, then reducing to 100 to 200 mg. per day over the next few days.

Alleviation of Anemia

Blood transfusion requirements for the anemia will vary from patient to patient; in some patients a state of equilibrium will become established at a reasonably satisfactory hemoglobin level, whereas other patients may require blood transfusions at intervals over a period of months or even years. Because of the risks of isoimmunization, hepatitis, and hemosiderosis, transfusions should be restricted as far as possible; hemoglobin should be maintained at a level which ensures that the patient is free from distress and is able to undertake a reasonable amount of activity.

Control of Hemorrhage

This is frequently the most important problem of treatment. If thrombocytopenia is sufficiently severe, there will be a bleeding tendency, either as ecchymosis and purpura or as retinal hemorrhages, gastrointestinal hemorrhage, menorrhagia, and bleeding into organs, especially cerebral hemorrhage. It is not possible to predict when bleeding may occur on the basis of the level of platelet count. At any given platelet count one patient may bleed while another will not, but the tendency to bleed will be greater at any level of platelets when there is a concomitant infection. In general, bleeding is common when the platelet count is less than 20×10^9 per liter, and rare when it is more than 50×10^9 per liter. Onset of hemorrhage may precipitate a further fall in platelets and increasing hemorrhage. Acute bleeding should be treated by transfusions with platelet-rich fresh plasma (e.g., 1 to 2 liters per day) or platelet concentrate, which should be continued until the bleeding ceases. Eventually, repeated transfusions will lead to production of antibodies with diminishing clinical response. Thus platelet transfusions must be used sparingly. Although it is desirable to use platelets from HL-A compatible donors, it is important not to use as donors of blood or platelets relatives who may become donors of bone marrow transplantation (see below). Menorrhagia should be treated by means of oral contraceptives.

Control of Infection

These patients are liable to infection; broad-spectrum antibiotics such as ampicillin are suggested for controlling gram-positive organisms and carbenicillin and cephaloridine for gram-negative organisms, unless the results of culture tests indicate some other specific antibiotics. It should be remembered that some antibiotics are recognized as aplastogenic to susceptible individuals, and they should be used for limited periods and with caution.

At all times the patient should try to avoid exposure to infections. He or she should be hospitalized as little as possible; when in the hospital, cross-infection should be avoided by patient isolation and barrier nursing, using plastic isolators or laminar air-flow units if available, especially when the neutrophil count is less than 0.2×10^9 per liter. To avoid self-infection by the patient's personal environment there is need for meticulous care with regard to skin cleanliness, oral hygiene, and prevention of upper respiratory tract infections.

Androgens

The efficiency of androgen therapy still remains debatable. It appears to be of value in hereditary aplastic anemias, both Fanconi and Diamond-Blackfan types. Response in chronic acquired aplastic anemia is more variable. Androgens undoubtedly benefit some patients, but this response may be only temporary with subsequent relapse despite continuing treatment, and ultimate prognosis seems to be little influenced by this form of therapy. Moreover, remission may not be induced for several months, by which time many of the poor-risk patients will have died. Nonetheless, a course should be tried in the first instance unless early marrow transplant is contemplated (see below). Of the available preparations, those administered by mouth are preferable. The most widely used at present is oxymetholone in a dose of 3 to 5 mg. per kg. per day; methandrostenolone (methandienone) in a dose of 2 mg. per kg. per day is an alternative (this use of methandrostenolone is not listed in the manufacturer's official directive in the U.S.A.). Therapy must be continued for several months at least, as delayed response is not uncommon. When there is a response, treatment should be continued until no further improvement is noted and should be reinstituted if withdrawal is followed by relapse.

Treatment should be stopped if jaundice occurs and liver function tests are abnormal. Acne, fluid retention, diarrhea, or hirsutism may be unpleasant side effects, but they are readily reversible when treatment stops. In children, however, androgens are liable to cause irreversible growth retardation.

Steroids

Corticosteroids do not have hematopoietic effect when administered alone but seem to act synergistically with androgens. They are also of some value in decreasing hemorrhagic manifestations, by lessening vascular fragility. Because of their potential side effects, if used at all, they should be used for short periods of time only and in low doses, e.g., 15 to 20 mg. of prednisone per day. Corticosteroids do, however, have a more definite place in immunosuppressive therapy (see below).

Immunosuppression

At least some cases of acquired pure red cell aplasia are due to an immunologic mechanism. These patients may respond well to treatment with azathioprine, 100 mg. daily, or cyclophosphamide, 150 mg. daily, together with prednisone, 20 to 40 mg. daily. (This use of azathioprine and cyclophosphamide is not listed in the manufacturer's official directive.) After remission it may be necessary to continue these drugs at a lower dosage which should be titrated in each individual case.

There is recent evidence that a proportion of cases of chronic acquired aplastic anemia may also have an immune basis, and here too it may be worthwhile trying a short course of immunosuppression. There is no reliable method available for identifying such cases in the first instance.

Splenectomy

This has a limited beneficial value in some patients. In aplastic anemia there is almost always a degree of hemolysis. In some patients splenectomy will reduce the hemolytic element and thus lessen transfusion requirements. If the operation is contemplated, it should be performed at a relatively early stage and not be delayed until the patient is moribund. However, it is a serious operation, especially in aplastic anemia, and not to be undertaken without considerable thought.

Bone Marrow Transplantation

Bone marrow transplantation from histocompatible siblings may result in a permanent cure provided that the difficulties of graft versus host reaction can be overcome. This requires the conditioning of the patient with high doses of cyclophosphamide for 4 days before grafting and continued immunosuppression with methotrexate for 100 days afterward. Reactions caused by the graft and by the immunosuppressive drugs may be life threatening, so that a decision to perform transplantation is not to be taken lightly. However, if this treatment is to be undertaken, it should be commenced as soon as possible after initial evaluation, as delay increases the risks of complications; also, if the patient requires blood or platelet transfusions, there is a likelihood of presensitization which makes the task of finding a compatible marrow donor increasingly difficult. Thus HL-A typing of the patient and the family should be performed when the patient is first seen; if transplantation appears to be feasible, the patient should be referred to a specialized marrow transplant unit with facilities for intensive medical and nursing care. Marrow transplantation is an important development in the treatment of aplastic anemia, but the hopes of the patient and the family must not be raised too high; its application is at present generally limited to patients who have HL-A compatible siblings, and even in this selected group only 50 to 60 per cent of the patients appear likely to have a favorable response.

Supportive Measures

The illness may be acute and rapidly fatal. More frequently it is chronic over a period of months and years. Although the prognosis is grave, the disease is not necessarily fatal; the longer the patient survives, the better the chance of his eventual recovery. There is every reason to persevere with treatment, especially to make every effort to tide the patient over episodes of hemorrhage or infection, and to counsel hope.

ANEMIA DUE TO IRON DEFICIENCY

method of
SYLVIA S. BOTTOMLEY, M.D.
Oklahoma City, Oklahoma

Iron deficiency is a common cause of anemia. It occurs in premenopausal women, especially during repeated pregnancies, and in infants who are otherwise healthy. In men and postmenopausal women, iron deficiency anemia is most commonly associated with chronic blood loss from the alimentary tract. Occasionally iron deficiency develops because of hemosiderinuria-hemoglobinuria and rarely because of malabsorption. The diagnosis is usually apparent when, together with the clinical setting, the laboratory values reveal microcytic, hypochromic red cells, a low serum iron with a normal to increased iron binding capacity, and absent iron stores. Early or mild iron deficiency, particularly that associated with recent blood loss, may not manifest these typical laboratory features (except for the absence of marrow iron stores). One must therefore have a high degree of suspicion that the lack of iron is the principal cause of anemia. Serum ferritin levels, which indicate iron stores, should be of value in assessing early iron deficiency.

The diagnosis of uncomplicated iron deficiency anemia is confirmed by a complete response to iron therapy but, more importantly, requires clarification of the underlying cause. In the occasional patient the underlying cause may be in remission or may become evident upon follow-up. When multiple factors contribute to anemia, the response to iron treatment may be diminished or absent until the other factors are corrected. The treatment of iron deficiency is appropriate management of the underlying cause and iron replacement. The effectiveness of iron replacement, although gratifying and predictable, depends upon the patient's compliance, the physician's attention, and the ability to supply iron in excess of that which may be lost with continued bleeding. Indiscriminate administration of iron for anemia may be harmful and can lead to delay in diagnosis.

Oral Iron Treatment

With rare exceptions iron deficiency anemia should be treated with oral iron. For maximal therapeutic effectiveness iron preparations should be readily soluble in the gastric and upper duodenal contents. In the adult they should supply 200 mg. of elemental iron per day and in children 4 to 6 mg. of elemental iron per kg. of body weight per day. The least expensive preparation for adults is ferrous sulfate, 300 mg. (containing 65 mg. of iron). Ferrous gluconate, 300 mg. (containing 37 mg. of iron), ferrous fumarate, 200 mg. (containing 67 mg. iron) or 300 mg. (containing 100 mg. of iron), and ferrous sulfate elixir, 40 mg. per ml. (containing 8 mg. of iron per ml.), are slightly more expensive. For children, pediatric drops of ferrous sulfate, 125 mg. per ml. (containing 8 mg. of iron), are most palatable. Enteric-coated or "prolonged release" preparations should not be used; not only are they more expensive but they disintegrate unpredictably in releasing divalent iron to the primary absorption site, the upper duodenum. Maximal absorption of iron occurs when it is ingested on an empty stomach, but minor side effects, such as gastrointestinal irritation, are more common. These are essentially eliminated in all patients if the iron is taken with or after meals, although then the amount of iron absorbed is reduced by approximately half. The patient's acceptance of prescribed oral iron therapy may take precedence over an optimal iron supply by reduction of the dose or the amount of iron absorbed (i.e., taken with meals); then a slower hematopoietic response can be expected. A gradual increase of the dose by 1 tablet every few days will be accepted by a patient who previously was considered to have true oral iron intolerance. Avoiding suggestion that side effects will occur will further enhance patients' acceptance. Iron should not be taken with antacids because they significantly impair iron absorption. Although ascorbic acid enhances iron absorption, large quantities are needed (i.e., 1400 mg. per 200 mg. of iron), gastrointestinal side effects of iron are enhanced, and the cost of therapy is increased. "Hematinic mixtures" contain insufficient iron, their cost is many-fold that of simple iron preparations, other components (e.g., vitamin B_{12}, intrinsic factor, and folate) enhance the risk of delayed diagnosis of unsuspected primary diseases, and they should never be used.

The initial reticulocyte response, after 5 to 10 days of iron therapy, is generally proportional to the degree of anemia but rarely exceeds 10 per cent. As a rough guide, the blood hemoglobin concentration should increase about 1.0 gram per 100 ml. per week, and after 3 weeks the hemoglobin should be approximately halfway between the initial and the normal level. A normal hemoglobin value should be obtained within 2 months. Patients with postgastrectomy states and with achlorhydria have a slower response. Since the rate of iron absorption progressively declines as the anemia is corrected, and since only 2 to 6 per cent of the iron ingested is absorbed once the hemoglobin is normal, iron therapy must be continued for an additional 6 months to replenish iron stores (500 to 1000 mg.).

No response or an incomplete response to the treatment regimen should in all cases be explained by one or more of the following: (1) Most commonly, the diagnosis is in error and reassessment of the anemia is necessary. (2) An additional illness exists and, if not evident, should be searched for (e.g., a chronic infection, pernicious anemia, thalassemia). (3) The patient has not taken the prescribed medication. (4) The dosage or the form of iron prescribed is inadequate; enteric-coated ferrous sulfate is frequently filled by pharmacists when ferrous sulfate has been prescribed. (5) There is continued blood loss which outstrips the iron supplied by the medication or the capacity of the marrow to respond. (6) Least likely, a malabsorption disorder of the intestine exists.

When prescribing iron tablets, patients should be warned to keep such medication out of the reach of children. The ingestion of even a small number of iron tablets by a young child may cause serious or fatal iron poisoning.

Parenteral Iron Treatment

Iron therapy by injection is rarely necessary to correct iron deficiency. There are a number of disadvantages to the use of parenteral forms of iron: (1) greater cost; (2) inconvenience and discomfort of repeated injections; (3) up to 30 per cent of the iron injected may not be utilized and may remain indefinitely in storage sites, making future histologic evaluation of iron stores unreliable; (4) side effects can be expected in 1 to 2 per cent of patients, including phlebitis, lymphadenitis, headache, nausea, fever, arthritis, urticaria, bronchospasm, and fatal anaphylaxis. Before parenteral iron administration is instituted, the basis for failure of response to oral iron therapy should be carefully analyzed and the diagnosis firmly established.

Parenteral iron therapy becomes necessary (1) in the patient whose blood loss exceeds the amount of iron which can be supplied by oral iron alone to avoid the need for transfusion (e.g., uncontrolled long-term bleeding from hereditary telangiectasia); (2) in intestinal malabsorption states; (3) in unreliable patients who do not adhere to oral iron treatment; and (4) rarely, in patients with intestinal lesions whose symptoms are aggravated by iron ingestion and, very rarely, when there is gastrointestinal intolerance of oral iron therapy.

Iron dextran contains 50 mg. of iron per milliliter. An initial dose of 0.5 ml. of the preparation is recommended to test for hypersensitivity. Measures to combat anaphylaxis should be available during initial injections. *Iron dextran* is preferably administered intramuscularly, deep in the upper outer quadrant of the buttocks by the Z-track technique to avoid skin staining and sterile abscesses. Up to 2.5 ml. (or 125 mg.) in each side may be administered daily or at less frequent intervals. The total iron deficit must be replaced and the quantity to be given is based on body weight, the level of the hemoglobin, and the amount required to replace iron stores. The total dose to be given may be derived from the table in the package insert, or by the following formula: hemoglobin deficit in grams per 100 ml. × body weight in pounds (or kg. × 2.2) = mg. of iron necessary to correct the anemia, plus 1000 mg. of iron to replenish iron stores. These doses do not compensate for that fraction of iron dextran given which may not be utilized. Iron dextran may also be administered undiluted intravenously in doses of 2 ml. per day, at a rate not exceeding 1 ml. per minute. Although total dose infusions diluted in 250 to 1000 ml. of isotonic saline are being given, this procedure is as yet not approved in the United States.

The response to parenteral iron therapy is no more rapid than effective oral iron treatment (i.e., an adequate iron intake in the absence of malabsorption), provided iron loss caused by active bleeding is sufficiently below that which can be absorbed from oral iron or below the maximal amount of iron which normal marrow can utilize (i.e., up to 200 mg. per day) for red cell generation.

Blood Transfusion

The need for blood transfusion in the treatment of iron deficiency should be carefully weighed against the severity and acuteness of the anemia and alternative measures. In addition to the expense, the hazards of transfusion reactions, sensitization, transmission of hepatitis, and circulatory overload remain significant. Usually, the severely, chronically anemic patient with a hemoglobin level in the range of 5 to 6 grams per 100 ml. and without associated disease remains stable for 5 to 7 days, when with prompt therapy an increase in hemoglobin can be expected to ensue. Packed red cells should be given when the anemic hypoxia compromises the function of vital organs, as in myocardial ischemia or cerebral insufficiency. In such situations red cells should be administered slowly (1 unit over 6 to 8 hours), and one should strive for a minimum quantity necessary to alleviate the major effects of the anemia. Excessive transfusion will blunt a hematopoietic effect of iron therapy for some time. Packed red cell transfusion may also be necessary if continued blood loss must be replaced in preparation for surgery, and in complex situations when other factors significantly contribute to the effects of severe anemia and limit a prompt response to iron therapy (e.g., carcinoma, infection, chronic renal disease). Whole blood should be given only in situations with superimposed severe hemorrhage and shock.

HEMOLYTIC ANEMIA—IMMUNE

method of
GERALD L. LOGUE, M.D.
Durham, North Carolina

A variety of different clinical syndromes can be caused by antibodies directed against one's own red cells. These syndromes may be classified on the basis of whether the antibodies are IgG or IgM and whether the antigen-antibody interaction occurs exclusively at reduced temperatures or at body temperature. An accurate diagnostic evaluation must precede specific therapy.

Warm-Reactive IgG Autoimmune Hemolytic Anemia

The most common form of autoimmune hemolytic anemia is caused by IgG autoantibodies which react at body temperatures. The direct antiglobulin test ("Coombs' test") will be positive, and if testing is available to define the immunoproteins coating the patient's red cells, immunoglobulin-G will be detected. Complement components, most notably the third component of complement, may or may not be detected on the cell surface. Currently the approach to therapy does not differ depending upon whether or not complement is found in association with the antibody.

In rare instances, IgG red cell antibodies may be present which are not detected by routine antiglobulin agglutination procedures. The diagnosis of these so-called "Coombs-negative" autoimmune hemolytic anemias rests on clinical grounds and, ultimately, upon more sophisticated antibody detection systems. The treatment of this form of hemolytic anemia will be identical to that of warm-reactive IgG disease.

Corticosteroid Therapy. Corticosteroids represent the primary therapy for this form of autoimmune hemolytic anemia. Prednisone in doses of 60 to 100 mg. (1 to 2 mg. per kg. per day) should be used initially. Sixty to 80 per cent of patients will respond clinically within 14 days. A decreased hemolytic rate will be evidenced by increasing hematocrit with continued increased reticulocyte counts until normal hemoglobin and hematocrit levels are achieved. The direct antiglobulin test will usually remain positive during the initial clinical response. Some patients with this type of autoimmune hemolytic anemia will have a relatively low reticulocyte count prior to therapy. The reticulocyte count often rises in these patients with initiation of therapy. Patients who have no response after 21 days represent a therapeutic failure and should be treated by other modalities.

Patients who are responsive to corticosteroid therapy usually obtain normal hemoglobin, hematocrit, and reticulocyte counts within 1 to 2 months. At that time gradual reduction in prednisone should begin. Weekly dose reductions of 10 mg. per day of prednisone are advised until a daily dose of 40 mg. per day is reached. The daily dose should then be reduced by 5 mg. per day every 1 to 2 weeks until a dose of 15 mg. per day is reached. A reduction of 2.5 mg. per day every 2 weeks is then advisable. At a dose range of 7.5 mg. per day, alternate day therapy may be given (i.e., 15 mg. every other day rather than 7.5 mg. per day). With some patients prednisone may be tapered and discontinued without disease relapse occurring, whereas others will require low dose therapy to maintain remission. Relapse of the hemolytic process necessitates an increase in prednisone dose, often to a level of 40 mg. per day, to recapture the clinical response. If more than 10 to 15 mg. per day of prednisone is required to maintain hematologic remission, the patient should be considered a therapeutic failure and other forms of treatment considered.

Splenectomy. If the patient's hemolytic process cannot be adequately controlled with corticosteroid therapy, splenectomy should be considered the next treatment of choice, unless there are major contraindications to surgery. The majority of patients with this type of hemolytic anemia will show a significant improvement or complete remission after splenectomy. Splenectomy is preferable to chronic administration of more than 10 mg. per day of prednisone for disease control. ^{51}Cr red cell organ sequestration studies are probably not useful in predicting which patients will respond to this treatment.

If splenectomy is necessary for disease control, it is preferable to accomplish it within 3 months of disease onset, as prolonged high dose corticosteroid administration increases the likelihood of surgical complications. Care must be taken to provide adequate parenteral corticosteroid support during and after the surgical procedure to prevent complications of adrenal insufficiency.

Cytotoxic Chemotherapy. Cytotoxic chemotherapy may be used in an attempt to induce immunosuppression in patients who have failed to respond adequately to corticosteroids and splenectomy or in patients in whom there are major contraindications to surgery. The goal of immunosuppression is to allow disease control to be maintained with acceptable doses of prednisone.

Cyclophosphamide, starting with doses of 100 to 150 mg. per day (1 to 2 mg. per kg. per day), may be used. (This use of cyclophosphamide is not listed in the manufacturer's official directive.) The patient is monitored for toxic side effects, including leukopenia, thrombocytopenia, or reticulocytopenia, and the dose is reduced if such side effects occur. The patient should be informed of the potential side effect of hemorrhagic cystitis from this agent and advised to maintain an adequate fluid intake to prevent this reaction. Alternatively, azathioprine in a dose of 2 to 2.5 mg. per kg. per day may be used. Response to this form of therapy often requires 1 to 3 months. (This use of azathioprine is not listed in the manufacturer's official directive.) If no beneficial response has been observed in 3 to 4 months, the cytotoxic chemotherapy should be discontinued. The patient should also be advised of the potential of developing a malignancy with long-term cytotoxic chemotherapy.

Treatment of Associated Disease. In many instances autoimmune hemolytic anemia is associated with other primary disease processes such as systemic lupus erythematosus (SLE), non-Hodgkin's lymphoma, or chronic lymphocytic leukemia. With some diseases such as SLE, the autoimmune hemolytic process may precede other clinical manifestations of the primary disease. Successful treatment of the underlying disease may be associated with remission of the associated autoimmune hemolytic anemia.

Transfusion Therapy. Patients with immune hemolytic anemia may have life-threatening, progressive anemia which requires transfusion of packed red cells. Mild symptoms such as weakness or decreased exercise tolerance are not indications for transfusion, but symptoms of coronary artery disease, congestive heart failure, or cerebrovascular insufficiency will require judicious transfusion of packed red blood cells.

It is often difficult or impossible to identify compatible blood for transfusion of these patients. This is because the patients' autoantibody often is a "panagglutinin" which reacts with all cells tested. In spite of this in vitro incompatibility, the transfused red cells will usually not undergo abrupt hemolysis. If other incompatibilities are not present, the transfused red cells will survive at the same rate as the patient's own red blood cells.

On the other hand, the blood transfusion service must take great care to be certain that the patient does not have blood group isoantibodies in addition to the autoantibody. Patients with autoimmune hemolytic anemia appear to have an increased tendency to develop such superimposed isoantibodies through sensitization from prior transfusion or pregnancy. If unnoticed, these isoantibodies may produce severe hemolytic transfusion reactions.

Cold Agglutinin Disease (CAD)

Cold-reactive IgM anti–red cell antibodies may be seen transiently following a variety of infections or may be seen as a chronic, progressive illness of the elderly. The former usually are not associated with hemolytic anemia, although an occasional severe hemolytic episode may occur if the patient undergoes undue cold exposure. The cold-reactive antibody which is observed following infections such as Mycoplasma pneumonia will usually disappear spontaneously within 2 to 4 weeks. In the chronic cold agglutinin syndrome, on the other hand, the cold-reactive antibody does not disappear spontaneously and will progressively increase over periods of months to years. This chronic cold agglutinin syndrome may be idiopathic or may be associated with other illnesses such as non-Hodgkin's lymphoma. In all instances overt hemolysis will be associated with a positive direct antiglobulin reaction caused by the presence of complement components on the patient's red cells. The relationship between the cold agglutinin titer and severity of hemolytic anemia is not rigid. Patients with cold agglutinin titers of 1/100 may have severe hemolysis, whereas those with titers of $1/10^6$ may not have significant hemolytic anemia.

The cornerstone of the treatment of hemolysis in the cold agglutinin syndrome is avoidance of exposure to cold. By rigidly adhering to a program of cold avoidance, including the wearing of warm clothing, earmuffs, and gloves when outdoors, many patients with CAD may require no other form of therapy. With this form of conservative management many such patients can be maintained with mild to moderate degrees of anemia (9 to 12 grams per dl. [100 ml.] of hemoglobin). The occasional patient with severe hemolysis may require hospitalization and adjustment of room temperature to greater than 85°F. (25.4°C.) while other therapeutic modalities are being considered.

If transfusion is necessary, the cross-matching should be carefully done at 37°C. (98.6°F.) and packed red cells administered through a 37°C. warming coil. Care must be taken not to expose the blood to temperatures above 37°C.

Patients with severe hemolytic anemia may be treated with chlorambucil, 4 to 8 mg. per day initially. (This use of chlorambucil is not listed in the manufacturer's official directive.) The patient is observed for toxic side effects, including leukopenia, thrombocytopenia, or reticulocytopenia, and the dose is reduced if such side effects occur. Monitoring of weekly blood counts is necessary with this form of therapy. Clinical response will usually require treatment for 1 to 2 months. If no response is seen in 3 to 4 months, this form of therapy should be discontinued.

Corticosteroid therapy has generally been thought to be of little benefit in CAD. Recent investigators, however, have suggested that some patients, especially those with antibodies of high thermal amplitude, will respond to such treatment. In patients with severe CAD, unresponsive to other forms of therapy, a 14 to 30 day trial of high-dose prednisone therapy may be in order. If no response is seen, this agent should be discontinued.

Other forms of therapy, including splenectomy, have not proved to be effective in this disease. Plasmapheresis has been used on occasion but is extremely dangerous and should be used only as a research tool. If the patient's whole blood is removed and exposed to reduced temperatures, hemolysis will rapidly ensue when the blood is reinfused.

If the CAD is associated with an underlying malignancy, successful treatment of the primary disease, such as with radiation therapy or chemotherapy, may be associated with remission of the autoimmune process. Relapse of the underlying primary disease may also be associated with relapse of the hemolytic anemia.

Paroxysmal Cold Hemoglobinuria (PCH)

Cold-reactive IgG autoantibodies directed against the P blood group system cause the illness PCH. This type of antibody usually appears following infections, and prior to the antibiotic era this reaction was most often seen with syphilis. In recent years the most common association has been with viral infections. The hemolysis occurs on exposure to cold and is complement mediated. As with CAD, the most effective form of therapy is protection from cold exposure. In many instances the antibody will disappear spontaneously. Corticosteroid therapy or splenectomy does not appear to be useful, but experience with these forms of therapy is limited.

Drug-Induced Immune Hemolytic Anemia

A variety of drugs may produce immune hemolytic anemia. These adverse reactions may be grouped into three categories: a drug-induced, autoimmune process produced predominantly by the drug methyldopa (Aldomet), and two immune types in which the antibodies produced are directed against the offending drugs. One form of this immune process may be associated with high-dose penicillin therapy and is caused by the reaction of an antibody with the drug which is tightly bound to the red cell. The second type of immune process is the so-called "innocent bystander" hemolytic reaction in which the antibody reacts with a drug that is not avidly bound to the patient's red cells. A large variety of drugs have been implicated in the innocent bystander reaction, including sulfonamides, sulfonylureas, quinine, organic insecticides, and a variety of antibiotics, including isoniazid, rifampin, and tetracyclines.

Approximately 10 per cent of patients receiving methyldopa (Aldomet) therapy will develop positive direct antiglobulin reactions. The vast majority of patients with this antibody will not have overt hemolytic anemia. If hemolysis occurs, it will often be mild and not require specific therapy. The rare patient who has severe hemolysis from a methyldopa-induced autoantibody may require therapy in the fashion described for warm-reactive IgG autoimmune hemolytic anemia. The antibody will usually disappear within 2 to 4 months after discontinuing the drug. Antibodies have persisted in some patients for more than 1 year.

The high-dose penicillin-induced form of immune red cell sensitization is usually not associated with overt hemolysis. In either form of immune drug reaction, the antibody is directed against the drug, and when this agent has been cleared the hemolytic process will cease. Thus the positive direct antiglobulin reaction associated with high-dose penicillin administration usually does not require specific therapy.

The "innocent bystander" immune hemolytic reaction is caused by activation of complement on the red cell surface and will be associated with a positive direct antiglobulin reaction caused by membrane-bound complement components. Thus this reaction is a cause of the "complement only" antiglobulin reaction. The hemolysis caused by complement activation in this reaction is predominantly intravascular. This hemolysis is often severe and may cause acute renal failure. Patients with this form of severe hemolytic anemia should be treated with measures to ensure maintenance of intravascular volume and urine flow as described for immediate hemolytic transfusion reactions. The hemolytic process will cease when the offending drug has been cleared from the patient's plasma.

HEMOLYTIC ANEMIA—NONIMMUNE

method of
DONALD R. HARKNESS, M.D.
Miami, Florida

In the absence of bleeding, shortened red cell survival indicates the presence of hemolysis. Rarely the marrow responds by production of sufficient numbers of erythrocytes to prevent a fall in red cell mass, and this is termed compensated hemolysis. More commonly anemia develops and uncompensated hemolytic anemia is said to be present. Indicators of increased red blood cell destruction include unconjugated hyperbilirubinemia, increased urobilinogen excretion in urine and stool, and increased endogenous production of carbon monoxide. If the hemolytic process is intravascular, there may also be increased serum lactic dehydrogenase, methemalbuminemia, decreased serum haptoglobins and hemopexin, hemoglobinuria, and hemosiderinuria. Some or all of the following signs of increased erythroid production may be present: reticulocytosis, polychromasia, anisocytosis, poikilocytosis, basophilic stippling, marrow erythroid hyperplasia, neutrophilia, thrombocytosis, and presence of nucleated red blood cells in the peripheral blood.

Most hemolytic anemias may be conveniently subdivided into two groups: acquired or extrinsic, and hereditary or intrinsic. The underlying pathogenesis of the hemolysis must be defined in order to institute appropriate therapy. It should be kept in mind that any process which causes a suppression of erythroid production, such as exposure to toxic substances (drugs, chemicals, alcohol), bacterial or viral infection, folic acid or iron deficiency, or uremia, may result in a precipitous fall in hemoglobin in persons with hemolytic disease. If the hemolytic process is moderate or severe, oral folic acid (1 mg. daily) is routinely prescribed. The use of packed red cell transfusions must be individualized.

ACQUIRED HEMOLYTIC ANEMIA

Mechanical Fragmentation

Cardiac Hemolytic Anemia. Intravascular hemolysis may occur after the insertion of artificial heart valves, after repair of septal defects, and, rarely, in patients with severe valvular heart disease in whom no surgical correction has been attempted. This complication is seen most frequently following aortic valve replacement. Red cell fragmentation may be striking on the peripheral blood smear. Usually the degree of anemia is mild, and treatment consists of supplemental oral iron to replace that which is lost in the urine. On occasion, however, the hemolysis is severe and requires reoperation. At surgery the initial prosthesis often is found to be positioned improperly or to be defective in such a way that a forceful regurgitant stream is created. In the case of septal repair, closure may be found to be incomplete or the material used to patch the defect may have failed to endothelialize.

March or Exertional Hemoglobinuria. This form of hemolysis is associated with physical activities, such as running or jogging on hard surfaces, striking hard objects as in karate or handball, or playing bongo drums. Trauma to the red blood cells is thought to result from compression of small blood vessels overlying bony prominences of the hands or feet. Hemolysis may be of sufficient degree to produce transient hemoglobinuria, which must be distinguished from myoglobinuria. In march hemoglobinuria, anemia seldom occurs, as only a small percentage of the erythrocytes are destroyed and the episodes are transitory. In runners the hemolysis may be prevented or diminished by wearing shoes with padded soles or by insertion of sponge rubber insoles.

Microangiopathic Hemolytic Anemia. Fragmentation of erythrocytes with intravascular hemolysis accompanies a large number of diseases which fall into two major categories: arteriolar disease (vasculitis) and disseminated intravascular coagulation (DIC). Both processes may be present in some instances.

Those diseases characterized primarily by vasculitis with which hemolysis may be associated include malignant hypertension, acute glomerulonephritis, polyarteritis, allergic vasculitis, eclampsia, Rocky Mountain spotted fever, thrombotic thrombocytopenic purpura (TTP), and the hemolytic-uremic syndrome. In most of these diseases the hemolytic anemia is mild and no specific therapy other than blood transfusion is available.

Thrombotic thrombocytopenic purpura (TTP), seen primarily in adults, is an idiopathic disease of abrupt onset characterized by fever, hemolytic anemia, thrombocytopenia, renal failure, and transient central nervous system manifestations. Coagulation studies are usually normal. Mortality is high (up to 80 per cent) despite the common use of high dose prednisone, splenectomy, dextrans, heparin, and blood transfusions. Recently, the use of exchange transfusions has been reported to cause dramatic improvement and significantly decreased mortality in a sizable number of patients. A patient with classic TTP has been treated successfully at our institution for nearly a year with the infusion of plasma or plasma products. After each infusion of fresh frozen plasma, outdated plasma, or the soluble material after preparation of cryoprecipitate, the hemolysis abruptly ceases. This suggests that some plasma factor is deficient in this patient. If verified in other patients with TTP, these observations offer both a new approach to therapy and a clue to the pathogenesis of this confounding disease.

The hemolytic-uremic syndrome, a disease occurring principally in children and resembling TTP, is characterized by acute renal failure and hemolytic anemia but without central nervous system involvement. Recovery is the rule. Therapy consists of renal dialysis alone or in combination with heparin therapy in doses of 25 to 35 I.U. per kg. per hour.

Disseminated intravascular coagulation (DIC) occurs in a variety of clinical situations in which the coagulation system is activated by introduction of thromboplastic substances into the bloodstream or activation of Hageman factor by endotoxin or antigen-antibody complexes. The list of diseases is long and includes endotoxic shock, septicemia, heat stroke, electrocution, abruptio placentae, amniotic fluid embolization, burns (even severe sunburn), and metastatic carcinoma. The hemolytic process is usually not severe. If necessary, hemolysis can be controlled by the intravenous administration of heparin in doses of 50 to 150 I.U. per kg. of body weight every 4 to 6 hours. Heparin therapy is more often required to stop or prevent bleeding than it is to treat the hemolysis. Ultimately the outcome nearly always depends upon the success with which the underlying disease is treated (see also pages 290 to 291).

Infection

Only in a few infections is clinically significant hemolysis present. The most important of these is malaria, in which hemolysis is a consequence of the multiplication of the parasite within the erythrocyte. On rare occasions a positive Coombs test is present. The drugs used for treatment of malaria may cause hemolysis in susceptible individuals (glucose-6-phosphate dehydrogenase [G-6-PD] deficient).

Hemolytic anemia has been reported in toxoplasmosis, *Clostridium welchii* infections, bartonellosis, typhoid fever, and relapsing fever. Immune hemolytic anemia may occur with viral infections, such as infectious mononucleosis and those caused by cytomegalovirus, and with Mycoplasma infections. Infections may lead to accelerated hemolysis and decreased marrow response in persons with various types of hereditary hemolytic anemias. Sometimes a previously undiagnosed person with hereditary spherocytosis, for instance, first comes to the physician's attention when anemia becomes more apparent at the time of an intercurrent illness.

In infection, therapy is directed against the underlying disease with no specific measures usually required for treatment of the anemia.

Nutritional

Although not a major contributing factor to the degree of anemia, there is a hemolytic component in anemias resulting from severe deficiencies of vitamin B_{12}, folic acid, and iron. In severe iron deficiency, red cell survival has been reported to be as low as half normal.

Hemolytic anemia has recently been reported in severe phosphate depletion such as may occur in diabetics, alcoholics, and patients receiving intravenous hyperalimentation. The hemolysis is assumed to result from decreased glycolysis secondary to the low intracellular inorganic phosphate which leads to a fall in both ATP and 2,3-DPG. Cells depleted of ATP become rigid and are removed from the circulation. Platelet, neutrophil, and central nervous system dysfunction have also been described, presumably caused by a similar alteration in metabolism. Although not reported in man, severe magnesium depletion could probably induce similar pathologic consequences because of the essential role of magnesium in cellular energy metabolism.

Therapy of the hemolytic anemia associated with nutritional deficiencies is dependent upon recognition and correction of the deficiency.

Chemical

Various drugs, chemicals, and plant and animal toxins can produce hemolysis by damaging the erythrocyte directly, by producing disseminated intravascular coagulation, by the peculiar susceptibility of erythrocytes in persons with hereditary abnormalities (e.g., G-6-PD deficiency, certain unstable hemoglobins), or by immune hemolysis. Arsine gas (AsH_3), copper sulfate, lead, chlorates, chloramine, formaldehyde, and hydroxylamine are examples of inorganic chemicals which produce hemolysis in normal persons. Several of these chemicals have produced hemolysis after diffusion into the bloodstream from the water used in hemodialysis. Aromatic organic chemicals such as benzene, toluene, phenols and phenylhydrazine, and their derivatives produce hemolysis, as does the administration of high doses of dapsone to normal persons. Exposures to 100 per cent oxygen and hyperbaric oxygen have also been implicated as causes of hemolysis. Intravenous introduction of very hypotonic solutions or distilled water induces red cell lysis.

Intravascular hemolysis sometimes occurs after bee stings and the bites of certain spiders and snakes. Presumably DIC plays a role in the hemolysis in these patients, but this is not known with certainty.

Therapy consists of recognition of the cause of the hemolysis and its removal.

Hypersplenism

Pancytopenia or selective cytopenias may result from sequestration in an enlarged spleen. Although hypersplenism may result from splenomegaly of any cause (e.g., cirrhosis, portal or splenic vein thrombosis, lipid storage disease, lymphoma-leukemia, myeloproliferative disease, inflammatory diseases), significant cytopenias are usually seen only with congestive splenomegaly (cirrhosis and portal or splenic vein thrombosis). Splenectomy corrects the cytopenias, but one must consider carefully the benefits versus the risks, because many of these patients are poor surgical candidates. Infarction of the spleen by selective splenic artery embolization with autologous clots or thrombogenic materials has been reported to be successful in several patients who were too ill to undergo laparotomy.

Spur Cell Anemia

Moderate to severe hemolytic anemia associated with bizarre spiculated erythrocytes occurs in a small percentage of patients with terminal alcoholic cirrhosis. Death from liver failure invariably occurs within 6 months of the onset of this syndrome. Spur cells arise from accumulation of large amounts of cholesterol on the membrane of the red blood cells, which are then destroyed in the spleen. Transfused cells rapidly acquire this morphologic aberration and are destroyed in similar fashion. Since most of these patients are seriously ill, splenectomy is not possible. Selective splenic artery thrombosis with autologous clots was successful in ameliorating the hemolysis in one patient.

Immune Hemolytic Anemias

Autoimmune. See pages 249 to 251.

Drug-Induced. See page 252.

Isoantibodies. TRANSFUSION REACTIONS. See pages 341 to 346.

ERYTHROBLASTOSIS FETALIS. See pages 274 to 280.

HEREDITARY HEMOLYTIC ANEMIAS

Membrane Abnormalities

Hereditary Spherocytosis. This disease is characterized by hemolysis of varying severity, splenomegaly, and jaundice; spherocytes are usually quite evident on the peripheral smear. Spherocytes are poorly deformable and are selectively destroyed in the spleen. Splenectomy is curative and is usually performed electively upon diagnosis, although preferably not before age 4 because of the possible increased risk of sepsis following removal of the spleen at earlier ages. Since hereditary spherocytosis is an autosomal dominant with high penetrance, family members should always be tested. Splenectomy is recommended even in persons with relatively mild hemolysis to prevent formation of gallstones and occurrence of aplastic crises associated with infections.

Hereditary Elliptocytosis. Also inherited as an autosomal dominant with high penetrance, this disease is characterized by the presence of elliptoid, oval, or cigar-shaped red blood cells. Only about 15 per cent of persons with hereditary elliptocytosis display hemolysis. Even within the same kindred, there may be considerable clinical variability. In those with hemolysis, splenectomy is indicated for the same reasons as in hereditary spherocytosis. Splenectomy is usually curative, but in a few patients hemolysis continues and the numbers of microovalocytes, bizarre-shaped red cells, and red cell fragments may increase following surgery.

Stomatocytosis. Stomatocytes are erythrocytes which have a linear "crease-like" area of central pallor on the peripheral smear rather than the circular zone seen in normal erythrocytes. On wet preparations these cells appear bowl-shaped. The presence of large numbers of stomatocytes is usually associated with mild or severe hemolytic anemia; there are probably several variants of this disease. In some patients the erythrocytes are osmotically fragile, contain increased amounts of Na^+ and decreased amounts of K^+, and have a marked increase in Na^+ and K^+ flux. In other patients only some of these abnormalities have been noted. Splenectomy has been beneficial in some patients and not in others. The mode of inheritance is autosomal dominant, and it is thought that this disease is also caused by an inherited abnormality of the red cell membrane as is presumed to be the case in both hereditary spherocytosis and hereditary elliptocytosis.

Hemoglobin Abnormalities

Sickle Cell Diseases. See pages 263 to 271.

Unstable Hemoglobins (Formerly Referred to as Congenital Heinz Body Hemolytic Anemias). Certain mutations in either the α or β chain confer instability upon the hemoglobin molecule and result in the formation of aggregates of denatured hemoglobin within the erythrocyte. These aggregates, called Heinz bodies, are removed by macrophages, primarily in the spleen, by a process called "pitting." This "pitting" process damages the membrane and causes a shortened survival. Hemolysis is very severe with some of these mutations, but mild in others; there is little or no hemolysis in persons with hemoglobin Zürich except after exposure to certain drugs.

The chronic hemolytic process leads to splenic enlargement, which may cause leukopenia, thrombocytopenia, and worsening of the anemia. In such patients splenectomy may be indicated and should correct both the neutropenia and thrombocytopenia and cause a moderate increase in hemoglobin.

Thalassemia. See pages 260 to 263.

Mutant Enzymes

Glycolytic Pathway. Hemolytic anemia has been reported with the homozygous inheritance of mutant forms of almost all the enzymes of glycolysis. Heterozygotes are usually unaffected. With the exception of pyruvate kinase deficiency, hemolytic anemia resulting from glycolytic enzyme deficiencies is rare. Experience is limited with these diseases, and for most no specific therapy is available.

The severity of the hemolytic process associated with pyruvate kinase deficiency is quite variable. In some kindreds severe hemolysis is present at birth, necessitating exchange transfusions, and these persons may require frequent transfusions. In the severer forms of pyruvate kinase deficiency splenectomy may decrease or abolish the need for transfusions and should be performed within the first year of life. In kindreds with less severe hemolysis, splenectomy is usually of little benefit. As in all forms of chronic hemolysis, these persons are subject to aplastic crises and cholelithiasis.

Enzymes of, or Related to, the Hexose Monophosphate Shunt. Persons with a very severe glucose-6-phosphate dehydrogenase deficiency may have chronic hemolytic disease which usually is not alleviated by splenectomy. Much more commonly (in as many as 200 to 300 million persons in the world) the enzyme deficiency is less marked and hemolysis occurs only upon exposure to a variety of chemicals and drugs, which in the presence of oxygen and hemoglobin generate H_2O_2 (e.g., sulfa drugs, nitrofurantoins, sulfones, antimalarials). Rarely hemolysis may be associated with severe metabolic disturbances (uremia, diabetic ketoacidosis), viremia, or bacterial sepsis.

G-6-PD deficiency is inherited as an X-linked recessive. In the United States this mild variant of G-6-PD occurs in 12 per cent of black males and is expressed in 1 per cent of black women. A somewhat more significant deficiency is commonly seen in persons of Mediterranean origin.

Occasionally drug-induced hemolysis may create sufficient intravascular destruction of erythrocytes to cause massive hematuria. In such instances it is necessary to institute therapy immediately in order to minimize damage to the kidneys. Therapy is the same as described on pages 341 to 346.

Drug-induced hemolysis has been reported in the rare persons whose red cells are deficient in glutathione peroxidase. Chronic hemolysis may be present with homozygous deficiency of glutathione reductase deficiency. Drugs may worsen the hemolysis in these persons, as well as in those with chronic hemolytic disease caused by severe G-6-PD deficiency.

MACROCYTIC (MEGALOBLASTIC) ANEMIA

(Other than Pernicious Anemia)

method of
THOMAS W. SHEEHY, M.D.
Birmingham, Alabama

The presence of megaloblastic anemia is almost pathognomonic of a deficiency of folic acid, vitamin B_{12}, or both. Usually the deficiency results from failure to ingest, absorb, utilize, or retain either one or both of these vitamins. Megaloblastic anemia develops as a complication of many clinical entities. Successful therapy and proper management of the anemia therefore entail a knowledge of factors contributing to the deficiency as well as the deficient vitamin. Treatment of the anemia without adequate diagnosis may result in serious consequences.

The basic human requirement of vitamin B_{12} is 0.10 microgram daily. Vitamin B_{12} is present in all foods containing animal protein, and the daily American diet contains 0.25 to 2.0 micrograms. Its extraction occurs in the stomach, where it is complexed with intrinsic factor. Specific receptor sites exist on the ileal epithelial cells. These bind B_{12} and initiate its absorption and intracellular transport to plasma where it is bound to the serum B_{12}–binding protein, transcobalamin II, and transported to storage sites. Total body stores are estimated at 2.5 to 5.0 mg., sufficient to last 3 to 10 years. Fortunately, serum B_{12} levels reflect the status of tissue stores.

The minimum daily requirement of folic acid is 50 micrograms. Folic acid is present in most food, especially green vegetables and fruit, but it is easily destroyed by heat. The American diet contains an abundance of food folates in the polyglutamate form. These are deconjugated in the proximal intestine, and the resulting monoglutamates are absorbed and transported to storage sites. Total body stores are estimated at 10 to 15 mg., of which half is present in liver. These are sufficient to last for 3 to 6 months if ingestion ceases or absorption fails. Unlike serum B_{12} levels, serum folate levels fall rapidly and long before tissue stores are depleted. However, tissue stores are reflected by red blood cell folate levels, and with folate deficiency both the serum and red blood cell levels are low. Red cell folate levels are also low with vitamin B_{12} deficiency, because vitamin B_{12} is essential to the transport of 5-methyltetrafolate across cell membranes. With B_{12} deficiency, serum folate levels are usually normal and serum B_{12} levels are depressed.

The following are among the major causes of *folate deficiency:*

1. Poverty, religious tenets, food faddism, and vegetarianism, all of which may lead to or be associated with subsistence on a diet devoid of adequate folate or vitamin B_{12}.
2. Malabsorption, with loss of mucosal surface area.
3. Pregnancy and lactation, which increase demand for folate.
4. Parasitism and bacterial overgrowth syndromes with competition for folate and vitamin B_{12}.
5. Sickle cell disease, malaria, and hemolytic disorders that lead to increased utilization and need for folate.
6. Drugs, with a variety of actions—e.g., alcohol impairs absorption, transport, release, and utilization when subsistence is based mainly on alcohol-derived calories. Folic acid antagonists (aminopterin), certain antihypertensives (triamterene) and anticonvulsants (phenytoin), and oral contraceptives interfere with its absorption and/or utilization.

Vitamin B_{12} deficiency usually results from impaired absorption. Pernicious anemia, atrophic gastritis, and complete gastrectomy lead to loss of intrinsic factor–secreting cells; surgical resection or disease of the distal ileum, such as regional enteritis or the sprue syndromes, leads to loss of specific receptor sites; stasis resulting from diabetes mellitus, scleroderma, or blind loops leads to bacterial overgrowth and competition for the vitamin.

Inadequate ingestion is an unusual cause of deficiency among the vegans of India or residents of tropical countries because of water contamination with animal products. In this country, deficiency may occur in strict vegetarians and among members of religious sects that prohibit ingestion of animal proteins.

A variety of congenital disorders may also lead to vitamin B_{12} deficiency. Among these are inability to synthesize intrinsic factor, failure of ileal enterocytes to bind the vitamin, and the lack of transcobalamin II to transport it.

Diagnosis

Treatment may be lifelong, and proper therapy is necessary to avoid serious complications; hence, a correct diagnosis is essential. The presence of a megaloblastic anemia, macroovalocytosis, hypersegmentation of white cells, thrombocytopenia, and even a megaloblastic bone marrow is not diagnostic for deficiency of either vitamin. Diagnosis is accomplished by obtaining serum vitamin B_{12} and folic acid levels before the institution of therapy. A serum vitamin B_{12} level of less than 100 picograms per liter is almost diagnostic of vitamin B_{12} deficiency. A serum folate level of less than 3 nanograms per ml. and a red blood cell folate below 150 nanograms per ml. indicate folic acid deficiency. Supporting evidence for a lack of vitamin B_{12} includes the absence of intrinsic factor in gastric juice, methylmalonic aciduria, and failure to absorb radioactive vitamin B_{12} given with intrinsic factor. The deoxyuridine suppression test (dU) appears to be the laboratory equivalent of a therapeutic trial. Although tedious, the therapeutic trial is still useful diagnostically, especially in areas where sophisticated laboratory support is absent. It involves ingestion of a low folate diet and parenteral administration of 100 micrograms of folic acid for 5 to 7 days. This is sufficient folate to induce a hematologic response with folate deficiency but not with vitamin B_{12} deficiency.

Principles of Therapy

These include (1) identification of the type of deficiency; (2) correction of inadequate intake; (3) treatment of correctable diseases leading to deficiency; (4) treatment of the anemia with restoration of the tissue stores; and (5) appropriate supplementation for life when necessary.

Therapy

Megaloblastic anemias develop slowly and are accompanied by physiologic adjustments. This allows most patients to tolerate their symptoms for long periods and usually permits treatment solely with vitamin therapy. Vitamin B_{12}–deficient patients, such as those with pernicious anemia, are given 1 mg. of cyanocobalamin intramuscularly daily for 5 days, and then 1 mg. every month or every 2 months indefinitely. Initially, folic acid–deficient patients are treated with 1 mg. of oral or parenteral folic acid daily for 10 days. Thereafter, supplemental vitamin therapy is given as indicated for the specific deficient states listed hereafter.

Transfusion. Occasionally, transfusion is necessary on an emergency basis for patients with unstable angina, myocardial infarction, congestive heart failure, pulmonary edema, and severe anemia. Here the administration of packed red blood cells may be lifesaving. When emergency transfusion is necessary, a three-way stopcock with a 50 ml. syringe placed between the needle and the transfusion pack permits rapid transfusion and avoids volume overload. Fifty ml. of packed red cells is injected, followed by withdrawal of an equal amount of patient blood. With this method, 1 or 2 units of blood can be given rapidly and immediate relief is often achieved. Volume overload is prevented by monitoring venous pressure frequently.

Less critically ill patients can be given 1 to 2 units of packed blood cells slowly. The decision to transfuse or not to transfuse is always based on sound clinical assessment of the patient's overall condition.

Platelet transfusions are seldom necessary and are given only with evidence of bleeding or retinal hemorrhage and platelet levels of less than 20,000 per cu. mm. Vitamin therapy leads to a prompt platelet rise which usually precedes reticulocytosis.

Dual Vitamin Therapy. Immediate therapy with parenteral cyanocobalamin and folic acid is indicated in the aforementioned conditions, as well as when the hematocrit is below 15 per cent, the platelet count is below 20,000 per cu. mm., or the patient is bleeding. Cyanocobalamin, 1 mg., and folic acid, 1 mg., are given intramuscularly on a daily basis until the results of serum assays reveal the correct deficiency. Thereafter, specific therapy should be 1 mg. of vitamin B_{12} daily for 5 days, followed by monthly injections of 1 mg.; or folic acid, 1 mg. daily intramuscularly or orally.

Treatment of Special Folate Deficiency States

Dietary Insufficiency. Inadequate ingestion resulting from alcoholism, poverty, or other causes may be difficult to treat for a variety of reasons. If the diet cannot be corrected and supplemental folic acid is available, 1 mg. should be given daily, orally, indefinitely.

Sprue Syndromes. Folic acid deficiency is common in these syndromes, but vitamin B_{12} absorption may also be impaired. Ordinarily, the administration of oral folic acid, 1 mg. daily, will lead to improvement in vitamin B_{12} absorption and to a slow but gradual rise in serum vitamin B_{12} levels. If vitamin B_{12} levels are low, some prefer to administer cyanocobalamin daily for a period of 7 days and then monthly until the absorption of radioactive B_{12} returns to normal.

Americans or Europeans with recently acquired tropical sprue should be treated with oral folic acid, 1 mg. daily for 1 year, and tetracycline, 250 mg. twice daily for 60 to 90 days. Their ability to absorb nutrients should be assessed during and after treatment.

Patients residing in endemic areas often have associated parasitism and iron deficiency. After eradication of the parasites, oral iron, 300 mg. daily, should be administered until the tissue stores are repleted. Tetracycline, 250 mg. twice daily, is given in conjunction with folic acid for 1 year, and the patient's ability to absorb nutrients is evaluated during treatment.

Gluten Enteropathy. Treatment requires a gluten-free diet for an indefinite period of time. Since vitamin B_{12} and folate absorption may be impaired in this entity, supplemental therapy, i.e., intramuscular cyanocobalamin, 1 mg. every month, and folic acid orally, 1 mg. daily, should be given until gluten-free diet has improved the patient's ability to absorb these vitamins normally.

Pregnancy and Lactation. Recent surveys in the United States have shown that 30 per cent of low income pregnant mothers have red blood cell folate levels suggestive of deficiency. The growing fetus acquires its folic acid from the mother. If she suffers from borderline depletion because of an inadequate diet or impaired absorption, increased fetal demand may precipitate anemia of both mother and child. Usually, anemia appears in the mother during the third trimester or during early puerperium if she continues to breast feed.

Treatment requires an adequate diet whenever possible and folic acid, 1 mg. orally daily during pregnancy and until lactation ceases.

Drugs. Alcohol is the most common cause of folate deficiency in the United States. Because of the unreliability of these patients and their propensity to ingest an inadequate diet, supplemental therapy is required, but conformity is difficult to achieve. When possible, 1 mg. of oral folic acid daily is prescribed.

Folic acid antagonists, such as aminopterin, block the utilization of folic acid and its conversion to folinic acid. Anemias associated with this type of drug can be reversed by the administration of folinic acid, 3 to 6 mg. daily intramuscularly.

Folate deficiency secondary to use of anticonvulsants or oral contraceptives can be overcome by the administration of 1 mg. of oral folic acid daily, even with continued ingestion of these drugs.

Treatment of Specific Vitamin B_{12} Deficient States

Dietary Deficiency. In this country, dietary deficiency caused by vegetarianism can be treated effectively by the intramuscular injection of 1 mg. of cyanocobalamin every month.

Blind Loop Syndromes. Bacterial competition for vitamin B_{12} can be ascertained in patients with massive intestinal diverticulosis, intestinal strictures, or surgically created blind loops by assessing their ability to absorb radioactive vitamin B_{12} before and after 7 days of tetracycline, 1 gram daily.

Whenever possible, surgical correction of the underlying disorder is indicated. If this is not feasible, indefinite maintenance with 1 mg. of cyanocobalamin intramuscularly every month is sufficient to correct and prevent recurrence of the anemia.

Postgastrectomy States. Here the basic defect is analogous to pernicious anemia, i.e., lack of intrinsic factor. Hence, treatment is the same—namely, prophylactic vitamin B_{12} therapy, 1 mg. of cyanocobalamin every month indefinitely.

Ileal Resection. Operative removal or mucosal disease of the distal 6 to 8 feet of the ileum reduces the ability to absorb vitamin B_{12}. Treatment consists of intramuscular administration of 1 mg. of cyanocobalamin every month indefinitely.

Parasitism. *Diphyllobothrium latum* (fish tapeworm) competes with intrinsic factor for vitamin B_{12} in the upper intestine. Treatment consists of eradication of the tapeworm and administration of vitamin B_{12}, 1 mg. of cyanocobalamin intramuscularly for 7 days, and then monthly for 1 year to replete tissue stores.

Other Causes of Megaloblastic Anemia

Although vitamin B_{12} and folic acid deficiency are responsible for the great majority of megaloblastic anemias, other causative factors must be considered. Megaloblastic bone marrow changes may occur with diseases such as orotic aciduria, acute myelogenous leukemia, or Di Guglielmo's syndrome, or with use of cytotoxic drugs, such as 5-fluorouracil, hydroxyurea, or cytosine arabinoside. Here again, serum folate and vitamin B_{12} levels are helpful, for in these conditions they are usually normal.

PERNICIOUS ANEMIA AND OTHER FORMS OF VITAMIN B_{12} DEFICIENCY

method of
BERNARD A. COOPER, M.D.
Montreal, Quebec, Canada

In pernicious anemia, megaloblastic anemia appears because of prolonged, severe deficiency of vitamin B_{12}. Of megaloblastic anemias caused by deficiency of vitamin B_{12}, pernicious anemia is unique only in that the cause of B_{12} deficiency is malfunction or absence of the gastric intrinsic factor. This mucoprotein, secreted by the gastric parietal cells, is required for the effective absorption of the low concentrations of vitamin B_{12} from the food.

Patients with pernicious anemia come to the attention of physicians for one of four reasons: (1) because of severe anemia, with consequent symptoms of cardiac insufficiency; (2) because of loss of appetite and a sense of illness, often leading to the clinical suspicion of gastrointestinal carcinoma; (3) because of neurologic abnormalities (subacute combined degeneration of the spinal cord), sometimes presenting with paraplegia; or (4) coincidentally, after blood examination which identified macrocytosis.

Megaloblastic anemia caused by deficiency of vitamin B_{12} requires lifelong therapy, whereas low levels of serum B_{12} without megaloblastic anemia have been observed in patients for many years without illness. Precise diagnosis is required. The following must be done before therapy: assays for serum vitamin B_{12} and folate, assay for erythrocyte folate level, and determination of serum potassium.

Schilling tests of vitamin B_{12} absorption should not be done initially, because they may be influenced by malabsorption of vitamin B_{12} which is transient and secondary to megaloblastic change, rather than its cause, and because of considerations described below.

Therapy

Patients Seen Because of Anemia, with Symptoms of Cardiac Insufficiency Caused by the Anemia. Such patients usually tolerate the anemia well until oxygen transport decrease and cardiac output increase compensatory to the anemia induce cardiac failure. Treatment should be directed to improving the hemoglobin level to one consistent with survival, while at the same time preventing death from cardiac failure and pulmonary edema. This should be accomplished by (1) slow transfusion (over 2 hours) of 1 unit of packed erythrocyte and (2) diuretic therapy, using 20 mg. of furosemide intravenously; (3) oxygen may also be given if required.

If the patient has not improved clinically after this therapy, additional transfusion and diuretic therapy occasionally may be required.

Specific Therapy for the Megaloblastic Anemia. Patients with severe megaloblastic change have been observed to develop hypokalemia during replacement therapy. Others have been observed to develop cerebrovascular occlusions, although the relationship of vascular occlusions to therapy of megaloblastic anemia has not been clearly demonstrated. Because of clear proof that the rate of clinical improvement from deficiency of vitamin B_{12} is not related to the quantity of vitamin B_{12} used for initial treatment when more than 1 microgram per day is given, the following program of therapy is recommended: *Days 1 and 2:* vitamin B_{12} (cyanocobalamin), 5 micrograms by subcutaneous injection daily. *Days 3 to 7:* vitamin B_{12}, 100 micrograms daily by subcutaneous injection.

Bone marrow morphology will be normoblastic by day 3. This therapeutic regimen will provide enough vitamin B_{12} for *all* patients with pernicious anemia. Occasionally, other necessary nutrients may be inadequate for an optimal rate of clinical improvement. Under such circumstances, the deficiency should be identified (e.g., iron, folate) and corrected.

During therapy, supplementary potassium chloride (40 mEq. per day) may be administered by mouth, although it may not be required when treatment is initiated with 5 micrograms of vitamin B_{12} per day. Serum potassium should be monitored daily for the first 4 days of therapy.

Occasionally, such patients will have such severe thrombocytopenia that life-threatening hemorrhage will ensue. Treatment for megaloblastic anemia in these patients should be with 100 micrograms per day of vitamin B_{12} from the start, with care to prevent hypokalemia. Platelet transfusions should be used to control hemorrhage until spontaneous platelet production is adequate. Adrenocortical steroids are of doubtful benefit in this type of thrombocytopenia.

Patients with Megaloblastic Anemia but Without Evidence of Cardiac Decompensation Caused by Anemia. Transfusion should not be given in these patients, as its benefits are minimal and its danger is not justified.

Following the taking of bone marrow and serum and blood samples for diagnosis, therapy with vitamin B_{12} should begin as above: *Days 1 and 2,* vitamin B_{12} (cyanocobalamin), 5 micrograms daily by subcutaneous injection. *Days 3 to 7,* 100 micrograms daily by subcutaneous injection.

Patients with Subacute Combined Degeneration of the Spinal Cord. Treatment of these patients should be identical with that for patients without severe neurologic abnormalities. The evidence appears to conclude that large doses of vitamin B_{12} do not provide more benefit than the type of dosage schedule recommended above. Some neurologists prefer to treat this disease with daily injections of 1000 micrograms of vitamin B_{12}. Aside from the possible danger of inducing hypokalemia and (perhaps) cerebrovascular occlusions, when treatment is initiated with this dosage no biologic harm is done by such therapy. The rate of correction of methylmalonate excretion in patients with deficiency of vitamin B_{12} is greater when these patients are treated with 1000 than with 100 micrograms of vitamin B_{12} per day, but there is no evidence that the rate of correction of this biochemical abnormality relates to the neurologic disease.

Follow-up of Patients

All patients with megaloblastic anemia and deficiency of vitamin B_{12} should have a Schilling or similar test of B_{12} absorption at some time after 1 week of therapy. Patients demonstrating malabsorption of vitamin B_{12} should have the test repeated with a source of intrinsic factor. Correction of malabsorption by porcine or human intrinsic factor documents pernicious anemia. Assays for vitamin B_{12} level in serum and preparations of reagents for Schilling tests sometimes are unreliable. Results of such tests must be evaluated with the clinical picture, and other tests ordered if disparities are noted.

All patients developing megaloblastic anemia or subacute combined degeneration of the spinal cord resulting from B_{12} deficiency probably should receive injections of vitamin B_{12} for life. At present, this should be administered as cyanocobalamin, 100 micrograms by subcutaneous injection every 4 weeks. More frequent injections are wasteful and unnecessary in pernicious anemia. Patients developing vitamin B_{12} deficiency caused by prolonged abstinence from all animal products may be treated with oral vitamin B_{12}, 5 micrograms per day. Patients developing such deficiency secondary to disease of the bowel should have B_{12} absorption monitored by Schilling test to determine if continued injections are required. All patients with pernicious anemia should be treated for life.

At this time, routine investigations of the gastrointestinal tract seeking gastric carcinoma in patients with pernicious anemia are not in fashion. Most physicians feel that clinical evaluation, history, and early identification of iron deficiency represent the best follow-up for these patients, with recheck routine hemograms three times per year.

THALASSEMIA

method of
BERNADETTE MODELL, M.B.B.Chir.
London, England

Pathophysiology

The basic problem in β-thalassemia is deficient β-globin chain synthesis, so that excess α-chains accumulate in poorly hemoglobinized red cells. There is maturation arrest, and the majority of cells die at a relatively early stage in the bone marrow, so that the anemia is primarily due to ineffective erythropoiesis. Compensatory bone marrow expansion is unparalleled in any other condition; the marrow mass may be increased as much as 30 times, and much of the pathology of the untreated disease arises from this. The cells that do emerge from the marrow contain α-chain inclusions and are often nucleated, so that they are trapped by the reticuloendothelial system and evoke abnormal reactions, especially in the spleen. The gross marrow expansion has widespread consequences; it has the general metabolic effects of a tumor, it distends and erodes the bones from within, and it causes an important vascular shunt and excessive gastrointestinal iron absorption. The patients therefore suffer from anemia, expansion and deformity of the bones, especially of the head and legs, pathologic fractures, anorexia and stunting of growth, and gross blood volume expansion caused by the vascular shunt through the marrow. There is usually secondary hypersplenism which, through deepening the anemia, exacerbates all aspects of the disease. Death from high output congestive cardiac failure, often complicated by infections, usually occurs in the untreated patient before 7 years of age. Excessive gastrointestinal absorption occurs in many patients and may contribute to death in patients who survive longer, either because they have thalassemia intermedia or because they are on treatment. Finally, there is an increased incidence of severe infections in patients with thalassemia major, both untreated and inadequately treated.

The anemia can be corrected by regular blood transfusion. Although this prevents most of the aforementioned complications by bringing the proliferating marrow within more or less normal bounds, it produces serious iron overload so that death from this cause occurs between 16 and 24 years of age. Death is usually due to resistant cardiac failure, sometimes complicated by hepatic failure, and may occur in the wake of an acute illness. There is often additional widespread endocrinopathy; failure of puberty is very common, and there may also be diabetes and hypoparathyroidism.

Thalassemia Intermedia

This is a milder condition in which the patient, although suffering much of the disorder described above, can maintain a mean hemoglobin of between 7.5 and 10.0 grams per 100 ml. and may survive without transfusion. It is a genetically heterogeneous group, occurring with an incidence of between 2 and 10 per cent among all groups of patients with homozygous thalassemia. Because they are untreated, some of these patients show the basic pathology of the disease in an almost unmodified form. Nevertheless, their prospects for long-term survival, normal sexual maturation, and reproduction have hitherto been better than those of transfusion-dependent patients.

Since the existing treatment of thalassemia is very trying for the patient and the outcome is still uncertain, it is important to identify those patients who have thalassemia intermedia at presentation, as they may be able to live an admittedly somewhat invalided life without transfusion and its serious consequences. Characteristically, patients with thalassemia intermedia present relatively late, i.e., after 18 months of age, with a relatively high hemoglobin (8.0 grams per 100 ml. or more), reticulocytes more than 4 per cent, and bilirubin more than 1.2 mg. per 100 ml. and can continue to maintain a hemoglobin of more than 7.5 grams per 100 ml. Secondary hypersplenism may mask thalassemia intermedia, causing it to mimic thalassemia major, even at an early stage; this should be especially suspected in patients coming from elsewhere who are more than 3 years old and who appear to require transfusion but have a history of no transfusion in the past.

Treatment of Thalassemia Major

Treatment of thalassemia major calls for (1) selection of the appropriate transfusion scheme to correct the anemia; (2) splenectomy, when indicated by an abnormally raised blood consumption or other criteria; (3) control of iron overload with deferoxamine; and (4) intensive treatment of acute illnesses.

Selection of Transfusion Scheme. High transfusion, i.e., keeping the mean hemoglobin within the normal range, is now the most common form of transfusion scheme. The *mean* hemoglobin is kept at 11.0 to 11.5 grams per 100 ml. by regular transfusions. This may be achieved by transfusing 1 unit every 2 weeks to raise the hemoglobin from 11.0 to 13.0 grams per 100 ml., or by transfusing 2 or 3 units every 6 weeks to raise the hemoglobin from 9.0 to 14.0 grams per 100 ml. These schemes appear equally satisfactory in terms of results for the patients. Children treated in this way do markedly better than those treated on lower transfusion schemes in the following ways: (1) normal appearance and health to 12 to 13 years, when the effects of iron overload may first be seen; (2) reduced incidence of infections; (3) reduced incidence of hypersplenism in some patients on high transfusion from the beginning; and (4) general relaxation of tension in the family.

The physical improvement appears to be due to suppression of the otherwise uncontrollably proliferating bone marrow. Marrow activity still remains above normal, however, and it is advisable to keep all patients on folic acid, 5 mg. daily, to prevent relative folate deficiency.

Indications for Splenectomy. Hypersplenism, i.e., excessive destruction of the blood elements by the spleen, is a very common complication of thalassemia. Its most important practical consequence is in increasing the blood requirement, and hence accelerating the progression of iron overload and increasing the trauma of the disease by increasing the frequency of transfusions. In medically less developed communities where blood is difficult to obtain, hypersplenism may make effective treatment impossible.

The effect of the spleen on blood consumption can be evaluated by using the chart shown in Figure 1. This describes the blood consumption (expressed as ml. of whole blood per kg. per year) of *splenectomized* patients in relation to transfusion scheme (expressed as *mean* hemoglobin maintained by transfusion). If an unsplenectomized pa-

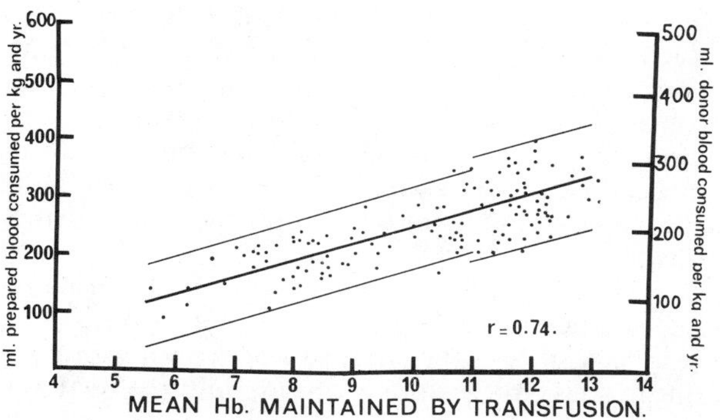

Figure 1. Standard relationship of blood requirement to mean hemoglobin maintained by transfusion in splenectomized patients (regression line ±2 SD). The left-hand scale shows volume of prepared blood from the blood bank, assuming 1 unit contains 500 ml. (volume of donor blood = 420 ml.). The right-hand scale shows volume of blood as received from the donor, assuming an Hb of 13 to 19 grams per 100 ml. (r = 0.74).

tient's observed annual blood consumption is compared with that of splenectomized patients, the effect of splenectomy on blood consumption can be accurately predicted. Since the spleen stores iron in the reticuloendothelial cells and its role in iron metabolism has not yet been clearly defined, it is uncertain at which point splenectomy will be of significant benefit to the patient on grounds of iron economy, and a somewhat arbitrary decision has still to be made. At present it seems reasonable to suggest splenectomy if the blood consumption is persistently raised to more than 1.5 times "normal" as shown on the chart. The chart also allows prediction of the effect on blood consumption of changing the transfusion scheme. It may often be found in this way that after splenectomy the transfusion scheme may be intensified while the blood consumption is nevertheless significantly reduced; i.e., removing the spleen may allow improved treatment within the existing framework. This is an important point in communities where blood is scarce.

The majority of patients in Britain are Cypriots with β-plus thalassemia major. Using the aforementioned criterion, the majority of patients in this group have become hypersplenic by 5 to 6 years of age, and peak age for splenectomy has been 5 years. It has been suggested that high transfusion from presentation may prevent the development of hypersplenism by suppressing the bone marrow. This appears to be true in approximately 50 per cent of patients, but in the others hypersplenism coexisting with high transfusion may increase the blood requirement and rate of iron loading to an exceptional extent. Therefore the evaluation of hypersplenism in high-transfused patients is of particular importance.

Thrombocytopenia occurs at a late stage in the development of hypersplenism and should not be considered a necessary condition for splenectomy. Since death from uncontrollable bleeding may occur in thalassemic patients with platelet counts in the range of 40,000 to 70,000 per cu. mm., thrombocytopenia of this order is an absolute indication for splenectomy. Leukopenia is less common and has not been reported to have such serious results.

Prophylactic antibiotics are indicated following splenectomy—e.g., penicillin, 125 mg. twice daily *indefinitely*—because of the evidence of continuing risk of serious overwhelming infections, usually with streptococci or pneumococci.

Control of Transfusional Iron Overload. INTRAMUSCULAR INJECTION OF DEFEROXAMINE (DESFERAL). The only established iron chelating agent is still deferoxamine (Desferal). It is given daily intramuscularly in a dose of approximately 20 mg. per kg. (i.e., 500 mg., 750 mg., 1.0 gram or 1.5 grams daily, according to weight), and 2 grams in each unit of blood at transfusion. This regimen brings about approximate iron balance after about 100 units of blood has been received (6 to 7 years of age) and reduces hepatic fibrosis. There is further retrospective evidence that it decreases mortality, increases incidence of puberty, and reduces incidence of cardiac arrhythmias in treated patients. The only complications noted so far have been occasional transient flushing, tachycardia, and tingling of the skin immediately following an injection. These are not hypersensitivity reactions but are probably due to the accidental intravenous injection of a bolus. Patients experiencing such a reaction are alarmed, but have not so far come to any harm and are usually able to continue treatment. No cataracts have been observed in thalassemic patients on daily deferoxamine, even after as long as 10 years. The addition of oral vitamin C, 200 mg. daily, doubles the iron excretion in response to deferoxamine in most patients. However, there are indications that larger doses (500 mg. to 1 gram) may increase iron toxicity in some patients. It should therefore be used with caution in seriously iron-loaded patients until further information is available.

SUBCUTANEOUS INFUSION OF DESFERAL. The limitations of the aforementioned method are the high solubility of Desferal, leading to short duration of action, and the restriction of the dose to the quantity that can be put into a singular intramuscular injection. Both these problems are overcome by the new method of continuous subcutaneous infusion from a lightweight portable syringe pump. Two to 4 grams is given over 12 out of each 24 hours. This method causes the mobilization over the long term of such substantial amounts of iron that it is the equivalent of venesection for hemochromatosis, and this approach has been rapidly taken up by many groups with a special interest in thalassemia. The important questions remaining to be answered are how acceptable this form of treatment will be to the majority of patients, and whether there are any unforeseen side effects of this intensified treatment. If the answers to both these questions are favorable, it is likely that transfusional siderosis can be effectively controlled by this method, giving realistic hope for the first time of a good long-term prognosis for thalassemia and other transfusion-dependent anemias.

Treatment of Acute Illness in Thalassemia Major. Hypoxia and acidosis probably exacerbate iron toxicity and may cause death from acute multiorgan failure. In addition, in splenectomized thalassemics there is a continuing risk of overwhelming infection. Therefore in all acute illnesses in thalassemic patients, some or all of the following steps should be taken according to the state of the patient: (1) raise the hemoglobin to 12 grams per 100 ml. or more as soon as safely feasible; (2) give Desferal intravenously, 60 mg. per kg. per 24 hours, to counter acute iron toxicity; (3) treat any sign of congestive cardiac failure rigorously; (4) treat any infection which causes toxicity as septicemia until proved otherwise, i.e., with intravenous antibiotics; (5) give hydrocortisone during the acute phase because of the possibility of adrenal failure; and (6) check the serum calcium and blood glucose because of the possibility of acute endocrine failure.

Treatment of Thalassemia Intermedia

Because this is such a variable condition, careful assessment of each individual patient is needed. The main threats to life in thalassemia intermedia are secondary exacerbating factors: (1) folic acid deficiency, (2) hypersplenism, (3) gastrointestinal iron loading, (4) overwhelming infection, and (5) uric acid nephropathy. In addition, there may be distressing metabolic bone disease, arthritis, and cholelithiasis.

Therefore in a patient with thalassemia intermedia who deteriorates, or in a new patient with a history suggesting deterioration, the following factors should be investigated:

Folate Deficiency. All patients should receive folic acid, 5 mg. daily.

Hypersplenism. This is very common in thalassemia intermedia, but the onset is often later than in thalassemia major—i.e., up to 18 years of age. Assessment is made as follows: (1) History: a fall in the mean hemoglobin not caused by folate deficiency is nearly always due to hypersplenism. (2) Size of the spleen: a spleen palpable more than 6 cm. is nearly always causing excessive red cell destruction. (3) Growth retardation: the onset of hypersplenism in thalassemia intermedia may be marked by slowing of growth. (4) Thrombocytopenia and leukopenia and a reduction in the numbers of nucleated red cells in the circulation. (5) Studies with autologous red cells tagged with ^{51}Cr: the red-cell lifespan may not be revealing, as it is nearly always somewhat shortened, even in nonhypersplenic patients, but organ studies of red cell pooling and the accumulation of radioactivity may be very helpful.

Assessment of the Extent of Iron Overload. If in response to 500 mg. of deferoxamine intramuscularly, more than 5 mg. of iron is excreted in the urine, or if the serum ferritin is more than 2000 nanograms per ml., treatment with daily intramuscular deferoxamine should be instituted.

Infections. Severe, overwhelming infections may occur both before and after splenectomy, and they should be treated vigorously, as for thalassemia major.

Hyperuricemia. This should be controlled with allopurinol.

Thalassemia intermedia is often a physically and emotionally crippling disease because of chronic invalidism, numerous physical problems, and chronic depression and anxiety of the patient and the family. The recent advances in the control of iron overload, detailed under the treatment of thalassemia major, raise the possibility that more severely affected patients with thalassemia intermedia might now be rightly treated as for thalassemia major with maintenance transfusion and long-term chelation therapy.

SICKLE CELL DISEASE

method of
DARLEEN F. POWARS, M.D.
Los Angeles, California

Introduction

Sickle cell disease is a treatable illness that affects more than 50,000 Americans and untold numbers of persons in other countries of the world. It is caused by a genetically induced abnormality of the beta chain of the hemoglobin molecule which results in the presence of a hemoglobin variant, Hb S. The most common form of sickle cell disease is sickle cell anemia (SS), followed by SC hemoglobinopathy and S-beta thalassemia variants. Simply stated, the clinical manifestations are related to the intraerythrocytic insolubility of hemoglobin S in the deoxygenated state. As a result, rigid red cells lack sufficient deformability to flow successfully through the smaller capillaries and sinusoids. The random obstruction in one or more of the organs of the body accounts for the wide clinical variability observed in the illness.

Prognosis of the patients with sickle cell anemia has greatly changed in the last 25 years. With current medical management, most young children with sickle cell anemia will survive into young and middle adulthood. Manifestations of the disease will vary considerably with the age of the patient. The younger child will show less specific organ involvement and more generalized problems (high fever and septicemia). The problems of the adult patient are largely the result of cumulative effect of many years of intermittent episodes of sickling on various organs of his body. Painful vaso-occlusive sickle cell crises, the hallmark of this disorder, without objective clinical findings are more frequent in older adolescent and young adult patients.

Because sickle cell disease is a lifelong disorder, medical care must adjust itself to the changing needs of the child and his family as he grows and develops into adulthood. During the early infant period, the emphasis of responsibility for and care of the patient rests with the parents. More than the normal child, the child with sickle cell disease, as he grows into maturity, must be taught to accept a changing pattern of responsibility for his own care so that he is not dependent on his parents, is emotionally stable, and is able to take his place in society. Although patients may have identical hemoglobinopathies, each has his own inherent pattern of illness with certain precipitating factors that are more important in him than in others. The care for each patient must be individualized.

Essential to the treatment plan is accurate laboratory support for the diagnosis, which cannot be made without hemoglobin electrophoresis or column chromatography. This diagnosis can be made even in the newborn infant.

Transfusion Therapy

Transfusion has historically been the mainstay of therapy. There is wide empirical agreement among most clinicians who treat patients with sickle cell anemia that transfusion therapy is beneficial and indicated under certain circumstances. In the past, most transfusion therapy has consisted of acid-citrate-dextrose (ACD) blood and/or red cells. Recently, the availability of citrate-phosphate-dextrose (CPD) blood which protects the oxygen-carrying capacity of the red cells by preserving 2,3-diphosphoglyceric acid has supplanted older forms of blood products. CPD anticoagulated packed red cells (buffy coat poor) may be used; frozen blood is preferred. Transfusions are given whenever the hemoglobin has decreased more than 2 grams per dl. (100 ml.) from the steady state or the packed cell volume has dropped more than 7 to 8 per cent. Thus 2 to 4 units of packed or sedimented fresh frozen red cells is administered to adolescents and adult patients, or 5 ml. per pound to infants and children, until a level of 8 grams per dl. is reached.

In the following clinical situations, transfusion therapy is recommended:

1. Aplastic sickle cell crisis with a peripheral reticulocyte count of 2 per cent or less, especially if the hemoglobin and/or hematocrit are decreasing.
2. Congestive heart failure or other cardiovascular insufficiency in the anemic patient.
3. As a general supportive measure in patients with severe infectious disease such as meningitis and septicemia.
4. In patients with pulmonary insufficiency associated with pneumonia, chest syndrome, or pulmonary infarct as a general supportive measure.
5. As an emergency lifesaving measure in a splenic sequestration crisis of infancy.
6. As a supportive measure prior to general anesthesia in surgery.
7. In most patients who have a hemoglobin level below 5 grams per dl. or packed cell volume of under 15 per cent.
8. In any patient in whom a hyperhemolytic crisis is accompanied by a decreasing hemoglobin. This problem is most regularly seen in adults who have an acute chest syndrome, because a large infarcting portion of the lung acts as a sequestrum for the red cells.

Transfusion therapy is *not* recommended in the following situations:

1. The individual patient will manifest a steady state "usual" hemoglobin concentration that will remain consistent throughout the various stages of his life. This should be determined during asymptomatic periods. Transfusion given simply because of anemia is not recommended.
2. Transfusion therapy does not reproducibly decrease the pain or shorten a generalized vaso-occlusive cryptogenic sickle cell crisis. Indeed, transfusion with older blood products in which there was a high acid load and a low oxygen carrying capacity may have actually increased the severity of the crises.

The following specific indications for transfusion therapy are under investigation in various medical centers throughout the country:

1. Prophylactic transfusion at the onset of pregnancy until delivery.
2. Hypertransfusion and/or exchange transfusion, followed by long-term prophylactic transfusion of children with cerebrovascular accidents (strokes).

In both these instances the aim is to maintain the hemoglobin S percentage at less than 25 per cent, the reticulocyte count at 2 to 3 per cent, and a hemoglobin level between 10 and 12 grams per dl. by transfusing CPD frozen packed red cells at approximately 3 week intervals.

3. Exchange transfusion therapy prior to surgery for patients who have a detached retina.

Specific Complications

Because the abnormal hemoglobin which causes the clinical manifestations cannot at present be modified, treatment must be aimed at the specific problems and complications. These problems can be categorized into (1) sickle cell crisis, (2) the young child, and (3) complications related to specific organ damage. In addition, (4) other conditions unrelated to sickle cell disease itself—e.g., pregnancy—require specific treatment because of the underlying disorder.

Sickle Cell Crisis. The most obvious manifestation of sickle cell disease is the vaso-occlusive or cryptogenic sickle cell crisis, which may last from a few hours to several days to weeks. These crises can be precipitated by many factors such as infection, fever, excessive fatigue, chilling, mild preclinical dehydration, and emotional stress. Frequently in patients over 10 years of age, no objective clinical findings can be identified. The only agreed-upon treatment is hydration. Hydration presumably decreases the internal erythrocytic mean corpuscular hemoglobin concentration (MCHC) and sufficiently increases the plasma volume and blood flow so that sickled cells can be dislodged from obstructed areas in the microvasculature.

If an experienced patient has mild or moderate pain, he should be encouraged to consume warm liquids, soups, and fresh juices at home. The patient is advised to imbibe 8 ounces of fluid every hour until his urine shows little color and to keep his urine as light as possible during this phase. Many patients have learned to evaluate their own approaching crisis by observing a deepening in the color of the urine.

More severe sickle crisis cannot be treated on an outpatient basis. The patient must be given intravenous hypotonic electrolyte fluids at 2500 ml. per square meter body surface per 24 hours. The following commercially available solutions are useful and safe in children:

Travenol, 5 per cent dextrose with electrolyte No. 48, which contains sodium at 25 mEq. per liter, potassium at 20 mEq. per liter, magnesium at 3 mEq. per liter, lactate at 23 mEq. per liter, and chloride at 24 mEq. per liter. In adult patients, in addition to the aforementioned preparation, (1) 5 per cent dextrose in 0.2 per cent sodium chloride (Na at 34 mEq. per liter and chloride at 34 mEq. per liter); (2) 5 per cent dextrose and 0.45 per cent sodium chloride (Na of 77 mEq. per liter); or (3) 5 per cent dextrose with electrolyte No. 75 (Travenol), with Na at 40 mEq. per liter, K at 35 mEq. per liter, Cl at 48 mEq. per liter, lactate at 20 mEq. per liter, and HPO_4^{-2} at 15 mEq. per liter, can be used effectively. We recommend that oral hydration be continued throughout at a modest rate to permit quicker removal of intravenous needles. On initiation of parenteral hydration, meperidine (Demerol) (0.5 mg. per lb. in children; 75 to 100 mg. in adults) is given parenterally. Frequently after a single injection of Demerol and aggressive intravenous hydration, the patient is sufficiently improved within 12 hours to be able to manage the remaining period of crisis at home. In more severe crisis, intravenous hydration is continued at 2500 ml. per square meter per 24 hours. Usually parenteral Demerol is necessary on an intermittent basis for approximately 72 hours. Of great symptomatic benefit is the use of a whirlpool of hot water three or four times a day for 20 minutes.

After a severe sickle crisis, generalized body aching is usually noted on about day 3 or 4. This muscle pain and tiredness in the whole body, similar to that experienced by anyone a few days after major trauma or unusual exercise, is frequently associated with some despondency. This should not be confused with continuing or recurrent sickle crisis. The patient should become ambulatory as soon as possible and should not be allowed to stay in bed more than 2 or 3 days, because stasis lung syndrome is a regularly observed major complication in any patient who remains in bed. Essentially no patient should be expected to die during a painful vaso-occlusive cryptogenic sickle cell crisis without complication. An optimistic, sympathetic, encouraging, positive approach to the patient in painful crisis is recommended. We do not recommend that parenteral narcotics be maintained in the home. In adult patients, aspirin or acetaminophen (Tylenol), or aspirin with ¼ grain (15 mg.) codeine, usually is sufficient analgesia to keep the patient comfortable.

Sickle Cell Anemia in the Young Child. The SS child less than 5 years old has three specific circumstances which require major decisions in treatment. These are (1) fever and the propensity to infection; (2) the hand-foot syndrome as a specific manifestation of infantile sickle cell crisis; and (3) splenic sequestration syndrome. The majority of children who die of sickle cell anemia will die as a result of either infection or splenic sequestration crisis.

FEVER. The risk of pneumococcal septicemia and/or meningitis in a child under 5 years old with sickle cell anemia is 10 per cent during that 5 year period. A fever usually over 103°F. (39.4°C.) is the early and only symptom of this condition. Studies by Pearson et al. and Powars et al. have shown that within the first 3 years of life, 20 per cent of all febrile episodes (102°F.[38.9°C.] or higher) in infants who are diagnosed at birth to have sickle cell anemia will reveal positive blood cultures for streptococcal pneumonia. If a temperature is greater than 102°F. (38.9°C.), the patient should be brought immediately into an emergency room or appropriate clinic with facilities for hospitalization. A blood culture and throat culture should be obtained and the patient given parenteral penicillin G at 200,000 to 250,000 units (125 to 150 mg.) per kg., preferably intravenously. Subsequent to the administration of the first dose of penicillin, the patient should be re-evaluated for such causes of fever as otitis media or an early pneumonia. If a clear-cut primary source of infection such as otitis media is found, antibiotic therapy may be modified to include ampicillin orally at a dose of 75 mg. per kg. in four divided doses, and the patient may be carefully monitored as an outpatient. The probably septic child should be admitted to the hospital and treated continuously with intravenous penicillin G at 100,000 units per kg. every 8 hours. After confirmation of sepsis by a positive blood culture, therapy should be continued for a minimum of 5 days. At 3 days of therapy, when blood and throat cultures are negative and the patient is well, therapy can be discontinued; but even in the face of negative cultures, when fever, cough, or lethargy persists, penicillin therapy should be continued for 5 to 7 days parenterally in the hospital.

Splenic Sequestration Syndrome. Splenic sequestration syndrome is diagnosed when a sudden increase in the size of the spleen, often to massive proportions, is associated with a rapidly decreasing hemoglobin. The patient may have an associated febrile illness and frequently has pneumococcal septicemia as a precipitating cause. This is an acute life-threatening emergency situation requiring rapid transfusions. Typed specific frozen packed red cells are best and should be given at 10 ml. per kg. The infant may be kept upright in an infant seat to improve respiratory function during the acute period, although an attempt to administer oxygen by mask may be made. Many infants with this degree of respiratory distress cannot tolerate masks or nasal catheters. Intermittent ventilatory assistance with 100 per cent oxygen can be helpful. A second transfusion of packed red cells is initiated at the third hour (10 ml. per kg.). Usually after the second transfusion, at about the sixth hour, the patient will begin to show significant improvement in respiratory rate and general well-being. Third and fourth supportive transfusions each of 10 ml. per kg. may be necessary. After successful transfusion therapy, the spleen will spontaneously decrease in size within 48 hours, and the sickled red cells that have been trapped in the spleen will then be released into the circulation. This will be manifest by a subsequent increase in hematocrit and the appearance of large numbers of distorted red cells. Because these cells have been partially damaged during the stasis within the spleen, they are usually quickly removed by the reticuloendothelial system. Within the next few days, bilirubin and urobilinogen in the urine will be elevated. The patient usually achieves a steady state by about the seventh to tenth day. Drugs such as digitalis that directly affect cardiac function are of no benefit in this condition. Some physicians have attempted to use furosemide (Lasix), 1 mg. per kg. intramuscularly, as a temporizing measure prior to transfusion therapy.

Hand-Foot Syndrome. The manifestations of vaso-occlusive sickle cell crises in the child under 5 are frequently different than at older ages. In such children the hand-foot syndrome is an excruciatingly painful swelling of the hands and feet as a generalized dactylitis. Roentgenologic and clinical findings of tenderness, redness, and fever are indistinguishable from those of acute bacterial osteomyelitis. However, uniform involvement of both hands and feet usually is not seen in acute infectious osteomyelitis. The major painful period lasts for 5 to 7 days, with a slower recovery phase of as much as 28 days. Treatment requires adequate hydration and identification of any underlying precipitating infectious disease. Forced oral hydration usually results in increased abdominal distention and vomiting; therefore parenteral intravenous hydration is necessary at 2000 ml. per square meter per 24 hours. The intravenous solution should be a hypotonic electrolyte solution such as 0.20 M sodium, with the sodium half in the form of sodium chloride and half sodium lactate. A commercially available hydrating solution is Travenol (5 per cent dextrose with electrolyte No. 48), which contains 25 mEq. of sodium, 20 mEq. of potassium, 24 mEq. of chloride, and 23 mEq. of lactate. This hypotonic electrolyte solution with some lactate allows for the administration of free water to the patient without excessive sodium overload. During this time of intravenous hydration, if the child is allowed to drink some milk, juices, and other liquids as desired, problems of overhydration and congestive failure are rarely encountered and underhydration or clinically significant hyponatremia is not seen. Fluid and electrolyte intake should be carefully monitored to prevent water intoxication and/or fluid overload. Moist heat in the form of a whirlpool or Jacuzzi apparatus is very useful. Home care should include an attachable Jacuzzi-like modification to the family's bathtub for symptomatic relief of the pain.

On occasion in patients with severe hand-foot syndrome, analgesic drugs are necessary. In the young infant we have found that oral codeine increases gastric distention and gastrointestinal disturbances. Acetaminophen (Tylenol), 5 mg. per kg. every 6 hours, may provide some slight relief but is usually not sufficient to ease the pain of severe hand-foot syndrome. Meperidine (Demerol), 0.5 to 1 mg. per pound (1 to 2 mg. per kg.)

every 4 hours intramuscularly, may be necessary for 3 to 5 days. Adequate pain relief is obtained when the child sleeps comfortably and wakes up hungry. This medication should not be given to the child for more than 3 to 4 days continuously without re-evaluation. By the end of 5 to 7 days the excruciating pain usually has lessened in degree, and the patient can be discharged for symptomatic care without drugs for analgesia. As long as the child needs drug analgesia, in-hospital parenteral hydration is necessary and parenteral analgesia is best. We caution, on a general basis, against the parenteral administration of narcotic agents in the home. For growing children with sickle cell anemia or sickle cell disease, use of such agents is rarely necessary and generally unwise.

Complications of Special Organ Systems. The organ systems most frequently involved with permanent damage are the bones, the kidneys, the brain, and the lungs. Rarely is permanent organ failure observed in the liver, pancreas, endocrine glands, or gonads. The number of painful crises that a patient may have had in the past does not necessarily predict that he will have significant clinical specific organ failure. On the other hand, when any organ system has been known to be involved in a vaso-occlusive process, this organ tends to be involved in subsequent episodes.

Cerebrovascular Accident. Other than death, a sickling episode in the brain is the single most devastating complication of sickle cell anemia. In children and young adolescents this is manifest by acute hemiparesis and often by seizures, with a cerebral infarct pattern on computerized tomography (CT) scan and no blood in the spinal fluid. Contrarily, in older adolescents and adults, cerebrovascular accidents are usually subarachnoid or intracerebral hemorrhage with acute headache, pain, coma, and a bloody spinal fluid. Management consists of those supportive measures ordinarily applied to any patient with a cerebrovascular accident. Initial support of vital functions is indicated, and long-term extensive rehabilitation may be necessary. Urea and mannitol have been shown to be of no avail, but oxygen is usually given. The treatment recommended earlier for a sickle crisis is to be followed. During the acute stage (first 96 hours), supportive transfusion or exchange transfusion therapy is given. Transfusion therapy is given with the somewhat wishful hope that normal red cells will intersperse themselves with the sickled red cells and decrease the degree and extent of the cerebrovascular obstruction. The stroke usually will progress during the first 4 or 5 days, at which time the neurologic status will stabilize. Subsequently, over the next 3 to 12 months there will be a gradual neurologic improvement, unless the patient has another cerebral insult. Discussion of long-term transfusion therapy in the further management of the patient who has had a stroke will be found on page 264. The long-term rehabilitation of the patient includes early ambulation and an aggressive program of pulmonary toilet. Many patients who do not die during the acute stroke episode die within the next 6 to 8 weeks of recurrent chest syndrome and pneumonia.

Orthopedic Complications. Diaphyseal bone infarcts are manifest by the acute and abrupt onset of pain, swelling, erythema, and excruciating tenderness, followed in a few days by x-ray evidence of periosteal elevation. During the acute stage, hospitalization is frequently necessary, and a diaphyseal bone infarct is treated as a localized sickle cell crisis with intravenous hydration, parenteral analgesia, and heat to the affected area, including whirlpool treatments. As with fractures, the acute pain lessens within 4 or 5 days, but there is a persistent remaining discomfort for 3 or 4 weeks. Ambulation and weight bearing are encouraged and cause no damage. The patient should be made to realize that there will be some pain in the area for approximately a month. Mild analgesics such as acetaminophen (Tylenol) and home whirlpool baths are sufficient to maintain the patient in comfort at reasonably normal activity outside the hospital during recovery.

Diaphyseal bone infarcts must be differentiated from Salmonella osteomyelitis. The two conditions are indistinguishable clinically. Because the treatment is diametrically different, an accurate diagnosis is essential. Bone culture is obtained by needle aspiration from the bone. At the same time, blood cultures and stool cultures are necessary with special emphasis on the identification of Salmonella species. Ampicillin, 150 mg. per kg. per day in four divided doses, is begun only *after* cultures are obtained. Minimal parenteral therapy includes 21 days of ampicillin intravenously at 150 mg. per kg. per 24 hours. Reasonable maximal therapy includes 42 days of intravenous ampicillin for severe and large infections, followed by months to years of oral antibiotics. In many patients with larger multiple bone involvements, recurrence of the problem is the rule, and thereafter the treatment must be for chronic Salmonella osteomyelitis. The necessity for surgical incision and drainage and/or debridement must be based on clinical judgment as to the extent of the involvement and the potentiality for areas of sequestration that antibiotics cannot reach.

Aseptic necrosis of the femoral and humeral heads and vertebral bodies regularly causes significant morbidity in patients with sickle cell anemia and SC disease who are more than 25 years of age. Vertebral body aseptic necrosis presents as recurrent episodes of acute back strain or lumbar dorsal strain and should be treated with analgesia, rest, and orthopedic braces. No successful surgical procedure has been devised. Aseptic necrosis of the femoral and humeral heads causes episodic severe pain of the joints involved. Roentgenography shows a destructive process that has clearly been present for some months. Symptoms are related to stretching of the joint capsule and adjacent structures as the femoral and/or humeral head collapses. There may be years of recurrent episodes, with quiescent periods during which bone structure will improve. Management must be conjointly directed by medical and orthopedic physicians. Rest and pain relief are needed during the acute episodes and joint rehabilitation during the nonpainful periods. The timing and indications for surgical intervention with replacement of all or part of the femoral or humeral head are controversial. Femoral head replacement in young patients, frequently men, in their late twenties or early thirties has not been uniformly successful, with a high rate of infection, no improvement of the patient's pain, and continued lack of normal joint mobility.

KIDNEY. Destruction and hyalinization of the glomeruli is a result of long-term sickling, and the resultant renal failure is manifested by hypertension, elevated blood urea nitrogen (BUN) and creatinine, and, in some instances, a nephrotic-like syndrome. Successful treatment of renal failure is dependent on sophisticated capabilitites for renal dialysis and renal transplantation. Early detailed attention to hydration, decrease in stressful and infectious complications, and management of hypertension can delay the appearance of end-stage renal disease in some instances. The reader is referred to the article on Chronic Renal Failure (pp. 535 to 540).

Patients with sickle cell anemia, sickle thalassemia, and SC disease will exhibit episodes of renal papillary necrosis, with acute painful calculus-like colic and evidence of blood and tissue in the urine. During the acute stage of renal papillary necrosis, intravenous urography is hazardous; the added viscosity of the contrast dye enhances the sickling there. Retrograde pyelography seems to be less dangerous and provides a reasonably accurate diagnosis. The patient is treated with intravenous hydration similar to that used in a generalized sickle cell crisis. Most urologists attempt to alkalinize the urine with sodium bicarbonate at 20 mEq. per liter intravenously. Hospitalization is always required for this condition. Aminocaproic acid has been used at an initial dose of 5 grams, followed by 1 gram hourly but not to exceed 30 grams per day in an adult. Because of the inherent hazards of this form of therapy, we do not routinely use this medication. Heparinization is not used. Bed rest is maintained for a few days, but soon the problems of possible lung stasis override the potential benefit for healing of the renal papillae. Episodes usually last 10 to 14 days and tend to recur.

Pyelonephritis and acute urinary tract infections are a regularly occurring problem of young women with sickle cell anemia, particularly during pregnancy. Treatment consists of antibiotics, usually ampicillin, and hydration. Milder episodes can be handled in the outpatient service. However, more severe disease necessitates hospitalization and the addition of gentamicin, 5 mg. per kg. intravenously in three divided doses daily for 14 days. The choice of antibiotics is ultimately dependent upon the specific culture and antibiotic sensitivity. Pyelonephritis in patients with sickle cell anemia is notoriously difficult to treat, recurs regularly, and predisposes to sickling in the renal papilla, so that one frequently encounters a combination of renal papillary necrosis along with the infection.

CHEST SYNDROME. Pneumonia and pneumonia-like illnesses comprise 45 per cent of the medical problems in hospitalized patients with sickle cell anemia. Etiologically, these syndromes are (1) bacterial infectious disease, usually the pneumococcus; (2) multiple micro-infarct–type illness with a diffuse bronchopneumonia or miliary pattern on x-ray; and (3) lobar infarctions with large areas of necrosis. Clinically, it is impossible to differentiate acute bacterial pneumonitis from the multiple micro-infarctive chest syndrome. Blood cultures are positive for *Streptococcus pneumoniae* more often in younger children than in adult patients. Cultures from pleural effusion are recommended and often provide a specific bacteriologic diagnosis. Therefore the physician usually finds himself in the position of treating this acute syndrome by suspecting that it may be bacterial in cause but being unable to obtain confirmatory evidence to support an absolute diagnosis. Because any infectious agent causes edema and stasis throughout the lung parenchyma, sickling is triggered in that area and enhances the clinical severity of the illness. This decreases effective vascular supply to the lung parenchyma, decreases the local availability of antibiotics, and prolongs morbidity.

We recommend the following therapeutic program for such a patient: (1) intravenous fluids given as for sickle cell crisis, and (2) intravenous penicillin G at 200,000 units per kg. (125 mg.) per 24 hours in four divided doses. (3) gentamicin, 5 mg. per kg. in four divided doses, is added to this regimen in adult patients with a significant possiblity of gram-negative rod bacterial pneumonia.

In patients with severe lobar involvement,

progression on x-ray is seen during the first few days of therapy. At about day 7, the patient will usually show a decrease of fever and some general improvement in well-being, and this will subsequently be followed by improving roentgenologic findings. The patient is treated with high dose antibiotics and fluids until there is clear resolution of pain, respiratory distress, and fever and an improving chest x-ray. At this time the patient is discharged and maintained on oral antibiotics until there is complete resolution on x-ray. In severe cases, the chest x-ray will not completely revert to its prior state for 6 weeks.

In patients with probable pulmonary infarction heparinization has been used, but there are no conclusive studies of the benefit of this treatment. We therefore do not recommend routine heparinization in patients with sickle cell anemia and chest syndrome. If heparin is given, a dose of 100 units per kg. every 4 to 6 hours maintains a partial thromboplastin time between 60 and 80 seconds.

Mycoplasma pneumonia takes an unusually severe form in patients with sickle cell anemia, with a prolonged protracted illness and both pleural and pericardial effusions. Presence of a cold hemagglutinin in the serum or specific complement fixation confirms this diagnosis. Therapy is erythromycin at a dose of 50 mg. per kg. per day, but not more than 4 grams per day, until resolution of the problem (often 28 days).

Ambulation is encouraged even in a patient with fever and chest pain, and respiratory therapists should provide frequent courses of therapy to force the patient to cough and expand his lungs.

Priapism. Priapism is a distressingly painful localized sickle crisis of the male sickle cell anemia patient between 12 and 30 years of age. This painful erection of the penis lasting for more than 6 hours cannot be relieved by an ejaculatory response. Prevention of priapism can be usually obtained by counseling young boys as they enter into puberty. They are advised that an erection of the penis should not be maintained for more than 2 hours and that ejaculation should be encouraged. Not all patients who have had priapism will be impotent. In point of fact, many patients seem to recover normal erectile sexual activity. We therefore strongly recommend against acute corpusectomy. Hypotonic electrolyte fluids are administered intravenously, as with any other sickle cell crisis. Whirlpool baths and heat are frequently used. Diazepam (Valium), 5 mg. every 8 to 12 hours, is given for sedation as an aid in decreasing anxiety, along with meperidine (Demerol), 0.5 mg. per kg. intramuscularly every 6 hours for analgesia. The episode usually lasts 5 to 7 days. There will be a 2 to 3 week period of general aching and discomfort with a return of erectile sexual function at 2 to 3 months.

Visual Problems. Retinal detachment is an acute ophthalmologic emergency in patients with sickle cell disease. This occurs more frequently in patients with variant hemoglobinopathies (SC) than in patients with sickle cell anemia and usually occurs after the third decade of life. Photocoagulation and scleral buckling for repair of the detached retina comprise the current recommended ophthalmologic therapy. Current opinion advises exchange transfusion to Hb A level of 60 per cent or more prior to photocoagulation. The aim of this exchange transfusion is to prevent ischemia of the anterior segment and further sickling.

Leg Ulcers. Stasis malleolar ulcerations begin in the second decade of life and persist through the third decade. Leg ulcers rarely occur in patients with variant hemoglobinopathies. No treatment has been shown to be regularly effective. We recommend a simple approach to the problem. The vital ingredient for successful management of leg ulcers is the availability of a conscientious nurse or physical therapist to aid the patient regularly in debridement, cleaning, and the general care of the leg involved. Cultures of the ulcer are obtained. Povidone-iodine (Betadine) solution is used for debridement. This is followed by a 30 minute whirlpool treatment of the entire leg. Subsequent to this, an Unna boot is applied. There are specific precautions in the application of the Unna boot. Each side of the dressing is cut as it is applied, to prevent shrinking of the boot as it dries and consequently to preserve remaining vascularity in the leg. The Unna boot is replaced once or twice a week, depending on the severity and progression of the ulcer for 3 to 6 months until healing has occurred. Leg ulcers consistently return in the same area. During intermittent times when the ulcer has re-epithelialized, the following prophylactic measures are instituted: (1) careful daily attention to foot and leg care with daily bathing and the use of a nonalkaline soap; (2) protective clothing over the area to minimize trauma (Jobst leotards); (3)reinstitution of ulcer care at the first indication of further breakdown of the tissue.

Clearly, the smaller the ulcer and the earlier treatment is instituted, the shorter will be the time of treatment. Large ulcers (over 5 cm. in diameter) that have eroded down to the bone may literally take years to heal. Skin grafts usually are not maintained.

Associated Conditions in Patients with Sickle Cell Disease. Medical and surgical conditions not directly caused by the disease pose specific management dilemmas in patients who have sickle cell anemia. The more common of these conditions will be discussed.

Pregnancy and Fertility. Pregnancy in

any woman with sickle cell anemia and probably in patients with SC disease carries an increased risk of morbidity and mortality to both the mother and infant. Approximately 30 per cent of all SS women will have a spontaneous abortion early in the first trimester of pregnancy. Usually it is not possible to prevent the abortion, because it occurs concurrently with the initial appreciation of pregnancy in the patient. Abortions usually are quick, spontaneous, and uncomplicated, posing relatively little added risk to the mother, and can be handled in the usual obstetric fashion.

Particularly susceptible to folic acid deficiency are young women who may be pregnant or have recently had an abortion or who may be on birth control medication. Folic acid, 1 mg. orally per day, is recommended.

The problems and complications of pregnancy increase in magnitude and severity during the last trimester. Major complications include a 25 per cent incidence of infections, pneumonia, sickle cell crisis, toxemia of pregnancy, and worsening of any specific organ problems that may already exist in the patient. A requisite of management is close obstetric supervision of the patient, with careful monitoring of the vital signs of the mother and fetus. Frequently, hospitalization is necessary during the last month of gestation so that cardiovascular balance by sodium restriction and treatment of toxemia can be maintained. We recommend a liberal but controlled use of transfusions following specific indications: (1) hematocrit below 15 per cent, (2) increasing cardiovascular insufficiency, (3) chronic renal disease, (4) an aplastic crisis, or (5) in association with severe infectious disease.

Transfusion therapy during labor and delivery should be based on observed blood loss and individualized according to the needs of the patient. During the labor, the patient should be admitted into an intensive care obstetrical unit with fetal monitoring capabilities. Intravenous hydration therapy as given for sickle cell crisis should be instituted. This prevents dehydration and sickling during the period of labor. We strongly recommend meperidine (Demerol) as a simple, relatively nontoxic anesthetic for the laboring mother. Delivery can be performed by the vaginal route in most situations. Elective cesarean section depends on the usual obstetric indications of cephalopelvic disproportion or fetal distress. Prostaglandin E_2 is *not* recommended for induction of labor because of some reports that this agent potentiates the sickling phenomenon. Liveborn infants are usually vigorous and pose no specific problems. The peripartum period is a high risk period for the mother. Uterine dystocia and postpuerperal infections are frequent.

Surgery and Anesthesia. Any necessary surgical procedure can be successfully performed on a patient with sickle cell anemia or SC disease. The major problem in surgical procedures lies with the anesthetic risk to the patient.

We recommend the following presurgical preparation prior to elective surgery and anesthesia. Three days prior to the elective procedure, the patient is admitted into the hospital for a complete cardiovascular and neurologic work-up. If the patient is severely anemic, transfusion of frozen citrate-phosphate-dextrose (CPD) blood is administered to raise the hematocrit to 25 to 30 per cent 2 days prior to surgery. Following blood transfusion, the patient is encouraged to ambulate and begin a program of respiratory therapy. This 48 hour period from transfusion to surgery allows for readjustment of cardiovascular status and time for assessment for any potentially unrecognized problems. The night before surgery at the time when oral intake is stopped, intravenous therapy is begun with a hypotonic solution of 1/5 isotonic saline and no added potassium at 2000 ml. per square meter of body surface. This prevents minimal dehydration during a prolonged period of enforced prohibition of oral intake. The anesthetic agent most commonly in use in the institution where the surgery is being performed is recommended. The patient is oxygenated optimally throughout the entire procedure. Following the surgical procedure, hypoxia is *not* used to awaken the patient. No tourniquets should be used for orthopedic or other surgical procedures.

Postoperative management is guided by the nature and type of surgery. Intravenous fluid maintenance is continued until there is no question that the patient can drink comfortably without pain.

Trauma. Fractures heal well in patients with sickle cell disease and should be managed by standard orthopedic procedures. Wounds heal well, and suturing should be based on usual practice.

Controversial Issues in Management

Anticoagulation Therapy. The use of anticoagulation therapy for treatment or prevention of sickle cell crisis has been associcated with an unacceptably high rate of excessive bleeding. Some investigators believe that heparin is beneficial in patients with large infiltrative pulmonary lesions that suggest pulmonary infarcts. Dosage must be adjusted for the individual patient by using the partial thromboplastin time as a guide. Dosage is ordinarily 150 units per kg. of body weight or 10,000 units per adult patient by intravenous injections every 4 to 6 hours. Anticoagulant therapy is continued from 2 to 6 weeks. After the initial treatment, subcutaneous heparin can be used with or without warfarin. More recently there has been increasing interest in agents such as aspirin and dipyridamole which inhibit platelet aggregation.

Alkalinization. It is known that red cells with Hb S will not sickle when deoxygenated if the pH of the surrounding fluid is above 8. Since it is not compatible with human life to increase the blood pH to this level, many attempts at more modest increases have been tried. Some benefit is generally reported in most studies in which alkalinization was attempted. In these studies, there was essentially no demonstrable pH change in the serum or the urine. Large amounts of fluid were required, and the patient became thirsty. The benefit from a program of alkalinization may be due to either the alkalinization itself or the increased hypotonic fluid intake. In view of the isosthenuria of patients with sickle cell anemia, alkalinization must be accompanied with adequate free water to allow for kidney excretion of sodium.

Oxygen. There seems to be no contraindication to use of oxygen as a supportive measure for patients with sickle cell anemia. Oxygen is frequently used in a wide variety of problems, particularly in vaso-occlusive crisis. It is our policy to allow the patient to decide if he believes that oxygen helps decrease his pain and aid in his feeling of well-being. Attempts to abort sickle cell crises with hyperbaric oxygen have given conflicting results.

Prophylactic Penicillin. Because there is a clear increase of major pneumococcal disease in patients with sickle cell anemia, the routine use of prophylactic penicillin has been suggested. Long-acting benzathine penicillin does not give a sufficient mean inhibitory concentration (MIC) against *Streptococcus pneumoniae* to be effective. Therefore in patients with sickle cell anemia, in order to prevent colonization with *S. pneumoniae,* prophylactic penicillin must be given orally daily at 250 mg. (400,000 units) twice daily. Studies are currently underway regarding the clinical benefit of prophylactic penicillin in younger children.

Antisickling Agents. Th^ best therapy for patients with sickle cell anemia would be an effective, safe, orally administered drug that could interfere with the sickling tendency of the red cells. There is no such drug that has been shown to be clinically effective. Table 1 lists those antisickling agents that are currently under investigation. The agents are listed according to their presumed and/or proved mechanism of action. Many of the agents which act by increasing oxygen affinity are cross-linking compounds with wide-ranging effects on other body proteins. Most of these agents will prove to be too toxic for general clinical use. A newer group of drugs which specifically interact with the red cell membrane to maintain flexibility may in the long run prove to be more useful. The alkylureas are a particularly important group, because they are the only known drugs that have been shown to actually unsickle the already deoxygenated sickle cell.

TABLE 1. **Antisickling Agents—1977**

Agents that act by increasing oxygen affinity (lowering P-50)
- CO
- $NaNO_2$
- Alkali
- Urea
- Cyanate
- Thiocyanate (cassava—African yam)
- Carbamyl phosphate
- Dimethyladipimidate (DMA)

Agents that do not significantly affect the P-50
- Zinc (slight effect)
- Para-aminobenzoic acid (PABA)
- HN_2
- Alkylureas (methyl-, ethyl, propyl-, butylurea)
- Procaine hydrochloride
- Amino acid salts
- Arachis oil

Antithrombotic agents
- Arvin
- Heparin
- Dicumarol
- Low molecular weight dextran
- Acetylsalicylic acid (aspirin)
- Dipyridamole
- d-2-(6′Methoxy-2′naphthyl)-propionic acid (naproxen)

Vasodilator
- Dipyridamole

Lower Hb S concentration inside the cell
- Hypotonic fluids
- Prevent Hb F "switch"
- Fe deficiency?

Agents that interact with red cell membrane
- Steroids
- Androgens
- Progesterone
- Phenothiazides
- Magnesium sulfate
- Zinc
- Prostaglandin inhibitors (indomethacin)
- Fagara zanthoxyloides root (2,4-dihydro-2, 2-dimethyl-2H-1-benzopyron-6 butyric acid; DBA) (Xanthorylol)
- Para-aminobenzoic acid

Miscellaneous
- Transfusion

NEUTROPENIA

method of
DAVID C. DALE, M.D.
Seattle, Washington

Introduction

Neutrophils are critical for the defense of the body against invasion by microorganisms. The blood serves to transport these cells from the bone marrow to sites of infection or inflammation in any of the body's tissues. Ordinarily, the number of blood neutrophils in a normal person remains relatively constant. The range for the normal neutrophil count is generally given as between 1800 and 7200 cells per cu. mm.; however, there is no precise upper or lower limit for the normal count.

The term "neutropenia" is used to describe circumstances when the blood neutrophil count is reduced. For practical purposes, neutropenia should be described as "mild" if the blood neutrophil count is 1000 to 2000 cells per cu. mm., as "moderate" if the count is 500 to 1000 cells per cu. mm., and as "severe" if the count is below 500 cells per cu. mm. These subdivisions of neutropenia are important, because the consequences of neutropenia vary dramatically, depending upon the degree to which the count is reduced.

Neutrophils function to phagocytize and kill microorganisms. Together with other types of phagocytic cells (monocytes and macrophages), they facilitate the removal of many foreign substances from the body. They are aided in their functions by immunoglobulins, complement, and a variety of other host factors. In many clinical situations neutropenia may be only the most obvious defect in the defense system of the susceptible host, and all the susceptibility to infections in neutropenic patients should not necessarily be attributed to their reduced neutrophil counts. This fact can be readily appreciated from the great variability observed clinically in the frequency of infections for various kinds of patients with neutropenia. Because of this variability the treatment of neutropenia depends greatly upon the clinical circumstances in which it is encountered.

General Approach to Management of Neutropenia

1. Concern should be directed principally to those patients with moderate and severe neutropenia. Mild degrees of neutropenia, transient or chronic, generally have no important clinical consequences.

2. Patient isolation. It is common practice in most hospitals to isolate patients with severe neutropenia in private rooms and to require visitors and staff to wear masks and growns when visiting these patients. The precise value of these procedures is not known. Thorough handwashing, avoidance of exposure of neutropenic patients to patients with obvious infections, and attention to good hygiene (e.g., regular bathing, dental care) are probably of far greater importance. Patient isolation by ultraviolet lamp barriers, laminar air flow rooms, or "life-island" isolators may be of value in delaying infection in severely neutropenic patients, but the expense of these techniques has limited their use. Most neutropenic patients can be managed without elaborate facilities.

3. Antibiotics. Most of the infections encountered in severely neutropenic patients are caused by organisms from the patient's own indigenous bacterial flora. It is thought that these organisms are prevented from invading the host by the intactness of the skin and mucous membranes and by a constant low grade exudation of neutrophils. In the severely neutropenic patient, some studies have shown that suppression of the gastrointestinal bacterial populations with antibiotics will reduce the risk of infections. The oral antibiotic regimen most commonly employed in these investigational studies is vancomycin, 500 mg. orally every 4 hours, gentamicin, 200 mg. orally every 4 hours, and nystatin, 5 million units orally every 4 hours. (The oral use of these agents for prevention of infection in this type of patient, however, has not yet been approved for general use.) This drug combination will not absolutely sterilize the bowel, but it will markedly reduce the amount of stool and make stool cultures negative while patients are receiving these drugs. In some institutions these drugs are given in concert with a cooked or sterilized diet and in combination with regular skin cleansing and topical antibiotics to the groin, axillae, and any apparently inflamed areas of skin. These oral antibiotics are largely not absorbed. A major problem is that they have unpleasant tastes, and patient compliance falls during chronic administration. The risk of emergence of antibiotic-resistant bacteria is relatively small. It should be noted that the oral administration of gentamicin has not yet been approved except for investigational purposes.

Systemic antibiotic therapy generally is not used for the prophylaxis of infections in neutropenic patients but is reserved for patients with fever and presumed infections. In most febrile, severely neutropenic patients presumed to have an infection, immediate antibiotic therapy with a combination of antibiotics covering both gram-positive and gram-negative organisms, including *Pseudomonas aeruginosa,* is recommended. Carbenicillin (75 mg. per kg. intravenously every 4 hours) and cephalothin (2 grams intravenously every 4 to 6 hours) are frequently advocated. Gentamicin (5 mg. per kg per day parenterally in patients with normal renal function) or tobramycin (5 mg. per kg. per day parenterally with normal renal function) is also frequently added. Antibiotic therapy can be adjusted when the results of blood cultures and other microbiologic reports are available. When transient severe neutropenia is encountered in the course of chemotherapy for neoplastic diseases, many specialists recommend continuation of broad-spectrum antibiotic therapy until the patient's neutrophil count has returned to greater than 200 to 500 cells per cu. mm. of blood. In patients with drug allergies, renal failure, substantial previous exposure to antibiotics, or evidence for fungal infections, the advice of a specialist in the treatment of infectious diseases is recommended.

4. Neutrophil transfusions. Methods have been developed recently for collecting neutrophils from normal persons for transfusion to severely neutropenic patients. The cells collected by any of several methods appear to have the ability to circulate, to migrate to sites of infection, and to kill bacteria. Several recent studies have established that severely neutropenic patients transfused with neutrophils and given appropriate antibiotics have a better chance of recovering from severe infections than patients treated with antibiotics alone. In patients with leukemia, the benefit is more apparent for patients having prolonged neutropenia, i.e., lasting for several weeks. Unfortunately, this is the category of patients with the poorest overall prognosis for the underlying disease. Patients with fever and neutropenia who do not have clear-cut bacterial infections as can be shown by positive cultures ordinarily have a relatively good prognosis when managed with antibiotic therapy without neutrophil transfusions. Research is in progress to define what kinds of patients will benefit most from this type of supportive care, how many cells need to be given, the appropriate dose interval for the transfusions, the best methods for collecting the cells, the risk of neutrophil donation to the donor, and the potential usefulness of prophylactic transfusions.

5. Splenectomy. The spleen serves to trap effete red blood cells and probably sequesters a substantial proportion of the blood neutrophils under some clinical circumstances. At present no accurate methods can be readily used to determine if the spleen is causing neutropenia by sequestering or destroying neutrophils. It has long been thought that under certain circumstances some splenic factor may suppress or perturb neutrophil production, but this theory remains unproved. In some diseases—e.g., myelofibrosis and chronic granulocytic leukemia—splenic production of neutrophils may contribute substantially to the blood neutrophil count. The decision to remove the spleen in a patient with neutropenia should not be based solely upon the level of the blood neutrophils. Splenectomy specifically for neutropenia probably should be limited to those patients with both splenomegaly and frequent infections.

6. Corticosteroids and other steroidal hormones. Because corticosteroids may increase the risk and mask the signs of infections and because they are of no specific clinical benefit to the vast majority of neutropenic patients, they should not be given without specific indications. Occasional patients with chronic idiopathic neutropenia or neutropenia resulting from an immunologic mechanism (as in lupus erythematosus or proved immune neutropenia) may benefit from corticosteroid therapy. In these instances the use of alternate day or intermittent therapy is recommended because of the lower risk of infection observed with this form of therapy. Androgen therapy with oxymetholone (1 to 2 mg. per kg. per day) or nandrolone (3 mg. per kg. per week) (this dose may be higher than that recommended in the manufacturer's official directive) may be beneficial in the management of aplastic anemia with neutropenia and certain related disorders (e.g., the neutropenia encountered with marrow aplasia in patients with paroxysmal nocturnal hemoglobinuria or Fanconi's anemia); but for most patients with neutropenia, androgens are of no proved benefit. These drugs cause masculinization and increase in libido and may cause a toxic hepatitis.

7. Lithium carbonate (usually about 600 mg. 3 times per day) will cause an increase in the blood neutrophil count in normal persons and has been tried as an experimental therapy in a variety of neutropenic patients with quite variable results. The side effects of this therapy are potentially numerous, and its therapeutic benefit is uncertain at present.

8. Other therapies. Occasional patients with folic acid or vitamin B_{12} deficiency may have neutropenia, and their counts will increase dramatically with the appropriate therapy. Occasional patients on chronic intravenous therapy will develop copper deficiency, and the associated neutropenia will respond to copper therapy.

Caring for the Patient with Neutropenia

1. Patients with idiopathic drug reactions causing neutropenia—e.g., phenylbutazone, chlorpromazine, penicillins, sulfonamides, propylthiouracil, and gold salts—usually present with fever, upper respiratory symptoms, and absent blood neutrophils after a period of days to months of therapy. In most of the patients, blood neutrophils will return in a period of 5 to 10 days if the offending drug is withdrawn. This kind of febrile, severely neutropenic patient should be treated with antibiotics as soon as possible, using the drugs mentioned above or similar broad-spectrum coverage. The antibiotics can then be adjusted

after microbiologic culture information becomes available. In patients with neutropenia caused by hematotoxic drugs (generally those agents used in cancer chemotherapy), the period of severe neutropenia is often 1 to 2 weeks, although there is considerable variability for the individual agents used. After a patient is given a hematotoxic drug, antibiotic therapy can be delayed until the neutrophils are below 500 per cu. mm. and sustained fever occurs under most circumstances. Treatment with antibiotics plus simple isolation techniques is usually sufficient to care for this patient until his counts improve.

2. Leukemia often presents with neutropenia, and neutropenia regularly occurs with chemotherapy. Chemotherapy to attempt to induce a remission in the leukemia and improve effective neutrophil production is the mainstay of this neutropenic problem. Supportive care consists of antibiotics, isolation, and platelet and possibly neutrophil transfusions.

3. Aplastic anemia is often accompanied by a severe neutropenia resulting from a failure of neutrophil production. These patients also may have monocytopenia and are often severely predisposed to infections. Supportive care with antibiotics is usually sufficient for the episodic infections. Long-term neutrophil replacement with transfusions is not currently feasible. Long-term improvement depends upon a spontaneous remission in the disease, successful treatment with androgens, or the availability of a bone marrow transplant donor.

4. Chronic neutropenia without splenomegaly is usually called "chronic idiopathic neutropenia" or "benign neutropenia." This is probably not a specific entity but a collection of patients with various disorders in neutrophil production and maturation. Only those patients with severe neutropenia need consideration of therapeutic intervention, because the patients with higher counts do quite well with no treatment. Splenectomy in the absence of splenomegaly is of no proved benefit. Long-term neutrophil transfusion support is not feasible. Treatment with alternate day corticosteroids (e.g., prednisone, 40 to 60 mg. every other day) has been beneficial in a few instances. Spontaneous remissions of chronic neutropenia, especially in children, have been reported. Lithium has been used in a few of these patients with quite valuable results.

5. Chronic neutropenia with splenomegaly is usually seen as a part of an inflammatory disease (sarcoidosis, infectious mononucleosis, hepatitis, and Felty's syndrome in patients with rheumatoid arthritis). It also occurs with congestive splenomegaly and in some patients in the late phases of myeloproliferative diseases. In all these conditions it is thought that the spleen may serve to sequester and possibly destroy neutrophils. In most patients, the low neutrophil count causes no increased infection susceptibility. If the spleen is removed, the neutrophil count may rise within a few minutes to a few hours after the splenectomy, indicating that the neutropenia was due to a disordered distribution of cells and not due to a failure in cell production. Splenectomy principally directed toward the neutropenia should be reserved for patients with problems of infections; in most cases splenectomy is done for management of thrombocytopenia or other problems and not for neutropenia alone.

6. Cyclic neutropenia is a rare disease causing recurring neutropenia at 3 week intervals. It can be diagnosed only by doing serial neutrophil counts for several weeks. Most patients tolerate the neutropenia with only a modest degree of morbidity. Antibiotic therapy is generally not indicated, even in the neutropenic periods, unless specific infections occur. Occasional patients have benefited from intermittent corticosteroid therapy (prednisone every other day), but these cases are rare. No other treatment is known to be clearly beneficial for this condition.

7. Neutropenia in severe infections, such as pneumococcal pneumonia, gram-negative bacteremia, and typhoid fever, is occasionally encountered. These patients have presumably exhausted their neutrophil reserves in responding to their infection. Their neutropenia is a marker for a poor prognosis. Specific antibiotic therapy directed to the infection is the mainstay of their care. It is not known if corticosteroid therapy or granulocyte transfusions are beneficial in these patients.

HEMOLYTIC DISEASE OF THE NEWBORN

(Erythroblastosis Fetalis)

method of
AARON R. RAUSEN, M.D.,
and RICHARD E. ROSENFIELD, M.D.
New York, New York

Introduction

Hemolytic disease of the newborn (HDN) can result from a variety of endogenous and exogenous causes (Table 1). The term is used most commonly to denote those instances caused by maternal alloimmunization. Although the principles of

TABLE 1. **Causes of Hemolytic Disease of the Newborn**

1. Maternal alloimmunization, Rh, ABO, Rh4(c), K1 (Kell), Rh3(E), others
2. Maternal autoimmunization, e.g., lupus erythematosus
3. Congenital (hereditary) hemolytic anemias:
   a. Red cell enzyme deficiencies, e.g., glucose-6-phosphate dehydrogenase, pyruvate kinase, triose-phosphate isomerase, hexokinase
   b. Red cell morphologic abnormalities, e.g., spherocytosis, elliptocytosis, stomatocytosis, pyknocytosis
   c. Hemoglobinopathies, e.g., α-thalassemia trait
4. Drugs and toxins, e.g., vitamin K (water soluble) in high dose to mother or infant, naphthalene, penicillin
5. Infections:
   a. Bacterial (usually perinatal)
   b. Viral (e.g., cytomegalic inclusion disease, congenital rubella, herpes simplex, coxsackievirus B4, viral hepatitides)
   c. Spirochetal (congenital syphilis)
   d. Protozoal (toxoplasmosis, malaria)
6. Metabolic disorders, e.g., galactosemia, osteopetrosis
7. Disseminated intravascular coagulation associated with infections, respiratory distress, congenital neoplasms, etc.

treatment of the anemia and unconjugated hyperbilirubinemia of HDN are similar in all cases, it is imperative, with appropriate differential diagnostic procedures, to establish the exact cause of HDN in each newborn infant. Additional therapeutic measures as well as altered genetic counseling and prognostic implications apply when HDN results from causes other than maternal alloimmunization. This discussion, unless stated otherwise, will be limited to the management of HDN caused by maternal alloimmunization.

Hemolytic disease of the newborn caused by maternal alloimmunization occurs in over 0.5 per cent of live births. Rh HDN still accounts for a number of stillbirths and seriously affected newborn infants, but protective administration of Rh antibody shortly after delivery has reduced its incidence by over 90 per cent. ABO HDN now accounts for most cases of HDN; it is usually of less severity than Rh HDN, is self-limited, and rarely causes death in utero or hydrops fetalis. Other maternal antibodies account for the remaining less than 5 per cent of cases, the most frequently encountered antibodies being against Rh4 (hr′ or c), K1 (Kell), and Rh3 (rh″ or E). Since anti-A and anti-B antibodies are naturally occurring, ABO HDN is common in firstborn incompatible offspring. The production of essentially all other antibodies requires exposure of the mother to significant quantities of incompatible red cells, so that firstborn offspring rarely have non-ABO HDN.

Optimal management of non-ABO HDN requires close liaison throughout pregnancy between obstetrician, pediatrician, blood bank, and the chemistry laboratory. This is especially true with Rh HDN. Here the population at risk can be defined, and prophylactic therapy given to women at risk can essentially eliminate the disease. An affected fetus can be detected well before delivery, and therapy can be given to the fetus as early as the twentieth gestational week, as well as to the infant after birth. This has all been accomplished since the discovery of the Rh factor and its relationship to erythroblastosis fetalis in 1941.

Antepartum Care

Diagnostic Tests. BLOOD TYPING. ABO and Rh typing are performed routinely early in pregnancy to determine those expectant mothers who are type O, or Rh-negative, or both. ABO HDN occurs almost exclusively in non-O offspring of type O mothers and non-O fathers. Over 90 per cent of type A or B fathers are heterozygous (i.e., A/O or B/O), so that half their offspring are spared. In contrast, most Rh positive fathers are homozygous. Although Rh subtyping may suggest heterozygosity, unequivocal evidence of Rh heterozygosity is assured only when a father has an Rh-negative child or parent.

Every pregnant woman should have her serum tested for Rh and other unexpected antibodies at least once early in pregnancy and again at delivery. When found, such antibodies are identified and assayed by titration, serially if necessary, to assist in managing the pregnancy.

AMNIOCENTESIS. During the first pregnancy complicated by unexpected Rh antibodies, amniocentesis is performed when the maternal titer is 1:16 or greater. The procedure is ordinarily first done at 28 weeks' gestation, but is performed at 20 to 24 weeks when there is a prior history of a severely affected offspring or stillbirth.

Amniocentesis is an outpatient procedure. The maternal bladder is emptied, and fetal position and heart sounds are determined. Placental location is determined by ultrasound, which minimizes the chance of placental trauma and fetal-maternal hemorrhage which might stimulate maternal antibody production. Avoidance of placental bleeding reduces the risk of hemorrhage for the fetus and allows for more valid amniotic fluid analysis. Under sterile conditions a 22 gauge, 4 inch lumbar spinal needle is inserted about 3 to 4 cm. below the umbilicus transabdominally into the uterus on the side containing fetal small parts. Five to 20 ml. of fluid is withdrawn and protected from light during processing to avoid photo-oxidation of bilirubinoid pigments. The supernatant obtained after centrifugation at $1000 \times g$ for 20 minutes is clarified by filtration through Whatman No. 4 filter paper.

Amniotic fluid varies in solute concentration, and tends to become more dilute as pregnancy progresses. Problems caused by this phenomenon are minimized by measuring the ratio of bilirubin pigments to total protein. Bilirubin pigments are determined spectrophotometrically as the difference in optical density (OD) at 450 nm. and 600 nm. in a cell with a 10 mm. light path. This determination correlates well with the ΔOD 450 nm. of Liley (Amer. J. Obstet. Gynec., *82*:1359, 1961). Total protein is determined by the Biuret method, and a bilirubin/protein ratio is derived as $\frac{\text{OD 450–600 nm.}}{\text{total protein}}$ g/100 ml. A value of less than 0.35 indicates little or no involvement, 0.35 to 0.55 moderate involvement, and greater than 0.55 severe involvement (Cherry et al.: Obstet. Gynec., *26*:826, 1965). Blood or meconium in amniotic fluid gives misleading results. Such specimens are discarded. Serial determinations performed every 7 to 21 days as needed allow for assessment of degree of involvement. An increasing ΔOD 450 nm. or bilirubin/protein ratio value indicates increasing severity of disease.

Results of amniotic fluid analyses determine management. A fetus with mild involvement is delivered after the thirty-eighth week of gestation. When a fetus is moderately involved, labor is induced between the thirty-fifth and thirty-eighth weeks of gestation. Decision within this period is based on degree of involvement, rate of progress of the disease, and risk of hyaline membrane disease as determined by the amniotic fluid lecithin/sphingomyelin (L/S) ratio. Severely affected fetuses are delivered immediately when the pregnancy is more than 34 weeks and the L/S ratio is at least 1.5 and preferably greater than 2.0 (Gluck et al.: Amer. J. Obstet. Gynec., *109*:440, 1971). When the fetus is deemed to be severely involved and at less than 34 weeks of gestation, intrauterine intraperitoneal transfusion is performed, using red cells compatible with the mother. When a fetus is at 32 to 34 weeks and severely involved and the mother is not toxemic but the L/S ratio is less than 2.0, we suggest administration of betamethasone intramuscularly (12 mg.) at least 24 hours prior to delivery when possible (Liggins and Howie: Pediatrics, *50*:515, 1972) to decrease the risk of respiratory distress syndrome.

Therapy. EARLY DELIVERY. When there is no obstetrical contraindication, labor is induced by dilute oxytocin infusion. A 6 to 8 hour trial on the first day and another such trial on the second day after rupture of membranes usually results in vaginal delivery. If unsuccessful, cesarean section is performed. The team that will care for the anticipated newborn premature infant must be involved throughout this obstetrical period in order to ensure optimal intensive general and hematologic care of the infant.

MATERNAL PLASMAPHERESIS. Recent reports from England (Fraser and Tovey: Clin. Haemat., *5*:149, 1976) suggest that intensive antenatal plasmapheresis can significantly lower Rh antibody levels in the blood of mothers carrying fetuses severely affected with Rh HDN. When performed in women whose fetuses developed severe disease relatively late in pregnancy, the procedure, when combined with intrauterine transfusion, appeared to result in an improved survival over what would have been expected with intrauterine transfusion alone (Fraser et al., Lancet, *1*:6, 1976). The Fraser and Tovey schedule for plasmapheresis involves 500 ml. per session once weekly from the tenth through the twentieth gestational weeks, and increases to as many as four sessions per week of 1 liter per session, interspersed with intrauterine transfusions later in pregnancy. Unpublished experience by Rubenstein (Rubenstein, P., personal communication) suggests that less intensive plasmapheresis of 500 ml. at precise weekly intervals will significantly reduce maternal antibody levels. Using this method of plasmapheresis in conjunction with intrauterine transfusion in over four dozen mothers with severely affected fetuses, Rubenstein has observed a survival rate in the order of 50 per cent. In our limited personal experience with this method, we have confirmed Rubenstein's observations concerning antibody levels and, like him, have observed sudden anamnestic increases in Rh antibody. At this time we reserve judgment concerning the role of maternal plasmapheresis in the management of the severely affected fetus.

INTRAUTERINE INTRAPERITONEAL TRANSFUSION. Severe fetal disease prior to 34 weeks of gestation is treated with intrauterine intraperitoneal red cell transfusion(s). The ideal fetal candidate is between 28 and 33 weeks of gestation, not hydropic, but severely involved by amniotic fluid criteria. A severely involved fetus at less than 28 weeks of gestation is a technically difficult candidate because of the small size and greater mobility of the target. Liggins' two-needle technique, whereby one needle transfixes the fetus, has enabled intraperitoneal transfusion to be accomplished successfully as early as 20 weeks. The more standard technique begins with the injection into amniotic fluid of 20 to 30 ml. of 75 per cent diatrizoate sodium (Hypaque) that is ingested by the fetus and localizes in the fetal small bowel in 6 to 8 hours, thus marking the fetal abdomen. After surgical preparation, under image intensification television fluoroscopy the relation of fetal abdomen to maternal abdomen is ascertained with metallic markers. With local anesthesia a 17 gauge thin-wall Tuohy needle (Becton, Dickinson & Co., T 466 LNRH) is inserted through the maternal abdominal wall into the fetal abdominal cavity. Entrance into a hollow cavity is confirmed by injection of saline, followed by 2 to 3 ml. of Hypaque, which by collecting under the diaphragm confirms the location of the needle in the peritoneal cavity. A polyethylene catheter with Luer end (Intramedic, Clay-Adams Inc., PE-50/C 38") is inserted through the needle and the needle withdrawn. Blood is then transfused. This should be fresh type O washed red cells compatible with maternal serum, suspended in a solution of 2.5 per cent glucose and 0.45 per cent NaCl. Particularly in the younger fetus, use of compatible, reconstituted previously frozen red cells should be considered. The viable lymphocyte content of such preparations is low, and thus the risk of graft versus host reaction may be minimized.

The volumes of intrauterine transfusion we recommend should prevent intraperitoneal pressure exceeding portal and umbilical venous pressure which could result in interruption of umbilical venous blood flow and death. Volumes as little as 20 ml. at 22 weeks and as much as 120 ml. at 33 weeks are usually well tolerated in the absence of significant fetal ascites. Transfusions are repeated at 10 to 21 day intervals until the thirty-fourth week of gestation, at which time pregnancy is interrupted. At delivery, care of the infant is similar to that of others with HDN. Depending on the percentage of transfused red cells and time since the last transfusion, the infant may manifest disease ranging from severe involvement requiring immediate resuscitation and exchange transfusion to no clinical involvement with no anemia, a preponderance of Rh negative red cells, and no development of hyperbilirubinemia. The majority of infants who receive intrauterine transfusion, however, do require at least supportive transfusions after birth and often several exchange transfusions to avert significant hyperbilirubinemia.

Care at Birth

When mild non-ABO HDN is suspected, at least one pediatrician versed in newborn care should be present at the birth to care for the infant and examine for pallor, petechiae, edema, and hepatosplenomegaly. Anticoagulated blood is obtained for determination of hemoglobin concentration, packed cell volume, and reticulocyte count; clotted blood is obtained for direct antiglobulin test, ABO and Rh types, and serum total and direct reacting bilirubin.

When severe non-ABO HDN is anticipated, a team of four skilled pediatricians is desirable to treat immediately perinatal asphyxia in the infant with hydrops.

Immediate Exchange Transfusion. In the case of the severely involved infant with marked anemia and cardiorespiratory distress, hepatosplenomegaly, edema, ascites, and elevated umbilical vein pressure, a combination of rapidly coordinated therapeutic maneuvers is performed to save the infant. Immediate assisted ventilation, abdominal paracentesis, catheterization of umbilical artery and vein to enable monitoring of blood pressure and gases, and correction of acidemia all aid cardiorespiratory function. A limited, cautious isovolemic 1 volume (200 to 250 ml.) exchange transfusion is then performed to raise the hemoglobin concentration to over 10 grams per 100 ml. Since blood volume usually is not increased even in severe hydrops and the elevated umbilical vein pressure is more related to increased portal pressure and ascites in severe hydrops, a deliberate volume deficit should not be induced. The aforementioned procedures frequently allow for survival and the subsequent use of standard 2 volume exchange transfusions to control hyperbilirubinemia.

Care After Birth

Exchange transfusion remains the cornerstone of treatment. The procedure replaces the infant's antibody sensitized red cells with those from a donor known to be compatible with maternal serum antibodies, corrects anemia, depletes the infant of his major source of bilirubin (damaged red cells), and removes a proportion of the total body bilirubin, thus preventing bilirubin encephalopathy.

Criteria for Exchange Transfusion. For non-ABO HDN, a positive direct antiglobulin (Coombs) test alone is no indication for exchange transfusion, because many such patients have disease so mild that exchange transfusion is unnecessary. However, with such an infant, when the cord hemoglobin concentration is less than 12 grams per 100 ml., the cord indirect bilirubin concentration is greater than 5 mg. per 100 ml., or the reticulocyte count exceeds 8 per cent, early exchange transfusion therapy is usually needed. A decision for exchange can be made when indirect bilirubin concentration exceeds, or is expected to exceed, 20 mg. per 100 ml. Prior maternal history, prematurity, or hepatosplenomegaly also sways the decision toward exchange transfusion. The level of bilirubin at which exchange transfusion is performed is altered downward if the infant has acidosis (current or prior), hypoalbuminemia, hypoglycemia, respiratory distress, or hypothermia, or if there is a maternal history of drug intake with an agent known to impair albumin binding of bilirubin. Multiple exchange transfusions are employed to control hyperbilirubinemia. Assessment of non-albumin-bound bilirubin and reserve albumin binding capacity helps in deciding when to perform exchange transfusion, particularly when factors exist that place the infant at risk with less than the usual level of indirect reacting bilirubin. The current mortality rate from exchange transfusion itself in centers where the procedure is frequently performed is less than 1 per cent for both term and premature infants. In each instance, the risk of exchange is weighed against the risk of brain damage.

Selection of Blood. Donor red cells should be compatible with hemagglutinins in the mother's plasma, and donor blood plasma should be compatible with the infant's red cells. Proper selection of compatible red cells often necessitates independent selection of suspending plasma which is ABO compatible with the infant's red cells. Fresh frozen plasma and plasma free of cryoprecipitate are adequate substitutes for fresh plasma. If extracted from acid-citrate-dextrose (ACD) or citrate-phosphate-dextrose (CPD) blood stored at 4°C., red cells up to 5 to 7 days old resuspended in fresh plasma are satisfactory. Banked whole blood should be less than 5 days old and preferably less than 3 days old to avert hyperkalemia. Frozen red cells are suitable. Although the average infant undergoing a single exchange transfusion does not require platelets or labile coagulation factors, fresh whole blood may be of benefit in the severely erythroblastotic infant with concomitant thrombocytopenia. We prefer CPD over ACD as the anticoagulant because of its lessened tendency to induce transient acidosis. Blood freshly collected in heparin (which must be used within 24 hours) avoids the hazards of citrate but adds (1) the risk of hemorrhage until neutralized by protamine sulfate at the end of the procedure and (2) the production of free fatty acidemia which enhances the kernicteric potential of a given concentration of bilirubin.

In an emergency, with no other available compatible blood, the mother's red cells suspended in compatible plasma from another source may be used. Incompatible blood is not recommended as a routine, but may be lifesaving if compatible blood is not available. In such a case additional exchange transfusions to control hyperbilirubinemia may be expected.

Technique of Exchange Transfusion. We employ the umbilical vein route. Expendable plastic equipment (Pharmaseal Laboratories, Glendale, California) has reduced many difficulties. Several details of technique that minimize risk deserve emphasis. These include maintenance of the infant's body temperature with servo-controlled radiant heat or a bunting; monitoring of cardiac status, preferably by electrocardiogram; emptying of stomach prior to exchange transfusion; anticipation of cardiorespiratory emergencies by presence of trained personnel with proper equipment; ability to readily suction and resuscitate; and warming of donor blood to 37°C. just prior to infusion by passage through special plastic recipient tubing traversing a blood warming apparatus (Fenwal Laboratories, Morton Grove, Illinois). Although some feel it unnecessary, to avoid hypocalcemia with citrated blood we infuse slowly about 1 ml. of 10 per cent calcium gluconate under electrocardiographic control after every 100 ml. of blood transfused. In infants, particularly prematures who already may be acidotic, we prefer to use CPD blood to minimize acidosis. If only ACD blood is available, we recommend adding THAM (tris hydroxymethyl aminomethane) to the unit of blood as a buffer. THAM-E (Abbott Laboratories, North Chicago, Illinois) is prepared as a 1.2 M solution by adding 250 ml. of 10 per cent dextrose in water to the bottle containing 36 grams of powder. Eight ml. is added to the blood immediately before exchange. The remaining THAM is discarded.

Hypoglycemia may occur before and after exchange transfusion, particularly in severely involved erythroblastotic infants and premature infants. It is detected by frequent blood glucose determinations and demands prompt treatment.

If x-ray control is available, it should be used to verify placement of the tip of the catheter into the inferior vena cava. When not available, in term infants the catheter should be placed no more than 5 or 6 cm. from the abdominal wall (and less in premature infants) to avoid the possibility of portal or mesenteric vein placement and the consequent risk of transient vascular occlusion and/or marked local pressure changes, leading to bowel wall compromise. Another risk of long catheterization is direct cardiac infusion with the danger of having the citrated blood traverse the foramen ovale and perfuse the coronary arteries.

A double volume exchange transfusion (170 to 200 ml. per kg. of body weight) removes about 85 per cent of the infant's starting red cell population. Bilirubin removal is less efficient, being in the range of 25 per cent of body bilirubin per double volume exchange. Efficiency of removal of red cells, bilirubin, and antibody is greatest at the beginning of the procedure. Irrespective of the infant's weight, we limit the total volume to 1 unit (450 ml.) for a single exchange. If the infant is not in distress, we use 20 ml. aliquots for exchange in infants with body weight over 2000 grams, 10 ml. volumes in infants 1200 to 2000 grams, and 5 ml. volumes in infants less than 1200 grams. The volume per individual exchange is reduced (but never less than 5 ml.) in sick infants. The procedure should take 40 to 60 minutes.

The unit of donor blood should not be suspended for administration, because this may result in completing the final portion of the exchange with a dilute suspension of red cells in plasma. This is avoided by placing the donor blood on its side, or with the outlet facing upward in a plasma expressor device (Fenwal Laboratories, Morton Grove, Illinois) so that red cell sedimentation in the up-ended bag will yield an adequate terminal hematocrit. When an infant is sick and there is a question of completing the exchange, the container is placed on its side.

Although we do not use supplemental albumin to augment bilirubin removal during exchange and bilirubin binding thereafter, this is an acceptable additive. We would recommend giving 25 per cent salt-poor albumin, either as a pre-exchange infusion of 4 ml. per kg. of body weight or as 50 ml. added to the unit of donor blood. Albumin should not be used in sick infants in whom resulting hypervolemia may not be tolerated.

To minimize septic complications the catheter is removed after each exchange transfusion. Subsequent catheter placement rarely is a problem. With uncomplicated exchange transfusions antibiotics are not routinely administered.

Postexchange Anemia. The most common cause of anemia after exchange transfusion is related to the use of low hematocrit donor blood, particularly at the end of the procedure. However, anemia may gradually develop owing to loss of donor red cells in vivo, and increase in the infant's blood volume, while there is still ineffective erythropoiesis. When the hemoglobin concentration falls below 6 grams per 100 ml., the infant may be transfused with compatible packed red cells, using 10 ml. per kg. of body weight. This is generally sufficient until adequate erythropoiesis resumes at as early as 4 weeks of age in the premature infant and by 8 weeks in the term infant. Iron therapy is not recommended because iron stores are high after prolonged hemolytic anemia in utero.

Anemia Without Exchange Transfusion. An infant with erythroblastosis who does not require exchange transfusion may develop severe anemia during the second through fourth weeks of life when erythropoiesis is minimal. Such nonexchanged infants must be evaluated frequently and given a simple transfusion with compatible erythrocytes when significant anemia develops. The indication for transfusion may be a hemoglobin concentration as high as 9 grams per 100 ml. in a 2 week old infant who displays a rapid decrease in hemoglobin concentration, or as low as 5 to 6 grams per 100 ml. in a 4 to 6 week old in whom reticulocytosis is not present. We recommend a transfusion of 10 ml. per kg. of compatible packed red cells.

Adjuncts in the Management of Hyperbilirubinemia. PHENOBARBITAL. Phenobarbital increases hepatic clearance of bilirubin mainly by inducing glucuronyl transferase; an effect on hepatic uptake and excretion of bilirubin has also been suggested. Other hepatic enzymes that influence the metabolism of drugs and endogenous steroid hormones are similarly affected. Several trials have demonstrated that serum bilirubin levels can be reduced by administering phenobarbital to the mother before delivery or to her infant immediately after delivery. It is less effective when given after hyperbilirubinemia has developed. Because of lack of sufficient data on both short- and long-term effects on the newborn, we do not employ phenobarbital therapy.

PHOTOTHERAPY. Visual light in the blue-green spectrum photo-oxidizes bilirubin into nontoxic water-soluble derivatives that do not bind albumin and are rapidly excreted from the body in bile and urine. Many physicians caring for newborns now use this therapy as an adjunct to avert significant hyperbilirubinemia. A suggested conservative approach is to reserve its use for those mild cases in which the rate of rise in serum bilirubin is relatively slow, and after exchange transfusion in an attempt to prevent the need for repeat exchange. Questions are still incompletely resolved regarding effects of phototherapy on other components of metabolism and its long-term effects on growth and development. Because of this we do not at present use phototherapy (except as a "prophylactic" measure in severely ill premature infants weighing less than 1200 grams, in whom the risks of exchange transfusion are real), but rely on exchange transfusion to forestall potentially neurotoxic bilirubin levels. In hospitals where exchange transfusions are performed infrequently and personnel are thus relatively inexperienced, we would advocate the use of adjunctive phototherapy. In such instances it would be prudent to institute exchange transfusion when the serum bilirubin level is just below the level warranting exchange in the infant not subjected to phototherapy.

Prevention of Rh HDN

Rh antibody injections for nonimmunized Rh negative women bearing Rh positive offspring are administered intramuscularly within 72 hours of delivery. This markedly decreases the incidence of primary immunization. The material used is gamma globulin prepared by Cohn fractionation of plasma from highly immunized Rh negative volunteers (Rho-GAM, Ortho Pharmaceutical Corporation, New Jersey). The standard dose recommended is 300 micrograms of antibody globulin. This dose should also be given to Rh negative women, with Rh positive husbands, who have undergone abortion after the eighth week of pregnancy. Postdelivery anti-Rh antibody administration still leaves perhaps 2 per cent primigravidas at risk who become immunized. This can be reduced at least in part by examining postpartum maternal blood for its content of fetal red cells. The Kleihauer-Betke test is advised for this evaluation (Oski and Naiman: *Hematologic Problems in the Newborn,* 2nd Ed. Philadelphia, W. B. Saunders Company, 1972, p. 63). Additional Rh antibody is administered to women identified to be at risk by having fetal-maternal bleeds exceeding 10 to 15 ml.

HEMOPHILIA AND ALLIED CONDITIONS

method of
HUSSAIN I. SABA, M.D.
Tampa, Florida

Hemophilia and allied conditions, collectively known as hemophilioid disorders, refer to a group of hereditary bleeding states which are associated with deficient activity of various procoagulants. It is now recognized that in the majority of patients deficient activity probably relates to the presence of an abnormal molecule rather than to a simple quantitative deficiency. These deficiencies are depicted in Table 1.

The three most common such disorders are classic hemophilia or hemophilia A (factor VIII deficiency), hemophilia B (factor IX deficiency), and von Willebrand's disease. Approximately 60 per cent of the patients have hemophilia A, 20 per cent have hemophilia B, and 12 per cent have von Willebrand's disease; the rest of the procoagulant deficiencies comprise 8 per cent. Although discussion will largely center on the three most common hemophilioid disorders, general principles of management apply to all related disorders. This discussion will also deal with the detection and management of circulating anticoagulants, or "inhibitors," now frequently encountered as treatment programs for hemophilioid disorders become more comprehensive.

CLASSIC HEMOPHILIA

Classic hemophilia is a deficiency of normal factor VIII molecules. The molecule consists of subunits bound together by weak chemical interactions. Low molecular weight units are responsible for the coagulant function of the molecules, and the high molecular weight units for antigenic properties. In approximately 90 per cent of patients with classic hemophilia, despite the low coagulant activity, the antigenic subunit is present in normal amounts. Only in 10 per cent are both the coagulant and antigenic components of the molecule reduced.

Depending on the amount of the coagulant activity measured by the factor VIII assay, the hemophiliac can be categorized into one of three groups: (1) *severe* hemophilia, with factor VIII activity less than 1 per cent; (2) *moderate* hemophilia, with 1 to 5 per cent activity; and (3) *mild* hemophilia, with 5 to 25 per cent activity. Patients with severe deficiency have intermittent *spontaneous* hemorrhage, especially into large joints and muscles, and a tendency to bleed with minimal trauma. With moderate deficiency, spontaneous hemorrhage is relatively rare, but bleeding can occur with surgery or trauma. With minimal deficiency, bleeding is seen only with considerable stress. In general, the PTT (partial thromboplastin time) test constitutes an excellent screening procedure for detecting all degrees of factor VIII deficiency. It may, however, miss some borderline, very mild factor VIII deficiencies. Hence, it remains important to obtain and evaluate a history of prior bleeding and, if significant, to carry out the most sensitive test—i.e., an assay for factor VIII.

Principles of Treatment

Great advances in the treatment of hemophilia have been made during the past decade, allowing hemophiliacs a better quality of life. Necessary surgical procedures are now possible, and occurrence of chronic disability can be minimized. The comprehensive care of hemophilia includes replacement therapy, correction of disability, and social care.

Replacement Therapy

The basis for replacement therapy in hemophilia and allied conditions is outlined in Table 1. Rational replacement therapy must be based on the understanding of physiologic and chemical characteristics of the deficient procoagulant, including the storage, stability, biologic (in vivo) half-life, and plasma concentrations needed for hemostasis under varying conditions.

Principles of Dose Calculation. Several methods have been in use. Two of the simple ones are described here.

1. Calculation of the patient's total plasma volume. Assuming total plasma volume to be approximately equal to 5 per cent of body weight, in a 70 kg. patient, the total plasma volume can be determined by multiplying the weight in kg. by 50 (70 × 50 = 3500 ml.). One unit of factor VIII is defined as the factor VIII activity in 1.0 ml. of fresh pooled human normal plasma. Assuming that the aforementioned 70 kg. patient has 0 per cent factor VIII activity in his plasma, then raising the factor activity to 100 per cent will require infusion of 3500 units of factor VIII; raising the level

TABLE 1. **The Hemophilioid Disorders**

PROCOAGULANT	COMMON SYNONYMS	USUALLY ACCEPTED BIOLOGIC HALF-LIFE IN VIVO (HOURS)	MINIMUM LEVEL FOR HEMOSTASIS %	HEREDITARY COAGULOPATHY	THERAPEUTIC AGENTS
I	Fibrinogen	72–96	50–100*	Congenital afibrinogenemia, hypofibrinogenemia	Fibrinogen concentrates, fresh frozen plasma
II	Prothrombin	100	30–40	Congenital hypoprothrombinemia	Stored plasma, prothrombin complex concentrates
V	Proaccelerin, accelerator globulin, labile factor	36	10–15	Factor V deficiency	Fresh frozen plasma
VII	Serum prothrombin conversion accelerator (SPCA), stable factor	3	10–15	Factor VII deficiency	Fresh frozen plasma, prothrombin complex concentrates
VIII	Antihemophilic factor (AHF), antihemophilic globulin	12–14	15–20	Classic hemophilia	Normal plasma, cryoprecipitate, glycine precipitate commercial products
IX	Plasma thromboplastin component (PTC), Christmas factor	15–24	10–20	Hemophilia B, PTC deficiency, Christmas disease	Stored plasma, prothrombin complex concentrates
X	Stuart factor	40	20	Stuart disease	Stored plasma, prothrombin complex concentrates
XI	Plasma thromboplastin antecedent (PTA)	20–50	?	PTA deficiency	Fresh frozen plasma
XII	Hageman factor	—	—	No hemorrhagic tendency	None necessary
XIII	Fibrin stabilizing factor, fibrinase	150	2–5	Factor XIII deficiency	Fresh plasma, fresh frozen plasma
Fletcher	Prekallikrein	—	—	No hemorrhagic tendency	None necessary

*Milligrams per dl. (100 ml.).

to 50 per cent, 1750 units of factor VIII; and raising the level to 25 per cent, 875 units of factor VIII.

2. The other simple formula which can be used to calculate the dose is as follows:

$$X = \frac{(Y)(Z)}{2}$$

where X = units of factor VIII required by infusion.
Y = % circulating normal factor VIII activity desired.
Z = weight in kg.

Example: In a hemophiliac weighing 64 kg. with 0 per cent factor VIII activity, the goal is to increase circulating factor VIII activity to 25 per cent of normal:

$$X = \frac{(25)(64)}{2} = 800 \text{ units of factor VIII required}$$

This simple formula gives virtually the same results as those requiring calculations or estimates of plasma volume.

For fresh frozen plasma: Assume that 1 ml. of fresh frozen pooled human plasma has 1 unit of factor VIII; therefore give 800 ml. of fresh frozen plasma.

For cryoprecipitate: Assume that 1 bag unit of cryoprecipitate contains 100 units of factor VIII; therefore give 8 bags of cryoprecipitate.

For commercial factor VIII concentrates: Follow instructions regarding factor VIII contents. The circulating half-life of factor VIII given with the first infusion is less than 8 hours, principally because of equilibration with extravascular space. With subsequent infusions the T½ of factor VIII is approximately 12 to 14 hours. This is the basis of giving a loading dose and then half of this loading dose every 12 hours to maintain the desired level during treatment. For example, in a 70 kg. severe hemophiliac undergoing major surgery, a loading dose of 3500 units of factor VIII would be given. Then half of this dose (1750 units) would be given every 12 hours to maintain circulating factor VIII activity at greater than 50 per cent.

Monitoring the Therapy. The aforementioned initial calculations for maintenance therapy may be only theoretical and must be monitored with appropriate laboratory tests. As mentioned above, the partial thromboplastin time (PTT), although generally useful, may not always reflect the precise level of circulating factor VIII. For this reason serial PTT testing during maintenance therapy should be backed on occasion with the more accurate factor VIII assay. Since the aim of maintenance therapy is to keep the circulating factor VIII activity above a certain level, the best time to carry out factor VIII assays is just prior to the next dose of factor VIII infusion.

Mode of Infusion. Although intermittent infusion as described above has been the most commonly employed procedure, more recently some have employed a *continuous* infusion technique. This mode of infusion avoids peaks and valleys in circulating factor VIII and theoretically maintains a constant level. When in certain critical situations it is necessary to maintain a factor VIII level above a certain minimum, this mode of infusion is preferred. It would still be wise to give an initial loading dose, followed by infusions of half of the loading dose at a continuous rate over the next 8 to 12 hours. Close monitoring with factor VIII assays, especially at the beginning of the treatment course, is also required here.

Side Effects of Therapy. These include fever and urticaria, principally with the use of plasma. Hepatitis is more common with the use of concentrate owing to pooling from many donors. There are some reports of hemolytic reactions caused by the presence of a high concentration of isoantibodies in infused concentrates.

Sources of Factor VIII Replacement. These include fresh frozen plasma; plasma fraction I-O; cryoprecipitate, "homegrown" and freeze-dried (available commercially); glycine precipitate; and animal antihemophilic globulin (AHG).

PLASMA. Because of the danger of hypervolemia, plasma should be used only to achieve circulating factor VIII activity of about 25 per cent. To attain this level, 15 to 20 ml. per kg. should be given as the initial dose and, when indicated, 3 to 6 ml. per kg. every 12 hours. Plasma infusion suffices for minor bleeding episodes such as small lacerations, relatively small tissue hematomas, and mild hemarthrosis. In some of these, a single loading dose may be sufficient. However, with catastrophic hemorrhage requiring a circulating factor VIII level of more than 25 per cent, cryoprecipitate or concentrates are required.

CRYOPRECIPITATE. This most widely used product is obtained by thawing fresh frozen plasma at 4°C. The cold insoluble precipitate can be prepared in most blood banks as a byproduct of component fractionation of whole blood. The amount of factor VIII in 1 unit of plasma is concentrated to one tenth the original volume. The factor VIII activity of "homegrown" cryoprecipitate may vary greatly. Since there is a variable but appreciable loss of factor VIII in the processing of cryoprecipitate, each bag of cryoprecipitate should be considered to contain no more than 100 units of factor VIII. One bag of cryoprecipitate per 4 kg. of body weight can raise the factor VIII level in the recipient up to a level of approximately 50 per cent. Commercially obtained cryoprecipitates (Kriobulin, Profilate) are also available. These products, unlike "homegrown" cryoprecipitates, are standardized and more stable. Two hundred fifty and 500 unit factor VIII activity bottles are available.

COMMERCIALLY OBTAINED GLYCINE PRECIPITATES. Several of these products* are available in the United States and in other countries. These concentrates are lyophilized standardized products which can be stored at 4°C. in the refrigerator. Vials of very high potency concentrates are available; therefore there is no volume problem in their infusion. These concentrates are very convenient for home care because of easy storage and reconstitution. After reconstitution these products are easily infused into the vein (without the use of intravenous tubing), using a needle and syringe equipped with a filter.

As indicated earlier, the main disadvantage of these concentrates is the risk of hepatitis. Some feel that this is such a potential handicap that their use at this time probably should be restricted to severe hemophiliacs who have had hepatitis in the past, or to those in whom emergency surgery or a continuous infusion is required.

ANIMAL AHG PRODUCTS. Although very high potency animal AHG products are available, they are now rarely used because of severe reactions.

Management of Specific Problems

Hemarthrosis. This is the most common problem encountered and is the major cause of disability. Early replacement of factor VIII is essential. If treated early, acute hemarthrosis can be successfully managed by one dose treatment, raising the factor VIII level to 25 to 30 per cent. Recurrent hemarthrosis requires intensive replacement to the level of 20 to 30 per cent for days to weeks along with temporary immobilization of the joint.

The question of joint aspiration in acute hemarthrosis is controversial. In a situation in which the joint swelling caused by accumulation of blood is very marked and there is intense pain, aspiration can be undertaken only following replacement therapy and with utmost care. Intensive trial of analgesics in acute hemarthrosis is emphasized, but one must refrain from using aspirin. Many patients can tell what kind of analgesic has helped them in the past.

*Hemofil (Hyland), AHF (Courtland), Fibro-AHG (Merck), Humafac (AHF), (Parke, Davis).

Soft Tissue Hematomas. Immediate attention should be given to soft tissue hematomas in critical areas. These include hematomas of the neck, mouth, and pharynx, where the danger of airway obstruction is considerable; retroperitoneal bleeding and hematoma, because of compression of abdominal organs; hematoma in the calf, because of danger of compression of nerve; and hematoma in the upper thigh and groin, with danger of extension under the inguinal ligament into the abdominal cavity. The aim of replacement therapy should be to raise the factor VIII level to 60 to 100 per cent and to maintain that level for at least 4 to 5 days.

Hematuria. This can occur in hemophiliacs without any history of trauma. Considerable blood loss is rare. Mild hematuria may resolve spontaneously; however, one-time treatment to raise the factor VIII level to 50 per cent is suggested. The use of epsilon-aminocaproic acid (EACA) is not advised, because it can cause development of clot and result in ureteral obstruction. A short trial of prednisone, 2 mg. per kg. for 2 days, then tapered and stopped after 5 days, can be beneficial in recurrent hematuria if replacement therapy is not desired. The mechanism of action of prednisone in this condition remains ill-defined.

Lacerations. As hemophiliacs with minor lacerations may not immediately lose more blood than the normal person, they often are not given replacement therapy at the time of initial management. However, most of these patients, if not given replacement therapy, have delayed bleeding and may then require hospitalization for infected or noninfected hematomas. Therefore replacement up to 30 to 45 per cent is advisable as one-time treatment before local measures and suturing. The replacement also ensures good healing.

Central Nervous System Bleeding. Hemophiliacs with a history of head trauma other than the most trivial should be given replacement therapy. This is suggested regardless of whether or not the patient has intracranial or extracranial bleeding. The factor VIII level should be raised to 100 per cent. Only then should investigative and surgical procedures, including arteriogram, lumbar puncture, and creation of a burr hole, be performed. After initial replacement, a factor VIII level of 50 per cent is maintained for 5 to 7 days.

Liver Biopsy. Liver biopsy can be performed in hemophiliacs if absolutely necessary. Raising the factor VIII level to 100 per cent just before the biopsy and then maintenance at a 50 per cent level for 3 to 5 days are suggested.

Traumatic Oral Mucous Membrane Bleeding and Dental Extraction. Epsilon-aminocaproic acid (EACA or Amicar) is beneficial in these problems.

Traumatic oral mucous membrane bleeding can be difficult to control and has required prolonged replacement therapy. This is relatively common in children and apparently is related to potent fibrinolytic enzymes in the salivary secretions. In this situation a one-time replacement to raise the factor VIII level to 30 to 50 per cent and then Amicar by mouth for 3 to 5 days does an effective job. The dose of Amicar in children is 10 to 12 grams per day (25 per cent syrup containing 1.25 gram per teaspoon). An alternative schedule is a loading dose of 200 mg. per kg., followed by 100 mg. per kg. every 4 to 6 hours.

In dental extraction Amicar has been used satisfactorily in a regimen of 100 mg. per kg. as a loading dose, and then 50 mg. per kg. every 6 hours orally. This is started 24 hours prior to surgery and continued for 5 to 6 days. Prior to surgery the patient also receives one-time replacement therapy to raise the factor VIII level to 50 to 100 per cent. For major dental surgery, replacement therapy is continued for 4 to 5 days as well.

Other Major Surgery. The factor VIII level should be raised to 100 per cent just prior to surgery and then maintained at 50 per cent or greater for a variable number of days, usually 7 to 8 days. Alternatively, a continuous infusion regimen can also be used in this situation, as bleeding can occur prior to the next dose in those patients placed on a replacement regimen of every 12 hours.

Orthopedic Measures. In hemophilia with recurrent joint bleeding, the early pathologic changes are small synovial tissue hemorrhages, frequently with accompanying acute inflammatory reaction. The permanent changes in the joints include synovial thickening as a result of tissue proliferation and irregular epiphyseal growth. These changes, along with hypervascularization of synovial tissue leading to its increased fibrinolytic activity, have been thought to be the cause of recurrence of joint bleeding. On this basis synovectomy, especially of the knee, has been suggested and in some cases has reduced disability. Destruction of synovial membrane has also been induced in these joints by local injection of osmic acid, thiotepa, and colloidal ^{198}Au. Other orthopedic maneuvers have included posterior capsulotomy, osteotomy, tenotomy, arthrodesis, and arthroplasty. These measures should be undertaken only by a skilled orthopedic surgeon familiar with hemophiliac problems and in consultation with a coagulationist, and only after nonsurgical measures have failed to provide relief.

Rehabilitation and Physical Therapy

A rational program of physical therapy is an important asset in the treatment of hemophilia. This should be done under the supervision of experts and at specialized centers. Physical therapy measures to prevent or minimize disability include positional therapy, including sleeping positions; kinesitherapy, mainly motion exercises in water; and isometric as well as isotonic contraction exercises.

Home Treatment and Social Care

At several centers patients have been trained in self-infusion replacement therapy after recognition of the symptoms of bleeding. Although these approaches have led to unnecessary treatment at times, over-all such programs have been found to be successful; they have led to reduction of days lost from work and from school, have reduced the frequency of visits to the outpatient department, and have reduced long waits in busy emergency rooms. Several factors should be taken into consideration before placing a patient on this regimen: (1) The patient should be intelligent and responsible. (2) The patient or a responsible family member should be trained to start intravenous infusions. (3) The possible development of factor VIII inhibitor should be checked periodically. (4) The patient should be in good contact with the physician handling the program.

Care should be available to handle psychologic problems associated with the disease, not only for the patient but also for the family. Psychosocial advice in regard to schooling, working situation, and general counseling also constitutes an important aspect of the psychologic management of these patients.

MANAGEMENT OF HEMOPHILIA-ALLIED CONDITIONS

The general principles of classic hemophilia management can be applied to hemophilia-allied conditions, as regards both replacement therapy and management of the specific problems.

Hemophilia B

The inheritance pattern and clinical presentation are similar to those of classic hemophilia. The disappearance of factor IX in vivo is relatively slow, the half-life being 15 to 20 hours. Despite the longer half-life, the booster dose should be given every 12 hours to maintain the desired level. The level of factor IX required for hemostasis in circulation is apparently similar to that of factor VIII.

Plasma should be used for mild to moderate bleeding episodes as prescribed for factor VIII deficiency. The concentrates should be reserved for more serious bleeding uncontrollable by infusion of plasma. Several of these are available commercially (Proplex, Konyne, PPSB). These concentrates, which contain other vitamin K dependent factors as well (II, VII, and X), should be used cautiously because of the development of hypercoagulable and disseminated intravascular coagulation (DIC)–like states reported by some investigators.

von Willebrand's Disease (vWD, Vascular Hemophilia)

Inheritance of von Willebrand's disease has been reported as both autosomal recessive and dominant. The bleeding diathesis is classically characterized by a prolonged bleeding time, abnormal adhesion of platelets to glass, a usually low level of factor VIII, and therefore sometimes prolonged PTT. The antibleeding factor (vWD factor, large molecular weight component of factor VIII molecule) is low or abnormal. Ristocetin, an antibiotic, fails to aggregate the platelets of vWD patients. The infusion of cryoprecipitate or factor VIII concentrate causes the rise of patient factor VIII coagulant activity by stimulation of de novo synthesis. Apparently the infusion of large molecular weight factor VIII molecules (vWD factor) stimulates the synthesis of low molecular weight factor VIII component. Both antigenic component (large molecular weight protein) and coagulant component (small molecular weight protein) are classically decreased in proportional amounts. A number of variant vWD families and patients have been discovered.

The coagulopathy includes generally superficial bleeding from skin and mucous membranes. Epistaxis, easy bruising, and menorrhagia are also important features. Hemarthrosis, as in hemophilia, is seen, but less frequently. Replacement therapy includes the infusion of cryoprecipitate. The hemostatic level to be achieved should be similar to that in hemophilia A. The most important parameter to be followed, however, should be the bleeding time. Cryoprecipitate infusion effectively corrects the bleeding time; nevertheless, sometimes high doses are required for the correction of the bleeding time and to produce effective hemostasis. In preparation for surgery, replacement should be started 48 hours prior to surgery. This is to allow the time for triggering de novo synthesis. Birth control pills have also been used in female vWD patients with some beneficial effect.

Congenital Afibrinogenemia and Dysfibrinogenemia

The half-life of fibrinogen is 4 days. Patients manifest coagulopathy by soft tissue hematoma, excessive bleeding from laceration, and ecchymosis, but rarely hemarthrosis. The diagnosis is made by prolonged thrombin-plasma clotting time and by immunoelectrophoresis of fibrinogen. Replacement therapy should be used judiciously and only with serious bleeding because of the possibility of development of antifibrinogen antibody. The aim should be to achieve a plasma fibrinogen level of 150 to 250 mg. per dl. (100 ml.). A booster dose should be given every 4 days; for surgical procedures, booster doses should be started preoperatively and continued for 5 to 7 days.

Factor II (Prothrombin) Deficiency

This congenital deficiency is most rare. Inheritance follows an autosomal recessive pattern. Any form of bleeding, including hemarthrosis, can occur. The half-life of factor II is 21 days. Most bleeding episodes are easily controlled with plasma.

Factor V Deficiency

The biologic half-life is 36 hours. Fresh frozen plasma is a good source. The 25 to 30 per cent level achieves effective hemostasis.

Factor VII Deficiency

The half-life is 3 hours; however, hemostasis can be achieved by giving booster doses of plasma every 8 hours. Four-hourly replacements should be given for surgical procedures. The usual priming dose of 10 ml. of plasma per kg. of body weight, followed by boosting with 4 ml. per kg., brings about effective hemostasis. Prothrombin complex, containing other vitamin K dependent factors along with factor VII, is available but seldom required.

Factor X (Stuart Factor) Deficiency

This very rare disorder is inherited as an autosomal recessive trait. Bleeding diathesis is generally mild. Most bleeding problems can be treated with plasma in doses of 15 to 20 ml. per kg. of body weight in adults and 10 to 15 ml. per kg. of body weight in children. A booster dose of 3 to 6 ml. per kg. of body weight every 8 to 12 hours can then be given.

Factor XI Deficiency

The inheritance of factor XI deficiency is probably autosomal dominant. Approximately one third of affected persons may not have bleeding diathesis. Those who have a bleeding diathesis can be managed with plasma in the dose indicated in factor X deficiency therapy.

Factor XII (Hageman Factor) Deficiency

Despite a grossly prolonged partial thromboplastin time (PTT), these patients do not have a bleeding diathesis and do not require replacement therapy.

Factor XIII (Fibrin Stabilizing Factor) Deficiency

This deficiency is inherited as an autosomal recessive pattern. A history of umbilical bleeding at birth is commonly present. Easy bruising, hematoma, poor wound healing, and characteristically delayed bleeding after dental extraction and minor surgery are usual patterns of this coagulation disorder. These patients are unable to make a stable clot at the bleeding sites. The screening test for factor XIII deficiency is one in which the clot is dissolved readily in 5 M urea or in 1 per cent monochloracetic acid. This should be confirmed by quantitative assay of factor XIII. The bleeding diathesis can be controlled by infusion of fresh frozen plasma. The plasma half-life is extremely prolonged (3 to 12 days). Infusion of 15 ml. per kg. every 4 to 5 weeks can be sufficient for effective hemostasis.

Fletcher Factor (Prekallikrein) Deficiency

First described in 1965, this deficiency is inherited as an autosomal recessive trait and is similar to Hageman factor deficiency. It is unassociated with a bleeding diathesis.

MANAGEMENT OF INHIBITORS

With the advent of more intensive study and management of hemophilia and its allied disorders, the problem of inhibitors is becoming more frequently recognized. Such recognition is important, because, once an inhibitor develops, treatment completely changes. The management may become very difficult.

The inhibitor against a specific clotting factor is recognized when patient plasma prolongs coagulation of an equal amount of normal plasma, whereas in deficiency states normal plasma replenishes the missing factor to at least 50 per cent, sufficient to correct any of the abnormal coagulation screening tests.

Inhibitors or circulating anticoagulants occur either spontaneously (in the absence of congenital bleeding diathesis) or in patients with hereditary bleeding disorders and previous use of replacement therapy.

Inhibitors Against Factor VIII

Both spontaneous type inhibitors and inhibitors developing in patients with classic hemophilia have been found. Spontaneous inhibitors against factor VIII have been reported in postpartum females; collagen vascular diseases, especially systemic lupus erythematosus (SLE) and rheumatoid arthritis; allergic reaction to drugs, especially penicillin and sulfonamides; allergic skin reactions (e.g., bullous erythema multiforme and pemphigus); inflammatory bowel disorders (e.g., ulcerative colitis or Crohn's disease); malignancy; and idiopathically. Patients with spontaneous inhibitors present with spontaneously occurring bruises, ecchymosis, hemorrhage, and hemarthrosis—features of classic severe hemophilia. In almost 50 per cent of these patients the inhibitor disappears spontaneously.

Inhibitors developing in hemophiliacs are seen in approximately 10 per cent of these patients. Although mainly seen in severe hemophiliacs, development of inhibitors does not appear to correlate absolutely with the number of transfusions previously given.

The immediately mixed PTT in factor VIII inhibitor patients can be normal unless the titer is very high. Therefore an incubated (1 hour at 37°C.) mixed PTT should be obtained to rule out factor VIII inhibitors. A control of known hemophiliac plasma, with no inhibitor, mixed with normal plasma, should also be run simultaneously. When the prolongation of patient's mixed incubated PTT is significant in comparison to the control, the diagnosis of inhibitor becomes very likely. The titer or unit of inhibitor can then be detected by assaying the residual factor VIII activity in the incubated mixture of normal plasma mixed with serial dilution of patient's plasma.

Treatment of Factor VIII Inhibitors. The factor VIII inhibitor is an immunoglobulin of IgG type. In many patients with this inhibitor a secondary anamnestic response is seen after replacement therapy. Some patients can be categorized in the low responder group in which the titer of inhibitors remains low. In the high responders, nevertheless, the anamnestic response causes a sudden high rise of inhibitor titer 3 to 10 days after replacement therapy, increasing the probability of spontaneous bleeding. Once the inhibitor titer rises to a high level and bleeding occurs, the replacement therapy with factor VIII, even in massive amounts, generally fails to neutralize the inhibitor in order to produce hemostasis.

Although at this time a unified approach remains unavailable, the following general principles can be applied in the management of these patients.

Conservative Therapy. Mild bleeding episodes in hemophiliacs with inhibitors can be managed conservatively with bed rest and analgesics. Although it is a time-consuming program, management of hemarthrosis, hematomas, and genitourinary bleeding in patients with inhibitors has been achieved.

In this conservative plan of management the following steps are applied: (1) a good physician and patient rapport; this is essential so that the patient realizes why replacement therapy may be contraindicated; (2) abstention from transfusing blood products in order to prevent antigenic stimulus and therefore the chances of anamnestic response (if anemia is marked, a transfusion is essential; it is given with washed packed red cells); and (3) prevention of iatrogenic trauma which increases the chances of bleeding. The last of these steps includes utmost care in drawing blood from the patient. Blood should be drawn only when absolutely necessary and only by expert personnel. A minimum of 8 to 10 minutes of pressure is applied at the venipuncture site after drawing blood in order to prevent hematoma. The reason for this is that once the hematoma starts in inhibitor patients, it can dissect very rapidly and extensively. No elective invasive procedure should be carried out.

Specific Therapy. If specific therapy is mandatory in a patient with factor VIII inhibitor, the following facts must be considered in order to modulate the therapy: knowledge of the titer of inhibitor, and knowledge from previous experience of whether the patient is a high responder or low responder.

Titer of inhibitors is very important. One unit of inhibitor is defined as the amount of antibody that will neutralize 1 unit of factor VIII in normal human plasma after 1 hour of incubation. Less than 5 units is considered low level, 5 to 25 units intermediate, and more than 25 units high level. In the treatment of low levels of inhibitor in low responders, a large repeated bolus of factor VIII concentrate can be tried to raise the factor VIII activity in these patients to 100 per cent level. If this is achieved, these patients are then placed on continuous infusion of factor VIII concentrate. Hemostasis may well follow despite the failure to achieve a desired level of factor VIII. In the treatment of low responders with moderate levels of inhibitor, hemostasis may be achieved with the aforementioned procedure in combination with repeated plasmapheresis. In patients with high inhibitor levels, the factor VIII replacement has been generally frustrating and unrewarding. Most of these patients bleed to death when they start bleeding, as all measures to induce hemostasis remain unrewarding.

Recently hemostasis has been achieved in these patients by the use of active prothrombin complex concentrates. The rationale for the use of these preparations has been the bypassing of the inhibitor and factor VIII reaction. These vitamin K dependent factor concentrates, apparently by virtue of the presence of activated factor(s), can directly convert the patient's prothrombin into thrombin, and thereby fibrin formation takes place, resulting in the arrest of bleeding. The two preparations of prothrombin complex concentrates that have been used are Proplex and Konyne. Judicious use of 1 or 2 bottles of these concentrates every 8 to 12 hours has arrested the bleeding in inhibitor patients.

Recent results have not been so rewarding, because further purification of these concentrates has been performed by the commercial companies and contamination of activated factors has been removed. This has been done in view of the controversy that these preparations with active factors have caused a DIC-like syndrome in factor IX deficient patients, for whom these products are primarily produced. More recently, Hyland Laboratory has produced a product (Autoproplex) of vitamin K dependent factors in which the factors have been deliberately activated. This product is especially designed to be used only in inhibitor patients to control their bleeding episodes and is on trial at many centers.

Inhibitors Against Factor IX

This inhibitor is also an immunoglobulin. In contrast to factor VIII inhibitor, the reaction of antifactor IX and factor IX is not time and temperature dependent. Therefore the mixed PTT (one part patient plasma and one part normal plasma) is prolonged immediately after mixing, and no incubation is required. Its spontaneous occurrence in non–hemophilia B patients is very rare. Problems of its management are similar to those of factor VIII inhibitor. Exchange transfusions with concomitant plasma transfusion have been used in some patients. At this time in severe bleeding problems, judicious use of prothrombin complex factors, following the same protocol as used for factor VIII inhibitor, can be tried.

Inhibitors Against Factor V

So far very few such patients have been described, and almost all have been of the spontaneous type—i.e., in the absence of hereditary deficiency of factor V. Some have occurred following the use of streptomycin. So far, significant bleeding has not been seen in patients with this inhibitor. Furthermore, it persists only for a few weeks after occurrence. The suggestion therefore is to follow the patient carefully and not to institute any specific treatment.

Inhibitors Against Factor XIII

Both spontaneous inhibitors and inhibitors in patients with congenital factor XIII deficiency have been reported. Isoniazid intake appears to be involved in most patients with this spontaneously occurring inhibitor. Severe bleeding diathesis has been reported. The inhibitor slowly disappears after withdrawing isoniazid.

Inhibitors in Systemic Lupus Erythematosus

Several inhibitors have been found to occur in systemic lupus patients. These include inhibitors acting directly against factor IX and factor XI. The other most common inhibitor seen in 5 to 10 per cent of patients with SLE is so-called "lupus anticoagulant." Its mechanism of action appears to be the inhibition of formation of prothrombin activating principle (V–X–Ca^{++}–phospholipid complex).

Bleeding in association with lupus inhibitors is not frequent, and it may be concomitant with qualitative and quantitative abnormalities of platelets. The titer of inhibitor fluctuates with the activity of disease and frequently disappears when the lupus is not active. Steroid and immunosuppressive agents in the dose used for active SLE have caused suppression and disappearance of this inhibitor. Frequently, questions arise of chances of bleeding in performing kidney biopsies in SLE patients with this inhibitor. Although a number of patients have undergone elective surgery in the presence of this inhibitor without excessive bleeding, abstention from elective surgery is suggested, especially in the presence of platelet and prothrombin abnormalities.

BLEEDING DISORDERS SECONDARY TO PLATELET ABNORMALITIES

method of
PHILIP W. MAJERUS, M.D.
St. Louis, Missouri

Thrombocytopenia

The treatment of thrombocytopenia depends upon its pathogenesis—increased palatelet destruction or decreased platelet production. The severity of thrombocytopenia determines the need to institute therapy. Generally patients with platelet counts of above 50,000 per cu. mm. have normal hemostasis even with major trauma; spontaneous bleeding rarely occurs with platelet counts above 25,000 per cu. mm. When platelet counts fall below 25,000 per cu. mm., therapy should be instituted, especially if hemorrhage is present or surgery is necessary. Bone marrow aspiration is essential to distinguish thrombocytopenia caused by increased platelet destruction (immune thrombocytopenias) from that caused by decreased production. Normal marrow cellularity with normal or increased numbers of megakaryocytes suggests the former. Ideally platelet survival studies would distinguish these types of thrombocytopenias, but they are impractical to do clinically. Great efforts to exclude toxic reactions to drugs or environmental agents as a cause of thrombocytopenia should be made before therapy is instituted. Intramuscular injections should be avoided in severely thrombocytopenic patients, and no drugs containing aspirin should be used.

Thrombocytopenia Secondary to Increased Platelet Destruction. These disorders include the immune thrombocytopenias: idiopathic thrombocytopenic purpura (ITP), some drug-induced disorders, some cases of thrombocytopenias secondary to lymphomas, chronic lymphocytic leukemia, or lupus erythematosus, as well as those caused by hypersplenism. In general the therapy of these disorders is similar (except for drug-induced immune thrombocytopenia), although the treatment described below is most directly applicable to ITP.

In children ITP occurs most commonly following acute viral illness, and is usually self-limited, abating within a few weeks or months. No therapy is necessary unless serious hemorrhage occurs.

In adults the disorder is more unpredictable in course and less likely to remit spontaneously.

General Measures. Patients should avoid strenuous activity, especially anything that would be likely to result in head trauma, because intracranial hemorrhage is the major life-threatening complication in this disorder. Aspirin therapy should not be used in thrombocytopenic patients, because aspirin interferes with the hemostatic function of the remaining platelets.

Corticosteroid Therapy. Initial therapy with prednisone, 60 to 100 mg. per day, is continued until the platelet count returns to normal levels or until 2 weeks have passed. When the platelet count is normal, the prednisone dosage is *slowly* reduced as monitored by the platelet count. This reduction can usually be accomplished over a 4 week period. If thrombocytopenia returns as prednisone is withdrawn, a second attempt at steroid therapy is undertaken. If this also fails (i.e., failure to achieve a normal platelet count or one over 75,000 per cu. mm. off corticosteroid therapy), splenectomy is performed. Although the majority of adult patients with ITP come to splenectomy, the trial of prednisone does spare 15 to 20 per cent of patients from splenectomy.

SPLENECTOMY. Splenectomy is performed for any of the following indications: (1) failure of corticosteroid therapy, (2) inability to tolerate corticosteroid therapy (i.e., duodenal ulcer, osteoporosis), or (3) major life-threatening hemorrhage. Patients who present with severe thrombocytopenia and large blebs of submucosal hemorrhage in the mouth and nose are considered for immediate splenectomy. Splenectomy results in a lasting remission in approximately two thirds of patients. If thrombocytopenia persists or recurs following splenectomy, prednisone therapy is again instituted as outlined above. Lower doses of prednisone may control thrombocytopenia after splenectomy.

IMMUNOSUPPRESSIVE THERAPY. Use of immunosuppressive agents is reserved for patients who fail to respond to splenectomy and corticosteroids or who require continued corticosteroid therapy after splenectomy. Azathioprine (Imuran), 100 mg. per square meter per day, or cyclophosphamide (Cytoxan), 100 mg. per square meter per day, is given, and blood counts are monitored at frequent intervals with modification of dosage if leukopenia or anemia develops. (This use of azathioprine and cyclophosphamide is not listed in the manufacturer's official directive.) The drug is discontinued if the leukocyte count remains below 3000 per cu. mm. Approximately two thirds of otherwise unresponsive patients will respond to this therapy, but response may be gradual over several months. When azathioprine (Imuran) is tapered, thrombocytopenia may recur (one half of patients who respond). Recently, vincristine, 1 to 2 mg. intravenously per week, has produced remissions in some refractory patients. (This use of vincristine is not listed in the manufacturer's official directive.) If a response occurs, therapy can be discontinued; in severe cases maintenance monthly or less frequently is required. Long-term immunosuppressive therapy should be avoided if possible because of reports of development of malignancies and opportunistic infections in patients receiving long-term immunosuppressive therapy.

Thrombocytopenia Secondary to Decreased Platelet Production. If a drug or other agent can be identified as the probable or possible cause of the suppressed platelet production, further contact with that agent should be avoided. Recently heparin has been shown to produce thrombocytopenia; thus patients receiving heparin should have platelet counts monitored. Supportive therapy with platelet transfusion is the mainstay of treatment of these patients.

PLATELET TRANSFUSION. Platelet transfusion is of little or no benefit in treating immune thrombocytopenia because of the shortened platelet survival in these patients. Rarely, in patients with serious hemorrhage, platelets are infused at the time of splenectomy *after* the splenic circulation has been clamped. Conversely, platelet transfusion is of major benefit in treating patients with thrombocytopenia secondary to bone marrow suppression by drugs (chemotherapy of malignant disease) or other chronic thrombocytopenias associated with aplastic anemia.

INDICATIONS. Platelet transfusions are clearly indicated for acute hemorrhagic episodes or prophylactically prior to major surgery. The efficacy of chronic prophylactic platelet transfusion therapy is less clear. This therapy has most often been used in patients with temporary thrombocytopenia produced by the toxic effects of chemotherapy or radiation therapy of malignancy or in patients with aplastic anemia. Although prophylactic platelet transfusion reduces the incidence of hemorrhage, recent studies indicate that a majority of patients acquire resistance to platelet transfusion because of the development of antibodies to the transfused cells. The major transplantation antigens are of importance in these reactions. Thus tissue-typing of potential sibling donors is desirable when chronic transfusion therapy is contemplated. Short of tissue-typing, unmatched sibling donors have been shown to be superior to random donors for chronic platelet transfusion therapy. When possible, a few donors or even a single donor should be used to minimize the number of potential sensitizing antigens. A single donor can donate 4 units of platelets once or twice weekly by thrombocytophoresis. When platelets are used to treat a single bleeding episode, danger of antibody formation is of less importance unless the need for future therapy is anticipated. Occasionally patients develop resistance to transfused platelets which is actually due to antibodies to leukocytes contaminating the platelets. This may be avoided by carefully removing leukocytes from the platelet concentrates.

DOSAGE. The platelet count should be maintained over 40,000 per cu. mm. if possible for the period of treatment when therapy is given before and after surgery. When platelets are given prophylactically to prevent bleeding in patients on chemotherapy, levels of 20,000 per cu. mm. are adequate. To maintain the higher level requires about 5 units of platelets per square meter of body surface area two or three times per week if the initial platelet count is zero.

Factors such as fever, infection, and hemorrhage may shorten platelet survival markedly, thus decreasing the response to therapy.

Thrombocytosis

The treatment of thrombocytosis depends on the magnitude of platelet count elevation and the underlying disease state. The most common causes of significant thrombocytosis (over 1,000,000 per cu. mm.) are polycythemia vera, primary hemorrhagic thrombocythemia, chronic granulocytic leukemia, myelofibrosis, iron deficiency anemia, cancer, and postsplenectomy thrombocytosis. If major hemorrhage occurs in the face of marked thrombocytosis, the platelet count may be acutely lowered to normal by thrombocytophoresis with reinfusion of the plasma and erythrocytes. It may be necessary to exchange 10 or more units of blood before the platelet count is controlled. Platelet exchange may now be carried out more conveniently using a cell separator when available. Since the platelet count may rise again promptly, it is necessary to institute other therapy to maintain a lowered platelet count. Nitrogen mustard, 10 mg. per square meter intravenously, is useful for this purpose and is effective within 7 to 10 days: alternatively, hydroxyurea, 3 to 6 grams orally, may be used. In less urgent situations when major hemorrhage is not a problem, busulfan (Myleran) therapy, 2 to 6 mg. per day, may be used to lower the platelet count over a period of several weeks. Caution must be exercised in using busulfan, because individual susceptibility to the toxic effects of this drug is great. Severe and even irreversible thrombocytopenia or pancytopenia may result from overdosage. It is important to exclude iron deficiency as the cause for the thrombocytosis, because iron therapy can easily reverse this form of thrombocytosis. When polycythemia vera is the underlying cause for thrombocytosis, the relatively high platelet counts (1,000,000 to 2,000,000 per cu. mm.) may be well tolerated as long as the hematocrit is maintained below 50 per cent by phlebotomy. Thus, although busulfan may be necessary during the early phase of therapy of polycythemia vera, once the hematocrit is normal it is no longer necessary to maintain the platelet count below 1,000,000 per cu. mm.

Qualitative Platelet Disorders

The most useful test to detect qualitative platelet disorders is the bleeding time. The most common acquired disorder follows aspirin ingestion. The drug acetylates platelet prostaglandin synthetase permanently, and so the defect persists for several days after aspirin. Other conditions (von Willebrand's disease, thromboasthenia, thrombocytopathy) are rare and difficult to diagnose, and there is no specific therapy to correct the platelet defects in any of them. Bleeding secondary to uremia (thrombocytopathy) is sometimes corrected by dialysis therapy. Platelet transfusions may be used effectively in these patients for the indications outlined above.

DISSEMINATED INTRAVASCULAR COAGULATION (DIC)

method of
HYMIE L. NOSSEL, Ch.B.
and KAREN L. KAPLAN, M.D.
New York, New York

Disseminated intravascular coagulation (DIC) includes a series of clinical syndromes in which excessive activation of the coagulation system occurs in vivo. It is inferred that thrombin action, accompanied by plasmin action, is responsible for most of the changes observed in the blood. The nature and severity of DIC are governed by (1) the nature, severity, and duration of the stimulus; (2) the ability of the reticuloendothelial system to clear activated coagulation factors from the circulation; and (3) the circulatory state of the patient in determining the localization and accumulation of fibrin and platelets within key target organs such as the kidneys.

The formation of abnormal amounts of thrombin and plasmin in the blood results in the formation of fibrin and proteolytic degradation products of fibrin (FDP) and in activation of platelets. The fibrin is removed from the blood much more rapidly than normal fibrinogen, and when the catabolic rate exceeds the rate of production, hypofibrinogenemia results. Alteration of platelets by thrombin may contribute to the development of thrombocytopenia. Increased concentrations of the different products of proteolyzed fibrinogen accumulate in the blood and permit diagnosis of the disorder. These products include fibrinopeptide A, fibrin in solution, and FDP. Localized accumulation of platelets and fibrin may occur in areas of vessel wall damage and may lead to physical damage to erythrocytes and impaired blood supply and damage to the organs supplied by the affected vessels.

Almost invariably DIC is associated with a prominent clinical disorder. Such disorders include (1) tissue damage, such as obstetrical accidents (retained dead fetus, premature placental separation, amniotic fluid embolism), massive trauma, and extensive burns; (2) generalized stimulus to clotting, including shock (hypovolemic, cardiogenic), acute infections (gram-negative sepsis most often, but also gram-positive sepsis, viremia, miliary tuberculosis, rickettsial disease, subacute bacterial endocarditis, and malaria), cancer (especially of prostate, pancreas and lung), leukemia, and anaphylaxis; and (3) liver failure.

Principles of Treatment

The principles of treatment are as follows: (1) Removal of any identifiable stimulus. (2) Correction of anoxia, hypovolemia, hypotension, or acidosis, all of which can aggravate the DIC. (3) Replacement therapy with appropriate blood products if the patient is bleeding and there is a hemostatic defect owing to consumption of coagulation factors. (4) Administration of anticoagulants to inhibit or reverse disseminated intravascular thrombosis in patients with evidence of ischemic organ damage and in patients with persistent DIC in whom the hemostatic defect cannot be corrected with blood products and in whom there is evidence of continuing thrombin action. It is important to emphasize that in patients with evidence of DIC, an additional hemostatic defect not caused by consumption of coagulation factors or inhibition by FDP may be present. It is therefore important to establish that the coagulation abnormality is consistent with the defect of DIC and is not due to vitamin K deficiency, liver disease, or renal disease.

Replacement Therapy

The blood fractions used will depend upon the nature and severity of the hemostatic defect. Fresh-frozen plasma should be used if the coagulation defect is most prominent, and platelet concentrates should be used if severe thrombocytopenia (less than 60,000 per cu. mm.) is present.

Anticoagulants

Anticoagulants, such as heparin, should be considered in the management of patients with DIC, consumption of coagulation factors, and bleeding if the stimulus is continuing and cannot be promptly removed. If there is evidence of ischemic organ damage—e.g., purpura fulminans, septic abortion with anuria—an attempt should be made to halt the thrombotic process with the use of heparin.

Heparin should be given by continuous intravenous infusion in a starting dose of approximately 100 units per kg. of body weight, followed by 10 to 15 units per kg. per hour. Two principles should be used in monitoring heparin therapy: (1) the patient should not be given an overdose of heparin which can induce bleeding; and (2) enough heparin should be given to arrest the thrombotic process.

Several practical difficulties are encountered in monitoring heparin therapy in a patient with DIC: (1) If the patient has a coagulation defect, it may be difficult to measure the effect of heparin using tests such as the activated partial thromboplastin time or whole blood clotting time. Under these circumstances, heparin should be assayed by the protamine titration method, aiming for a heparin level of between 0.2 and 0.3 unit per ml. (2) The effectiveness of heparin can be monitored by demonstrating that the consumption of fibrinogen has been reversed as manifested by (a) decrease in fibrin monomer complexes assayed by the protamine sulfate test; (b) decrease in fibrin degradation product (FDP) levels; (c) increase in the fibrinogen level in plasma following neutralization of the heparin in vitro with protamine sulfate; and (d) normalization of the Reptilase clotting time, which is prolonged by FDP but not by heparin.

HEMOCHROMATOSIS AND HEMOSIDEROSIS

method of
MARCEL E. CONRAD, M.D.
Birmingham, Alabama

In normal adults, the quantity of iron absorbed is equal to the amount that is excreted. Consistent deviations from this balance lead to iron deficiency on one hand and to iron overload on the other. If this balance is upset by increased iron absorption, by injection of iron, or by blood transfusion, iron accumulation occurs in various tissues with eventual damage to these organs.

Idiopathic hemochromatosis is a hereditary disorder of iron metabolism in which absorption consistently exceeds body loss. It usually becomes manifest during the fifth or sixth decade of life as hepatic cirrhosis, diabetes mellitus, cardiac insufficiency, or pigmentation of the skin. The unexplained occurrence of one or more of these findings should arouse suspicion of the underlying diagnosis. Likewise, blood relatives should be investigated to determine if they are accumulating excessive amounts of iron.

Secondary hemochromatosis refers to a group of disorders in which tissue damage occurs as a result of generalized and massive iron overloading in association with a known cause. The causes of secondary hemochromatosis are prolonged and excessive consumption of iron (Bantu), excessive parenteral administration of iron, repeated blood transfusion for causes other than blood loss, and certain anemias with impaired hemoglobin synthesis (thalassemia, sideroblastic anemias).

Hemosiderosis is the term utilized for the presence of excessive body iron without tissue damage. In addition to including disorders in which there is an increase in total body iron, it is used to indicate a selective deposition of iron in one or more body organs such as in the lungs with pulmonary siderosis, in the kidneys with chronic intravascular hemolysis, and in the liver of certain cirrhotics.

The occurrence of excessive iron overloading is suggested by an elevated serum iron concentration such that the total iron binding capacity of serum is almost completely saturated. The generalized nature of the iron overload can be demonstrated by stainable iron in specimens of liver, skin, bone marrow, and gut. The massive nature of the iron overload is established by the number of phlebotomies that are required to deplete body stores of excess iron. Serum ferritin determinations are elevated in clinical hemochromatosis, but may be normal in family members with preclinical iron overloading.

Treatment

The clinical course of untreated hemochromatosis is characterized by tissue destruction, malfunction of involved organs, and death. Since it seems that this is caused by the excess iron deposition, rational treatment consists in the removal of iron. This is accomplished most effectively by vigorous bloodletting. The rate of phlebotomy depends upon the patient's size, medical condition, and ability to maintain an acceptable blood hemoglobin concentration. Most adult hemochromatotics tolerate removal of 2 or even 3 pints of blood weekly on an outpatient basis and maintain a circulating hemoglobin concentration greater than 10 grams per 100 ml. Slower rates of phlebotomy unduly prolong the exposure of tissue to an increased iron concentration, whereas more rapid bleeding may cause hypoalbuminemia and a moderately severe anemia. Vigorous phlebotomy can be continued until the labile iron store is depleted. This usually constitutes about three fourths of the total excess body iron. Depletion of this readily available iron pool can be detected by an inability to maintain the circulating hemoglobin concentration, the development of reticulocytopenia, and depression of the serum iron concentration to iron-deficient values. However, excessive quantitites of iron can still be found in stains of tissue specimens, and cessation of phlebotomy is followed by rapid return of the hemoglobin concentration and serum iron concentration to prephlebotomy values. Continued bloodletting at a slower rate permits depletion of the less easily mobilized iron store. Once these stable stores are emptied, a more prolonged period of anemia and hypoferremia ensues. This should be confirmed by iron stains of liver and bone marrow specimens. Most patients with symptomatic idiopathic hemochromatosis have a 20 to 50 gram store of body iron when they seek medical attention (normal, 4 grams of total body iron). As each gram of hemoglobin contains 3.46 mg. of iron, each 500 ml. phlebotomy depletes the body of 0.2 gram of iron. Therefore bloodletting of at least 50 liters is usually required to eliminate excess iron. Once a normal body store of iron is achieved, reaccumulation of massive quantities of iron should be prevented. Since hemochromatotics accumulate about 3 mg. of iron from a normal diet daily in excess of body losses, quarterly bloodlettings of 500 ml. are necessary throughout life to maintain normal iron balance. Dietary restriction of iron is impractical, and chelating agents have been of little value in the treatment of hemochromatosis.

In the iron-overloading anemias the rate of bleeding which can be tolerated must be individually determined because of variability in the degree of impairment of hemoglobin synthesis. Many patients with either pyridoxine-responsive anemia or sex-linked hypochromic anemia can be bled 1 or 2 pints of blood weekly with maintenance of a circulating hemoglobin concentration of 9 to 10 grams per 100 ml. In pyridoxine-responsive anemia the daily administration of large doses of pyridoxine (100 to 300 mg.) permits an increased rate of phlebotomy. Patients with thalassemia major do not tolerate bloodletting. On the contrary, they frequently require periodic transfusions because of the severity of anemia. The repeated use of iron-chelating agents such as deferoxamine (Desferal) in patients with thalassemia major may prolong life. (This use of deferoxamine is not specifically mentioned in the manufacturer's official directive.) The recommended dosage is 0.5 to 1.0 grams daily administered intramuscularly. In addition, 2 grams can be administered intravenously with, but separate from, each unit of blood transfused at a rate not to exceed 15 mg. per kg. per hour.

In most disorders with limited or focal iron overloading, there is insufficient evidence to advocate phlebotomy. However, recent evidence suggests that patients with porphyria cutanea tarda have improvement in cutaneous manifestations and porphyrin excretion following venesection, with a reduction in hepatic siderosis.

Usually, the diabetes mellitus, cirrhosis, and cardiac manifestations associated with generalized massive iron overloading improve significantly following vigorous bloodletting. Appropriate supportive therapy of these complications is necessary.

HODGKIN'S DISEASE: CHEMOTHERAPY

method of
GIANNI BONADONNA, M.D.
Milan, Italy

The past 20 years have brought significant improvements in the survival rate of Hodgkin's disease. Although the incidence of Hodgkin's disease is limited compared to that of other tumors, the importance of this disease in the progress of cancer treatment stems from its almost unique responsiveness to both radiotherapy and chemotherapy. For more than 25 years, Hodgkin's disease has represented the most effective model for trials with local, regional, and extensive irradiation, as well as with all available growth-inhibiting compounds. Much of the progress achieved in control of this disease was derived from accurate staging procedures and from aggressive treatment modalities designed specifically with curative intent. Modern treatment of Hodgkin's disease requires experience in the field of clinical oncology and a particular skill in the use of available therapeutic modalities. Although treatment can be successfully coordinated by a practicing physician, patients usually achieve maximum benefit from the improved staging procedures and treatment plans by referral to specialized centers. There, medical oncologists, pathologists, and radiation therapists can provide facilities for proper staging, intensive therapy and adequate supportive treatment. More important, since long-term disease-free survival or cure depends on the initial treatment selection, prospective treatment plans derived from an integrated interdisciplinary approach are more easily performed in qualified institutions. In fact, although both chemotherapy and radiotherapy are effective tools, the contemporary therapeutic approach to many stages of the disease is gradually moving toward the use of combined treatment modalities. In undertaking the treatment of Hodgkin's disease, physicians must have adaptability and the capacity to accept new ideas and new discoveries.

Diagnostic Evaluation and Staging

Diagnosis requires removal of one or more lymph nodes. In a case of mediastinal adenopathy in the absence of peripheral nodes, biopsy should be carried out through mediastinoscopy. To perform the initial diagnosis of Hodgkin's disease, laparotomy is almost never required. Owing to the considerable difficulty often encountered in making a correct histologic diagnosis of lymphomatous lymph nodes, it is highly advisable that all specimens be reviewed by an expert hemopathologist. The Lukes-Butler histopathologic classification is currently used in clinical practice because of its simplicity and prognostic significance. The four histologic subgroups are the following: lymphocytic predominance (LP) (10 to 12 per cent), nodular sclerosis (NS) (45 to 55 per cent), mixed cellularity (MC) (30 to 35 per cent), and lymphocytic depletion (LD) (8 to 10 per cent). This last subgroup can be further subdivided into diffuse fibrosis and reticular type.

The Ann Arbor modification of the Rye staging system is the classification currently in use (Table 1). Stages I, II, and III indicate different extents of involvement limited to the lymph node system, whereas stage IV signifies spread to noncontiguous extranodal sites. The small group of patients presenting with extranodal involvement (lung, muscle, skin, bone) contiguous to involved nodes are classified in the appropriate lymph node system stage, followed by the subscript E. Splenic involvement is also denoted separately by the subscript S. It is always important to record the systemic symptoms because of their prognostic and therapeutic implications. It should be remembered that in the Ann Arbor classification pruritus alone is no longer considered a systemic symptom.

Determining the extent of disease according to this system has proved to be of considerable importance in assessment of the prognosis and in selection of the proper treatment. To record all the data necessary to properly stage each patient, a number of procedures are recommended, as listed in Table 2. The adoption of the Ann Arbor classification implies a dual system of stage designation: according to clinical staging (CS) only, and according to pathologic staging (PS). CS rests on the history and physical examination, initial biopsy, laboratory tests, and radiographic evidence. PS adds definitive additional histopathologic information obtained through marrow biopsy (with Jamshidi needle or open-surgical technique), peritoneoscopy, and/or laparotomy. Although it is usually both feasible and desirable to complete the diagnostic workup before starting treatment, there are known situations which

TABLE 1. **Ann Arbor Staging Classification**

Stage I	Involvement of a single lymph node region or of a single extralymphatic organ or site (I_E)
Stage II	Involvement of two or more lymph node regions on the same side of the diaphragm, or localized involvement of an extralymphatic organ or site (II_E) and of one or more lymph node regions on the same side of the diaphragm
Stage III	Involvement of lymph node regions on both sides of the diaphragm, which may also be accompanied by localized involvement of an extralymphatic organ or site (III_E) or spleen (III_S) or both (III_{SE})
Stage IV	Diffuse or disseminated involvement of one or more extralymphatic organs with or without associated lymph node involvement

Fever >38°C. (100.5°F.), night sweats, and/or weight loss >10 per cent of body weight in the 6 months preceding admission are defined as systemic symptoms, and denoted by the suffix letter B. Asymptomatic patients are denoted by the suffix letter A. Biopsy-documented involvement of stage IV sites is identified by the following symbols: marrow = M+; liver = H+; lung = L+; pleura = P+; bone = O+; skin = D+.

TABLE 2. **Diagnostic Workup**

Necessary Procedures for Proper Staging

CS
1. Detailed history with special attention to the presence or absence of systemic symptoms
2. Careful physical examination, emphasizing peripheral node chains, size of liver and spleen, Waldeyer's ring, and bony tenderness
3. Adequate surgical biopsy, reviewed by an experienced hemopathologist
4. Required laboratory tests: complete blood count, erythrosedimentation rate, serum copper, Bromsulphalein at 45 minutes, serum alkaline phosphatase, serum uric acid
5. Chest roentgenogram (PA and lateral); whole lung tomography if mediastinal/hilar adenopathy is present
6. Bilateral lower extremity lymphography with identification of suspicious nodes for surgeon

PS
7. Needle bone marrow biopsy (preferably bilateral)
8. Staging laparoscopy with multiple (4 to 6) liver biopsies; spleen biopsies can also be obtained
9. Staging laparotomy if 6 and 7 are negative, if no other extranodal site is positive, and if therapeutic decisions will depend on the identification of splenic involvement; at the end of laparotomy, one open iliac crest bone marrow biopsy can be performed

Ancillary Procedures Required Under Certain Conditions

1. Intravenous pyelography and/or inferior cavography to supplement equivocal lymphographic findings
2. Skeletal survey (thoracolumbar vertebrae, pelvis, proximal extremities) in presence of areas of bone tenderness and/or pain
3. Skeletal scintigram in presence of persisting bone pain and when skeletal roentgenogram is negative
4. Hepatic and splenic scintigrams in presence of palpable organs and when peritoneoscopy or laparotomy is not feasible
5. Gallium or bleomycin scans when the results of other conventional diagnostic procedures are not conclusive

call for a modified approach. For example, in the presence of massive mediastinal and/or hilar adenopathy producing a compressive syndrome, it is recommended that 1500 to 2000 rads be delivered in about 2 weeks in order to shrink the lymph node masses before performing lymphography and surgical abdominal exploration.

The ancillary procedures, to which upper gastrointestinal series and barium enema can be added, include a list of radiologic and radioisotopic tests which have too low a yield in Hodgkin's disease to be justifiable as routine examinations. They should be added selectively when specifically indicated either by inconclusive findings from conventional procedures or by the nature of the patient's symptoms and signs.

It should be recalled that skeletal roentgenograms for the diagnosis of metastases have well-known limitations, and only in a minority of patients can malignant bone lesions be detected when asymptomatic. I suggest that routine radiographic skeletal survey for patients with Hodgkin's disease be abandoned, and replaced by skeletal scintigraphy and specific localized radiographs of lesions demonstrated by scintiscans. The results of gallium and/or bleomycin scans cannot be used as definite evidence of Hodgkin's disease without biopsy confirmation. Finally, it is desirable to estimate the delayed hypersensitivity skin reaction by injecting natural intradermal antigens and dinitrochlorobenzene (DNCB).

The Ann Arbor staging classification specifies that both CS and PS apply only to the patient at the time of disease presentation and prior to the first treatment. Since, unfortunately, patients are still often seen after errors have been made in both staging and therapeutic management, reassessment and determination of correct stage may be helpful in selected cases. In addition, a significant number of patients come to the physician in relapse and require careful evaluation to determine further treatment strategy. Table 3 outlines the recommendations proposed at Stanford in 1972 to designate patients in relapse.

Laparoscopy and Laparotomy

The need for the laparotomy staging procedure in all patients with no overt stage IV disease on a clinical basis remains controversial. There is no doubt that through this surgical procedure, which includes splenectomy and multiple biopsies of liver and retroperitoneal and mesenteric nodes, staging accuracy and knowledge of the natural history of the disease have definitely improved. In previously untreated patients, laparotomy can detect occult splenic involvement in 20 to 30 per cent of patients with CS I and II, and in 50 to 70 per cent of those with CS III. Hodgkin's disease in the spleen is more often encountered in patients with systemic symptoms as well as in patients with unfavorable histology (mixed cellularity and lymphocytic depletion). Occult liver involvement is expected to occur in 3 to 6 per cent, positive celiac nodes in 10 to 15 per cent, and mesenteric nodes in less than 5 per cent. The comparative evaluation of radiologic-histologic findings of retroperitoneal nodes well opacified by lymphography has shown that, in experienced hands, lymphographic diagnosis is correct in more than 90 per cent of cases.

TABLE 3. **Designation for Patients in Relapse**

Local recurrence: A recurrence in an area previously treated

Regional recurrence: A recurrence outside the previously treated areas but confined to the same side of the diaphragm where disease was found initially

Transdiaphragmatic recurrence: recurrence of disease in lymph nodes (or spleen) but on the other side of the diaphragm than originally noted

Extralymphatic recurrence: Appearance of disease in extranodal or extrasplenic sites

In recent years the National Cancer Institute, Bethesda, and the Istituto Nazionale Tumori, Milan, have shown that laparoscopy (or peritoneoscopy) can replace laparotomy in establishing the diagnosis of liver involvement in a large majority of patients. In our series of 146 previously untreated patients, laparoscopy detected hepatic lymphoma in seven patients (5 per cent). Subsequent laparotomy revealed that the liver was positive in three additional patients, and in two patients systemic symptoms were present. By combining laparoscopy and needle marrow biopsy, 8 per cent of the patients were found to have stage IV disease, compared to 2 per cent of those subjected to laparotomy and open iliac crest marrow biopsy which were performed in patients with negative findings on liver and marrow by the first procedures. It is important to emphasize that in no patient with stage IA or IIA was occult hepatic lymphoma detected by both surgical procedures.

Who should undergo laparotomy with splenectomy? This procedure was first advocated and is still performed in many centers to detect occult splenic involvement, because many specialists believe that patients with Hodgkin's disease of the spleen represent a high-risk group for concomitant or subsequent hepatic and marrow disease. On this basis, laparotomy should be performed only if management decisions depend on the identification of occult abdominal disease and particularly of a positive spleen. Since a combined treatment approach, as described later, is presently suggested for many patients with Hodgkin's disease, laparotomy is becoming less important as a routine staging procedure. To detect patients with stage IV disease laparoscopy and needle marrow biopsies can substitute for laparotomy with open marrow biopsy in the large majority of patients. Therefore from the point of view of establishing occult extranodal lymphoma either in liver or marrow, laparotomy should always be preceded by the aforementioned combined procedure. Staging laparotomy probably remains a necessary procedure in CS IA and IIA, as the 5 year survival rate of patients with no occult disease below the diaphragm, treated with total or subtotal megavoltage radiotherapy alone, approaches 90 per cent. Laparotomy is also indicated in the presence of splenomegaly when radiotherapy is planned as the first treatment modality. In fact, splenectomy, besides reducing the tumor burden, avoids the risk of excessive radiation exposure to the left kidney and to the left lower lobe of the lung. Other indications for laparotomy are patients with equivocal lymphography and women asking to preserve their ovarian function during pelvic irradiation. On the other hand, clinicians should know that (1) laparotomy findings prove to be almost invariably negative when clinically the disease is confined either to the upper part of one side of the neck or to the mediastinum, especially if the histology is lymphocytic predominance or nodular sclerosis; and (2) 60 to 80 per cent of the patients with CS III were shown to have splenic involvement. This was particularly true in those with systemic symptoms and/or mixed cellularity and lymphocytic depletion histology. Thus in both groups of patients the results of laparotomy can be largely anticipated in terms of splenic involvement on the basis of past experience with surgical staging. In summary, although the definite role of staging laparotomy remains a dilemma, its use is not recommended as a routine procedure to stage Hodgkin's disease in clinical practice.

Laparotomy plus splenectomy is associated with known morbidity such as pneumococcal or *Hemophilus influenzae* sepsis (particularly in the splenectomized child), varicella zoster infection, and bowel obstruction resulting from adhesions among the intestinal loops. These findings seem to represent a further good reason for a more extensive use of laparoscopy, a consistently less traumatic procedure, in view of the fact that chemotherapy is becoming more often employed, with or without radiotherapy, regardless of positive or negative splenic involvement.

Therapy

During the past decade, the treatment of Hodgkin's disease has evolved into a fairly established strategic approach based primarily upon stage and presence or absence of systemic symptoms. However, the management of certain stages of the disease is presently in a state of flux, and this creates difficulties for the practicing physician. The knowledge that both extensive radiotherapy and combination chemotherapy when given alone have reached a plateau in the cure rate of early and late stages, respectively, has prompted a number of studies aimed at improving results in terms of both decreased relapse rate and increased survival. Unfortunately, the combined radiotherapy-chemotherapy approach is presently still in the experimental phase. Therefore only general guidelines can be provided.

Single Agent Chemotherapy. Table 4 lists the anticancer drugs most effective in Hodgkin's disease, their usual conventional dose when administered alone, the response rate observed in advanced disease, and the most important side effects. Single agent chemotherapy in Hodgkin's disease has been replaced in the past few years by combination chemotherapy because of its proved superiority in the incidence of complete remissions, duration of response, and survival. However, single agent chemotherapy can still be employed in a few circumstances, such as in elderly patients with concomitant severe illnesses, those living in isolated areas, and patients with psychologic disturbances.

Should one of the aforementioned situations occur, sequential single drug therapy can be planned. Treatment is usually started by using one of the alkylating agents (nitrogen mustard, cyclophosphamide). Chemotherapy is continued until the patient relapses or excessive toxicity occurs. Once the initial response is obtained, maintenance treatment with an oral alkylating agent is required to keep the patient in either complete or partial remission with minimal bone marrow toxicity. If and when the disease becomes

TABLE 4. **Single Agents Most Effective in Hodgkin's Disease**

NOTE: It is recommended that the administration of drugs listed in this table be under the supervision of a qualified physician experienced in their use. The manufacturer's official directive (official package circular) should be consulted for current dosage recommendations and other pertinent information before prescribing for patient's use.

DRUG	USUAL DOSE ROUTE, INTERVAL	RESPONSE RATE (%) *Overall*	*Complete Remission*	MAJOR TOXICITY
Alkylating agents				
Nitrogen mustard (Mustargen)	12–15 mg./m.² I.V. monthly	65	15	Bone marrow
Cyclophosphamide (Cytoxan, Endoxan)	1500 mg./m.² I.V. monthly 300–500 mg./m.² I.V. weekly 60–100 mg./m.² P.O. daily	55	15	Bone marrow, cystitis, alopecia
Chlorambucil (Leukeran)	3.5–8 mg./m.² P.O. daily	60	15	Bone marrow
Vinca alkaloids				
Vinblastine (Velban)	3–6 mg./m.² I.V. weekly	65	30	Bone marrow, neuropathy
Vincristine (Oncovin)	1–1.2 mg./m.² I.V. weekly	60	15	Neuropathy, constipation
Antibiotics				
Doxorubicin (Adriamycin)	60 mg./m.² I.V. q. 3 weeks	40	10	Bone marrow, alopecia, stomatitis, cardiomyopathy after 550 mg./m.²
Bleomycin (Blenoxane)	5–10 units/m.² I.V. or I.M. weekly	40	10	Fever, stomatitis, skin lesions, lung fibrosis after 200 mg./m.²
Nitrosourea derivatives				
Bis-chloroethyl-nitrosourea (Nitrumon)	150–250 mg./m.² I.V. q. 6 weeks	50	10	Bone marrow (delayed), local pain on administration
Chloroethyl-cyclohexyl-nitrosourea (Lomustine)	80–130 mg./m.² P.O. q. 6 weeks	70	20	Bone marrow (delayed)
Streptozotocin*	500 mg./m.² I.V. × 5 days q. 3 weeks 1500 mg./m.² I.V. weekly	45	6	Renal tubular acidosis, glycosuria, aminoaciduria, azotemia, hypoglycemia
Corticosteroid				
Prednisone	25–100 mg./m.² P.O. daily	60	5	Diabetes, hypertension, osteoporosis, peptic ulcer
Miscellaneous				
Procarbazine (Matulane, Natulan)	75–150 mg./m.² P.O. daily	70	20	Bone marrow
Imidazole carboxamide (Dacarbazine, DTIC)*	150–250 mg./m.² I.V. for 5 days q. 3–4 weeks	55	10	Bone marrow, local pain on administration
Epipodophyllotoxin VM 26*	30 mg./m.² I.V. daily 100 mg./m.² I.V. weekly	40	0	Bone marrow, alopecia

*Investigational—or investigational for this use.

refractory to the alkylating agents, vinblastine is tried next and then procarbazine if symptoms and signs persist or recur. When all these agents have been given an adequate trial and chemotherapy is still indicated because of further progression, one of the new antibiotics (doxorubicin hydrochloride [Adriamycin] or bleomycin) can be given. Bleomycin can be particularly useful in the presence of concomitant marrow suppression, because this drug does not produce leukopenia and thrombocytopenia. Also, vincristine and imidazole carboxamide (investigational in the United States of America) can be used in the presence of low marrow reserve, as they are moderately myelosuppressive agents. On the contrary, doxorubicin hydrochloride (Adriamycin) and both nitrosourea derivatives are potent myelosuppressive drugs. In particular, the latter compounds produce a delayed leukopenia and thrombocytopenia (about the fourth week). Adrenal steroids are administered mostly in the presence of bone marrow depression, hemolytic anemia, fever, anorexia, and cachexia. Any given drug usually produces a different response rate whether it is administered as the first chemotherapeutic agent or after previous treatment with other compounds. However, it is important to remember that there is cross-resistance only among the alkylating agents and between the two nitrosourea derivatives.

Combination Chemotherapy. The MOPP regimen (Table 5) should be considered the most simple, effective, and safe drug combination to be used in clinical practice for the primary treatment of patients with stages III and IV. The numerous combinations designed by deletion, substitution, or addition of various components of the MOPP

TABLE 5. **MOPP Regimen: Single Cycle**

DRUGS	ROUTE	DOSE (MG./M.^{2})	DAYS 1	2	3	4	5	6	7	8	9	10	11	12	13	14	15 → 28
Mustard	I.V.	6 mg.	↑							↑							No therapy
Vincristine	I.V.	1.4 mg.	↑							↑							
Procarbazine	P.O.	100 mg.	→	→	→	→	→	→	→	→	→	→	→	→	→	→	
Prednisone*	P.O.	40 mg.	→	→	→	→	→	→	→	→	→	→	→	→	→	→	

All drugs are administered in mg./m.^{2} of body surface.
*Every fourth cycle.

regimen have failed to prove their superiority when retrospectively compared to MOPP. In patients previously untreated with chemotherapy or in those relapsing from primary irradiation, the expected incidence of complete response after MOPP (disappearance of all symptoms and signs of disease with return to normal of roentgenographic, radioisotopic, and biochemical studies) approaches 80 per cent. This can usually be obtained by giving a minimum of six monthly cycles; in patients with stage IV, complete remission can be achieved irrespective of the site(s) of extranodal involvement (marrow, liver, lung). In a few patients, especially those with nodular sclerosis type, as many as 12 cycles are required before the patient can be considered in true complete remission. Once complete remission is obtained, it is advisable to administer two additional cycles of MOPP as consolidation treatment. The achievement of the status of true complete remission is the most important factor affecting the prognosis. In complete remitters, about 65 per cent continue to remain free of disease at 5 and 10 years, a length of time compatible with cure. The remaining patients relapse, usually within the first 3 years of achieving complete remission. At this point MOPP treatment can be resumed, and a second prolonged remission can be obtained in about half the patients. MOPP treatment is more effective in patients without systemic symptoms than with them. The most recent results reported by the National Cancer Institute showed that all "A" patients remained in complete remission at 5 years, compared to 60 per cent of "B" patients. Of those achieving complete remission, about 80 per cent were alive at 5 and 70 per cent at 10 years.

Remission Maintenance. Once a complete remission, confirmed by a second biopsy of pretreatment extranodal sites (e.g., liver and bone marrow) has been achieved, there seems to be no real advantage in prolonging the treatment either with the same combination or with single agents. In fact, long-term results of all available studies have failed to prove that maintenance therapy

TABLE 6. **Combination Chemotherapy Regimens in MOPP Resistant Patients**

ACRONYM	DRUGS	DOSE SCHEDULE	NEW CYCLE BEGINNING ON DAY	RESPONSE RATE(%) *Overall*	*Complete Remission*
1. ABVD	Adriamycin	25 mg./m.^{2} I.V., days 1 and 15	29	61	61
	Bleomycin	10 units/m.^{2} I.V., days 1 and 15			
	Vinblastine	6 mg./m.^{2} I.V., days 1 and 15			
	DTIC*	375 mg./m.^{2} I.V., days 1 and 15			
2. B-DOPA	Bleomycin	4 units/m.^{2} I.V., days 2 and 5	22	80	60
	DTIC	150 mg./m.^{2} I.V., days 1 to 5			
	Vincristine	1.5 mg./m.^{2} I.V., days 1 and 5			
	Prednisone	40 mg./m.^{2} I.M., days 1 and 6			
	Adriamycin	60 mg./m.^{2} I.V., day 1			
3. BVDS	Bleomycin	6 units/m.^{2} I.V., day 15	29	50	30
	Vinblastine	6 mg./m.^{2} I.V., days 1 and 15			
	Doxorubicin†	30 mg./m.^{2} I.V., day 1			
	Streptozotocin‡	1500 mg./m.^{2} I.V., days 1 and 15			
4. CVB	CCNU§	100 mg./m.^{2} P.O., day 1	29	85	26
	Vinblastine	5 mg./m.^{2} I.V., days 1 and 8			
	Bleomycin	8–10 units/m.^{2} I.M., days 1 and 8			

*DTIC: Dimethyl-triazeno-imidazole-carboxamide.
†Adriamycin.
‡Investigational.
§CCNU: Chloroethyl-cyclohexyl-nitrosourea.

definitely improves either median duration of initial remission or survival. On the contrary, prolonged maintenance therapy can increase susceptibility to infections.

Management of MOPP-Resistant Patients. It is important to know that patients relapsing after a complete remission induced by MOPP are not necessarily resistant to MOPP. Retreatment with MOPP induces a prolonged disease-free survival in 60 per cent of patients whose initial complete remission was longer than 1 year, whereas this can be achieved in about 20 per cent of those with an initial complete response of less than 12 months. Therefore an alternative treatment is indicated for patients (1) not entering the first complete remission with MOPP, (2) relapsing within 12 months from an initial complete response, or (3) showing either no response or relapse after treatment with MOPP. In recent years, many combinations were designed with the specific intent to provide a successful treatment in MOPP failures. The results of most drug regimens are still based on very few patients. Table 6 outlines the dose schedule and the reported response rate of four combinations (ABVD, B-DOPA, BVDS, and CVB) whose efficacy was tested in a number of MOPP-resistant patients. At the Istituto Nazionale Tumori, ABVD was tested both as primary and as secondary treatment. In patients not previously treated with chemotherapy, ABVD produced a comparable incidence and duration of complete remission when randomly tested with MOPP. In 18 MOPP failures, 6 cycles of ABVD produced complete remission in 11 patients (61 per cent), with a median duration in excess of 13 months and a median survival in excess of 28 months, respectively. ABVD is given every 2 weeks, and all four drugs are injected intravenously, preferably through the tubing of an intravenous infusion.

Drug Toxicity. The most prominent side effects of all drugs useful in Hodgkin's disease are listed in Table 4. Combination chemotherapy produces different side effects related to the types of drugs included in the regimen. However, prolonged intermittent multiple drug regimens, especially in untreated patients, proved to be surprisingly well tolerated, thus allowing the administration of a high percentage of optimal doses. The acute side effects are first represented by nausea and vomiting a few hours after the drug injection. Prolonged vomiting often occurs after ABVD because of doxorubicin hydrochloride (Adriamycin) and imidazole carboxamide. This can sometimes be controlled by prochlorperazine (Compazine). During MOPP treatment, patients should be advised to avoid alcohol, narcotics, tranquilizers, antihistamines, or sympathomimetic agents because of the monoamine oxidase inhibitory effect of procarbazine. Vincristine produces a typical peripheral neuropathy. If symptoms and signs are mild (loss of deep tendon reflexes, paresthesias of fingers and toes) the drug dosage need not be reduced. When occasionally foot drop and/or difficulty in ambulating or severe constipation occurs, vincristine should be temporarily discontinued. Vinblastine can produce the same pattern of toxicity, although the incidence of neuropathy is definitely less than with vincristine. This type of toxicity occurs particularly in elderly patients. All combinations produce different degrees of hair loss (MOPP, 30 per cent; ABVD, 70 per cent). In regimens including doxorubicin hydrochloride (Adriamycin) and/or bleomycin, complete alopecia is often observed. Hair loss is completely reversible once therapy is completed. Bleomycin also produces skin hyperpigmentation as well as various degrees of cutaneous thickening of palms and soles. These lesions (15 to 30 per cent) are usually irreversible. Mild oral mucositis

TABLE 7. **Dose Adjustments Recommended in Presence of Myelosuppression**

LEUKOCYTE COUNT BEFORE STARTING A NEW COURSE	PLATELET COUNT BEFORE STARTING A NEW COURSE	DOSAGE WHICH CAN BE ADMINISTERED
⩾ 4000	⩾ 130,000	100% of all drugs
3999–3000	129,000–90,000	100% of PRD, BLM, DTIC 50% of HN2, ADM, VLB, CCNU, PCZ
2999–2000	89,000–60,000	100% of PRD, BLM 50% of VCR, DTIC 25% of HN2, ADM, PCZ
1999–1500	59,000–40,000	100% of PRD, BLM 25% of VCR, DTIC
< 1500	< 40,000	100% of PRD, BLM

HN2: Nitrogen mustard; ADM: Adriamycin; VLB: vinblastine; CCNU: chloroethyl-cyclohexyl-nitrosourea; PCZ: procarbazine; VCR: vincristine; DTIC: imidazole carboxamide; BLM: bleomycin; PRD: prednisone.

can be observed in 3 to 10 per cent of patients treated with regimens including one or both antibiotics. Irregular menses are produced in 20 to 35 per cent of menstruating females. At times, cessation of menses is permanent (see also Long-Term Complications, p. 301).

One of the most important dose limiting factors is represented by hematosuppression. This requires a dose adjustment schedule (Table 7). In general, attenuation of doses is preferable to discontinuation of treatment for several weeks. Two other major dose limiting factors are caused by lung fibrosis induced by bleomycin, and by cardiomyopathy secondary to doxorubicin hydrochloride (Adriamycin). After total doses exceeding 200 mg. per square meter of body surface area bleomycin produces in 10 to 15 per cent of patients a reticulomicronodular pattern located usually at the lower lung zones and at the level of costophrenic angle. The initial signs could evolve into a coarse streaking reticulation. In more advanced stages this becomes confused with patchy infiltrates. Histology reveals the presence of hyperplasia and endoalveolar migration of type II pneumocytes and macrophages, fibrinous edema, hyaline membranes, and newly formed reticular and collagen fibers within the alveolar septa. The total incidence of cardiac failure induced by Adriamycin ranges from 1 to 2 per cent. This markedly increases (20 to 30 per cent) after cumulative doses exceeding 550 to 600 mg. per square meter. The clinical picture is usually characterized by cardiomegaly, biventricular failure associated or preceded by an increased ratio of pre-ejection period to left ventricular ejection time, and low QRS voltage. The only preventive measure consists in stopping drug administration before the cumulative dose of 550 mg. per square meter is reached. Clinicians should also be aware that a history of prior cardiovascular disease or prior radiotherapy to areas encompassing the heart are risk factors, and cardiomyopathy may occur in these instances after total doses below 450 mg. per square meter. Recent studies employing endomyocardial biopsies revealed that patients treated with more than 250 mg. per square meter may develop a focal noninflammatory myocytolytic process and that ongoing active degenerative changes occur months after cessation of therapy.

Combined Treatment. Even in theoretically optimal conditions provided by surgical staging procedures, both radiotherapy and chemotherapy, when given alone, have probably reached a plateau in their capability to cure early and advanced Hodgkin's disease. For this reason in the past few years radiotherapy and chemotherapy have been sequentially combined in an attempt to improve disease-free survival. In fact, the failure of optimal radiotherapy to obtain a long-term disease-free survival in 25 to 60 per cent of patients with Hodgkin's disease spread above and below the diaphragm and/or with constitutional symptoms is most likely due to the presence of occult foci beyond the fields of irradiation. Therefore in patients with nodal extension intensive combination chemotherapy can play an essential role in the eradication of micrometastases. The optimal sequence has not yet been determined.

We have recently employed the "sandwich" technique (MOPP, 3 cycles → radiotherapy → MOPP, 3 cycles) in patients with pathologic stages IIB, IIIA, and IIIB. Radiotherapy consisted of subtotal or total nodal irradiation with 3000 to 3500 rads. Complete remission was obtained in 80 per cent of patients (with no systemic symptoms, 100 per cent; with systemic symptoms, 71 per cent). Neither disease-free nor overall survival can be fully determined at present. However, the short-term results would indicate that this combined treatment modality is superior to optimal radiotherapy alone. Treatment was surprisingly well tolerated and was usually devoid of prolonged hematosuppression, provided that 4 to 6 week intervals were observed between the end of initial chemotherapy and the start of radiotherapy as well as between the completion of irradiation and the beginning of further chemotherapy.

Other authors have employed radiotherapy followed by 6 cycles of MOPP. In this case, some patients relapse during radiotherapy or soon thereafter, and subsequent chemotherapy is made difficult and at times impossible by prolonged marrow suppression. In those treated with the opposite sequence we have found that in about 20 per cent of patients the course of radiotherapy to the pelvic nodes had to be either discontinued or prolonged because of persisting marrow suppression. The combined treatment modality has also been recently studied in stage IV patients. In those achieving complete and partial remission greater than 75 per cent after chemotherapy (MOPP or ABVD), we have delivered, after a 4 to 6 week interval, low-dose radiotherapy (2000 to 2500 rads) to the sites of major pretreatment involvement, including lung, bone, and liver. The rationale for administering local radiotherapy stems from the observation that relapses after chemotherapy were observed to occur preferentially in areas of originally bulky disease. At the end of the irradiation program complete remission was about 90 per cent, and practically all complete responders remain continuously free of disease 3 years after completion of radiotherapy.

Practicing physicians should be aware that, at present, the combined modality as primary treatment for patients with both nodal and extranodal lymphoma should not yet be regarded as conventional therapy. Therefore this approach should be best confined to qualified centers and research institutions. In fact, the initial promising results showing a significantly decreased relapse rate must also be confirmed in terms of statistically improved overall survival. Furthermore, not enough data are available in terms of acute and delayed toxicity to make these treatments routinely available in clinical practice. It remains to be fully assessed whether vigorous and effective treatment applied at the time of first relapse after primary radiotherapy can produce survival results comparable to those being obtained with an aggressive combined modality approach at the expense of less morbidity.

Treatment of First Relapse After Irradiation. In patients relapsing from primary irradiation, a combined modality approach is almost always indicated. In particular, when the disease recurs in a treated lymph node chain, at the margin of the radiation field, or in the presence of extensions to previously untreated nodal areas (same side or opposite side of diaphragm), the recommended treatment is radiotherapy supplemented by six cycles of MOPP. In patients showing extension to spleen and/or to extranodal sites, the most useful treatment is represented by split-course MOPP chemotherapy (usually three cycles), followed after 1 month by low-dose radiotherapy (2000 to 2500 rads in 3 to 4 weeks) to regions of bulky lymphadenopathy, as well as some extranodal sites such as liver, lung, and bone, and then, after another 4 week interval, by three to six more cycles of MOPP. It should be remembered that in patients with extranodal disease prior irradiation does not decrease per se the incidence of complete responders after intensive chemotherapy when results are compared to those achieved in previously untreated patients. If marrow relapse associated with pancytopenia occurs after extensive irradiation, it is advisable to start treatment with nonmyelotoxic agents such as bleomycin, prednisone, and vincristine.

Special Therapeutic Problems. HODGKIN'S DISEASE IN CHILDREN. Treatment for children remains controversial. Patients with stages I and IIA are usually treated with 3500 to 4000 rads to mantle and para-aortic fields, whereas stage IIB, IIIB, and III_S patients are given subtotal or total nodal irradiation (3500 to 4000 rads) followed by 6 cycles of adjuvant MOPP. Recently the "sandwich" technique has been more often utilized. With this strategic approach about 90 per cent remain continuously free of disease and 95 to 98 per cent survive for 5 years without evidence of disease. However, the severity of late effects of chemotherapy and especially of radiotherapy (growth inhibitory effects) demands minimal effective treatment for Hodgkin's disease in children. Therefore in children with favorable PS IA (unilateral upper neck node, unilateral inguinal mass, any histology; mediastinal adenopathy, nodular sclerosis), involved field radiotherapy alone with 3000 to 3500 rads can probably cure at least 90 per cent of patients. In children with either an unfavorable disease presentation or PS II or III and III_S (A and B), the "sandwich" therapy (MOPP, 3 cycles → involved field radiotherapy → MOPP, 3 cycles) represents the treatment of choice. Stage IV patients are managed as described for adults. Recent information indicates that the risk of serious bacterial infections appears less related to splenectomy per se than to combined chemotherapy plus or minus radiotherapy. However, despite the fact that the overall incidence of occult splenic involvement is higher in children than in adults, splenectomy must be avoided in children under 5 years of age.

OBSTRUCTION AND COMPRESSION. These complications usually occur at the level of the superior vena cava, trachea, or ureters as a result of large adenopathies, as well as of the spinal cord because of epidural compression from extranodal disease. They are often medical emergencies, and the therapeutic decision should be made without delay. In the presence of localized disease associated with large mediastinal-hilar adenopathies producing edema of the upper trunk and dyspnea, the combination of diuretics, nitrogen mustard (10 to 12 mg. per square meter of body surface area), and full dose radiotherapy represents the treatment of choice and provides a prompt relief of symptoms. The drug should be injected through the tubing of a running intravenous infusion into a leg vein to avoid extravasation produced by retrograde venous pressure. In patients with generalized disease, combination chemotherapy is indicated. Systemic treatment can be supplemented with local radiotherapy. In patients resistant to MOPP, radiotherapy can be combined with vinblastine (10 to 12 mg. per square meter) and/or Adriamycin (25 to 50 mg. per square meter), or preferably with 1 or more cycles of a non-cross-resistant combination such as ABVD. The same strategic approach can be used in the presence of unilateral or bilateral ureteral obstruction. The treatment for rapidly progressive extradural cord compression is represented by emergency laminectomy followed by local radiotherapy and corticosteroids. In the slow progressive syndrome, surgery can be avoided if early diagnosis is made and corticosteroids, nitrogen mustard, or vinblastine plus radiotherapy are started immediately. Once the compressive syndrome is controlled, subsequent therapy is that appropriate for the patient's stage. When cranial nerves or brain stem are involved, the approach of choice is radiotherapy delivered to the base of the skull, as well as corticosteroids.

Pleural Effusion. This complication can be produced either by lymphatic obstruction in the mediastinum or by pleuropulmonary involvement of Hodgkin's disease. In the first case, appropriate radiation therapy to the mediastinum usually resolves the effusion. When cytology of the pleural fluid and/or pleural biopsy indicate the presence of visceral disease, combination chemotherapy provides the most successful treatment. In patients previously treated, repeated intrapleural instillations of nitrogen mustard (10 to 12 mg. per square meter in 20 to 30 ml. of isotonic saline solution) or bleomycin (30 to 60 units) can be attempted after maximal removal of pleural fluid. In those resistant to standard drugs, intrapleural quinacrine (Atabrine) should be administered. (This use of quinacrine is not listed in the manufacturer's official directive.) After removal of about two thirds of the fluid, the drug is instilled at a dose of 200 to 300 mg., to a total dose of 1000 to 1200 mg. Quinacrine produces fever and local tenderness.

Miscellaneous Complications. Constitutional symptoms promptly disappear as soon as the disease responds to chemotherapy or irradiation. Occasionally, indomethacin (Indocin) at a dose of 50 to 200 mg. per day is indicated to control high fever. If possible, the drug should not be administered at the time of maximal pyrexia to avoid hypotension induced by rapid abatement of fever.

Hyperuricemia produced by prompt lysis of large tumor masses can lead to uric acid nephropathy. This dangerous complication can be avoided by administering allopurinol (Zyloprim), 100 to 200 mg. four times a day, prior to and during the initial period of chemotherapy or radiotherapy; i.e., until the bulky disease is no longer present. Allopurinol can be supplemented with adequate fluid administration. Occasionally, alkalinization of the urine is required.

Coombs-positive hemolytic anemia is not rare in intermediate and advanced stages of the disease. It can be best managed by combination chemotherapy. When radiotherapy is employed, prednisone, 50 to 100 mg. a day, should be added and continued until control is achieved. Then it can be gradually tapered. Splenectomy is the treatment of choice for hypersplenism associated with pancytopenia. After removal of the spleen the tolerance to anticancer drugs is usually increased.

Long-Term Complications. The intensive treatments described have led to both increased survival and cure rates in all stages of Hodgkin's disease. Therefore it is not surprising that some long-term side effects from treatment, as observed in laboratory animals, are also being observed in humans. It is well known that practically all antitumor agents may cause structural and numerical damage to chromosomes, and that they are mutagenic, teratogenic, and carcinogenic. Fortunately many of these effects appear to be of relatively minor importance. As far as intensive radiotherapy is concerned, the risk of paramediastinal pneumonitis, pericarditis, and retarded vertebral body growth in children has been documented. The delayed toxicity of bleomycin and doxorubicin hydrochloride (Adriamycin) has been described before. The clinical sequelae of drug-induced chromosomal aberrations have not yet been well established, and the risk of cytogenetic damage does not warrant abandoning the current successful therapeutic approach. Contraception is highly recommended in patients receiving chemotherapy, thus circumventing the possible teratogenic effects of cytotoxic agents. Whenever possible, chemotherapy should be avoided during pregnancy, especially in the first trimester. Long-term chemotherapy induces sterility in at least half of men and women. This is also considered to be an acceptable risk, but it should be explained to patients before starting treatment.

The potential carcinogenicity of antitumor agents after long-term treatment continues to be the most troublesome of the various side effects observed in laboratory animals. There is an increasing number of reports of a second tumor which, with few exceptions, has been acute nonlymphocytic leukemia. There is also a suggestion that the incidence of second malignancies is higher in patients treated with combined radiotherapy-chemotherapy than in those receiving either chemotherapy or radiotherapy alone. However, the true incidence of treatment-induced neoplasms must be confirmed on a larger series of patients. On the basis of available data, it is difficult to evaluate the role of chemotherapy in this apparently increased incidence of second neoplasms. Physicians should be aware that, in general, cancer patients are at higher risk of developing a malignancy than is the general population, and that Hodgkin's disease patients possess defects in cell-mediated immunity which may favor the growth of second neoplasms. Furthermore, it is possible that acute nonlymphocytic leukemia may be a part of the natural history of Hodgkin's disease which is only recently becoming evident because of the increasing numbers of long-term survivors.

At present, the magnitude of the problem concerning the long-term complications appears limited, and not sufficient to prevent the appropriate use of effective therapeutic modalities.

HODGKIN'S DISEASE: RADIATION THERAPY

method of
LEONARD R. PROSNITZ, M.D.
New Haven, Connecticut

General Considerations

Hodgkin's disease has happily progressed from being considered uniformly fatal to being now curable in the majority of patients, even probably in those with advanced disease. It is one of the few malignant diseases for which both very effective radiotherapy and chemotherapy are available. Therapy of Hodgkin's disease is not completely settled but is rapidly evolving toward what one hopes will be the most effective type of treatment with the least complications. Often this may involve combined modality therapy—both combination chemotherapy and radiation. In this disease the multidisciplinary approach with participation of both medical oncologist and radiotherapist from the onset is particularly important and should not be just a principle to which only lip service is paid.

Clinical Evaluation and Staging

Selection of appropriate therapy is totally dependent on accurate staging of the patient. The Ann Arbor classification is the most widely accepted staging system (Table 1). In the history, particular attention should be given to the presence or absence of fever, sweats, or weight loss. Itching and alcohol pain are other generalized symptoms of interest, although not officially considered as "B" symptoms. If present initially, their reappearance after treatment almost always signifies a relapse.

TABLE 1. **Staging for Hodgkin's Disease—Ann Arbor System**

Stage I:	Involvement of a single lymph node region (I) or a single extralymphatic site (I_E).
Stage II:	Involvement of two or more lymph node regions on the same side of the diaphragm (II) or localized involvement of an extranodal site and one or more lymph node regions on the same side of the diaphragm (II_E).
Stage III:	Involvement of lymph node regions on both sides of the diaphragm (III), which may include the spleen (III_S), or localized extranodal involvement (III_E), or both (III_{SE}).
Stage IV:	Diffuse or disseminated involvement of one or more extranodal sites with or without lymph node involvement.

A and B subclasses indicate absence or presence of any of the following systemic symptoms: fever, sweats, or weight loss of 10 per cent of body weight.

CS and PS refer to clinical staging and pathologic (surgical) staging, respectively.

TABLE 2. **Laboratory Investigation of Hodgkin's Disease**

Required:
- CBC, platelets
- BUN, liver function studies, uric acid
- Chest x-ray
- Lymphangiogram
- Bone marrow aspirate and biopsy ("B" patients, stages III and IV A&B)

Optional:
- Sedimentation rate, serum copper
- Chest tomograms, IVP
- Liver-spleen scan, bone scan
- Laparotomy
- Immunologic testing
- Gallium scan
- CT scan
- Ultrasound

In addition to the usual physical examination, a number of laboratory studies are appropriate. They are listed in Table 2 as "required" and "optional." In our view a lymphangiogram is essential at present even if a laparotomy is to be done. The lymphangiogram locates suspicious nodes for the surgeon to biopsy which are often quite hard to find at laparotomy. It helps the radiotherapist in designing treatment portals. It also provides a very useful means of following abdominal lymph nodes. Bone marrow examination is usually not required in stage IA and IIA patients unless there are special clinical circumstances—e.g., an elevated alkaline phosphatase or unexplained bony pain. The yield of positive marrows in IA and IIA patients is very low—less than 1 per cent.

Among the "optional" tests laparotomy is the most important, and we believe that it should be done in the great majority of patients. Many studies have shown that stage I or II patients by all clinical and laboratory testing except laparotomy will have a 30 per cent incidence of abdominal disease when a staging exploration is done. This information is used to substantially change treatment plans.

Gallium scanning has not proved especially helpful in evaluating the abdomen because of its lack of specificity. Computerized tomography (CT) scanning and ultrasound are currently under investigation to determine their role in lymphoma staging.

Once the anatomic extent of disease is determined, the patient can then be classified in the Ann Arbor system. Some confusion exists as to the use of the "E" (extranodal) terminology. This classification was originally set up to handle patients who had localized extension of nodal disease to extranodal sites—e.g., a mediastinal mass extending into adjacent lung—but were still curable with local measures only, i.e., radiotherapy. Technically, a patient with mediastinal and neck masses and multiple pulmonary nodules would be stage II_E; but such a patient should really be called stage

IV, being incurable with radiotherapy alone. The "E" terminology should be restricted to those situations in which all the disease can safely and appropriately be treated with radiotherapy alone.

In addition to staging, the type of Hodgkin's disease should be subclassified by an experienced hematopathologist. The Rye classification into four subtypes of Hodgkin's disease—lymphocytic predominant, nodular sclerosis, mixed cellularity, and lymphocyte depletion—is the accepted one. Within a given stage it is not clear if the histopathologic type alters the prognosis. Lymphocyte predominant and nodular sclerosing types tend to occur in the earlier stages, the converse being true for mixed cellularity and lymphocyte depletion. There are also certain anatomic distributions that tend to be associated with certain histologic types, but a detailed discussion of this is beyond the scope of this article. Suffice it to say that the histologic type of Hodgkin's disease per se does not influence the choice of therapy.

Radiotherapy Techniques

When management is with radiation alone, tumoricidal doses must be used—generally 3500 to 4500 rads in 4 to 5 weeks' time, five treatments weekly. Linear accelerators are preferable to cobalt for carrying out the therapy because of the sharply defined beam edge. Extended field treatment, i.e., the use of large fields to irradiate several groups of lymph nodes in continuity, is indicated. The mantle field treats cervical, supraclavicular, infraclavicular, mediastinal, and axillary nodes to the level of the diaphragm. Individual lead blocks to protect lungs, heart, and trachea must be made. Both anterior and posterior fields are treated daily. Blood counts should be followed carefully during treatment. Our policy is to treat involved nodes to 4500 rads and clinically uninvolved areas to 3500 rads. This is accomplished by simply "shrinking" the field to cover just the involved areas after 3500 rads. We have not found a posterior spine block necessary, and it may shield tumor in the mediastinum. If the total dose is kept to the levels mentioned, the dose rate is kept at 200 rads a day or less, and both fields are treated daily, spinal cord damage is not a problem.

The commonly used abdominal fields are the para-aortic nodes and splenic pedicle ("spade" field) and the inverted Y which covers the para-aortic and pelvic nodes in continuity. There should be a 3 week rest between mantle and abdominal fields to allow for bone marrow recovery. Care must be taken to separate the abdominal field and the mantle field on the skin in order to avoid overlap at depth with possible damage resulting to the spinal cord. For the abdominal fields, doses of 3500 to 4000 rads, 150 to 200 rad fractions in 4 to 5 weeks' time, are used. Again, both the anterior and posterior fields are treated daily.

Complications of Therapy

During the course of treatment a number of *acute side reactions* are encountered, most of them relevant to the mantle field. They are listed below, along with suggestions for management:

1. Fatigue will be present in most patients. No treatment is necessary.

2. Nausea, anorexia, and vomiting occur quite variably. If nausea does occur, it typically develops an hour or so after treatment, lasts several hours, and then disappears. Antiemetics are useful, particularly when given prophylactically at the time of treatment. Diarrhea may occur with the abdominal treatment, but it is unusual.

3. Sore throat develops by the second or third week of mantle treatment and disappears after the larynx is blocked. No therapy is very helpful.

4. Dry mouth, alteration of taste, and increased dental caries are common problems, even though only some of the salivary glands are irradiated and the doses are relatively low. Good dental prophylactic measures should be carried out before radiotherapy is begun. Spontaneous recovery of taste and relief of dryness will take place in the weeks following radiation.

5. Hair loss over the occipital area of the skull and reddening of the skin of neck and shoulders are invariable accompaniments of treatment, and patients should be warned to expect them. A number of lubricating creams or ointments may be used on the skin for symptomatic relief.

6. Bone marrow depression may occur, and periodic blood counts should be obtained during treatment, but this is rarely a problem. Marrow depression may be a problem if the rest interval between mantle and abdominal field radiation is too short.

Of more significance are the following *long-term complications* that may arise. Their prevention is far more important than their treatment, as generally the latter is not helpful.

1. Radiation pneumonitis: A self-limited, irritative cough in the weeks following mantle radiation is very common. Apical lung and perihilar scarring is also very commonly seen on the chest x-ray, although usually it is not symptomatic except for the aforementioned cough. Symptomatic pneumonitis may be seen if large mediastinal masses and consequently large lung volumes are irradiated to high doses. This may be prevented by a number of measures such as careful shaping of lung blocks and split course techniques to allow the mass to shrink so that the lung blocks can be increased in size. Fortunately, in most patients the pneumonitis resolves spontaneously, although fatalities have occurred. In severe cases, corticosteroids may be used, although their value is unclear.

2. Pericarditis usually occurs in the setting of large mediastinal masses when the entire heart

receives doses of 4000 rads or more. Shrinking the field after part of the dose and reshaping the lung blocks to protect the cardiac apex are effective preventive measures. The overall incidence is 3 to 10 per cent. Spontaneous resolution is the rule, but occasionally pericardial stripping is necessary.

3. Hypothyroidism is related to both radiation and the large iodine load from lymphangiography. Changes in thyroxin and/or thyroid-stimulating hormone (TSH) levels may be seen in 30 to 50 per cent of patients, although clinical hypothyroidism is much less frequent. At present this is not preventable, but fortunately it is easily treatable with thyroid extract. The percentage of patients with chemical changes increases with time, so this complication should be looked for carefully.

4. Spinal cord damage: Transverse myelitis should be exceedingly rare if care is taken to avoid overlapping fields and if the dose levels mentioned are used. A transient radiation effect on the spinal cord (Lhermitte's sign—paresthesias in the extremities when flexing the neck) occurs in one third of patients but rarely or never progresses to permanent cord damage.

5. Growth retardation is regularly seen in children, particularly in the shoulders and clavicles following mantle field irradiation. Little can be done to prevent it. In special circumstances a smaller radiation field should be considered.

6. Reduction in fertility is a problem only when the pelvis is being irradiated. If the ovaries have been repositioned surgically, special blocks may be used to protect them. With optimal shielding, however, the ovaries will still receive 10 per cent of the tumor dose, and sterilization will occur in about 50 per cent of patients who receive a gonadal dose of 400 rads. Special testicular shields may also be constructed which will limit the dose to less than 3 per cent of the tumor dose. With gonadal doses in men below 100 rads, recovery of fertility after a number of months will usually take place.

7. Second malignancies are very rare with radiation alone but may occur in 1 to 3 per cent of patients treated with both radiation and chemotherapy.

Treatment Recommendations and Prognosis

Stage IA, IIA, II_EA (Pathologically Staged). Our treatment program for these patients is irradiation to the mantle portal and, after a rest interval of 2 to 3 weeks, radiation to the para-aortic nodes and splenic pedicle to the level of the aortic bifurcation. These portals are used regardless of the anatomic sites above the diaphragm. If there is high cervical involvement, a supplemental field may be added to cover Waldeyer's ring. In the presence of an equivocal or positive lymphangiogram despite a negative staging laparotomy, or when there is uncertainty as to the adequacy of the laparotomy, the pelvic nodes may be included.

These patients have an overall 5 year survival of 90 to 95 per cent and a 5 year relapse-free survival of 75 to 80 per cent when treated in this fashion with radiation alone. If a less extensive treatment field is used, the overall survival thus far has been about the same but a higher relapse rate is seen. Presumably in the long run this will be reflected in a decrease in overall survival. The addition of chemotherapy to a group with a 75 to 80 per cent cure rate with radiation alone does not seem justified at present.

Stage IB, IIB, II_EB (Pathologically Staged). This is a comparatively rare subgroup of patients, but it clearly does exist. The recommended treatment is total nodal irradiation—mantle and a full inverted Y field, including the pelvis. Again, a 75 to 80 per cent 5 year disease-free survival is obtained. When this type of radiation was compared with total nodal radiation and nitrogen mustard, vincristine sulfate, procarbazine, and prednisone (MOPP) chemotherapy for these patients, no differences were seen in relapse-free or overall survival.

Stage IIIA. How these patients should be treated is one of the more controversial subjects in the management of Hodgkin's disease. In our institution management with total nodal radiation alone has been unsatisfactory, as 60 per cent of stage IIIA patients so treated have relapsed within 5 years. On the other hand, one large randomized trial has shown radiation alone to be superior to MOPP chemotherapy alone; a relapse-free survival of 60 to 70 per cent at 4 years was obtained. Our recommendation is that these patients be treated by combined modality therapy, with combination chemotherapy followed by total nodal radiation. The chemotherapy should comprise 6 months of MOPP or an equivalent program. About 90 per cent of patients will have a complete response to the chemotherapy. Radiotherapy should then be given to the mantle and inverted Y fields. The dose of radiation should be reduced to 2000 to 2500 rads if there has been a good response to chemotherapy. Our experience with more advanced disease indicates that excellent local control is achieved with reduced radiation doses if the patient has received effective chemotherapy as well.

An alternative treatment for stage IIIA patients would be total nodal radiotherapy in full doses (3500 to 4500 rads), followed by 6 months of combination chemotherapy. The dose of the latter usually has to be attenuated after radiotherapy. With either one of these treatment programs, we anticipate relapse-free survivals of around 70 to 75 per cent at 5 years or perhaps longer. Other forms of treatment that have been advocated include total nodal irradiation plus liver irradiation if the spleen is involved, which it is in 75 per cent of IIIA patients. This approach has been largely confined to one institution, and good data have not been published comparing it to other treatment modalities. In our series, the liver was infrequently the site of failure when treating patients with total nodal irradiation alone.

When dealing with minimal amounts of disease below the diaphragm—e.g., a patient who is CS II/PS III on the basis of para-aortic nodes only without splenic involvement—total nodal irradiation alone probably suffices.

The precise treatment program that will result in the best cure rate with the least morbidity remains unknown for stage IIIA disease.

Stages IIIB and IV. These stages represent generalized disease and are not curable with radiotherapy alone. Primary reliance for treatment must fall on combination chemotherapy (cf. Hodgkin's Disease: Chemotherapy, pp. 293 to 301. However, radiation therapy appears to have a significant role to play in conjunction with chemotherapy. Multiple agent chemotherapy with MOPP or a comparable program will induce a complete remission in 60 to 80 per cent of stage IIIB and IV patients. Relapse rates, however, have ranged from 30 to 70 per cent. Long-term maintenance with drugs may delay the onset of relapse but does not appear to prevent it entirely.

A treatment program employing both combination chemotherapy and low dose radiotherapy (1500 to 2000 rads) to all areas of disease known to be present before the onset of chemotherapy has been found to be very effective in preventing relapse. In this program, 6 months of drug treatment are given, then low dose radiation, followed by another 4 months of drug treatment. A complete remission rate of 75 per cent has been obtained, and—more important—the relapse rate is only 10 per cent among the complete responders. The 5 year relapse-free survival of stage IIIB and IV patients treated in this fashion is 67 per cent.

The radiotherapy techniques are to treat *all* the areas involved with disease prior to initiating chemotherapy to 1500 to 2000 rads, but only the involved areas. The lone exception is the bone marrow, which, of course, cannot be radiated in its entirety. The dose rate should be 150 to 200 rads daily. Organs such as liver or lungs may be safely irradiated with 1500 rads at a rate of 150 rads per day. Modified mantle and/or inverted Y fields are used to cover the lymph nodes, depending on the pretreatment anatomic distribution of disease.

Management of Relapse and Follow-up Care

Patients who relapse following radiotherapy should be carefully restaged with the appropriate diagnostic tests that have already been described. Usually laparotomy is not indicated, particularly if it has been done on the initial staging evaluation. Patients may be assigned a staging classification with the letter R as a prefix to indicate the stage at relapse.

Relapse after radiotherapy may occur in a nodal area previously irradiated, an unirradiated nodal area, extranodal sites, or some combination of these three. Such patients should be treated as if they had generalized disease, with a program as described for the management of stage IIIB and IV disease. Even if the disease appears confined to unirradiated nodal sites, retreatment with radiotherapy alone will usually fail, with generalized disease occurring sooner or later. Treatment should commence with combination chemotherapy for a period of 6 months; low dose radiation is then given to the sites of pretreatment involvement. Even if such a site has been previously irradiated to 4000 rads, reirradiation with an additional 1500 rads usually will not present a problem. The spinal cord, however, should be protected if it has been previously treated.

Patients who relapse after radiotherapy respond to the combined modality program in the same way as previously untreated stage IIIB or IV patients. Two thirds of these patients can be rendered disease-free for prolonged periods of time and may be cured of their disease.

In order to detect relapse early, close follow-up of patients after initial radiotherapy is important. Generally, patients are seen at a minimum of every 3 months for the first 3 years after completing treatment. In addition to chest films, abdominal x-rays allow one to follow the abdominal nodes until the lymphangiogram dye is all absorbed. The sedimentation rate and serum copper are good indicators of disease activity, although somewhat nonspecific. Normal values, however, are reassuring in that they indicate that there is, in fact, no disease activity.

ACUTE LEUKEMIA IN ADULTS

method of
JANET CUTTNER, M.D.
New York, New York

When to Treat

As a general rule most patients with acute leukemia require immediate treatment. There is a subgroup of patients with acute myelogenous leukemia who have what is called "smoldering" leukemia. This entity occurs usually but not exclusively in the elderly. These patients classically present to their physicians with symptoms of anemia. The platelet count is usually low normal but rarely below 50,000 per cu. mm. The white blood count is usually elevated but not more than 50,000 per cu. mm. Bone marrow aspiration reveals less than 25 per cent myeloblasts. These patients may do well for several weeks to many months without any therapy other than an occasional blood transfusion. They should be followed and have blood counts performed every 3 to 4 weeks, and a bone marrow aspiration should be performed monthly. When progressive disease develops, as manifested by platelet counts below 50,000 per cu. mm., progressive granulocytopenia, and greater than 40 per cent blasts in the bone marrow, chemotherapy is indicated. In our experience patients who are not treated for several months but who then progress respond as well as newly diagnosed patients who are treated immediately.

Patients with acute lymphocytic leukemia rarely present in a "smoldering" form and almost always require therapy soon after the diagnosis is made.

Where to Treat

Adults with acute leukemia must be treated in hospitals that are able to adequately support the patient with platelet and granulocyte transfusions over an extended period of time, usually several weeks. The patient should be treated by a hematologist or medical oncologist, and there should be adequate nursing facilities and bacteriologic and pharmacologic support. Adequate support, especially with platelets and granulocytes, is of paramount importance in the treatment of these patients, who may be severely granulocytopenic and thrombocytopenic for several weeks until the bone marrow recovers from the aggressive chemotherapy. Centers specializing in the treatment of acute leukemia are obviously ideal for these patients to receive their initial treatment. There are some community hospitals which have fairly extensive support facilities and trained hematologist/oncologists and can give primary care to these patients.

Complications of Treatment

The most common complications of acute leukemia are bleeding and infection. It is essential that the physicians treating leukemic patients be aware of these problems and treat the patient expectantly. Complications can occur at any time, that is, from presentation until such time as the patient enters a bone marrow remission. The following complications may occur at presentation and must be treated on an emergency basis prior to induction chemotherapy.

Infection. Any patient with acute leukemia who presents with fever must be considered to have an infection and must be treated very quickly. A very careful physical examination should be performed, looking for a source of infection. Blood, urine, nose and throat, and any other appropriate cultures should be taken immediately, and a chest x-ray should be done on an emergency basis. If no source of infection is apparent, which is quite common, the patient should be treated expectantly with broad-spectrum bactericidal antibiotics. At present we have found that cephalothin (Keflin) with either gentamicin or tobramycin is a very effective combination. If Pseudomonas infection is strongly suspected or found, carbenicillin should be added. If the patient becomes afebrile, we usually continue treatment for a total of 10 days. If the blood cultures are positive, the antibiotics may be changed when sensitivities become available. If the patient remains febrile, a new search must be made for sources of infection.

Disseminated Intravascular Coagulation. The classic type of leukemia which is associated with disseminated intravascular coagulation (DIC) is acute promyelocytic leukemia. We do know, however, that DIC can be seen with other types of acute myelogenous leukemia. These patients usually present not only with petechial hemorrhages but also with large ecchymoses. They may also present with epistaxis, gingival bleeding, or retinal hemorrhages. The diagnosis is made by the finding of a low fibrinogen (less than 100 mg. per 100 ml.) and positive fibrin split products. The prothrombin time and partial thromboplastin time are usually prolonged as well. The initial treatment is low dose heparin. By that I mean 12,000 units of heparin divided into 8-hourly doses given over a 24 hour period intravenously. If the fibrinogen does not start to rise, the heparin dose can be cautiously increased by 4000 units per 24 hours. It is important to realize that the cause of DIC is the release of procoagulant material by the leukemic cells. The use of heparin is only a stopgap measure. The treatment of the leukemia is the definitive treatment of the DIC.

Leukostasis. These patients present with an initial white count greater than 100,000 per cu. mm. and have a high incidence of intracerebral bleeding. They should be treated with antileukemic chemotherapy as soon as possible. If the uric acid is within normal limits and they do not require other emergency treatment, they should be given allopurinol, 600 mg. daily, intravenous fluids, and alkalinization with bicarbonate. This is followed by treatment with cytosine arabinoside and daunorubicin which will lower the white count very quickly (see Induction Chemotherapy). If one cannot institute therapy immediately and has the facilities available to perform leukopheresis, this can be a lifesaving procedure. We have been able to mechanically remove large numbers of white cells from these patients for 1, 2, or 3 days prior to the institution of chemotherapy.

Hemorrhage. Thrombocytopenic bleeding should be treated with platelet transfusions. For the average adult the use of platelet concentrates, at least 10 units of platelets per day for several days, will be required to stop bleeding. Patients with a platelet count of 20,000 per cu. mm. or less have a high incidence of spontaneous bleeding and should receive platelet transfusions.

Urate Nephropathy. This is a rare complication prior to the institution of chemotherapy. It occurs in patients with a very elevated white blood count or with organomegaly. This has to be treated prior to the institution of any antileukemic chemotherapy. If the patient has an adequate urine output, the treatment of choice is fluids, alkalinization with bicarbonate, acetazolamide (Diamox), and allopurinol initially in a dose of 900 to 1200 mg. a day. If the patient develops renal shutdown, emergency hemodialysis should be performed and can be a lifesaving procedure. This is usually required on a very short-term basis until the allopurinol and alkalinization become effective. No patient who presents with hyperuricemia of a significant degree should receive antileukemic chemotherapy until the uric acid level is normal.

What to Do Prior to Induction Chemotherapy

All patients should receive allopurinol in a dose of 300 mg. a day. Patients who present with severe anemia should be transfused with packed red cells prior to therapy. We prefer to have a hemoglobin level of at least 9 grams per 100 ml. If the patient is thrombocytopenic and bleeding, he should receive platelet transfusions. If the patient is being treated in a center where granulocyte transfusions are available, we routinely tell a family member to mobilize other family members and/or friends to go to the blood bank to be tested, so that we will be able to give the patient donor platelets and granulocytes should this become necessary. If the patient is in a center where laminar air flow rooms are available, he should be transferred to this unit immediately upon admission so that he will not be exposed to hospital bacteria. If such a unit is not available, the patient should be treated in a single room where reverse isolation techniques can be utilized.

Induction Chemotherapy

The following treatment can be used for acute myelocytic leukemia, acute myelomonocytic leukemia, acute promyelocytic leukemia, acute monocytic leukemia, and acute erythrocytic leukemia. The use of a 7 day continuous intravenous infusion of cytosine arabinoside in a dose of 100 mg. per square meter on days 1 through 7 and daunorubicin (investigational) given as a single rapid injection at a dose of 45 mg. per square meter on days 1, 2, and 3 is a highly effective regimen. A complete remission rate between 55 and 70 per cent can be obtained with this regimen. A higher remission rate is seen in younger patients, especially those who receive maximum support during induction with platelets and granulocytes. A repeat bone marrow aspiration is performed 2 weeks after the start of induction chemotherapy, that is to say, on day 15. If the bone marrow is acellular, a repeat bone marrow aspiration is performed 5 days later. If the bone marrow aspiration is hypocellular and contains approximately 20 per cent blasts but the remainder of the marrow cells are lymphocytes, plasma cells, and normal bone marrow precursors, a repeat bone marrow should be performed in another 5 days. If the bone marrow aspiration shows a cellular marrow which contains mainly blasts, a second course of induction chemotherapy, consisting of a 5 day continuous infusion of cytosine arabinoside and 2 days of daunorubicin, is given. Approximately 50 per cent of the patients will require a second course of chemotherapy. When a complete remission is obtained, i.e., 5 per cent or less blasts in the bone marrow with good evidence of megakaryopoiesis, granulopoiesis, and erythropoiesis, and when the peripheral blood count shows a platelet count greater than 100,000 per cu. mm. and a total granulocyte count greater than 1500 per cu. mm., the patient may be discharged from the hospital and is ready for maintenance chemotherapy.

Another form of induction therapy that has been reported to give good results is a 7 day continuous infusion of cytosine arabinoside given as above, plus a 3 day course of doxorubicin hydrochloride (Adriamycin) in a dose of 30 mg. per square meter given intravenously on days 1, 2, and 3.

Acute Lymphocytic Leukemia. Induction therapy for acute lymphocytic leukemia consists of vincristine given at a dose of 2 mg. intravenously weekly for 3 weeks, plus prednisone given at a dose of 40 mg. per square meter daily for 21 days, followed by L-asparaginase (investigational) given at a dose of 500 I.U. per kg. for 10 days intravenously. A repeat bone marrow aspiration should be performed on the day prior to beginning L-asparaginase and after the completion of the course of L-asparaginase. The criteria for documenting complete remission are the same as for acute myelocytic leukemia (see above). If the patient is not in remission after this treatment, daunorubicin (investigational) in a dose of 45 mg. per square meter intravenously for 3 days, plus a second course of vincristine and prednisone in the doses outlined above, may be tried.

Supportive Care

In supportive care one must have the availability of giving red cell, platelet, and granulocyte transfusions. The patient's hemoglobin should be kept above 9 grams per 100 ml. by the use of packed red cell transfusions. Platelet transfusions should be given prophylactically to patients whose platelet count is less than 20,000 per cu. mm. If donor platelets are available, these are usually more effective than the use of platelet concentrates. The use of broad-spectrum bactericidal antibiotics should be instituted when the patient spikes a temperature of 101°F. (38.3°C.) or greater which persists for at least several hours. The most common types of infections are caused by gram-negative organisms such as *Escherichia coli* or *Pseudomonas aeruginosa.* A commonly used antibiotic combination is intravenous cephalothin (Keflin) and either gentamicin or tobramycin. If Pseudomonas infection is documented, carbenicillin is added to the regimen. If fever persists in spite of good antibiotic coverage in the presence of granulocytopenia, granulocyte transfusions are indicated. Granulocyte transfusions must be ABO compatible to the donor and recipient. Granulocyte transfusions should be given for 4 consecutive days.

If fever persists in a patient who is getting broad-spectrum antibiotics and granulocyte transfusions, one must look for other types of infections. Fungal sepsis with either *Candida albicans* or *Candida tropicalis* must be searched for. Candida infections of the mouth are common and do not require systemic therapy. Candida esophagitis causes very severe pain on swallowing both solids and liquids. If esophagoscopy is performed, one can see fungal plaques in the esophagus. Candida esophagitis can be treated with great success with a short course of intravenous amphotericin B. If a systemic infection with Candida is documented, a longer course of amphotericin B is indicated. Another fungal infection that can be seen in this group of patients is caused by Aspergillus. These patients usually have a pneumonia, and the diagnosis can usually be made only by a lung biopsy. The treatment is very difficult, but intravenous amphotericin B plus rifampin appears to show promise.

Maintenance Therapy

Maintenance treatment of acute myelocytic leukemia (AML) consists of monthly 5 day courses of cytosine arabinoside in a dose of 100 mg. per square meter given subcutaneously every 12 hours for ten doses. In addition in the first month the patients will receive 6-thioguanine in a dose of 100 mg. per square meter by mouth every 12 hours for ten doses. On alternate months they will receive vincristine, 2 mg. intravenously on the first day of maintenance, and then dexamethasone, 8 mg. per square meter not to exceed 16 mg. orally on days 1 through 5. Daunorubicin (investigational) in a dose of 45 mg. per square meter on the first 2 days of maintenance is given in addition to the cytosine arabinoside on the third, seventh, and eleventh courses of maintenance chemotherapy. Doses of chemotherapy may have to be reduced if severe granulocytopenia or thrombocytopenia is produced with the aforementioned dose. One must first reduce the dose by 75 per cent and then by 50 per cent if necessary. A maintenance course should be delayed until the platelet count is 100,000 per cu. mm. and the absolute granulocyte count is greater than 1500 per cu. mm. A bone marrow aspiration should be performed prior to maintenance every month for at least the first year and then every 2 months. Both 6-thioguanine and cytosine arabinoside can cause liver function abnormalities, and initially at least this will have to be distinguished from hepatitis that the patient may have got from blood, platelet, and granulocyte transfusions received during induction. Dose reductions are in order if liver function abnormalities are found with these drugs. This may include giving courses of chemotherapy every other month instead of monthly.

The use of immunotherapy in the form of MER, which is the methanol extraction residue of bacille Calmette Guérin (BCG), is under investigation. These vaccines are given in addition to the chemotherapy. Recent evidence, which must be considered preliminary at present, indicates that MER may be an important adjuvant therapy in AML. MER is given as an intradermal injection; it can produce fever, chills, and ulceration that heals with scar formation. MER is given intracutaneously in five sites, which are usually the upper extremities, dorsal surface of the thighs, and the anterior chest in the midaxillary line. The patient is given five subcutaneous injections of 200 micrograms each. MER has an advantage over BCG in that it is a killed vaccine, and because of this there are no changes in potency.

All patients with acute lymphocytic leukemia (ALL) should receive central nervous system prophylaxis in the form of intrathecal methotrexate given immediately after induction and weekly for 3 more weeks, plus cranial radiation in a dose of 2400 R. The dose of intrathecal methotrexate is 12 mg. per square meter, not to exceed 15 mg. The methotrexate is diluted with either Elliot's B solution or Ringer's lactate. A volume of cerebrospinal fluid equal to the volume of methotrexate to be instilled should be removed just prior to the instillation of the methotrexate. The maintenance therapy consists of daily 6-mercaptopurine (6MP) in a dose of 90 mg. per square meter, plus weekly oral methotrexate (MTX) in a dose of 15 mg. per square meter. In addition, patients should receive reinforcement therapy consisting of monthly vincristine in a dose of 2 mg. intravenously, plus 7 days of prednisone in a dose of 40 mg. per square meter. An alternative maintenance therapy would be 5 day courses of oral 6MP in a dose of 200 mg. per square meter. This is followed by a 9 day rest period, and then a second course is given, followed by a 9 day rest period. This alternates with two 5 day courses of methotrexate in a dose of 7.5 mg. per square meter for 5 days again with a 9 day rest period and a repeat course of methotrexate. Every 8 weeks' reinforcement is given with 2 weekly injections of vincristine and 14 days of prednisone.

Complications

The most common complication in ALL is central nervous system leukemia. It is heralded by the presence of headaches, nausea and vomiting, and the finding of papilledema. The treatment is intrathecal methotrexate in the same doses as previously described. The intrathecal methotrexate is usually given every 4 days until there is clearing of the blasts in the cerebrospinal fluid. Once this complication is under control, intrathecal methotrexate should be given every 4 weeks in addition to the maintenance chemotherapy. Central nervous system leukemia is not common in acute myelocytic leukemia. If it occurs, the treatment of choice would be intrathecal cytosine arabinoside in a dose of 30 mg. per square meter, not to exceed 50 mg. every 4 days until there is clearing of the blast cells in the cerebrospinal fluid, and then monthly. (The use of intrathecal cytosine arabinoside is not listed in the manufacturer's official directive.) Another complication which is seen mainly in acute lymphocytic leukemia is testicular infiltration. The diagnosis is made by testicular biopsy. The treatment is either orchiectomy or radiotherapy. Skin infiltration can be seen with either ALL or AML, but is more common with ALL. Again the diagnosis is made by a skin biopsy. Skin infiltration usually responds to treatment with either radiotherapy or systemic chemotherapy.

Postrelapse Therapy

In acute lymphocytic leukemia a second remission can frequently be obtained with either vincristine and prednisone or vincristine, prednisone, and daunorubicin (investigational) in the doses described for induction therapy. Maintenance therapy with cytosine arabinoside and cyclophosphamide can then be used. In acute myelocytic leukemia repeat induction therapy with cytosine arabinoside and daunorubicin can be tried if the patient has not received more than a total dose of daunorubicin of 450 mg. per square meter. This will result in a second remission in approximately 20 per cent of the patients. If the patient is being treated in a research center, at this stage the patient would be offered treatment with one of the newer Phase I or Phase II drugs.

ACUTE CHILDHOOD LEUKEMIA*

method of
RONALD L. CHARD, Jr., M.D.,
JOHN R. HARTMANN, M.D.,
IRWIN D. BERNSTEIN, M.D.,
W. ARCHIE BLEYER, M.D.,
and F. LEONARD JOHNSON, M.D.
Seattle, Washington

The prognosis of acute leukemia in children has improved markedly over the past decade. In acute lymphoblastic leukemia (ALL) 90 to 95 per cent of children achieve a remission, at least 50 per cent are surviving 3 to 5 years relapse-free, and very possibly 80 per cent of these may be cured. In acute nonlymphocytic leukemia (ANLL; i.e., acute myeloblastic and its variants) 70 to 80 per cent of the patients can be expected to achieve a remission. Median remission durations are from 12 to 14 months, and only 15 to 20 per cent are surviving 5 years relapse-free.

This success has greatly increased the physician's responsibility. Cure, not palliation, is the goal. Early diagnosis, adequate staging, and a prompt aggressive approach with multidisciplinary therapy are mandatory to achieve these results.

There are many factors responsible for these improvements. First has been the recognition of biologic sanctuaries of leukemic cells such as the central nervous system. This has led to effective presymptomatic therapy of the central nervous system, which in ALL has reduced this complication from 50 per cent to less than 10 per cent. Second and third, two of the more important factors, are aggressive multiple-agent chemotherapy and prompt and intelligent use of supportive

*Some agents mentioned in this article are considered investigational. Before using any of the drugs mentioned, the physician should be well informed of their actions and of the information in the manufacturer's official directives.

therapy for the prevention of infection, bleeding, and hyperuricemia. Fourth has been an increasing overall awareness that the initial diagnosis, treatment, and total-therapy planning are best done in a center specializing in the care of children with malignant disease. Following this the referring physician is all important in delivering much of the follow-up care, including the administration of and monitoring of the maintenance treatment, with guidance from the center. In this way the child and parents have the benefit of being in their own home and community. Fifth is the observation that front-end prognostic factors, age and initial white blood count, are strong determinants of treatment results. This has led to the development in ALL of different treatment programs for these different prognostic groups of patients dependent on these factors.

It is important to remember that early death, in the first few weeks, does not occur because of lack of response to therapy, but because of the early complications of the disease: hemorrhage secondary to thrombocytopenia, infection secondary to granulocytopenia, and metabolic disorders secondary to a large tumor cell burden. Management of these problems will be discussed before going on to specific antileukemic therapy.

Essential Supportive Care

Bleeding. The threat of severe hemorrhage is usually present during the first 7 to 21 days of treatment. This is most commonly due to thrombocytopenia. A few patients will also have disseminated intravascular coagulation, but usually this is of only a few days' duration. Because some degree of thrombocytopenia will occur during induction therapy, aspirin should be assiduously avoided. As thrombocytopenia is usually of short duration—1 to 3 weeks—aggressive use of platelet transfusions is advised. We routinely administer platelet transfusions when the platelet count falls to less than 15,000 per cu. mm. or with any sign of clinical bleeding. Six units per square meter is an adequate dose level to follow, or one can estimate the requirement on an expected rise in the platelet count of 12,000 per unit per square meter.

In the use of packed red blood cells, 10 to 15 ml. per kg. is the proper volume for a single transfusion in the nonbleeding patient. In the patient with severe anemia (hemoglobin 6.0 or less), 5 to 7 ml. per kg. should be used for the initial transfusion to prevent volume overload and congestive heart failure.

Infection. Infection and/or severe fever to 39°C. (102.5°F.) or more in a newly diagnosed, agranulocytic leukemic child is an emergency. Treating the patient is much easier than documenting the infection. We advocate immediate cultures of blood, urine, stool, throat, and cerebrospinal fluid (CSF) if indicated, and then the prompt institution of broad-spectrum intravenous antibiotics: carbenicillin, 500 mg. per kg. per day, one fourth every 6 hours; gentamicin or tobramycin, 5 mg. per kg. per day, one third every 8 hours; and a cephalosporin (cephalothin or cefazolin), 150 to 200 mg. per kg. per day, one fourth every 6 hours. This combination should cover all the gram-positive, most gram-negative (especially Pseudomonas), and some anaerobic bacteria. If the cultures are negative and there is little change in the febrile course, the antibiotics are stopped after 4 days. If the cultures are negative but there is a rapid defervescence with no return of fever, all antibiotics are continued for a minimum of 7 days. If the cultures are positive, appropriate specific therapy is instituted and must be continued for a minimum of 7 days with intravenous therapy.

Metabolic Complications. Many patients will have an elevated serum uric acid at the time of diagnosis. The production and excretion of large amounts of uric acid may occur with the institution of antileukemic therapy producing renal failure if the physician is not aware of this problem. This can be prevented by (1) hydration to a state of diuresis; (2) allopurinol, 200 to 400 mg. per square meter per day divided into three daily oral doses; and (3) alkalinization of the urine with sodium bicarbonate, 150 mEq. per square meter per 24 hours, to increase the solubility of uric acid. Hyperkalemia also occurs with leukemic cell breakdown, and it is essential to monitor the patient's potassium during the initial days of therapy. Cell destruction also produces increased phosphate levels, which, along with alkalinization of the urine, leads to hypocalcemia, presenting as neurologic disturbance and tetany. If this should occur, prompt discontinuation of sodium bicarbonate is indicated as well as careful administration of a 10 per cent calcium gluconate infusion.

SPECIFIC ANTILEUKEMIC THERAPY

Acute Lymphocytic Leukemia

Prognostic Factors. Multivariant analysis of a study conducted by the Children's Cancer Study Group from 1972 to 1975 has now confirmed the relationship of age and initial WBC with prognosis. Six hundred and eleven children received the same induction therapy and were stratified by initial WBC for CNS randomization treatment, and then all received the same maintenance therapy. Induction utilized prednisone, vincristine, and L-asparaginase. The

CNS treatment phase indicated that intrathecal methotrexate alone, as used in this program, was inferior to any arm utilizing radiation therapy and that cranial radiation, 2400 rads, plus intrathecal (IT) methotrexate was as effective as craniospinal radiation in prevention of CNS relapse and less toxic to the marrow. Maintenance consisted of daily 6-mercaptopurine, weekly oral methotrexate, and monthly pulses of 5 days of prednisone with a single dose of vincristine. Multivariant life-table analysis indicated three distinct groups of patients from their response to this program:

1. Low risk: Age at diagnosis, 3 to 7 years; WBC at diagnosis, <10,000 per cu. mm. Ninety per cent of 175 patients are surviving, and 75 per cent have never relapsed at 40 months from diagnosis.

2. Average risk: Age, 3 to 7 years; WBC, 10,000 to 50,000 per cu. mm. Age, <3 years and ≥7 years; WBC <50,000 per cu. mm. Seventy per cent of 330 patients are surviving; 60 per cent have never relapsed at 40 months from diagnosis.

3. High risk: All patients regardless of age, WBC >50,000 per cu. mm. Of 106 patients, 39 per cent are surviving and only 36 per cent have never relapsed at 40 months from diagnosis.

A subsequent study by the Children's Cancer Study Group, started in January 1975 and closed in February 1977, involving 796 patients is showing the same three groups of patients by response at 20 months of follow-up.

Various other factors such as organomegaly, lymphadenopathy, and mediastinal mass have been reported to correlate with prognosis. In the Children's Cancer Group study, the presence of a mediastinal mass did not add significantly to the predictive value of WBC and age alone. Cell size and cytochemical stain characteristics have been felt by some to have prognostic effect; others have shown no effect. Cell surface markers have now also been shown to be definite prognostic indicators. Patients whose leukemic cells express T and B cell surface markers do poorly. Those with no identifying cell surface markers (null cells) usually do well. It has not yet been shown whether the cell surface marker overrides the initial WBC and age as prognostic factors. This is currently under study.

Therapy. It is clear that not all children with ALL should be treated in the same manner. Low risk patients should be treated with minimum effective therapy. Average risk patients require more intensive therapy. In the high risk group experimental approaches with intensive multiagent chemotherapy will be necessary to improve remission duration and survival. In all patients, however, the general strategy of therapy is similar. An initial induction phase is necessary to reduce the leukemic cell population to the point at which all signs and symptoms associated with leukemia disappear and normal function and hematologic status return. The finding that over 50 per cent of patients induced into and maintained in bone marrow remission for over 18 months develop central nervous system leukemia has led to routine presymptomatic or adjuvant treatment of the craniospinal axis after remission has been successfully induced. A study by the Children's Cancer Study Group in a large number of patients has confirmed that craniospinal irradiation and cranial irradiation plus intrathecal methotrexate are equally effective in reducing the incidence of central nervous system relapse during hematologic remission to less than 7 per cent. After successful induction into remission and adjuvant central nervous system therapy are completed, it is necessary to maintain the patient on multiagent chemotherapy for between 3 and 5 years to prevent leukemic relapse. The ideal duration of maintenance therapy is yet to be determined, but preliminary studies suggest that continuation of therapy beyond 3 to 5 years of continuous complete remission does not alter overall relapse rates and has the disadvantage of prolonging drug-related toxicity. It is our own practice (if the patient is not on a study) to continue therapy for 5 years. Seventy to 80 per cent of patients who have therapy discontinued after 3 or more disease-free years will remain in remission indefinitely and are, it is hoped, cured.

Therapy, outlined in Table 1 for the three different groups of patients that have been identified, will be briefly discussed.

Low Risk Group. 1. Induction with daily prednisone, weekly intravenous vincristine, and three times per week intramuscular L-asparaginase for nine doses. L-Asparaginase is added to prednisone and vincristine because it increased the induction rate from 86 per cent to 94 per cent, which was statistically significant, in a large group of patients studied by the Children's Cancer Study group. There is also evidence that its addition prolongs remission duration. In addition, intrathecal methotrexate, 12 mg. per square meter, is given with the initial diagnostic tap and again on days 15 and 29. It is recommended that all patients have a spinal tap at diagnosis to rule out CNS involvement at that time. Toxicity of a single dose of intrathecal methotrexate every 2 weeks should be minimal during induction therapy and may further decrease development of this complication later. On day 29 a bone marrow is done, and, if in remission, the central nervous system prophylaxis is started.

2. Central nervous system prophylaxis: Pred-

TABLE 1. **Treatment of Acute Lymphoblastic Leukemia**

	LOW RISK	AVERAGE RISK		HIGH RISK
	Age 3–7 yrs. WBC <10,000/cu. mm.	Age 3–7 yrs. WBC 10,000–50,000/cu. mm.	Age <3 ≥7 WBC <50,000/cu. mm.	All ages WBC >50,000/cu. mm.
Remission induction (29 days)	Prednisone, 40 mg./m.^{2} P.O. q.d. days 1–29 Vincristine, 1.5 mg./m.^{2} I.V. days 1, 8, 15, 22 (maximum 2.0 mg.) L-Asparaginase, 6000 I.U./m.^{2} I.M. days 3, 5, 7, 10, 12, 14, 17, 19, 21 Intrathecal methotrexate, 12 mg./m.^{2} days 1, 15, 29 (maximum 12 mg.)	Prednisone, vincristine, and L-asparaginase as in low risk and added cyclophosphamide (Cytoxan), 100 mg./m.^{2} P.O. q.d. days 1–29		See text
Central nervous system prophylaxis (29 days)	Cranial radiation, 2400 rads in 12 treatments Intrathecal methotrexate, 12 mg./m.^{2} on days 8, 15, and 22 Prednisone, taper over 10 days 6-Mercaptopurine, 75 mg./m.^{2}/day			
Maintenance	6-Mercaptopurine, 75 mg./m.^{2} P.O. q.d. Methotrexate, 20 mg./m.^{2} P.O. weekly Vincristine, 1.5 mg./m^2 I.V. every 28 days (maximum 2.0 mg.) Prednisone, 40 mg./m.^{2} P.O. daily for 5 days after vincristine	Alternating courses of POMP and POCA for 1 year (see text), then maintenance as in low risk group		See text

nisone is tapered over 10 to 14 days. Daily 6-mercaptopurine, 75 mg. per square meter, is started. Intrathecal methotrexate, 12 mg. per square meter, is continued, but now on a weekly basis (i.e., days 8, 15, and 22 of CNS prophylaxis or days 36, 43, and 50 from time of starting induction therapy). Cranial radiation to 2400 rads is begun. This is usually well tolerated at a dose fraction of 150 to 200 rads per day.

3. Maintenance therapy: Two weeks from completion of CNS therapy or 1 week from the last intrathecal methotrexate injection, maintenance begins. Daily 6-mercaptopurine is continued, and weekly oral methotrexate, 20 mg. per square meter per dose, is started. The patient also receives his first dose of maintenance every-28-day vincristine, 1.5 mg. per square meter intravenously, and 5 days of oral prednisone, 40 mg. per square meter per day, with abrupt discontinuation. The patient receives monthly prednisone and vincristine for 12 months, and then this is discontinued. After this, remission is maintained with daily oral 6-mercaptopurine and weekly oral methotrexate. The most recent study by the Children's Cancer Study Group indicates that at least in this group of patients 1 year of pulse doses of prednisone and vincristine is as good as 3 years. The duration that maintenance therapy should be continued is unknown at this time, but it is fairly clear that a total of 3 years of continuous maintenance is the minimum. Studies are now underway to try to answer this difficult question; it is hoped that by 1980 a more definitive answer will be available.

AVERAGE RISK GROUP. 1. Induction is the same as that for the low risk patients; i.e., prednisone, vincristine, L-asparaginase, and intrathecal methotrexate.

2. Central nervous system prophylaxis is also the same as in the low risk patients; i.e., discontinuation of prednisone, starting daily 6-mercaptopurine with weekly intrathecal methotrexate for three doses and cranial radiation at 2400 rads.

3. Maintenance therapy: Only 60 per cent of the average risk patients remained relapse-free at 40 months on daily 6-mercaptopurine, weekly oral methotrexate, and monthly pulses of prednisone and vincristine. In an attempt to improve this result a change has been made in the first year of maintenance therapy for this group of patients. Two weeks following completion of prophylaxis

therapy patients will receive alternating courses of prednisone, vincristine, methotrexate, and 6-mercaptopurine (POMP) and prednisone, vincristine, cytosine arabinoside, and doxorubicin (Adriamycin) (POCA). Treatment is initiated with two 14 day courses of POMP (prednisone, 40 mg. per square meter orally on days 1 through 4; vincristine, 1.5 mg. per square meter intravenously on day 1 [maximum 2.0 mg.]; methotrexate, 5 mg. per square meter orally on days 1 through 4; and 6-mercaptopurine, 500 mg. per square meter orally on days 1 through 4, followed by a 10 day rest), followed by two 21 day courses of POCA (prednisone, 40 mg. per square meter orally on days 1 through 4; vincristine, 1.5 mg. per square meter intravenously on day 1 [maximum 2.0 mg.]; cytosine arabinoside, 100 mg. per square meter on days 1 through 4; and doxorubicin [Adriamycin], 40 mg. per square meter intravenously on day 1; the 4 days of treatment are followed by a 17 day rest). Then alternating cycles of two courses of POMP and two courses of POCA are given until the patient has received a total of five cycles of each combination. Ideally, this program should take 50 weeks, but interruptions in therapy caused by myelosuppression, infection, or other complications may delay its completion. After the five cycles of each combination are given, the patient is placed on the low risk maintenance regimen shown in Table 1. (*Note:* Physicians using the aforementioned agents and others mentioned in this article should be well informed of the action of these drugs before use and should be familiar with the information in the manufacturers' official directives.)

In a recent study by the Children's Cancer Study Group utilizing this program versus daily 6-mercaptopurine, weekly methotrexate, and monthly prednisone and vincristine in patients with an initial WBC greater than 20,000, although the POMP-POCA program was not significantly superior at the end of 1 year, preliminary results during the second year of maintenance are indicating that the POMP-POCA patients are experiencing fewer relapses.

High Risk Group. Treatment results in this group of patients when using previous leukemia programs have been unsatisfactory as already described. Our feeling is that patients with an initial WBC greater than 50,000 and positive cell surface markers, either T or B cells, should be considered and treated as having a diffuse lymphoma. The best treatment program for disseminated lymphoma to date is the Sloan-Kettering LSA_2-L_2 protocol, which utilizes an induction of prednisone, vincristine, daunomycin, high-dose cyclophosphamide (Cytoxan), and radiation therapy to lesions greater than 5 cm.; consolidation with cytosine arabinoside and 6-thioguanine; and then intensive therapy with L-asparaginase. The maintenance program involves cycles of (1) 6-thioguanine plus Cytoxan→ (2) hydroxyurea plus daunomycin→ (3) oral methotrexate plus CCNU or BCNU→ (4) cytosine arabinoside plus vincristine→(5) intrathecal methotrexate→ back to cycle No. 1. Studies are now underway by several cooperative groups and cancer centers in which this program is randomly being studied versus programs utilizing multiple doses of high dose cyclophosphamide and high dose methotrexate infusions with citrovorum rescue for childhood lymphomas and high risk leukemia patients. It is our strong recommendation that all these patients be referred to a treatment center because of the increased treatment toxicities necessary to achieve satisfactory results, and because of the need for *all* these patients to be available to cooperative groups and centers, so that new information leading to improvements in treatment and further staging can be obtained as rapidly as possible.

It is beyond the scope of this article to discuss the treatment of bone marrow relapse, central nervous system leukemia, and extramedullary relapse (gonads, kidneys). However, it should be pointed out that recurrence of leukemia is by far the worst prognostic factor known, and patients who relapse should be treated in consultation with an experienced pediatric oncologist.

Acute Nonlymphocytic Leukemia (ANLL) (Acute Myelocytic, Monomyelocytic, Monocytic, Histiocytic, and Erythrocytic)

Although lagging far behind results in ALL, definite improvements have been made in both induction rate and remission duration in childhood ANLL. This has been accomplished by the use of multiple drug induction programs. Early death from hemorrhage and infection is more common in this disease than in ALL because of the necessary marked increase in marrow aplasia produced by induction treatment. As initial supportive therapy needs are much greater and required for a longer period of time, before embarking on such a course of therapy one must be certain of the ready availability of component blood replacement facilities, especially platelets, and expertise in handling infection in the agranulocytic patient.

Prognostic factors also appear to be important in this disease. A recent study by the Children's Cancer Study Group confirmed that patients with an initial WBC less than 20,000 have a significantly higher induction rate than patients with an initial WBC greater than 20,000.

Therapy. 1. The most effective induction program so far utilized by the Children's Cancer Study Group utilizes a five drug induction program called "D-ZAPO": daunomycin, 30 mg. per square meter intravenously days 1, 2, and 3; 5-azacytidine, 50 mg. per square meter intravenously every 12 hours for eight doses or 100 mg. per square meter per day for 4 days; cytosine arabinoside, 25 mg. per square meter intravenously every 8 hours for 12 doses or 75 mg. per square meter for 4 days; vincristine, 1.5 mg. per square meter intravenously on day 1; and prednisone, 40 mg. per square meter per day orally or intravenously for 4 days in three daily divided doses. This five drug cycle is repeated every 14 days for four courses. It has produced a complete remission rate of approximately 75 per cent.

2. Remission is then maintained with daily oral 6-thioguanine, 75 mg. per square meter per day, and every-28-day 4 day pulses of cytosine arabinoside, 75 mg. per square meter intravenously or subcutaneously, plus 5-azacytidine, 100 mg. per square meter per day subcutaneously or intravenously, and vincristine, 1.5 mg. per square meter intravenously on the first day of each pulse. One must pay close attention to the patient's WBC and platelet count for 1 to 2 weeks following each pulse of maintenance therapy, as significant thrombocytopenia (platelet count less than 100,000 per cu. mm.) and/or neutropenia (absolute granulocyte count less than 1000 per cu. mm.) can and does occur. If this occurs, the daily 6-thioguanine should be discontinued until the platelet count is greater than 100,000 per cu. mm. and the absolute granulocyte count greater than 1000 per cu. mm. In two consecutive studies by the Children's Cancer Study Group, the replacement of cyclophosphamide by 5-azacytidine in induction and remission and the addition of daunomycin to the other four agents in induction has given superior results. With this remission therapy one can expect a median remission of 12 to 14 months and a relapse-free survival at 3 and 5 years of 20 per cent and 15 per cent, respectively.

Because of these improved, although still disappointing, long-term results and the recent reports of the relative success of bone marrow transplantation in patients with ANLL who have failed chemotherapy and have a red cell ABO and white cell Human Leukocyte Antigen identical sibling, a study is now under development to use bone marrow transplantation during first remission in the child with ANLL who has a donor. In those patients with an appropriate sibling match, we are comparing transplantation with conventional chemotherapy for quality of survival. Every patient with this disease should be referred to a center and ABO, HLA, Mixed Leukocyte Culture family blood typing done as early as possible to establish whether bone marrow transplantation may be considered.

Prognostic factors also appear important for remission duration. In a recent study by the Children's Cancer Study Group, females had significantly longer remissions than males, patients with initial WBC of less than 20,000 per cu. mm. had significantly longer remissions than those with initial WBC greater than 20,000 per cu. mm., and children between the ages of 5 and 10 years did significantly better than those less than 5 years or older than 10 years.

Immunotherapy, using various immune stimulants (BCG, MER, C-Parvum) with or without leukemia cells, is now being evaluated for ability to increase remission duration when added to chemotherapy treatment for childhood ANLL. Results of small nonrandomized trials have suggested some effect, but to date larger randomized controlled trials have not confirmed these earlier reports.

Psychological Support

The emotional impact of the diagnosis of leukemia is devastating to a family. Frequently, after the name leukemia is mentioned, little else is recalled in the initial discussions of the prognosis and treatment. It is very important to remember that every phase of the discussion about the illness, its treatment, and side effects must be repeated many times before parents really begin to understand. We have found that it is extremely important to tell the patient the name of the diagnosis and the positive things that can be done. The patient is always informed of side effects of the drugs so that symptoms caused by therapy are not thought to be due to worsening disease. After the disease and its treatment have been discussed with the patient, we believe it is best to discuss the disease thereafter only at the patient's request and not to introduce the subject spontaneously. The patient's as well as the family's questions are always answered frankly and truthfully. Children should always be informed as to whether there will be any pain with any procedure before the procedure is done. In this manner the patient as well as the family rapidly develops trust and confidence in the physician. We have found that the assistance of nurses, social workers, psychiatrists, and hospital chaplain has been essential in the total care of the psychosocial management of these patients and their families. Parent groups have also been shown to be of great assistance in many instances.

The patient and parents, as well as the physician, must be fully aware of drug toxicities. Listed in Table 2 are the drugs discussed and their major side effects.

TABLE 2. **Major Side Effects of Antileukemic Agents**

DRUG	TOXICITY
Prednisone	Hypertension Peptic ulceration Excessive weight gain Diabetes
Vincristine (Oncovin)	Neurotoxicity Alopecia Tissue necrosis with extravasation
L-Asparaginase	Allergic reaction Liver Pancreatitis Coagulation problems
6-Mercaptopurine	Marrow suppression Liver
Methotrexate	Marrow suppression Liver Gastrointestinal ulceration Pulmonary infiltration
Cytosine arabinoside (Cytosar)	Marrow suppression Nausea and vomiting Mucositis
5-Azacytidine	Marrow suppression Nausea and vomiting Liver Dermatitis
6-Thioguanine	Marrow suppression Gastrointestinal Liver
Daunorubicin (daunomycin) and doxorubicin (Adriamycin)	Marrow suppression Nausea and vomiting Cardiac Mucositis Tissue necrosis with extravasation
Cyclophosphamide (Cytoxan)	Marrow suppression Nausea and vomiting Hemorrhagic cystitis

THE CHRONIC LEUKEMIAS

method of
ARTHUR SAWITSKY, M.D.,
and KANTI R. RAI, M.D.
New Hyde Park, New York

Introduction

Survival data in the chronic leukemias have not changed materially for the past 50 years, and the median survival in chronic myeloid leukemia (CML) is still 30 months, whereas that of chronic lymphocytic leukemia (CLL) is generally reported to be about 70 months. However, the survival curve is not symmetrical, and an appreciable number of long-term survivors, even to 10 to 20 years, tends to blunt the impact of early death in half of these patients. These data suggest that differing biologic sets or populations of patients must exist within the overall groups called CML and CLL. Such a consideration makes it necessary to use a staging or clinical classification system so that the treatment plan may include evaluation of biologic differences within each of these diseases, thereby enabling individualized treatment planning.

Chronic Lymphocytic Leukemia

The diagnosis of CLL is not considered difficult; it is based upon the presence of abnormally high numbers of lymphocytes in the peripheral blood and bone marrow. Prolymphocytic leukemia, leukemic reticuloendotheliosis (hairy cell leukemia), and chronic lymphosarcoma cell leukemia have been recognized as separate clinical entities and are excluded from the group we call CLL.

Clinical Staging of CLL. From a study of a large number of patients with CLL, we have found that survival can be correlated with a few simple clinical signs. Patients who were diagnosed to have CLL because of peripheral blood and bone marrow lymphocytosis alone were called Stage 0 and had a median survival time of 12 years; those with lymphocytosis and palpable lymphadenopathy were called Stage I and had a median survival time of 8 years; those with lymphocytosis and hepatic and/or splenic enlargement were called Stage II and had a median survival time of 6 years. Patients with lymphocytosis and a hemoglobin of 11 grams per dl. (100 ml.) or less were called Stage III, and those patients whose platelets were below 100,000 per microliter were called Stage IV. The median survival for these Stage III and IV patients was 1.5 years.

Approach to Therapy Utilizing the Staging System. Since no single therapeutic schedule has been shown to increase the duration of survival in patients with CLL (although many different ones have enthusiastic proponents), there has been understandable reluctance to treat patients with CLL aggressively. However, the use of clinical staging techniques, to separate patient groups into expected short-term (Stages III and IV) and long-term survivors (Stages I and II), allows for some meaningful comparisons and evaluation of the proposed treatments in biologically homogeneous populations of patients. In addition, clinical staging is of value in recognizing Stage 0 patients, who have an expected median survival of 12 years. These patients should not be treated regardless of the demonstrated lymphocytosis. Treatment should be considered for patients with clinical progression to Stage I or beyond. All patients in Stage III or IV are candidates for active treatment, even though their symptoms might be minimal at the time of observation. Using a staging technique similar to the one we have described provides a more defined guide for approaches to therapy than the vague classification of benign and aggressive disease. The latter description of clinical status plays a more helpful role in patients with Stage I or Stage II disease, in which the evidence of aggressive or progressive behavior is indication for treatment, whereas a benign or stable state in such patients dictates judicious restraint.

Method of Treatment. It is currently accepted that CLL lymphocytes have a long life span and are functionally inadequate. Therefore more and more such lymphocytes accumulate in the patient during the course of the disease, and therapy is generally directed toward reduction of the lymphoid cell mass. In over 90 per cent of CLL patients, reduction in cell mass leads to reduction in organomegaly and lymph node masses with a parallel reduction in clinical signs and symptoms and an increase in the patient's performance status, but with the continued presence of an absolute lymphocytosis in the peripheral blood and bone marrow. This improved clinical status may be striking, and hemoglobin, white cell numbers, and platelet values may have also returned to normal and may remain stable for varying periods of months or even years. Such improved status is termed a partial remission (PR). In about 10 per cent of patients, not only are signs and symptoms of disease abolished but also the lymphocytosis, and peripheral blood and bone marrow are returned to normal both qualitatively and quantitatively. These patients are in complete remission (CR). In our experience patients who approach or attain complete remission status (CR or PR) survive longer than patients who show minimal improvement or no response. However, vigorous and aggressive treatment must be balanced against treatment-induced bone marrow toxicity.

PHASE OF OBSERVATION. A patient should not be assigned to a treatment plan until he or she has been observed at 10 to 14 day intervals for a minimum of 4 to 6 weeks. The exception to this general rule is the patient who is in obvious need of supportive or antitumor therapy. During the observation period, clinical staging and laboratory and x-ray data are obtained. If there are no signs or symptoms of obvious clinical progression, the observation period is further extended.

Patients with stable disease and showing no progression are not assigned to any specific treatment modality, but monthly observation is continued for the first 6 months. With a continued stable clinical state, the time between office visits is lengthened.

Patients with bulky and localized lymph nodes and/or organomegaly and active or progressive disease are considered for x-radiation as initial treatment. Patients with generalized disease are assigned to an alkylating agent, and presently our initial drug of choice is chlorambucil.

ALKYLATING AGENTS. The lymphocyte in CLL is initially responsive to almost all alkylating agents. Chlorambucil (CLB), the first drug of choice, is relatively devoid of disturbing side effects, and toxicity usually develops slowly.

The usual recommended starting dose for chlorambucil is 0.1 to 0.2 mg. per kg. per day given orally, and the total daily dose varies from 6 to 10 mg. About 60 to 70 per cent of patients will respond to this dosage, and the first significant benefit is usually seen after 5 to 6 weeks. The rate of fall in peripheral white cell count determines the CLB dose. Most often white cell reduction precedes platelet or red cell toxicity, but occasionally bone marrow toxicity manifested by progressive thrombocytopenia or anemia is seen before any observable clinical benefit. More usual is a rise in red blood cells and platelets as the severe peripheral lymphocytosis abates.

More recently, we have used CLB in an intermittent high dosage manner. This method has a theoretical advantage over the conventional low dose schedule in that it allows time between doses for the recovery of normal elements of the bone marrow long before the regeneration of the more slowly proliferating leukemic lymphocytes. In this method chlorambucil is given as a single starting dose of 0.4 mg. per kg. on day 1, repeated on day 29 and every 28 days thereafter, depending on peripheral blood values reflecting bone marrow function. When there is objective evidence of inadequate response without toxicity, the dose of CLB is augmented by increments of 0.2 mg. per kg. every 28 days, or the interval between doses is shortened to 3 weeks. (This dosage of chlorambucil is not listed in the manufacturer's official directive.)

Although the overall survival of patients on daily and intermittent dosage schedules is similar, we prefer the intermittent schedule because of good patient acceptance, minimal toxicity, and ease of administration.

CORTICOSTEROIDS. We prefer to withhold prednisone or other corticosteroids in our initial treatment plan, unless (1) an immune-type of hemolytic anemia or thrombocytopenia is demonstrated; (2) a thrombocytopenia associated with purpura is present; or (3) there is an anemia with a hemoglobin of less than 11 grams per dl. at the beginning of treatment.

Virtually all patients treated with prednisone or other corticosteroids respond with subjective improvement, and a majority of patients also show almost immediate regression in lymph node and organ size. Thrombocytopenia and anemia become less severe and may even approach normal values. A concomitant absolute peripheral lymphocytosis of significant degree, even to doubling the peripheral blood count, is occasionally observed; but with continued treatment the severe lymphocytosis abates and then may fall well below pretreatment levels. Unfortunately patients treated with prednisone alone do not maintain this improved status. In a recent study by Cancer and Leukemia Group B of 19 patients with Stage III or IV disease who were treated with prednisone alone, none achieved complete remission, and only 11 per cent achieved a partial remission (PR) status, compared to complete remission (CR) in 10 per cent of 38 patients treated by intermittent dosage of CLB plus prednisone, with 47 per cent of this group achieving CR + PR. In addition, patients treated with prednisone alone relapsed after a median of 7 months, compared to 16 months for the CLB plus prednisone group.

Whenever we use prednisone singly or in combination, we prefer to use an intermittent dosage schedule. Prednisone is initially given at a dose of 0.8 to 1.0 mg. per kg. per day in three divided doses orally for 2 weeks; the dosage is reduced by 0.2 mg. per kg. per day every 2 weeks. Prednisone is then stopped abruptly after 6 weeks of administration. Prednisone is again started on the eighth week (day 57) at a level of 0.5 mg. per kg. per day in three divided doses for 7 to 10 days each month.

We have found that fluid retention, cushingoid changes, and other complications are minimized with this schedule. In our experience the frequency of infection has not been exacerbated in CLL patients so treated with prednisone.

Patients with autoimmune manifestations such as hemolytic anemia or immune thrombocytopenia may require corticosteroid therapy without interruption for prolonged periods.

Autoimmune Manifestations of CLL. About 10 to 20 per cent of patients with CLL manifest some evidence of a disordered immune response. A positive direct antiglobulin test (direct Coombs' test) is reported in about 15 per cent of patients with or without anemia. An acute hemolytic anemia may sometimes be the cause which brings the patient to the physician, but more often the hemolytic anemia complicates the course of the disease. Less frequent is the presence of immune thrombocytopenia, diagnosed because of a bone marrow with at least adequate numbers of megakaryocytes and usually a readily palpable spleen. On rare occasions erythema multiforme or erythema nodosum may be present.

Initial treatment of the anemia and/or thrombocytopenia is the administration of prednisone in a dosage of 1.0 to 1.5 mg. per kg. per day in divided doses. Response may not be seen for 7 to 10 days after initiation of treatment, but a lack of response after 2 weeks of therapy with sufficient prednisone indicates treatment failure. Under the latter circumstance splenectomy may become necessary. Splenic sequestration with radiolabeled autologous or homologous red cells may be demonstrable, but such studies are not required. The final decision on splenectomy will rest on the patient's age, general condition, and response status to antileukemic therapy. Occasionally x-radiation of an enlarged spleen has proved beneficial.

Radiation Therapy. Lymphocytes are extremely radiosensitive, and the use of x-rays to reduce bulky lymphoid masses is one of the oldest methods of treatment for CLL. Radiation using radioisotopes such as radiophosphorus, although effective, has been found to be difficult to manage and is no longer generally recommended in CLL.

Splenic radiation may be considered as a means of control of the disease in those patients in whom the major presenting lymphoid mass is the spleen. In such patients splenic radiation may produce reduction in spleen size and a prolonged stable disease state.

Other forms of radiotherapy have been proposed for the control of patients with CLL, such as total body irradiation and mediastinal radiation, but these are best left to experimental programs for further evaluation.

Special Considerations. Herpetic virus infections, both herpes simplex and herpes zoster, are common viral diseases in the CLL patient either at the time of diagnosis or during the course of the disease. Secondary infection of the vesicles and pain resulting from the herpes zoster may be troublesome. The potential for herpes zoster universalis is real, and active control of the viral disease with convalescent serum or antimetabolite is indicated. For similar reasons smallpox vaccination is to be avoided, and severe vaccinial reactions may follow such a procedure.

Supportive Treatment. Patients with CLL are frequently in a good general clinical status. Fatigability, the hallmark of myeloproliferative syndromes, when present in CLL usually means anemia. Fever, a common sign of active and progressive myeloid leukemia, is virtually always a sign of complicating infection in the patient with CLL. The higher the fever, the more likely is infection the cause. Patients with CLL have an increased predilection for infections toward the late stages of their disease. Infective organisms usually include staphylococci, pneumococci, Pseudomonas, Klebsiella species, *Pneumocystis carinii,* cytomegalovirus, and Monilia. Although tuberculosis is always a threat, it has not proved troublesome in our experience.

Patients no longer responsive to usual treatment schedules should be referred to centers where experimental treatment programs are available.

Chronic Myeloid Leukemia

Attempts to produce criteria for clinical staging of patients with chronic myeloid leukemia (CML) that correlate with patient survival have not met with the same degree of success as in CLL. Three forms of CML are recognized, and each correlates with a survival pattern. These are an infantile form; the "typical" adult form, which may be seen occasionally in childhood and in which a Ph′ chromosome is present; and a third form, in the adult, in which no Ph′ chromosome can be found.

The diagnosis of CML is based upon the presence of abnormally high numbers of leukocytes in the peripheral blood, with a preponderance of myelocytes, metamyelocytes, and segmented neutrophils, and a hypercellular bone marrow with myeloid proliferation. Splenomegaly is usually present. The bone marrow myeloid cell karyotype shows a deletion of the long arm of the G22 chromosome, with translocation usually to the long arm of the C9 chromosome. This abnormality (Ph′ chromosome) is found in about 85 per cent of patients with CML. In these patients the blood neutrophil leukocyte alkaline phosphatase activity (LAP) is absent or abnormally low. The clinical course and survival of patients who have Ph′ positive CML characteristically have a higher response rate to conventional therapy and a median survival of 36 to 40 months, compared to an 18 month median survival for patients who are Ph′ negative.

Clinical Phases of CML. There are three clearly discernible clinical phases of CML. At the time of diagnosis the patient generally shows activity of the disease in the blood, bone marrow, and spleen. With therapy all measurable evidence of disease usually abates (except for the presence of the Ph′ chromosome), and the patient is considered to be in a stable phase. With the passage of time, the disease becomes manifest again in the blood and the marrow, and the patient is considered to be in relapse. Usually the status of relapse is indistinguishable from the status at diagnosis. The third clinical phase is of the terminal blastic crisis, which is morphologically similar to acute myelocytic leukemia. The three clinical phases therefore are (1) relapse, or status at diagnosis; (2) stable phase (these two phases are called the chronic or the nonblast phase); and (3) acute blastic transformation.

Approach to Therapy Based on the Clinical Phase of the Disease. Although patients with CML tend to respond to all types of cytotoxic therapy, i.e., chemotherapy or radiation therapy, with a reduction in spleen size and a corresponding fall in leukocytes, those patients who are Ph′ positive do so more readily and more completely than do the Ph′ negative patients. Despite the high frequency of good control by any method and the production of a better quality of life during the course of disease, the median survival of patients with CML remains short. The duration of the initial stable phase is variable and in any one patient may last for months or years. But each clinical relapse is progressively less responsive to further therapy, and each new stable phase obtained is of a shorter duration than the previous one. The choice of treatment depends rather upon its convenience to patient and physician than upon any significant qualitative difference between the types of therapy available. Once a response has been obtained, it is our experience that there is no real difference whether the stable phase is maintained with continuous chemotherapy or by the use of an intermittent drug schedule given only for indications such as a rising blood count or increased spleen size.

Ultimately a terminal phase ensues, characterized by a persistent leukocytosis in spite of treatment as well as persistent or progressive anemia and/or thrombocytopenia. An increased number of blast cells enter the peripheral blood. Low grade fever without apparent infection is present but may not be recognized to be of leukemic origin until the laboratory blood values signal relapse. An increasingly short doubling time of the peripheral white blood cell count in patients off therapy is indicative of a poor prognosis. A marked basophilia of 15 to 20 per cent or a developing anemia and/or thrombocytopenia are all associated with active disease and poor prognosis. We have found that a hyperploid karyotype is also a poor prognostic sign and may herald blast crisis. The treatment of the blast phase of CML, although not very promising, is presently similar to the treatment of acute leukemia.

Method of Treatment. PHASE OF OBSERVATION. In general, no cytotoxic therapy is given at the initial visit; a weekly or biweekly visit is recommended, and the erythroid, platelet, and white cell levels are monitored. If the peripheral blood values allow and the white blood cells remain stable and under 75,000 per microliter, no specific therapy is undertaken. Platelet counts in the range of 1 million to 1.5 million per microliter are not infrequent, but we do not consider such values as indicators for treatment.

Once a patient becomes symptomatic or

shows signs of increasing leukocytosis or a change in physical findings indicative of active disease, treatment is undertaken.

Chronic Phase. Chemotherapy is our treatment of choice for the chronic (nonblast) phase of CML. Of the various drugs available, none is superior to busulfan. The initial daily dose of busulfan is 0.11 mg. per kg. or 4 mg. per square meter of body surface, with a maximum initial daily dose of 8 mg. The dose of busulfan is gradually reduced as the peripheral white blood cell count falls toward normal. The usual method is to reduce the dose by 50 per cent with a 50 per cent reduction in the peripheral white blood count. Our aim is to bring the peripheral white cell count to below 15,000 cells per microliter. Platelet count must be monitored concomitantly, and an inappropriate fall in platelet count requires a more drastic reduction of daily dose than does the fall of white count.

With improvement in the peripheral blood count there is improvement in the patient's sense of well-being and general performance. Spleen size decreases dramatically, but many patients will continue to show a residual splenomegaly even while otherwise manifesting complete clinical stability. Bone marrow remains hypercellular, and the leukocyte alkaline phosphatase activity (LAP)—characteristically low or absent at the time of diagnosis—remains low even during remission or a period of stable disease, except for about 30 per cent of patients in whom low normal or even normal LAP activity may be noted. Sudden or rapidly rising LAP values may herald the onset of blast crisis.

Toxicity and side effects of busulfan: There is little or no initial toxicity to busulfan in the early phase of treatment, and little or no fall in white blood cell or platelet count may be observed. This may lull both physician and patient into a false sense of confidence, and too infrequent laboratory monitoring of peripheral blood cell values may be prescribed. There is a wide range among patients in the rate of fall of cellular elements and consequent bone marrow hypoplasia, but marrow hypoplasia may be severe, irreversible, and associated with toxic death. Thrombocytopenia may also be severe and may be limiting for effective drug therapy. Anemia and general wasting may also occur. Since there is no clear relationship between the degree of drug-induced marrow hypoplasia and remission duration or survival (although such relationships have been drawn by some authors), overtreatment is not recommended. With prolonged use of busulfan some patients develop an increase in skin pigmentation. The association of anemia, skin pigmentation, and general wasting has led to a consideration of impaired adrenocortical activity, and rarely adrenocortical failure has been reported following the use of busulfan. Dyspnea associated with interstitial pulmonary fibrosis may occur in patients who have received busulfan for protracted periods, and this pneumonitis may be first manifested months after discontinuing the busulfan treatment. Treatment with corticosteroids may improve some patients, and there is sometimes gradual improvement following cessation of busulfan. Other side effects of long-term busulfan therapy are related to cellular changes in epithelial cells—e.g., cytomegaly, multinucleated cells, nuclear vacuolization, and inclusion bodies have been demonstrated in many parenchymatous organs and in the endocrine glands.

Other forms of therapy during the chronic phase: Other chemotherapeutic agents that have been advocated for use in the CML include dibromomannitol (which acts like busulfan), 6-mercaptopurine, hydroxyurea, cyclophosphamide, and nitrosourea. These agents have been used singly and in combination.

Radiation Therapy. Radiation therapy, using splenic radiation (5 to 15 treatments of 100 to 150 rads each), has been found to control the disease. With this regimen slight anorexia and nausea may occur. Regression of the enlarged spleen is readily noted by the end of the first week, and the peripheral white count falls concomitantly. In general, hematologic control frequently ensues and the patient feels quite well. Occasionally splenic radiation is followed by severe bone marrow hypoplasia, which in two of our patients was irreversible and resulted in death. These latter occurrences are unusual, but the phenomenon of splenic radiation being followed by bone marrow toxicity and hypoplasia is well established.

Although radiophosphorus has been used to treat chronic myeloid leukemia in the past, we have not used that modality since 1960.

Special Considerations. Left upper quadrant pain resulting from splenic infarction is not uncommon during the course of CML. This event is usually self-limiting; with bed rest, analgesia, and reassurance, splenic infarction does not produce severe consequences.

Hyperleukocytosis with peripheral white blood cells in excess of 150,000 cells per microliter is more common early in the course of CML. Excessive numbers of white blood cells may be associated with cerebral leukostasis, and therefore such a medical emergency requires that this degree of leukocytosis must be reduced. Such patients usually have a high serum uric acid, and cytotoxic therapy will augment uric acid production and may threaten renal function. Therefore proper hydration of the patient must be established, and the urine should be alkalinized, although the latter is not always fully necessary. Allopurinol should be given at a level of 100 mg. three times per day, and hydroxyurea should be started at a level of 0.5 gram twice daily for the first day and then given as 1.0 gram twice daily for the next 2 days. Daily leukocyte and platelet counts must be obtained to monitor the drug dosage. If no fall in leukocytes occurs, the hydroxyurea dosage should be increased to 3.0 grams daily and the dosage maintained at that level until a falling leukocyte count dictates decreasing the drug dose. When the leukocyte count falls below 50,000 cells per microliter, hydroxyurea may be discontinued.

New Approaches in Treatment. Two major developments in the treatment of the chronic phase of CML are still under investigation. One of these concepts considers the spleen as the major site of the leukemic cell origin; the treatment is directed at splenectomy at the time of initial diagnosis, followed by intensive chemotherapy to ablate the Ph′ clone from the bone marrow. The second concept is to enhance the host immune mechanism during the period of remission with the hope of prolonging the duration of remission. This adjuvant immunotherapy largely utilizes bacille Calmette Guérin (BCG) (or its methanol-extractable residue, MER). Continued investigations on these two methods of treatment will be required before we can recommend such therapy for general application. If a physician considers that a patient might benefit from these, such a patient should be referred to institutions where these research approaches are under clinical trials.

Treatment of the Terminal Phase. About 75 per cent of patients with chronic myeloid leukemia eventually die of blast crisis. The median survival of patients in blast crisis is measured in weeks, and a survival of 3 or 4 months is to be expected. The other 15 to 25 per cent of patients die of bone marrow failure with myelofibrosis, increasing spleen size, hepatomegaly, hemorrhage, and infection. Although splenectomy is sometimes the only choice in this latter group, it is rarely of real benefit.

The treatment of blast crisis is very unsatisfactory today. A large number of different therapeutic regimens have been tried. Remissions are relatively infrequent and of short duration. The best results that we have obtained have been with a combination of orally administered prednisone, 0.75 mg. per kg. per day, 6-mercaptopurine, 3 mg. per kg. per day, hydroxyurea, 30 mg. per kg. per day, and intravenous vincristine, 1.5 mg. per square meter (maximum dose of 2 mg.), given weekly for 4 weeks. When remission is obtained, maintenance therapy has depended upon oral hydroxyurea, 7 mg. per kg. per day, 6 mercaptopurine, 0.7 mg. per kg. per day, and prednisone, 0.25 mg. per kg. Although this combination has resulted in approximately a 35 per cent complete and partial remission rate, unfortunately these remissions have been of a very transient nature, with a median remission duration of only 2 to 3 months.

Occasional patients will develop meningeal leukemia while in the blast phase of CML. We have treated these patients with either intrathecal methotrexate at a dose of 15 mg. twice weekly for 1 to 2 weeks or intrathecal cytosine arabinoside at a dose of 30 mg. per square meter (maximum dose of 50 mg.) twice weekly for 2 weeks. (The intrathecal use of cytosine arabinoside is not listed in the manufacturer's official directive.) When intrathecal cytotoxic agents are used, peripheral blood counts must be monitored for any hematotopoietic toxicity. Occasionally in a patient in blast crisis, extramedullary myeloblastic tumors may be found. These may involve lymph nodes, bony tissue, and skin, and these tumor masses are very sensitive to local radiotherapy.

Supportive Therapy. Although the overall survival of patients with CML has not increased appreciably during the past 50 years, there is still a need for an optimistic approach to the care of these patients. They require emotional support for their illness, and a frank appraisal of what is known about the disease, the efforts that are currently being made for innovative treatment, and the increasing success of treatment of other types of leukemia and malignancy should all help in producing a mood of cautious optimism. A significant number of patients are long-term survivors. We are currently following eight patients for 10 years or more who are either on therapy or have been off therapy for more than 5 years. Even so, karyotype studies of bone marrow aspirations from these long-term survivors continue to show the presence of a Ph′ chromosome in 90 per cent of the metaphases.

Initial treatment must be directed toward hydration and prevention of uric acid complications. The use of allopurinol to reduce serum uric acid levels is well established. Packed red cell transfusions are usually given for anemia. Such supportive therapy is usually not required until late in the disease. Platelet transfusions are indicated only during periods of marrow hypoplasia or ablation and should not be used for minor degrees of thrombocytopenia. Upper quadrant pain is frequently a manifestation of splenic infarction, but splenic rupture is almost never encountered and splenic infarction tends to be self-limiting. Sedation, analgesia, and bed rest are usually all that are required to treat this complication. Antibiotic support when needed usually follows the usual indications for such therapy.

NON-HODGKIN'S LYMPHOMAS

method of
MELVIN R. MOORE, M.D.
Atlanta, Georgia

Malignancies of the immune system, collectively referred to as the non-Hodgkin's lymphomas, comprise a diverse group of diseases with marked variation in clinical presentation, course, and prognosis. Therapeutic decisions are based on histopathologic designation and extent of disease involvement (stage). The importance of a meticulous pretherapy evaluation cannot be overemphasized. Since treatment planning depends on a clear understanding of the disease process and since early treatment may limit later therapeutic options, consultation by an experienced oncologist or hematologist should be sought prior to initiating therapy.

Histopathology

In 1956 Rappaport introduced a classification of non-Hodgkin's lymphomas based on the pattern of malignant invasion in the lymph node (nodular vs. diffuse) and the cell type involved in the malignant process. This classification (Table 1) was found to be highly predictive of clinical presentation and prognosis and is currently used in treatment planning. Favorable histologies (NM, NLPD, NLWD, DLWD), with median survival in excess of 7 years, are seen in approximately 40 per cent of patients; unfavorable histologies (NH, DU, DH, DM, DLPD), with median survival ranging from 3 years to 6 months, are seen in the remaining 60 per cent. Histopathologic type also correlates with patterns of presentation. Lymphocytic lymphomas have a relatively high incidence of bone marrow involvement, liver involvement, and widespread lymph node disease. Histiocytic lymphomas are more often localized and have a predilection for primary occurrence in extranodal sites such as bone and gastrointestinal tract.

Newer histologic classifications are based on the concept of Lukes and Collins that malignant disorders of the lymphatic system should be classified by the functional characteristics of the abnormal cell. Using in vitro techniques to identify surface markers, tumors can be classified as being derived from B lymphocytes, T lymphocytes, or null cells (neither B nor T). The concept of differentiation stressed in the Rappaport system is replaced by morphologic characteristics that correlate with the degree of stimulation that a normal lymphocyte demonstrates during the blastogenic response to antigen or mitogen. The Lukes classification has demonstrated that all nodular non-Hodgkin's lymphomas and the majority of diffuse non-Hodgkin's lymphomas are B cell diseases, and that lymphomas classified as histiocytic in the Rappaport scheme are in fact usually derived from B lymphocytes. The extensive clinical-pathologic correlations that will be necessary to make this functional classification of non-Hodgkin's lymphomas clinically useful have not yet been reported.

Stage

In the non-Hodgkin's lymphomas, stage and survival are less well correlated than in Hodgkin's disease. It is important to distinguish patients with localized (Stage I) or regional (two or more lymph node regions on the same side of the diaphragm—Stage II) disease from patients with more extensive (Stage III and IV) involvement. Patients with primary extranodal lymphomas

TABLE 1. **The Non-Hodgkin's Lymphomas***

NODULAR				DIFFUSE		
Abbreviation	*Relative Incidence*	*Median Survival*	CELL TYPE	*Abbreviation*	*Relative Incidence*	*Median Survival*
—	—	—	Undifferentiated	DU	4%	0.6 yr.
NH	7%	3.0 yrs.	Histiocytic	DH	28%	1.1 yrs.
NM	19%	7.5 yrs.	Mixed histiocytic and lymphocytic	DM	10%	1.5 yrs.
NLPD	18%	7.5 yrs.	Lymphocytic, poorly differentiated	DLPD	10%	1.8 yrs.
NLWD	1%	>7.5 yrs.	Lymphocytic, well differentiated	DLWD	3%	>7.5 yrs.

*Adapted from Jones, S. E.: JAMA *284*:633, 1975.

(e.g., bone and gastrointestinal tract) or localized extranodal disease should be classified and treated according to the remainder of involvement and are designated by the subscript E after the stage (e.g., I_E, II_E). Only 15 per cent of carefully staged patients with favorable histologies (NM, NLPD, NLWD, DLWD) present with Stage I and II disease, whereas approximately 34 per cent of patients with unfavorable histologies (NH, DU, DH, DM, DLPD) are Stage I or II.

An orderly progression of staging procedures to be pursued until Stage III (lymphatic disease on both sides of the diaphragm) or Stage IV (extralymphatic disease) is documented would include (1) careful history and physical examination, (2) blood studies (complete blood count [CBC], differential, platelet count, SMA-12, Coombs' test, serum protein electrophoresis), (3) chest x-ray (whole lung tomography if chest x-ray is positive), (4) bipedal lymphangiography, (5) bilateral core needle bone marrow biopsies, (6) cytology of any effusion, (7) percutaneous liver biopsy, and (8) laparoscopy with directed liver biopsies. Additional studies such as radionuclide scanning, upper gastrointestinal series, barium enema, and intravenous pyelogram will be indicated in selected patients. Immunologic testing (in vivo and in vitro) is of interest but will not affect therapy. Staging laparotomy should be viewed as an experimental procedure and not used for routine staging.

Therapy

Although presentation in early stages is relatively rare in the non-Hodgkin's lymphomas, it is essential that Stage I and II patients be recognized, as long-term disease-free survival may be achieved by the use of radiation therapy. The addition of systemic therapies, such as combination chemotherapy or total body irradiation (TBI), to local radiation therapy in an attempt to eradicate subclinical disease and prevent relapses in Stage I and II patients is under active investigation but has not yet been proved beneficial.

Response rates to chemotherapy and TBI are excellent in patients with Stage III and IV lymphomas with favorable histologies (NM, NLPD, NLWD, DLWD). In spite of these excellent responses, there is currently no evidence that aggressive early therapy improves survival in such patients or that cure is attainable. Patients with Stage III and IV lymphomas with favorable histologies should be viewed as having a chronic illness and treated palliatively to ensure minimum morbidity from the treatment and disease and maximum survival.

Patients with Stages III and IV lymphomas with unfavorable histologies (NH, DU, DH, DM, DLPD), particularly those with histiocytic and undifferentiated tumors, do not respond well to TBI, single agent chemotherapy, or the standard combination chemotherapy used for favorable histology patients (cyclophosphamide, vincristine, and prednisone). Paradoxically, a variety of more intensive combination chemotherapeutic regimens, employing doxorubicin hydrochloride (Adriamycin), bleomycin, high dose methotrexate, and cytosine arabinoside in addition to the standard agents listed above, have not only improved complete remission rates but also resulted in long-term disease-free survivals in up to 50 per cent of Stage III and IV patients with unfavorable histologies. Thus the outlook for this 40 per cent of all patients with non-Hodgkin's lymphoma who present with Stage III and IV disease with unfavorable histology has dramatically improved through the introduction of aggressive combination chemotherapy.

Stages I and II, Favorable Histology (NM, NLPD, NLWD, DLWD). After careful staging, this group of patients should receive at least involved field radiation therapy to a dose of about 4500 rads (Table 2). My own preference is for *extended field radiation therapy* to include lymph node areas contiguous to those that are involved. More extensive radiation therapy, TBI, chemotherapy, and immunotherapy are being tested as adjuncts to local radiation therapy, but have not yet been proved beneficial. If additional therapy is planned, six cycles of combination cyclophosphamide, vincristine (Oncovin), and prednisone (COP) as described below or TBI may be employed.

Stages I and II, Unfavorable Histology (NH, DU, DH, DM, DLPD). This group of patients should receive *radiation therapy to an extended field* as described above for Stages I and II with favorable histology (Table 2). Additional therapy is not of proved benefit in this group of patients. If additional therapy is planned, COP or TBI may be used only for DM and DLPD. Patients with NH, DU, and DH histology would require aggressive combination chemotherapy, consisting of bleomycin, doxorubicin hydrochloride (Adriamycin), cyclophosphamide, vincristine, and prednisone (BACOP) for 6 months as described below. Given the present state of knowledge, I would suggest that radiation therapy be used alone in the initial treatment of all patients with Stages I and II non-Hodgkin's lymphoma (exceptions to this generalization would include diffuse undifferentiated lymphoma and mediastinal T-cell or null cell lymphoma of adolescents).

Stages III and IV, Favorable Histology (NM, NLPD, NLWD, DLWD). Two simple relatively nontoxic regimens are available for the initial management of advanced lymphomas of favorable histology (Table 2). The first is *single oral alkylating*

TABLE 2. **Therapy of the Non-Hodgkin's Lymphomas**

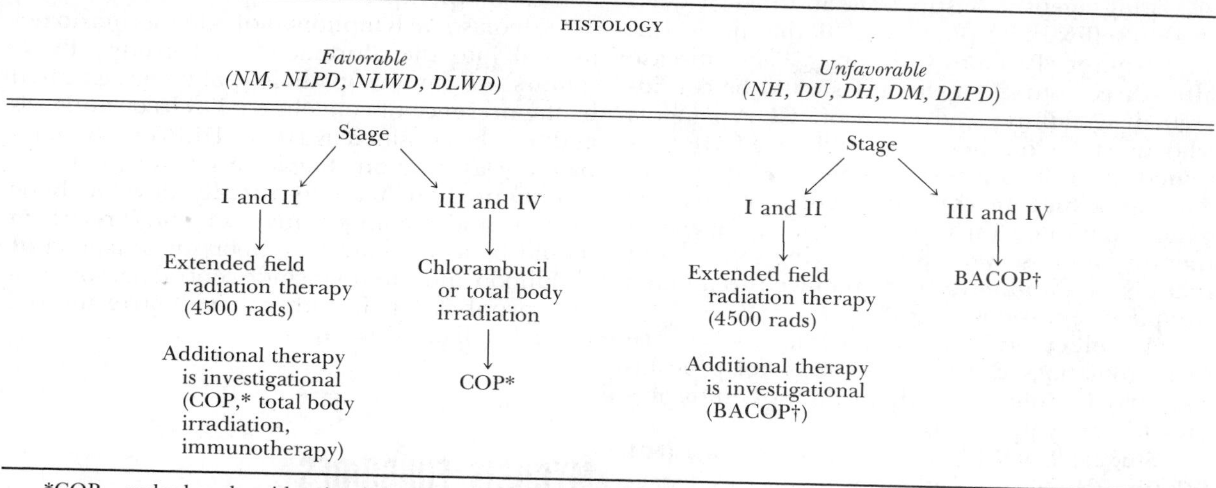

*COP—cyclophosphamide, vincristine (Oncovin), prednisone.
†BACOP—bleomycin, doxorubicin hydrochloride (Adriamycin), and COP.

agent therapy, using a drug such as chlorambucil. Immediately prior to therapy patients are given allopurinol, 100 mg. orally three times daily to prevent urate nephropathy. Allopurinol may be discontinued after 1 month of chemotherapy and serum uric acid levels monitored. Chlorambucil is given initially in a dose of 12 mg. orally every day. Complete blood counts (CBC) and platelet counts are obtained weekly for the first 4 to 8 weeks (at least monthly thereafter), and the dose of chlorambucil is decreased to 6 mg. per day orally when the absolute granulocyte count is <2000 or platelet count <150,000. Treatment should be interrupted when the absolute granulocyte count falls below 1500 or platelet count below 100,000. Therapy should be reinstituted at a lesser dose when blood counts improve, attempting to keep the absolute granulocyte count and platelet count at approximately 2000 and 150,000, respectively. Patients whose disease is documented to progress while receiving doses of chlorambucil adequate to produce modest leukopenia may be considered drug failures. The second therapy recommended for initial management of Stage III and IV favorable histology lymphomas is *TBI*. After allopurinol is begun, TBI is administered in 15 rad fractions given twice weekly. Therapy is continued until a cumulative dose of 150 rads is reached or blood count depression (particularly thrombocytopenia) is encountered. The advantages of TBI include low morbidity and the relatively brief duration of therapy. Difficulty encountered in repeating courses of TBI because of thrombocytopenia raises the possibility of long-term bone marrow suppression resulting from this modality. At present TBI is an acceptable alternative to single oral alkylating agent chemotherapy in the primary management of Stage III and IV non-Hodgkin's lymphomas of favorable histology.

When progressive disease is documented in patients on single oral alkylating agents or following TBI and in patients with particularly rapidly progressive or symptomatic disease at the time of diagnosis, *COP therapy* is recommended. The method of administration of these three agents varies greatly. I prefer giving cyclophosphamide as an oral dose of 300 mg. per square meter of body surface area daily on days 1 through 5, vincristine as an intravenous dose of 1.4 mg. per square meter (not to exceed 2 mg. total dose) on day 1, and prednisone as an oral dose of 100 mg. per square meter daily on days 1 through 5. Courses of therapy should be given at 21 day intervals. CBC and platelet counts are obtained weekly for the first few courses. If the nadir of absolute granulocyte counts is <750 or platelets <75,000, the dose of cyclophosphamide should be decreased by 50 per cent and slowly escalated in subsequent courses if blood counts permit. If the absolute granulocyte count is <1500 or platelets <100,000 when a cycle of therapy is due, treatment should be delayed by a week to allow for further marrow recovery. Patients expected to have compromised bone marrow reserve (e.g., prior TBI, prior chemotherapy, age >65) may begin at 50 per cent cyclophosphamide dose with escalation as blood counts permit. The occurrence of peripheral neuropathy (foot drop or wrist drop) is an indication to withhold vincristine until motor strength is fully recovered. Additional toxicities that may be expected include nausea and vomiting, alopecia, hemorrhagic cystitis (discontinue cyclophosphamide and substitute another alkylating agent), constipation, and loss of deep tendon reflexes. Response to COP therapy is usually prompt. Patients with progressive disease after three courses of therapy should be considered drug failures and taken off COP. Patients who are stable on therapy should have COP continued until disease progression is documented. Patients achieving complete remission may be either continued on COP therapy or taken off therapy and observed after receiving six cycles of therapy in addition to those required to attain a complete remission.

A select group of patients who are asymptomatic and whose disease is not progressing may be followed without therapy until progression or symptoms occur.

Stages III and IV, Unfavorable Histology (NH, DU, DH, DM, DLPD). Patients with advanced stage and unfavorable histology, unlike those with favorable histology, have highly malignant disease with shortened survival (Table 1) and should receive aggressive chemotherapy at the time of diagnosis (Table 2). One of the more successful programs is the BACOP regimen reported by Schein et al. This regimen consists of cyclophosphamide, 650 mg. per square meter intravenously on days 1 and 8; doxorubicin (Adriamycin), 25 mg. per square meter intravenously on days 1 and 8; vincristine (Oncovin), 1.4 mg. per square meter intravenously on days 1 and 8; bleomycin, 5 mg. per square meter intravenously on days 15 and 21; and prednisone, 60 mg. per square meter orally on days 15 through 28. Courses are repeated at 28 day intervals. The addition of Adriamycin adds the possibility of cardiomyopathy to the toxic effects that may be encountered. Total cumulative dose of Adriamycin should not exceed 550 mg. per square meter, and therapy should be monitored by systolic time intervals or ejection fractions calculated by echocardiography. Pulmonary fibrosis is seen in patients receiving bleomycin. Total cumulative dose should not exceed 300 mg., and pulmonary function tests should be monitored. In addition, fever and dermatologic toxicity (erythematous pruritic nodules) are commonly observed in patients receiving bleomycin. BACOP therapy is significantly more toxic and difficult to manage than COP and should be administered only by an experienced hematologist or medical oncologist. Patients achieving a complete remission on BACOP as documented by careful pathologic restaging have a high likelihood of remaining in unmaintained complete remission. Patients not attaining a complete remission may continue on BACOP or may benefit by the addition of local radiation therapy to residual disease or a trial of cyclophosphamide, vincristine, high dose methotrexate, and cytosine arabinoside combination chemotherapy.

Mediastinal lymphomas of adolescents do not fit well into the aforementioned group. These tumors are immunopathologically characterized by the presence of convoluted T cells or null cells and may be classified as DU or DLPD in the Rappaport classification. Regardless of stage at presentation, these patients rapidly develop bone marrow and meningeal involvement. Treatment should be as in acute lymphoblastic leukemia of childhood and should include central nervous system prophylaxis (intrathecal methotrexate and cranial radiation therapy).

MYCOSIS FUNGOIDES

method of
WILLIAM E. CLENDENNING, M.D.,
and FREDERICK D. WAX, M.D.
Hanover, New Hampshire

Mycosis fungoides is a distinctive T-cell lymphoma which begins in the skin. It is characterized by abnormal lymphocytes which have hyperchromatic, hyperconvoluted nuclei. These cells have the immunologic properties of T lymphocytes. This lymphoma commonly presents as a nonspecific dermatitis which persists for an average of 2 to 10 years before a pathologic diagnosis of lymphoma can be established. The variable presentations of this first stage (I) of mycosis fungoides include eczematous and psoriasiform dermatitis, parapsoriasis en plaque, poikiloderma atrophicans vasculare, alopecia mucinosa, and lymphomatoid papulosis. The second stage (II) is characterized by infiltrated plaques and the third stage (III) by nodules, tumors, and ulcers. Perhaps 10 per cent of patients present with cutaneous tumors, without preceding dermatitis or plaques. This is called the d'emblée form of the disease. Another 10 per cent begin with a generalized erythroderma. A leukemic variant, in conjunction with generalized erythroderma, has been known as the Sézary syndrome. In the third stage of the disease, lymph nodes and other internal organs, particularly the lungs, liver, and spleen, may be involved.

Once a pathologic diagnosis is established, the median survival for all patients is less than 5 years. Associated lymphadenopathy, characterized pathologically by nonspecific hyperplasia, is associated with a median survival of 34 months.

However, when lymph nodes show specific involvement, the median survival decreases to 18 months. If lymph node involvement is combined with tumors and ulcerations in the skin, survival is further reduced to 1 year. Visceral involvement is associated with a median survival of less than 1 year.

Staging

The studies needed to determine the extent of the disease are similar to those done in the work-up of other lymphomas. A complete history and physical examination are performed. Laboratory tests should include a complete blood count (including differential with special examination of the peripheral smear for atypical lymphocytes), liver function studies, tests of renal function (including creatinine clearance), and uric acid. A chest x-ray and liver-spleen scan are routinely performed, as is a bone marrow biopsy. A lymphangiogram is important, but if this is technically impossible, an intravenous pyelogram may be substituted. Biopsy of a peripheral lymph node is indicated. If no palpable nodes are present, a blind biopsy of an axillary node is recommended. Staging laparotomy with splenectomy, liver biopsy, and abdominal node biopsy may be considered, particularly if there is evidence for hepato- or splenomegaly. The patient can then be staged according to the extent of cutaneous (T), lymph node (N), and visceral (M) disease. This TNM classification system is used for registration and for selection of appropriate treatment protocols. This type of evaluation is being done on a national basis at several medical centers in the United States where there are members of the Mycosis Fungoides Cooperative Study Group. It is suggested that, whenever possible, patients with mycosis fungoides be referred to one of the participating centers for staging and therapeutic recommendations. Randomization of therapy is often desirable and justifiable at our present state of knowledge if agreed to by the patient through informed consent.

Therapy

Stage I or II Without Lymphadenopathy. 1. Electron beam: Patients are treated by total skin irradiation with 2.5 MeV electrons for a total dose of 3000 rads over a 30 to 40 day period. Acute side effects include a temporary increase in erythema and edema of the skin, as well as scalp and body hair loss. Chronic radiation changes of the skin may develop, characterized by telangiectasis, atrophy, and hyperpigmentation. Complete temporary remissions have been reported in up to 100 per cent of Stage I and 60 per cent of Stage II patients. With long-term follow-up, some apparently permanent remissions are recorded.

2. Topical nitrogen mustard: The patient applies, usually daily, a solution made by diluting 10 mg. of nitrogen mustard (mechlorethamine) in 60 ml. of tap water. Application is done, after a cleansing bath, to the entire body, using gauze sponges. Less solution is used in sensitive intertriginous areas, and care is taken to avoid contact with the eyes. There is a high incidence of the development of contact allergy associated with this therapy. Therefore various preparatory regimens for the induction of immunologic "tolerance" have been suggested for use prior to the institution of therapeutic paintings. None have established value. If allergic contact sensitization develops, the patient may tolerate more dilute solutions or topical carmustine (BCNU) may be substituted. Prolonged remissions have been reported with this method.

3. A combination of electron beam followed by topical nitrogen mustard.

4. Topical corticosteroids: Potent fluorinated corticosteroid creams are used, often with plastic wrap occlusion to promote penetration. These often relieve pruritus temporarily and may produce some regression of lesions. They are useful adjuncts to other regimens.

Any Stage with Lymphadenopathy Pathologically Showing Only Benign Hyperplasia. 1. Electron beam, topical nitrogen mustard, or both as described above.

2. Adjuvant chemotherapy: This may be done following a course of electron beam or in conjunction with topical nitrogen mustard paintings. Various single and multiple drug regimens are currently under study; following are two examples. *(a)* Methotrexate, 500 mg. per square meter of body surface area intravenously with citrovorum factor rescue. This is given every 3 weeks with increments of 100 mg. per square meter to 750 mg. per square meter for a total of six courses. (See Chemotherapy, below, for specifics of methodology.) *(b)* Low dose CHOP. This consists of cyclophosphamide (Cytoxan), 500 mg. per square meter intravenously, doxorubicin (Adriamycin), 40 mg. per square meter intravenously, and vincristine (Oncovin), 1.4 mg. per square meter intravenously on the first day, with prednisone, 60 mg. per square meter, on each of the first 5 days of a 21 day cycle. Six courses are given.

Any Stage with Pathologically Confirmed Lymph Node Involvement, Visceral Involvement, or Erythroderma, with or without a Leukemic Peripheral Blood Picture. 1. Electron beam, topical nitrogen mustard, or both.

2. Chemotherapy: This may be used alone

or in conjunction with electron beam, topical nitrogen mustard, or both. A variety of regimens have been tried. Three "induction" regimens currently under study by the Mycosis Fungoides Cooperative Group are as follows: *(a)* Methotrexate, 500 mg. per square meter intravenously, infused in 5 per cent dextrose in water over 6 hours. This is followed in 2 hours by citrovorum factor, 5 per cent of the methotrexate dose (mg. per mg.) intravenously. Citrovorum factor is repeated intravenously or orally every 6 hours for the next 72 hours. The urine is kept alkaline by the use of acetazolamide (Diamox), 250 mg. twice daily orally, and by oral sodium bicarbonate, 2 grams every 4 hours as necessary if the urine pH falls below 6.8. This therapy is repeated every 3 weeks, with increases in the dose of methotrexate by 50 per cent (250 mg. per square meter) in subsequent courses up to a maximum of 1000 mg. per square meter. *(b)* Methotrexate, 250 mg. per square meter intravenously with citrovorum factor rescue, is given by the same protocol as in *(a)*, but with no subsequent increase in dose. This is given on day 1. Doxorubicin (Adriamycin), 45 mg. per square meter, is given by intravenous push into a rapidly running infusion of isotonic saline on day 15. Bleomycin sulfate (Blenoxane), 5 to 8 mg. per square meter intramuscularly, is given on days 15 and 22 (5 mg. per square meter is given for the first course, and, if tolerated, 8 mg. per square meter for subsequent courses). Courses are repeated at 28 day intervals for a minimum of six courses. *(c)* Methotrexate, 500 mg. per square meter intravenously with citrovorum factor rescue, is given as outlined in *(a)* on day 1. Doxorubicin (Adriamycin), 60 mg. per square meter, is given by intravenous push on day 22. Bleomycin sulfate (Blenoxane), 30 mg. per square meter, is given intramuscularly on day 29. Courses are repeated at 42 day intervals for a minimum of six courses.

Following "induction" therapy, "maintenance" chemotherapy may be given for 18 months provided prohibitive toxicity and/or relapse do not occur. One such regimen is cyclophosphamide (Cytoxan), 750 mg. per square meter intravenously every 3 weeks, and methotrexate, 15 mg. per square meter orally twice weekly.

Other Therapy. 1. PUVA: Oral 8-methoxypsoralen, followed in 2 hours by graded longwave ultraviolet light (UVA), has recently been reported to cause temporary remission of the cutaneous lesions of mycosis fungoides. Further studies are intended or in progress, as this modality may become a useful adjunct, particularly in the earlier stages of the disease when definite pathologic diagnosis is difficult.

2. Prednisone, 30 to 60 mg. daily, and/or chlorambucil, 0.1 mg. per kg. daily, is an occasionally useful oral chemotherapeutic regimen for elderly or otherwise debilitated patients who cannot tolerate a more vigorous chemotherapeutic program.

3. Daily low doses of intravenous nitrogen mustard (various schedules reported) are helpful in some patients with advanced disease.

4. Single tumors, which may present particular difficulty through their location or because of ulceration, can receive "spot" radiation, using 100 to 140 Kv conventional x-ray. Intralesional injection of nitrogen mustard, with or without triamcinolone, can also be considered for such lesions as 5 to 100 micrograms of nitrogen mustard per ml. of isotonic saline, with 1 mg. of triamcinolone.

MULTIPLE MYELOMA

method of
BRIAN G. M. DURIE, M.D.
Tucson, Arizona

Multiple myeloma is a monoclonal plasma cell malignancy arising from a single transformed cell of the B-lymphocyte series. The major clinical features include bone pain and various manifestations of anemia, renal insufficiency, hypercalcemia, hypogammaglobulinemia, and, less frequently, systemic amyloidosis. Definitive diagnosis requires documentation of a serum and/or urine monoclonal immunoglobulin (M-component) by protein electrophoresis and immunoelectrophoresis. This M-component, present in more than 95 per cent of patients, must be accompanied by at least some of the characteristic features of myeloma—the most important being more than 10 per cent (usually more than 30 per cent) plasma cells in the bone marrow or plasmacytoma on tissue biopsy, lytic bone lesions or diffuse osteoporosis on x-ray, and presence of urine monoclonal free light chains (Bence Jones protein) *in addition to* a serum M-component and the other secondary manifestations of myeloma already listed. It is important to exclude other causes of M-component production, including lymphomas, chronic lymphocytic leukemias, solid tumors, and both bacterial and viral infections.

Staging Evaluation

Clinical staging is an important prerequisite for adequate therapy. It has now been amply demonstrated that stage of disease (or tumor burden) and M-component type substantially affect prognosis. Other important data, necessary for prompt treatment of any presenting complications, are bone marrow aspiration to assess degree of infiltration and reduction of normal marrow elements; uric acid determination; measurement of normal immunoglobulin levels; and culture or other diagnostic procedures necessary to evaluate infection.

Initial Supportive Therapy

The use of cytotoxic chemotherapy has clearly made a favorable change in the prognosis of patients with multiple myeloma. However, because of the high incidence of medical complications at the time of diagnosis, initial therapy is necessarily multidisciplinary, often requiring close interaction between hematologists-oncologists, internists of several disciplines, radiation therapists, and orthopedic surgeons.

Bone Pain and Pathologic Fractures. Although diffuse bone pain usually responds to chemotherapy, severe localized pain at sites of lytic lesions or compression fractures may require localized radiotherapy. Extended field radiotherapy should be avoided, as it limits tolerance to systemic chemotherapy. Unless pain is unusually severe and cannot be controlled with conventional analgesia or there is an imminent catastrophe such as spinal cord compression or fracture of a long bone (e.g., femur), radiotherapy is deferred until the effect of chemotherapy can be assessed. However, surgical decompression followed by radiation may be necessary, after emergency myelography, to relieve acute cord compression. Open surgical fixation plus radiation is necessary for pathologic long bone fractures (especially femur) and is additionally recommended as a prophylactic measure if fracture appears imminent at the site(s) of large lytic lesions. The usual dose of local irradiation is 2500 rads, which can frequently eradicate local disease. It is recommended that prednisone (40 to 60 mg. per square meter of body surface) be administered along with radiation to reduce tissue swelling and enhance the tumoricidal effect. It is of the utmost importance to encourage physical activity as soon as feasible, using analgesics, lumbar corsets, and walkers as necessary.

Renal Insufficiency, Hypercalcemia, and Hyperuricemia. Renal insufficiency with a serum creatinine >2 mg. per 100 ml. occurs in approximately 20 per cent of patients with myeloma. It is usually associated with some combination of other factors, including hypercalcemia, hyperuricemia, dehydration, Bence Jones proteinuria, infection, and amyloidosis. With aggressive supportive measures these complications can usually be reversed or controlled. Adequate hydration is essential. Alkalinization of the urine is helpful in the presence of significant Bence Jones proteinuria and hyperuricemia. Hypercalcemia requires aggressive fluid replacement, usually intravenously with 5 per cent dextrose in half isotonic saline solutions if possible, with furosemide (Lasix)-induced diuresis to promote calcium excretion and prevent fluid overload. Occasional patients will require additional measures to reduce the serum calcium to a safe level. Mithramycin (20 micrograms per kg.) intravenously is a rapid, effective agent for reduction of hypercalcemia; however, it must be used with caution in the presence of significant thrombocytopenia or neutropenia. Prednisone (alone) is relatively ineffective and requires several days to produce an effect.

Allopurinol in a dosage of 300 mg. orally daily is effective for the prevention and control of hyperuricemia. An intravenous preparation is available for emergency use in comatose patients. Occasional patients, especially those with pronounced Bence Jones proteinuria, may require peritoneal or hemodialysis to correct renal insufficiency for the period necessary to reduce Bence Jones protein synthesis with chemotherapy and correct other metabolic complications. Rare patients have required long-term dialysis.

Infection. Reduced levels of normal immunoglobulins and sometimes neutropenia or abnormal neutrophil function (resulting from effects of serum M-component) make myeloma patients susceptible to infection. Infections are usually due to common gram-positive organisms (e.g., pneumococcus). Prompt institution of bactericidal antibiotics (generally penicillin or a cephalosporin derivative) is warranted when the patient has fever or other symptoms suggesting infection and after appropriate cultures have been obtained. Chemotherapy is normally deferred until infection(s) are adequately controlled. Prophylactic injections of gamma globulin are of limited value. Vaccination with live organisms must be avoided.

Anemia. Initial severe anemia may require prompt transfusion with packed red blood cells, with care taken to avoid fluid overload in this largely elderly group of patients. With complete or partial response to induction chemotherapy, the hemoglobin almost always increases to >9 to 10 grams per 100 ml. Patients who are nonresponders or are relapsing with symptomatic anemia may be benefited by androgens, using oral fluoxymesterone in a daily dose of 0.25 mg. per kg. for women and 1.0 mg. per kg. for men—both for at least 3 months. (This use of fluoxymesterone is not listed in the manufacturer's official directive.) A very few patients will continue to require periodic transfusion.

Chemotherapy

Alkylating agent chemotherapy is the mainstay of therapy for multiple myeloma. The standard alkylating agents are melphalan and cyclophosphamide, which appear to have equal efficacy. Combinations of these agents, along with carmustine (BCNU), doxorubicin (Adriamycin), vincristine, and prednisone, have recently been evaluated with respect to possible superior cell kill with induction chemotherapy. As yet it remains unclear whether or not response rate or remission duration and/or survival are improved with combination therapy induction.

However, the following treatment program has provided encouraging results in trials by the Southwest Oncology Group:

Vincristine, 1.0 mg. intravenously on day 1.

Melphalan, 0.15 mg. per kg. per day for days 2 through 5.

Cyclophosphamide, 3.0 mg. per kg. per day for days 2 through 5.

Prednisone, 1.5 mg. per kg. per day for days 2 through 5.

The white blood count, differential, and platelet count should be measured 14 and 21 days after the initial treatment course. As soon as the granulocytes have recovered to more than 2000 per cu. mm. and the platelets to more than 100,000 per cu. mm., another course of combination chemotherapy should be given. Doses of melphalan and cyclophosphamide should be increased in 20 per cent increments to the maximum level associated with mild toxicity. In those few patients presenting with initial granulocytopenia or thrombocytopenia, maximum doses are given for at least two treatment courses. The dose of vincristine should be increased to 1.5 mg. intravenously with the second treatment course and repeated at this level with subsequent courses in the absence of neurotoxicity.

Periodic evaluation of certain laboratory tests is necessary to document an objective response to chemotherapy. Response is confirmed when serum myeloma protein production falls by more than 75 per cent after calculations have considered the changing serum myeloma protein concentration, the plasma volume, and the catabolic rate of the myeloma globulin; the daily excretion of Bence Jones protein must also decline to less than 0.2 gram daily.

About two thirds of patients respond to this treatment combination. A 75 per cent reduction in myeloma protein production occurs in half of the responding patients within 3 months. In responding patients, bone pain and impaired performance usually improve within several weeks. Responding patients will also maintain their hematocrit at about 27 ml. per 100 ml. and their serum calcium below 11.5 mg. per 100 ml., may recalcify lytic bone lesions, and may demonstrate an elevation of depressed normal immunoglobulins.

Treatment courses should be continued for 12 months. Patients in whom serum and urine myeloma proteins have disappeared may be followed without any chemotherapy until there is unequivocal evidence of rising myeloma protein production or an increase in the size and number of lytic bone lesions. Reinstitution of chemotherapy will recontrol the myeloma in most patients for many months until relapse develops. Patients who have not reduced tumor mass markedly or patients relapsing despite alkylator-prednisone therapy should be offered at least two courses of a doxorubicin (Adriamycin) combination at 3 week intervals:

Vincristine, 1.5 mg. intravenously on day 1.

BCNU (bis-chloroethylnitrosourea), 0.6 mg. per kg. intravenously on day 2.

Doxorubicin (Adriamycin), 0.6 mg. per kg. intravenously on day 2.

Prednisone, 1.5 mg. per kg. per day for days 2 through 5.

Combination chemotherapy improves the survival of patients with multiple myeloma, but this benefit is restricted largely to patients who develop quantitative evidence of disease control. The median survival correlates closely with the severity of certain disease complications at the time of diagnosis and the degree of tumor reduction with chemotherapy. Thus patients considered to have far advanced myeloma with little myeloma protein reduction have a short median survival (i.e., about 1 year); those with mild disease and a marked degree of tumor reduction have a longer median survival (i.e., about 4 years).

POLYCYTHEMIA VERA

method of
NEAL J. WEINREB, M.D.,*
and LOUIS R. WASSERMAN, M.D.*
New York, New York

Polycythemia vera is a chronic, proliferative disorder of the bone marrow and other hematopoietic tissues. An initial phase of nonphysiologic erythrocytosis is associated with simultaneous or sequential proliferation of other hematic and stromal cells, resulting in leukocytosis,

*Aided in part by U.S.P.H.S. Grant #CA-10728 from the National Cancer Institute to the Polycythemia Vera Study Group.

myeloid immaturity, thrombocytosis, and hepatosplenomegaly. As the disease progresses over a period of 5 to 20 years, erythrocytosis often subsides and anemia may ensue as a transition occurs to a "spent" phase characterized by myelofibrosis and a shift of blood cell formation to extramedullary sites. During either the erythrocytotic or the "spent" phase, overt malignant transformation to acute leukemia may sometimes occur as a terminal event.

It has been difficult to determine whether the natural history of the disease is as depicted above or whether the sequence described is significantly influenced by therapeutic interventions. Although it is generally accepted that survival is increased and complications reduced in treated as compared with untreated patients, previous studies of polycythemia vera have resulted in conflicting conclusions concerning survival, natural history, incidence of leukemic transformation, and optimal therapy. The Polycythemia Vera Study Group was established in 1967 under the sponsorship of the National Cancer Institute for the purpose of resolving the many dilemmas confronting the physician treating a patient with polycythemia vera. This group of investigators from 25 institutions is currently conducting a prospective, randomized, cooperative study of three commonly used treatments for polycythemia vera: phlebotomy only, chemotherapy with chlorambucil plus supplementary phlebotomy, and radiotherapy with intravenous radioactive phosphorus plus supplementary phlebotomy. The details of treatment described below adhere to the protocols of the Polycythemia Vera Study Group. Definitive differences in overall survival are not yet apparent among the three treatment groups. However, preliminary results of the study suggest that the decisions concerning choice of therapy should be determined according to individual patient characteristics at the time of initial evaluation (e.g., age, history of past thrombosis), and that, with careful follow-up and regulation of erythremia and thrombocytosis, life expectancy in patients with polycythemia vera may approach that of comparably aged, nonpolycythemic controls.

General Principles of Treatment

Careful Differential Diagnosis. Polycythemia vera must be distinguished from relative or spurious erythrocytosis, and from erythrocytoses related to hypoxia (altitude, chronic pulmonary disease, cyanotic heart disease, smoking, high oxygen affinity hemoglobinopathy), or autonomous erythropoietin overproduction. Patients with polycythemia vera have an increased red cell mass and some combination of splenomegaly (by palpation, roentgenogram, or scan), leukocytosis, thrombocytosis, and increased leukocyte alkaline phosphatase activity. Arterial oxygen saturation is usually normal in patients with polycythemia vera.

Reduction of Blood Volume. During the uncontrolled erythremic phase of polycythemia vera, morbidity and death are frequently related to thromboembolic and/or hemorrhagic complications. The propensity to thrombosis and hemorrhage is largely a consequence of expansion of the circulating red cell and total blood volumes with resultant vascular distention, hyperviscosity, stasis, inefficient oxygen delivery, and tissue hypoxia. The primary objective in the treatment of polycythemia vera is reduction of an elevated red cell volume to the normal range and subsequent maintenance of red cell volume *normalcy.* Although it is desirable to periodically measure the true red cell volume during remission as well as at time of relapse, from a practical viewpoint patient management is most often related to the serial measurement of the packed cell volume (PCV, hematocrit). In most instances, the red cell volume will be normal when the PCV is maintained in a range of 40 to 47 per cent. Current techniques for control of red cell volume include removal of circulating red blood cells by therapeutic phlebotomy and/or suppression of erythrocyte overproduction with cytotoxic chemotherapy or radiotherapy.

Reduction of Platelet Count. Thrombocytosis and qualitative defects in platelet function are frequently observed in polycythemia vera, and may contribute to thromboembolic and hemorrhagic morbidity and mortality, even when erythremia is effectively controlled. Rapid, transient relief of symptomatic thrombocytosis has been noted after plateletpheresis. Sustained control of thrombocytosis in polycythemia vera is usually achieved with myelosuppressive therapy. The role of platelet deaggregating agents (e.g., aspirin, dipyridamole) in polycythemia vera is not yet defined. Small doses of aspirin are sometimes effective in relieving symptoms of erythromelalgia.

Management of Hyperuricemia. A majority of patients with polycythemia vera have hyperuricemia and/or hyperuricosuria. Allopurinol, 100 mg. three times per day orally, is usually effective in lowering the serum uric acid concentration to below 7.0 mg. per dl. (100 ml.), thus preventing the deleterious consequences of chronic, sustained hyperuricemia (gouty arthritis and urate nephropathy). Allopurinol may often be discontinued during remission, particularly in patients treated with myelosuppressive therapy. In our experience, neither cutaneous sensitization to allopurinol nor hepatotoxicity has occurred with significant frequency in patients with polycythemia vera.

Treatment of Pruritus. Pruritus of varying severity occurs in 40 per cent of the patients and may sometimes be the most discomforting symptom of polycythemia vera. The treatment of pruritus has been generally unsatisfactory. Cyproheptadine, 4 mg. orally four times daily, is effective in some patients but often causes marked drowsiness. Cholestyramine resin is reported to be of some benefit; but in our limited experience with this agent (four patients), responses have been marginal and gastrointestinal side effects substantial.

Hazards of Surgery. Surgery is contraindicated in erythremic patients with polycythemia vera; the risk of operative and postoperative morbidity and mortality in such patients was observed to exceed 80 per cent. Emergency surgery should be preceded by phlebotomy of sufficient volume to reduce the red cell volume to normal. Operative or postoperative bleeding in patients with polycythemia vera is sometimes related to platelet dysfunction. Platelet transfusions may be of value in such instances. Even in well-controlled patients with polycythemia vera, the risk of surgical complications, particularly bleeding, approaches 20 per cent. In some instances, surgical bleeding may be attributable to unrecognized pre-existent, disseminated intravascular coagulation. Preoperative screening for abnormalities in bleeding time, fibrinogen concentration, fibrin split products, and other coagulation parameters may identify the patients at greatest risk. It is our practice to hospitalize all patients with polycythemia vera who require surgery, including minor procedures and dental extractions.

Therapeutic Regimens

Phlebotomy. Venesection is the most rapidly effective means of controlling erythrocytosis. Sustained suppression of erythropoiesis is often achieved after a series of phlebotomy treatments as a result of depletion of body iron reserves. Depending on individual circumstances, phlebotomy may be used as the primary treatment for polycythemia vera, or as supplementary therapy for immediate control of relapses in patients treated with myelosuppressive agents.

After initial diagnosis, most patients can tolerate repeated phlebotomies of 300 to 500 ml. every other day until such time as packed cell volume (PCV) is reduced to 40 to 47 per cent and the red cell mass is normal. Elderly patients and those with compromise of the cardiovascular system should be phlebotomized more cautiously (200 to 300 ml. twice weekly). Nearly 500 patients have been managed according to this approach by member investigators of the Polycythemia Vera Study Group, with a negligible occurrence of thromboembolic complications during the period of initial phlebotomy. Upon completion of the initial series of phlebotomies, the red cell mass should again be measured to confirm that plasma volume expansion is not masking continued erythrocytosis.

When a normal red cell mass and PCV have been achieved, the patient can be followed at 4 to 8 week intervals. Additional phlebotomy should be ordered whenever the PCV exceeds 47 per cent unless the red cell mass is found to be normal at this hematocrit. We prefer to maintain the PCV at the *lower* limit of normal. The patient must be instructed to avoid the use of iron-containing preparations such as vitamins and tonics.

Phlebotomy as the sole form of therapy in polycythemia vera is advocated by those who believe that morbidity and mortality are primarily reduced by correcting just the increased blood volume. The use of myelosuppressive agents that may alter the cytogenetic characteristics of the stem cell, and may be leukemogenic, is thus avoided. Phlebotomy alone is the treatment of choice in young patients, including rare cases of polycythemia vera in children and adolescents, women of child-bearing age, and males below age 40; in patients with indolent polycythemia; and in patients in whom the diagnostic criteria are insufficient to establish the diagnosis with assurance (unclassified erythrocytosis). Phlebotomy is also indicated in the infrequently seen polycythemia vera in pregnant women, although in such patients the PCV often declines, sometimes to anemic levels, during the time of child-bearing, only to relapse to elevated levels several weeks postpartum.

Phlebotomy treatment has several drawbacks. Depletion of iron stores is sometimes associated with symptoms of iron deficiency, especially fatigue and anorexia, and, less often, glossitis and dysphagia. Phlebotomy will not control progressive, painful splenomegaly, hyperleukocytosis, and thrombocytosis. Although the platelet count in polycythemia vera does not invariably increase after venesection, when symptomatic thrombocytosis occurs, phlebotomy management should be modified to include intermittent use of myelosuppressive therapy to reduce the platelet count to normal. (Chlorambucil as outlined below; or melphalan, 10 mg. orally per day for 5 days, and then 2 mg. orally per day until the platelet count is less than 250,000 per microliter; or radioactive phosphorus as outlined below.)

In elderly patients, particularly in those with a previous history of cardiovascular or cerebrovascular disease, phlebotomy as the sole therapy for polycythemia vera is usually inadvisable because these patients are particularly susceptible to the early occurrence of thromboembolic complications (sudden death, myocardial infarction, stroke, and thrombophlebitis). A phlebotomy regimen can be managed successfully only in patients who can be checked by their physician at regular intervals. Phlebotomy treatment may also be unacceptable in some patients with extremely refractory erythrocytosis who require frequent venesections. However, these patients may be equally resistant to myelosuppressive therapy as well.

Under Public Health Service (PHS) regulations, blood that is withdrawn from polycythemic patients who otherwise qualify as blood donors (i.e., the patient is not receiving medication) is acceptable as a source of whole blood, provided that the blood is conspicuously labeled to indicate the donor's disease. The decision to use polycythemic blood for transfusions rests with the physician in charge of the blood bank and with the physician attending the prospective recipient. There is no evidence that transfusion of polycythemic blood is at all harmful. At our institution, blood from polycythemic patients has been used for at least 30 years without any known detrimental effects. Patients with polycythemia vera may be particularly suitable as platelet donors. The routine processing and transfusion of blood components derived from qualified polycythemic donors should be encouraged.

Myelosuppressive Therapy. The two types of myelosuppressive agents used most frequently are drugs and radiation. Enthusiasm for this form of therapy has been tempered by a concern for the possible leukemogenic and carcinogenic role of ionizing radiation and radiomimetic drugs in polycythemia vera. However, myelosuppressive therapy is often recommended for patients above the age of 40, because the additional beneficial effects on thrombocytosis, leukocytosis, hyperuricemia, and symptomatic hepatosplenomegaly that are not attainable with phlebotomy alone may reduce the early occurrence of thrombohemorrhagic complications and augment survival time. With myelosuppressive therapy, the period of induction may extend over several weeks before the desired effect is achieved. During this time, the PCV should be kept in the normal range by use of phlebotomy. The problem of hematologic toxicity (depletion of marrow and circulating blood elements) must be carefully avoided in any myelosuppressive regimen.

RADIATION. Radioactive phosphorus (^{32}P), which has been used successfully for over 30 years, is the current agent of choice for radiotherapy of polycythemia vera. The dosage schedule recommended by the Polycythemia Vera Study Group is as follows: 2.3 millicuries (mCi) per square meter of body surface area is administered intravenously for the initial dose, with a maximum dosage not to exceed 5 mCi. The patient is seen at 4 week intervals. The PCV is maintained below 47 per cent with phlebotomy. This dose usually results in normalization of PCV and platelet count within 4 to 8 weeks. If, however, after 3 months, remission is not achieved and the patient requires supplementary phlebotomy, administration of ^{32}P is repeated and the dosage increased by 25 per cent to a total not to exceed 7 mCi. Should the patient continue to be refractory, a third and fourth dose may be administered, each time after 12 week intervals, with dose augmentation to a maximum of 7 mCi. In the rare event that a patient does not respond after four doses in 1 year, no further ^{32}P is given and an alternative therapy is selected. ^{32}P is not given whenever the white blood cell count (WBC) is less than 3000 per microliter or the platelet count is less than 100,000 per microliter.

The intravenous route is preferred because absorption of orally administered ^{32}P is unpredictable. Remissions after ^{32}P therapy are frequently of long duration, often in excess of 1 to 2 years. After relapse, subsequent remissions that follow reinduction with radiophosphorus tend to be successively shorter in duration. With the recommended dosage schedule, thrombocytopenia sometimes occurs, but significant leukopenia has rarely been a problem. There are no other significant side effects. ^{32}P therapy is predictable and reliable, and enjoys a high degree of patient acceptability because of generally lengthy treatment-free intervals and fewer visits to the physician's office.

In previous retrospective studies, 10 to 15 per cent of patients with polycythemia vera treated with radiophosphorus developed acute myeloblastic leukemia at an average period of 10 to 12 years from the time of initiation of therapy. At this time, a relationship between the total dosage of ^{32}P administered and the likelihood of developing acute leukemia is not clearly defined. Development of acute leukemia in patients with polycythemia vera treated either with phlebotomy only or with alkylating agents is also well documented.

ALKYLATING AGENTS. The Polycythemia Vera Study Group uses either chlorambucil (Leukeran) or melphalan (Alkeran) for chemotherapy of polycythemia vera. Busulfan (Myleran), although often effective in inducing lengthy remissions without need for maintenance therapy, is not ordinarily recommended because of inordinate risk of persistent leukopenia and thrombocytopenia, skin hyperpigmentation, and pulmonary toxicity. Cyclophosphamide (Cytoxan), 75 to 100 mg. orally per day every other month, is sometimes particularly effective in shrinking hepatosplenomegaly in polycythemic patients with marked extramedullary hematopoiesis. Other agents that have been used effectively include hydroxyurea (Hydrea), procarbazine (Matulane), dibromomannitol, pipobroman (Vercyte), and pyrimethamine (Daraprim). (With the exception of pipobroman, this use of the aforementioned agents is not listed in the manufacturer's official directive.)

Chlorambucil (Leukeran): The initial dosage of chlorambucil during the induction period is 10 mg. orally per day. (This use of chlorambucil is not listed in the manufacturer's official directive.) The patient is seen at 3 week intervals. Therapy is withheld should the PCV be below 42 per cent, the WBC less than 3000 per microliter, or the platelet count less than 100,000 per microliter. The dosage is reduced by 2 to 4 mg. per day if the WBC is 3000 to 5000 per microliter or the platelet count 100,000 to 150,000 per microliter. Supplementary phlebotomy is performed if the PCV is greater than 47 per cent. After 6 weeks, if the PCV continues above 47 per cent or the platelet count exceeds 600,000 per microliter, the daily dosage may be increased by 2 mg. in the absence of leukopenia. Further increases in the dosage may be allowed in refractory patients at subsequent 3 week intervals provided there is no evidence of hematologic toxicity. When the PCV, WBC, and platelet count are stable in the normal range for a period of 8 weeks without supplementary phlebotomy, maintenance therapy, chlorambucil, 6 to 10 mg. orally per day for 1 month, *every other month,* is started. Most patients remain in remission on alternate month maintenance therapy. Some patients require continuous drug therapy for maintenance of remission. The drug schedules above may sometimes have to be modified to suit the individual patient.

In the experience of the Polycythemia Vera Study Group, chlorambucil is as effective as ^{32}P in inducing and maintaining remission. The incidence of thrombocytopenia is comparable, but significant leukopenia is observed more commonly with chlorambucil. The frequency of patient visits and blood counts is greater for patients treated with chlorambucil, and patient reliability in taking the proper dosage of the prescribed medication is a significant factor. Occasional gastrointestinal intolerance of chlorambucil and transient pruritic skin lesions responding to withdrawal of the drug have been described. Alopecia has not been a common problem. Aspermia and infertility in male patients treated with chlorambucil is a significant complication which should be fully discussed before beginning therapy.

Melphalan (Alkeran): Melphalan is also effective for the treatment of polycythemia vera and may replace chlorambucil in patients exhibiting drug idiosyncrasy. In patients in relapse, melphalan achieves remission somewhat more rapidly than chlorambucil. However, hematologic toxicity (leukopenia and thrombocytopenia) occurs twice as frequently with melphalan, emphasizing the need for careful monitoring of blood counts. The initial dose of melphalan is 4 to 8 mg. orally in the morning for 5 days, after which the dosage is reduced to 2 mg. three times *weekly* for 4 weeks (this use of melphalan is not listed in the manufacturer's official directive). Treatment is then stopped for 4 weeks. Blood counts are performed at 1 to 2 week intervals, and therapy is adjusted in accordance with the results until a probable maintenance dosage has been established.

Choice of Therapy

There is no evidence that any of the aforementioned treatments is clearly optimal for all patients with polycythemia vera. Results from the Polycythemia Vera Study Group are still preliminary and are based, at this time, on an average of 4 years of patient follow-up. The following conclusions therefore represent only our personal convictions based on the evidence available to date:

1. Patients younger than 40 years old, men and women alike, patients with indolent polycythemia, and patients with "unclassified erythrocytosis" are best managed with phlebotomy alone, unless marked, symptomatic thrombocytosis necessitates addition of intermittent myelosuppressive therapy.

2. Phlebotomy therapy only is generally not indicated in elderly patients, particularly those with a predisposition to thromboembolic disease.

3. Expectations that alkylating agents would be less leukemogenic than ^{32}P have not been fulfilled with the dosage schedules commonly used. Acute leukemia has been documented in a number of patients with polycythemia vera treated solely with alkylating agents, and the period between initiation of therapy and onset of acute leukemia appears, in some instances, to be shorter than that expected with ^{32}P therapy. We therefore believe that, when myelosuppressive therapy is to be used, radioactive phosphorus, which is advantageous in terms of ease of administration, long duration of unmaintained re-

mission, and patient convenience, is generally the preferred treatment for most newly diagnosed patients, with alkylating agents reserved for refractory cases.

4. Identification of effective, nonleukemogenic chemotherapy for polycythemia vera continues to be a necessary research objective.

THE PORPHYRIAS

method of
JOEL M. LAMON, M.D.,
and DONALD P. TSCHUDY, M.D.
Bethesda, Maryland

The porphyrias are a clinically heterogeneous group of diseases which can be defined as primary disorders of porphyrin metabolism, in contrast to secondary porphyrinuria, which occurs in the presence of other well defined disorders. They have been classified into erythropoietic and hepatic types, but for purposes of this discussion we will categorize them as producing cutaneous or acute attack disease (Table 1). Seven porphyrias have been described. They include porphyria cutanea tarda (PCT), congenital erythropoietic porphyria (CEP), erythropoietic protoporphyria (EPP), erythropoietic coproporphyria (ECP), acute intermittent porphyria (AIP), variegate porphyria (VP),* and hereditary coproporphyria (HCP).* The specific diagnosis of one of these diseases is based on demonstration of a characteristic pattern of metabolites of the heme biosynthetic pathway in urine, red cells, and stool.

The cutaneous porphyrias are photosensitive syndromes which present a spectrum of symptoms and clinical disease. This group includes all forms of porphyria except AIP. A bullous dermatosis with skin fragility and hypertrichosis is typical of VP, HCP, and PCT. Urinary uroporphyrin and coproporphyrin measurement will disclose the chemical abnormality in these diseases. A more massive urinary uroporphyrin excretion occurs in CEP and is associated with severe photosensitivity. EPP produces a remarkable syndrome of rapid onset and variably severe photosensitivity characterized by erythema, burning, and pruritus over

*Listed as both an acute attack and cutaneous porphyria.

TABLE 1. **The Porphyrias**

	TESTS TO ORDER*	ENZYME DEFICIENCY	INHERITANCE
Porphyrias producing cutaneous disease (excretion of porphyrins: uro-, copro-, and proto-)			
Porphyria cutanea tarda (PCT)	Urine uro- and coproporphyrin	Uroporphyrinogen decarboxylase	Autosomal dominant and acquired
Variegate porphyria (VP)	Urine ALA, PBG, uro-, and coproporphyrin Stool protoporphyrin	?	Autosomal dominant
Hereditary coproporphyria (HCP)	Urine ALA, PBG, and coproporphyrin Stool coproporphyrin	Coproporphyrinogen oxidase	Autosomal dominant
Congenital erythropoietic porphyria (CEP)	Urine uroporphyrin (isomer I) Plasma uroporphyrin	Uroporphyrinogen III cosynthase	Autosomal recessive
Erythropoietic protoporphyria (EPP)	Red cell protoporphyrin Stool protoporphyrin	Ferrochelatase	Autosomal dominant
Erythropoietic coproporphyria (ECP)	Red cell coproporphyrin Stool coproporphyrin	?	?
Porphyrias producing acute attacks (excretion of porphyrin precursors: ALA and PBG are increased during an acute attack)			
Acute intermittent porphyria (AIP)	Urine ALA, and PBG	Uroporphyrinogen I synthase	Autosomal dominant
Variegate porphyria (VP)	Urine ALA, PBG, uro-, and coproporphyrin Stool protoporphyrin	?	Autosomal dominant
Hereditary coproporphyria (HCP)	Urine ALA, PBG, uro-, and coproporphyrin Stool coproporphyrin	Coproporphyrinogen oxidase	Autosomal dominant

*This is a simplification of porphyrin excretion in the porphyrias. A more complete discussion of porphyrin abnormalities is available elsewhere.

the sun-exposed areas. Protoporphyrin excess can be appreciated only in the red cells and stool.

The clinical picture of acute attack porphyria (AIP, VP, and HCP) may contain any one or a combination of several neurologic dysfunctions during the acute phase of the illness. Symptoms may include abdominal, back, or extremity pains and paresthesias, numbness, weakness, loss of motor function with subsequent muscle atrophy, nausea, palpitations, and constipation (diarrhea is less frequent). Signs that are supportive of the diagnosis are urinary retention, diaphoresis, sinus tachycardia, hypertension, axonal degeneration or demyelination (by electromyogram [EMG] examination) with muscle atrophy, organic brain syndrome, and seizures. The demonstration of elevated porphobilinogen (PBG) in the urine is diagnostic during an acute attack. Elevated urinary aminolevulinic acid (ALA) is also characteristic, but not diagnostic. Screening procedures (Watson-Schwartz and Hoesch tests) detect elevated urinary PBG. Quantitative 24 hour urinary measurements of PBG and ALA are mandatory following a positive interpretation of either screening test. Therapeutic considerations of these disorders can be divided into prophylaxis, treatment of symptoms and complications, and attempts to reverse the fundamental disease process. In the acute attack types of porphyria, prophylaxis is particularly important and may avoid life-threatening complications.

The Cutaneous Porphyrias

Porphyria Cutanea Tarda (PCT). This disease is typical in older males, and a background of excessive alcohol intake is frequent. Both sporadic and family aggregations of PCT have been seen, and a deficiency of uroporphyrinogen decarboxylase has been described recently. An autosomal dominant inheritance was confirmed using this enzyme lesion as a marker of disease. In addition to alcohol, estrogen and iron have been implicated in the pathogenesis of the disease.

Treatment should include abstinence from alcohol and iron-containing medication and discontinuance of estrogen therapy or oral contraceptives if possible. We have found phlebotomy (as have other clinicians) to be uniformly successful in the treatment of PCT. The basis of its therapeutic effect is through iron depletion. Phlebotomy of 1 unit of whole blood is performed at approximately monthly intervals. Determinations of hemoglobin, hematocrit, and quantitative urinary uro- and coproporphyrin are performed at each visit. Clinical remission usually occurs after there has been a decline of uroporphyrin excretion to less than 500 to 1000 micrograms per 24 hours (normal, <60 micrograms per 24 hours). Phlebotomy is postponed when hemoglobin is less than 11 grams per 100 ml. A fall in red cell mean corpuscular volume (MCV) is a clue to iron depletion. A relatively frequent phlebotomy schedule, such as every 2 weeks, may lead to excess iron depletion. The reduction in urine uroporphyrin excretion seems to occur slowly, and the monthly schedule has avoided unnecessary anemia. One should expect to achieve almost complete depletion of iron stores before urine uroporphyrin excretion falls. There is no contraindication to phlebotomy of affected menstruating females. However, since their disease is typically related to oral contraceptives, these should be discontinued along with the institution of phlebotomy.

Chloroquine therapy has been successful, but it has caused some morbidity related to liver toxicity and gastrointestinal side effects. (This use of chloroquine is not listed in the manufacturer's official directive.) New regimens using chloroquine at a low dose for an extended period of time have been reported to be successful and safe. In most instances phlebotomy remains the treatment of choice.

Variegate Porphyria and Hereditary Coproporphyria (VP and HCP). These two porphyrias have cutaneous symptoms similar to PCT. A bullous dermatosis on the sun-exposed areas of the body, especially the dorsa of the hands, and increased fragility of the skin are typical. Patients are seen who have only the cutaneous manifestations without acute attack symptoms. Because of the clinical similarity of the cutaneous manifestation to PCT, these two disorders must be considered in atypical PCT—i.e., in young people and in people without evidence of iron excess, estrogen use, or toxin exposure. A positive family history for similar cutaneous disease may be present in VP, HCP, or PCT. Stool protoporphyrin elevation is unique to VP among this group, stool coproporphyrin is elevated in HCP, and PCT has an isocoproporphyrin in the stool.

The cutaneous disease is frequently mild. The major therapeutic maneuver is avoidance of sun exposure, as iron depletion by phlebotomy has not been a successful therapy. To our knowledge beta-carotene has not been used. In both VP and HCP, the major concern has been acute attack phenomena, which are discussed below.

Congenital Erythropoietic Porphyria (CEP). This is a rare, autosomal recessive form of porphyria. These patients often excrete ten-fold more urinary uroporphyrin than PCT patients. This uroporphyrin is predominantly the series I isomer, which is nonfunctional in heme biosynthesis. A hypochromic anemia associated with both ineffective erythropoiesis and hemolysis is observed. Skin deformities also occur that are related to the bullae and skin fragility.

Splenectomy has had variable degrees of success in decreasing hemolysis and porphyrin production. Recently beta-carotene (Solatene) orally has proved to be an effective photoprotective agent for these people. Red cell transfusion has resulted in a fall in uroporphyrin excretion and a decrease of sun sensitivity. Vitamin E treatment has been reported to decrease urinary porphyrin excretion; however, it did not alter the photosensitivity or the hemolytic anemia. Resolution of the skin disease and the anemia and disappearance of the splenomegaly have all been reported to be responsive to light shielding to wavelengths below 510 nm.

Erythropoietic Protoporphyria (EPP). This photosensitive porphyria is unique for the absence of findings in the urine. Penetrance of this autosomal dominant condition is variable, with mild and subclinical disease typically recognized following the diagnosis of a more severely affected family member. The recent appreciation of hepatobiliary dysfunction as a sequela of longstanding and chemically severe EPP has stimulated more interest in therapeutic intervention.

Beta-carotene (Solatene) is an effective treatment of the photosensitivity. The patients take this medication during the sunny months of the year. An effective dosage is achieved by each patient's titrating his medication to compensate for photosensitivity. Most patients notice carotenodermia, but this has not been a problem for them. The chances of untoward effects of beta-carotene therapy are minimal.

Despite this effective sunscreening, the chemical abnormality of the disease is not altered. Because of the newly recognized sequelae of cholelithiasis, liver dysfunction, and even cirrhosis with liver failure, attempts at altering the accumulation of protoporphyrin in the body are being investigated. Cholestyramine has been used in an effort to interrupt the enterohepatic circulation of protoporphyrin. Exchange transfusion has been used to halt the production of red cell protoporphyrin. The feasibility and efficacy of these endeavors for preventive treatment of hepatobiliary disease remain to be seen.

Erythropoietic Coproporphyria (ECP). ECP is too rare for a specific discussion. This diagnosis would be made by the chemical evaluation of suspected cutaneous porphyria, and treatment is the same as for EPP.

The Acute Attack Porphyrias

Acute Intermittent Porphyria (AIP). Although AIP is clinically more common in females, males are equally affected by the uroporphyrinogen I synthase (uro I syn) deficiency, which is detected by a red cell enzyme assay. As noted in Table 1, elevation of urinary PBG and ALA (porphyrin precursors) is the characteristic chemical abnormality in the acute attack porphyrias, which also include VP and HCP. In a family containing a person who has urinary PBG elevation and red cell uro I syn deficiency, we categorize four groups of people. First are those with active disease. This includes the index case and other family members who have acute attack symptoms and elevated urinary PBG. Second are those people who are asymptomatic but who have elevated urinary PBG. Red cell uro I syn deficiency is a concomitant of these first two groups, but is not necessary to establish the diagnosis. The third category consists of those family members with deficient red cell uro I syn activity, but who are asymptomatic and have no urinary abnormalities. Approximately 50 per cent of blood relatives in such a family will fall in one of these three categories. The fourth category consists of the other 50 per cent who will be normal with respect to AIP.

Prevention of illness in persons with known disease is of fundamental importance in the acute porphyrias. Drugs that are known to precipitate porphyric attacks should be avoided. The most common include barbiturates, griseofulvin, phenytoin, sulfonamides, meprobamate, chlorpropamide, tolbutamide, antipyrine, and estrogen. We also avoid compounds related to these known precipitating agents. It is prudent to avoid the use of drugs whose effect on AIP is unknown. Some common drugs that are considered safe are meperidine, phenothiazines, diazepam, glucocorticoids, penicillins, erythromycin, aminoglycosides, tetracyclines, propoxyphene, and propranolol. Starvation can also precipitate an acute attack, and this is considered to be secondary to carbohydrate restriction. Alcohol should be avoided. Whether infections, trauma, or surgical procedures are primary causes of a porphyric attack or whether they are the reasons for carbohydrate deprivation or for use of contraindicated medication is not clear. Utmost precaution should be taken in known porphyrics while ensuring prompt treatment for intercurrent illness.

Chlorpromazine (Thorazine) is a useful agent in treating abdominal pain, presumably in part through its ganglionic blocking activity. One should follow closely the porphyric patient who is taking chlorpromazine, being careful to avoid producing extrapyramidal side effects. Diazepam is safe for the management of acute seizure disorders related to porphyria. For seizures not related primarily to the porphyria, the choice of therapy is difficult. Not only phenobarbital and phenytoin but also primidone and carbamazepine can induce delta-aminolevulinic acid synthetase in rat liver. Bromides have been used with success in this situation. Propoxyphene is tolerated well, and for severe pain meperidine is effective. The risk of analgesic dependence is significant in these patients, and this should be kept in mind, especially after the resolution of an acute attack. Propranolol may be useful for some of the autonomic problems, including hypertension and tachycardia. Recent reports claim a beneficial effect of this drug on the abdominal pain and porphyrin metabolism.

Although some women experience cyclic attacks occurring just prior to the onset of menstruation, and although estrogen can precipitate a porphyric attack, most women experience no major problems with the disease during pregnancy, including some who have experienced earlier attacks. The premenstrual attacks which some women experience have been responsive to the suppression of ovulation in a small series. Androgens and, in recent years, oral contraceptives have been useful in this group. Oral contraceptives should be avoided in AIP, except for this special situation. Since experience with this type of therapy in cyclic attacks is limited, it is not yet clear whether all patients of this type will respond to suppressive therapy.

Active treatment for an acute attack is largely supportive. Aggressive physical and occupational therapy should be provided for those patients who experience motor neuropathy. Respirator support may be indicated, and the patient may be dependent on a respirator for many weeks. Although the prognosis is bleak in this situation, the goal of therapy is cessation of the attack and full return of function. A high carbohydrate diet (about 300 grams per day) is recommended for all acute porphyria patients; however, during an acute exacerbation one should provide as much in excess of this level as possible. Four hundred to 600 grams of carbohydrate a day have been given during the acute phase. The therapeutic response to carbohydrate is variable; some patients show rapid improvement, whereas others are not affected. The mechanism of the carbohydrate effect is not understood. Hematin, the iron-protoporphyrin molecule derived from red cells, has been used in recent clinical trials with promising results. During a course of intravenous therapy, the urinary ALA and PBG abnormalities have uniformly decreased. The correlation of clinical improvement has been effective only in some patients. Established neuropathy appears to be refractory to hematin. More clinical trials are necessary.

Variegate Porphyria and Hereditary Coproporphyria (VP and HCP). The background and therapeutic considerations of these two acute attack porphyrias are virtually identical to those of AIP. The red cell uro I syn assay is normal in these patients. They may or may not experience cutaneous symptoms. When they are asymptomatic, their urinary PBG and ALA may be normal; however, during an attack the urinary PBG is elevated. Propranolol has been used to treat the acute abdominal pain of VP as well as the associated tachycardia. (This use of propranolol to treat abdominal pain is not listed in the manufacturer's official directive.)

THERAPEUTIC USE OF BLOOD COMPONENTS

method of
PETER A. TOMASULO, M.D.
Milwaukee, Wisconsin

Introduction

The separation of blood into its components by centrifugation, washing, and biochemical purification allows more than 15 therapeutic products to be prepared from each donation. The risk of transfusion is reduced by using only that product which is needed. Purification allows delivery of blood components in concentrations high enough to be effective without producing volume overload. Careful choice of the appropriate blood product makes the other components of the blood available for proper processing. One voluntary donation of a unit of blood can be used to meet the multiple needs of different patients. Using good medical judgment to choose only the necessary component leads to the efficient use of a complex tissue in short supply.

Blood products should be administered to supply specific deficient components. Blood is not a tonic. Neither whole blood nor any of its components will shorten convalescence, heal wounds, or nonspecifically make patients feel better. In fact, one should generally assume that the nonspecific effects of blood transfusion are undesirable.

Oxygen Carrying Capacity

The component of blood which carries oxygen is the erythrocyte. The erythrocyte can be administered as whole blood, packed cells, buffy-poor packed cells, saline-washed packed cells, or frozen washed packed cells. Each red cell preparation has different characteristics and specific indications for administration. Patients should usually be transfused with group and type-specific red cells. During relative blood shortages, it is perfectly acceptable to give crossmatch-compatible group O red cells to patients of other blood types.

Group AB patients can receive red cells from group A, group B, or group O donors safely. Whenever nongroup-specific blood is administered, it should be transfused as packed red blood cells. Removing the plasma reduces the quantity of transfused isohemagglutinins capable of producing mild destruction of recipient cells.

Patients with acute massive blood loss and shock sometimes (but only rarely) require transfusion before a routine crossmatch can be performed. Uncrossmatched group O $Rh_o(D)$ negative blood may be given in this situation. Group O $Rh_o(D)$ negative red blood cells will neither sensitize the host to ABO antigens nor be destroyed by ABO isohemagglutinins. The transfusion is generally safe, but the administration of uncrossmatched blood in an emergency is not usually necessary. Because blood typing requires only 10 minutes, group-specific blood can be provided quickly. Complete compatibility testing requires 1 hour, but "emergency" crossmatches can give some assurance of safety in 10 minutes. Perfusion of critical organs can generally be maintained by transfusing electrolyte or protein solutions until the crossmatch is completed.

Any red cell transfusion has the potential to produce a fatal reaction. This risk should not be assumed unless the transfusion is absolutely necessary. No patient whose oxygen-carrying deficit can be corrected without blood transfusion should receive red cells. Iron deficiency anemia, the anemia associated with vitamin B_{12} or folate deficiency, and/or the anemia associated with mild acute blood loss can generally be corrected without blood transfusion. Many chronic anemias are not associated with symptoms. Patients with renal failure and chronic hemolytic anemias have hematocrits as low as 15 to 20 per cent without significant disability. Patients with rheumatoid arthritis and other inflammatory diseases often have milder depression of the hematocrit without symptoms of anemia. Most patients with longstanding anemia do not require red cell transfusion. One should never transfuse a patient merely to correct an abnormal laboratory value.

Patients with significant anemia of undetermined origin should be evaluated both clinically and with the aid of the laboratory prior to transfusion. Examination of the peripheral blood smear yields important information and documents the patient's condition prior to transfusion. This procedure and certain others should always be performed prior to transfusing any patient with an anemia of unproved cause.

Packed Red Blood Cells. Packed red cell concentrates can supply oxygen-carrying capacity for almost all anemic patients. This product is prepared by sedimenting whole blood and removing 80 per cent of the supernatant plasma. The volume of the unit is 250 ml. Its hematocrit is approximately 70 per cent, and it has the same oxygen-carrying capacity and the same amount of iron (250 mg.) as a unit of whole blood.

Removing the supernatant plasma reduces the risk of volume overload and citrate toxicity. In addition, if blood is sedimented immediately prior to transfusion, the quantity of transfused potassium, sodium, and ammonia will be reduced. This may be significant for patients with liver disease, neonatal patients, and patients with renal and heart disease. Occasionally, the slow flow rate of a packed red cell unit becomes a problem. This can be handled by adding 30 to 50 ml. of isotonic saline to the bag via Y-tubing (dextrose in water and buffered electrolyte solutions should not be added to packed red cell units).

Whole Blood. There are no clinical situations that absolutely require the use of whole blood. Whole blood transfusions should be given to patients suffering from acute blood loss (surgical or traumatic) of sufficient magnitude to cause hypovolemic shock. Whole blood should be given when an increase in both the intravascular volume and the oxygen-carrying capacity is needed. In either situation, packed red cell concentrates and electrolyte or protein solutions can also supply the patient's needs.

Blood donors routinely lose up to 14 per cent of their blood volumes in 5 or 10 minutes without untoward effects. The replacement of a 500 ml. blood loss at elective surgery is hardly ever necessary, and acute elective surgical blood loss of less than 1500 ml. should be replaced with packed cells in most instances. Patients with low hematocrits resulting from bleeding are not likely to be hypovolemic unless they are bleeding acutely. Certainly an anemic patient who has not bled for 48 hours should receive packed cells instead of whole blood.

Leukocyte-Poor Red Cell Preparations. Many patients with chronic illnesses need long-term support with red cell transfusions. Sensitization by soluble and cellular antigens may occur after any transfusion. In addition to the problems in red cell crossmatching, patients who have received great quantities of blood may have regular recurrent febrile nonhemolytic reactions. These can be ameliorated and often eliminated by appropriate use of leukocyte and platelet-poor red cell concentrates. Not all chronically transfused patients have febrile reactions; if they do develop, they may be sporadic. Chronically ill patients should not be treated with white cell–poor products in anticipation of febrile non-hemolytic transfusion reactions. Up to 25 per cent of the red cells may be lost when white cells and plasma are removed. The blood resources of most communities cannot tolerate this unnecessary waste, and for the individual patient the loss of red cells incurred in making buffy-poor preparations may actually mean an exposure to more units of blood. Leukocyte-poor products should be used only after febrile nonhemolytic reactions have been shown to be recurrent.

BUFFY-POOR PACKED RED BLOOD CELLS. Approximately 80 per cent of the white blood cells and platelets can be removed from blood by inverted centrifugation. Leukocyte-poor (buffy-poor) packed red cells have been shown to be effective in preventing febrile nonhemolytic transfusion reactions in highly sensitized subjects. Leukocyte-poor packed red cells should be administered to frequently transfused patients who have had two or more successive febrile nonhemolytic transfusion reactions.

SALINE-WASHED LEUKOCYTE-POOR RED CELLS. A few patients will continue to have febrile reactions even when buffy-poor packed cells are used. These patients should receive saline-washed, buffy-poor units. Washing leukocyte-poor blood removes most of the white cells, platelets, and plasma remaining after inverted centrifugation. This product is more effective than buffy-poor blood in treating patients with febrile reactions. Washing is time-consuming, and some additional red cells are lost. Washed units must be transfused within 24 hours of preparation, because an open system is used. The short shelf life is necessary to prevent bacterial growth.

FROZEN RED CELLS. Freezing blood with a cryoprotective agent such as glycerol allows the storage of blood for extended periods of time. This blood must be repeatedly "washed" to remove the glycerol. Washing removes plasma proteins, white cells, and platelets. Patients with febrile nonhemolytic transfusion reactions rarely have problems severe enough to justify the use of frozen blood, but this product contains the smallest quantity of potentially sensitizing non–red cell antigens.

Frozen red cell concentrates are most helpful in the therapy of patients with rare red cell types. Because the frozen units can be stored for years, persons with rare blood types should be encouraged to donate blood for freezing in anticipation of possible future autotransfusion.

Saline-washed and frozen packed red cells are nearly free of all tissue antigens. There is controversy about the benefits of these products for potential transplant recipients. The cost of preparing these units is high; because an "open" system is used, the shelf life is only 24 hours. Frozen red cells may be less likely to cause hepatitis than packed red cells, but this has not yet been definitely established.

Hypovolemia

Acute hypovolemia initially can be treated by infusing saline or other electrolyte solutions. In many situations, it will be necessary to add protein to the infusate to make the effect more longlasting. The purified albumin preparations are the products of choice to increase the intravascular volume in these situations. Fresh frozen plasma has been used to expand the vascular volume, but this has disadvantages (see below).

Plasma Protein Fraction and Albumin. Plasma protein fraction is a 5 per cent protein solution consisting of albumin and a small amount of globulin. Albumin is a more highly purified product and is available in 5 and 25 per cent solutions. The use of albumin solutions has increased dramatically in recent years. These products are relatively safe. Fewer than 2 per cent of all transfusions are accompanied by reactions, and none are longlasting or severe. When adequately heat treated, these products are free of the risk of hepatitis.

The concentrated (25 per cent) albumin preparation increases intravascular volume by drawing fluid from the extravascular space. The 25 per cent solution must be given with considerable caution when the recipient is elderly or suffering from cardiac dysfunction because of its dramatic effect on intravascular volume.

The principal indications for albumin therapy are acute hypovolemia associated with surgery, trauma, severe burns, or respiratory distress syndrome; dialysis; and such chronic conditions as malabsorption and nephrotic syndrome. In the opinion of many, albumin solutions are overused clinically, particularly in the treatment of chronic disorders. These products should not be used merely to "treat" a low serum albumin value or for nutritional purposes. Oral administration of amino acids and proteins and intravenous administration of amino acids lead to increased protein synthesis even in patients with liver dysfunction.

Clotting Factor Deficiencies

Many clotting factor deficiencies are not associated with an increased risk of hemorrhage. Soluble clotting factors can be reduced to approximately 25 per cent of normal levels without increasing the bleeding potential. Platelet counts over 15,000 or 20,000 per cu. mm. are generally sufficient to prevent spontaneous hemorrhage, and counts over 50,000 per cu. mm. provide essentially normal hemostasis even in stress situations. Abnormal laboratory values alone are not indications for therapy. Laboratory evaluation should be begun when the clinical examination of the patient suggests a pathologic bleeding state. Evaluation of clinical and laboratory information will lead to a documentation of the deficiency and an understanding of its cause. Only after this investigation can therapeutic decisions be made.

Every product available to treat clotting deficiencies has the potential to cause hepatitis. A platelet concentrate or a pool of cryoprecipitated factor VIII (cryoprecipitate) made of 10 units each may be five to ten times more likely to cause hepatitis than is 1 unit of packed red cells. The commercial concentrates of clotting factors are prepared from large pools of plasma and therefore are more likely to contain the hepatitis virus than cryoprecipitate or platelet concentrate. The factor IX complex concentrates have been linked with serious thrombotic syndromes. None of these products should be administered without specific clinical indications.

Platelet Concentrates. Patients with severe thrombocytopenia, abnormal bleeding, and decreased platelet production may respond favorably to platelet transfusion. Patients who have received great quantities of blood rapidly (more than 12 units in a few hours) may develop abnormal bleeding resulting from dilutional thrombocytopenia. Platelet transfusions are efficacious in these patients if the blood loss can be controlled. Many thrombocytopenic states are characterized by rapid platelet destruction. Patients with very short platelet life spans do not respond as well (either by increasing the count or by decreasing the volume of blood lost) to platelet transfusions. If a patient with a shortened platelet survival has a life-threatening hemorrhage, attempts should be made to provide hemostasis with large doses of platelets in spite of the early platelet destruction.

Platelets are thought to contain the antigens of the ABO system, but ABO mismatched platelets are as effective as ABO-compatible platelets and should be used when compatible platelets are not available. Units of platelets may contain up to 0.5 ml. of red cells, and therefore $Rh_o(D)$ negative children and $Rh_o(D)$ negative women of childbearing age should receive platelets from $Rh_o(D)$ negative blood, or they should receive $Rh_o(D)$ immune globulin if they receive random donor platelets. It is impossible for any blood center to supply all the $Rh_o(D)$ negative patients with platelets from $Rh_o(D)$ negative blood. Sensitization can be prevented with $Rh_o(D)$ immune globulin. Sepsis, splenomegaly, and previous transfusion are known to decrease the effectiveness of platelet transfusions.

In a nonsensitized patient, 1 unit of platelets per 10 kg. of body weight will provide an increment (1 hour post-transfusion) of approximately 50,000 platelets per cu. mm., therefore in a 70 kg. man, a transfusion of an 8 unit platelet concentrate will ordinarily provide a significant increment and effective hemostasis. It is impossible to prevent sensitization to platelet antigens, and therefore all recipients of multiple platelet transfusions will develop antiplatelet antibodies. These antibodies will lead to progressively smaller platelet increments and shorter platelet survivals. It is unlikely that platelet transfusions can be effective without producing an increment in the platelet count. For this reason, all platelet transfusions should be accompanied by an immediate pretransfusion platelet count and platelet counts 1 and 12 or 24 hours after transfusion.

When the increments and platelet life span begin to decrease in a patient requiring repeated platelet transfusions, new therapeutic modalities should be considered. Patients who have become refractory to platelets prepared from random donors will usually respond to platelets prepared from HLA-matched donors. The use of modern cell separators makes possible the production of platelet concentrates from single donors who are matched to the recipient. Using donors matched for the HLA antigens or donors matched for cross-reacting HLA antigens, it is possible to provide hemostatically effective platelets for most patients refractory to random donor platelets. HLA matching donor and recipient does not permanently prevent refractoriness, however; even with matched donors, increments will eventually decrease. Presently, there is no evidence to suggest that early use of HLA-matched platelets is of special benefit, and there are theoretical considerations suggesting that early exposure to the HLA-matched products may lead to more difficult problems with refractoriness in the long run. This subject is presently being investigated.

Fresh Frozen Plasma. This product contains normal levels (1 unit per ml.) of all the soluble clotting factors. Fresh frozen plasma (FFP) can be used to treat any of the hereditary clotting deficiencies. Short-term hemostasis can be provided for some patients with diminished hepatic synthetic function and for patients suffering from vitamin K deficiency. Vitamin K deficiency often can be treated by oral or parenteral vitamin K. Transfusion is not always necessary. Using FFP as a therapeutic source of factor VIII and factor IX for hemophiliacs is the least wasteful therapy available, but the large volumes required to provide hemostatic protection make other products more attractive.

FFP may be used to treat hypovolemia, but

there are disadvantages. Although FFP is inexpensive, this product requires 1 hour to thaw, contains isohemagglutinins, can cause nonhemolytic transfusion reactions, and has the same potential as 1 unit of packed red cells to cause hepatitis.

Patients receiving great quantities of stored blood are often routinely given fresh frozen plasma "to replace protein coagulation factors." There is very little evidence that such a routine is ever indicated in patients with normal hepatic function, and the practice is even questionable in patients with defective hepatic synthetic function. Patients receiving more than 10 or 12 units of blood in a few hours should be examined closely for the development of abnormal and/or excessive bleeding. Thrombocytopenia is much more likely to occur than is protein deficiency. If the clinical and laboratory data suggest that abnormal bleeding has occurred because of protein deficiencies, then fresh frozen plasma might be administered. Other products may be more appropriate. The physician should be aware that other hemorrhagic syndromes may develop in patients receiving great quantities of blood. Fresh frozen plasma is not routinely indicated for all situations.

Cryoprecipitated Factor VIII. One unit of cryoprecipitate (15 ml.) contains between 75 and 110 units of factor VIII coagulant activity and approximately 200 mg. of fibrinogen. This product should be a therapy of choice for almost all hemorrhagic episodes in hospitalized patients with classic hemophilia (factor VIII deficiency).

Antihemophilic Factor Concentrate. Several commercially prepared lyophilized factor VIII (AHF) concentrates are available. The American National Red Cross has also developed a partially purified concentrate. These products can be quickly transfused to factor VIII–deficient patients, and high levels of factor VIII can be easily maintained for prolonged periods. The product is prepared from a large plasma pool, and therefore is very likely to be contaminated with the infective agent for hepatitis. Although many patients with hemophilia are relatively "immune" to hepatitis because of their frequent exposure to blood products, this risk should not be ignored, especially in children or in infrequently treated adult hemophilic patients. Both AHF concentrates and cryoprecipitate are convenient for "home" therapy.

Factor IX Concentrates. A number of lyophilized preparations containing factors II, VII, IX, and X are available. These products may be more likely to cause hepatitis than the factor VIII concentrates, and rarely have been associated with severe thrombotic syndromes. The use of factor IX concentrates should be reserved for those patients with severe (less than 1 per cent clotting factor activity) Christmas disease and a history of many transfusions. The use of this material to reverse warfarin (Coumadin) therapy or to correct the coagulopathy of severe liver disease is not recommended. Fresh frozen plasma can be used to treat hemorrhagic episodes of many patients with factor IX deficiency, but because of volume considerations the lyophilized factor IX concentrates will be necessary for severe hemorrhages and for home therapy situations.

The factor IX complex concentrates are now being used experimentally to treat hemorrhagic episodes in patients with hemophilia A and circulating anticoagulants directed against the factor VIII molecule. The rationale for this therapy is not presently apparent, but the preliminary results suggest effectiveness.

Calculating Clotting Factor Doses. One ml. of normal plasma contains 1 unit of factor VIII and 1 unit of factor IX activity. The half-life of both factor VIII and factor IX is approximately 8 to 10 hours. Because factor IX is a small molecule, it distributes in a volume twice the size of the intravascular volume. This fact must be considered when treating a patient with Christmas disease.

The level of clotting factor activity must be chosen to fit the clinical situation (approximately 30 to 50 per cent for most hemorrhages). The plasma volume is calculated by the following formula:

$$\text{Weight (kg.)} \times 70 \text{ ml. blood per kg.} = \text{blood volume}$$

$$\text{(Blood volume)} \ (1 - \text{HCT}) = \text{plasma volume}$$

Knowing the plasma volume, it is a simple matter to determine the number of units of factor VIII or factor IX to infuse (e.g., plasma volume equals 3000 ml.; 30 per cent level would be 900 units of factor VIII). The first dose of factor IX given should be one and a half to two times the calculated amount to reach a chosen intravascular level (1500 to 1800 units for 30 per cent level). Factor VIII and factor IX levels should be monitored with laboratory assays whenever possible. Treatment should be administered early in bleeding episodes.

Products for Defense

Granulocyte Concentrates. Granulocyte concentrates can be prepared from single donors either by differential sedimentation or by nylon fiber filtration. Both methods of preparation have been shown to produce products which are effective against infection in leukopenic patients with marrow dysfunction. Granulocytes should be administered to infected patients with absolute granulocyte counts (bands and segmented neutrophils) less than 500 per microliter. The concentrates should consist of at least 1×10^{10} granulocytes and should be administered each day the patient is infected and profoundly leukopenic. White cell concentrates should be ABO compatible and crossmatched for red cell antibodies. White cell counts and differentials should be obtained immediately prior to the transfusions and 1 hour after each granulocyte transfusion. Increments observed will be small if detectable at all. The granulocyte transfusions should be administered at a rate not greater than 10^{10} cells per hour. Patients should be carefully observed during the infusions. HLA typing and/or other immunologic crossmatching techniques may be necessary for safety and effectiveness of granulocyte transfusions. These issues are now being evaluated. The administration of granulocytes prophylactically is also being studied. Considerations relating to cost and donor availability may require that white cells be transfused only to critically ill patients who meet very specific treatment criteria.

Rh_0(D) IMMUNE GLOBULIN. Rh_0(D) immune globulin is a highly concentrated preparation of antibody to the Rh_0(D) antigen (which confers Rh "positivity" to red cells). When administered in the proper dose, it can prevent sensitization of an Rh_0(D) negative mother by fetal-maternal hemorrhage from an Rh_0(D) positive infant. The dose depends on the size of the fetal-maternal hemorrhage. It is often necessary to determine the size of the fetal-maternal hemorrhage by counting the fetal cells in the maternal circulation. This is done by staining the mother's blood for fetal hemoglobin and counting the fraction of cells that are positive. It is rarely necessary to use more than 1 vial. Rh_0(D) immune globulin should be administered to Rh_0(D) negative children and women of the childbearing age whenever there is exposure to Rh_0(D) positive red cells by transfusion or pregnancy.

IMMUNOGLOBULIN. Treatment of patients with immunoglobulin deficiency can be accomplished either by transfusion of plasma or by injecting gamma globulin intramuscularly on a monthly basis. The first dose of gamma globulin should be 0.25 gram per kg. and further administration schedules can be determined to control symptoms and infections in the individual patient. Patients with IgA deficiency probably will not benefit from therapy with immunoglobulin preparations.

Filters

All products issued from the blood bank, including fresh frozen plasma, should be administered through filters. Plasma protein fraction and albumin preparations are exceptions to this rule. The usual pore size is 170 microns. This filter is adequate in almost all clinical situations. This filter should be used for platelets, granulocytes, plasma, and red cells. In patients who are massively transfused, there can be a build-up of cellular aggregates in the microvasculature. Microfilters (40 microns) have been developed to prevent this accumulation of aggregates. The indications for microfilters, even in cases of massive transfusion, have not been clearly established. The routine use of microfilters is not recommended. Microfilters should not be used for platelet or granulocyte transfusions.

UNTOWARD REACTIONS TO BLOOD TRANSFUSION

method of
ALFRED J. GRINDON, M.D.
Atlanta, Georgia

A blood transfusion may be followed by an untoward reaction as frequently as 3 per cent of the time. Although most of these reactions will be without serious consequence, acute hemolytic transfusion reactions may be catastrophic, and post-transfusion hepatitis still contributes significantly to the morbidity and mortality of blood transfusion. Therefore it is important to be able to recognize the different types of reaction to transfusion, and the steps that should be taken for the prevention and therapy of transfusion reactions.

Acute Hemolytic Transfusion Reaction

This type of reaction is to be feared the most, not only because it has the most dramatic consequences but also because of its inevitable association with error and iatrogenic disease. Most serious hemolytic transfusion reactions are associated with intravascular hemolysis (rather than the slower extravascular hemolysis), as a result of transfusion of blood into a recipient who has an antibody with which the transfused red cells are clearly incompatible. The cause is usually incorrect patient sample identification or incorrect patient identification, and the three major consequences of acute hemolytic transfusion reaction are shock, disseminated intravascular coagulation, and renal shutdown.

Prevention. The key to prevention of the hemolytic transfusion reaction is an adequate patient identification system. Although transfusion therapists justifiably hesitate to transfuse red blood cells that are weakly incompatible with the recipient's serum (for instance, in a patient with autoimmune hemolytic anemia), the cause of serious and often fatal intravascular hemolysis is usually the transfusion of grossly incompatible blood (such as Group A blood to a Group O recipient) because of an error in identification. It is vitally important to have patient samples for compatibility tests drawn by responsible people and labeled at the patient's bedside from information contained on the patient's armband, and finally to have the unit of blood, labeled with accurate patient identification obtained from the sample, compared carefully again with the armband at the patient's bedside at the time of transfusion. All hospitals have developed systems to obtain this kind of protection, but unfortunately neglect of these systems is often tolerated. Even simple safeguards, such as performing elective transfusion during the day when the regular skilled staff is available, are often overlooked. Hospital boards and transfusion committees should concentrate their efforts on reviewing the documentation purporting to show that these systems have been adequately implemented, if they seek to prevent hemolytic transfusion reactions.

Treatment. Successful treatment of an acute hemolytic transfusion reaction depends upon rapid diagnosis. The signs and symptoms of this type of reaction are widely recognized; what is less readily recognized is that *any* untoward event occurring during or shortly after a blood transfusion (including unexpectedly increased bleeding in an anesthetized patient) suggests this possibility. Any time such a reaction is suspected, the transfusion must be stopped (but the intravenous line left open with a slow saline drip) and samples of blood drawn from the patient and returned to the blood bank with the unused portion of the transfusion or the empty container. Usually the blood bank can determine within 5 minutes whether or not potentially serious hemolysis is taking place, simply by examining the serum for the presence of hemoglobin and performing a direct antiglobulin (Coombs') test. These tests may become positive with the hemolysis of as little as 30 to 40 ml. of red cells. If these determinations are negative, it is unlikely that dramatic measures will have to be taken. If there is evidence of hemolysis, treatment should be instituted promptly.

The major consequences of acute hemolytic transfusion reactions are hypotension and shock, disseminated intravascular coagulation (DIC), and renal shutdown. Attempts must be made to maintain blood volume with volume expanders and salt solutions if necessary, rather than vasopressors which might compromise renal blood flow. DIC is considered on pages 290 to 291 and will not be discussed at length here. Nevertheless, it is important to recognize that shock and DIC are occasional components of hemolytic transfusion reactions, and these developments as well as renal shutdown must be anticipated.

Because the causes of renal shutdown following acute hemolytic transfusion reaction are still incompletely understood, the treatment has remained empirical. The traditional approach has been to maintain urinary output with the use of the osmotic diuretic mannitol. This drug is given initially in a trial dose of 100 ml. of 20 per cent solution over a few minutes if the urine output drops below 60 ml. per hour. This dose is then repeated to maintain urine flow at this level. It can be given up to a total dose of 200 grams in 24 hours. For patients whose urine output has fallen and who prove refractory to trial doses of mannitol, furosemide (Lasix), 40 to 80 mg. intravenously, should be tried. If oliguria persists despite these measures, acute renal failure should be suspected and the patient managed for this condition. Although conclusive evidence is lacking, there are at least suggestive data that renal shutdown may be preventable or even reversible in whole or in part with the rapid and vigorous use of diuretic therapy.

This traditional approach has recently been questioned by some who feel that mannitol has not proved helpful, and that the drugs of choice are furosemide or ethacrynic acid. Because so few clinical data on the efficacy of differing modes of treatment are available and because skilled transfusionists have used mannitol over the last 15 years as the mainstay of therapy, my preference is to use this drug except when there is a question about the patient's ability to tolerate a transiently expanded blood volume (e.g., in incipient congestive heart failure).

Other less well accepted modes of therapy have been tried. Because acute renal shutdown may involve shunting of blood from one part to another of the renal arterial system, some workers have suggested the use of adrenergic blocking drugs. It is currently accepted that those vasopressors that restrict renal blood flow are contraindicated. Similarly, others have felt that the underlying problem was related primarily to the antigen-antibody interaction, with activation of complement, the coagulation sequence, and vasoactive polypeptides, and that therefore the use of heparin was indicated. Although this approach is rational, it carries considerable risk, and is not generally used. Still other workers have felt that one of the primary mechanisms for renal shutdown was the precipitation of hemoglobin in renal tubules, and that therapy should therefore be directed toward the solubilization of hemoglobin by alkalinization of the urine. None of these three approaches has been widely accepted, and the mainstay of therapy has remained the maintenance of diuresis, with the use of mannitol (or other diuretics).

Delayed Hemolytic Transfusion Reaction

Delayed hemolytic transfusion reactions are seen when red cell antigens are transfused to which the recipient has immune memory (as a result of previous transfusion or pregnancy) but low or absent levels of circulating immunoglobulin. Although the crossmatch may be compatible, the immune system is stimulated and a rapid "secondary" or "anamnestic" immune response takes place. Days to weeks after transfusion, the transfused red cells are hemolyzed because of the rapid production of circulating antibody. This hemolysis occurs relatively slowly in the reticuloendothelial system; although probably much more common than is usually recognized, it is not usually dangerous. There have been only two reported cases of renal shutdown following delayed hemolytic transfusion reactions. When the diagnosis of delayed hemolysis is made, the patient should be monitored to ensure that urinary output does not fall and that anemia does not become severe. The patient may require additional transfusion.

Transfusion Reactions Not Associated with Hemolysis

Volume Overload. Volume overload is one of the more frequent causes of untoward reaction to transfusion. It is seen typically when the anemic patient with a normal or greater than normal blood volume is transfused more rapidly than necessary with the use of whole blood. Signs and symptoms are those of right-sided congestive heart failure. One of the more subtle but useful signs is the development of tachypnea during the course of a transfusion.

Volume overload is prevented by the use of packed red cells rather than whole blood when indicated, and by slow transfusion (from 2 to 4 hours per unit) of these packed cells in infants, the elderly, and those with a history of congestive heart failure. In this group, one could also consider monitoring of central venous pressure and transfusion in an upright position.

Treatment is generally that of acute pulmonary edema. An approach to treatment that might be considered in a patient at risk who needs transfusion is a modified exchange transfusion, with the infusion of 2 units of red cells alternating with the withdrawal of a unit of whole blood. This procedure limits the amount of volume expansion at any one time.

Allergic Reactions. Another common type of transfusion reaction is the development of urticaria shortly following the initiation of transfusion. Urticaria occurring as an isolated phenomenon can be readily treated by the administration of an antihistaminic such as diphenhydramine (Benadryl), 50 mg. orally or intramuscularly. Following such treatment the urticaria disappears rapidly, and transfusion can be continued. There is no need to evaluate such patients further for more serious transfusion reactions. On occasion, urticarial reactions can have a bronchial component, manifested by wheezing. Such reactions are more serious because the threat of airway obstruction is present. If the patient is not in distress, antihistaminics as described above should be tried. If all symptoms resolve promptly with the administration of antihistaminics, nothing more need be done, and the transfusion can be continued. If the reaction does not respond to the administration of antihistaminics, the use of aqueous epinephrine, 0.5 ml. of 1:1000 solution intramuscularly, should be considered.

The most severe of the allergic reactions are those anaphylactic reactions caused by IgG antibodies to IgA, in patients lacking IgA. Treatment of this type of reaction is with aqueous epinephrine, 0.5 ml. of 1:1000 solution intramuscularly. If the diagnosis of anaphylactic reaction caused by antibodies to IgA can be made, the treatment of choice is to prevent further transfusion of material containing IgA. This is accomplished either by transfusion of the patient's own blood (after storage in liquid or frozen state) or by obtaining blood from special rare donors, on file with the American Association of Blood Banks or the American Red Cross, who are known to be deficient in IgA. Some of these patients have been successfully managed by transfusion with well washed red blood cells, but transfusion reactions have been reported following the transfusion of deglycerolized (previously frozen) red cells.

Febrile, Nonhemolytic Transfusion Reactions. Febrile, nonhemolytic transfusion reactions are caused by reaction to transfused foreign antigens other than those on red blood cells. Such antigens can be found on granulocytes, lymphocytes, platelets, or the plasma proteins. Typically, these reactions have been associated with the transfusion of "buffy coat" containing both granulocytes and lymphocytes. The signs and symptoms can be diverse, but characteristically include an elevated temperature. Since fever is also one of the hallmarks of the acute hemolytic transfusion reaction, all patients who develop fever during or after the course of a blood transfusion must have the transfusion stopped and the reaction investigated, before assuming that the reaction is merely of nonhemolytic type. Once the possibility of hemolysis has been eliminated, treatment can be begun. The treatment for the febrile nonhemolytic reaction is purely symptomatic, using analgesic and antipyretic medication (other than aspirin, in a bleeding patient). Since desperately ill patients may not have the cardiovascular reserve to cope with such reactions, attention should be directed toward prevention. Most of these reactions can be prevented by transfusion of leukocyte-poor red cells, from which 60 to 80 per cent of the white cells have been removed. If the patient continues to have febrile reactions following the infusion of leukocyte-poor red cells, consideration should be given to the transfusion of red cells that have been washed, with the removal of 80 to 90 per cent of the white cells present in the original unit. The washing can be done in a manual or automated fashion, but in either case it is relatively expensive, and washed red cells should be provided only for those patients who have febrile transfusion reactions to leukocyte-poor blood. For those patients who continue to have transfusion reactions following the infusion of washed red cells, the use of red cells which have been frozen, thawed, and subsequently washed in the deglycerolization process may be an improvement. Again, improved removal of white cells from the blood, and therefore fewer febrile reactions, is associated with an incremental cost.

Septic Reactions. Septic reactions have fortunately become rare following the development of systems of closed plastic containers for the preparation of blood components. Therefore prevention of such reactions is no longer focused upon aseptic techniques for blood and component manipulation in the blood bank, but rather upon continued attention to meticulous technique both in drawing blood from donors and in transfusion practice. Products prepared in an open system, such as deglycerolized red cells, must be transfused within 24 hours of preparation. A unit of blood that has been removed from refrigeration for transfusion purposes must be administered promptly to the patient for whom it is intended, and should not hang at the patient's bedside for more than 4 hours during the course of a transfusion. Blood that has been out of refrigeration for more than 30 minutes must not be returned to refrigeration and subsequently reissued for transfusion, because under these conditions cold-growing gram-negative organisms may proliferate. The complication most to be feared is not the infusion of viable organisms (except for those patients at risk to develop septicemia, such as those with valvular heart defects), but rather the infusion of large amounts of bacterial pyrogen, associated with the presence of massive numbers of bacteria. The signs and symptoms of this type of reaction are those of endotoxin shock, and the diagnosis is confirmed by finding bacteria in a Gram stain of the product being transfused. The treatment is that of gram-negative septicemia and endotoxin shock, and may be found on pages 4 to 7.

Pulmonary Infiltrate with Leukoagglutinin. This recently described type of transfusion reaction is caused by a humoral immune response to leukocyte antigens. It is characterized by dyspnea, hypoxemia, and a radiographic appearance of pulmonary edema in a patient who has no other manifestation of right-sided heart failure. The diagnosis is based upon the radiographic appearance associated with a normal pulmonary wedge pressure or central venous pressure. The treatment must be directed to correction of the hypoxia, with a high oxygen atmosphere. Corticosteroids have not been shown to be effective.

Problems Associated with Massive Transfusion. HEMORRHAGIC DIATHESIS. Some untoward reactions are seen only with the transfusion of massive amounts of blood (for instance, the exchange of one blood volume in 24 hours). One of these problems is the development of a hemorrhagic diathesis. This is caused most often by dilutional thrombocytopenia, because of the lack of viable platelets in the transfused stored blood. The goal of therapy in this situation is to maintain the platelet count above a level compatible with surgical hemostasis, such as 50,000 platelets per microliter. In an otherwise healthy patient, 10 to 12 units of blood must be transfused over a brief period of time before the platelet count reaches this level. Since the platelet count in fresh whole blood approximates 250,000 per microliter, if 1 unit of fresh blood or its equivalent were given with every 4 units of stored blood, the resulting mean platelet count would approximate 50,000 per microliter. The number of platelets in 2 platelet concentrates is equivalent to that found in 1 unit of fresh whole blood. Therefore in a massive transfusion situation, it would seem reasonable to provide 2 platelet concentrates for every 5 units of stored blood, after the patient has received an initial 10 to 12 units of blood. It must be recognized that this is a formula approach which ideally is modified by application to the individual patient's problem. One should look for signs of thrombocytopenia in a patient who has been massively transfused; if such signs are present and are confirmed with a platelet count, the diagnosis of thrombocytopenic bleeding is followed by the transfusion of platelet concentrates. Often, however, time is not available for this approach.

The hemorrhagic diathesis following massive transfusion is occasionally attributed to coagulation factors other than platelets. However, only factors V and VIII are labile and depleted in blood or plasma stored at 5°C. Further, only low levels of factor V are needed for hemostasis, and such levels are usually found in stored blood. Even though higher levels of factor VIII may be needed, the rapid production of factor VIII makes acquired depletion in massive transfusion extremely unlikely in patients who were not hemophilic to begin with, or in whom there is no evidence of consumption of coagulation factors.

Disseminated intravascular coagulation (DIC) is sometimes seen in patients who are being massively transfused. Although labile clotting factors such as platelets, factor V, factor VIII, and fibrinogen may be consumed in such a process, the best approach to the treatment of DIC is to correct the underlying process, rather than to consider replacement with missing blood components. Although some workers recommend the use of heparin, this therapy remains controversial and difficult to recommend in an actively bleeding patient.

COLD BLOOD. The rapid infusion of large amounts of blood that has just been taken from 5°C. storage can lead to the development of dangerous cardiac arrhythmias in the recipient. Therefore with such rapid transfusion consideration should be given to warming the blood. Many devices for this purpose are available; the best of these warm the blood as it passes through a coil on the way to the body. The simple expedient of placing coiled transfusion tubing in a monitored 37°C. water bath is very effective. Those devices that warm the whole unit of blood before beginning a transfusion (such as microwave ovens) are potentially dangerous, and must be used with great care. Meticulous daily quality control is an important part of the use of these instruments.

POTASSIUM, AMMONIUM, HYDROGEN ION, CITRATE. The administration of large amounts of plasma containing elevated levels of potassium, hydrogen ion, ammonium ion, and citrate usually represents no problem for the recipient. Patients with renal failure who already have a markedly elevated serum potassium can be given relatively fresh (less than 1 week old) red cells, packed just before transfusion. The infusion of large amounts of blood with a pH of 7.1 to 7.2 will not cause severe acidosis if the patient is kept out of shock with vigorous volume replacement. If hypovolemic shock develops, the use of sodium bicarbonate or other alkalinizing agents will not reverse the subsequent acidosis. The mild acidosis resulting from massive transfusion need not be treated.

The infusion of large volumes of citrate over a short period of time has been associated with the signs and symptoms of hypocalcemia. This problem can be aggravated by pre-existing liver disease or hypothermia. In an otherwise normal person hypocalcemia will not develop until an infusion rate approximating 1 unit of blood every 5 minutes is achieved. At this rate one should begin thinking about the possibility of hypocalcemia. Electrocardiographic changes suggestive of hypocalcemia can be treated by the administration of 10 ml. of a 10 per cent calcium gluconate solution for every 1000 ml. of blood transfused.

2,3-DIPHOSPHOGLYCERATE (DPG). The storage of blood in acid-citrate-dextrose (ACD) solution leads to a depletion of DPG and, following transfusion of such blood, a shift in the oxyhemoglobin dissociation curve in vivo. Some workers feel that this shift may cause a diminution in tissue oxygenation, particularly following the transfusion of large volumes of stored blood. Because today blood is commonly stored in citrate-dextrose-phosphate (CDP) solution (in which DPG is much better maintained), because DPG is rapidly regenerated in stored red cells once they are transfused, and, finally, because there are many compensatory mechanisms operating at the tissue level to maintain oxygenation, it is not clear that this is ever more than a theoretical risk in humans. At this time there is no reason for the transfusionist to be concerned about DPG levels in transfused blood.

MICROAGGREGATES. Particulate debris accumulates in blood stored at 5°C. This debris can readily pass the 180 μ filter in the ordinary blood transfusion set, but is effectively trapped and removed by one of a number of "microaggregate" filters having a pore size of less than 40 μ. Transfused microaggregates are filtered by the pulmonary circulation, so that they are not usually found in the arterial circulation following transfusion. Some workers feel that this entrapment of microaggregates may lead to pulmonary insufficiency in patients receiving large volumes of stored blood. Except for patients undergoing cardiopulmonary bypass, insufficient data exist to necessitate the use of these filters in patients who are being massively transfused.

Delayed Reactions. In addition to delayed hemolytic transfusion reactions, there are many other types of reaction which occur in a delayed fashion. The most significant of these is post-transfusion hepatitis. The two most important steps to take for the prevention of post-transfusion hepatitis are the use of a sensitive test for the detection of HB_sAg and the use of blood from volunteer donors. Despite these measures, transfusion-associated hepatitis persists. Post-transfusion hepatitis can be caused by several agents in addition to the hepatitis B virus, and even for hepatitis B the testing methods are not so sensitive as to eliminate hepatitis. Unfortunately, no specific therapy is available for the treatment of this disease.

It is important to recognize that blood transfusion is a potential vector in the transmission of diseases such as malaria, cytomegalovirus disease, and syphilis. Specific treatment for malaria and syphilis will be found on pages 34 to 37 and 560 to 562, respectively.

Transfusion hemosiderosis can develop in patients who require chronic transfusion therapy. The use of iron chelating therapy to prevent or ameliorate this disease has been largely unsuccessful. Patients in chronic transfusion programs should be provided with relatively fresh blood to minimize the frequency of transfusion.

Recipients of blood transfusion become sensitized to red cell antigens at the rate of approximately 1 per cent per unit of blood transfused. There is no definitive treatment, except to see that subsequent transfusions lack the offending antigen. In the special situation in which Rh negative recipients may receive Rh positive platelet concentrates, Rh immune globulin could be given to prevent sensitization to the Rh antigen. One intramuscular dose of Rh immune globulin may be adequate to prevent sensitization from as many as 20 units of Rh positive platelet concentrate.

Post-transfusion purpura is a rare form of sensitization, in which the recipient develops an immune response not only to transfused platelets but also to his own platelets. These patients have been treated successfully with exchange transfusion.

SECTION 5

The Digestive System

BLEEDING ESOPHAGEAL VARICES

method of
TELFER B. REYNOLDS, M.D.
Los Angeles, California

Initial Assessment

Even in patients with obvious chronic liver damage, upper gastrointestinal hemorrhage is often due to diffuse gastritis, Mallory-Weiss tear, or peptic ulcer so that emergency panendoscopy is needed before a diagnosis of bleeding esophageal varices is assured. In some actively bleeding patients, it is difficult to be certain of the bleeding site even at endoscopy; skill and experience on the part of the endoscopist are important in this regard. Need for emergency endoscopy is less if the patient has nonalcoholic liver disease, if the hemorrhage occurs in a hospital setting in the absence of intake of potential mucosal irritants, or if bleeding varices have been identified on a previous occasion. We prefer endoscopy to barium swallow in upper gastrointestinal hemorrhage because it is more accurate in assigning a bleeding site and does not interfere with subsequent angiography.

For therapy of upper gastrointestinal bleeding it is essential first to stabilize vital signs by blood transfusion. Five per cent albumin solution, fresh frozen plasma, isotonic sodium chloride, or Ringer's lactate may be used while whole blood is being crossmatched. Blood should be sent to the laboratory for hemoglobin, hematocrit, and routine hepatic and renal function tests (bilirubin, serum proteins, transaminases, prothrombin, urea nitrogen, and creatinine). Essentials of the history and physical examination are performed as rapidly as possible. While vital signs are being stabilized, the stomach should be lavaged with cold saline solution to prepare for endoscopy.

If Bleeding Has Stopped Spontaneously

If lavage and endoscopy indicate that bleeding has ceased and that varices were the probable bleeding site, we leave a nasogastric tube in place for a few hours to check for recurrent bleeding. Hematocrit is measured at appropriate intervals. One dose of magnesium sulfate or magnesium hydroxide is given down the tube to aid in expelling blood from the intestine. Neomycin therapy is begun (1 gram every 8 hours) in anticipation of possible development of hepatic encephalopathy. Single injections of 75 mg. of vitamin K and 5 mg. of folic acid are given to correct possible deficiencies. Transfusion with whole blood or packed red cells is continued until a hematocrit of approximately 30 per cent is attained. Whole blood is preferred if there are clinical signs of hypovolemia (unstable blood pressure, venous constriction, cold extremities); otherwise, packed cells are used. Plasma volume usually is increased in chronic liver disease, and portal pressure varies directly with plasma volume; hence it is desirable to avoid undue increase in plasma volume while correcting anemia.

If There Is Active Bleeding at a Moderate Rate

If bleeding continues at a modest rate while the stomach is being lavaged, we add vasopressin infusion to the aforementioned regimen. Twenty units of aqueous vasopressin is added to 200 ml. of isotonic saline or 5 per cent glucose solution and infused intravenously over a 20 to 30 minute period. (This use of vasopressin is not listed in the manufacturer's official directive. See package insert before giving intravenously.) Pallor, abdominal cramps, and defecation often result. This treatment lowers portal pressure by reducing splanchnic flow into the portal bed and sometimes results in cessation of variceal bleeding. The infusion can be repeated once if it seems incompletely effective.

If variceal bleeding continues at a moderate rate for more than 2 to 4 hours, we resort to balloon tamponade. Our choice is the triple lumen Linton tube (Davol, Inc., Providence, R.I. 02901) with a single, pear-shaped balloon that compresses the region of the esophagogastric junction. Usually it is possible to insert the tube through the nose. One should be certain that it is not doubled back on itself and has been passed far enough for the balloon to be in the stomach before it is inflated in order to avoid injury to the esophagus. After inflating the balloon with 600 ml. of air, it is pulled and anchored to a wire face mask that resembles a baseball catcher's mask. Alternatively, the tube can be attached to a 2 pound weight via an overhead pulley system in an orthopedic bed. Tension on the tube may be quite uncomfortable for the patient initially, and it may be necessary to begin with a 1 pound weight and gradually increase it. If possible, patients should be in an intensive care setting when balloon tamponade is used. The gastric lumen of the tube should be irrigated regularly to keep it clear of clots and to evaluate bleeding.

If Bleeding Is Profuse or Prolonged

When initial assessment by gastric lavage and/or endoscopy indicates rapid and continued bleeding, then we tend to use balloon tamponade immediately, sometimes accompanied by a vasopressin infusion.

If tamponade therapy is successful, the traction is released and the gastric balloon deflated after 8 to 12 hours, leaving the tube in place to check for recurrence of bleeding. If bleeding starts again, the balloon is reinflated and traction is reinstituted and maintained for an additional 12 to 24 hours. The longer the tube is in place, the greater the incidence of complications from its use.

If tamponade therapy fails to stop the bleeding, our practice is to deflate the balloon and reinflate it with 800 ml. of air, hoping to compress a little more area in the upper stomach, and to increase the traction on the tube (to as much as 3 pounds). If bleeding still continues, as it does in occasional patients, we ask for consultation with the radiology department for consideration of angiography and selective vasopressin infusion. Selective left gastric angiography may disclose a previously unsuspected arterial or capillary bleeding site (Mallory-Weiss tear, gastritis, ulcer) that will call for surgical consideration. If no contrast extravasation is shown in the arterial phase and if venous phase films show portal collateral flow and mucosal staining, then the diagnosis of bleeding varices is confirmed. The catheter is then moved to the superior mesenteric artery for constant infusion of vasopressin at 0.1 to 0.4 unit per minute. (See manufacturer's official directive before giving intravenously.) Side effects from vasopressin are minimal when it is given into the splanchnic bed, even for prolonged periods.

Surgical Therapy

With the aforementioned therapeutic approach to hemorrhage from esophageal varices, bleeding is not always controlled, and mortality still approaches 50 per cent in patients with alcoholic liver disease, being highest in those who are "decompensated" with jaundice, ascites, and encephalopathy. When should surgery be considered as emergency therapy? It is our practice not to subject patients to emergency surgery if bleeding ceases spontaneously or seems controlled by some combination of the measures detailed above. Similarly, we do not advise surgery in patients who have obviously "decompensated" liver disease. Our earlier experience showed a discouragingly high operative mortality in patients who had more than one of the following four criteria: (1) serum bilirubin above 3 mg. per 100 ml., (2) serum albumin below 3 grams per 100 ml., (3) ascites, and (4) encephalopathy. More recently, operative mortality was found to be high in patients who had abundant alcoholic hyalin on liver biopsy, so we try to obtain rapid processing and interpretation of a liver biopsy to help in assessing operative risk in alcoholic patients who are surgical candidates. In general, we limit emergency surgery to patients in whom conservative measures fail to control bleeding or who rebleed after initial control *and* who are considered reasonably good operative risks by the aforementioned criteria. The type of surgery performed is end-to-side, distal splenorenal, or H-graft mesocaval shunt.

Newer Forms of Therapy

A new form of therapy for the patient whose bleeding fails to respond to conservative measures and who is considered too ill for surgery is selective transhepatic catheterization of the left gastric (coronary) vein with injection of sclerosing agents. This technique has not yet been widely used or evaluated, and our liver unit has had limited experience with it.

CHOLECYSTITIS AND CHOLELITHIASIS

method of
CHARLES K. McSHERRY, M.D.
New York, New York

The past decade has witnessed a vast expansion of our knowledge of the mechanisms of gallstone formation. The result of this research has been the achievement of chemical dissolution of gallstones by chenodeoxycholic acid. The oral administration of this primary bile acid expands the bile acid pool size within the enterohepatic circulation and increases the cholesterol solubilizing capacity of gallbladder bile. In addition, chenodeoxycholic acid decreases the hepatic excretion of cholesterol in bile. The net effect of these metabolic changes is the gradual absorption of cholesterol from the stone surface and its eventual dissolution. The prerequisites for the successful dissolution of cholesterol gallstones are a functioning gallbladder as evidenced by oral cholecystography and the absence of radiographically visible calcium in the gallstones.

At this writing, the safety and efficacy of chenodeoxycholic acid therapy in humans are under investigation by the National Cooperative Gallstone Study with funds supplied by the National Institutes of Health. The protocol envisages 1000 patients with gallstones treated with chenodeoxycholic acid over a 2 year period. The study is expected to resolve such questions as the incidence and severity of hepatotoxicity, the duration of therapy necessary to achieve stone dissolution, and the incidence of recurrent biliary calculi after the cessation of bile acid therapy. Hepatotoxicity occurs in animals administered chenodeoxycholic acid, presumably because of increased amounts of lithocholic acid in the enterohepatic circulation. This latter bile acid is formed by bacterial dehydroxylation of chenodeoxycholic acid in the large intestine. In humans, efficient hepatic sulfation of lithocholic acid is presumed to minimize the hepatotoxic effects of this bile acid. Recurrence of gallstones is anticipated in perhaps as many as one third of the patients after chenodeoxycholic acid has been discontinued. Until such time as the aforementioned issues have been resolved or more effective and safe compounds introduced, surgical therapy must be considered the treatment of choice for gallstone disease.

Other developments that have had a significant impact on the surgical treatment of calculous biliary tract disease, especially in the jaundiced patient, include the increased use of preoperative endoscopic retrograde cholangiopancreatography (ERCP) and the introduction of the Chiba or "skinny" needle for percutaneous transhepatic cholangiography. ERCP via a duodenal fiberscope permits cannulation at the ampulla of Vater of the common bile duct or pancreatic duct, or both, and the injection of contrast media. The information provided by these radiographs is both specific and diagnostic. As performed by capable endoscopists, the technique is associated with few untoward effects. Some patients may have abdominal pain and fever. Serum amylase levels may be elevated, and bacteremia has been reported.

Percutaneous transhepatic cholangiography using the Chiba needle also provides specific diagnostic information and is especially helpful in evaluating patients with postcholecystectomy bile fistulas and jaundice in whom common duct injury is suspected. The Chiba needle has resulted in a high success rate in visualizing the biliary tree, and the potential complications of bile peritonitis and hepatic bleeding have been significantly reduced.

Chronic Cholecystitis

Our experience at The New York Hospital–Cornell Medical Center with 10,008 patients with nonmalignant biliary tract disease operated upon from 1932 to 1974 indicates that 80 per cent had "chronic" and 20 per cent "acute" disease of the gallbladder. Patients with chronic cholecystitis exhibit considerable variation in both the severity and duration of symptoms. Typically, these patients complain of upper abdominal pain that usually becomes localized to the right side. The pain is often described as "crampy" and occurs within a brief interval after eating. The pain may radiate to the back or, less commonly, to the shoulder. The duration of the pain is variable, and it may subside spontaneously or after vomiting. The differential diagnoses often include angina, hiatus hernia with reflux esophagitis, and peptic ulcer disease.

The appropriate management of patients with suspected chronic cholecystitis and cholelithiasis must begin with radiographic confirmation of the diagnosis. Oral cholecystography accurately establishes the presence or absence of gallbladder disease in 95 per cent of subjects in whom the study has been performed properly. The major problem in the interpretation of the oral cholecystogram is the significance of nonopacification of the gallbladder. Extrinsic causes of nonopacification include interference with the transport of contrast agent to the small intestine, malabsorption, liver disease, biliary intestinal fistula, or an excessive amount of contrast agent, which may produce vomiting and diarrhea and thereby decrease absorption. Intrinsic causes include obstruction of the cystic duct and chronic cholecystitis. In the absence of extrinsic causes, nonopacification of the gallbladder on two studies is indicative of disease in 97 per cent of the patients.

Intravenous cholangiography is of limited value for investigating disease of the gallbladder. Since intravenous cholangiography does not depend on the concentrating ability of the gallbladder for opacification, it will produce filling of the gallbladder in chronic cholecystitis but not in obstructive gallbladder disease. However, the degree of opacification of the gallbladder achieved is often inadequate to reliably exclude the presence of stones or other lesions. Intravenous cholangiography is indicated in the investigation of diseases of the extrahepatic ducts in the nonjaundiced patient. It should be employed for suspected gallbladder disease only when the oral examination is impracticable—e.g., because of time limitations in emergencies or coexistent disease of the alimentary tract, or when oral intake is contraindicated.

In our published experience with 8020 patients with chronic cholecystitis, cholecystectomy alone or in combination with common duct exploration was performed in 7416 instances and cholecystostomy alone or in combination with common duct exploration in 90 patients. Clinicians are in agreement that cholecystectomy provides immediate and permanent relief from symptoms in most patients with gallstones. In the absence of severe coexisting medical conditions, the patient who has cholelithiasis is best managed by elective cholecystectomy. Cholecystostomy is usually reserved for those patients in whom associated disease is of such severity that life expectancy is adjudged to be 2 years or less. Cholecystostomy may be performed under local anesthesia with minimal additional operative stress imposed upon the already compromised patient. This procedure is also indicated in those patients with obliteration of the normal anatomic landmarks in the hepatoduodenal ligament secondary to severe inflammation. In these patients elective cholecystectomy 6 to 8 weeks later is feasible after subsidence of the inflammatory response.

Cholecystectomy is not without hazard. The incision and technique employed to remove the gallbladder vary with the experience and training of the surgeon. Serious postoperative complications related to technique are often the result of one of the following events: partial or complete interruption of the common duct or its main tributaries, the right and left hepatic ducts; impairment of the blood supply to the liver; and transection of unobserved anomalous ductal and vascular channels between the liver and gallbladder or cystic duct.

The operative mortality for elective cholecystectomy at The New York Hospital–Cornell Medical Center is 0.5 per cent. The principal cause of postoperative death has been cardiovascular disease, especially myocardial infarction. The incidence of nonfatal complications is 6.9 per cent, the majority of which affect organs or systems other than the biliary tree. Pulmonary disorders, particularly pneumonitis and atelectasis, were the most frequent complications. Retained or overlooked common duct stones are believed to occur in 2 to 3 per cent of patients who have had cholecystectomy. Several safeguards may be employed to minimize this distressing complication. Operative cholangiography is perhaps the most important adjunct for demonstrating calculi in the ductal system during operation. That this technique does indeed reduce the incidence of retained calculi has been documented by many investigators. The routine use of operative cholangiography has been advocated but is probably not feasible at present because of insufficient x-ray facilities in the operating rooms of many hospitals. The flexible fiberoptic choledochoscope has been introduced in more recent times, and there is every indication that the proper use of this instrument will also reduce the incidence of retained common duct stones.

Asymptomatic Gallstones

One of the more frequent and complex problems in biliary tract disease is the management of patients with asymptomatic or "silent" cholelithiasis. Such stones are usually found in the course of medical evaluation for unrelated disease or as an incidental finding at laparotomy. Evidence from several reported series of patients suggests that approximately 50 per cent of these patients develop symptoms and another 25 per cent the complications of gallstone disease, e.g., acute cholecystitis, common duct obstruction, usually within 5 years. Although malignant tumors of the gallbladder are infrequent compared with those elsewhere in the gastrointestinal tract, their relationship to gallstones is statistically impressive. Carcinoma of the gallbladder most commonly occurs in elderly patients with cholelithiasis of long duration.

Although many factors enter into the decision of cholecystectomy versus nonoperative therapy in the individual patient with asymptomatic gallstones, the most important are the risks of surgical therapy and the general physical condition of the patient. Opinion is unanimous among surgeons that the morbidity and mortality of cholecystectomy are greatly reduced in the absence of the complications of cholelithiasis. Clearly, however, the most important consideration is the general condition of the patient. The natural history of calculous biliary tract disease must be weighed against the risks of surgery and such factors as the presence or absence of cardiovascular disease, diabetes, and pulmonary disorders.

Acute Cholecystitis

In the experience with nonmalignant biliary tract disease at The New York Hospital–Cornell Medical Center, 20 per cent of patients are operated upon for acute cholecystitis. Clinically this entity is characterized by the presence of systemic and local signs of inflammation and pathologically by an acute inflammatory process in the gallbladder. The pathogenesis of acute cholecystitis is initiated presumably by calculous obstruction of the cystic duct. This is followed by inflammation of the mucosa and increased fluid sequestration within the lumen which produces gallbladder distention. If the obstruction is unrelieved, the blood supply to the gallbladder may be compromised, as a result of which necrosis and perforation of the gallbladder are the sequelae. Gangrene and perforation occur in 10 to 15 per cent of patients with acute cholecystitis. The perforation is usually walled off by omentum and adjacent viscera. Progression of the disease beyond this stage leads to subhepatic abscess or biliary-enteric fistula. A consequence of the latter may be gallstone ileus.

Patients with acute cholecystitis complain of severe pain in the epigastrium and right hypochondrium that is often intensified by movement and respiration. Initially the pain may be intermittent or colicky but then becomes constant. Vomiting, fever, and, less frequently, chills are also reported by these patients. The physical examination usually discloses marked tenderness and rigidity in the right upper quadrant and epigastrium. The distended gallbladder may be palpated at the liver edge in approximately 25 per cent of the patients. Minimal jaundice is occasionally noted and is usually due to the associated inflammation of the bile ducts and liver rather than biliary obstruction. Laboratory studies disclose a leukocytosis, and there is often a slight elevation of the serum amylase, bilirubin, and alkaline phosphatase. Plain x-rays of the abdomen are usually unrevealing unless the biliary calculi are radiopaque; rarely gas-producing microorganisms in the gallbladder will cause "emphysematous" cholecystitis. The diagnosis of acute cholecystitis is best confirmed by intravenous cholangiography. Visualization of the common bile duct but not the gallbladder is the finding one anticipates with acute cholecystitis. Visualization of the gallbladder virtually excludes this diagnosis.

The initial treatment of patients with acute cholecystitis consists of cessation of oral intake and, in the patient who has been vomiting, nasogastric intubation. Appropriate electrolyte solutions are administered parenterally to correct existing deficiencies and to maintain normal hydration. Antimicrobial therapy is instituted in all patients with fever and leukocytosis. Cephalothin or ampicillin, 1 to 2 grams every 6 hours via the intravenous route, provides sufficient broad-spectrum activity for most patients. In patients with suspected gram-negative septicemia, clindamycin and gentamicin are also administered after blood cultures have been obtained.

The therapy of acute cholecystitis has been the subject of considerable debate and controversy for many years. The focal point of this debate relates to early versus delayed operation. Advocates of delayed operation argue that 75 to 90 per cent of patients with acute cholecystitis respond to the measures outlined in the preceding paragraph and are well within 2 to 14 days of the onset of the attack. Such patients are subjected to an elective cholecystectomy 2 to 3 months later, at which time there is less edema and inflammation and presumably less hazard.

The proponents of early cholecystectomy, i.e., within 24 to 48 hours of the onset of acute cholecystitis, cite the failure of medical therapy in some patients, the danger of perforation, and the fact that all patients must eventually undergo cholecystectomy as reasons for proceeding without undue delay in interrupting the disease process. Our experience supports this approach to acute cholecystitis. Removal of the acutely inflamed gallbladder and, if necessary, common duct exploration are quite safe and almost always possible. Indeed, cholecystectomy early in the disease process is often less difficult than a dissection through scar tissue performed some months later. Occasional patients require cholecystostomy for technical considerations irrespective of the time that has elapsed from the onset of acute cholecystitis to surgical treatment.

At The New York Hospital–Cornell Medical Center, 1988 patients with acute cholecystitis were operated upon during the years 1932 to 1974 with an overall mortality rate of 3.3 per cent. In this group, 1420 patients subjected to cholecystectomy alone had a mortality rate of 1.3 per cent. Of 280 patients that had cholecystostomy performed, the mortality rate was 8.9 per cent. Cholecystectomy or cholecystostomy plus choledochotomy was performed in 288 patients with a mortality rate of 7.6 per cent. These statistics suggest that a major factor in the operative mortality for acute cholecystitis is the extent or severity of the disease process.

The Hyperplastic Cholecystoses

The hyperplastic cholecystoses are a group of benign lesions of the gallbladder characterized by excessive proliferation of its normal tissue components. These lesions are believed to be degenerative in nature and can be distinguished from chronic cholecystitis, which is a true inflammatory response. Included in the hyperplastic cholecystoses are such lesions as adenomyomatosis, cholesterolosis, neuromatosis, lipomatosis, fibromatosis, and hyalinocalcinosis (calcified gallbladder). Occasionally more than one type of cholecystosis may appear simultaneously in the same gallbladder. Although unproved, it is believed that all the cholecystoses have a common cause. These lesions are to be differentiated from true papillomas of the gallbladder, which are neoplastic lesions with malignant propensities.

Many of these lesions are discovered in roentgenograms in patients who do not have symptoms of biliary tract disease. In other patients, perhaps more commonly in those with cholesterolosis and hyalinocalcinosis, symptoms are identical to those described by patients with chronic cholecystitis and cholelithiasis. Our approach to the symptomatic patient with hyperplastic cholecystoses is to evaluate carefully the entire gastrointestinal tract, and in the absence of lesions that could mimic gallbladder disease we recommend cholecystectomy. At present we hesitate to recommend cholecystectomy for asymptomatic patients. Our experience with the results of cholecystectomy in symptomatic patients has, in general, been good.

Choledocholithiasis

Common duct calculi are usually a manifestation of longstanding stones in the gallbladder. The older the patient and the longer calculi have been present in the gallbladder, the higher the incidence. Over a 42 year period (1932 to 1974) with 10,008 patients treated surgically for calculous biliary tract disease, we explored the ductal system at the time of the primary operation in 1427 patients (14.3 per cent). In 847, calculi were recovered, an incidence of 59.3 per cent.

In addition to calculi, other causes of obstructive jaundice that must be considered in the differential diagnosis are carcinoma, stricture, sclerosing choledochitis, congenital anomalies, and parasitic infections. A thoughtful history and complete physicial examination will serve to differentiate most of these conditions. Serum liver function tests and barium roentgenograms of the stomach and duodenum are often helpful in establishing the cause of jaundice. As described in the introduction to this article, endoscopic retrograde cholangiography or percutaneous transhepatic cholangiography is employed to provide the specific anatomic and pathologic information necessary to plan the operative approach to these patients.

A matter of primary concern in the management of patients with common duct obstruction resulting from calculi is the control of infection in the liver and biliary tree. Almost every organism commonly found in the gastrointestinal tract has been cultured from bile. In most instances, bacteria are transported from the gastrointestinal tract to the liver via the portal circulation. In the presence of obstruction to the flow of bile, the opportunity is provided for growth and increased virulence of these microorganisms. The clinical manifestations of infection range from a mild cholangitis to rapidly progressing and overwhelming septicemia. In the latter situation, decompression of the ductal system, usually accomplished by T-tube drainage of the common duct, offers the most benefit. High dose broad-spectrum antimicrobial therapy, using, for example, ampicillin, clindamycin, and gentamicin, is a valuable adjunct to surgical drainage.

CIRRHOSIS

method of
JOHN T. GALAMBOS, M.D.
Atlanta, Georgia

Introduction

Once cirrhosis is well established, the process is not reversible by any treatment. Depending on the cause, however, the development of cirrhosis may be prevented or its clinical manifestations ameliorated by removal of the offending agent or suppression of the underlying pathogenic mechanism (Table 1).

Therapy of Asymptomatic Cirrhosis

There are many patients who have well established cirrhosis but are asymptomatic. These patients require no specific treatment but are watched for the development of early signs of deterioration or complications. The feeding of excessive amounts of dietary protein or large amounts of vitamins has no demonstrable beneficial effect in a person who eats a reasonably nutritious diet. It is not known whether the administration of antacids between meals would prevent bleeding from esophageal varices.

When the offending agent is known, cirrhosis may be prevented. If cirrhosis is established, the clinical course may be significantly affected by avoidance or removal of the offending agent. In infancy when cirrhosis caused by galactosemia is once established, it is no longer responsive to therapy; however, it is readily preventable by avoiding galactose in the diet. The most common source of galactose is milk (lactose or milk sugar). Similarly, infants who have fructose intolerance can be protected by avoiding in their diet table sugar (fructose, disaccharide of glucose and fructose) or fructose itself present in fruits.

TABLE 1.

DISORDERS	THERAPY
Galactosemia	Avoidance of galactose (lactose)
Glycogen storage disease IV, lack of debrancher enzyme	None
Fructose intolerance	Avoid sugar (sucrose) and fruits (fructose)
α_1-Antitrypsin deficiency	None
Wilson's disease	Penicillamine, K sulfide, genetic counseling
Hemochromatosis	Phlebotomies
Congestive cirrhosis	Surgical or medical therapy of underlying disease; avoidance of estrogens
Alcoholic cirrhosis	Absolute → relative abstinence and improved nutrition
Cryptogenic cirrhosis	Nonspecific therapy of chronic hepatitis

Wilson's disease is the most common type of cirrhosis which—if recognized in time—can be prevented by specific drug therapy. This can be done when the disease masquerades as a chronic hepatitis or it can be identified in asymptomatic individuals. Preclinical Wilson's disease is usually detected during the examination of family members of patients with known Wilson's disease. Both in the cirrhotic and noncirrhotic patient with Wilson's disease, the therapy of choice is D-penicillamine, given in doses of 1 to 4 grams (usually between 1.5 and 2 grams) a day. At the initiation of therapy, potassium sulfide may be administered with meals to avoid the absorption of excessive copper from dietary sources. The higher dose chelation therapy of Wilson's disease should proceed until the liver copper and total body stores of copper are reduced to normal; this is likely to last from 5 to 7 years or longer. Lifelong copper chelation is probably desirable in these patients, but the minimum effective dose of D-penicillamine is not established.

Hemochromatosis must be clearly separated from hemosiderosis, commonly seen in patients with alcoholic cirrhosis, particularly those who have undergone portacaval shunt surgery. Therapy consists of weekly phlebotomies of 500 ml. of blood until the serum iron has decreased and a mild iron deficiency anemia is achieved; thereafter a mild iron deficiency is assured by phlebotomies at less frequent intervals. The average patient will require close to 100 phlebotomies.

Congestive cirrhosis can best be prevented, but when hepatic fibrosis is developing, it may still be improved by the removal of the underlying cause. This can be done by surgery on the heart or pericardium, or by preventing prolonged congestion after hepatic vein occlusion. After hepatic vein occlusion, it is important that a portacaval shunt be performed promptly, particularly in young women who are on antiovulatory medications. The longer the delay, the more extensive the parenchymal destruction, the more advanced the fibrosis, and the worse the prognosis for life. If hepatic vein occlusion also involves the vena cava, then a portal pulmonary shunt must be constructed to decompress the markedly congested liver. In patients with sickle cell anemia, therapy may not be effective in preventing the development of a congestive type of cirrhosis, but this is a rare complication of this hemoglobinopathy.

Secondary biliary cirrhosis may develop in patients who have nonresectable obstruction of the biliary tree. In these patients the cirrhosis is not preventable, but usually it is the cause of the destruction which limits survival. However, patients who have partial obstruction of a major bile duct can develop cirrhosis even if the serum bilirubin elevation is minimal or intermittent. The danger signal is the progressive risk of the alkaline phosphatase which heralds the probability of cirrhosis and calls for earlier surgery.

Therapy of Symptomatic Cirrhosis

Liver failure caused by cirrhosis can be grouped into four separate categories: (1) failure of the hepatic parenchyma ("decompensated" cirrhosis, usually caused by activity of the underlying chronic hepatitic process), (2) failure of the blood flow (portal hypertension with varices), (3) failure of lymphatic and renal function (ascites), and (4) failure of the nervous system (encephalopathy or myelopathy). Each of the four types of failure may develop alone or in various combinations.

"Liver Cell" Failure (Chronic Hepatitis). These patients exhibit the usual clinical signs of "liver disease" with malaise, anorexia, and sometimes nausea and vomiting. They usually have jaundice, liver palms, and spider angiomas, and exhibit changes attributable to altered sex hormone metabolism such as testicular atrophy, changes in hair distribution, or amenorrhea. If looked for, evidence of malnutrition is found, although these patients may appear "adequately nourished" or even obese, or may show overt signs of anutrition, often with multiple vitamin deficiencies. In some patients evidence of a deficiency of a single vitamin, such as pellagra or peripheral neuropathy, dominates the clinical picture. Treatment of these patients with nicotinic acid or thiamine, respectively, is insufficient. Multivitamins should be given in addition. Cirrhotic patients, particularly those with alcoholic cirrhosis, commonly manifest marked decrease of their height/creatinine (24 hour urinary excretion) ratio. This index of decreased muscle mass, as well as the fasting serum amino acid pattern, in these cirrhotic patients may be as profound as that seen in kwashiorkor.

Parenchymal failure is treated first by removal of the offending agent, such as ethanol, drugs, copper, or iron. Bed rest is a cornerstone of therapy. This is based on empirical observations rather than on controlled clinical trials.

The diet may include 1 gram of protein per kg. of body weight. Caution must be exercised in forcing large amounts of dietary protein on the sick patient. Many of these patients are in nitrogen balance on as little as 35 to 40 grams of protein per day and cannot efficiently handle larger amounts of protein in their diet. A simple way to estimate the ability of a cirrhotic patient to handle dietary protein is to measure the urinary urea excretion. The 24 hour excretion of urea nitrogen (N) is a simple and readily available test. When the cirrhotic patient is not gaining muscle weight, he should excrete two thirds to three fourths of the dietary N (protein) as urea N. The measurement of urinary N excretion gives a rational basis for the selection of the maximum amount of dietary protein the patient can utilize efficiently. The cirrhotic patient's appetite is best in the morning; therefore as much high quality protein (eggs) should be provided at breakfast as the patient can tolerate. During the day, however, frequent small feedings are better accepted than the regular meals. The easiest method is to give the patient liquid nourishment between the usual meals with small servings at meal time. The replacement of ice water with fruit juices or sweetened drinks will provide additional carbohydrate calories. In malnourished patients additional large amounts of "therapeutic vitamin" capsules are given. Initially, large amounts of thiamine may be required in addition to supplying the vitamin B complexes as well as ascorbic acid. If the patient has nutritional macrocytic anemia, he should receive a single injection of 1000 micrograms of vitamin B_{12} in addition to 1 mg. of folic acid twice daily. Because alcoholic patients have impaired ability to utilize dietary folic acid and eat little food containing folic acid, it is desirable to give folic acid even when megaloblastic anemia is not present. During years of poor intake, many of these patients became vitamin B_{12} depleted in spite of having no difficulty absorbing the vitamin. Iron should be given to anemic patients only if the serum iron is low. Many anemic alcoholic patients with cirrhosis have high iron stores in their marrow and liver. Phytonadione (vitamin K_1), 10 mg. daily, is given parenterally for 3 days if the prothrombin time is prolonged.

DRUGS. There is no drug which specifically helps parenchymal necrosis. However, in two clinical syndromes corticosteroids are apparently helpful:

1. Cryptogenic cirrhosis with cholestasis. These patients may show rapid decrease of serum bilirubin concentrations after administration of corticosteroids (prednisolone, 10 to 15 mg. four times daily). Progressive decrease of the prednisolone dose during the succeeding 3 to 4 weeks is desirable, and the drug can usually be discontinued in 4 to 6 weeks.

2. Cryptogenic cirrhosis with chronic hepatitis. Patients whose liver biopsy shows an active chronic hepatitis (parenchymal necrosis and inflammation) usually show a good clinical improvement when moderate doses of corticosteroids are administered (prednisolone, 10 mg. two to four times daily). Their jaundice, serum glutamic oxaloacetic transaminase (SGOT), and serum gamma globulin levels decrease, and their appetite and serum albumin increase. The corticosteroid dose is gradually reduced during the next 2 to 4 weeks but is maintained for prolonged periods of time (prednisolone, 10 to 15 mg., with azathioprine [Imuran], 50 mg. daily). (This use of Imuran is not listed in the manufacturer's official directive.) The maintenance dose depends on the patient's course. This apparently rewarding clinical response is not seen regularly in all patients.

Bleeding Varices with Portal Hypertension. The most catastrophic event in the life history of a cirrhotic patient may be a massive hemorrhage from the stomach or esophagus. It must be remembered, however, that variceal bleeding need not be massive; intermittent or, indeed, prolonged low grade bleeding can occur from this source. Treatment consists of blood replacement, correction of clotting factor deficiencies, and control of hemorrhage. The prolonged one stage prothrombin time is corrected by injection of vitamin K_1 oxide and with the administration of fresh blood or fresh frozen plasma. If bleeding is massive, it is desirable that every other unit of blood be less than 24 hours old or, preferably, less than 6 hours old. Blood which has been in the blood bank for several weeks should not be used unless no other is available. Blood should be evacuated from the gastrointestinal tract by the administration of cathartics by mouth and by enemas.

Control of Variceal Bleeding. VASOPRESSIN THERAPY. If the variceal bleeding does not stop after the administration of fresh blood, plasma, and vitamin K_1, then infusion of vasopressin should be tried. (This use of vasopressin is not listed in the manufacturer's official directive. See package insert before giving intravenously.) This can be given in either continuous or intermittent infusion. It can be infused either in the peripheral vein or in the supermesenteric artery. Particularly when the bolus therapy is used, precautions must be taken to prevent side effects. Electrocardiographic (EKG) leads are attached to the patient, and the EKG is monitored. The administration can proceed as 20 to 30 units of vasopressin in 50 to 100 ml. of 5 per cent dextrose in water rapidly infused (see package insert). The aim is to administer the vasopressin as fast as possible to (1) induce facial pallor, (2) elevate the peripheral blood pressure, and (3) produce abdominal cramps or bowel movement, but *not* so fast as to produce myocardial ischemia manifested by depression of S-T and T segments on the EKG. In this way an effective *dose* and *rate of administration* are established. This dose can be administered in the same manner every 3 hours for a day or more as a therapeutic adjunct to reduce the rate of blood loss or to stop bleeding altogether. If vasopressin infusions effectively reduce the transfusion requirements, continued treatment is warranted. When continuous infusion is applied, then 0.2 to 0.5 unit of vasopressin per minute is infused intravenously, or if this does not prove effective, then in the supermesenteric artery.

Because of the antidiuretic effect of vasopressin, it is advisable that intermittently 20 per cent mannitol be infused rapidly to induce water diuresis and prevent excessive water retention. The infusion of 250 to 500 ml. of 20 per cent mannitol in 90 minutes every 12 hours during continuous vasopressin infusions has been successful in preventing the development of hyponatremia.

If the patient has large amounts of ascites and the infusion of vasopressin does not control the variceal bleeding, the removal of ascitic fluid may transiently lower the portal pressure long enough to permit cessation of bleeding. Constant monitoring of the hematocrit and central venous pressure is essential once a large amount of ascitic fluid has been removed, because loss of circulating volume can occur not only by hemorrhage but also by reaccumulation of the ascitic fluid. Blood and fresh frozen plasma are given to maintain (1) a central venous pressure of 4 to 8 cm. water, (2) a hematocrit between 30 and 35 per cent, and (3) a stable blood pressure.

BALLOON TAMPONADE. If bleeding continues unabated despite infusions of fresh blood and vasopressin, compression of the gastric fundus with or without compressing the distal esophagus with the *Sengstaken-Blakemore* (S-B) or Linton tube is indicated. This device is dangerous and may be used only if preparations are made for the prevention or control of life-threatening complications. The balloons must be tested for leakage before they are inserted in the patient. The amount of air required to inflate the gastric balloon sufficiently to prevent its sliding into the esophagus is determined before intubation (usually 200 to 300 ml. of air is required). One *must make sure* that the gastric balloon is in the stomach before it is distended to the previously determined size; otherwise it will rupture the esophagus. The tube is then pulled snug up against the diaphragm. The best way to keep the gastric balloon in position is to put a football helmet on the patient and tie the tube with about 1 pound pull to the face guard. The esophageal balloon is distended then, and the pressure is kept at about 30 mm. of mercury. (This pressure is constantly monitored with a sphygmomanometer.) If the patient's portal pressure has been recently determined, the esophageal balloon pressure is kept a little above the previous portal pressure. An additional nasogastric tube is placed just above the balloon to aspirate swallowed secretions. Once the balloon is distended, it is kept in place for at least 12 hours. To prevent pressure necrosis of the esophageal mucosa, deflate the balloon for a few minutes each hour after the first 5 hours. As a practical matter, spontaneous fluctuations of pressure in this balloon are wide enough to prevent tissue necrosis. If bleeding stops, the esophageal balloon is deflated after 12 hours. If bleeding does not recur, the gastric balloon is deflated 4 to 6 hours later. Prolonged compression of the gastric fundus leads to mucosal necrosis. The tube is not removed for another 24 hours, because the greatest probability for the recurrence of bleeding is within these 24 to 36 hours. The third lumen of the tube can be used for aspiration of blood from the stomach and for the administration of sucrose in water, electrolytes, and medication.

CARE OF THE SENGSTAKEN-BLAKEMORE TUBE. The use of the tube is potentially hazardous and can be more dangerous than the bleeding itself if the tube is not attended constantly and cared for properly.

1. Make certain that the gastric balloon is large enough so that it cannot slide into the esophagus.

2. Make certain that the pressure in the

esophagus is never much over the estimated portal pressure, and the balloon is deflated periodically to prevent necrosis of the esophageal mucosa. If the mucosa becomes necrotic or if excessive pressure is allowed to develop in the balloon, the esophagus can easily be ruptured!

3. Someone should be in *constant* attendance, and a pair of scissors should be readily available to cut and remove the tube if it slides up and obstructs the airway.

4. Suction is used to prevent aspiration of swallowed secretions from the obstructed esophagus.

Before the tube is removed, make sure that bleeding has stopped and let the patient swallow 1 to 2 ounces of mineral oil, which will lubricate the tube and make removal a little easier.

Because of blood clots it is not likely that gastric aspiration can effectively evacuate blood from the stomach. Saline purgatives are given as required through gastric tubes (see Encephalopathy, p. 359). The gastric contents are tested for HCl. If Topfer's reagent is used, the bloody fluid would prevent the recognition of the red color which indicates a pH of 3.5 or less. Therefore a piece of white filter paper (toilet paper or paper towel will do just as well) is inserted in the gastric aspirate. Within a minute the leading edge of reasonably clear gastric juice ascends on the paper. A drop of Topfer's reagent is placed at the junction of dry and wet paper. If the indicator solution turns red, it can be easily seen now. A red color indicates that the pH is low, and the patient should be given antacids in sufficient amounts and frequency to maintain an intragastric pH above 3.5.

Emergency Shunt Surgery. In general, emergency operation to stop upper gastrointestinal hemorrhage caused by portal hypertension is a last, desperate measure. In contrast to the poor outcome experience reported in most European and American medical centers, an occasional report of a better outcome has been described. Nevertheless, emergency shunt should be reserved for certain specific clinical situations:

1. When the bleeding cannot be controlled or sufficient blood is not available to replace continued blood loss. Under these circumstances, accurate evaluation of the splanchnic circulation and estimates of hepatic blood flow should be obtained by splenic, superior mesenteric, and hepatic arteriography. In those patients who are candidates for the *selective* (Warren) shunt (see below), the emergency operation should consist of the selective procedure. If, however, there are contraindications present for the Warren shunt, then a *total* shunt should be performed; if possible, a mesocaval or mesorenal H-graft interposition shunt may give less postoperative encephalopathy than the portacaval shunt.

2. In a patient who had been adequately evaluated before the bleeding, whose cirrhosis is inactive (chronic alcoholic or hepatitic process is minimal or absent), whose laboratory liver tests indicate little active liver injury (bilirubin less than 2 mg. per dl. [100 ml.] and albumin over 3 grams per dl. [100 ml.]), and for whom a skilled vascular surgical team is available. This patient is a better surgical risk at the onset of hemorrhage than he will be for weeks or months after a massive or prolonged bleeding.

Elective "Therapeutic" Shunt Operation. There are two types of shunts: (1) a *total* (conventional) shunt, which consists of decompression of the portal system; and (2), a *selective* shunt, which consists of selective decompression of varices only without altering portal pressure. There are two types of total shunts: (a) A shunt that decompresses both the intra- and extrahepatic portal systems (the prototype is the side-to-side portacaval shunt); there are at least a dozen modifications of this procedure. (b) A shunt resulting in decompression of the extrahepatic portal system only; i.e., the end-to-side portacaval shunt. This is modified by further increasing the intrahepatic portal pressure and blood flow by arterialization of the hepatic stump of the portal vein.

Regardless of the type of *total* shunt performed, any procedure that reduces the resistance of the extrahepatic portal system results in reduction of the splanchnic blood volume, reduction of the portal pressure, and, consequently, reduction of the portal flow to the liver—that is, if portal flow was hepatopetal to begin with. In contrast, the *selective* Warren shunt was designed to reduce the pressure in the varices and drain the varices through the short gastric veins into the spleen and from the spleen into the renal vein. At the same time, the second phase of the operation consists of disconnecting the varices from the portal vein by identifying and ligating all communicating vessels between the two sets of veins.

In a controlled randomized trial in which currently over 50 patients have been followed for sufficiently long periods to identify significant trends, it is clear that the effectiveness of the *selective* Warren shunt in preventing recurrent bleeding is the same as that of a *total* shunt. Furthermore, the operative mortality and the technical difficulties of the *selective* Warren shunt as compared to, for example, an *H-graft* interposition total shunt, are not significantly different. On the other hand, the frequency of postoperative encephalopathy is significantly lower after the *selective* Warren shunt than after a *total* shunt. This is because the hepatic functional capacity (as measured by the liver's ability to handle nitrogen: maximum rate of urea synthesis) is depressed very little by the *selective* Warren shunt but is significantly impaired by a *total* shunt. The likely explanation is that the *total* shunt diverts portal flow from the liver, which results in deterioration of the hepatic functional capacity, leading to portal systemic encephalopathy. The currently accumulating evidence will make it increasingly difficult to justify the performance of a *total* shunt in patients who are candidates for the *selective* Warren shunt. These patients are candidates for the Warren shunt when they have portal hypertension and a significant portal flow to their liver. Current contraindications to the Warren shunt are ascites (if it is currently present; however, if ascites was removed by therapy, the patient becomes a candidate for the Warren shunt); acquired or congenital anatomic abnormalities that would prevent the construction of the selective Warren shunt; and portal vein thrombosis or reversal of portal flow, which makes a selective shunt a moot question, as it can no longer preserve a nonexistent portal flow to the hepatic parenchyma. Evidence for reversal of portal flow can be obtained during hepatic arteriography when, instead of opacifying the hepatic venous outflow alone, the contrast material exits from the liver through the portal vein. Under carefully controlled conditions, reversal of portal flow can also be demonstrated during wedged hepatic venography, but the errors of this procedure are great owing to the use of excessive force in injecting contrast material through the wedge catheter. The best method to demonstrate hepatopetal flow is the venous phase of the superior mesenteric arteriogram. Once reliable techniques have been developed to estimate hepatic blood flow and portal flow in a cirrhotic patient under conditions which do not impose an unacceptable hazard to the patient, then these techniques will replace the angiographic estimate of portal perfusion of the liver.

Ascites (Failure of Lymphatic and Renal Function). A common temptation is to remove anything that is abnormal and do this as rapidly and efficiently as possible. As a rule, more harm can be inflicted on the patient by overzealous efforts to remove ascitic fluid (either by the use of potent diuretics or by paracentesis) than by ignoring it. Before undertaking the therapy of ascites in a cirrhotic patient, one must remember that in many of these patients vigorous diuresis to "get them to their *dry* weight" may also result in reaching their *dead* weight. When diuretics are given for the removal of ascitic fluid, one should constantly watch for the early signs and symptoms of untoward side effects. The principles of therapy are as follows:

1. Sodium restriction. Ideally, restriction to 20 mEq. per day of sodium is most effective; however, most patients have a poor enough appetite that severe sodium restriction also restricts the variety of foods that may be offered, and limitation to 50 to 85 mEq. per day is usually an adequate restriction. Most patients will not consume all their diet—i.e., all the "permitted" sodium.

2. If the patient has severe anemia or low circulating blood volume, this must be corrected before diuretic therapy is started.

3. Bed rest with bathroom privileges, daily weights, and measured fluid intake and output are necessary only if ambulatory therapy was ineffective.

4. Blood pressure is measured supine and erect two to three times a day.

5. The patient's pulse and neck veins when he is in a 30 to 45 degree position are examined daily.

6. The hematocrit, serum electrolytes, blood urea nitrogen (BUN), and creatinine are examined two or three times a week, depending on the diuretic response.

Note: Bed rest and sodium restriction alone may induce satisfactory diuresis.

7. Finally, diuretics are administered.

DIURETIC DRUGS. Various potent diuretics are available. Spironolactone (Aldactone) is given first. The average adult usually requires 150 mg. per day of spironolactone to prevent continued excessive potassium loss. If no diuresis occurs in 48 hours, determine the sodium/potassium ratio of the first morning's urine (spot urine). If this ratio is much less than 1, increase the spironolactone dose to 200 to 300 mg. per day. If the first morning's urine sodium/potassium ratio is close to or over 1, add to your therapy intermittently 20 or 40 mg. of furosemide. Be very careful in giving potassium to a patient who is on spironolactone. Very rapid rises of serum potassium may develop—a rise from low to high levels has occurred in 24 to 48 hours.

The aim is to induce a slow, gradual weight loss. One ought to avoid rapid diuresis which may appear as a dramatic clinical "triumph" but can be hazardous and often is debilitating to a patient.

It must be kept in mind that the maximum capacity of the lymphatics to mobilize ascitic fluid into the circulation and replace the diuretic loss is limited. As a general rule, one is on the safe side to assume that this limit is around 400 ml. a day, although it may be higher in some patients. As diuresis progresses, an increase of hematocrit and blood urea nitrogen (BUN) and a decrease of plasma volume can be anticipated. This is corrected with an intravenous infusion of plasma. Regardless of the patient's serum albumin concentration, the infusion of salt-poor albumin is ineffective in inducing diuresis because the low serum albumin concentration is not a cause but a result of the accumulation of ascites. When diuresis is rapid, extreme care must be exercised not to precipitate severe hyponatremia and hypovolemia.

Diuretic therapy must be discontinued in patients who develop symptoms of encephalopathy or who have evidence of progressive renal failure.

THERAPY OF LOW SERUM SODIUM CONCENTRATION. A decrease in serum sodium concentration may result from one of three mechanisms: sodium depletion, overhydration, or potassium depletion. Ascites is the result of an isotonic expansion of the extracellular fluid and an accumulation in the abdominal cavity. Therefore when a cirrhotic patient has ascites, one can safely assume that his total body sodium is increased regardless of serum sodium concentration. Correction of low serum sodium is done by osmotic diuresis, potassium administration, and water restriction.

1. If the patient's serum sodium concentration is below 125 mEq. per liter, daily total liquid intake should be restricted to the previous day's 24 hour urine output plus 300 ml. More stringent fluid restriction is necessary if serum sodium is below 120 mEq. per liter.

2. Potassium replacement. If the patient has not only low serum sodium but also low chloride concentration, he should be given potassium chloride. Although other potassium salts are more palatable, they are usually useless. The serum potassium concentration is a poor index of total body potassium; nevertheless, if serum potassium increases over 5.5 mEq. per liter or BUN is high and rising, potassium administration must be stopped. At least 40 to 100 mEq. of KCl is given daily by mouth in divided doses or intravenously. The former is preferable, as intravenous KCl can be painful.

3. Diuretic therapy is reduced or discontinued, and 500 ml. of 20 per cent mannitol is infused daily in 90 minutes. This osmotic diuretic induces water loss in excess of electrolyte loss relative to intake and helps to promote the reestablishment of more normal serum osmolarity.

4. Plasma or plasma protein fraction (PPF) is infused to correct plasma volume depletion.

"VIGOROUS" THERAPY OF ASCITES. Although ascites should be considered a symptom and the major problem is the underlying liver disease, certain circumstances make it necessary to rapidly mobilize the ascitic fluid. Vigorous therapy may be necessary in a patient whose umbilical hernia may rupture or who has very tense ascites which interferes with breathing and eating, or in patients with modest ascites in whom a selective shunt operation would be considered if the ascites could be removed. In these patients diuresis is usually induced by (1) restricting sodium intake to 10 to 20 mEq. per day; (2) increasing oral spironolactone administration to the point that the first morning urine sodium/potassium ratio is close to 1; and (3) infusing 500 ml. of plasma or plasma protein fraction (PPF) daily in 3 hours, followed by 20 to 40 mg. of furosemide intravenously, followed by the infusion of 500 ml. of 20 per cent mannitol in 90 minutes. If the patient also has tense ascites, 800 to 1000 ml. of ascitic fluid is removed. This will give sufficient relief. Negative pressure breathing will improve the rate of return of ascitic fluid.

PARACENTESIS. Ascitic fluid can effectively be eliminated by paracentesis. This, however, will usually result in the rapid reaccumulation of ascitic fluid, oliguria, and reduction of circulating plasma volume. This can be prevented by reinfusion of ascitic fluid; the infusion of 5 per cent albumin in isotonic sodium chloride; or plasma or PPF to maintain an adequate circulating plasma volume. For ascitic fluid reinfusion therapy a peritoneal dialysis set can be used. Diuretic therapy is continued. This type of therapy is usually successful for the short term; however, it is neither necessary nor warranted in the majority of patients.

The most efficient ascitic reinfusion is the surgical insertion of an "artificial thoracic duct." This is one of the "peritoneal subclavian" shunts. In selected patients with truly refractory ascites, the LeVeen shunt proved to be very effective in two thirds to three fourths of the patients in whom this has been applied. There is a lack of long-term experience with these shunts, but they have been well tolerated for over a year in a number of patients. The procedure consists of two small incisions, one to insert the valve in the peritoneal cavity and the other in the neck to insert it in the subclavian vein. The tubing is channeled subcutaneously between the abdomen and the neck. In some patients the rapid return of ascitic fluid induced massive diuresis. However, the increased central venous pressure may cause transient pulmonary edema. Vigorous diuretic therapy in these patients rapidly corrects the hypervolemia. Furthermore, the increased venous pressure reduces the rate of return of ascitic fluid and automatically controls this problem. With the advent of the "peritoneosubclavian" shunt, portal decompressive surgery to reduce the rate of ascites production will probably not be required.

Encephalopathy (Hepatic Coma).* Although the precise mechanism of hepatic coma not induced by drugs is not known, it is well documented that these patients have major defects in their nitrogen metabolism. These cirrhotic patients are not able to handle ammonia or make urea at a normal rate. Because of their limited ability to metabolize a nitrogen load, the principal therapy is limited nitrogen (protein amino acid, ammonia) intake.

The therapy of hepatic coma depends on the precipitating factor.

SPONTANEOUS. If symptoms appear without any apparent precipitating cause, the treatment consists of (1) reduction of protein intake while ensuring 1000 carbohydrate calorie intake to suppress gluconeogenesis; (2) neomycin, 1 gram every 6 hours; and (3) the avoidance of sedatives or narcotics. As symptoms subside and handwriting improves, a 20 gram protein, low ammonia diet is permitted. If this is tolerated for 3 days, the daily protein intake is raised gradually to 40 or maybe 50 grams. Once this amount is tolerated, the dose of neomycin is reduced by 1 gram per day each 3 to 4 days as long as symptoms of coma do not recur (handwriting remains normal and asterixis is absent). In some patients a 40 to 50 gram protein diet is tolerated without serious symptoms when only 2 to 3 grams per day of neomycin is given. These patients can continue like this for months or years without demonstrable intellectual deterioration. It is preferable to use neomycin to permit a diet of at least 35 to 40 grams of protein per day rather than to eliminate protein from the diet. Sufficient amounts of lactulose (a nondigestible disaccharide) are given to induce two soft bowel movements a day but not so much as to cause an osmotic diarrhea. Note that for those patients who are lactose intolerant (which may include over two thirds of black Americans), lactose, a much cheaper "nondigestible" disaccharide, can be used instead of lactulose.†

COMA SECONDARY TO GASTROINTESTINAL BLEEDING. When symptoms of coma appear in a patient with gastrointestinal bleeding, the prognosis for the coma is better than that with spontaneous coma. Blood must be evacuated from the stomach and intestines by the following methods: (1) Aspiration and ice water lavage of gastric contents. Constant mechanical suction alone is not effective, because the small bore nasogastric tube easily becomes plugged with clots. Intermittent lavage with a 50 ml. syringe improves the efficiency of constant suction. (2) Sixty ml. of milk of magnesia and 2 grams of neomycin are placed in the stomach each 2 hours, and suction is omitted for 40 minutes. Suction is then reinstituted for 70 minutes; the stomach is lavaged for 10 minutes every 2 hours until gross blood is removed. Once the patient develops diarrhea, milk of magnesia is discontinued. (3) Tap water enemas (or saline, if the patient has no ascites) are given each 6 hours until return is clear or the patient is fatigued. After cleansing enemas, 1 gram of neomycin in 100 ml. of water is given as a retention enema. Careful attention is paid to changes in serum electrolytes and urine output to prevent excessive water retention as the result of enemas and gastric lavage. The major problem is the control of hemorrhage itself.

IATROGENIC HEPATIC COMA. Therapy of various symptoms may predispose to or precipitate coma:

1. Total shunt (portal decompressive surgery). The therapy for this type of coma is the same as that for spontaneous coma.

2. Diuretic therapy. Symptoms of coma may develop after the administration of various diuretics for the therapy of ascites. This may occur at times even if significant diuresis did not take place. The mechanisms of this type of coma are not known, although altered inorganic ion metabolism (detectable or undetectable by changes of serum electrolyte or pH concentrations) has been considered at fault. Some diuretics increase renal venous ammonia concentrations. In these patients diuretics should be discontinued, and any abnormalities in serum electrolytes and circulating plasma volume should be corrected. Patients are then treated as if in spontaneous coma.

3. Narcotics and sedatives. These drugs are poorly tolerated by ill cirrhotic patients and can easily precipitate coma. Frequently, symptoms of coma such as irritability, restlessness, and insomnia are treated with sedatives that accelerate the progression of the symptoms of coma. Therapy consists of cessation of the administration of offending agents. If neurologic symptoms persist, the patient is treated as having spontaneous coma.

THE UNRESPONSIVE PATIENT. When symptoms of hepatic coma progress to unconsciousness, a small bore plastic tube is placed in the stomach for hydration and carbohydrate feeding. The daily water volume depends on renal function. At least 1000 carbohydrate calories are ad-

---

*Hepatic coma refers to the entire spectrum of neurologic disturbances: from disturbed handwriting and asterixis; through personality changes, intellectual deterioration, and alteration of consciousness; to unresponsiveness.

†It is generally accepted current practice to restrict protein in the diet of patients who are prone to develop encephalopathy. It is commonly overlooked that some foods contain excessively high amounts of ammonia. These high ammonia containing foods must be restricted in the diet of cirrhotic patients. These foods are strong cheeses, salamis and sausages, Jell-O and gelatin, commercial hamburgers, and onions. For details see Rudman et al.: Amer. J. Clin. Nutr., *26*:487, 1973.

ministered, for example, as a constant drip of 1200 ml. of 20 per cent sucrose or as glucose polymers (Polycose) per day. *Do not use glucose;* it has twice the osmolarity per calories of sucrose. It is customary to add vitamins B and C in the sugar solution. Oxygen may be administered by nasal catheter. One gram of neomycin is infused in the gastric tube every 4 hours.

OTHER FORMS OF THERAPY. Intravenous glutamic acid, arginine, and small or massive doses of corticosteroids have no proved value.

Exchange transfusions, cross-circulation with volunteers or primates, or pig liver perfusion are not indicated in the treatment of hepatic coma in a cirrhotic patient.

CONSTIPATION

method of
EDDY D. PALMER, M.D.
Hackettstown, New Jersey

Definition

Defining constipation is difficult because of wide normal variations in bowel habits from person to person and in any person from time to time. Basically, the definition has to do with transit time through the colon, but an important facet is simply whether the person views his bowel activity as normal or abnormal. There is a wide range of acceptability among people of all ages for their bowel activities. Except in rather unusual circumstances, if a person's bowel activities from month to month are not viewed as a problem by the person, they should not be viewed as such by the doctor.

It should be noted that even though the bowels move every day, the person may be several days behind in evacuating the distal colon. Thus by definition there is constipation even though there is a daily bowel movement. It must also be noted that the definition of constipation is not concerned with the hardness of the stools. Fecal impactions, which represent a late stage of constipation, are regularly soft and putty-like.

Classification

Therapy cannot be intelligently planned until the constipation has been typed. There are four types:

1. Pharmacologic constipation. This type is brief, resulting from a wide variety of prescribed drugs; it is well known to every clinician and requires no further mention.

2. Chronic hypotonic constipation. This type is most often found in babies and young children, in adults with hypothyroidism, occasionally in those who have diabetes, and in association with certain neurologic diseases. The constipated stool is putty-like, largely increased, and never hard and subdivided. Transit is delayed everywhere along the course of the colon, but mainly in the ascending colon and rectum. Feces can almost always be felt on digital examination. On barium enema, the colon is found to be mildly dilated and elongated, with half-hearted haustral activity. Physiologically, the problem is muscular hypotonicity with somewhat slow water absorption.

3. Dyschezia or habit (rectal) constipation. This type is caused by "bad habits" that usually begin in childhood and continue for a variable period. Colonic transit is normal to the rectum, with failure then of the person to recognize the defecatory urge or simply failure to respond to it (e.g., laziness, no opportunity, fear of pain during defecation). In children soiling is common and is explained by an overflow phenomenon. Feces are always palpable on digital examination.

4. Chronic hypertonic constipation. This is by far the most common type in adults; it results from excess colonic muscular activity, especially in the descending colon and sigmoid, with hypersegmentation and prominent creasing, rather than propulsion of the mass. There is retention, progressive dehydration of the feces, and overproduction of mucus. Scybala are observed only in this type. The rectum is usually empty except for fragments, but the sigmoid is often full and prominent on abdominal palpation.

This type of constipation is characteristic of the irritable colon syndrome, in which it often alternates (sometimes quickly) with diarrhea.

A fifth category might be mentioned, comprising further stages or sequels of constipation—impactions, fecalomas, and obstipation.

Therapy

The basis for treatment should clearly be dictated by the physiologic defect responsible, although, as any clinician knows, theory that is clear cut in the books often seems to become confused in the patient. Because most constipation is chronic, the effort must be to handle the problem as far as possible by natural means or changes in habits; but to be realistic, it must be admitted that at times prolonged use of rather vigorous medications is required to assure satisfactory relief. The clinician must be concerned over the long-term potential whenever he prescribes strong drugs for constipation.

Hypotonic constipation calls for stimulation.

1. Exclude hypothyroidism, diabetes, and systemic neurologic diseases.

2. Establish a regular routine of prune juice (or prunes, figs, or dates) and bran (twice a day).

3. Establish a regular routine of physical exercise, when practicable.

4. If these moves prove insufficient, add an oral stimulant laxative at bedtime. There are many satisfactory ones from which to choose, including senna concentrate (Senokot), bisacodyl (Dulcolax), and sodium lauryl sulfate, 1,8-dihydroxyanthraquinone (Anavac).

Dyschezia or habit constipation requires retraining; if not of very long standing, it may be curable in the adult. It is almost always curable in the child (who these days seems to present this problem far more often than the adult).

1. Exclude or treat anal disease, the pain of which often is responsible for failure of the patient (child or adult) to respond to the defecatory urge.

2. For adults and parents of young patients, discuss with them the need to respond to the defecatory urge. Help with arranging habits to permit response (difficult yet possible in some adult patients, such as traffic policemen). Impress all with the importance of keeping the rectum empty.

3. When severe diastasis recti, pulmonary incompetence, or general debility is part of the patient's problem (in generating sustained abdominal pressure for defecation), advice regarding use of an abdominal binder during defecation is in order.

4. For children, current thinking dictates return to simple heavy mineral oil as the only medication. One ounce is given at bedtime nightly, at least 1½ hours after supper. This is done regularly, with adjustment of the dose downward only if there should be significant leaking with soiling of underclothes. It is usually necessary to continue the nightly mineral oil for about 2 months before trying the child on his own. Thereafter, the oil may be continued or not, as the bowel rhythm dictates.

For adults, the same regimen is recommended. A current trend is prescription of a bowel stimulant, apparently with the thought of increasing the defecatory urge so that the patient is really forced to get to the bathroom. If there is sufficient remaining rectal response "reflex," this approach can be effective; nevertheless, a trial of mineral oil is recommended first.

Hypertonic constipation is by far the most difficult constipation problem. There is a tendency for the patient to be impatient with slow results of treatment. The patient usually complains of other colonic symptoms (mainly hypogastric discomforts and gas), so that often treatment cannot be directed solely at the constipation.

1. Explain in detail that the constipation is being caused by an overly responsive, hypertonic colon; explain why scybala are being formed, why there is oversecretion of mucus, and what is causing the discomfort.

2. Prescribe a hydrophilic bulk laxative such as psyllium hydrocolloid (Effersyllium), psyllium hydrophilic mucilloid (Metamucil, Konsyl), or others twice a day, and depend on this as the most important medication. Bran in the diet helps.

3. Add at the start an antispasmodic-sedative combination, such as belladonna alkaloids with phenobarbital (Donnatal), dicyclomine (Bentyl) with phenobarbital, or others; there are many to choose from. The antispasmodic-sedative should be continued for about 6 weeks and then discontinued, and the results assessed. In all probability it will be found necessary to use this type of medication off and on, to help the hydrophilic laxative during the worst episodes.

4. Use of more vigorous preparations, such as large doses of milk of magnesia or magnesium citrate, can ideally be avoided; but realistically, it must be admitted that from time to time they may have a place in management. Similarly, enemas should rarely be used but can never be discarded entirely for this type of problem.

Constipation in the geriatric patient, whatever its type, presents a special clinical problem, because it tends to be erratic, becoming very severe at times and associated with an increasing risk of impaction. It calls for more radical treatment from time to time than might seem appropriate in a younger patient. Patients cannot be re-educated to change their habits at this age. The type of medication must be changed rather frequently, to care for the problem as it presents itself at the moment. Two points must be emphasized. First, certain old people must be observed closely if severe constipation or obstipation is to be recognized, for they may be uncommunicative and may not report such matters. Second, the opposite problem must be guarded against when considering therapy; some old people complain about constipation that they don't have, because of confusion, search for attention, or simple misunderstanding. In general the stimulant laxatives should be depended on (e.g., Senokot, Dulcolax, Anavac). Prune juice often is a help. Milk of magnesia, in the dose required, is worth trying.

DYSPHAGIA AND ESOPHAGEAL OBSTRUCTION

method of
JOSEPH A. RINALDO, JR., M.D.
Detroit, Michigan

Dysphagia is any interference with the smooth passage of food from the mouth to the stomach resulting from a mechanical obstruction or a disorder of motility. It is always a serious problem until proved otherwise.

Prompt and adequate therapy depends on early diagnosis, an awareness of the full range of diagnostic methods, and a resolution to manage the treatable lesion as aggressively as is feasible.

A careful history should establish the site of obstruction and the presence or absence of pain, reflux, or regurgitation, as well as weight loss and possible aggravation of the symptoms by bending or lying down. The clinician must suggest to the radiologist the suspected site of the lesion, because the technique for examining the pharyngoesophageal region is different from that for the distal esophagus. The clinician should always ask specifically for films of the esophagus if he has any suspicion that the patient has dysphagia. Flexible esophagoscopes and gastroscopes now make these studies quite tolerable, and esophageal pressure studies can be obtained in several centers. When esophageal manipulations are necessary, they should be done by a specialist who has used the methods frequently.

Psychophysiologic Dysphagia

Psychophysiologic dysphagia is usually caused by either an anxiety or a conversion reaction, and once adequate diagnostic studies have been completed, interview therapy by the general physician or a psychiatrist is needed. Many patients will obtain considerable relief from reassurance that there is no serious illness. However, since this is a diagnosis of exclusion, the physician should keep an open mind for several months and should reinvestigate if the patient's symptoms are not relieved.

Congenital Dysphagia

Esophageal atresia is treated surgically.

Dysphagia lusoria (anomalous right subclavian artery) almost never needs any treatment. A description of the problem is usually sufficient to relieve the patient.

Neuromuscular Dysphagia

Cerebrovascular disease, myasthenia gravis, amyotrophic lateral sclerosis, and *myotonic dystrophy* all cause dysphagia referred to the oropharyngeal area. Treatment is for the primary condition (see elsewhere in this volume). If the condition is of limited duration, nutritional support can be obtained by tube feeding, gastrotomy, or intravenous hyperalimentation.

Hypertrophy of the cricopharyngeus muscle is a rare condition in which there is narrowing of the esophageal inlet resulting from thickening of this muscle and perhaps from failure of the muscle to relax with swallowing. It is important to call the radiologist's attention to this lesion and to have cineradiographic studies of the area done. Treatment is esophagomyotomy of this muscle.

Achalasia should be suspected from the history and the radiographic study. Esophageal pressure examination will confirm the diagnosis. Nonsurgical treatment is brusque dilation using pneumostatic dilators or the Stark dilator. Surgical treatment is esophagomyotomy. Both methods have strong proponents and produce about equal results. We prefer the use of dilators; however, these instruments should be used only by an expert. Mercury or other metal bougies do not work, as achalasia is not a stricture but a failure of the inferior esophageal sphincter to relax.

Diffuse esophageal spasm is a diagnosis made by esophageal pressure examination. A description of the condition to the patient and some mild sedation are usually adequate for treatment. Nitroglycerin, 0.4 mg. sublingually, will relieve acute episodes of substernal pain. Occasionally long esophagomyotomy is necessary, but consultation with one of the authorities in this field is desirable before recommending this treatment.

Diverticula can be either proximal or distal. *Zenker's diverticulum,* which is just proximal to the cricopharyngeus muscle at the pharyngoesophageal junction, requires treatment only if retained food is being regurgitated. Treatment is excision. The older method of fixation of the diverticulum has been discarded. Myotomy of the cricopharyngeus muscle may be desirable, because it is felt that failure of this muscle to relax may be the cause of Zenker's diverticulum.

Midesophageal diverticulum rarely needs any treatment.

Epiphrenic diverticulum occasionally requires excision. It is wise to perform an esophageal pressure study, because it is felt that failure of the esophageal sphincter to relax is a factor contributing to the formation of the diverticulum. For this reason esophagomyotomy is recommended at the time of excision.

Collagen Diseases

Dysphagia is often associated with systemic sclerosis because of hypotonicity and esophageal stricture. A small hiatal hernia is frequently present. The temptation is to repair the small hiatal hernia, but this never helps. If stricture is present, it should be dilated. One should not assume that dysphagia in systemic sclerosis is always the result of hypomotility, because dilation of a stricture will often give relief.

If reflux occurs, it is necessary to minimize it by avoiding those activities that provoke reflux and to reduce the effect of acid gastric juices (see Peptic Esophagitis, below). There is no effective treatment for systemic sclerosis per se. Because of the chronic nature of the illness, a depressive reaction is frequently present. Acknowledgment of this depression and interview therapy by the primary physician are extremely important in helping the patient adjust to the chronicity of the illness.

Structural Dysphagia

Uncomplicated *hiatal hernia* rarely causes dysphagia. When dysphagia occurs, it is due to such complications as *narrow squamocolumnar ring (Schatzki), esophageal stricture, hypertonic inferior esophageal sphincter,* and *diffuse esophageal spasm.* Treatment of each of these is outlined under the appropriate diagnostic heading. Rarely, none of these complications is found when the hiatal hernia patient has dysphagia. Hiatal hernia repair may or may not relieve the symptoms under these circumstances.

Upper *esophageal web (Plummer-Vinson syndrome, Paterson-Kelly syndrome)* is usually easily ruptured at the time of esophagoscopy. Middle and lower esophageal web may be treated by dilation or excision.

Inflammatory Dysphagia

Peptic esophagitis is often associated with gastroesophageal reflux and complicates hiatal hernia and systemic sclerosis. Gastroesophageal reflux can be reduced by eating small meals, never lying down until at least 3 hours after eating, avoiding bending, and avoiding lifting. The head of the bed should be elevated by placing a ¾ inch plywood wedge with a base of 24 inches and a height of 6 inches under the mattress. This is more effective than blocks under the head of the bed. Antacids should be given in doses of 30 to 45 ml. 1 and 3 hours after meals and at bedtime. If this is ineffective, bethanechol chloride (Urecholine), 10 to 25 mg. before meals and at bedtime, should be tried. Anticholinergics should be avoided.

Acute corrosive esophagitis should be treated immediately by neutralization of the offending agent. Esophagoscopy will determine the extent of the lesion. If there is inflammation, prednisone, 10 mg. twice daily, is indicated for 3 weeks. A mercury bougie should be introduced daily for 1 week, then every other day for the next week, and then at less frequent intervals for a year. The patient may need dilation of the esophagus for many years thereafter.

Bacterial or *fungal esophagitis* should be treated with the specific antibiotic or antifungal agent. *Monilial esophagitis* is more common than was once realized. It has been treated successfully with nystatin (Mycostatin), 1 teaspoonful (500,000 units) three times each day.

Narrow squamocolumnar ring (Schatzki) is sometimes missed radiographically because of the failure to fill the esophagus and the stomach adjacent to the ring. Rings over 23 mm. in diameter do not require dilation; rings under 12 mm. do. Dilation of the ring with a bougie is the treatment of choice.

More extensive *stricture* should be treated by progressive dilation. If gastroesophageal reflux occurs after the stricture is adequately dilated and it is associated with a hiatal hernia, then repair of the hernia may be indicated. Under these circumstances simple reduction of the herniated stomach is not enough, and an additional procedure to bolster the inferior sphincter is indicated. Several methods are now available, all variants of fundal plication. On rare occasions the inflammatory and fibrotic reactions are so severe that reaction of the distal esophagus is necessary to obtain relief.

Neoplasms of the Esophagus

Benign neoplasms can usually be excised locally. *Malignant neoplasms* of the proximal esophagus are usually treated with radiotherapy; those of the distal two thirds of the esophagus are treated by excision. Care must be taken to provide adequate nutrition during the diagnostic and treatment periods. The possible nutritional modalities include parenteral hyperalimentation, tube feeding (see below), or gastrotomy. A variety of stents may be forcibly inserted through the lumen when the patient has a nonresectable neoplasm. As mentioned before, interview therapy designed to assist the patient in adjusting to the chronic illness is indicated.

Tube Feeding

This is an extremely useful adjunct in treatment of some esophageal lesions. One should try 240 polyethylene tubing that has had its tip gently flamed to smooth the edges without occluding the lumen. A continuous flow pump can then be used to instill the food that has been liquefied. It is possible to provide the patient with a well-balanced diet in this way. Enough water must be given to the patient to ensure adequate urine flow.

DIVERTICULA OF THE ALIMENTARY CANAL

method of
GRANT V. RODKEY, M.D.
Boston, Massachusetts

Esophagus

Esophageal diverticula are relatively common among patients of older age groups, and may occur in the upper, mid, or lower segments of that structure. Pharyngoesophageal and epiphrenic diverticula are of the pulsion type, whereas those of the midesophagus are usually secondary to adhesions and traction from previously inflamed adjacent lymph nodes.

Symptoms are largely limited to those diverticula which are of the pulsion type, and are chiefly dysphagia, regurgitation, and substernal pain. Rarely local perforation may occur or hemorrhage may complicate the disease.

Treatment of these lesions is essentially surgical. Pharyngoesophageal diverticula are now believed to develop chiefly as a secondary manifestation to spasm of the cricopharyngeal sphincter. Thus small diverticula may be managed by extramucosal posterior myotomy of the cricopharyngeus muscle through a left cervical approach. Larger diverticula should be excised with layer closure of the esophagus, carefully avoiding stenosis, and combined with posterior myotomy. Complications may include infection, esophagocutaneous fistula, and unilateral cord palsy secondary to injury of the recurrent laryngeal nerve. However, with modern surgical techniques the incidence of such complications should be minimal, and all patients with symptomatic pharyngoesophageal diverticula should be advised to have surgical repair.

Epiphrenic diverticula may be associated with neuromuscular dysfunction of the lower esophagus, hiatus hernia, or stricture. If symptoms are significant, transthoracic excision of the diverticulum with concomitant repair of associated defects of the esophagus, cardia, or diaphragmatic hiatus is indicated.

For all practical purposes, traction diverticula of the midesophagus do not produce symptoms and do not require specific treatment.

Stomach

Diverticula of the stomach are uncommon, but not rare. They usually occur at a point near the cardia on the posterior wall of the stomach, but in a small proportion of cases may be found in the prepyloric area. When they occur, they are usually solitary lesions.

Symptoms from gastric diverticula are ill defined, in part because of the frequency of concomitant structural or functional disorders of the upper digestive tract. The diverticula have been thought to be capable of causing epigastric or retrosternal pain, and they are occasionally the site of ulceration and hemorrhage. If the severity of symptoms requires treatment and other diseases have been excluded by careful study, including endoscopy, surgical excision of the diverticulum is the only effective therapy. However, the experienced surgeon will exercise extreme caution to be sure that he does not overlook some accompanying occult lesion which has been the real cause of the symptoms.

Duodenum

In contrast to those of the stomach, duodenal diverticula are frequently present and are often multiple, although it is rare for more than three or four to be present in a single patient. They usually arise on the mesenteric (pancreatic) side of the duodenal loop, and are intimately attached to pancreas lying on the posterior surface of that organ or protruding into the head of the gland. They are usually to be found in the second and third portions of the duodenum and commonly occur near the papilla of Vater. Pseudodiverticula may occur in the first portion of the duodenum as a sequel to peptic ulceration or scarring, or to previous surgery (e.g., pyloroplasty). Duodenal diverticula are usually discovered during x-ray examinations of the gastrointestinal tract with contrast medium, and are easily overlooked at the time of surgical exploration unless their presence has been noted previously.

Symptoms from duodenal diverticula undoubtedly do occur occasionally, but their precise definition is difficult unless there is hemorrhage or local inflammation with perforation—both extremely rare occurrences.

From a practical point of view, one should usually regard duodenal diverticula as an incidental finding not responsible for dyspeptic symptoms. However, it is of extreme importance to the surgeon doing surgery on the biliary tract to be wary of diverticula near or at the lower termination of the common bile duct, lest unrecognized perforation of the thin-walled portion of the duodenum occur.

If symptoms are clearly attributable to diverticula of the duodenum, the only therapy to be recommended is surgical excision. This is not a simple problem, and operation may be followed by acute pancreatitis or by duodenal leakage, peritonitis, and fistula. The operation should be undertaken thoughtfully and only by experienced surgeons.

Small Intestine

Diverticula extending into the mesentery of the small bowel, contained by a covering of serosa, submucosa, and mucosa, and analogous in structure to duodenal diverticula are occasionally encountered. Their frequency is considerably less than that of duodenal diverticula, and when they are present they are more often found in upper jejunum than in lower segments of the intestine. Diverticula of the small bowel are usually multiple, and they may involve long segments of the bowel or its entirety. Diagnosis is usually made on the basis of a barium meal followed through the intestine by means of serial films.

Symptoms caused by small bowel diverticula of this type are vague. Acute inflammation, perforation, hemorrhage, and obstruction rarely occur but are clearcut indications for surgical intervention. More frequently, symptoms of intestinal dysfunction—flatulence, abdominal pain, bloating, weight loss, megaloblastic anemia, or steatorrhea—may occur. Even these are rare, and when present they may represent a variant of the so-called "blind loop syndrome." Relief of symptoms may be obtained by intermittent short courses of antibiotic therapy (i.e., tetracycline, 250 mg. four times daily for 2 to 3 days), or by varying the diet pattern. Parenteral vitamin supplements may infrequently be required.

If significant symptoms are present from diverticulosis of the small bowel, surgical treatment may have to be considered. The only effective way to deal with these lesions is resection of a segment of the bowel; but if a large proportion of the small bowel is affected (as it usually is if symptoms are severe), this therapy is inappropriate.

Meckel's diverticulum of the ileum is a congenital remnant of the omphalomesenteric duct which may be manifested in a variety of ways. These include a blind pouch projecting from the antemesenteric border of the ileum (usually within 2 or 3 feet of the ileocecal valve) or a mucus-lined tract extending from ileum to umbilicus or to adjacent small bowel mesentery.

Symptoms caused by Meckel's diverticulum fall mainly into three categories: (1) those consequent to the present of heterotopic tissue—mainly gastric mucosa—in the diverticulum; (2) those resulting from mechanical factors set up by the presence of the diverticulum; and (3) those secondary to acute inflammation of the diverticulum. Rarely, Meckel's diverticulum may be the site of origin for tumors, either benign or malignant.

Symptoms relevant to the presence of heterotopic tissue in the diverticulum are chiefly those of gastrointestinal hemorrhage, often massive and secondary to acid-peptic digestion of mucosa adjacent to the base of the diverticulum. Most of these cases occur in children. The blood presenting in the stool in these patients usually varies from dark to light red, depending upon the rate of hemorrhage.

Mechanical effects of Meckel's diverticulum which cause symptoms are those of small bowel obstruction or, infrequently, intussusception.

Inflammation of Meckel's diverticulum is the third most frequent manifestation of its presence, and the signs and symptoms are those of appendicitis. Perforation and peritonitis may occur if diagnosis is delayed.

Finally, occult neoplasms of Meckel's diverticulum may become manifest by hemorrhage, obstruction, or metastases, or may be discovered incidentally in the course of laparotomy for another illness.

The treatment of all complications of Meckel's diverticulum is surgical excision. Indeed, such a diverticulum should be removed whenever it is discovered during the course of operation of another cause, the patient's condition permitting.

Appendix

It is not generally appreciated that the appendix may be the site of diverticulosis. The condition is rare, and its clinical significance, if any, is obscure. Diagnosis is always an incidental finding at laparotomy, and it seems reasonable to advise incidental appendectomy in such instances. If diverticulitis of the appendix occurs, the symptoms and pathologic findings are indistinguishable from those of acute appendicitis and the treatment is identical.

Colon

Diverticula of the colon should be classified as congenital or acquired. Congenital diverticula occur in the region of the cecum; are composed of serosa, muscularis, submucosa, and mucosa; and occur with comparable frequency among all population groups. They may be discovered as incidental findings on barium enema or may become manifest because of complications of acute inflammation or (rarely) hemorrhage. The symptoms of diverticulitis of the cecum mimic those of appendicitis, although progression of symptoms may be more leisurely, and nausea occurs less frequently than with appendicitis. Treatment is limited to patients with acute diverticulitis, and consists of operation with excision of the lesion. This may be accomplished by local excision if the pathology is recognized. Sometimes it is not possible to exclude the diagnosis of cancer of the cecum at operation, and in such cases a right colectomy should be performed. In a few instances, inflammation may involve only the posterior wall of the cecum and may be difficult to discover unless the cecum is detached from its peritoneal fixation and rolled forward for inspection. Excision of the diverticulum and performance of cecostomy at the site is an alternative method of managing some of these lesions. Diverticula of the cecum discovered incidentally during laparotomy for another illness should be treated by excision or by simple inversion.

Colonic diverticula of acquired origin rarely occur among Orientals, but are common among

Western populations. They are composed of serosa, submucosa, and mucosa only; arise first in the sigmoid region and tend to proliferate proximally from this point; and seem to represent intermuscular or perivascular herniations as an expression of increased intraluminal tension arising from neuromuscular dysfunction and altered patterns of peristalsis. Although they may appear earlier, they do not commonly occur before age 40. They become progressively more frequent with advancing age. These diverticula have narrow mouths and tend to collect inspissated feces. Mechanical irritation and bacterial digestion may frequently induce pathologic changes in the diverticula which may be manifested by symptoms of local inflammation or perforation, local or general peritonitis, hemorrhage varying from microscopic to massive, small or large bowel obstruction, cystitis, pelvic abscess, or fistula formation. Because of the comparable age groups involved, differentiation between diverticulitis and carcinoma of the colon may be difficult.

Despite the potential hazards of diverticulosis of the colon, most patients with this disease may be managed without surgical intervention. Medical therapy consists of a diet of normal or high fiber residue (except during attacks of acute diverticulitis), supplemented by 1 to 2 teaspoonfuls of powdered psyllium seed husk (Metamucil) per day. Anticholinergics and mild sedation should also be a part of the regimen.

During attacks of acute diverticulitis, the bowel should be put to rest by giving intravenous fluids, restriction of oral intake, and use of nasogastric suction as required. Systemic antibiotics (cephalothin [Keflin], 6.0 grams per day, or other broad-spectrum agent) should be given parenterally until the acute phase of the inflammation subsides and gastrointestinal function returns.

For less severe attacks of diverticulitis, manifested by left lower quadrant tenderness but without systemic illness, the patient may be managed with a liquid or very low residue diet, antibiotics or phthalylsulfathiazole (Sulfathalidine), 2.0 grams every 6 hours by mouth, and physical rest. Interestingly, many of these patients may gain relief of symptoms of diverticulitis following a barium enema, perhaps because of filling of the diverticula by the barium.

The complications of diverticulitis that may require surgical intervention include persistent or recurrent local inflammation, abscess formation, free perforation with peritonitis, obstruction, fistula formation, and hemorrhage. In the case of hemorrhage, it has been established that bleeding may often originate in the right colon even though diverticulosis is chiefly left-sided. Also, massive hemorrhage may occur because of so-called "angiodysplasia" (arteriovenous malformations), which may occur in the right colon with or without associated colonic diverticulosis. If facilities for selective mesenteric angiography are available, all patients with massive lower gastrointestinal hemorrhage should be studied by this method as early as possible. Intra-arterial or systemic infusion of vasopressin will control acute hemorrhage in a significant proportion of these patients after the bleeding source has been identified. If bleeding persists despite vasopressin infusion, surgical resection of the appropriate segment of bowel is indicated.

If angiographic studies are not available, massive lower intestinal bleeding associated with diverticulosis should be treated by subtotal colectomy and ileosigmoidostomy, as accurate localization of the bleeding point during operation is usually not possible.

The aim of surgical treatment for the remaining complications of diverticulitis is the extirpation of the diseased segment and restoration of intestinal continuity. However, the complicating factors may make a primary resection unwise, and in such circumstances staged resections (preliminary transverse colostomy, resection, and final colostomy closure; or sigmoid resection, end colostomy, and rectal turn-in with delayed reanastomosis) have been found to contribute to lowered mortality. Appropriate parenteral nutrition and antibiotic therapy should be adjuncts to operation. Technical problems involved in the surgical treatment are too complex for consideration here, but they tax the skill of the most expert surgeons and should never be considered lightly.

Simultaneous occurrence of diverticulitis and carcinoma of the colon may cause confusion in diagnosis, especially in those patients in whom a partial obstruction is seen on barium enema examination. These patients should be carefully studied, and early operation should be recommended unless carcinoma can be clearly excluded.

With a view to reducing the morbidity required by staged resections for complications of diverticulitis, serious consideration should be given to elective operation in patients with the following manifestations:

1. Recurrent attacks of diverticulitis, especially in patients under 50 years of age.
2. Marked narrowing or deformity of the colon by x-ray with stasis of the proximal bowel.
3. Persistent palpable mass.
4. Dysuria, frequency, or pneumaturia.
5. Repeated serious episodes of hemorrhage.

Fortunately, diverticulitis does not affect the

extraperitoneal rectum, and it should be possible to restore continuity of the bowel in those cases not complicated by a low-lying carcinoma.

Hazardous complications, prolonged morbidity, and serious economic losses may be averted by judicious selection of patients in the categories described for elective primary colonic resections. Clinical judgment in such patients is enhanced by close cooperation between internist and surgeon.

CROHN'S DISEASE

method of
DAVID H. LAW, M.D.
Albuquerque, New Mexico

Principles of Treatment

Although the mortality rate is less than 15 per cent, this disease is chronic, causing great morbidity. Since there is not yet a medical cure and surgery is fraught with recurrences, management involves a supportive medical approach, and the physician should not be dismayed or discouraged by the lack of a specific therapy. With appropriate, thoughtful treatment, the great majority of patients can be helped to lead productive, full lives. To accomplish this, there are four categories of medical therapy: general symptomatic and supportive treatment, nutritional treatment, antimicrobial therapy, and anti-inflammatory treatment.

Symptomatic Treatment

For the usual patient with symptomatic disease, some control of life pattern is necessary, with a guarantee of adequate physical rest and sleep, attempt toward normalization of work patterns, and establishment of a healthy, trusting relationship with the physician. The morbidity and chronicity of this disease necessitate the open, uninhibited discussion of personal, social, and economic as well as medical problems by the patient. Psychotropic agents are used for psychiatric problems and, of themselves, play no role in the treatment of Crohn's disease. Phenobarbital, 30 to 60 mg. three times daily, diazepam (Valium), 2 to 5 mg. three times daily, or chlordiazepoxide hydrochloride (Librium), 5 to 10 mg. three times daily, may provide additional rest and relaxation for the irritable, nervous, and tense patient.

Abdominal pain and cramps may require analgesics, but because of the chronicity of the disorder we strongly advise against the use of narcotics. We use propoxyphene hydrochloride (Darvon), 32 mg. every 4 to 6 hours, or acetaminophen (Tylenol), 325 mg. every 4 to 6 hours.

For the more than two thirds of the patients who manifest diarrhea, the use of an absorbent bulk agent such as psyllium hydrophilic mucilloid (Metamucil), 1 teaspoon in a glass of water two to three times a day, may help produce formed stools. This should not be used in the presence of partial bowel obstruction. Pharmacologic antidiarrheal preparations frequently are necessary. We have used diphenoxylate hydrochloride, 2.5 mg., with atropine sulfate (Lomotil), 1 to 2 tablets three to four times per day, paregoric, 5 to 15 ml. three to six times per day, or deodorized tincture of opium, 8 to 12 drops three to six times per day as necessary. One must guard against abuse of these drugs with ensuing dependence.

Patients with an accentuated gastrocolic reflex and diarrhea may be helped by anticholinergic agents 30 minutes before meals—propantheline (Pro-Banthine), 15 mg. three to four times a day, or glycopyrrolate (Robinul), 1 to 2 mg. three times a day. One must be alert to the fact that these anticholinergic drugs and codeine-morphine congeners may play a role in the pathogenesis of toxic dilatation of the colon.

It is now recognized that patients who have undergone ileal resection or who have extensive ileal disease may manifest watery diarrhea on the basis of impaired bile salt absorption, with deconjugation of residual bile salts in the colon and resultant catharsis. In such patients, a binding resin, cholestyramine (Questran), 4 grams three to four times per day, may provide remarkable relief. It may, however, lead to an increased steatorrhea with malabsorption of some drugs and fat-soluble vitamins, especially in patients with more than 100 cm. of ileum resected or severely involved with disease. For patients with stasis of intestinal contents from a "blind loop syndrome" secondary to operation, internal fistula formation, or partial obstructions, low dose tetracycline, 0.5 to 1.0 gram per day for 7 to 10 days, may terminate diarrhea and steatorrhea related to altered intraluminal bacterial flora.

Nutritional Therapy

Our ability to provide nutritional therapy in particular situations has improved dramatically in recent years. There are no data, however, suggesting that a specific diet is indicated in all patients with Crohn's disease. Diet must be individualized to the patient's tolerances and needs, stressing high calorie and high protein intake. For certain patients who demonstrate disaccharide intolerance with diarrhea, cramps, and bloating, elimination of milk and milk products from their diet may constitute a simple, effective therapeutic trial. The decision to exclude or limit milk and milk product foods should be made only on such clinical grounds, because these are effective nutritional products if tolerated.

The patient with steatorrhea from bowel resection or extensive disease may respond to a standard low fat diet supplemented by a medium-chain triglyceride preparation. The latter is available as the oil or in a commercial formula (Portagen), which may be used as a sole diet source as it is a complete dietary formula containing all essential vitamins and minerals. For patients with partial or recurrent small bowel obstruction episodes, standard low residue diets should be used. When severe small bowel insufficiency exists or when the patient needs complete "bowel rest" with marked quantitative reduction of the fecal stream, two avenues of diet therapy remain. These approaches may be of great assistance in the management of certain patients with fistulas, abscess, or obstructive complications of the disease by permitting improved nutrition or even positive nitrogen balance, and at the same time permitting healing or resolution of disease processes. The *chemically defined diets* or elemental diets (e.g., Vivonex HN) are bulk-free preparations of pure L-amino acids, simple sugars, and all essential nutrients. Six packets of the flavored, water-soluble powder provide 1800 calories and the usual total adult daily nutritional requirements. Enzymatic digestion is not required, and rapid absorption in the upper intestine is the rule with minimal fecal residue and resultant "bowel rest." No fat is contained in the formula, and steatorrhea therefore is minimized. Many patients complain of an unpleasant aftertaste which limits long-term use of the agent unless it is administered by way of a nasogastric feeding tube.

There have been a number of newer low residue products introduced on the commercial market in recent years. These are of variable compositions and are chemically defined; most are essentially fat-free and may be used as a supplement to other regular diets or as a sole source of calories. Most of these products are presented to the patient in an approximate 25 per cent weight-to-volume solution which possesses a high osmolarity, approximating 800 mOsm., which may in itself cause abdominal discomfort and diarrhea. This can be minimized by initiating feedings with dilute solutions at half strength and by slowing the rate of administration. In situations in which these diets are to be the sole source of nutrition over a prolonged period of time, we have utilized a small pediatric feeding tube (No. 8 French) and a variable speed pump to control the rate of delivery. Among the other commercial solutions we have used are the following: Flexical (containing 34 grams fat per 1000 calories), Precision High Nitrogen Diet, and Warren-Teed Low Residue.

The use of *total parenteral nutrition* is an even more recent form of bowel rest which at the same time permits a totally adequate nutrition. Using an indwelling deep venous catheter placed in the superior vena cava, hyperalimentation can be accomplished with up to 3000 to 5000 calories per day in the form of concentrated glucose (20 to 50 per cent) and 10 to 20 grams nitrogen per day as protein hydrolysates (C.P.H., Amigen, Aminosol) or, preferably, as pure L-amino acids (FreAmine II). All required vitamins, macronutrients, and trace elements also can be provided, and patients can be maintained in positive nitrogen balance over a period of weeks to months while their bowels are at total rest and medical or surgical treatment is provided. Extreme care and scrupulous supervision are necessary to minimize complications of this important form of therapy. This technique may provide the margin between a patient's starving to death and his being in positive nitrogen balance with healing and replacement of lean body mass and blood proteins. Recent studies have strongly suggested that total parenteral nutrition with the bowel at rest may result in closure of fistulous tracts, resolution of edematous and inflamed obstructing lesions of the bowel, and remission of diffuse, active mucosal disease. Further controlled evaluation is needed.

Finally, even in the normally ingesting patient, we must provide those nutrients which may be depleted by ileal disease and diarrhea: vitamin B_{12}, 100 micrograms per month intramuscularly, if absorption is impaired; iron orally as a gluconate (Fergon), 1 to 2 tablets three times daily, or parenterally as iron dextran (Imferon) (dosage is calculated according to insert instructions); potassium and magnesium supplements if diarrhea is severe; and vitamin supplementation either parenterally as a preparation of fat- and water-soluble vitamins (M.V.I.), 5 ml. per day intravenously (½ ampule), or as the B-C vitamin complex only (Berocca-C), 2 to 10 ml. intravenously per day. There are no adequate data concerning the actual requirements of these specific nutrients during the course of active inflammatory bowel disease, but they are assumed to be greater than normal. Possible vitamin A and D toxicities should be remembered with long-term parenteral vitamin A and D use.

Antibiotic Therapy

The use of antibiotic therapy in patients with Crohn's disease should be limited to specific infectious complications. When frank abscess (intra-abdominal, perirectal, or incisional) exists, use of systemic broad-spectrum antibiotics is indicated. It usually must be combined with drainage of collected pus. For patients obviously ill with high fever, leukocytosis, peritoneal signs, and toxicity with evidence of infection, we have used ampicillin (Polycillin, Totacillin, Amcill), 4 to 6 grams per day intravenously for 10 to 14 days, or intravenous penicillin, 10 to 15 million units per day, and either kanamycin (Kantrex), 500 mg. intramuscularly twice daily for a similar period, or gentamicin (Garamycin), 3 mg. per kg. per day intramuscularly. If apparent infection fails to respond, one must consider the possibility of Bacteroides or Pseudomonas infection. Whenever possible, antibiotic use should be tailored to documented or anticipated sensitivities of the infecting agent. With extensive mucosal disease, elevated temperature, and white blood cell count but an absence of obvious localized infection, we use a less vigorous program: oral ampicillin, 2 to 4 grams per day for 10 to 14 days.

Anti-Inflammatory Therapy

Anti-inflammatory therapy is the final category of treatment, and it constitutes a group of agents that, for the most part, are reserved for the more severely ill patient who has failed to respond to general supportive, nutritional, and antibiotic treatment when appropriate.

Three classes of agents have been used, and it should be stressed that to date there are no statistically significant data supporting the long-term efficacy of any of them. There are testimonials, and in our experience patients have appeared to respond to each class of drug; however, their long-term use is empirical and not without significant hazard.

The poorly absorbable sulfonamide preparation salicylazosulfapyridine (Azulfidine) has been shown to be effective in long-term management of ulcerative colitis, and its use has been extended to patients with Crohn's disease. The recently completed National Cooperative Crohn's Disease Study clearly demonstrated a short-term effectiveness in the management of Crohn's disease for this drug in doses of 1 gram per 15 kg. of body weight. Indeed, at 6 weeks the drug was as effective as prednisone in the doses tested, and the effectiveness was maintained over a period of several months at half dose. Its modes of action are unknown but are felt to be anti-inflammatory as well as antimicrobial. Dosage of 2 to 4 grams three times per day after meals, tapering to a maintenance dose of 1 gram two to four times a day, may be associated with remission, and we feel it is worthwhile, especially in patients with colonic involvement. We use this agent prior to trials of therapy with adrenal corticosteroids or immunosuppressive agents unless the patient is extremely ill or has marked systemic manifestations of the disease such as iritis-uveitis, arthritis, or skin lesions. If nausea occurs, the use of enteric coated EN-tabs may be attempted or the dose may be diminished; if skin rash or bone marrow depression occurs, the drug must be stopped.

Adrenal corticosteroid therapy in the form of cortisone congeners or ACTH may be associated with marked relief of acute symptoms, both systemic and intestinal. In our experience, it is especially effective in patients with extensive small bowel involvement and a gross malabsorption syndrome, in patients with nonobstructive bowel disease in the acute inflammatory stage, and in patients with distal colonic involvement. Again, the National Cooperative Crohn's Disease Study demonstrated a clear efficacy for prednisone (0.25 to 0.75 mg. per kg.) in the acute management of symptomatic Crohn's disease. We use oral prednisone, 40 to 60 mg. per day, given as a single morning dose for a period of 2 to 4 weeks, with tapering of the dose over a period of several weeks to 15 to 20 mg. per day. If long-term treatment is contemplated, we attempt to schedule every-other-day doses of double the daily dose—i.e., 30 to 40 mg. every other day—in the hope of diminishing adrenal suppression and minimizing complications. This is particularly important in the management of children, who may suffer growth retardation both from the disease and from chronic daily steroid treatment. Although the vast majority of patients demonstrate an initial good response, relapse rate is over 50 per cent at 6 months when treatment is discontinued.

If oral treatment is not feasible or if the patient fails to respond, we consider it worthwhile to use intravenous ACTH, 40 units delivered in 500 ml. of 5 per cent dextrose over an 8 hour period twice daily every day. This may be tapered gradually to 40 units intramuscularly two or three times a week and administered on an outpatient basis.

With localized rectal disease and the symptoms of proctitis, rectal fissures, and perirectal and rectal fistulas, steroid enemas may be useful. Commercial kits of methylprednisolone, 40 mg. (Medrol Enpak), or 100 mg. hydrocortisone retention enemas (Cortenema) may be given twice daily, or the local pharmacy may make up an equivalent hydrocortisone and prednisolone solution to be administered by the patient. Eventually steroid suppositories may be substituted: hydrocortisone acetate, 25 mg. (Cort-Dome) suppositories, high potency.

There have been enthusiastic reports about the use of cytotoxic agents in the treatment of a variety of diseases whose pathogenesis might involve immune factors. Crohn's disease has been treated with nitrogen mustard, 6-mercaptopurine, and azathioprine. None of these agents are approved by the Food and Drug Administration for this use, and there are inadequate studies to statistically evaluate their long-term effect. Although the National Cooperative Crohn's Disease Study failed to show efficacy in the short-term treatment of the group of patients they studied, there still may be a subset of patients with severe disease who will respond over a period of several months. On the basis of uncontrolled reports, it seems as though azathioprine (Imuran), 1.5 to 4.0 mg. per kg., may result in quite remarkable improvements over a 1 to 2 month period in some patients who are severely ill with Crohn's disease and apparently refractory to other treatment. Currently, such treatment can be recommended only on an experimental or study basis.

Surgical Treatment

Although most patients with Crohn's disease eventually undergo some form of surgery, there is a high incidence of recurrence following all types of procedures. Operations should be reserved for specific indications which fail to respond to appropriate medical therapy. These include free perforation; symptomatic abscess formation; unrelenting obstruction; persistent fistula formation (especially to bladder, abdominal wall, and peritoneum); uncontrolled hemorrhage or toxic dilatation of the colon (both rarities); and systemic manifestations which are refractory to nonoperative treatment (pyoderma gangrenosum, debilitating arthritis, uveitis-iritis, progressive pericholangitis, and, in children, failure to grow). If the patient is considered an invalid socially, economically, or medically and a resectable lesion is found, operation should be considered. We suggest resection of involved bowel with end-to-end anastomosis when feasible, remembering the sequelae of the short bowel syndrome secondary to massive resections.

HEMORRHOIDS, ANAL FISSURE, AND ANAL FISTULA

method of
RALPH B. SAMSON, M.D.
Columbus, Ohio

Prior to therapy of any type, a thorough history and physical examination is performed on all patients, including proctosigmoidoscopy unless severe pain prevents this examination. Barium enema is obtained on all patients with a change in bowel habit or bleeding that cannot be accounted for by proctosigmoidoscopy, and as a routine in all surgical patients over the age of 40. We feel that upper gastrointestinal barium studies, with a small bowel follow-through, should be obtained in all patients with a history or findings suggestive of inflammatory bowel disease.

It is our belief that most symptomatic anorectal problems are a result of inflammation and infection in the crypts and glands of the anal canal. Hemorrhoids are tumors made up of collections of varicose veins, radicles of the inferior, middle, and superior hemorrhoidal veins, which occur beneath the mucous membrane of the lower rectal segment and beneath the skin of the anal canal and perianal margins. Uncomplicated varicosities in the perianal and anal canal are relatively asymptomatic unless complicated by associated inflammation and/or infection in the anal glands.

Not all patients with symptoms of hemorrhoids require surgery. Each patient needs individual evaluation. An early acute inflammatory process, resulting in edema, small thrombi, and moderately severe pain, frequently responds to palliation. If, however, these acute processes recur at rather frequent intervals, surgery may be indicated; if they occur over a long period of time, resulting in chronic changes in the hemorrhoidal complex with scarring, surgery may be a necessity.

External Hemorrhoidal Thrombosis

External hemorrhoidal thrombosis is the most common, urgent, and painful hemorrhoidal problem. This intravascular coagulation is usually induced by a mild acute inflammatory process in the crypt and gland directly above the thrombosed external hemorrhoid. The treatment options are as follows.

Palliation. 1. Bed rest.

2. Hot sitz baths, if there is much edema or sphincter spasm, two or three times a day. Hot applications may be of value.

3. Mild analgesia, such as propoxyphene and acetaminophen (Darvocet-N 100).

4. Diazepam (Valium), 5 mg. three times daily, when sphincter spasm is present and severe.

5. Bulk laxative, psyllium hydrophilic mucilloid (Metamucil), 1 teaspoon once or twice daily, with 8 to 10 glasses of water daily.

Operative Treatment. Office excision of the involved thrombosis is undertaken when it is quite painful and when it involves only one quadrant of the anal canal. It also must be limited to the external hemorrhoidal area and not extend above the mucocutaneous junction. The intravascular clot, or clots, must be removed with a rather generous elliptical excision down to the muscle. All clots must be removed if recurrence is to be avoided.

TECHNIQUE. 1. Infiltrate the involved area with a small amount of 1 per cent lidocaine

(Xylocaine) with epinephrine 1:100,000, using a No. 25 or 27 gauge needle.

2. Fully excise the thrombosis, including all small intravascular clots.

3. Palpate the area with a gloved finger to be certain that all clots have been removed. An ellipse of skin overlying the thrombus should be removed to prevent the incision from filling with blood postoperatively.

4. Control all bleeding sites; cautery is most useful.

5. Apply a small piece of Gelfoam to the incision site to control ooze; a No. 11 size is most appropriate.

6. Apply a small pressure dressing to overlie the Gelfoam and hold it in place.

7. On the first postoperative day have the patient begin hot sitz baths and instruct him to cleanse the perianal area locally with wet cotton, avoiding toilet tissue. Instruct the patient to apply a small pledget of cotton in the anal opening and change it frequently. Keep the area as clean and dry as possible.

8. Avoid rough particles in the diet, such as nuts, seeds, corn, and popcorn, while healing occurs. Also, avoid all alcoholic beverages.

9. A mild analgesic, such as propoxyphene and acetaminophen (Darvocet-N 100), is given.

10. Diazepam (Valium), 5 mg. three times daily, for sphincter spasm is recommended.

11. The patient is instructed to return in 2 weeks for re-evaluation.

If the area of thrombosis involves more than one third of the circumference of the perianal region, it is probably wiser to hospitalize the patient for a formal operation.

Internal Hemorrhoids

Internal hemorrhoids are asymptomatic unless prolapse is present, resulting in bleeding or excessive mucus production. Complete prolapse may occur with straining or with bowel movements, necessitating manual reduction of the prolapsed mucosa and hemorrhoids. At times, when edema becomes severe and manual reduction is no longer possible or is not performed immediately following prolapse, superficial ulceration or, in time, interference with blood supply and gangrene may occur. Hemorrhoidectomy, in such a case, becomes a necessity. Ordinarily, hemorrhoidectomy is an elective procedure. However, when severe anemia occurs, or when acute prolapse with thrombosis and interference with blood supply results, it is no longer an elective procedure but becomes urgent.

If internal hemorrhoids are only moderate in size upon examination, if they prolapse but reduce spontaneously, if there is no other coexisting surgical pathology, and if the patient does not give a history of repeated episodes of thromboses, nonoperative outpatient management may be indicated.

Palliation. 1. Rule out other causes of anal pathology and rectal bleeding. Sigmoidoscopy and barium enema with air contrast films should be performed.

2. Eliminate any dietary indiscretion; recommend a bulky diet with roughage (in the acute phase, bran is contraindicated).

3. Correct constipation, if present, by using a bulk laxative, and stress adequate fluid intake, 8 to 10 glasses of liquids daily.

4. Instruct the patient in local anal hygiene, as outlined previously.

5. Apply hot compresses or hot sitz baths twice daily.

6. Apply a local ointment such as cod liver oil, lanolin, talc, and petrolatum (Desitin) if inflammation is rather minimal. If it is more severe, 1 per cent hydrocortisone creme (Cort-Dome Creme) is used.

Barron's Ligation. Barron's ligation is quite suitable for removal of moderate-sized internal hemorrhoids with reducible prolapse. It effectively controls bleeding from such hemorrhoids with little or no external component. Also, Barron's ligation can control the symptoms of large prolapsing internal hemorrhoids in patients who, because of age or other medical problems, are not candidates for adequate surgical removal. Thrombosed external hemorrhoids, following ligation, are a rather frequent complication. Each hemorrhoidal ligation is often followed by a variable period of pain or discomfort, usually subsiding completely after 6 or 7 days when the ligated portion sloughs away. There is a risk (1 to 2 per cent) of severe bleeding for approximately 6 to 16 days following treatment. No rectal instillations, suppositories, or enemas should be given while the patient is under treatment, particularly until the sloughing of the ligated portion occurs.

TECHNIQUE. 1. After digital lubrication of the anal canal, insert a medium size Hirschman anoscope.

2. Center the bevel over the internal hemorrhoid to be ligated.

3. Ask the patient to strain slightly.

4. As the hemorrhoid bulges into the anoscope, grasp it with an alligator or special allis type forceps, which is inserted through the drum of the Barron ligator.

5. Settle the drum on the hemorrhoid.

6. Slide the rubber ring over the hemorrhoid in such a position that the mucocutaneous junction is at least 0.5 cm. distal to the ligature.

If the mucocutaneous junction is in the rubber ring, severe pain will follow and removal of the ligature will be necessary. On an outpatient basis, treatment should be given to only one hemorrhoid group at a time and should be repeated only at intervals of 2 to 3 weeks.

Postoperative care consists of hot sitz baths as needed, mild analgesia, and bowel management as described after excision of thrombosed hemorrhoid.

7. Prescribe diazepam (Valium), 5 mg. three times daily as necessary, for any levator spasm which may result. Explain to the patient that there will be a bearing-down sensation for 24 to 48 hours after the ligation and some slight distress after that for perhaps 2 weeks.

Injection Treatment. In our practice Barron's band ligation has replaced, in most instances, injection treatment of internal hemorrhoids. Certainly, prolapsing internal hemorrhoids are more adequately treated by Barron's band ligation. At present, we use injection treatment only for small bleeding areas which are so small that the Barron ligating rubber ring cannot adequately be applied. Injection treatment therefore is rarely used.

TECHNIQUE. 1. Using a solution of 5 per cent phenol in cottonseed oil which has been autoclaved, and using a 20 gauge tonsil needle through a medium Hirschman anoscope, the area to be injected is cleansed of gross soilage.

2. The needle is introduced into the submucosa (be sure the needle is freely movable beneath the mucosa and is not in the muscle).

3. Aspirate to be certain that the needle is not in the lumen of a blood vessel.

4. Inject 0.5 to 1 ml. of the solution. The area should be distended, but blanching should not occur. Two to three areas may be injected at the same time, if necessary.

Excisional Hemorrhoidectomy

Formal operative hemorrhoidectomy is reserved for prolapsing internal hemorrhoids with large external components and/or a history of repeated external thrombosis with evidence of cryptoglandular disease. Frequently, these patients have associated anal lesions, in addition to the varicosities, such as hypertrophied papillae, deep crypts, and scarring of the anal canal as a result of previous episodes of symptomatic hemorrhoids.

There are several techniques for the surgical excision of internal and external hemorrhoids. The operation is best performed under caudal or local infiltration anesthesia.

Procedure. A procedure conservative of anoderm and perianal skin but removing all pathologic tissue, including internal, anal, and external hemorrhoids, along with the chronically infected crypts, anal glands, and scar, is the procedure of choice. This permits closure by suture of all wounds and earlier healing. Such an operative procedure has been described many times under the general title of closed hemorrhoidectomy. We prefer a modification of the Ferguson technique. Closed hemorrhoidectomy, in our opinion, reduces postoperative pain; healing occurs by first intention, and hospitalization is minimized to 4 to 5 days. The majority of patients can return to their usual occupation in 2 to 3 weeks.

Postoperative Hemorrhoid Care. 1. The patient is given ice chips only by mouth until he voids; then a regular diet is allowed as soon as tolerated.

2. The patient is allowed up to void with aid after 6 hours.

3. Hot compresses are applied continuously after surgery until commencement of sitz baths, and then as necessary.

4. The dressing is removed 8 to 10 hours after surgery.

5. Sitz baths are given twice daily or as necessary, starting the day after surgery.

6. The patient may be up, as desired, on the first postoperative day.

7. If no bowel movement occurs by the second postoperative day, a small oil retention enema is given. If no bowel movement occurs by the third postoperative day, a saline enema is given.

8. Pain medication is given as needed, particularly in the first 24 hours. We prefer meperidine, 75 to 100 mg.

9. A bulk laxative is given. Our preference is Methylcellulose (Mucilose granules), 1 teaspoonful twice daily with a full glass of water.

10. Sulfacetamide, 1 gram four times daily, unless diarrhea occurs.

11. Propoxyphene hydrochloride with acetaminophen (Darvocet-N 100), 1–2 tablets every 3 to 4 hours, is given beginning on the first postoperative day.

The patient is to wear dry cotton in the area with a small amount of zinc stearate powder at all times. This anal hygiene and sitz baths are continued at home. The bulk laxative is also continued at home. Upon discharge the patient is instructed to take sulfacetamide, 1 gram three times daily, for approximately 6 days.

The patient is discharged from the hospital on the fourth or fifth postoperative day when normal bowel action has occurred. He is seen and examined in the office approximately 14 days after surgery. The first examination consists primarily of inspection of the wounds to ensure that no infection has occurred, as well as a gentle digital examination of the canal to ensure that normal caliber is being maintained. Patients are permitted to return to work on the fourteenth to sixteenth postoperative day unless their occupation entails heavy lifting; in such a case we suggest postponing working until 21 days after surgery.

Anal Fissure

Anal fissure may be acute or chronic. An acute anal fissure may result from trauma from a large hard stool and may actually be an acute tear of the anoderm, or it may occur from the trauma of frequent loose movements, possibly as a result of the enzymatic action of the loose stool on the anal skin. Anal fissure characteristically occurs posteriorly in the anal canal but not uncommonly is found anteriorly. A chronic anal fissure occurs as a result of recurrent cryptoglandular disease proximal to the area of fissure. The chronic fissure bed is believed to represent the posterior portion of a previous abscess and is fed by a deep gland in the crypt just above. The large papilla, which is commonly found with chronic anal fissure, is also a result of the chronic inflammatory process. Stenosis, so often associated with chronic anal fissure, results from spasm induced by the painful anal wound and scar tissue formed along the course of the lymphatic drainage of this chronically infected area. Treatment by conservative methods of any but superficial fissure is rarely successful because of the spasm, fibrosis, and chronic infection.

Conservative Management. 1. Bowel management with a soft bulky stool by means of the previously outlined diet and bulk.

2. Meticulous hygiene of the anal canal and perianal area, as described.

3. Hot sitz baths, as necessary, for relief of sphincter spasm and the acute inflammatory process.

4. Local application of a soothing, healing ointment which covers and clings to this area, such as Desitin ointment.

5. A local anesthetic ointment, preferably without a "caine" (such as diperodon, 1.0 per cent in petrolatum, propylene glycol, sorbitan [Diothane]) to be applied as necessary.

If relief from the symptoms of acute anal fissure does not occur rather promptly, or if exacerbation of symptoms recurs repeatedly, then surgical treatment is indicated.

Surgical Treatment. Excision of the entire fissure, cryptoglandular area, and hemorrhoids just above and adjacent to the fissure should be carried out en bloc. If a ring of fibrous scar is present, causing anal stenosis, it should be cut through, but normal elastic anal sphincter should not be incised. When the fissure occurs in the posterior aspect of the anal canal, healing and relief of pain occur much earlier if a graft of normal skin is applied immediately to the denuded area. This is performed by suturing a flap graft of skin to the mucosa, forming a new grafted posterior aspect of the anal canal.

In the anterior aspect of the canal, mobilization of perianal skin is not easily accomplished. Therefore after excision of pathology and repair of the mucosa, the external area is left open for adequate drainage.

An alternative surgical approach, substituting for excision, is lateral subcutaneous internal sphincterotomy, as advocated by some surgeons. Even with this method, the large area of scar, the sentinel tag externally, and the internal papilla apparently must be removed at times for adequate complete healing.

Perianal Abscess

The primary symptom of perianal abscess is pain—constant, throbbing, unrelenting pain. At times hot sitz baths may provide temporary relief. Examination may or may not show redness and swelling in the perianal region. However, there is definitely increased pain with palpation. When a patient presents with these symptoms and induration in the perianal area is present, even though no fluctuation is noted, a perianal abscess must be considered present until proved otherwise. Never wait for fluctuation. If symptoms and induration are present, explore. This can usually be done in the office under local analgesia. Do not put the patient on antibiotics prior to incision and drainage, for they mask signs and symptoms and frequently make it much more difficult to diagnose an abscess.

Technique. 1. Use a small needle; a No. 25 or 26 is usually adequate. Infiltrate 1 per cent lidocaine well into the skin and subcutaneous tissue and into the palpable mass.

2. If the abscess is deep and fluctuation and redness over the area are not evident, use a No. 18 or larger needle; insert into the area of the mass after the local infiltration and aspirate. If pus is obtained, maintain this needle in place.

3. Use a No. 11 blade and plunge along the needle into the abscess cavity.

4. Open the tract adequately.

5. Remove an ellipse of skin and subcutaneous tissue.

6. Insert a small wick drain of ½ or 1 inch iodoform gauze. Do not pack the cavity; simply insert the wick drain to keep the skin edges well apart.

7. Remove the drain in approximately 48 to 72 hours.

8. After drainage, if this abscess is large or is marked by cellulitis, give antibiotics (ampicillin, 500 mg. every 6 hours for 3 to 4 days).

9. Hot sitz baths are provided four times a day for the first 48 hours, and then twice a day if symptoms subside.

10. Have the patient wear a small piece of cotton to absorb the drainage from the wound.

11. Instruct the patient in anal hygiene as previously outlined.

12. Give a bulk laxative, if indicated.

13. The patient is instructed to return for re-evaluation in 10 to 14 days unless symptoms are exacerbated. At the time of re-evaluation, the abscess and possible fistulous tract are probed, the internal opening is searched for, and a complete proctologic examination is completed, including sigmoidoscopy. The patient is permitted to return to work in 24 to 48 hours after incision and drainage, or as soon as his symptoms permit.

Anal Fistula

A perianal abscess is usually the acute phase in the development of an anal fistula. The abscess and the fistula usually result from cryptoglandular infection. The infection follows the anal glands beneath the mucosa to form the anal abscess, which then either spontaneously ruptures or is surgically incised, resulting in a fistula extending from the infected crypt and anal gland to the perianal tissue or back into the anal canal or low rectum. Internal fistulas may develop as a result of intermuscular abscess of the upper anal canal and lower rectal wall.

Cure of anal fistula is dependent on identifying its point of origin. Goodsell's rule reminds us that when the external opening is located posterior to a transverse line dividing the anal orifice, the primary, or internal, opening is in the posterior midline. When the secondary, or external, opening is anterior to the line bisecting the anal canal, the primary opening lies in a straight radial direction from the external opening. When the external opening of the draining fistulous tract is more than 2 cm. from the anal verge, the internal opening is most often in the posterior midline.

Surgery for anal fistula necessitates complete removal and repair of the primary or internal opening of the fistula. This defect in the canal is the source of the continued contamination of the perirectal tissues which causes the fistula to persist. The surgical procedure necessary to correct anal fistula depends on the location of the internal opening and the extent of the involvement of the anal sphincter and perirectal area. Most fistulas, even though they involve a rather large amount of the anal sphincter mechanism, can be repaired without producing anal incontinence. In a rare neglected fistula, particularly the anterior fistula in the female, which involves all, or most, of the anal sphincter mechanism plus the perineal muscles, anal incontinence can possibly result from fistulectomy, necessitating a later operation after healing has occurred to repair the incontinent sphincter mechanism.

Anal fistula resulting from inflammatory bowel disease, granulomatous disease of the intestinal tract, or ulcerative colitis is best treated conservatively. In most instances, adequate drainage of the abscess, to promote a chronic fistulous tract, is preferable to radical fistulectomy, for incontinence can result in these patients with severe diarrhea. Postoperative care after fistulectomy is identical to that outlined for hemorrhoidectomy.

GASTRITIS

method of
ANGELO E. DAGRADI, M.D.
Long Beach, California

Inflammatory disease of the stomach is generally categorized as acute or chronic. The disorder is commonly restricted to the mucosal layer, but in certain types the deeper strata of the gastric wall are also involved. The inflammatory changes may involve the stomach diffusely, or they may be localized and patchy in distribution.

Accurate diagnosis of this disease depends upon microscopic examination of an adequate specimen of mucosa, obtained from an area of involvement by means of gastroscopy. Visual inspection of the mucosa by endoscopy is somewhat less accurate; radiographic examination and clinical diagnosis based upon symptomatology are the least accurate. The latter methods, however, being the more practical, are the ones most commonly employed.

Acute Gastritis

Exogenous Gastritis. Symptoms include nausea, vomiting, diarrhea, malaise, and fever. These occur alone or in combination, and in relation to ingestion of chemical or bacterial toxins (ethanol, staphylococci, drugs, seafoods) or systemic viral infection. The disorder is self-limited. Treatment is directed toward control of nausea and vomiting and correction of fluid and electrolyte loss. It is guided by the severity of the symptoms and includes the following measures:

1. Bed rest.
2. Withholding oral feedings (NPO).
3. Antiemetics such as prochlorperazine (Compazine), 10 mg., or hydroxyzine (Vistaril), 25 mg., intramuscularly at 4 hour intervals.
4. Intravenous fluid replacement, using isotonic saline solution or 5 per cent glucose and saline, with the addition of 20 to 40 mEq. of potassium chloride to each liter of solution.
5. When nausea and vomiting have subsided and fluid and electrolyte losses have been corrected, or in those patients in whom symptoms have not been severe and oral feedings can be

tolerated, carbonated drinks, such as ginger ale or Seven-Up, are usually beneficial. Subsequently, freshly prepared chicken broth, soda crackers, and tea may be fed to the patient and, gradually, the normal dietary regimen resumed.

Hemorrhagic-Erosive Gastritis. This disorder is manifested by hematemesis and/or melena of varying degrees of severity. Precipitating factors include ingestion of certain drugs—e.g., ethanol and/or salicylate-containing medications, reserpine, steroid hormones, colchicine, phenylbutazone, indomethacin—and certain systemic diseases, including uremia, hepatic failure, and stress. Bleeding may recur intermittently during any given episode, and it frequently will occur again at a future time if the person is re-exposed to the original causative agent. The diagnosis is made by gastroscopy during the bleeding episode, or by surgery, or at autopsy.

Treatment is directed to the correction of blood loss, control of bleeding, and prevention of recurrence. This involves the following measures:

Estimation of Severity of Blood Loss. 1. Vital signs (blood pressure, pulse, respiration) each 15 minutes until stable.

2. Bed rest.

3. Irrigation of stomach with ice water via nasogastric tube until returns are clear of blood and clots.

4. Hematocrit determination every 6 hours.

5. Placement of central venous catheter for monitoring venous pressure.

Institution of Measures to Correct Blood Loss. 1. Expansion of plasma volume by intravenous administration of saline and/or glucose solution, human serum albumin, or dextran if shock is present.

2. Type and cross-match blood and transfuse.

Upper Gastrointestinal Panendoscopic Examination to Establish Bleeding Source.

Control of Bleeding. 1. Correction of clotting abnormalities by administration of fresh whole blood and/or fresh frozen plasma, vitamin K, and vitamin C.

2. Ice water lavage of the stomach through a large bore Ewald tube (40 F.). With the patient placed on a table in the head-down prone position, irrigation is continued until returns are free of blood and clots. Gastric cooling by this method effectively slows or stops bleeding of upper gastrointestinal origin.

3. Anticholinergic drugs such as atropine sulfate, 0.4 mg. (1/150 grain), or propantheline bromide (Pro-Banthine), 15 mg. intramuscularly every 4 to 6 hours, may permit arteriovenous shunts in the submucosa to open, diverting blood from the mucosal capillaries.

4. Topical hemostatic agents: (a) Levarterenol bitartrate (Levophed), 8 to 16 mg. in 100 to 200 ml. of iced isotonic saline solution, is instilled into the stomach via a nasogastric tube, left in place for a half hour, and then removed by irrigation. (This use of levarterenol is not listed in the manufacturer's official directive.) Similar aliquots may be reinstilled and the process repeated four times. If hemostasis does not occur by then, this approach should be terminated. (b) Thrombin-Gelfoam cocktail. This is made by mixing, in a Waring Blender, a glassful of absorbable gelatin powder (Gelfoam), an ampule of topical thrombin (10,000 units), and 180 ml. (6 ounces) of milk or molar lactate solution. This is ingested by the patient or instilled into the stomach via a nasogastric tube.

5. Direct infusion of vasospastic drugs, via selective angiography, into vessels supplying the bleeding lesions; e.g., vasopressin at rate of 1 ml. per minute (0.2 to 0.3 units per ml.).

If bleeding is controlled, the patient is graduated from a full liquid to a soft bland and, finally, a bland diet. Liquid antacids, in doses of 30 ml. (1 ounce), are administered on even hours, alternating with 90 to 120 ml. (3 to 4 ounces) of milk on the odd hours. This type of management should be continued for 3 to 4 weeks. If bleeding continues unabated or recurs repeatedly and 10 or more units of blood has been administered, surgical intervention should be considered. Vagotomy with pyloroplasty or partial gastrectomy may succeed in controlling the hemorrhage. If this fails, total gastrectomy may be required.

Prevention of Recurrence. Prevention requires studied avoidance of ingestion of the inciting agents.

Corrosive Gastritis. Severe and extensive destruction of the stomach may be produced in consequence of the ingestion, by accident or by intent, of corrosive chemicals. The most common chemicals ingested are lye (e.g., Drano, Liquid Plumber) and muriatic acid (HCl). The mouth, pharynx, and esophagus are injured concomitantly to varying degrees. Serious involvement of the esophagus is most commonly produced by alkaline corrosive agents, whereas the injurious effect of acid corrosives is usually greatest to the stomach.

Symptoms following ingestion include vomiting, retching, hematemesis, and severe pain in the upper abdomen, substernally, and in the mouth and pharynx. Peripheral vascular collapse may ensue.

Treatment involves the following measures:

1. Correction of shock state by intravenous administration of fluids, human serum albumin, and whole blood.

2. Control of pain and sedation: (a)

Meperidine hydrochloride (Demerol) intramuscularly in doses of 50 to 100 mg. every 4 hours. (b) Diazepam (Valium), 5 to 10 mg. intramuscularly every 4 hours.

3. Topical anesthesia to burned mucosal surfaces. Lidocaine hydrochloride (Xylocaine) 2 per cent viscous is administered in doses of 15 ml. every 2 to 4 hours, to be swished around in the mouth and swallowed.

4. The presence of chemical injury to esophagus or stomach can be determined by early endoscopic examination. If severe damage to the esophagus is visualized, further advance of the endoscope into the stomach may be dispensed with at the discretion of the endoscopist.

5. Control of secondary infection and inflammatory cicatrization. In those patients in whom injury has been caused to the esophagus and/or stomach, a broad-spectrum antibiotic is given, such as cephalothin (Keflin), 3 to 6 grams intravenously daily, or tetracycline, 250 mg. orally every 6 hours, along with steroid hormones such as hydrocortisone sodium succinate (Solu-Cortef), 250 mg. every 6 hours, or methylprednisolone sodium succinate (Solu-Medrol), 10 to 40 mg. intravenously every 6 hours, or prednisone, 5 mg. every 6 hours, given orally for 7 to 10 days.

6. Prevention of esophageal stenosis. A 30 F. Maloney, mercury-weighted, soft rubber bougie is passed perorally through the esophagus once daily during the first 2 weeks. Subsequently bougies of gradually increasing caliber are used until 42 F. is reached. Early institution of oral feedings is also helpful for preventing cicatricial stenosis, as ingested food is itself a good esophageal dilator. A liquid diet is instituted early in the course of the disease, followed by progression of the diet through full liquid, soft bland, and bland over a period of 10 days, as tolerated.

7. Evaluation of residual injury. Evaluation is done in 4 to 6 weeks following the injury and involves upper gastrointestinal radiologic and endoscopic examinations.

8. Treatment of gastric outlet obstruction if this complication should eventuate (partial gastrectomy or gastroenterostomy).

Phlegmonous Gastritis. A suppurative infection of the gastric wall, caused by pyogenic organisms (e.g., *Staphylococcus aureus,* pneumococcus, colon bacillus, *Clostridium welchii*), may occur in patients with gastric carcinoma, benign gastric ulcer, peritonitis, or septicemia. This fortunately rare condition presents as an acute abdomen (abdominal pain, tenderness, rigidity), occasionally with hematemesis, and with systemic symptoms (chills, fever, shock, septicemia).

Treatment includes the following measures:

1. Correction of peripheral vascular collapse.

2. Vital signs every 4 hours.

3. Blood cultures.

4. Broad-spectrum antibiotics, administered intravenously and tailored to the nature of the specific offending agent(s), as established by blood culture and culture of abscesses evacuated by surgery.

5. Surgical intervention. This is the definitive method by which this condition is diagnosed. Surgery is done because it is commonly impossible to exclude other acute abdominal catastrophes in the differential diagnosis and because it is valuable for evacuating and draining purulent collections.

Chronic Gastritis

This disorder possesses gastroscopic, pathophysiologic, and histologic characteristics which can be correlated. It is encountered frequently during gastroscopy, presenting with varying degrees of severity and extent of involvement, and may or may not be associated with overt symptoms. The mucosal alteration is kaleidoscopic, mutating from superficial gastritis to superficial atrophic gastritis and eventually to total atrophy; each phase is capable of developing a hemorrhagic component, occasioning hematemesis and/or melena.

Chronic Superficial Gastritis. This is encountered in the postoperative stomach, especially following Billroth II gastrectomy, in which it results from the chronic irritation caused by reflux into the stomach of biliary and pancreatic secretions. It is also noted to occur commonly in chronic alcoholic patients, following x-irradiation of the stomach, and following long-term ingestion of various drugs. Patients afflicted by this disorder may describe symptoms of "chronic indigestion," characterized by postprandial distress and aggravated by the ingestion of highly seasoned foods, greasy foods, and hot liquids, and especially by distention of the inflamed stomach by food. Relief is obtained by the exercise of dietary discretion and by ingestion of carbonated liquids and powders which contain bicarbonate or carbonate ions.

Bile reflux gastritis will respond frequently to the administration of cholestyramine (Questran) in doses of 2 to 4 grams administered three to four times daily between meals and at bedtime. In the absence of side effects (constipation, nausea, epigastric pain), a prolonged trial may prove beneficial. The diet should be supplemented with fat-soluble vitamins because of the tendency for these to become depleted in consequence of the sequestration of bile salts by the medication.

Chronic Atrophic Gastritis (Gastric Mucosal Atrophy). This represents the end-stage of the gastric inflammatory process. Severe destruction of the glandular elements has occurred (disappearance of chief cells, parietal cells, and those neck-gland cells responsible for formation of intrinsic factor), with replacement by a mucosa consisting of mucus-secreting (goblet) cells (intestinalization). This is commonly quite thin but in certain instances is very thick, producing large folds that demonstrate a mamillated appearance grossly and at gastroscopy (hyperplastic atrophy or Menetrier's disease).

Problems occurring during this stage of the disease process arise from the following factors:

1. Anacidity due to loss of parietal cells. (a) Diarrhea and flatulence (gastrogenous diarrhea). This disorder frequently responds to the oral administration of acid—1 to 3 Acidulin Pulvules or 30 drops of a 10 per cent solution of hydrochloric acid in 60 ml. of water administered three times daily with meals. (b) Iron deficiency anemia. Iron-dextran (Imferon), administered intramuscularly in doses of 50 to 100 mg. twice weekly, will occasion reticulocyte response and return of red blood cell and hemoglobin levels to normal.

2. Loss of chief cells. Pepsin may be added to correct deficiency of this proteolytic enzyme in consequence of loss of chief cells.

3. Loss of neck-gland cells producing intrinsic factor. This eventuates in failure to absorb vitamin B_{12} and occasions development of megaloblastic (pernicious) anemia when the hepatic stores of B_{12} eventually become depleted. Patients demonstrating severe and extensive gastric mucosal atrophy on gastroscopy and anacidity on gastric analysis should undergo evaluation for the presence of pernicious anemia. This includes examination of the peripheral blood, including cell indices, bone marrow, and Schilling test. Treatment requires intramuscular injections of cyanocobalamin (vitamin B_{12}) in doses of 1000 micrograms daily for 1 week, followed by 1000 micrograms once monthly for the remainder of the patient's lifetime.

4. Chronic loss of protein due to the inflammatory process in patients with Menetrier's disease (protein-losing gastropathy). Treatment includes intravenous administration of human serum albumin or of whole blood and intramuscular administration of anabolic steroid hormones such as testosterone or nandrolone phenpropionate (Durabolin). In rare instances, the protein loss has been sufficiently severe and intractable to require such drastic therapy as total gastrectomy as a lifesaving measure.

5. Propensity of severe and extensive atrophic gastritis to undergo neoplastic transformation (polyps, carcinoma) and to develop gastric ulcer. These patients should be examined by gastroscopy at least once yearly with performance of target biopsy of all visualized suspicious lesions.

GASEOUSNESS

method of
HARRIS R. CLEARFIELD, M.D.
Philadelphia, Pennsylvania

Although symptoms related to gaseousness provoke relatively little research interest, the problem is one of the most common disorders encountered by the practitioner. Belching, flatulence, and abdominal discomfort either may represent the primary complaint or may be associated with some other symptom complex. The construction of a therapeutic program requires understanding of the various mechanisms leading to gaseousness.

Pathogenesis

The "gas" which one belches is generally similar in composition to atmospheric air—79 per cent nitrogen and 21 per cent oxygen. Several ml. of air are ingested in the process of swallowing food or saliva. Factors which decrease the efficiency of the swallowing mechanism or increase the frequency of swallowing are likely to result in increased air accumulation in the upper gastrointestinal tract. An additional source of upper gastrointestinal gas is the constant neutralization of gastric acid by alkaline pancreatic-biliary secretions, resulting in the release of CO_2. If alkaline duodenal secretions are refluxed back into an acid-secreting stomach, carbon dioxide may contribute to the gastric air bubble as well.

The volume of flatus passed daily usually ranges between 500 and 1500 ml., with marked variation depending upon dietary and other factors. Air swallowing has often been considered the significant determinant of flatus volume, but more recent studies indicate the additional important role of bacterial fermentation. The nitrogen in swallowed air is not absorbed from the intestinal tract and is therefore passed rectally. Nonabsorbed foods, principally cellulose products, and nonhydrolyzed sugars, such as lactose in lactase-deficient patients, are fermented by colonic bacteria, leading to hydrogen and carbon dioxide release. Methane, oxygen, and trace gases such as H_2S play no significant role in the symptoms of gaseousness. If bacterial overgrowth in the small intestine occurs, fermentation and gas production will be increased.

The transit time for intestinal gas is rather rapid, approximately 20 to 30 minutes from stomach to anus. The midabdominal crampy pain frequently associated with gaseousness was thought to be directly related to the quantity of air being propelled through the intestines, but studies have failed to show an increased total gas content in such patients. It appears that the discomfort may result from abnormal motility patterns induced by normal or slightly increased volumes of gas in susceptible persons.

Symptoms and Syndromes Related to Gaseousness

Belching. Belching is a common symptom, resulting from the accumulation of swallowed air into a gastric air bubble. If a sensation of distention is perceived, spontaneous or induced belching may afford relief. The symptoms may become troublesome if excess air swallowing occurs. Some patients induce belching by purposely swallowing air in an attempt to gain relief from organic or functional disorders. This habit may become repetitive. An occasional patient presents with extremely loud belching (esophageal belching), a complaint which is almost always associated with a high degree of anxiety or other emotional disorders.

Magenblase Syndrome. A significantly enlarged air bubble may be experienced as epigastric or left upper quadrant pressure. The discomfort may radiate to the precordial area and strongly suggests the possibility of angina—thus its designation as pseudoangina. It generally occurs with or after eating, is relieved by belching, and is not related to exertion, which should help distinguish it from a cardiac cause.

Splenic Flexure Syndrome. If the splenic flexure is redundant or if motility disorders in the descending colon prohibit the forward passage of gas, trapping in the splenic flexure leads to distention and pressure under the diaphragm. The symptoms resemble those of the magenblase syndrome, except that the pressure distress is more laterally located in the left upper quadrant. Discomfort may radiate to the precordial area and thus also simulate angina. Symptoms often occur after eating, because the distended stomach presses upon the splenic flexure in these patients. Relief is obtained by belching or passing flatus. The discomfort is frequently reproduced by performing an air-contrast barium enema after ingestion of a carbonated beverage to distend the stomach.

Hepatic Flexure Syndrome. If air trapping occurs in the hepatic flexure, discomfort in the right upper quadrant may occur. This type of distress may be misinterpreted as biliary colic and may lead to cholecystectomy if gallstones are demonstrated by contrast studies. If the surgery is performed for the wrong reason, the pain may recur postoperatively and receive another erroneous diagnosis, the "postcholecystectomy syndrome," which is simply the persistence of a functional disorder after biliary surgery, with the gallstones playing no role in the pain production.

Abdominal Bloating. This is a difficult but common complaint to deal with, because abdominal x-rays often fail to correlate the gas content with the degree of distention perceived by the patient. In some instances the distention is largely due to gastric gas accumulation, but in other patients an involuntary relaxation of the abdominal musculature occurs, perhaps as an effort to obtain relief from intestinal spasm or other motility disorders. Thus "bloating" is not simply a problem of excess intestinal gas accumulation, but rather a combination of gas (which may be normal or increased in quantity) and motility disturbances.

Flatulence. The passage of flatus can be likened to belching, in that each is a normal response to gas accumulation and neither has been subjected to studies which would permit a distinction between normal and abnormal volumes or frequency. The increased degrees of "social consciousness," concern, and discomfort are the motivating factors which prompt flatulent patients to seek medical attention.

Gaseousness Associated with Organic Disease. Patients with hiatal hernia, peptic ulcer, abdominal neoplasm, and other organic disorders may present with symptoms of gaseousness as the primary complaint. As noted previously, patients with abdominal discomfort may consciously or involuntarily swallow excess quantities of air and experience associated motility disturbances. Hiatal hernia has often been labeled as a cause for belching, but one might theorize that excess belching could weaken the lower esophageal sphincter and thus lead to hiatal hernia. One should be cautious of easily accepting a diagnosis of functional gaseousness as a new complaint in a patient over 50 years of age, because such problems often begin at an earlier time in life. Late onset of functional disturbances raises the question of underlying organic disease.

Gaseousness Associated with Other Functional Disorders. Although belching, flatulence, and bloating often occur as isolated complaints, it is not uncommon to encounter these symptoms in patients with spastic colon, functional diarrhea, or pyloroduodenal spasm. The approach to the motility disorder must include attention to the factors which predispose to gaseousness, as failure to consider both problems often leads to treatment failures.

Therapy

Investigation. Although gaseous symptoms of recent onset may be treated symptomatically, as detailed below, distress of more chronic nature should be evaluated more thoroughly, with appropriate barium contrast studies, sigmoidoscopy when indicated, and hematologic/biochemical determinations. The investigation serves a dual purpose, as it reassures the patient that a serious organic disorder, such as cancer, is not responsible for the symptoms, and may identify, for the physician, the presence of associated disorders, such as hiatal hernia or ulcer, which may contribute to the discomfort. The reassurance derived from a thorough investigation often reduces the patient's anxiety to the point that routine therapeutic measures are considerably more effective.

Diet. Complex and rigid dietary approaches have often been based on folklore, rather than scientific evidence. Patients who find themselves unable to follow a rigid diet may add guilt to their emotional burden. The following observations can be easily remembered and yet not interfere with a reasonably full and esthetically satisfactory diet:

1. The mechanics of eating are important. Faulty dentures should be repaired so that adequate mastication is possible. Meals should be eaten slowly and preferably in a relaxing atmosphere, rather than gulped "on the job" or in a frantic eating place. The daily food intake should be evenly distributed into three meals, rather than a hurried or absent breakfast and lunch followed by a large dinner. Liquids should be taken sparingly at meals, as more air is swallowed with liquids than solids, and liquids tend to distend the stomach to a greater degree.

2. Carbonated beverages, chewing gum, and sucking on hard candies should be eliminated, because they increase air swallowing directly (carbon dioxide) or indirectly by stimulating saliva production and increased swallowing.

3. If patients with crampy pain and flatulence consume milk or other dairy products on a regular basis, a trial of total withdrawal or a lactose tolerance test is often useful in identifying lactase deficiency.

4. Indigestible carbohydrates, such as beans, salad, or fresh fruit (except bananas), should be restricted. Bran is popular now for the therapy of constipation and irritable colon, but symptoms of gaseousness may prove troublesome. If bran is added to the diet, it should be done in small increments.

5. There is no need to insist on a totally bland diet, because seasoning to taste makes mealtimes more enjoyable. Meats, fish, poultry, boiled vegetables, canned fruit, wheat products, and eggs should permit a wide selection of foods.

Anticholinergic Therapy. The major indication for anticholinergic therapy is disordered intestinal motility, leading to crampy distress. If this symptom is prominent, agents such as tincture of belladonna, propantheline (Pro-Banthine), glycopyrrolate (Robinul), or dicyclomine (Bentyl, an antispasmodic) may prove useful. The dosage should be gradually increased until improvement or side effects occur, for one of the most common causes of failure of this therapy is inadequate dosage. However, the dry mouth which occurs with adequate therapy may predispose to excess air swallowing; the decreased gastric emptying and decreased lower esophageal sphincter pressure which may result in increased heartburn or belching; and bladder and eye complications should be considered. Therefore the potential value and hazards of this approach require evaluation prior to use.

Antacids. Heartburn may prove sufficiently distressing to stimulate air swallowing. The use of 10 to 15 ml. of a standard antacid 1 hour after meals may prove beneficial, in addition to other antireflux measures. Also, the use of an antacid 1 hour after meals may serve to reduce the carbon dioxide generation that occurs in the duodenum. The antacid-simethicone preparations are popular, although evidence is currently lacking for the efficacy of simethicone products in the treatment of gaseous disorders.

Sedative and Antidepressive Therapy. Sedative and antidepressive therapy, when indicated, may prove useful in the overall program. Combination sedative-anticholinergic preparations are convenient, but this advantage may be offset by the lack of flexibility in adjusting both components, particularly when an attempt to reach a suitable anticholinergic effect is desired, because excess sedation may result.

Psychotherapy. The prompt psychiatric referral of a patient with severe gaseous symptoms is usually met with hostility. Even though an anxiety-depressive reaction may appear to warrant formal psychotherapy, the reassurance of a careful investigation, symptomatic measures, and office discussions relating to "life stresses" is often sufficient.

Attention to Associated Disorders. Postnasal discharge leads to increased swallowing and therefore may be an additional cause for aerophagia. Air swallowing is also a problem for some smokers and constitutes yet another reason for discontinuing the habit. Treatment of associated peptic ulcer disease, reflux esophagitis, and other disorders may result in decreased gaseousness.

ACUTE VIRAL HEPATITIS

method of
RAYMOND S. KOFF, M.D.
Boston, Massachusetts

Hepatitis A virus, hepatitis B virus, and non-A, non-B hepatitis viruses (presently lacking further designation but occasionally referred to as hepatitis "C", "D", and so on) are responsible for most cases of the acute systemic illness known as acute viral hepatitis. Seroimmunologic techniques permit the identification of acute viral hepatitis as hepatitis A, hepatitis B, or, by exclusion, non-A, non-B hepatitis. The last-named disorder appears to be distinct from infection with Epstein-Barr virus, cytomegalovirus, herpes simplex virus, and other identified viruses which have been infrequently implicated in acute viral hepatitis. Although hepatic involvement is a feature of several of these infections, evidence of hepatitis is usually overshadowed by extrahepatic manifestations of viral illness.

Agents and Epidemiology

Hepatitis A. This 27 nm. viral particle is probably an RNA virus of the enterovirus family. It has been found in the stool of infected patients, regardless of the route of inoculation (oral or parenteral), prior to the onset of symptoms and during the first few days of clinical illness. This limited period of fecal shedding correlates with the known limited period of infectivity of feces in hepatitis A. Viremia is transient. Fecal-oral transmission is the predominant mode of spread, and there is no evidence of a chronic carrier state or persistent reservoir of infection in human beings or nonhuman primates. The endemicity of hepatitis A is dependent on person-to-person propagation (horizontal transmission), although common-source vehicles of infection, such as water, bivalve mollusks, and other foods, have been implicated in occasional outbreaks and in sporadic cases. Nonhuman primates may be infected transiently and may serve as a source of infection for animal handlers.

Antibody to hepatitis A (anti-HA) is a neutralizing antibody present in convalescent sera and immune serum globulin (ISG). Anti-HA develops at or shortly after the rise in serum transaminases, and reaches peak levels within several weeks. Its persistence following hepatitis A infection is responsible for homologous immunity.

Recent serologic data suggest that in the United States hepatitis A is no longer a disease primarily of children. Young adults and the middle-aged who have escaped childhood infection remain at risk. However, most infections are anicteric or asymptomatic. Even when clinically evident, the disease is relatively short-lived and generally mild (the case fatality rate is approximately 0.1 per cent), and no important sequelae are known with the exception of rare instances of pancytopenia.

Hepatitis B. Hepatitis B virus is a 42 nm. double-shelled particle containing circular, double-stranded DNA. The particle is composed of distinct antigenic material in an outer coat—the hepatitis B surface antigen (HB_sAg)—and in an inner core—the hepatitis B core antigen (HB_cAg). These antigens elicit specific antibodies: anti-HB_s and anti-HB_c. The latter develops early after hepatitis B infection, whereas the former may not be detected until late in the convalescent phase. A nonparticulate "e" antigen and a specific hepatitis B DNA polymerase are present in serum early after infection and may be correlated with the presence of infectious virus in blood. Their persistence following the acute phase of illness may be related to the development of chronic hepatitis.

Circulating HB_sAg can be detected transiently in the blood of 80 to 90 per cent of infected patients regardless of whether or not the complete virus is present. Free HB_cAg is not detected in blood. In 5 to 10 per cent of patients HB_sAg persists for many months to years. These patients may be asymptomatic carriers or may develop chronic hepatitis.

Hepatitis B affects all age groups and is, on the average, more severe than hepatitis A. The case fatality rate is approximately 1 per cent. The disease is transmitted parenterally or by close intimate contact with patients with acute disease or carriers. The latter appear to serve as a persistent reservoir of infection and may be responsible for the high prevalence of hepatitis B in certain regions. It is clear, however, that not all carriers are equally contagious. Vertical transmission has been established from acutely infected or carrier mothers to their newborns. With the exception of equipment shared for inoculations and contaminated, inadequately treated blood products, common-source vehicles of infection do not play a role in hepatitis B transmission.

Non-A, Non-B Hepatitis. There are no known serologic markers by which non-A, non-B hepatitis can be identified, and the nature of the responsible agents remains uncertain. Probably more than one agent is involved. Available evidence indicates that non-A, non-B hepatitis is now the major cause of transfusion-associated viral hepatitis and is implicated in the multiple episodes of viral hepatitis often observed in parenteral drug abusers. Non-A, non-B hepatitis also may be important in sporadic hepatitis cases in which no recognized route of transmission can be identified.

The disease produced by non-A, non-B hepatitis has a variable incubation period and a wide spectrum of severity, resembling either hepatitis A or B. Anicteric cases outnumber icteric cases, but fulminant hepatic failure also has been described. Non-A, non-B hepatitis resembles hepatitis B in that it (1) appears to be blood-borne (a carrier state seems probable), (2) often produces a prolonged illness lasting many months, and (3) may progress in some instances to chronic hepatitis. Limited studies suggest that secondary cases among household contacts of acutely ill patients are uncommon.

Prevention and Postexposure Prophylaxis

Prevention of viral hepatitis is dependent upon (1) rapid diagnosis, identification, and notification of patients; (2) determination of the probable causative agent; and (3) attempts to interrupt the route of transmission resulting in spread of infection to susceptibles. Postexposure prophylaxis requires the use of standard immune serum globulin (ISG) or hepatitis B immune globulin (HBIG). Neither ISG nor HBIG has any value in hepatitis once the disease is established.

Hepatitis A. Since hepatitis A is usually spread by fecal contamination, meticulous personal hygiene is critical. The patient is not permitted to handle food or water directly, or indirectly, by contaminating cutlery, crockery, or glassware to be used by others. The patient and household contacts are reminded of the necessity of careful handwashing after personal contact and of avoiding shared food, water, or toilet items. The patient's clothing and linens which are likely to be fecally soiled should be laundered separately in a hot water washing machine. The use of disposable dishes, cups, and cutlery is encouraged, and separate toilet facilities are desirable.

The value of reinforcing these hygienic practices is limited by the fact that the patient with hepatitis A has been shedding virus for at least 2 weeks before the illness is clinically apparent and peak viral excretion occurs 2 to 10 days prior to elevation of serum transaminases. Thus household and other intimate contacts may have had multiple exposure opportunities by the time the diagnosis of hepatitis A is made. As a result the basic prophylactic measure after exposure to hepatitis A is the administration of ISG. ISG when given intramuscularly within 2 weeks after exposure, in a dose of 0.02 ml. per kg. of body weight, will prevent symptoms and jaundice, although subclinical infection may occur. ISG is indicated for close contacts, such as household members, but is not routinely given to casual contacts. ISG may also be of value in prophylaxis when exposure to a common-source vehicle of infection is recognized.

Larger amounts of ISG are not more efficacious than the standard dose but may provide protection for 4 to 6 months. A dose of approximately 5 ml. of ISG is recommended for extended visits to endemic areas. Readministration at 4 to 5 month intervals may be necessary to maintain protection. This dose and schedule are also recommended for handlers of newly imported nonhuman primates. Handlers are also encouraged to use gowns and gloves and to limit their access, when possible, to newly imported animals.

Hepatitis B. Hepatitis B is a potential hazard for medical and dental personnel, and for employees of institutions for the mentally handicapped, who are exposed to patients with acute hepatitis B or some HB_sAg carriers. High risk personnel include those employed in oncology and hemodialysis-transplantation units, clinical laboratory workers, and both oral and general surgeons. For these personnel a program of continuous education concerning hepatitis transmission, periodic reviews of safety standards and hygienic practices, and surveillance for hepatitis B infection is recommended. The wearing of gloves and protective clothing is encouraged to avoid contamination with blood or other potentially infective body fluids.

Equipment used for tissue penetration—e.g., ear-piercing or tattooing needles, dental and medical needles, and similar instruments exposed to blood or serum—must be disposable or treated by heat sterilization before re-use. Meticulous care should be taken in discarding disposable equipment to avoid inadvertent "needle-sticks." Nondisposable contaminated equipment may be sterilized by autoclaving at 121°C. for 15 minutes, boiling for 20 minutes, or exposing to dry heat at 170°C. for 60 minutes. Syringe techniques must be scrupulously monitored to be certain that a contaminated needle is not used to re-enter a multiple dose container.

For delicate equipment which cannot withstand the aforementioned heat sterilization, such as fiberoptic endoscopy instruments, vigorous soap and water washing and rinsing to remove organic contaminating material is the primary goal. The effectiveness of chemical or gas sterilization is uncertain.

The incidence of post-transfusion hepatitis B has been greatly diminished by the screening of blood donors for HB_sAg. The avoidance of blood from paid donors will further reduce the incidence of all forms of transfusion-associated hepatitis. Blood products that are associated with a high risk of hepatitis should be used sparingly and only for specific indications.

HBIG, containing very high titers of anti-HB_s, is licensed for postexposure prophylaxis of persons exposed to hepatitis B–contaminated blood or other fluids by "needle-stick." The recommended dose is 5 ml., which may be repeated 1 month later. It should be given as early as possible after exposure. HBIG will provide protection for several months but may interfere with the development of immunity. It has been effective in reducing the frequency of infection in intimate contacts of patients with acute hepatitis B. The efficacy of HBIG in persons inadvertently transfused with HB_sAg positive blood or blood products, or in newborns of infected mothers, is not yet established.

Postexposure prophylaxis is not necessary for persons with pre-existing anti-HB_s as they are generally not at risk for reinfection unless an extremely large inoculum is received. A hepatitis B vaccine, presently under development, is not yet available in the United States.

Non-A, Non-B Hepatitis. Measures directed at disease prevention have been hampered by incomplete understanding of the epidemiology of these disorders and by the absence of serologic markers of infection. It seems clear, however, that the incidence of non-A, non-B viral hepatitis associated with blood transfusion may be reduced by the use of volunteer rather than paid blood donors. Limited data also suggest that standard ISG administered at the time of transfusion may reduce the risk of non-A, non-B hepatitis. This observation is compatible with the notion that specific neutralizing antibodies to non-A, non-B hepatitis viruses are present in ISG. Further study is necessary before prophylaxis with ISG can be recommended.

Treatment

Typical Acute Hepatitis. Patients are usually managed at home. Hospital admission is necessary if (1) persistent nausea and vomiting lead to dehydration; (2) alterations of personality, mental status, or sleep rhythm develop, suggesting early hepatic encephalopathy; (3) evidence of prothrombin prolongation (>6 seconds over control) occurs; or (4) the diagnosis is uncertain.

Diet and Drugs. At home the patient is encouraged to maintain oral intake of liquids and a palatable unrestricted nutritious diet. Alcohol is prohibited during the acute phase. Since nausea may worsen during the day, a large breakfast is encouraged. Vitamin supplements are not given unless specific deficiencies exist. Unless absolutely essential, drugs are avoided. Corticosteroids are not used.

Activity. Strenuous or prolonged physical activity is restricted, but bed rest is not required except as dictated by the severity of the patient's fatigue and malaise. Increasing activity is permitted when improvement is evident to the patient (milder symptoms) and physician (improved liver chemistries). Persistent minor abnormalities of liver chemistries do not preclude the gradual resumption of normal activities.

Evaluation. During the acute phase of the illness the prothrombin time, serum bilirubin, and serum transaminases are performed twice weekly. Liver size is determined, and mental status is carefully assessed. In the uncomplicated typical case, improvement is evident by the end of the second to third week of observation, and follow-up studies may be performed at weekly and then monthly intervals until it is clear that the illness is over. In those patients in whom HB_sAg remains positive at 3 months after onset, or in whom transaminase abnormalities persist, follow-up studies are continued in light of the possible development of chronic hepatitis.

Severe Acute Hepatitis (Bridging Necrosis and Fulminant Hepatitis). Patients whose symptoms and laboratory studies continue to worsen or reach a plateau without improvement after 2 to 3 weeks of illness may have bridging hepatic necrosis. These patients may develop encephalopathy, fluid retention manifested by edema and ascites, and significant prolongation of the prothrombin time. Hospitalization is necessary to establish the diagnosis, by liver biopsy if possible, and to manage the complications of this disorder, which are similar to those described below for fulminant hepatitis. "Enteric precautions" are routinely observed within the hospital for hepatitis A, but they are less critical in hepatitis B. Overemphasis on isolation techniques may interfere with the repeated careful observation of the patient and diminish the benefits of hospitalization.

Fulminant hepatitis is characterized by the development of hepatic encephalopathy and striking prolongation of the prothrombin time in the setting of acute hepatitis. Progressive jaundice and diminution of liver size are usual but not inevitable. Approximately 65 to 95 per cent of patients succumb, with the highest mortality in those over age 40 and in those with underlying disease. Survivors usually have complete hepatic resolution. Complications contributing importantly to mortality include cerebral edema, gastrointestinal bleeding, respiratory failure, cardiovascular collapse, and renal failure. The goal of treatment is "buying time" to permit hepatic regeneration and restoration.

Management in an intensive care unit is recommended, because excellent nursing care with careful and continuous observation and monitoring of vital functions, with immediate therapeutic intervention when necessary, may enhance survival rates. Maintenance of an open airway is a prime concern, and assisted ventilation after placement of an endotracheal tube should be performed early if respiratory failure seems imminent, rather than after prolonged hypoxemia. The development of "shock lung" is a poor prognostic sign. Positive end-expiratory pressure (PEEP) has been used, but its effectiveness is unclear. Water, glucose, and electrolyte balance are achieved with intravenous fluids, and serum potassium and inorganic phosphorus should be maintained at normal levels. A nasogastric tube is useful for keeping the stomach decompressed and monitoring for bleeding. Standard hyperalimentation fluids are not used. Protein ingestion is halted, and either lactulose, 50 ml. every 6 hours, or neomycin, 1 gram every 4 to 6 hours, may be given by nasogastric tube to the comatose patient or orally in patients who are alert enough that the risk of aspiration is small.

Indwelling catheters are used sparingly and with meticulous care. Infections are treated promptly but not prophylactically. Fresh frozen plasma is used to correct bleeding resulting from defective hemostasis, but should not be used prophylactically. Heparin and coagulation factor concentrates are avoided. Cimetidine, an H_2 receptor blocker, may reduce the frequency of gastrointestinal bleeding.

Treatment of cerebral edema with mannitol, glycerol, or dexamethasone may be attempted but is generally disappointing. Intracerebral pressure monitoring may prove useful in the evaluation of therapy. Heroic procedures—e.g., exchange transfusion, cross-circulation, total body washout—are avoided, because the recovery of consciousness associated with these procedures has been transient and none of these maneuvers has been shown to enhance survival rates. The efficacy of L-dopa is uncertain.

Corticosteroids are probably of no benefit in severe viral hepatitis. In bridging necrosis there is some evidence that they may be harmful. In fulminant hepatitis available data do not show a clear-cut advantage or disadvantage, and more data are needed to determine the ultimate utility of steroids in this disorder.

THE MALABSORPTION SYNDROME

method of
DAVID H. ALPERS, M.D.
St. Louis, Missouri

Recognition of Malabsorption

Patients may present with any one or a combination of the following symptoms: weight loss, abdominal distention, borborygmus, edema, diarrhea, foul-smelling stools, paresthesias, ecchymosis or bleeding, glossitis and cheilosis, peripheral neuropathy, dermatitis, muscle weakness or tenderness, or fatigue. It is important to remember that malabsorption may be global, involving all nutrients, or quite specific, involving only one substance—e.g., iron or calcium. The presenting symptoms may vary quite widely, depending on the substance(s) being malabsorbed. In addition, the proper diagnostic test must be carefully selected to fit the symptoms. Finally, just as there is no constant set of symptoms or diagnostic studies, therapy must be tailored to the specific disease and deficiencies which ensue.

Many of the symptoms of malabsorption are found in malnutrition. Deficiency of protein can lead to edema, ecchymosis, and abdominal distention. Caloric deficiency causes weight loss, diarrhea, and fatigue. Vitamin deficiency can lead to neuropathy, glossitis, paresthesias, or other specific symptoms for each vitamin not ingested. Furthermore, malabsorption, if present, must be separated into those disorders caused by small intestinal disease with normal digestion, and those with malabsorption as the result of maldigestion (pancreatic insufficiency, bile acid deficiency).

Generalized Malabsorption–Acute

Occasionally patients present with severe malnutrition and require rather acute treatment. The goal should be to provide calories and protein, and to treat whatever deficiencies are present.

1. Total parenteral nutrition (see below).
2. Albumin intravenously, 25 grams once or twice daily.
3. Packed red cells as needed.
4. Calcium intravenously as needed to maintain normal ionized calcium with drip of 10 per cent calcium gluconate, which is about 10 per cent elemental calcium by weight.
5. Magnesium intravenously as needed to maintain serum magnesium at 1.5 mEq. per liter with 25 per cent magnesium sulfate (2 mEq. per ml.), up to 2 mEq. per kg. of body weight over 4 to 6 hours.
6. Potassium intravenously 40 to 80 mEq. per 24 hours or as needed to maintain potassium at 3.5 mEq. per liter.

Carbohydrate Malabsorption

Nonspecific Therapy. LOW AVAILABLE CARBOHYDRATE DIET (Table 1). This diet will be useful for patients with the short bowel syndrome (because it is low in osmolarity), with lactose intolerance (because it is low in lactose), and in the dumping syndrome (because it is low in osmolarity and prevents hypoglycemia).

Specific Therapy. LOW LACTOSE DIET FOR LACTOSE INTOLERANCE (Table 2). Avoid foods with labels showing lactose, milk solids, milk products, or whey. Avoid all cream sauces or soups.

LOW GLUCOSE-GALACTOSE DIET. This diet is used for glucose-galactose malabsorption. The diet will consist of fructose-containing liquids (Galactomin, Cho-Free with fructose) for infants, and will avoid starches, lactose, and glucose-containing foods for adults. This condition is exceedingly rare.

LOW SUCROSE DIET. This diet is used for sucrase deficiency. It avoids foods rich in sucrose—mostly vegetables (e.g., beets) and fruits. A complete diet can be found in the article by Hediger: J. Amer. Diet. Assoc. *46*:197, 1964.

Protein Malabsorption and Loss

In general, mild to moderate malabsorption of protein produces no symptoms per se. Therefore little therapy is necessary, for restriction of protein does not improve total absorption, although it may increase the percentage of proteins absorbed. However, severe protein malabsorption, severe protein-losing enteropathy, or a combination of both processes may lead to hypoal-

TABLE 1. **Low Available Carbohydrate Diet**

FOODS ALLOWED	FOODS NOT ALLOWED
Complex carbohydrates	Milk products
Starches	Dextrose-containing foods or liquids
Rice	
Protein (not predigested)	Sucrose-rich foods or liquids
Fats	

TABLE 2. **Low Lactose Diet for Lactose Intolerance**

FOOD ITEM	FOODS ALLOWED	FOODS NOT ALLOWED
Beverages	Alcohol Carbonated beverages Coffee, tea Nondairy substitutes Fruit juices Ices	All types of milk Buttermilk Yogurt Ice cream Sherbets
Meats and fish	All except those listed in opposite column	Frankfurters or sausage made with fillers which contain a batter or bread made with milk
Fruits	All	None
Breads and cereals	Bagels, kosher breads, graham crackers	Any bread or cereal made with milk—many crackers contain lactose
Fats	Vegetable oils, bacon, lard, mayonnaise, pure vegetable oil margarine	Butter, commercial salad dressing, sour cream, whipping cream
Desserts	Angel food cake, fruit pies, marshmallows, pure chocolate candies	Cakes, candies, cookies, doughnuts, puddings, etc., made with milk

buminemia, edema, poor wound healing, and increased susceptibility to infection. Many intestinal diseases which produce severe malabsorption are also associated with some protein loss—e.g., Crohn's disease, nontropical sprue, Whipple's disease. When symptoms occur, specific therapy may be needed.

Nonspecific Therapy for Protein Loss. LOW FAT DIET. See below. In diseases which are associated with lymphatic obstruction (lymphangiectasia, severe congestive failure), decreased fat absorption and lymphatic flow will decrease protein loss.

Specific Therapy for Protein Loss or Malabsorption. FAT MALABSORPTION. See below.

PROTEIN SUPPLEMENTS. *Oral:* Gevral or Casec protein, 8 oz. glass (15 grams protein) two or three times daily. *Intravenous:* albumin, 25 to 50 grams daily, to keep serum albumin at 2.5 grams per 100 ml. or greater. If protein loss is severe, the primary diseases must be treated, as intravenous albumin will be lost from the body as fast as it enters. If doubt exists about the presence of protein loss, ^{51}Cr albumin (Chromalbin) excretion can be measured.

Fat Malabsorption

Malabsorption of long chain fatty acids is most important in the production of symptoms. The unabsorbed fatty acids are modified in the colon to produce toxic short chain or hydroxylated fatty acids, leading to diarrhea and foul-smelling stool. Improvement of fat malabsorption is important, even if the underlying disease cannot be adequately treated.

Nonspecific Therapy. LOW FAT DIET (Table 3). The main objective is to limit the daily intake of fat by at least half of the patient's usual intake, or to the lowest amount tolerated by the patient. The average intake of fat in an American diet runs from 70 to 150 grams per day. Thus a 40 gram fat diet is low, but a 75 gram fat diet may be adequate fat restriction for some people (Table 4).

MEDIUM CHAIN TRIGLYCERIDES (MCT). MCT require less emulsification with bile acids and less pancreatic lipase for hydrolysis, and the fatty acids are absorbed without micelles because of their greater water solubility. Thus they are useful in a wide variety of disorders causing fat malabsorption. However, they contain only 7 calories per gram, and excessive amounts (over 300 calories per day) cause diarrhea. Their use is therefore as a supplement, not a major caloric source.

MCT oil is given as 30 ml. orally three or four times daily, either undiluted or mixed with a strong-flavored juice (e.g., tomato).

Specific Therapy. Many diseases present with fat malabsorption, but may have significant malabsorption of other nutrients. These disorders are all

TABLE 3. **Low Fat Diet for Fat Malabsorption**

FOOD ITEM	FOODS ALLOWED	FOODS NOT ALLOWED (DEPENDING ON DEGREE OF RESTRICTION)
Milk	Skim milk	All other milks
Meat	Lean meats, especially beef, lamb, veal	Sausage, luncheon meats, frankfurters, liver, brain
Poultry	Chicken, turkey	Duck, goose
Fish	All shellfish, flatfish (flounder, cod, crappie)	All other fish, even tuna packed in water
Nonmeat protein	Cheese, especially peas, beans	Soy beans, nuts, peanut butter

Avoid all fruit or creamed foods, all desserts made with cream, all commercial salad dressings, and sour cream.

TABLE 4. **Comparison of Various Levels of Fat Restriction**

DIET	FOODS ALLOWED
40 grams fat	Vegetables, fruits, bread, cereal, *plus* skim milk Two servings of lean meat, 3 oz. each One egg One tsp. margarine
60 grams fat	In addition to foods allowed above: Two cups of 2% milk *or* Two servings of lean meat, 4 oz. each One egg or more margarine, 1 tsp./meal
75 grams fat	In addition to foods allowed above: Whole milk instead of 2% milk *or* two slices of bacon *or* 4 oz. of ice cream *or* two servings of lean meat of 6 oz. each instead of 4 oz.

discussed here, but could be applicable to other problems of malabsorption.

NONTROPICAL SPRUE. GLUTEN-RESTRICTED DIET (Table 5). This diet avoids protein found in wheat, barley, and oats. Rice and corn are allowed. Foods with unclear labels should be avoided, such as those foods containing "cereals," "thickeners," and "starch," in which the additives are not defined. The Food and Drug Administration does not require the listing of the source of flour or starch. The most reliable cookbook can be obtained from the Dietary Department of the University of Michigan Medical Center in Ann Arbor (Hjortland, M., and Birk, A.: Low Gluten Diet with Tested Recipes, 1969).

CORTICOSTEROIDS. For severe life-threatening illness, 60 mg. of prednisone per day is given, decreasing as needed. As an adjunct to diet, 5 to 20 mg. of prednisone per day is given as needed for control of symptoms. Steroids are not usually necessary, but may be helpful in the occasional critically ill patient, or in the patient who cannot adequately follow dietary restrictions.

TABLE 5. **Gluten-Restricted Diet for Nontropical Sprue**

FOOD ITEM	FOODS ALLOWED	FOODS NOT ALLOWED
Beverage	Milk Wine, liquors Most carbonated beverages	Ovaltine, root beer, instant tea, ale, beer, gin, vodka, whiskey
Meat	All except those listed in opposite column	Breaded meats, sausage, frankfurters
Nonmeat protein	Egg, beans, peas, nuts	
Breads and cereals	Flours made from rice, corn, potato, soy, arrowroot	Wheat, rye, oats, barley, buckwheat, and all foods made from these flours
Fruits, vegetables	All	None

SHORT BOWEL SYNDROME DUE TO DISEASES OF ILEUM (REGIONAL ENTERITIS) OR RESECTION OF ILEUM. When resection or disease of the ileum involves less than the terminal 100 cm., malabsorption of bile acids predominates over fat malabsorption. These patients have a bile acid (chenodeoxycholic acid)–induced secretion of water and electrolytes from the colon (cholerrheic diarrhea) and respond to bile acid binding substances (cholestyramine). When more than 100 cm. of ileum is diseased, fat malabsorption predominates, and bile acid pools are now so low that not enough bile acid enters the colon to induce diarrhea. These patients will not improve with bile acid binders, which will merely serve to worsen the steatorrhea by binding the remaining bile acids.

1. *Cholestyramine,* 4 grams orally four times daily, with three doses given by lunch time. *Caution:* this drug may bind other medications (digoxin, thyroxine, vitamin D) which are in general sterols or negatively charged.

2. *Antispasmodics* to decrease transit time. Deodorized tincture of opium, 5 to 15 drops four times daily; or opium, 30 mg., belladonna, 15 mg., one capsule given four times daily.

STAGNANT LOOP SYNDROME. *Broad-spectrum antibiotics*—e.g., tetracycline, ampicillin, or erythromycin, 250 mg. four times daily.

Often it is helpful to give antibiotics for 12 days, and discontinue for 2 days in cyclic fashion.

PANCREATIC INSUFFICIENCY. 1. *Enzyme replacement:* Pancreatin (Viokase) or pancrelipase (Cotazyme), 3 to 6 tablets with meals.

2. *Bicarbonate,* 0.5 gram tablets, 6 to 24 per day. This is not often needed, as enzyme replacement along with low fat diet usually alleviates symptoms.

TROPICAL SPRUE. Because of the frequency of spontaneous remissions, the value of short-term therapy is debatable. However, it is still advisable to use broad-spectrum antibiotics and hematinics if needed, realizing that the observed response may not be due to the therapy. In endemic areas long-term treatment with antibiotics seems to be useful.

BROAD-SPECTRUM ANTIBIOTICS. Tetracycline, 250 mg. four times daily. This may be most helpful when used on a long-term basis (4 to 6 months).

HEMATINICS. Folic acid, 1 to 2 mg. orally daily, and vitamin B_{12}, 1000 micrograms intramuscularly every 1 to 2 weeks, should both be given, as both are often lacking. Do not use folic acid alone, as it can exacerbate vitamin B_{12} deficiency. If iron deficiency is present, oral iron can be added (see below).

WHIPPLE'S DISEASE. ANTIBIOTICS. The optimal regimen has not yet been determined. Penicillin, alone or with streptomycin, and tetracycline have been successfully used.

Procaine penicillin, 600,000 units intramuscularly twice daily until clear improvement occurs (1 to 2 weeks), followed by penicillin G, 500 mg. twice daily, or tetracycline, 250 mg. four times daily, until the biopsy returns to normal (4 to 12 months). Streptomycin, 500 mg. twice daily intramuscularly for 10 to 14 days at onset if needed.

CORTICOSTEROIDS. These are not usually needed, but may be added (40 to 60 mg. of prednisone) if the patient is very ill and a rapid response is important. Once remission begins, these can be rapidly tapered.

Vitamin Malabsorption

Water-soluble vitamin deficiencies are easy to recognize and treat, because standard serum assays are available for vitamin B_{12}, folic acid, and vitamin C, and inexpensive oral or parenteral preparations are available. Fat-soluble vitamin deficiency can be readily detected, but therapy is more difficult. Commercial preparations of fat-soluble vitamins are water miscible, by virtue of the addition of a detergent. If ingested by a patient with decreased intraluminal micelles, the vitamins will leave the aqueous phase in the lumen, and be malabsorbed. Further, reliable parenteral preparations are not available, as intramuscular injections are made in oil, from which absorption is irregular. Intravenous preparations of vitamins A and D are feasible but not widely available. Finally, response to therapy with vitamins A and especially D is slow and difficult to evaluate. The therapy listed below is for acute deficiency states. Prophylaxis can be achieved at much lower doses, comparable to those found in commercial multivitamin preparations. Folic acid and vitamin B_{12} are not included in these preparations, however.

1. *Folic acid:* 1 mg. orally daily.
2. *Vitamin B_{12}:* 1000 micrograms intramuscularly each month.
3. *Ascorbic acid:* 200 to 2000 micrograms orally daily. Excessive doses of ascorbic acid (>3 grams daily) may result in diarrhea and must be used cautiously in patients prone to acidosis.
4. *Thiamine (B_1):* 10 mg. orally or intramuscularly daily.
5. *Riboflavin (B_2):* 10 to 60 mg. orally daily.
6. *Vitamin A:* 5000 to 30,000 I.U. daily orally or intramuscularly. Beware of hypervitaminosis A and continue therapy at this level for only 1 to 3 weeks. Follow therapy with serum vitamin A, and reduce the dose when normal serum levels occur. Usually 3000 to 5000 units per day will suffice for maintenance.
7. *Vitamin D:* 50,000 I.U. orally daily of ergocalciferol (Calciferol) (D_2). Beware of hypervitaminosis D, and decrease to 50,000 I.U. two to three times weekly. Follow therapy with serum 25-OH vitamin D, or with 24 hour urinary calcium determination. Fifty thousand I.U. daily is an excessive dose but is the only one readily available at present.
8. *Vitamin K:* Vitamin K_1 (water-miscible), 10 mg. orally or intramuscularly per day for hemorrhage. Vitamin K_3 (menadione sodium bisulfate—water-soluble), 10 mg. orally per day.

Mineral Malabsorption

Calcium deficiency is usually seen in disorders in which both calcium and vitamin D are malabsorbed. Therefore sometimes both substances must be replaced. In addition, when magnesium deficiency is present, replacement of magnesium is necessary before hypocalcemia can be corrected. There is no evidence that any form of iron other than simple salts is more effective in enhancing absorption.

1. *Calcium:* Normal replacement ranges from 1 to 2 grams of calcium per day. Os-Cal, 1 tablet four times daily, contains 250 mg. Ca per tablet. Ca gluconate, 600 mg., contains about 55 mg. Ca per tablet. Ca carbonate (Titralac), 5 ml., contains 500 mg. Ca. Urinary calcium should be checked after institution of calcium therapy.
2. *Magnesium:* Most salts are relatively insoluble. The best tolerated is Mg gluconate, 0.5 gram four times daily.
3. *Potassium:* 10 per cent KCl solution, 1 tablespoonful three times daily. Each tablespoonful contains 20 mEq. of KCl.
4. *Iron:* Ferrous sulfate, 325 mg. orally four times daily before meals and at bedtime.

Calorie Malabsorption

Food Supplements (Table 6). Liquid food supplements were originally designed to provide an entire day's caloric, vitamin, and mineral intake. Because of side effects (nausea, diarrhea) and either unpalatable taste or taste fatigue, they have not proved useful for total caloric replacement except for a very limited period. They are used to supplement the appropriate diet. Furthermore, these preparations are very heterogeneous. Some are high in carbohydrate, others in fat, and still others in protein. "Elemental" diets such as Vivonex, in which all food types are completely hydrolyzed to basic nutrients (amino acids and sugars), are usually not necessary, even in pancreatic insufficiency, and are most trouble-

TABLE 6. **Percentage of Calories in Food Supplements**

	% CHO	% PROTEIN	% FAT	LACTOSE	OSMOLARITY	CALORIES/ML.
Balanced feeding (liquid)						
Meritene	46	24	30	+	615	1
Sustacal	54	24	22	+	625	1
Isocal	50	13	27	—	350	1
Precision Isotonic	60	12	28	—	300	1
Flexical	61	9	30	—	805	1
Portagen	55	14	31	—	354	1
High carbohydrate (liquid)						
Polycose	100	—	—	—	570	2.0
Hycal	100	—	—	—	1300	2.5
Precision-LR	90	9	1	—	525	1
Vivonex	90	9	1	—	600 (unflavored)	1
Citrotein	74	24	2	—	496	0.5
High protein (liquid without milk)						
Casec	0	95	5	—	NA	0.4
Gevral	25	73	2	—	127	0.4

some to take because of high osmolarity and bad taste. Some products contain lactose, and should not be used when lactase deficiency is suspected. The Ca, P, Na, and K content of these products varies widely, and not all patients can tolerate high sodium or potassium diets. If supplements of Ca or Mg are being given, the content of these ions in the diet or in supplements must be considered.

Total Parenteral Nutrition (TPN). This method usually provides 3000 to 4000 calories per day in 3 to 4 liters of fluid. Requirements for caloric and protein retentions include H_2O 35 ml. per kg., 0.5 to 1.5 grams of protein per kg., and 25 to 40 calories per gram of protein for positive balance. Each liter of TPN fluid contains 39 grams of protein and 1000 calories, along with 40 to 50 mEq. Na and 30 to 40 mEq. K. Phosphate, calcium, magnesium, and vitamins are also provided. Folate, vitamin B_{12} (1 vial Folbesyn), and Fe^{++} in the form of iron dextran (Imferon), 10 mg. per week, should be added. One or 2 tablespoons of corn oil per week by mouth supplies essential fatty acids. One unit of fresh frozen plasma per week can be used to supply trace metals. A typical daily TPN program is shown in Table 7.

It should be stressed that this program must be adjusted for the needs of the individual patient. Because the solution is hypertonic, fluids must be given through a central venous line. TPN should be started with 1 liter daily, increasing to 3 or 4 liters daily. Side effects to be watched for include fluid retention, hyperglycemia, hypoglycemia, hypokalemia, hypocalcemia, hypomagnesemia, hypophosphatemia, sepsis, and complications of catheter insertion. When discontinuing TPN, this should be done by gradually decreasing to 1 liter daily.

TABLE 7. **Basic Daily Program for Total Parenteral Nutrition**

	BOTTLE 1	BOTTLE 2	BOTTLE 3
Freamine 8.1%	500 ml.	500 ml.	500 ml.
$D_{50}W$	500 ml.	500 ml.	500 ml.
KPO_4	30 mEq.		30 mEq.
KCl		40 mEq.	
Na acetate	40 mEq.		40 mEq.
NaCl		40 mEq.	
Ca gluconate		1 ampule	
50% $MgSO_4$		2 ml.	
Multivitamins			1 ampule

INTESTINAL OBSTRUCTION

method of
CORNELIUS E. SEDGWICK, M.D.
Boston, Massachusetts

Intestinal obstruction must always be considered an acute surgical emergency. Early diagnosis and prompt surgical intervention are imperative if low morbidity and mortality rates are to be achieved. The surgeon should not temporize once the diagnosis has been established. Frequent clinical observation is more important than laboratory tests and radiographs. Nonoperative measures to deflate the bowel with nasogastric tubes, medication to relieve pain, antibiotics to control fever, and replacement of fluids and electrolytes which may lead to improvement in the patient's condition must be used only as adjunctive therapy to surgical intervention.

Only occasionally does conservative nonsurgical therapy suffice. Preoperatively, the patient must be brought into as satisfactory a state as possible. This should be accomplished in a maximum of 10 hours, particularly in patients with small bowel obstruction. More time, if necessary, can be allowed in a patient with partial bowel obstruction. Preoperative preparation includes the following:

1. *Insertion of nasogastric tube.* A long tube is more effective if it can be placed in the small bowel. Otherwise, a large caliber nasogastric tube for gastric aspiration and suction may be more effective. The nasogastric tube not only helps to deflate the upper gastrointestinal tract but may prevent aspiration and pulmonary complications.

2. *Central venous pressure monitoring.* A central venous pressure line is established so that monitoring of fluid may be accomplished. The basic pathophysiology is third space loss of vascular volume. Blood pressure, pulse, and urinary output are also indications of shock or impending shock. Electrolytes and fluid are administered, using central venous pressure monitoring as a guide as well as levels of blood pressure, pulse, and urine output.

3. *Catheter.* An indwelling catheter is placed in the bladder, and urinary output is monitored hourly.

4. *Antibiotics.* In the toxic state prophylactic intravenous antibiotics should be given. A combination of ampicillin, gentamicin, and clindamycin is given until a specific organism is identified.

5. *Hyperalimentation.* Total parenteral nutrition is now gaining widespread use in the nutritional support of critically ill patients, including those with small bowel obstruction. Two methods can be employed: (a) Intravenous hyperalimentation (IVH) as described by Dudrick, which employs amino acids and hypertonic dextrose together with electrolytes, minerals, and vitamins. These nutrients are delivered into a central vein (usually the superior vena cava, which is cannulated via the infraclavicular route). (b) Lipid system, a fat emulsion of soybean oil and egg yolk phospholipid, is administered through a peripheral vein with a solution of 5 per cent dextrose and 3 per cent amino acids.

By the use of either of these methods, fluid and electrolyte disorders, vitamin deficiencies, and nutritional depletion can be corrected while wound healing is promoted. It is important to assess and categorize malnutrition and then institute the appropriate form of therapy.

All the problems related to catheter insertion (pneumothorax, hemothorax, subclavian vein thrombosis), metabolic complications (hyperglycemia, hypokalemia, phosphate, calcium, and magnesium imbalances), essential fatty acid deficiency, and catheter sepsis must be kept in mind. Intravenous nutritional support can be carried out with minimal complications now that the preparation and administration of solutions have been made both safe and easy.

Intravenous nutritional support must be kept in mind as the primary mode of therapy under the following specific circumstances:

1. Patients with prolonged ileus after an operation to relieve intestinal obstruction, particularly when malnutrition has been pre-existent.

2. Recurrent and subacute intestinal obstruction often leads to an inadequate dietary intake over several weeks or months. Such patients need to be repleted preoperatively while diagnostic procedures are being carried out, and documentation of objective response to nutritional support is desirable before undertaking any elective operation.

3. An increasing number of patients are now able to survive with the short gut syndrome for long periods of time because of the availability of intravenous hyperalimentation. This treatment can now be carried out safely by these patients at home. A small number of such patients gradually will become able to tolerate special forms of orally administered diets while adequate intravenous nutritional support is carried out and the intestinal mucosa is allowed to hypertrophy and regenerate.

The greatest hazard in bowel obstruction is strangulation and necrosis. The most common causes are adhesive bands, hernia, colonic neoplasm, and inflammatory bowel disease. A distended right colon associated with chronic bowel disease indicates an impending perforation. Fecal impaction and sigmoid volvulus may be diagnosed and treated by rectosigmoid examination alone. Most other causes require early recognition and prompt surgical intervention to prevent necrosis of bowel. Laparotomy must be performed through an adequate incision. It is best to eviscerate the bowel from the abdominal cavity quickly and to determine the cause of obstruction promptly.

Inspecting a small segment of bowel, replacing it in the abdominal cavity, and continuing this procedure along the bowel is traumatizing and should be condemned. When the bowel is completely removed from the peritoneal cavity, the junction of the dilated proximal bowel and the collapsed distal bowel is quickly discovered.

Obstruction may be relieved by excision of an adhesion, by bypass anastomosis, or by resection. If the viability of the bowel is in doubt, a reasonable procedure is to cover the bowel with warm soaks, wait several minutes to see if the circulation is restored, and, if not, to proceed with resection. It may be necessary to decompress the bowel so that the abdomen may be closed more easily and also to reduce intestinal pressure on the diaphragm. This is usually accomplished with an intestinal suction tube through a small opening in the bowel.

Large bowel obstruction is most often due to neoplasm, inflammatory disease, diverticulitis, or chronic ulcerative colitis. The decision for proximal decompression or primary resection may be difficult. Certainly in most instances, the purpose of emergency surgical intervention is decompression. Proximal transverse loop colostomy is satisfactory for left colon and rectal lesions. In extremely ill and debilitated patients, tube cecostomy under local anesthesia may be lifesaving. Tube cecostomy will decompress the bowel if adequate irrigation (500 ml.) is performed carefully each day.

Postoperative management consists of maintaining stable pulse, blood pressure, and urinary output. Fluid and electrolyte replacement is monitored by the central venous pressure. Administration of antibiotics is continued. Colonic decompression is continued with nasointestinal intubation and colostomy irrigation until peristalsis and bowel function return to normal limits. Great attention must be given to the prevention of pulmonary complications. I believe simple deep breathing exercises are the best method to prevent these complications.

ACUTE PANCREATITIS

method of
STUART H. DANOVITCH, M.D.
Washington, D.C.

Therapy of acute pancreatitis is predicated on accurate diagnosis. Recent emphasis on detecting an elevated urinary clearance ratio of amylase to creatinine in acute pancreatitis has been helpful in sorting out patients presenting with nausea, vomiting, and abdominal pain. Clearance ratios in excess of 6 or 7 per cent are not characteristic of other causes of hyperamylasemia such as mumps, ectopic pregnancy, mesenteric vascular disease, macroamylasemia, or perforated viscus. In conjunction with serum lipase and amylase measurements, diagnostic precision is improved, and some diagnostic laparotomies, otherwise justified, may be avoided.

Fortunately the outcome of acute pancreatitis is favorable in 90 per cent of instances, but the mortality rate in the other 10 per cent of patients with a hemorrhagic, necrotizing lesion approaches 60 to 70 per cent. Initial therapy is conservative and nonoperative, and although the efficacy of many of the therapuetic maneuvers has not been substantiated by randomized trials, they are for the most part prudent and safe. The overriding therapeutic concern is to put the gland to rest and permit it to heal.

Medical Therapy

1. Nothing by mouth.
2. Intermittent nasogastric suction—in milder cases this may not be necessary.
3. Relief of pain. Use meperidine HCl, 50 to 100 mg. intramuscularly every 4 to 6 hours, unless the patient is hypotensive.
4. Fluid replacement. This is critical. Patients with milder disease may require only 5 per cent dextrose in ½ isotonic saline solution with suitable potassium and vitamin supplementation, totaling 3000 ml. daily. More severely ill patients will require colloid replacement, including plasma, albumin, and blood, as well as intravenous fluids, occasionally totaling 10 liters a day. Copious fluid loss from vomiting, intra-abdominal and retroperitoneal exudation, and diaphoresis is common. Urine output should be maintained at 50 ml. per hour.
5. Central venous pressure or pulmonary capillary wedge pressure monitoring is mandatory for patients with hypotension or requiring fluid replacement in excess of 5000 ml. per day.
6. Nasal oxygen is required for hypoxia, a recently emphasized complication of acute necrotizing pancreatitis.
7. Small doses of insulin may be needed if the blood sugar exceeds 300 to 350 mg. per dl. (100 ml.).
8. Ten per cent calcium gluconate should be given intravenously at a rate of 1.0 ml. per minute to correct serum calcium concentration <7.0 mg. per dl. Ten to 30 ml. every 6 hours may be needed.
9. Antibiotics are not used routinely, as they do not alter the outcome. They are appropriate for coexisting pneumonia or urinary tract infection or suspected pancreatic abscess or infected pseudocysts. Choices include a cephalosporin plus gentamicin or clindamycin when anaerobes are suspected.
10. Anticholinergics are of no proved efficacy, and they may contribute to both an ileus and tachycardia, thereby masking progress. I avoid them.

Clinical Observations

The following need close monitoring to assess progress:

1. In patients with hemodynamic instability, blood pressure and pulse are recorded every 2 hours.
2. Temperature, every 4 hours.
3. Hourly urine output.
4. Hematocrit, every 6 to 12 hours.
5. Serum glucose, sodium, potassium, chloride, carbon dioxide content, calcium, and phosphorus, every 12 to 24 hours.
6. Daily serum amylase, lipase, white blood cell count and differential, blood urea nitrogen (BUN), creatinine, plain and upright abdominal films.
7. At least daily assessment of the patient to determine abdominal distention, tenderness, bowel sounds, masses, or intraperitoneal fluid, plus chest examination.
8. Chest x-ray, arterial blood gases, and ECG as indicated.

Progress is indicated by improvement in the aforementioned parameters. Such progress should be apparent in 36 to 48 hours, and failure to occur raises the possibility of a need for alternative therapy.

Unconventional Therapies

In patients with severe disease, peritoneal lavage with renal dialysate in a continuous in-and-out fashion without an equilibration period has been said to be salutary for experimental pancreatitis in laboratory animals and, anecdotally, has been reported to be beneficial in man.

Similarly, surgery with lavage of the abdomen and drainage of the pancreatic bed of necrotic debris may be required in patients not responding to conventional therapy. Decompression of the digestive tract with a cholecystostomy, gastrostomy, and introduction of a feeding jejunostomy, plus placement of sump drains into the lesser sac and lateral gutters, are done.

Complications requiring close attention include shock, oliguria with renal failure, hypoxia, pleural or pericardial effusions, cardiac arrhythmias, pseudocyst, pancreatic abscess, and sepsis. Hypocalcemia less than 7.0 mg. per dl. and extreme hematocrits greater than 54 per cent or less than 25 per cent similarly are bad signs.

Feeding and rehabilitation begin with favorable response to treatment, including (1) disappearance of pain with no analgesic need, (2) reappearance of bowel sounds and passage of flatus, (3) defervescence, (4) stabilization of blood pressure and slowing of pulse, and (5) return of appetite without nausea and vomiting. Normalization of laboratory abnormalities (WBC, amylase, lipase) is not required prior to refeeding.

Diagnostic evaluation to ascertain the cause of pancreatitis can now be done. Alcoholism, trauma, cholelithiasis, hypercalcemia, hyperlipidemia, cancer, viruses, drugs and toxins (diuretics, steroids, oral contraceptives, azathioprine, sulfasalazine, isoniazid), and hereditary factors all must be considered.

No chronic medication or dietary manipulation is indicated in the usual patient convalescing from pancreatitis.

CHRONIC PANCREATITIS

method of
KENNETH W. WARREN, M.D.,
Boston, Massachusetts
and PABLO HERNANDEZ M, M.D.
Caracas, Venezuela

Introduction

Chronic pancreatitis is an inflammatory disease of the pancreas characterized clinically by a wide diversity of symptoms and signs, including pain, weight loss, disturbances of intestinal function (diarrhea and steatorrhea), cysts and pseudocysts, diabetes, jaundice, ascites, narcotic addiction, and alcoholism. Pain is the principal symptom, and its presence is often the reason for medical and, later, operative treatment. The significant clinical features in a series of 530 patients with chronic pancreatitis are shown in Table 1.

TABLE 1. **Significant Clinical Features in 530 Patients with Chronic Pancreatitis**

CLINICAL FEATURES	PATIENTS No.	%
Pain	527	99
Weight loss	417	79
Previous operation	370	70
Alcoholism	216	41
Narcotic addiction	185	35
Cholelithiasis	150	28
Pancreatic cysts	143	27
Pancreatolithiasis	114	22
Diabetes	96	18
Jaundice	73	14

TABLE 2. **Etiologic Antecedent in 530 Patients with Chronic Pancreatitis**

ANTECEDENT	PATIENTS No.	PATIENTS %
Chronic alcoholism	216	41
Cholelithiasis	150	28
Trauma	15	3
Congenital factors	3	0.6
None	196	37
Alcoholism and cholelithiasis	52	10

Etiology

The cause of chronic pancreatitis is unknown. Certain clinical antecedents, such as cholelithiasis, alcoholism, trauma to the pancreas, and obscure congenital factors, are known to be associated with chronic pancreatitis, but precise etiologic relationships are difficult to prove (Table 2).

Medical Treatment

Patients who have a moderate degree of chronic pancreatitis associated with infrequent episodes of pain but with no exocrine pancreatic insufficiency or diabetes may be treated medically.

A bland, low-fat diet with liberal amounts of proteins and carbohydrates is prescribed. Fat, between 85 and 100 grams a day, is permitted. Exocrine pancreatic insufficiency is treated with pancreatic extracts, preferably pancreatin (Viokase) or pancrelipase (Cotazym) alone or in combination, in doses of 8 to 20 tablets a day. Medical treatment may occasionally fail, because pancreatic enzymes are rapidly and irreversibly inactivated by gastric acid, and the enzymatic degradation is even more rapid and complete under the proteolytic action of pepsin. For these reasons, it is appropriate to use antacids even when gastric function is normal. Analgesic medication with non-narcotic agents may be used. Acetaminophen and propoxyphene, alone or in combination with aspirin or caffeine, have been effective. Diabetes should be controlled with diet, hypoglycemia agents, or insulin in accordance with the inherited disease. Alcohol is absolutely interdicted. Ample psychologic support is often helpful to these patients.

Surgical Treatment

Surgical treatment is mandatory when pain cannot be relieved by medical treatment without risk of narcotic addiction; when other clinical symptoms (weight loss and jaundice) or pseudocysts are present; or when such complications as obstruction of the duodenum, common bile duct, or portal vein appear. Of course, surgical treatment is also indicated if biliary tract disease is present and if malignancy is suspected. Once it has been decided that operative treatment is necessary, the next question applies to the type of operation which should be performed. We believe that, independent of etiologic factors, the surgical procedure must be chosen on the basis of pathologic findings in combination with radiographic studies of the pancreas. The pathologic changes produced by chronic pancreatitis range from swelling and mild induration of the gland to fibrosis, atrophy, patchy or widespread necrosis, cystic changes, and pancreatolithiasis. Several of these alterations may be seen in the same gland, and different phases in the progression of the disease may be observed in the same patient. The head of the pancreas, for example, may be normal macroscopically, but the body and tail may be involved by far-advanced disease. The core of these observations is that partial or complete obstruction of the pancreatic ducts is apparently responsible for recurrent attacks of pancreatitis, and the treatment therefore depends on relief of this obstruction.

Indirect Procedures. Surgical treatment of cholelithiasis and choledocholithiasis is necessary. Relief will occur, however, only if pancreatitis is at an early stage. Poor results will be obtained if advanced changes (cysts or calculi) are present. Other indirect procedures, such as diversion of the biliary tree or operations directed at the autonomic nervous system for relief of pain, are of doubtful benefit.

Direct Procedures. Operations on the pancreas itself are more effective, because the pathophysiologic problem in chronic pancreatitis is obstruction of the pancreatic ducts. The objective of the surgical procedure therefore is to relieve obstruction.

SPHINCTEROTOMY AND RETROGRADE DILATATION OF THE PANCREATIC DUCTS. This procedure is reserved for patients with mild or moderate degrees of pancreatitis whose obstruction is in the proximal part of the duct of Wirsung and duct of Santorini. Sphincterotomy alone gives satisfactory results in 50 per cent of these patients, whereas sphincterotomy combined with transduodenal exploration, manipulation, extraction of calculi, and intubation of the pancreatic duct to improve the flow of pancreatic secretions into the duodenum produces good results in 75 per cent of patients. Sphincteroplasty is more effective than sphincterotomy. In 3 per cent of patients, the main pancreatic duct is the duct of Santorini, and obstruction within this duct must also be removed. This procedure will be ineffective, however, if pathologic changes are consistent with advanced chronic pancreatitis and extensive pancreatolithiasis.

TRANSPANCREATIC EXPLORATION AND MANIPULATION OF THE PANCREATIC DUCTS. When more than one point of obstruction is evident in the pancreatic duct, retrograde exploration may be combined with transpancreatic incision of the duct of Wirsung in the neck or body of the gland. In this way, several areas of the stricture can be dilated and incised. If all points of stricture can be released, the pancreatic duct can be drained transduodenally. When this is not possible, anastomosis may be made between the duct and gastrointestinal tract.

PANCREATOJEJUNOSTOMY OR PANCREATOGASTROSTOMY. For patients who have advanced pancreatitis with pancreatolithiasis or a dilated duct, or both, we prefer to make a large longitudinal opening in the duct of Wirsung and anastomose this to a defunctionalized loop of jejunum or to the posterior wall of the stomach. The stoma should be sufficiently large to permit maintenance of permanent patency, and the pancreatic duct epithelium and the jejunal or gastric epithelium must be carefully apposed. A T tube is used to splint the anastomosis.

EVACUATION AND DRAINAGE OF PANCREATIC CYSTS OR ABSCESSES. Of the patients with advanced chronic pancreatitis, 25 per cent also have associated pancreatic cysts. Internal drainage gives the best results. The type of drainage depends on the location and the pathologic findings. The more frequent derivations used are cystogastrostomy, cystojejunostomy, and cystoduodenostomy. External drainage is reserved for patients who are desperately ill, or for those with small cysts or cysts in an unusual location (for example, the posterior aspect of the head of the pancreas or the uncinate process).

PANCREATIC RESECTION. Pancreatic resections are reserved for those patients with longstanding and extensive chronic pancreatitis with progressive calcifications and fibrosis that destroy both exocrine and endocrine parts of the gland. In such patients, ductal decompression has not been successful and symptoms have persisted. Therefore we resort to pancreatic resection, the extent of which depends upon the part of the gland involved by the disease. The procedures we have used are distal pancreatectomy, pancreatoduodenectomy, radical distal pancreatectomy, and total pancreatectomy.

No single operation is preferred for chronic pancreatitis. Each patient must be considered individually and treated according to the pathologic findings when the pancreas is exposed and examined in the operating room. It is only on the basis of this individual consideration that a proper surgical approach can be obtained and applied to pancreatic problems.

PEPTIC ULCER

method of
JAMES A. WHITAKER, M.D.,
and ALLAN R. COOKE, M.D.
Kansas City, Kansas

Despite the multitude of therapeutic regimens in treating peptic ulcer—e.g., diets, manipulation of living habits, drugs, or combinations of these regimens—there is a lack of adequately controlled double blind trials to evaluate therapy in this disease. Thus treatment is largely empirical.

Regardless of the method chosen to manage a particular patient with a peptic ulcer, the goals of therapy should be the same. One aims to relieve pain, hasten the healing of the ulcer, prevent complications, and, finally, prevent recurrences. Most attention had been focused on the first two of these goals in evaluating therapy, but the last two are of greater importance for long-term management. Studies directed specifically at therapy for preventing complications and recurrences are needed.

Regimens That Hasten the Healing of a Peptic Ulcer

Admission to the Hospital with Bed Rest. Patients with gastric ulcer heal their ulcers faster when treated as inpatients than when managed as outpatients. Bed rest at home has not been studied. Inpatient bed rest has not been studied carefully for duodenal ulcer. Patients with duodenal ulcer can be managed as outpatients. Because of the high cost of hospitalization, patients with gastric ulcer, after initial investigations, can be managed as outpatients.

Cessation of Cigarette Smoking. Smokers have an increased incidence of peptic ulcer (gastric and duodenal) and have increased morbidity and mortality from their ulcers. It has also been well established that gastric ulcers consistently heal more quickly when smoking is discontinued. Smoking should be discouraged.

Carbenoxolone. Carbenoxolone is a glycyrrhetinic acid derivative, used widely in Europe for several years. Evidence from a large number of clinical trials strongly supports its efficiency in hastening the healing of gastric ulcers. It is about as effective as bed rest, but does not hasten healing in those patients at bed rest in hospital. Recurrence rates for gastric ulcers upon stopping the drug vary, but range from 38 to 50 per cent in various series. Most studies in patients with duodenal ulcer have failed to show a significant effect on healing rates. The drug has aldosterone-like side effects with salt and fluid retention and hypokalemia and causes a modest increase in blood pressure. This will no doubt diminish its widespread acceptance. It is given in a dose of 100 mg. three times daily. This agent is awaiting Food and Drug Administration (FDA) approval before it can be released for general use.

H_2 Receptor Blockers. It has long been known that conventional antihistaminics (H_1 blockers) do not block the stimulatory effects of histamine on gastric acid secretion. Black, in 1972, at Smith, Kline and French Laboratories, introduced a new group of drugs which block the effect of histamine on gastric acid secretion. These drugs inhibit acid secretion in response to all stimuli, which suggests that histamine may be involved in all modes of stimulation of acid secretion. These agents are called *H_2 receptor antagonists* to distinguish them from the usual antihistamines or H_1 receptor antagonists.

The first agent of this group widely studied in patients was metiamide. It was found to inhibit meal-stimulated acid secretion by about 80 per cent when given in a single 300 mg. oral dose. However, because a small number of patients developed reversible agranulocytosis while on this agent, its commercial development was stopped. A similar agent, *cimetidine,* has been developed, which is as potent as metiamide but does not appear to depress the bone marrow. It does not contain the thiourea group in metiamide, the moiety thought to be responsible for the myelosuppressant effect. In at least four case-controlled double blind trials, cimetidine was found to reduce and shorten the duration of pain and to hasten the healing of duodenal ulcer. In most of the studies there was a good correlation between symptomatic relief and ulcer healing. A large double blind clinical trial is currently underway in the United States to evaluate its use in reflux esophagitis and gastric and duodenal ulcers. Recurrences when the drug is stopped, however, have not been closely looked at; nor are long-term studies available at this time.

Side effects in acute studies appear to be minimal, with mild increases in serum creatinine and serum glutamic pyruvic transaminase (SGPT) being seen occasionally in patients on doses of 1.6 grams daily or more. Eighty per cent of cimetidine is excreted unchanged in the urine, and thus dosages may have to be altered in patients with compromised renal function. Dosage is 0.8 to 1.6 grams daily in divided doses after meals and at bedtime.

Other Therapeutic Measures

Dietary. Hourly milk therapy and bland diets do not reduce gastric acidity, and milk probably increases net acid secretion. Four controlled studies have shown no benefit of a bland diet on the clinical course of peptic ulcer. We believe a patient should be allowed to eat a normal diet and modify it according to preference. Food should be avoided after dinner at night to reduce nocturnal acid secretion. Regular consumption of coffee (and perhaps colas) and alcohol should be avoided. Decaffeinated coffee is as potent a stimulant of acid secretion as regular coffee.

Antacids. Antacids have been widely used in the management of peptic ulcers. The rationale for their use is based on the facts that the adage "no acid, no ulcer" is generally valid, that peptic activity decreases as gastric acidity decreases, that experimental ulcer formation is inhibited by antacids, and that acid-reducing operations actually cure the ulcer. There are no convincing data at present that antacids improve healing, prevent recurrences, or prevent complications. Several uncontrolled studies suggest that antacids relieve pain, but even this has been questioned recently.

The effectiveness of an antacid depends upon its potency, the patient's parietal cell mass, gastric secretory response to eating, and the rate of gastric emptying. In fasting patients, a liquid antacid is emptied rapidly from the stomach, providing intragastric buffering for only 20 to 30 minutes. Postprandially, however, gastric acidity rises slowly during the first hour, and rapidly in the second hour. Antacids given at 1 hour after a meal will prevent this rise (Fig. 1). Thus a dose given at 1 and 3 hours after a meal has a prolonged buffering effect that may last until the next meal. Fordtran and coworkers have shown that buffering capacities of commercially available antacids can vary 17-fold. Thus the

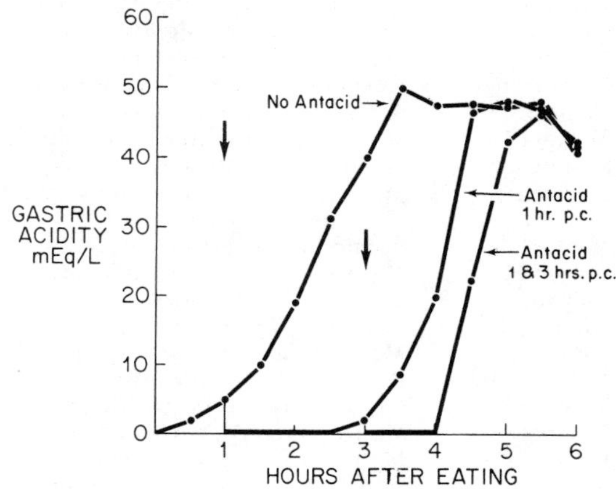

Figure 1. Average gastric acidity in a group of patients with duodenal ulcer after a steak meal, and the effect of 80 mEq. antacid given 1 hour after the meal or 1 and 3 hours after the meal. (From Sleisenger, M. H., and Fordtran, J. S. [eds.]: Gastrointestinal Disease. Philadelphia, W. B. Saunders Company, 1973, p. 732.)

secretory rate of the patient, as well as buffering capacity of the antacid selected, should be considered when selecting the dose of antacid to be administered.

DOSE. For gastric ulcer, Fordtran recommends about 40 mEq. hourly (10 ml. of aluminum and magnesium hydroxide with simethicone [Mylanta] or 15 ml. of magnesium and aluminum hydroxide [Maalox]) (see Table 1) during waking hours, until healing. Healing of the ulcer should be obvious in 3 weeks, about 90 per cent complete in 6 weeks, and complete in 12 weeks. If the ulcer fails to heal in this time, there should be no question of adequate antacid therapy. After healing is complete, approximately 80 mEq. 1 hour after meals and at bedtime is recommended for an indefinite period. This is done in the hope of preventing recurrences, which occur in 50 to 60 per cent of patients who have been on unspecified or irregular therapy.

For duodenal ulcer, Fordtran recommends 80 mEq. hourly while awake until the patient is pain free and then 80 mEq. 1 and 3 hours after meals and at bedtime for 6 weeks. In patients with recurrences, antacid therapy is recommended indefinitely.

We believe this regimen is a good guideline if one thinks intensive antacid therapy aids in the healing of peptic ulcer. Many physicians would use antacids only for the relief of pain, and even this is questioned. Compliance is a variable factor, making intensive long-term antacid therapy difficult to maintain, and thus patient education in proper use of antacids is recommended. Also, significant side effects can occur with the large doses recommended above. These side effects are diarrhea (magnesium); constipation, acid rebound, and hypercalcemia (calcium); binding of phosphorus, tetracycline, atropine, and iron (aluminum hydroxide); sodium overload (see Table 2); and milk-alkali syndrome. Because of the many disadvantages of calcium, some experts would not recommend calcium-containing antacids, particularly if large doses are to be used.

Although antacid tablets are more convenient than liquids, they are less effective buffers and must be chewed thoroughly for maximal effectiveness. As a result, they are not recommended for management of patients with active ulcer disease.

Because antacids seem to relieve ulcer pain, because they are rational by virtue of their ability to reduce gastric acidity, and because they are time honored, they will continue to be prescribed. However, as stated above, their effectiveness is unproved.

TABLE 1. **Antacid Potencies—The Number of mEq. in 10 ml. of Antacid Titrated to pH 3.0 with 0.1 N HCl, 60 RPM, 37° C.**

ANTACID	CONTENTS	0 TIME *mEq.*	0 TIME %*	120 MIN.† *mEq.*
Ducon	Al and Mg hydroxides, Ca carbonate	20.2	29	70.4
Mylanta II	Mg and Al hydroxides, simethicone	4.3	10	41.4
Titralac	Glycine, Ca carbonate	32.9	85	38.7
Camalox	Al and Mg hydroxides, Ca carbonate	12.7	49	35.9
Aludrox	Al hydroxide gel, Mg hydroxide	6.4	23	28.1
Maalox	Mg and Al hydroxide gel	5.5	21	25.8
Creamalin	Hexitol stabilized Al hydroxide gel, Mg hydroxide	11.1	43	25.7
Di-Gel	Al and Mg hydroxides, simethicone	5.6	23	24.5
Mylanta	Mg and Al hydroxides, simethicone	4.1	17	23.8
Silain-Gel	Mg and Al hydroxides, simethicone	3.3	14	23.1
Marblen	Mg and Ca carbonates, Al hydroxide, Mg phosphate, Mg trisilicate	17.2	75	22.8
WinGel	Al and Mg hydroxides, hexitol stabilized	8.4	37	22.5
Gelusil M	Mg trisilicate, Al hydroxide, Mg hydroxide	11.1	49	22.3
Riopan	Mg and Al hydroxides	3.5	16	22.1
Amphojel	Al hydroxide gel	3.9	20	19.3
A-M-T	Mg trisilicate, Al hydroxide gel	6.5	36	17.9
Kolantyl Gel	Bentyl, Al hydroxide, Mg hydroxide, methylcellulose	5.7	34	16.9
Trisogel	Mg trisilicate, Al hydroxide gel	7.2	43	16.5
Malcogel	Mg trisilicate, Al hydroxide gel	3.9	25	15.9
Gelusil	Mg trisilicate, Al hydroxide	4.1	31	13.3
Robalate	Dihydroxyaluminum aminoacetate	3.4	30	11.3
Phosphaljel	Al phosphate gel	2.5	59	4.2

*Percentage of total buffer capacity at 120 minutes. Indicates the rapidity of onset of action.

†The value in this column is a measure of buffer capacity of the antacid in milliequivalents per 10 ml. after 120 minutes. (Modified from Sleisenger, M. H., and Fordtran, J. S. [eds.]: Gastrointestinal Disease. Philadelphia, W. B. Saunders Co., 1973, p. 726.)

TABLE 2. **Sodium Content of Some Antacids per 10 ml. Dose**

ANTACID	SODIUM CONTENT (mEQ.)
Ducon	0.64
Mylanta II	0.74
Titralac	1.10
Camalox	0.22
Aludrox	0.43
Maalox	0.22
Creamalin	0.26
WinGel	0.31
Gelusil M	0.62
Riopan	0.06
Amphojel	0.46
A-M-T	0.84
Kolantyl Gel	0.53
Gelusil	0.59

Anticholinergics. Anticholinergics act by competitive inhibition of acetylcholine release from nerve endings and in optimal doses decrease basal and stimulated gastric acid and pepsin secretion by about 50 per cent, a reduction similar to that of vagotomy. When administered 30 minutes before eating, they act for about 4 to 5 hours, although the pH over a 24 hour period is mostly above 2. To achieve this response they must be given in an "optimal" dose, which is just below the appearance of side effects (dry mouth, blurred vision, and urinary retention).

Despite many clinical trials there remains continued controversy about the usefulness of anticholinergics in increasing the healing rates of duodenal ulcer and in preventing recurrences. This unresolved problem is in part due to the virtual impossibility of conducting studies under "blind" conditions because of the obvious side effects. Only one study has been done in gastric ulcer in which an anticholinergic plus antacid was tested against antacid alone. This study indicated a lower recurrence rate with the drug combination. These results need confirmation.

For the aforementioned reasons anticholinergics are not recommended by most physicians, and we do not use them routinely. If used, they are usually given to younger, otherwise healthy patients as a nocturnal dose when side effects would be unnoticed. Usual dosage is 1 tablet 30 minutes before meals and 2 at bedtime, with stepwise increase of this dose until side effects are noticed. One dose or half dose less than that which causes side effects is the "optimal" dose. Typical dosage schedules are as follows: poldine, 4 mg. 30 minutes before meals and 8 mg. at night; oxyphencyclimine, 5 mg. 30 minutes before meals and 10 mg. at night. However, it must be emphasized that each patient must have his dose individualized. Contraindications include gastrointestinal hemorrhage (as anticholinergics will mask the tachycardia of volume depletion), gastric retention and pyloric obstruction, reflux esophagitis, achalasia, urinary retention and prostatism, and glaucoma.

Gastric Irradiation. Gastric irradiation has been popularized primarily by Palmer at the University of Chicago. A standard dose is delivered to the acid-bearing portion; gastric secretion decreases in approximately 90 per cent of the patients, and histamine-fast achlorhydria, which occurs in 10 per cent of the patients, may last 6 months or longer. About a 50 per cent reduction in acid secretion which persists for greater than 1 year was achieved in 40 per cent of about 1500 patients treated in this manner. This can be useful therapy in patients with complicated medical problems which make them especially high risk surgical candidates.

Other Treatments Not Generally Recommended

Sedation. Sedation has not been found to be of value in peptic ulcer and is not recommended for routine use. Some physicians believe that sedatives may be useful in the anxious patient.

Estrogens. Estrogens have been found to moderately increase healing rates in duodenal ulcer but not in gastric ulcer. Since they have serious side effects, they are not recommended.

Antisecretory Hormones. Secretin, glucagon, vasoactive inhibitory peptide, and urogastrone all inhibit acid secretion and theoretically may be useful in treating peptic ulcer. However, all are inactive orally, which is a major limitation. Only secretin has been studied in a clinical trial; it was found to be ineffective in pain relief (even though gastric acid was reduced significantly) and healing of duodenal ulcer. The other hormones have not been tested clinically. Thus, on present data, these hormones are not recommended.

Prostaglandins. Prostaglandins are potent inhibitors of acid secretion. Their structure has been modified to make them effective orally and long acting. An example is 16,16-dimethyl prostaglandin E_2, which in a dose of 1 microgram per kg. caused about 80 per cent inhibition of pentagastrin-stimulated acid secretion. Their major side effect has been diarrhea, although good inhibition of acid secretion can be attained effectively with doses that cause a minimum of diarrhea. In a few trials, prostaglandins have been found to hasten healing of gastric ulcers. The evidence is not sufficient to draw conclusions. At present, they are not recommended.

Zinc Sulfate, Colloidal Bismuth and Sodium Amylosulfate. These agents may be useful in increasing healing rates in peptic ulcer. Sodium amylosulfate was found to aid in healing gastric ulcers but not duodenal ulcers. The evidence is insufficient at present to draw firm conclusions. We currently do not recommend these.

Cabbage Juice, Vitamins A and C, Cholestyramine, Soya Bean Milk, Gastric Freezing. These have all been proved to be worthless in ulcer therapy. Metoclopramide requires further study. At present we do not recommend it.

Interdictions

As mentioned before, alcohol and caffeine-containing beverages should be avoided. Potentially ulcerogenic drugs, particularly unbuffered aspirin, should be discontinued and substitutes used if available.

Addendum

Recently in a placebo-controlled trial, 30 ml. of Mylanta II given 1 hour and 3 hours after meals and at bedtime was found to accelerate the healing of duodenal ulcer. This study indicates that antacids in large doses are effective in treating duodenal ulcer.

TUMORS OF THE STOMACH

method of
R. S. SHAPIRO, M.D.,
and W. R. SCHILLER, M.D.
Toledo, Ohio

The diagnosis and treatment of gastric tumors represent a challenge for both physicians and surgeons, because the symptoms of gastric malignancy are often absent or nonspecific and far advanced disease is usually present by the time classic symptoms appear.

Benign gastric lesions can often be differentiated from malignant ones by x-ray and endoscopic examinations. These include benign tumors of blood vessels, nerves, lymphatics, fat, and smooth muscle. Usually they can be adequately treated by segmental resection of the portion of stomach containing the lesion. Double contrast examinations of the stomach have increased the accuracy in detection of small lesions, and the use of transendoscopic brush cytology has further improved the accuracy in evaluation of questionably malignant lesions. Japanese clinicians report that screening examinations of persons with a high risk of developing gastric carcinoma are effective in detecting the smaller, curable lesions. Included in this group of high risk persons are those with such premalignant gastric lesions as atrophic gastritis, pernicious anemia, achlorhydria, intestinal metaplasia, and polyps of the villous and adenomatous varieties.

Gastric Polyps

Adenomatous gastric polyps are often an incidental finding on gastrointestinal roentgenograms or endoscopy and usually produce no symptoms. However, they occasionally may be responsible for abdominal pain or gastrointestinal bleeding, and their malignant potential appears to increase with size. The risk of malignancy is significant for polyps larger than 2 cm., especially if sessile. Evaluation should include barium upper gastrointestinal x-rays and endoscopy with brush cytology and biopsy. Asymptomatic adenomatous polyps smaller than 2 cm. or on a long stalk can be treated adequately by endoscopic removal or observed by periodic examinations. However, some benign polyps may require removal because of bleeding or herniation through the pylorus. All symptomatic polyps, sessile polyps, or those larger than 2 cm. should be removed with a margin of normal gastric wall. Multiple polyps of this type may require partial gastric resection. On the other hand, hypertrophic gastric polyps are not premalignant, and removal can be evaluated according to the presence of symptoms in each individual case. Any polyp with histologic invasion should be treated by gastric resection.

Gastric Ulcers

Approximately 5 to 10 per cent of gastric ulcers are malignant de novo. Symptoms and location are usually of no value in determining malignancy. X-ray appearance is occasionally diagnostic of cancer but is more often equivocal. Endoscopic brush cytology is the single most reliable test of malignancy. A negative endoscopic biopsy does not exclude carcinoma because of the small size of tissue sampled. Persistence of symptoms or failure to achieve a 50 per cent reduction in ulcer size in 4 weeks or a 90 per cent reduction in 6 weeks despite medical treatment should lead to surgical removal. The cooperative Veterans Administration study on gastric ulcers demonstrated a high incidence of ulcer recurrence, and increased incidence of gastric cancer was found in those patients whose ulcers failed to heal by 12 weeks.

Muscular Tumors

Muscular tumors constitute the largest group of benign gastric neoplasms. Although usually asymptomatic, they may produce pain or bleeding. These lesions are intramural in location and may grow both intraluminally and toward the serosa, producing a so-called "dumbbell" appearance. They may grow to a large size, especially in the fundus. Radiographically, the smooth filling defect is occasionally mistaken for a lymphoma. Endoscopy is useful in establishing the nature of the lesion and in obtaining a histologic diagnosis. Local resection is all that is required for cure. Recurrence is exceedingly rare.

The clinical presentation of gastric leiomyosarcoma is similar to that of its benign counterpart. Malignancy often cannot be ascertained except by careful histologic study of multiple sections obtained after removal of the specimen. Leiomyosarcomas begin intramurally and may ulcerate or invade adjacent organs by direct extension. Distant metastases are rare. A wide en bloc excision of tumor and adjacent invaded organs is the treatment of choice. Local excision, if possible, should be performed to prevent bleeding and obstruction even if all gross tumor cannot be removed. Although results of treatment are better than for carcinoma, extensive local spread has often occurred by the time the diagnosis is made.

Gastric Lymphomas

Lymphomas of the stomach may mimic symptoms of other upper gastrointestinal maladies. It is often impossible to distinguish them from carcinoma by gross examination, although they do have a characteristic microscopic appearance. It is important to make the distinction because of the better prognosis and radiosensitivity of gastric lymphomas. In addition, gastric lymphomas must be distinguished from pseudolymphoma and benign lymphoid hyperplasia. Endoscopy with biopsy may be very helpful in evaluation of these lesions. Jacobs observed achlorhydria in about one third of patients with gastric lymphoma, whereas all patients with pseudolymphoma had normal gastric analysis.

Primary gastric lymphomas arising from neoplastic submucosal lymphatics must be differentiated from disseminated lymphoma metastatic to gastric lymphatics, which has a poor prognosis. Patients with this widely disseminated type of lymphoma which also involves the stomach should not undergo aggressive surgical therapy but instead should receive systemic chemotherapy.

Work-up of localized gastric lymphoma should include (1) careful physical examination, including all lymph node areas; (2) upper gastrointestinal (UGI) series; (3) gastroscopy with brush cytology and biopsy; (4) liver function tests and liver-spleen scan; (5) bone marrow biopsy; and (6) lymphangiography and gallium scanning in selected patients.

Laparotomy should be performed on all patients except those with a disseminated lymphoma and those whose medical condition precludes operation. Resection should include an en bloc removal of primary tumor, spleen, omentum, adjacent lymph nodes, and invaded organs. This most often requires a subtotal gastric resection, but occasionally a total gastrectomy is necessary. A resection should be performed, if possible, even if gross tumor remains, because lymphomas are quite radiosensitive and prolonged survival and even cure may follow resection and irradiation. The use of routine postoperative irradiation in patients without evidence of residual disease is controversial, but most investigators now favor its use. In patients treated by a combination of surgical resection and radiotherapy, Burnett and Herbert reported a 5 year cure rate of 67 per cent, whereas in patients treated by gastrectomy alone only 43 per cent survived 5 years. Furthermore, Wolferth and associates reported a 66 month median survival time in patients who received both curative resection and radiotherapy, compared to 39 months in patients treated by surgery alone.

Although attempts have been made to correlate survival to histologic cell type, there has been little success, primarily because of difficulties in classification. In general, however, lymphocytic lymphoma is thought to have a good prognosis, whereas reticulum cell sarcoma has a poorer outlook.

Adenocarcinoma

The diagnosis of gastric carcinoma is often made too late. There is evidence that identification of early lesions may be expected to improve survival. Prognosis appears to depend on the depth of invasion and the presence and extent of lymph node and distant metastases.

Work-up should be aimed at establishing a histologic diagnosis and searching for possible distant metastases. In a series of autopsies performed upon patients with gastric cancer, metastases were found in the liver in 70 per cent; peritoneum, omentum, and mesentery in 43 per cent; lungs and pleura in 33 per cent; and bones in 11 per cent. Evaluation for metastases should take these facts into account, and therefore preoperative work-up should include (1) complete physical examination, (2) upper gastrointestinal x-rays, (3) chest x-ray, (4) gastroscopy with brush cytology and biopsy, (5) liver function tests and liver scan, and (6) carcinoembryonic antigen (CEA) determination.

Prior to operation, anemia, dehydration, and electrolyte imbalances should be corrected by the administration of blood and fluids. Nasogastric decompression should be provided for several days to patients with evidence of obstruction. Mechanical and antibiotic bowel preparation should be accomplished to permit resection of invaded colon. In addition, the patient's nutritional status should be investigated. Significant weight loss and low serum protein and albumin levels are common and may be corrected by a course of enteral or intravenous hyperalimentation. Such nutritional support enhances the specific and nonspecific immune responses to stress and allows for improved healing of wounds. The overall result is a diminution of the morbidity and mortality of major surgery on these patients.

The operation of choice for gastric carcinoma depends on tumor size, location, and the degree of extragastric spread. An adequate operation should consist of an en bloc resection of primary tumor, regional lymph nodes, and invaded adjacent organs. At least a 5 cm. proximal and 2 to 3 cm. distal tumor-free margin should be obtained with the aid of frozen sections to verify normal resection margins. For small lesions involving the body or antrum of the stomach, a radical omentectomy, and removal of regional lymph nodes along the greater and lesser curvatures, splenic vessels, left and right gastric arteries, and retroduodenal area. Small lesions of the gastric fundus and cardia may be handled by esophagogastric resection, splenectomy, and pyloroplasty.

Total gastrectomy is no longer routinely performed because of its increased morbidity and mortality. In addition, studies have failed to establish its superiority over radical subtotal gastrectomy for most lesions. However, total gastrectomy should be performed for extensive lesions and linitis plastica when subtotal gastric resection is inadequate to control the primary lesion. This situation may be encountered in about 10 to 20 per cent of all gastric carcinomas. The high mortality and morbidity previously seen following total gastrectomy have been reduced with the aid of intensive preoperative supportive therapy, improvements in the methods of reconstruction of gastrointestinal continuity, and appropriate postoperative medical therapy. The use of intravenous hyperalimentation via the subclavian vein both pre- and postoperatively has been useful. The overall 5 year survival for carcinoma of the stomach remains in the range of 10 to 15 per cent. Of those resected for cure, approximately 35 per cent can be expected to survive 5 years, although it must be remembered that half of all patients are incurable at the time they are first seen.

Reconstruction of gastrointestinal continuity with esophagoduodenostomy or esophagojejunostomy (with or without enteroenterostomy) is associated with a high incidence of malnutrition and reflux esophagitis. The use of a 30 cm. Roux-en-Y esophagojejunostomy has been effective in limiting reflux esophagitis. A variety of pouch reconstructions have been attempted in an effort to replace the gastric reservoir. These have included the use of colon and jejunum. Colonic interposition was found to be less satisfactory because of excessive stasis and reflux. Of the various types of jejunal interposition, the Hunt-Lawrence pouch is the most popular. In some studies done following total gastrectomy for excision of gastric cancer, the Hunt-Lawrence pouch was shown to limit malnutrition, weight loss, anemia, and dumping. Other studies, however, done following total gastrectomy for nonmalignant conditions show that it offers little over Roux-en-Y constructions in terms of caloric intake, weight gain, malabsorption, or dumping.

The recognition and treatment of postgastrectomy vitamin B_{12}, folic acid, and iron deficiencies are important. Total gastrectomy removes the endogenous source of intrinsic factor; therefore 100 micrograms of vitamin B_{12} should be given intramuscularly each month. Patients with folic acid deficiencies should receive 1 mg. of folic acid orally per day. Those with iron deficiency should receive orally 300 mg. of ferrous sulfate three times daily. Knowledge of the etiology and treatment of postgastrectomy physiologic alterations has improved significantly. The dumping syndrome is often controlled by dietary restriction of carbohydrates and by avoiding liquids with meals. Milk and milk products especially seem to be associated with the dumping syndrome. Blind loop syndrome resulting from bacterial overgrowth in the afferent loop is often corrected by a 2 week course of oral tetracycline. Surgical revision may occasionally be required.

A palliative resection to prevent bleeding and obstruction should be performed, if possible, even if all gross tumor cannot be removed. Other alternatives include anterior gastrojejunostomy to bypass the neoplasm and feeding gastrostomy or jejunostomy. However, experience has shown that resection provides the best palliation and occasionally a chance for prolonged survival.

Postoperatively, patients should be followed periodically for evidence of residual or recurrent tumor. This may be treated by radiotherapy and chemotherapy, which are presently available for the treatment of advanced disease. Although the results of radiotherapy alone are discouraging, the combination of radiotherapy and 5-fluorouracil has been reported by several investigators to have a significant palliative effect. To date, only 5-fluorouracil, mitomycin, and the nitrosoureas have been shown to have significant antitumor activity against gastric carcinoma. Mitomycin is used infrequently because of its bone marrow toxicity. Combination chemotherapy has improved the response rate somewhat over single drug regimens. The most encouraging combinations have been 5-fluorouracil and BCNU and 5-fluorouracil and CCNU, although they are still investigational.

TUMORS OF THE COLON AND RECTUM

method of
ROSCOE E. MILLER, M.D.,
and GLEN A. LEHMAN, M.D.
Indianapolis, Indiana

Large bowel tumors are found in approximately 10 per cent of adults over 50 years of age. More than 90 per cent of such lesions are benign; colorectal carcinoma remains the most common visceral malignant neoplasm.

Accurate identification of large bowel tumors has been greatly advanced by the increasing use and availability of quality air contrast barium enemas and fiberoptic colonoscopy. Nevertheless, sigmoidoscopy, digital rectal examination, and stool occult blood testing remain essential in the evaluation of patients with colorectal symptoms.

Management of such tumors is largely dependent upon their size and location, their degree of suspicion of malignancy, and the general health of the patient.

Benign Tumors

Benign colorectal tumors may be divided into those of (1) mucosal origin (polyps) and (2) submucosal origin. The latter group comprises less than 5 per cent of all colonic tumors and includes leiomyomas, lipomas, and carcinoid tumors. The carcinoid tumors require complete endoscopic or surgical removal because of their rare associated malignant potential. Other submucosal lesions generally require no therapy unless bleeding, obstruction, or suspicion of carcinoma persists.

Polyps are further categorized as (1) pedunculated—with a stalk; and (2) sessile—without a stalk.

Hyperplastic polyps account for more than 50 per cent of polyps less than 5 mm. in diameter. These sessile lesions are generally found only at sigmoidoscopy or fiberoptic colonoscopy. All polyps of such small size, no matter what their final pathology, may be removed in toto by biopsy or fulgurated without histologic examination. Hyperplastic polyps are not believed to have any malignant potential. If these small lesions are seen at barium enema and are beyond sigmoidoscopy range, neither colonoscopy nor surgery is indicated; a repeat barium enema in 1 to 2 years appears warranted.

Adenomatous polyps are true neoplasms of the colonic mucosa. Although discussed here under the heading of benign tumors, these lesions may undergo malignant degeneration. Adenomas may be clinically grouped according to size.

Small (<5 mm.) adenomatous polyps are managed just as are hyperplastic polyps (see above).

Medium-sized (6 to 10 mm.) polyps, whether pedunculated or sessile, are best managed by total excisional biopsy at fiberoptic colonoscopy or sigmoidoscopy. An acceptable alternative, especially if fiberoptic colonoscopy is not readily available or the patient has significant associated disease (e.g., emphysema, past myocardial infarction), is expectant observation with a follow-up air contrast barium enema in 6 to 12 months. The incidence of invasive carcinoma in this group probably does not exceed 1 per cent, although in situ carcinoma may occur in up to 6 per cent. After a follow-up examination shows no change, the asymptomatic patient can be followed by air contrast barium enema at 12 to 18 month intervals.

Large polyps (>11 mm.) carry a significant risk of invasive carcinoma and should therefore be removed in toto at fiberoptic colonoscopy or sigmoidoscopy. Pedunculated lesions greater than 3 to 4 cm. or sessile lesions greater than 2 cm. are frequently difficult to remove at endoscopy and may therefore require laparotomy or transanal operative excision.

When the removed polyp shows in situ carcinoma, no further resection is needed. If invasion beyond the muscular mucosa exists but 1 to 2 cm. of uninvolved stalk is present with the specimen, no further resection is probably indicated. Stalk invasion without a free margin is an indication for segmental resection. Extensive stalk invasion or invasion occurring in a sessile lesion generally requires a standard cancer operation.

Once a benign or malignant lesion has been removed by endoscopy or surgery, a follow-up air contrast barium enema and sigmoidoscopy are indicated in 6 to 12 months and at 1 to 3 year intervals thereafter. If the original lesion was beyond sigmoidoscopic range, but no new lesion is seen on a quality air contrast barium enema, controversy presently exists among radiologic, endoscopic, and surgical experts as to the necessity of follow-up fiberoptic colonoscopy.

Villous adenomas are the second type of true neoplasms. The majority of these polypoid lesions are less than 4 cm. in diameter, being either sessile or pedunculated. Their management is the same as that outlined for adenomatous polyps. Approximately 20 per cent of these tumors grow to greater than 4 cm. in size and give a typical frond-like radiographic appearance. Rarely, severe watery diarrhea and hypokalemia accompany these large tumors. Large villous adenomas have up to a 50 per cent invasive carcinoma rate, thereby indicating a need for surgical removal. In the high risk surgical patient in whom multiple endoscopic biopsies reveal no cancer, fulguration and close follow-up at 3 to 6 month intervals is an acceptable alternative.

Villoglandular polyps with mixed features of villous adenoma and adenomatous polyps are managed similarly according to their size and degree of associated malignancy.

Juvenile polyps are hamartomatous lesions composed of inflammatory and connective tissue elements. These are not true neoplasms and have no premalignant potential. The majority of these polyps are pedunculated and occur in children. If asymptomatic, juvenile polyps require no therapy, as most will regress or slough. If symptoms of bleeding, obstruction, or intussusception occur, complete removal of such polyps by sigmoidoscopy or colonoscopy is indicated. No follow-up x-ray or endoscopy is usually necessary if the patient remains asymptomatic.

Inherited polyposis syndromes are uncommon but important manifestations of colonic tumors. *Familial polyposis* and *Gardner's syndrome* are autosomal dominant diseases with virtually 100 per cent malignant potential. Both diseases are characterized by generalized colonic adenomatous polyps. (Additionally, patients with Gardner's syndrome may have small bowel, stomach, bone, or subcutaneous tumors.) When diagnosed, the most accepted therapy is total colectomy with ileostomy. A less desirable alternative approach is subtotal colectomy with ileoproctostomy, with frequent follow-up and fulguration of residual polyps. Even if asymptomatic, children and siblings of polyposis patients over 10 years of age require stool occult blood testing and sigmoidoscopy annually. Air contrast barium enema should be performed to further evaluate members with positive symptoms or screening studies. A few authorities recommend that fiberoptic colonoscopy or air contrast barium enema be done at 1 to 3 year intervals for screening purposes.

Peutz-Jeghers syndrome is an autosomal dominant disease characterized by hamartomatous polyps of the stomach, small bowel, and colon, with very low malignant potential. Additionally, diagnostic melanin pigment spots occur on the lips and buccal mucosa. Symptomatic lesions (bleeding, obstruction, intussusception) require endoscopic or surgical removal.

Malignant Tumors

Adenocarcinoma comprises more than 98 per cent of malignant colonic tumors. Once the diagnosis has been established, surgical extirpation of the carcinoma and the associated lymphatic drainage is the standard means of therapy. Surgical resection, using the "no touch" technique, offers the best chances of long-term survival. Primary colonic anastomosis and preservation of the anal sphincter are not possible with lesions of the mid and lower rectum. In such patients colostomy acceptance and management are greatly facilitated by visitation with members of an ostomy society.

Evaluation for metastases preoperatively should include liver function tests and a chest x-ray. If bone pain, central nervous system symptoms, or hepatic chemistry abnormality exists, appropriate scans (bone, brain, liver, including computerized tomography scans), bone x-rays, and/or liver biopsy are recommended. If metastases are found preoperatively, resection or diverting colostomy is still necessary if the tumor is causing significant bleeding or obstruction. Controversy still exists as to whether or not patients benefit from resection of all primary tumors in the presence of metastases so as to decrease the tumor mass.

Fulguration has a very limited role in the therapy of rectal cancer. Small lesions occurring in the elderly or high risk operative candidates may be ablated by this means, although recurrence rates are high. In patients with distant metastases, bleeding or obstruction may be controlled with local fulguration. Fulguration is to be condemned in good risk patients with operable lesions.

The value of preoperative radiation for rectosigmoid cancer is currently being further evaluated. Initial reports indicate slightly improved 5 year survival rates from a preoperative dose of 2000 to 4600 rads given over 2 to 5 weeks. Completion of current studies is necessary before this method can be advocated for all patients with rectosigmoid cancer. Palliative radiation can aid in the control of obstruction or bleeding from inoperable rectal tumors. In some patients radiation may shrink the tumor and convert an "inoperable" case into an operable one.

If metastases are documented, chemotherapy is generally recommended. A variety of single and combined drug programs have been tested, but none appear to be superior to 5-fluorouracil alone. Approximately 15 per cent of patients will show transient tumor regression and slightly improved survival rates at the expense of chemotherapy side effects.

The importance of adequate nutrition in cancer patients is now more recognized. Negative protein balances occurring especially in the perioperative period may be avoided by intravenous hyperalimentation or judicious use of elemental diets. The side effects of chemotherapy are tolerated more readily in the well nourished patient.

Despite all the aforementioned therapeutic modalities, the 5 year expected survival for all patients with cancer of the colon and rectum as a group is approximately 50 per cent. Totally asymptomatic patients with large bowel carcinomas have a greater than 85 per cent 5 year survival. It seems evident that the major advances in treatment of these neoplasms must be oriented toward earlier detection or prevention. Fiberoptic colonoscopy and air contrast barium enema are sensitive detectors for carcinoma but are not practical means to screen large numbers of patients (except those with specifically high risk such as chronic ulcerative colitis, familial polyposis, or past colonic carcinoma patients). Carcinoembryonic antigen is of no screening value, but will help detect recurrence of tumor after resection. Sigmoidoscopy and stool occult blood testing are more practical screening tools, but also have limitations.

The limited human data available on prevention of colonic carcinoma suggest that removal of all benign colonic polyps and consumption of a diet low in fats are associated with a lower subsequent carcinoma incidence. The importance of dietary fiber has received great attention in recent years, but has not been convincingly shown to decrease subsequent carcinoma development. Additionally, recent studies indicate that disulfiram (Antabuse) and certain vitamin A analogues decrease the incidence of chemical toxin-induced colonic carcinoma in experimental animals.

ACUTE VIRAL AND BACTERIAL DYSENTERIES

method of
RALPH A. GIANNELLA, M.D.
Lexington, Kentucky

The acute viral and bacterial dysenteries are worldwide in distribution, spare no population group, and affect all ages. In the developing world, acute diarrheal disease is the most important cause of death in malnourished infants and children. Although acute diarrheal disease is a less serious problem in the United States, it remains an important cause of morbidity in infants, the elderly, and debilitated patients, and is second only to the common cold as a cause of illness in the population at large.

Many species of bacteria and viruses cause acute diarrhea either by direct person-to-person spread or by ingestion of contaminated food or water. The past several years have witnessed major advances in the definition of new causative agents of acute diarrhea, in our understanding of the specific diarrheal syndromes, and in our understanding of the diarrheal process in general.

Pathogenesis

The pathogenesis of acute bacterial diarrheal disease is currently classified into the following categories: (1) *Toxigenic*—those bacteria that cause diarrhea by the elaboration of an enterotoxin which stimulates the small intestinal mucosa to actively secrete fluid. There is no mucosal damage. (2) *Invasive*—those bacteria that penetrate the mucosa of the small and/or large intestine, cause an acute inflammatory reaction, and interfere with normal salt and water transport mechanisms. (3) *Mixed*—bacterial pathogens which both invade the mucosa and elaborate enterotoxins.

The "toxigenic" bacteria, *Vibrio cholerae, Vibrio parahaemolyticus, Escherichia coli, Staphylococcus aureus, Clostridium perfringens,* and *Bacillus cereus,* may all cause diarrhea by a similar mechanism. The elaborated enterotoxins activate the mucosal enzyme adenyl cyclase, thereby enhancing the intracellular concentrations of cyclic AMP. Cyclic AMP then stimulates the outpouring of fluid by the small intestine. The mechanism(s) by which invasive bacteria cause diarrhea are as yet undefined. Thus far, a number of viruses have been found to cause diarrhea in man. In infants and children, reovirus-like agents (also called duovirus, orbivirus, and rotavirus) appear to be the most important cause of so-called "winter diarrhea." In adults, a number of parvoviruses have been shown to cause diarrhea—e.g., Norwalk, Montgomery, Hawaii agents. These are currently named after the location of initial isolation of the viruses. The mechanism by which these viruses cause diarrhea is currently unclear, but several of these agents invade the intestinal mucosa and alter mucosal histology.

Therapy

The objectives of therapy include (1) rehydration and prevention of dehydration, (2) abbreviating the course of the illness, if possible (i.e., antimicrobials), and (3) symptomatic therapy. Fortunately, most episodes of acute diarrhea are self-limited and in fact abate before a specific diagnosis can be made. Thus in most patients specific therapy is not possible or not warranted, and the indiscriminate use of antibiotics is to be deplored.

Since most episodes of acute diarrhea are self-limited, concerns of diet are usually of minor importance. Cessation of oral intake is not usually necessary—except in the case of *severe* vomiting—and may be detrimental to gut function if prolonged. If diarrhea is severe or persists beyond 1 day, avoidance of fat and milk products is recommended, because malabsorption and disaccharide intolerance (usually lactose) may occur, especially in infants. It should be remembered that in some patients (especially infants and children) lactose intolerance may persist for days or weeks after cessation of diarrhea. This is usually manifested as intolerance for milk products.

Fluid Therapy. In most patients with acute infectious diarrhea, the most important aspect of therapy is the replacement of fluid and electrolytes lost in stool and vomitus and the prevention of dehydration. This can best be accomplished by the oral route by the ingestion of carbonated beverages, apple juice, clear soups, or Karo syrup plus water, or with commercially available electrolyte solutions (Pedialyte, Lytren, Gatorade). These commercially available solutions are not ideal for oral rehydration because of their low content of electrolytes or inadequate or excessive glucose concentrations. They are, however, superior to plain tap water.

A more appropriate oral solution is an isotonic balanced glucose-electrolyte solution containing sufficient electrolytes and adequate but not excessive concentrations of glucose. Ingestion of such a balanced solution, by virtue of its glucose content, will enhance intestinal absorption of salt and water and may actually reduce stool output. Such a solution ("GE-SOL") can be made as follows: sodium chloride, 3.5 grams; sodium bicarbonate, 2.5 grams; potassium chloride, 1.5 grams; and glucose, 20.0 grams per liter of tap water. This solution yields approximately, in mM. per liter (±5 per cent):

Na^+	90
K^+	20
HCO_3^-	30
Cl^-	80
Glucose	111

On *rare* occasions, a child, usually malnourished, will be unable to absorb glucose, and ingestion of a glucose-electrolyte solution will aggravate the diarrhea. This can be detected by the finding of a high concentration of glucose in stool and by a reduction in stool volume on cessation of glucose-electrolyte oral therapy.

Patients with *mild dehydration* may be rehydrated by oral ingestion of glucose-electrolyte solutions. Patients with *moderate or severe dehydration* are best hospitalized and rehydrated with intravenous fluids. The volume of fluid administered is determined by the degree of dehydration and by the magnitude of continuing losses in stool and vomitus, and can be monitored by clinical signs and adequacy of urine output. In such patients, the composition of intravenous fluids should approximate the composition of the diarrheal fluid. Isotonic saline alone is not adequate, because potassium and base (HCO_3^-) lost in fecal output must be replaced as well. Solutions of the following general composition are recommended: sodium (120 to 130 mEq. per liter), potassium (10 to 15 mEq. per liter), chloride (80 to 95 mEq. per liter), and bicarbonate (40 to 50 mEq. per liter).

Antimicrobials. As already stated, most episodes of acute infectious diarrhea spontaneously abate without specific therapy. Thus, in general, antibiotics should not be used. In the common "food-poisoning syndromes," caused by the ingestion of the enterotoxins of *C. perfringens, S. aureus, B. cereus,* or *V. parahaemolyticus,* antibiotics are ineffective and the illness usually abates within 24 hours. Viral diarrhea, of course, does not benefit from antibiotic therapy.

In salmonellosis (nontyphoidal), it is generally agreed that antibiotics should *not* be used in the usual case of *uncomplicated* Salmonella gastroenteritis. Antibiotic therapy does *not* shorten the duration of the illness, and does prolong the fecal excretion of the organisms and enhances the appearance of antibiotic-resistant strains. However, if the patient appears "toxic" with high fever, leukopenia, or striking leukocytosis, or if the clinician is concerned about septicemia or the development of focal lesions, antibiotic therapy should certainly be instituted after blood and stool cultures are obtained. Antibiotics should be selected on the basis of antibiotic sensitivity testing and a general knowledge of the antibiotic susceptibility patterns of the Salmonella strains prevalent in the community. In general, ampicillin, trimethoprim-sulfamethoxazole, or chloramphenicol is used. A detailed discussion of antibiotic treatment of salmonellosis is found on pages 65 to 67.

In the case of shigellosis, most authorities agree that antibiotic therapy does shorten the duration of the illness, but that all patients do *not* require antibiotics. In the majority of the cases, especially those caused by *Shigella sonnei,* the illness will spontaneously remit, and antibiotics are not required. In the moderate or severe case, however, antibiotics should be used. In the United States, most Shigella isolates are resistant to sulfonamides, and many isolates are resistant to tetracyclines. In general, ampicillin is the drug of first choice, but in certain communities many shigellae are already resistant to this drug as well. In adults,

2 grams of ampicillin per day by mouth (500 mg. four times a day) is usually recommended. In children, 50 mg. per kg. per 24 hours given in four doses by mouth is usually recommended. If antibiotic therapy is to be used, in vitro antibiotic testing should be performed to delineate which antibiotic is appropriate.

Symptomatic Therapy. In general, in "invasive" diarrheas, salmonellosis and shigellosis, drugs which interfere with intestinal motility (diphenoxylate with atropine, codeine, tincture of opium, paregoric) are best avoided. Although they may help control the diarrhea, they may allow proliferation of the organisms within the paralyzed gut, enhance mucosal invasion and inflammation, and prolong the illness. In viral or "toxigenic" diarrheas, however, these agents may make the patient more comfortable. Diphenoxylate with atropine (Lomotil), 1 or 2 tablets every 2 to 4 hours (this dose is higher than that listed in the manufacturer's official directive), codeine, 15 to 30 mg. every 6 hours, or paregoric, 4 to 8 ml. every 4 hours, can be used. In the mild or moderate case, bulk forming agents, such as kaolin and pectin, usually suffice.

NONSPECIFIC CHRONIC ULCERATIVE COLITIS

method of
RICHARD O. BICKS, M.D.
Memphis, Tennessee

The goals of treating chronic ulcerative colitis are threefold: (1) controlling symptoms, (2) inducing a remission, and (3) preventing recurrences. The therapy should be prolonged, comprehensive, and individualized. Since neither the etiology nor the pathogenesis of the disease is known, empirical therapy is often based on comparative studies and anecdotes. The physician who sees only sporadic cases should make himself familiar with the complications of both the disease and its therapy. Otherwise, prompt referral is indicated. The physician must also be prepared to recognize the patient's emotional response to his illness and must devote long hours to coping with anxiety, frequently infantile behavior, dependency, and demands on his time. Early hospitalization is recommended for all patients except those who have proctitis only. This allows a better evaluation of patient response to therapy, as well as a better doctor-patient relationship. Diagnosis must be established by rigorously ruling out the numerous specific causes of bloody diarrhea, especially Crohn's disease.

General Medical Measures

Diet. The colitis patient is frequently afraid to eat because of ensuing cramps and diarrhea and has also usually been given bad advice about dietary restrictions. There is nothing in food that has been identified as the etiologic agent of ulcerative colitis. There is a need for increased caloric intake, particularly of protein, vitamins, and minerals, and the diet should be restricted only in terms of the personal idiosyncrasies of the individual patient. Specific entities such as lactose sensitivity should always be looked for; if found, a lactose-free diet should be instituted. Rigid elimination diets give the physician something to do and almost always ensure lack of patient cooperation. The only exception is when the patient is acutely ill; then formula diets (Precision L-R, Isocal) are indicated. The most sensible advice that one can give the patient is to eat whatever he wants, avoiding only food that increases his symptoms.

In severely ill patients with fever, weight loss, abdominal cramps, and diarrhea, the use of both central and peripheral hyperalimentation is helpful. Great care is needed with central hyperalimentation because of the incidence of electrolyte imbalance and infection. In the acutely ill hospitalized patient, "putting the colon to rest" allows adequate nutrition to be maintained. Peripheral hyperalimentation with the newer liquid solutions is less frequently employed but represents a remarkable advance. These solutions of glucose, amino acids, and lipids can be prepared with the cooperation of the hospital pharmacist. Fluoroscopy is needed to place the catheters and meticulous care given to prevent infection. Attention to metabolic complications such as hypophosphatemia and hypomagnesemia is imperative.

Intravenous fluids, particularly glucose, if used to maintain adequate nutrition, should always be accompanied by vitamins. Special attention should be paid to potassium, calcium, and magnesium depletion in hospitalized patients. These electrolytes should be measured at frequent intervals. In the acutely ill patient with fulminating colitis, hypokalemia can lead to toxic dilatation of the colon, so that potassium supplements, particularly in patients receiving corticosteroids, are a crucial aspect of therapy. Here oral potassium supplements such as Kay Ciel, Slow K, or Kaochlor liquid (potassium chloride) are indicated, along with the use of intravenous fluids containing 20, 40, or even 60 mEq. of potassium chloride per liter; however, the intravenous infusion is painful and causes a chemical phlebitis.

Sedation and Tranquilization. Numerous psychiatric studies have been reported concerning the personality of the patient with ulcerative colitis. Certainly reactive depression, anxiety, hostility, and dependence are frequently found, but I do not recommend psychiatric referral except when clear-cut psychiatric syndromes are identified. The sympathetic and knowledgeable physician who can give the patient understanding and emotional support does a far better job. The judicious use of minor tranquilization such as diazepam (Valium), 5 to 10 mg. before each meal and at bedtime, or chlordiazepoxide (Librium), 5 or 10 mg. before each meal and at bedtime, often helps the patient cope with anxiety and emotional fatigue. Adequate sleep should be encouraged so that the patient awakens refreshed. Habituating or addicting sedation should be avoided. One should not insist on rigid instructions of physical rest, particularly to the wage-earning head of a household, as he will probably not comply. This will only add to the patient's anxiety and confusion.

Antispasmodics and Anticholinergics. The colitis patient complains frequently of tenesmus, cramps, and abdominal pain. Mild sedative-antispasmodic mixtures such as tridihexethyl and meprobamate (Pathibamate), chlordiazepoxide and clidinium (Librax), and hyoscyamine sulfate and phenobarbital (Donnatal) frequently relieve these symptoms. Cramps and diarrhea can be well managed with diphenoxylate (Lomotil), 1 or 2 tablets before each meal and at bedtime. Pure anticholinergics such as glycopyrrolate (Robinul), 1 to 2 mg. before meals and at bedtime, or propantheline (Pro-Banthine), 15 mg. before meals and at bedtime, have more side effects of blurred vision and delayed urination and probably should be employed less frequently. The use of deodorized tincture of opium or codeine should be reserved for short-term situations. The dose of deodorized tincture of opium is 10 drops in water after each loose watery bowel movement, and that of codeine is 15 to 30 mg. before each meal. These are very important drugs in the management of the pain, cramps, and tenesmus that frequently incapacitate the patient. Their short-term use for several days will frequently help the patient through an exacerbation of symptoms, but can precipitate colonic dilatation.

Antibiotics. Systemic antibiotics, intramuscularly, intravenously, or by mouth, are not indicated in the usual colitis patient. However, in the severely ill hospitalized patient with fever and leukocytosis, bactericidal antibiotics are indicated. My choice is a combination of penicillin, 1.2 million units every 6 hours, and gentamicin (Garamycin), 80 mg. intramuscularly every 8 hours. In the penicillin-sensitive patient, erythromycin can be substituted or streptomycin used instead of gentamicin. These should not be continued for more than 5 to 7 days or until signs of toxicity subside. Growth of resistant organisms will probably occur in that time period. Oto- and nephrotoxicity should be watched for during the use of drugs to combat gram-negative infections. Bacteriostatic broad-spectrum antibiotics should be avoided because of bowel side effects and because they are generally ineffective. The treatment of intercurrent infections of the skin, respiratory tract, and genitourinary tract should avoid antibacterials that have diarrheal side effects and should be based on appropriate sensitivity studies.

Blood. Anemia secondary to chronic infection and blood loss is a frequent complication of ulcerative colitis. Oral iron (ferrous sulfate, 325 mg. after meals four times daily) should be attempted, but this frequently causes indigestion, gas, and cramps. Iron dextran (Imferon injections) is needed to replenish depleted iron stores. These shots are painful and stain the skin unless given by a special "Z" track technique. The dose is calculated from the hemoglobin level. In hospitalized patients who are chronically and acutely ill, blood transfusions are used to maintain hematocrits in the range of 35 per cent.

Antimicrobial Therapy. Salicylazosulfapyridine (Azulfidine) is a bowel cleansing agent that has been used in the treatment of ulcerative colitis since its introduction many years ago. The drug's actions are unknown. It seems to help prevent recurrences but probably does not induce a remission or control symptoms. It remains one of the mainstays of therapy. Graduated doses, beginning with 1 gram daily in divided doses and working up to 4 to 8 grams daily, are optimal. Treatment is usually begun with 0.5 gram twice daily after meals, and increased in increments of 0.5 to 1 gram daily as tolerated to a total of 4 to 8 grams daily. Side effects are frequent. Headache, nausea, vomiting, allergy to sulfonamides, and severe hematologic complications occur in about 20 per cent of patients. The other forms of sulfa drugs, such as sulfisoxazole or sulfathalidine, are ineffective. I prefer to use corticosteroid therapy to control symptoms and induce a remission, and employ salicylazosulfapyridine to prevent exacerbation. Lifetime therapy is probably indicated if the patient can tolerate the drug.

Corticotropin (ACTH) and Corticosteroids. These drugs are the cornerstone of modern medical therapy of ulcerative colitis. In proctitis they are the treatment of choice and can be given rectally in the form of a foam (Proctofoam-HC) or retention enemas (Cortenema, Rectoid) initially twice daily for 10 days, then once at bedtime for another 10 days, then phasing out to every other night, twice per week, and, finally, once to twice a month to retain remission. There is some absorption of steroids through the inflamed rectal mucosa, but the side effects are minimal. This use of local steroid therapy is the method of choice in disease limited to the rectum.

Oral steroids are usually given in the form of prednisone (Deltasone, Meticorten) in an initial dose of 40 to 60 mg. daily. There is usually a prompt response, with increased appetite, decrease in cramps and diarrhea, defervescence, and a clinical sense of well being. Healing is slow and frequently takes months, and the prompt clinical response must not be confused with a remission. Depending on the patient's age, body build, and severity of symptoms, the dose is lowered cautiously in 5 to 10 mg. increments until the lowest possible dose is found that will maintain clinical control. The average length of time the high doses (over 20 mg. daily) are given is 4 to 6 weeks, and the average maintenance dose is 10 to 20 mg. of prednisone daily. Maintenance oral steroid therapy should be continued until proctoscopic evidence of healing is obtained. This can take as long as 3 to 6 months. Some patients are exquisitely sensitive to oral prednisone, and small doses seem to be adequate in maintaining a remission. When relapses occur after oral corticosteroid dosage is reduced, full initial dosage must be reinstituted. It must be emphasized that corticosteroid therapy is a part of the comprehensive medical therapy to be used along with all the measures mentioned previously.

Complications of steroid therapy are numerous and frequent. Fluid retention, moon facies, acne, striae, altered carbohydrate metabolism, hypokalemia, muscle cramps, and demineralization of the bones are some of the more common complications. Altered resistance to infections seems less frequent, although skin infections are very common. Dietary sodium restriction (1.0 to 2.0 grams) will help prevent fluid retention. Alternate day steroid dosage does not work in the management of ulcerative colitis. A family history of diabetes should always be sought; if it is present, the patient should be monitored for altered carbohydrate metabolism by testing for both glycosuria and hyperglycemia. Oral steroids should be used cautiously in all patients, but their use in the older age groups is particularly dangerous. Long-term therapy in postmenopausal females frequently leads to demineralization of the bone and osteoporotic fractures of the lumbar spine. Hydrocortisone (Solu-Cortef) and ACTH can be given intravenously to patients who are acutely ill. Toxicity, characterized by fever, anemia, and acute exacerbation of colitis, can be best managed by hospitalization and intravenous ACTH, 20 units every 12 hours for a total daily dose of 40 mg., or hydrocortisone (Solu-Cortef), 100 mg. intravenously every 8 hours for a total daily dose of 300 mg. There is probably very little difference between these preparations as to clinical efficacy and response. As a rule of thumb I prefer to use intravenous ACTH in patients who had not received steroids previously, so that if surgery becomes necessary, the problems of delayed wound healing and increased demand for steroids during the stressful operation and postoperative period will not be a consideration. However, if the patient has been on oral steroids previously, I prefer to use intravenous hydrocortisone in the dose mentioned above. If the patient receives these intravenous medications, antispasmodics and anticholinergics should be stopped and only judicious use of narcotics should be employed, as toxic colonic dilatation is frequent under those circumstances.

Steroids are nonspecific therapy for ulcerative colitis and act essentially as potent anti-inflammatory agents. Older patients are particularly susceptible to complications. The duration of steroid therapy depends on the response of the patients, their age, the extent of the disease, and the time needed to obtain proctoscopic evidence of healing. In general, it should be possible to wean people off oral steroids after 6 to 9 months of continuous therapy. It is my practice to give all patients injections of ACTH Gel (Acthar-Gel), 100 units daily for 5 days on cessation of oral steroids that had been given for more than a year. However, this may be inadequate to restore normal adrenal function, and the patient may develop an addisonian crisis during a stress such as trauma, overwhelming infection, or unrelated surgery. Such relative or actual adrenal cortical insufficiency may also occur in a patient on maintenance doses under similar circumstances.

Special Clinical Situations

Ulcerative Proctitis. The involvement of the distal rectum with the disease process practically never progresses to the full-blown picture of ulcerative colitis. This should be confirmed by colonoscopy. This clinical subset is best managed by the use of steroid foam or retention enemas (Proctofoam-HC, Cortenema, Rectoid). Rectal retention enemas are given twice daily for 10 days during an acute exacerbation, then at bedtime for another 10 days, and then every other night for another week or two, finally phasing out to maintenance therapy of once or twice per month. An uncommon patient with proctitis will require oral steroids for a short length of time in the doses mentioned above to induce a remission.

Fulminating Ulcerative Colitis. This clinical syndrome is characterized by fever, toxicity, increase in rectal discharges, cramps, diarrhea, anemia, and dehydration. The patient is acutely ill and must be hospitalized. Correction of electrolyte imbalance, potassium depletion, and anemia with the use of blood and the use of intravenous steroids are indicated. Antispasmodics and anticholinergics should not be used, because they can precipitate toxic dilatation of the colon. In this clinical situation intramuscular bactericidal antibiotics are used. Fulminating colitis is an absolute indication for the use of high doses of intravenous corticotropin or hydrocortisone. All adjunctive measures should be employed, including blood transfusions. Although no time limit can be set and treatment must be individualized, surgical consultation should be obtained. Serial white counts, electrolytes, and flat films of the abdomen should be obtained on a daily basis.

Toxic Megacolon. This is the most feared complication of ulcerative colitis. It may appear de novo as part of a fulminating episode, or even rarely as the initial presenting syndrome in an acutely ill patient. It can be precipitated by potassium depletion, by anticholinergic medication, or as a sequela of barium enema or colonoscopy. The patient is both acutely and chronically ill with high fever and tachycardia. The striking finding is that of abdominal distention with a quiet abdomen. Low-pitched groans are heard on auscultation. A false sense of security is present, because the diarrhea and discharges associated with the disease have stopped. Hospitalization is urgent. High dose intravenous steroids, blood, intramuscular or intravenous antibiotics, hyperalimentation, and careful observation are mandatory. Daily white blood cell counts, measurement of electrolytes, and flat films of the abdomen with an upright chest film must be obtained. It must be remembered that both the intravenous steroids and antibiotics can mask the physical signs of perforation. Daily measurements of the diameter of the dilated colon should be made from a flat film of the abdomen. The importance of the upright chest film in looking for free air under the diaphragm cannot be overemphasized. Skilled surgical consultation should be obtained immediately after the diagnosis has been made. I arbitrarily allow the patient 96 golden hours to respond to intensive medical management. All patients with toxic dilatation have a total colitis and if they survive this complication, or the colon returns to normal size, almost all will have a colectomy within a year. It is preferable to have an elective surgical procedure performed. Any failure to respond or suspicion of perforation (whether demonstrated or not) should be an indication for emergency surgery.

Systemic Complications. Chronic ulcerative colitis is associated with systemic complications of iritis, uveitis, polyarthralgias, ankylosing spondylitis, pyoderma, erythema multiforme, and chronic liver disease. All these complications are indications for steroid therapy. Failure to respond, with the possible exception of ankylosing spondylitis, is an indication for surgery. With ankylosing spondylitis, measurement of histocompatibility antigen HLA B27 is helpful, because in my experience this particular systemic complication does not always clear up after colectomy.

Risk of Cancer. The incidence of cancer in ulcerative colitis is about five times higher than in the general population. However, this occurs in a special group of patients whose disease involves the total colon, has its age of onset in adolescence, and, regardless of activity, has existed for more than 10 years. I do not recommend prophylactic colectomy, but I recognize that this is a controversial subject. Serial rectal biopsies may show the changes which will help make a decision. As the neoplasms associated with ulcerative colitis generally are multifocal and highly malignant, even a yearly barium enema examination may not help. Serial colonoscopy with biopsy may be a partial solution to this problem. Here the decision should be individualized, but I feel that with increasing surgical skills the pendulum has now swung to increasing frequency of surgical intervention.

Failure of Growth in Adolescence. This is a rare situation in which age of onset of a usually total colitis in the adolescent may lead to failure of growth and development. Comprehensive medical management should be employed, as in adult cases, employing all modalities of therapy. The indication for colectomy will be discussed below. Again, the decision here should be individualized, recognizing that total colectomy may not favorably affect the growth pattern of the affected child.

Ulcerative Colitis in Pregnancy. I urge all my fertile female patients not to get pregnant while their disease is active and especially while they are taking steroid therapy for colitis. If colitis appears during the first trimester, the choice of continuing this pregnancy and the risk of the medical treatment to the developing fetus are explained to both marital partners and decisions made by mutual understanding of the risks involved. In my experience the only potential fetal problem has been relative adrenal insufficiency, if the pregnancy is allowed to go to term. After the development of the placenta in the second trimester, the need for steroid medications drops dramatically. A pediatrician should be available at the time of delivery to evaluate the baby. Ulcerative colitis appearing in the postpartum period is handled as a usual case. Postpartum exacerbations and prophylaxis are treated as in the ordinary patient.

Indications for Surgery. Surgical therapy of ulcerative colitis has been increasing in frequency. The surgeon can now make a well functioning ileostomy, using Turnbull's modification of Brooke's procedure. Patients are in a better nutritional state with hyperalimentation and blood transfusions. Enterostomal therapists and ileostomy clubs have helped patients with both the mechanical and the emotional problems associated with ileostomy. The operation of choice is total colectomy. This is frequently done as two separate procedures, with a subtotal colectomy and ileostomy performed first and the rectal stump removed later. There are some absolute indications for surgery. These include either free or walled-off perforation, extramural abscess, demonstration of cancer, and toxic megacolon which has been unresponsive to therapy after 96 hours. Systemic manifestations unresponsive to steroids in adequate doses, the presence of stricture in ulcerative colitis (cancer until proved otherwise), obstruction, or an inflammatory mass are also indications for surgery. The most controversial problem concerning surgical intervention is definition of the patient with chronic invalidism and failure of medical management. This decision should obviously be individualized, depending on the patient's life style, age, loss of employment time, side effects of medications, and need for prolonged steroid management. In my experience the more difficulty the patient has had from his ulcerative colitis, the better postoperative adjustment is made. Elective surgery should preferably be done at a time when the disease is under control after adequate medical and emotional preparation.

Conclusion

Chronic ulcerative colitis can be managed successfully by an interested and knowledgeable physician. The problems are threefold: (1) controlling the symptoms, (2) inducing a remission, and (3) preventing the recurrence. Maintaining adequate nutrition, physical and emotional rest, judicious use of antispasmodics, and correction of electrolyte imbalance and anemia are basic therapeutic maneuvers. Sulfasalazine (Azulfidine) probably helps maintain the remission but produces a high incidence of side effects and thus needs careful monitoring. The cornerstone of medical therapy is adrenal corticosteroids intravenously, orally, or rectally, depending on the severity and extent of the disease. A sympathetic, knowledgeable physician who can offer comprehensive medical therapy, as well as emotional support and awareness of the side effects of drugs and the complications of the disease, can reduce the medical mortality to practically zero.

Surgery is now indicated in about one third of all patients. Absolute surgical indications include perforation, obstruction, presence of cancer, toxic megacolon existing for more than 96 hours, and probably systemic manifestations of the disease unresponsive to corticosteroid therapy. The procedure of choice is total colectomy, usually done in one stage. Preoperative evaluation of the patient in terms of adrenal function, anemia, and electrolyte imbalance is important. The cooperation of enterostomal therapists and well adjusted members of ileostomy clubs is very helpful. Colectomy "cures" chronic ulcerative colitis, but it also substitutes another disease, the ileostomy. All the physician's skills are needed to help the patient with an ileostomy adjust and manage.

Experienced consultants should be utilized in special situations such as failure of growth and development in adolescence, babies born of mothers on high doses of steroids, and occurrence of ulcerative colitis during pregnancy.

The modern treatment of nonspecific ulcerative colitis, although hazardous and not curative, has made it possible for the physician to help the patient toward the goal of minimal morbidity and zero mortality from the disease.

SECTION 6

Metabolic Disorders

BERIBERI

(Thiamine [Vitamin B_1] Deficiency)

method of
DONALD S. McLAREN, M.D., Ph.D.
Edinburgh, Scotland

This is a fascinatingly diverse vitamin deficiency. It affects two systems—the nervous and cardiovascular—has both acute and chronic forms, has diverse causes in the Orient and the West, and affects infants and adults differently. Thiamine pyrophosphate (TPP, cocarboxylase) is involved in carbohydrate metabolism, mainly as coenzyme in the decarboxylation of alpha-ketoacids such as pyruvate in the tricarboxylic acid cycle, and to a lesser extent as a cofactor of transketolase in the pentose phosphate pathway.

Classic dietary deficiency beriberi occurs in the rice-dependent parts of Asia where heavy milling of the grain removes thiamine and other nutrients. Parboiling (boiling before husking), if practiced, disperses the nutrients throughout the grain, preserving thiamine and preventing beriberi. Infantile beriberi, a highly fatal disease presenting in acute cardiac, aphonic, and pseudomeningeal forms, occurs in babies exclusively breast fed by mildly deficient mothers. In adults the most common clinical manifestations are chronic polyneuropathy (especially wrist and foot drop) and acute cardiac failure (usually high output, left and right sided). Acute cerebral beriberi (the Wernicke-Korsakoff syndrome) is uncommon, for reasons that are unclear.

In North America and Europe thiamine deficiency is usually secondary to chronic alcoholism, but it may complicate debilitating conditions such as malabsorption, hyperemesis, or malignant disease; also, it has been precipitated by prolonged hypertonic glucose infusions, chronic hemodialysis, and starvation treatment of obesity if thiamine supplementation is omitted. Among several neurologic disorders described in chronic alcoholism, only the Wernicke-Korsakoff syndrome, alcoholic cerebellar degeneration, and some cases of tobacco-alcohol amblyopia (Carroll: Amer. J. Ophthal., *27*:713, 1944) respond specifically to thiamine (Victor et al.: *The Wernicke-Korsakoff Syndrome,* Blackwell, 1971). In alcoholics the polyneuropathy responds best to multivitamin therapy, as do most instances of nutritional amblyopia. Acute cardiac beriberi usually occurs as a separate entity.

Therapy

In all forms of beriberi described above, thiamine deficiency does not occur in isolation. Multivitamins, minerals, a balanced diet adequate in energy and protein content, and attention to underlying causes such as alcoholism or malabsorption are an integral part of the treatment in all patients. Optimal response to thiamine may be impaired if other accompanying deficiencies remain uncorrected (Zieve et al.: J. Lab. Clin. Med., *72*:268 and 761, 1968). Specific thiamine therapy in large doses is indicated in three conditions, in each of which it may serve as a therapeutic test to clinch a diagnosis which is never easy to make, and may be lifesaving in the acute forms. These are (1) cardiac beriberi, (2) cerebral beriberi, and (3) infantile beriberi.

Cardiac Beriberi. Complete bed rest is an important adjuvant to therapy. Generalized edema often subsides with rest alone. Conversely, exercise may intensify the symptoms and precipitate a recurrence following recovery, or may turn an asymptomatic or subacute deficiency state into fulminating heart failure. This is predominantly right sided, with systolic hypotension, venous distention, and little pulmonary congestion. Thiamine hydrochloride, 100 mg., is given intramuscularly or occasionally intravenously, with dramatic improvement seen within hours if the diagnosis is correct. Rarely, fatal anaphylactic reactions have followed intravenous injection, unrelated to dose size. This possibility must be considered when the vitamin is given intravenously, particularly if it was received parenterally some considerable time previously. Thereafter 25 mg. is given orally twice a day for 3 days and 10 mg. twice daily into convalescence. Initially the pulse slows, cardiac output is brought down to normal, peripheral vascular resistance increases, and venous pressure decreases. The electrocardiogram usually shows few changes, but in a few patients increase in voltage of the QRS complex, correction of inverted T waves, and shortening to normal of S-T segment prolongation occur with treatment. Occasionally a normal electrocardiogram will develop T wave inversions in some precordial leads during recovery. The enlarged heart usually returns to normal within several days. If alcoholic cardiomyopathy with interstitial fibrosis is present, response is poor and relapse frequent. Few hemodynamic studies have been made during recovery. In one patient normal peripheral vascular tone was restored in 37 minutes and low succeeded high output failure. In two patients with Wernicke's encephalopathy but no heart failure, abnormal initial values of cardiac index and peripheral resistance were made to approach normal within 1 hour of thiamine administration (Akbarian et al.: Amer. J. Med., *41*:197, 1966). Traditionally cardiac glycosides have been regarded as ineffective; more recently reports suggest that digitalis and G-strophanthin (ouabain) may be beneficial, but a thorough trial has not been made. Methoxamine, a sympathomimetic amine with a predominantly peripheral action, has failed to produce vasoconstriction. Vasopressin (Pitressin), once advocated for the fulminant case, is contraindicated because of its coronary vasoconstrictor properties in adult man.

Cerebral Beriberi (Wernicke-Korsakoff Syndrome, Nutritional Cerebellar Degeneration). Treatment of the patient with severe disease is exactly the same as for a patient with acute cardiac beriberi: 100 mg. of thiamine intramuscularly, followed by smaller doses during recovery. In patients who show only ocular and ataxic signs, the prompt administration of thiamine prevents the development of an irreversible and incapacitating amnesic psychosis. Strict bed rest is necessary at first to prevent precipitation of cardiac symptoms. All the ocular signs, with the exception of horizontal nystagmus, which often persists permanently, respond within a few hours and usually clear completely. In contrast, the ataxia usually responds only after several days, and recovery is incomplete in more than 50 per cent of patients. The global confusional state normally clears in a period varying from a few days to 2 months and then reveals the disorder of memory and learning (Korsakoff's psychosis), which, in a group of more than 100 patients studied by Adams and coworkers, showed an equal chance for the recovery to be absent, slight, significant, or complete. Recovery from the polyneuropathy is always slow and usually incomplete in severe cases. The extent to which the patient will ultimately recover is unpredictable during the acute stage. Failure to appreciate this may result in premature commitment of the patient to a mental hospital. The eventual disposition of the patient is made on the basis of the severity of the residual amnesic psychosis and the social circumstances, but only after one is certain that no further improvement in memory is possible. The mortality is about 20 per cent in the acute phase of the disease.

Infantile Beriberi. Infants with chronic beriberi respond slowly and often incompletely as far as the neurologic signs are concerned when 10 mg. of thiamine is given twice a day. With severe heart failure, convulsions, or coma, the initial dose should be 25 mg. given slowly intravenously, but the outlook is poor.

HYPO- AND HYPERVITAMINOSIS A

method of
FRANK REES SMITH, M.D.
New York, New York

Vitamin A is essential for normal growth, for the maintenance of epithelial integrity, and for vision. Vitamin A is provided in the diet preformed as the alcohol, retinol, or from provitamin A carotenoids, in particular β-carotenes. Carotenes are active only after being cleaved to retinal, then oxidized to retinol during the absorption process in the intestine. Retinol is esterified in the intestine and is transported to the liver by means of the chylomicrons. Vitamin A is stored in the liver and released as needed as the free alcohol, retinol, bound to a specific carrier protein, retinol-binding protein. In the fasting state, normally, approximately 5 per cent of the vitamin A activity in serum is in the form of retinyl esters present in lipoproteins; 95 per cent of the activity is as retinol bound to retinol-binding protein. Deficiencies of vitamin A may be a consequence of inadequate intake, of inability to absorb the fat-soluble vitamin, of impaired hepatic storage, or of impaired hepatic release. Disturbed visual function is the most common manifestation of deficiency, with a loss of night vision being the earliest sign, followed by Bitot's spots, corneal xerosis, and, finally, keratomalacia and blindness. The major risk of hypovitaminosis A is to the eye, and vitamin A deficiency is a major cause of blindness on a world scale.

Units. The previous expression of dietary vitamin A activity in international units (I.U.) is being replaced by that of retinol equivalents (R.E.). One retinol equivalent is equal to 1 microgram of retinol (3.33 I.U.) or 6 micrograms of β-carotene (10 I.U.). In the suggested dietary allowances which follow, it is assumed that half the vitamin A activity ingested is as retinol and half as β-carotene (thus the apparent discrepancy between R.E. and I.U.).

Hypovitaminosis A

Prevention. Adequate dietary allowances of vitamin A are as follows: infants to 6 months of age, 420 R.E.; infants 6 months to 1 year of age, 400 R.E. (1400 to 2000 I.U.); children, 400 to 700 R.E. (2000 to 3500 I.U.); adults, 800 to 1000 R.E. (4000 to 5000 I.U.). During pregnancy 1000 R.E. (5000 I.U.) is recommended, with an increase to 1200 R.E. (6000 I.U.) during lactation. These amounts of vitamin A can be provided with a normal diet. In the following circumstances, however, additional vitamin A supplementation should be considered: (1) children with protein-calorie malnutrition, malabsorption syndromes, cystic fibrosis, or chronic liver disease; (2) adults with longstanding malabsorption who have not been able to replenish hepatic stores of vitamin A, those with severe liver disease, and those on unusual, unbalanced diets. Treatment, of course, should be directed toward the underlying abnormalities. Vitamin A supplementation may be used at two to five times the normal dietary intake when there is a clear rationale for the therapy. Supplementation should not be given indefinitely. Serum vitamin A should be monitored in view of the hazards of vitamin A toxicity.

Treatment. In children with protein-calorie malnutrition, a functional defect in hepatic retinol release may exist so that treatment with adequate protein and calories is essential. The presence of corneal xerosis suggests the danger of keratomalacia, so these children should receive 30,000 micrograms of an aqueous dispersion of retinol intramuscularly immediately, and then daily oral supplements of 10,000 micrograms of water-miscible retinol for another 5 days. With milder signs of vitamin A deficiency or with serum vitamin A concentrations below 15 micrograms per dl. (100 ml.), daily oral supplements of 2000 micrograms of retinol should be adequate. In patients with active fat malabsorption, the amount may be doubled. Clinical improvement and serum levels should be followed and the dose adjusted accordingly.

Hypervitaminosis A

The prolonged use of high potency vitamin A preparations, particularly in teenagers and young adults, or in children of overzealous parents, may produce acute or chronic toxicity. Acute toxicity is characterized by an increase in intracranial pressure with papilledema, visual difficulties, headache, nausea, and vomiting. Additional signs such as dermatitis and arthritis may be present. With this clinical presentation in young people, the physician should always ask specifically about vitamin A supplementation. The diagnosis of hypervitaminosis A may be confirmed by finding serum vitamin A concentrations in excess of 80 micrograms per dl. The determination of the amount of vitamin A as retinyl ester may also be helpful, as fasting levels of greater than 5 per cent are suggestive of toxicity. Vitamin A toxicity is thought to occur when the capacity of serum retinol-binding protein to transport vitamin A is exceeded, and thus the vitamin is presented to cell membranes in a form other than bound to retinol-binding protein.

Additional signs of vitamin A toxicity include alopecia, cortical hyperostosis, and cryptogenic cirrhosis. Toxicity has been seen in patients ingesting daily doses ranging from as little as 5500 R.E. (18,500 I.U.) to 18,000 R.E. (60,000 I.U.) over as short an interval as 1 to 3 months. Infants and children develop symptoms after taking lower doses of vitamin A for shorter times.

Treatment of vitamin A toxicity is primarily the prompt withdrawal of vitamin A supplementation. Signs and symptoms clear within days to weeks. Permanent sequelae have not been reported, although the course of vitamin A-induced liver disease is not known.

DIABETES MELLITUS IN THE ADULT

method of
MARTIN G. GOLDNER, M.D.
Palo Alto, California

The aim of all therapy is to remove the cause of illness and to restore full health. In chronic diseases such as diabetes mellitus, in which complete cure is not yet at hand, the realistic therapeutic aim must be (1) to adjust the patient, physically and emotionally, to his health impairment; (2) to employ all available therapeutic means to minimize signs and symptoms of the disease; and (3) to attempt to prevent and delay the progress of the disease and the development of complications—in brief, to establish the best possible control of the disease.

Therapy for chronic diseases—more than that against acute illnesses—must be directed not only *against* the disease, but *toward* the patient. He is the one who has to live with his disease. He has the right to expect that whatever management is undertaken will give the greatest benefit with the smallest risk to enable him to enjoy the widest possible range of activities of living. This aim is realizable to a large extent in the care of diabetes mellitus, particularly the diabetes of the adult. It requires that physician and patient enter the management as equal partners with mutual trust, a relationship described rather poorly as that of "consumer" and "provider," and much better as that of "manager" and "counselor." In fact, when treatment often is not much more than reorientation of life style and eating habits, the patient should be the manager and the physician the trusted advisor.

MODALITIES OF TREATMENT

The very first step in the management of diabetes in the adult—short of emergency treatment—should be *education*, the patient getting acquainted with the nature of his disease and learning how far he will be able to manage it, and when to call for help. Only a patient knowledgeable about his disease and its risks, and about the means of treatment, their range of effectiveness, and their limitations, can be expected to make the best possible use of these modalities. The well educated patient will understandingly accept necessary restrictions in his activities of living, which the less informed would neglect only too easily and reject as arbitrary impositions by a domineering physician. Likewise, the less informed will easily take license, whereas the informed will know the limits of his freedom. And, foremost, proper education will give the patient the understanding to recognize when and where self-care must come to an end, and when to surrender the management into the hands of his physician, such as will occur under the threat of serious complications or intercurrent diseases.

The physician, in turn, must respect the patient's desire and right to know and to partake in decision-making; he must observe closely the old Hippocratic rule of "nil nocere"—never suggest greater restrictions than necessary, and always permit as much freedom as possible.

Diet, insulin, and the oral hypoglycemic agents are, next to education, the main modalities of treatment.*

Diet is the backbone of the management of diabetes. It attempts to adjust the patient's nutrition to his limited capacity to utilize carbohydrates.

To the extent to which it succeeds, it alone will provide the best possible control; if it fails, it must not be abandoned, but must be supplemented with other modalities.

Since the caloric requirement of the diabetic does not differ from that of a comparable healthy person, dietary adjustment cannot be done only by caloric restriction and elimination of carbohydrates. It must rather make use of replacing the readily absorbable refined sugars by slowly absorbed fiber-containing starchy nutrients and of changing the number of daily meals and their carbohydrate content, so as to facilitate their utilization. The diabetes of the adult, which is characterized by maturity onset, moderate or mild insulin deficiency, and a rather stable and not ketoprone course, and which is commonly associated with obesity or even precipitated by it, is most responsive to dietary management. This type of diabetes constitutes the largest segment of the diabetic population—some 50 to 80 per cent. Thus the vast majority of all diabetics can benefit from dietary management alone.

The usefulness of *drug treatment* depends to a large extent on the favorable ratio between its efficacy and its potential harmfulness. A certain amount of risk may be acceptable for an essential or lifesaving drug, whereas the greatest possible safety must be expected from an agent with limited effectiveness. With comparable safety, the more effective agent would be preferable; with comparable effectiveness, certainly the agent with greater safety should be chosen.

The hypoglycemic potency of *insulin* is such as to make it effective in all types of diabetes and at all times. Its clinical indication is limited only by the fact that it is not needed in the management of the diet-responsive type of diabetes. There is as yet no evidence that a patient managed satisfactorily on diet will derive greater benefits from additional insulin injection or, for that matter, from medication with any other agent with hypoglycemic activity.

Among the *side effects* of insulin hypoglycemia, hypersensitivity, resistance, and lipoma and lipoatrophy are noteworthy. Insulin hypoglycemia is not a true side effect but results from

*It is too early to assess the impact of promising studies with somatostatin, glucagon, and islet-cell transplants upon the clinical management of diabetes.

overdosage. It frequently presents problems of management and may limit "strict" control. *Local skin reaction* is common, particularly at the start of insulin treatment. This hypersensitivity reaction usually disappears with continuing treatment. Generalized allergic reactions with mucous membrane swelling occur rarely. They can be managed by switching to another brand of insulin or by desensitization with repeated intracutaneous injections of insulin. Discontinuation of insulin treatment has to be recommended only in very rare instances. *Insulin allergy* may be associated with insulin resistance. Insulin resistance is defined clinically as a daily insulin requirement of 200 units or more. It may be caused by a variety of metabolic factors, and frequently may occur and disappear spontaneously. If large enough doses of insulin are given, the resistance can be overcome (see coma treatment on p. 419). *Insulin granulomas* are simple foreign body granulations caused by too frequent traumatization of the same area. They may give the impression of insulin resistance, but here the injected insulin is absorbed too poorly from the scar tissue to be fully effective; change of the injection site will show that properly absorbed insulin is effective indeed. *Insulin lipomas* and insulin lipoatrophy are unusual side effects of insulin, occurring almost without exception on the injection site only. There is no known treatment for this lesion, which is not serious but may have unpleasant cosmetic implications. Often the condition is confined to specific areas and insulin injections will be tolerated well at other areas.

These possible side effects are related to the one general shortcoming of insulin, that it must be injected and that it is ineffective if given orally.

The oral hypoglycemic agents have the single and great advantage of being effective if taken by mouth. There is no doubt that they exert a hypoglycemic effect that is often strong enough to reduce diabetic hyperglycemia to normoglycemia. But their potency is limited both in magnitude and in type of disease. In optimal doses they may equal the potency of 30 to 40 units of insulin. Increasing doses would not increase the efficacy, and even this magnitude of potency can be achieved only if the diabetic insulin deficiency is not absolute. In juvenile diabetes and in surgical diabetes they are ineffective. The maturity onset type of diabetes, however, will be found to be to a large extent responsive to the oral agents. Through natural progression of the disease or complicating conditions of this type of diabetes, however, the insulin deficiency may deteriorate and the oral agent may fail to be effective. Similarly, such drug escape may also occur without direct cause after prolonged use of any of these agents. In contrast to the efficacy of insulin, it may be said that the oral hypoglycemic agents are effective in some types of diabetes mellitus only, and only at some times.

Drug reactions of the oral hypoglycemic agents are relatively rare and minor—e.g., as transitory skin rashes or epigastric distress. More serious are some specific side effects related to the metabolism of these agents. Most oral agents are excreted through the kidneys; some are metabolized and inactivated in the liver. Impaired renal function may delay excretion; impaired liver functions interfere with inactivation. In both instances accumulation of active compounds may precipitate episodes of protracted hypoglycemia. In addition, chlorpropamide has been found to have a most interesting side effect. It can potentiate the action of the antidiuretic hormone and thus precipitate occasionally rather serious water retention. The hypoglycemic guanidine derivatives present a rather serious risk. They may precipitate or aggravate lactic acidosis.* Finally, there is the highly contested but as yet not disproved finding of the University Group Diabetes Program (UGDP) that treatment with diet and oral hypoglycemic agents is accompanied by a greater risk of lethal cardiovascular complications than dietary management alone or diet plus insulin treatment.

All these risks ought to be weighed against the great convenience of oral administration whenever clinical use of these agents is considered.

WHAT CONSTITUTES CONTROL?

The control of diabetes is usually measured by the degree of control of the diabetic hyperglycemia and/or glycosuria. One of the most frequently used criteria is to consider "control" as "good" if 70 per cent or more of all fasting blood glucose values taken during an evaluation period are 110 mg. per 100 ml. or less; as "poor" when 70 per cent or more of these blood glucose values are 130 mg. per 100 ml. or higher; and as "fair" when values are in between. Glycosuria is a less reliable measure, because it depends on the renal threshold for glucose. With normal threshold, however, absence of glucose from the daily urine tests would suggest "good" control, whereas conversely continuous marked glycosuria associated with ketonuria indicates "poor" control. "Fair" control is signified by occasional mild (trace) or moderate (1+ to 2+) glycosuria.

It is evident that the reliability of these criteria

*At this writing, it appears likely that the hypoglycemic guanidine derivatives will be withdrawn from the market.

depends much on the frequency with which the respective tests are performed. Moreover, measuring only one parameter of the disease, implies a close positive correlation between blood sugar control and all other manifestations of the disease, which as yet is still uncertain. The unfortunate and not infrequent occurrence of degenerative vascular complications in patients under apparently "good" control may result from the unreliability of too infrequent monitoring; but it may signify also that the relationship between blood sugar control and the degenerative diabetic complications is not as close as assumed. This question may find its definitive answer in the near future when transplant surgery or medical technology will make possible continuous blood sugar monitoring and corresponding delivery of insulin without interfering with normal activities of living. Until then the degree of blood sugar control may have to be reviewed together with other pertinent factors, such as feeling of well-being, capacity to perform normal activities of living, and weight equilibrium. Not infrequently the patient may feel best in these respects when the blood sugar control is not better than "fair."

With ideal control as yet unattainable and the value of strict control in doubt, it may be more realistic and in line with the described aims of management to achieve "optimal" clinical control of both the tangible and the intangible factors of the disease.

INSTITUTING MANAGEMENT OF UNCOMPLICATED DIABETES

Dietary Management

Today's diet for diabetics is basically not much different from the so-called "prudent" diet for healthy nutrition. It provides adequate calories and essential nutrients as required for the maintenance of the ideal weight of the patient with due consideration of age, sex, height, and the degree of daily activities. Such diet permits the obese patient to lose weight gradually and the underweight to gain weight slowly until the calculated ideal weight has been reached. As a reducing diet, this procedure lacks the initial drastic weight loss of the presently popular starvation diets, but it is less risky, particularly for the diabetic, and its results are more persistent. Periods of starvation diets are followed more often than not by renewed gain of weight.

The diabetic maintenance diet takes into account the limited capacity to utilize carbohydrates. Their intake therefore is limited both in quality and in quantity. Refined sugars are eliminated, but a wide variety of starchy foods are utilized to provide an almost normal supply of carbohydrates. Their slow absorption, particularly if they are rich in fibers, copes with a slowly responding insulin apparatus. Thus postprandial hyperglycemia and glycosuria can be avoided, whereas an equivalent amount of glucose would result in marked hyperglycemia and urinary sugar loss. This diet, moreover, provides a healthy ratio between saturated and unsaturated fats, but restricts the total lipid intake to a level not more than acceptable for appetizing and satisfying meals. The diet consists generally of 50 per cent of its calories in carbohydrates, 20 per cent protein, and 30 per cent in fats, and is well fortified with all essential vitamins and minerals.

With a basic caloric need of 20 calories per kg., and 10 calories per kg. added for moderate activity, a diabetic with an ideal weight of 70 kg. would require 2100 calories daily for weight maintenance. With regard to distributions of nutrients, this diet would contain 250 grams of carbohydrates, 70 grams of protein, and 40 grams of fat. What transforms it to a specific diabetic diet is (1) the type of carbohydrates contained by nutrients, (2) a fixed distribution of the amount of carbohydrates over the various meals, and (3) a fixed number of daily meals and regular mealtimes.

Although the healthy person may have his mealtimes at random and distribute his food allotment at will, the diabetic must avoid these irregularities. At best, five fixed mealtimes should be observed, but at least four daily meals—breakfast, lunch, dinner, a bedtime feeding, and an in-between feeding, either in the midmorning or the midafternoon. The midmorning feeding may be most convenient for the school child who is used to a midmorning recess and snack; adults may prefer the mid- or late afternoon feeding. The bedtime feeding, recommended to every diabetic, becomes a must when dietary management has to be supplemented with drug management. The recommended distribution of the carbohydrates over the recommended number of meals might best be breakfast 1/6, lunch 2/6, dinner 1/6, bedtime 1/6, and midmorning or midafternoon 1/6—but must be left to individual adjustments.

There is no shortcut to translating these general rules into the individualized dietary regimen. Fortunately, there is no need for rush in the case of uncomplicated diabetes. One of the best ways to proceed is as follows:

1. Give permission to continue to eat and drink as before for the 1 or 2 week period until the next scheduled visit.

2. Give instructions to keep a complete record of the daily food intake, noting both the

amounts and the time everything is eaten or drunk.

3. Give instruction in urinalysis, testing to be done and recorded before each meal.

Compliance with this procedure will provide not only a record of the day-by-day caloric intake and the distribution of the nutrients, but also the most useful assessment of the individual patient's food predilection. In addition, it may surprise the patient—and occasionally the physician—that the "free diet" which most people believe they indulge in fluctuates rather little from day to day (with the possible exception of weekends and holidays). This discovery does much to facilitate the acceptance of a calorically restricted diet, particularly if food predilections are maintained whenever possible and the changes concern mainly the meal times, the distribution of nutrients over different meals, and the necessity of continual adherence to them.

The use of special "diabetic food preparations," such as diabetic candies, cakes, and beverages, is discouraged as much as possible so that the patient's diet differs as little as necessary from the diet of the rest of the family. Fresh fruit and vegetables should be stressed, with water-packed or frozen preparations preferred over canned goods, which are sweetened. Sugar substitutes should best be avoided, not so much because of their potential risks, but because they may not be needed in as liberal a diet as the described one.

With the diet plan agreed upon and with instructions given about appropriate diet manuals and about food equivalents, a second 2 week period is used, continuing the detailed diet diary and recording the daily urine tests, but now under observation of the prescribed diet. This forms the basis for the final adjustment. If some of the daily tests are repeatedly negative and others positive, the tolerance may be improved by withdrawing some carbohydrates from the meal preceding the positive test and adding them to a meal preceding a negative test. With some juggling around, a satisfactory balance will be established. The multiple urinalyses may then be reduced to one daily, with a schedule such as the following: first day, before breakfast; second day, before lunch; third day, before dinner; fourth day, before bedtime; and so on.

If, however, significant glycosuria persists before each or most meals, the attempt of dietary management alone has failed and drug supplementation must be started.

Insulin Management

Insulin management is always an addition to dietary management, never a substitute for it. It must be considered if a trial with diet alone has failed, or if a patient presents with signs of a keto-prone type of disease, even though ketosis itself may not yet be present. Marked glycosuria with signs of dehydration and significant weight loss may suggest starting immediately with combined diet and insulin management. It should, however, be kept in mind that insulin management should be undertaken with the intention of "once on insulin, always on insulin"; it should never be instituted precipitously, and rarely as a temporary measure only (as during complicating illnesses).

The first step of insulin management is thorough *instruction of the patient in the types of insulin, and the technique of the injection of insulin.*

Insulin is available in preparations of various strengths and different lengths of action. With regard to strength, the U-100 preparation, containing 100 units in 1 ml., appears to be the most useful one. It simplifies measuring the required units using a syringe with decimal calibration. It has largely replaced the formerly widely used strengths of U-20, U-40, or U-80, which frequently caused errors in measuring. Fast-acting preparations are the "regular" or "crystalline" insulin, which begin to be effective about 10 to 20 minutes after subcutaneous injection, lasting about 4 to 6 hours, with peak activity at about 2 to 3 hours. The long-acting preparations become effective about 1 or 1½ hours after administration, maintain optimal efficiency for several hours, and fade gradually over 2 to 3 hours. Their duration of activity varies from about 12 and 18 hours for Semilente and NPH insulin to 18 to 26 hours for Lente and 24 to 36 hours for protamine zinc and Ultralente insulin.

Short-acting insulin is helpful to properly utilize single meals; as many as three daily injections would be needed for the control of fasting hyperglycemia and the additional increases of the blood sugar level after each of the daily meals. Yet, even then the nocturnal blood sugar fluctuations would hardly be affected.

Not a few physicians and patients are willing to accept the inconveniences and risks of multiple daily injections in the hope that this may simulate closely the action of endogenous insulin and be the best way to prevent or delay the development of the degenerative chronic complications of diabetes.

Long-acting insulin affects mainly the fasting or "basic" hyperglycemia and thus also the blood sugar level during the night (when the patient is fasting). The postprandial hyperglycemia is influenced only secondarily, because this is superimposed upon a lowered baseline level.

Most clinicians and patients prefer the long-acting insulin preparations, which may be given only once daily. If properly spaced, they provide a continuous lowering of the fasting glycemia. Assuming that the rising limb of its action curve equals in time the fading-out period, a second day's injection would begin to substitute gradually for the decreasing activity of the first day's dose, thus achieving a rather stable blood sugar level. As mentioned above, the limiting factor for the effective dose is the risk of nocturnal hypoglycemia.

The initial dose of insulin depends on the speed and the degree of safety with which one wishes to achieve satisfactory results. No insulin-sensitivity tests or predictions based on the amount of glycosuria or degree of hyperglycemia can eliminate trials and errors. Those who start with relatively high doses, i.e., more than 30 units, invite risks. Such risks may be acceptable under close supervision in a hospital. But the main purpose of insulin, as well as diet management, is to manage the disease as much as possible under the patient's normal activities of living. Hospital control therefore would require readjustments when the patient returns home, minimal as they may be. Ambulatory management must be undertaken with as little risk as possible and therefore should start with a minimal dose, which may be built up gradually to the maintenance dose. Twenty units of a long-acting preparation is a dose large enough to have a noticeable effect and small enough to be relatively free of risk. This dose may be tried for about 1 week; if unsatisfactory, it may be raised by 5 units at 3 to 4 day intervals until satisfactory urinalyses are obtained and an estimation of the fasting blood sugar level indicates that there is no risk of hypoglycemia. Ten units of regular insulin is an adequate starting dose.

When the dose of long-acting insulin cannot be raised safely any further, and when additional insulin is required, short-acting preparations must be used in addition. Doses of 10 units or slightly higher may be given before breakfast, or prior to that meal which is followed persistently by significant glycosuria. Mixing of insulin is inadvisable, as it may alter the action curve of either preparation. Proper measuring requires learning to aspirate the exact dose into the syringe without admixture of any air bubbles. Although not dangerous, it may obscure the exact measuring of the dose and cause too little insulin to be injected.

Correct subcutaneous injection and frequent change of the injection site are of greater importance. Intracutaneous or intramuscular injections are less readily absorbed than subcutaneous injections. Repeated subcutaneous injections into the same site call forth connective tissue reactions. Small subcutaneous granulomas develop, which delay absorption but make the area less sensitive to the needle prick. Consequently uninformed patients prefer to use the same site continuously and are puzzled that insulin treatment has become ineffective or that "insulin resistance" has developed. Changing the injection site usually restores the efficiency of the previously effective dose and reveals the true nature of this so-called resistance. To prevent this phenomenon, regular change of the site is mandatory.

Another false impression of insulin resistance may be brought about when doses larger than 1 ml., i.e., more than 100 units, must be given. Depots of such size are commonly absorbed much more slowly than smaller depots, and may be partly inactivated in situ; thus no full benefit is derived from this large dose. It will prove to be fully effective if injected in divided dosage at two different sites.

For self-injection the most convenient area is the outer aspect of the thigh. Drawing three imaginary lines vertically from a few centimeters below the groin to a few centimeters above the knee and imagining on them seven different points, one may use each line for seven injections, switch to the next line after 1 week, and return to the same site only once every 3 weeks. One may use both thighs and increase further the injection interval. If more than one injection is required, both areas may be used simultaneously, one for the long-acting and the other for the short-acting insulin; after 3 weeks the two preparations may be switched.

Oral Hypoglycemic Agents

Many physicians consider the oral hypoglycemic agents as convenient medication in those instances in which the patient is unable or unwilling to adhere to dietary management or in which only small doses of insulin would be required to establish satisfactory control. Many patients, having heard about the availability of oral medication, are anxious to use it without being aware of its limitations. In such instances informed consent must be considered most necessary. Patients should be informed about the possible risks and the considerable limitations. They should be forewarned that they may need insulin in the case of progression of the disease or of intercurrent complications. It cannot be emphasized strongly enough that the oral hypoglycemic agents are neither a substitute for diet nor one for insulin.

Oral hypoglycemic agents are available as sulfonylurea derivatives or guanidine derivatives, in short-acting and long-acting preparations, as indicated in Table 1. Even when used and found to be effective, their usefulness should be re-evaluated at intervals because of the previously mentioned drug escape. With regard to the guanidine derivatives, special attention must be given to the risk of lactic acidosis (see footnote, p. 413).

TABLE 1. **The Oral Hypoglycemic Agents**

DRUG	STRENGTH (MG.)	ACTION CURVE (HOURS)	RECOMMENDED DAILY DOSAGE (MG.)
Sulfonylurea			
Tolbutamide	500	12	500–3000
Chlorpropamide	100, 250	60–90	100–500
Acetohexamide	250, 500	12–24	250–1500
Tolazamide	100, 250, 500	14–24	100–1000
Biguanides*			
Phenformin	25	4–6	25–200
Phenformin TD	10, 50	8–14	50–200

*Withdrawn from market in the United States of America.

Combined use of several oral preparations or use of an oral preparation together with insulin should be discouraged. It complicates rather than simplifies the management.

MANAGEMENT OF THE ACUTE DIABETIC COMPLICATIONS

Diabetic Ketoacidosis

Ketoacidosis, with or without coma, once the most feared and usually fatal acute complication, has become gratifyingly rare since the introduction of insulin. It is eminently preventable and avoidable; it is equally well treatable, but still has a high rate of mortality.

Ketoacidosis develops if the diabetic insulin deficiency falls below a critical level. Omission of the prescribed dose may be the precipitating cause, but most commonly it results from a combination of factors such as fever, intercurrent infectious diseases, severe trauma and shock, or gastrointestinal upset with vomiting, diarrhea, and resulting dehydration. Most of these conditions can be life threatening in themselves; all inhibit normal insulin activity and call for increased insulin secretion or dosage. Because of loss of appetite and inability to eat, the uninformed patient all too often will be inclined to decrease or omit his insulin injection, thus compounding the risk. He must be impressed that *the most important preventive measures are* (1) to increase his insulin dose by about one half; (2) to substitute for the regular meals soft or liquid feedings of equivalent carbohydrate content and to force the intake of these substitutes; and (3) to call for medical help as soon as possible.

Diabetic ketoacidosis does not develop suddenly. It takes its course over hours; there is time enough to cope with it in its early stage and to reverse the course. Prevention, unfortunately, will not be possible in the instances in which ketoacidosis is the very first manifestation of a hitherto undiagnosed diabetes—not infrequently among juvenile diabetics, less likely in adults.

Treatment must be fast, circumspect, and closely supervised and monitored, requiring teamwork in a hospital setting. Presence of coma is a clear sign of the seriousness of the condition, but absence of coma with the otherwise classic syndrome of severe dehydration, rapid and deep respiration, nausea, and vomiting gives no reassurance of lesser emergency. Treatment ought to start even prior to the removal to a hospital, and intensive care monitoring must not cease when the acidosis appears to be broken and blood sugar homeostasis is restored; it must continue to protect the patient against any possible reaction to the frequently unavoidable overdosage of medications during the emergency treatment period, especially insulin hypoglycemia and hyperpotassemia.

The essentials of treatment are, of course, insulin in adequate dosage and fluid and electrolyte replacement in proper amounts, followed by glucose administration to supply substrate for energy. The sooner the shift from fat to glucose metabolism can be achieved, the greater are the chances for full recovery (see Table 2).

Insulin should be given and recorded properly prior to the transfer to the hospital. Only if there is reasonable doubt about the diagnosis in a comatose patient may an intravenous injection of glucose be given first, to rule out the possibility of a hypoglycemic coma. The insulin preparation of choice is the fast-acting preparation. About 50 units should be given intravenously, simultaneous with 100 units subcutaneously. The large doses are necessitated by the insulin resistance, usually associated with ketoacidosis, and the intravenous administration by the dehydration and shock often attending ketoacidosis and interfering with subcutaneous absorption.

A *venoclysis with isotonic salt solution* or Ringer's solution is started as early as possible to deliver about 4 liters during the first 12 hours of treatment. The rate of the infusion must depend on the patient's condition. The average fluid deficit of the adult patient in diabetic coma is about 8 to 12

TABLE 2. **The Essentials of Treatment of Diabetic Acidosis**

WHAT	WHY	WHEN	HOW	BEWARE
Insulin	To stop ketogenesis To start glycogenesis	Immediately	50 units I.V. plus 100 units S.C.; double previous dose every hour until response	Hypoglycemia Hypopotassemia
Isotonic saline solution	To replace fluids To replace Na, Cl	Immediately	3000 to 6000 ml. I.V., 120 drops per min.	Overhydration Renal failure
Plasma	To combat shock	If response to saline is poor	Intravenously	Hepatitis (late)
Glucose	To supply energy To prevent insulin hypoglycemia	As soon as glycosuria decreases	Intravenously, 5% in saline	Increase of loss of glucose, electrolytes, and water
Bicarbonate	To combat acidosis	If aforementioned measures are ineffective	500 ml. 4% sodium bicarbonate solution, Ringer's, Hartman's solution	Alkalosis, if renal function is impaired
Potassium	To replace loss of K	Late, not before blood sugar level is falling	Best by mouth	Hyperpotassemia, if renal function is impaired

liters. *Plasma* may have to be given in order to combat severe shock.

Blood samples are drawn as soon as possible for chemical analyses; a detailed protocol is started to record all pertinent clinical and laboratory findings as well as medication given and procedures performed. *Urinalysis* may be omitted if no urine can be obtained short of catheterization. Improved diuresis may have to be awaited.

Careful *search for precipitating or contributing causes* of the emergency must be carried out. In the elderly patient a fulminant infection, a cardiovascular accident, a gastrointestinal disease, or trauma may be suspected. An electrocardiogram will serve also as a baseline for monitoring possible hypo- and hyperpotassemia; gastric lavage may be instituted to relieve gastric dilatation and to prepare the stomach for the resumption of oral feeding.

Insulin administration is continued at hourly intervals in ever-increasing doses (best by doubling the preceding dose, injections being given subcutaneously) until significant improvement is noted. There is no limit to the amount of insulin which may have to be given. Occasionally, as much as 3000 units has been required to break the insulin resistance of ketoacidosis. Such great accumulation of insulin, of course, brings with it the serious risk of an ultimate and protracted insulin hypoglycemia.

An alternative method of insulin management of ketoacidosis uses continuous intravenous infusion of small doses of insulin (5 to 10 units per hour). Good results have been reported; yet in a condition which still has a mortality rate of 3 to 10 per cent, the concern must be great that the most resistant cases may not be treated adequately and quickly enough if this procedure is employed.

Glucose administration becomes mandatory as soon as indications appear that insulin is becoming effective, the blood sugar level decreases, and the ketonemia subsides, with corresponding urine tests. An intravenous infusion of 5 per cent glucose in isotonic saline solution is substituted for the running venoclysis. The next insulin dose is cut in half or omitted entirely, depending on the subsequent tests. The purpose of the glucose infusion at this rather early point is a dual one: (1) to protect against hypoglycemia and (2), most importantly, to provide substrate for the energy metabolism which now begins to shift back to carbohydrate utilization in an organism with depleted glucose stores. Glucose infusion is continued until the patient has become alert and is ready for oral alimentation.

With this rapid and aggressive coma treatment, there is usually no need for *bicarbonate administration,* but attention must be focused on possible overhydration and the fluctuations of the blood potassium level.

Overhydration and its most serious manifestation, cerebral edema, must be suspected if an apparently responding patient begins to relapse again into stupor and coma while blood sugar and CO_2 combining power are approaching normal. Mannitol infusion or reintroduction of hyperglycemia may be attempted to restore normal osmotic pressure.

Hypopotassemia is the result of the reflux of extracellular potassium into the intracellular space under the influence of insulin. It is evidently a phenomenon of recovery. Frequently the patient will already be able to receive oral alimentation at this time. Potassium should then be offered by mouth in the form of tomato juice or grapefruit juice or meat broth reinforced with potassium salts. If this is not yet possible, recourse must be taken to intravenous infusion (potassium phosphate as buffered solution, 40 to 80 mEq. of 5 per cent glucose in water), provided there is no renal impairment and good urinary flow. Hyperpotassemia must be avoided; it may present a greater risk than hypopotassemia.

With the life-threatening complication under control, the main task is to re-establish maintenance treatment and to manage whatever precipitating and complicating condition may have been present. A patient who has been on insulin management prior to the emergency can be expected to have about the same insulin requirement as before. This dosage of long-lasting insulin should be injected before breakfast on the morning following discontinuation of emergency insulin treatment. If the last dose of fast-acting insulin was given less than 4 hours earlier, the first dose of long-lasting insulin may be cut in half and the full dose given 24 hours later. A patient who had managed his disease on diet alone must now continue with insulin treatment; his disease has become keto-prone and insulin dependent. Insulin management should be instituted as prescribed above.

Insulin Hypoglycemia

Insulin hypoglycemia is a risk of insulin treatment, but also of the oral hypoglycemic agents, particularly the long-acting forms of chlorpropamide and acetohexamide. If not treated early, it develops rapidly into the full-blown picture of seizures and coma. Fortunately it is preventable as well as easily treatable. The informed patient will be alerted to take an extra feeding whenever he experiences the characteristic early symptoms of lightheadedness, double vision, or excessive perspiration and agitation. The patient ought to know that reactions to short-lasting insulin preparations may occur about 2 to 3 hours after the meal prior to which the injection was given, that reactions to the long-lasting preparations may develop late at night, particularly when the bedtime feeding was light or omitted entirely, and that the reactions to the oral hypoglycemic agents are usually late and protracted.

Occasional reactions can be prevented by awareness of the following factors:

1. Increased exercise decreases the need for insulin. Thus in the case of unusually heavy exercise (competitive sports and others), the dose of insulin should be reduced temporarily by at least 10 units.

2. Certain common drugs such as aspirin or phenylbutazone may enhance the hypoglycemic activity of both insulin and the oral agents; therefore symptoms may be expected and dealt with very early.

3. The commonly recommended fruit juice or lump of sugar relieves a short hypoglycemic episode but may call forth increased endogenous insulin secretion and thus a rebound reaction. Such remedies do not adequately relieve the protracted hypoglycemic reaction after long-acting insulin or oral agents. Here they must be supplemented by a soft or solid meal such as cereals and milk, or a sandwich.

Glucagon injections have been recommended for the management of hypoglycemic reactions. Yet the need for injection is an inconvenience, particularly for self-care, and supplementation with a carbohydrate-containing meal is necessary nevertheless.

Repeated insulin reactions call for a revision of the maintenance diet. Most instances of so-called "brittle diabetes," with its fluctuations between hypoglycemic reactions and episodes of hyperglycemia and glycosuria, can be brought under control by careful revision. Commonly, it is not the disease which is brittle but the patient!

The treatment of hypoglycemic coma is intravenous glucose administration. It must be done quickly because of the risk of irreversible brain damage caused by punctate intracerebral hemorrhages. It should be done on the spot prior to removal to a hospital.

Nonketotic Hyperosmolar-Hyperglycemic Coma

Nonketotic hyperosmolar-hyperglycemic coma develops more rapidly and more insidiously than diabetic ketoacidosis. Its victims are usually elderly patients suffering from the relatively mild form of the rather stable, nonketotic, and non-insulin–requiring maturity-onset diabetes. The precipitating cause is severe dehydration resulting from fever, vomiting, diarrhea, or a combination of these factors. Their insulin reserve is still adequate to prevent overproduction of ketoacids, but not sufficient to promote full glucose utilization. The glycemia rises to extremely high values (800 to 1000 mg. per 100 ml. or more); the osmolality increases to above 36 mOsm. per liter, in part because of the relative insulin deficiency and in part because of dehydration and secondarily impaired renal function. In order to *prevent* this life-threatening complication, every elderly diabetic should be made aware of this possible serious complication, no matter how mild his disease may be, and should know that whenever he experiences bouts of vomiting or diarrhea he must (1) force fluids, preferably warm tea or water, and (2) call for medical help immediately. Chances are fair that aggravation of the syndrome can be prevented.

Treatment of the fully developed syndrome consists of the attempt to overcome the hypovolemic shock. Infusions of isotonic saline will both expand the extracellular fluid space and indirectly decrease the blood sugar level. Half-isotonic saline may be used for water replacement if the patient has not recovered fast enough to take fluids by mouth. Insulin will be required in small doses to restore blood sugar homeostasis. The patient usually is very sensitive to insulin.

Frequently the condition is complicated by lactic acidosis, in which case the already serious prognosis is made worse.

Lactic Acidosis

Lactic acidosis is not a specific diabetic complication, but rather is related to shock and renal failure, which are often the contributing causes of either ketoacidosis or hyperosmolar coma. Treatment must be directed against the precipitating causes. Prognosis is always most serious.

Lactic acidosis may also be precipitated or facilitated by the orally effective hypoglycemic guanidine derivatives (phenformin). Therefore medication with these substances, even if tolerated well under normal conditions, should be discontinued immediately if intercurrent illnesses occur. To prevent the risk of this complication and aggravation of the underlying diabetes, substitution of the oral agent must be instituted; this is best done by insulin (see footnote, p. 413).

MANAGEMENT DURING INTERCURRENT ILLNESSES AND DURING SURGERY

Almost without exception, intercurrent illnesses as well as nonsurgical or surgical trauma are stressful experiences which are bound to aggravate underlying diabetes. Most commonly the patient's normal alimentation and his normal activities of living are interfered with. Energy intake may be decreased, and energy output is frequently increased. In such instances it is most important to substitute for the inability to eat by appropriate means (parenteral feeding), to monitor carefully the glycemia and glycosuria as well as possible ketonuria, and to start or increase insulin treatment. Fast-acting insulin should be used in anticipation of possible rapid changes occurring in the patient's condition and the need for readjustment of the diabetic management.

Careful attention must be given to the possibility of drug interaction between insulin and the agents employed to treat the intercurrent disease.

Increased insulin sensitivity may occur in certain diseases of endocrine deficiency such as myxedema or adrenal or pituitary insufficiency. The absence or decrease of a hormonal insulin antagonist may give the impression of improvement of a diabetes complicated by these states of endocrine deficiency. A similar picture of apparent improvement of diabetes may be seen in the case of progressive renal disease. Here likewise, the insulin requirement decreases.

THE CHRONIC DIABETIC COMPLICATIONS

The marked extension of life expectancy of the diabetic during the past decades, owing to insulin and also to the antibiotics, has exposed the patient to the hazards of aging and degeneration. This fact alone could account for the high incidence of hypertensive-arteriosclerotic-cardiovascular disease in the aged diabetic population. But the rate of coronary heart disease, stroke, and peripheral vascular occlusion among diabetics is considerably higher than in the nondiabetic population, and onset is usually earlier. The disease-specific diabetic *microangiopathy* is most likely the contributory aggravating or precipitating cause of this greater severity and wider systemic involvement of degenerative vascular complications in diabetes. Impairment of the capillaries and small vessels interferes with the normal blood supply of all tissues, including the larger vessels and nerves, and makes them particularly vulnerable to a variety of insults such as infection, trauma, toxins, and of course the processes of aging. Diabetic microangiopathy is most likely the common cause—though in varying degrees—of diabetic retinopathy, nephropathy, and neuropathy as well as angiopathy. It seems to develop in the early stages of diabetes, progressing slowly and insidiously, and leading to clinical symptoms after a duration of the disease of 10 years or longer. Its relative independence from the carbohydrate anomaly of the disease is suggested by the facts that (1) the characteristic capillary changes can be observed histologically at a very early stage in skin, retina, muscle, and almost any other tissue, and (2) not infrequently diabetic neuropathy or peripheral angiopathy may precede the discovery of diabetes both in the juvenile and in the adult. It should not be suprising therefore that even the best diabetic control, as available today, fails all too often to prevent or to delay these chronic complications.

In the absence of a specific therapy or cure for these complications, it is mandatory to follow strictly the previously described criteria of optimal control of the underlying diabetes. In addition, all possible measures must be taken to protect the vascular bed against avoidable damages from within and without. This will include, on the one hand, appropriate elimination or restriction of lipid and salt intake and abstinence from nicotine; and, on the other hand, strict hygiene to protect against infection and traumatization of the peripheral vascularity. All modalities useful for the treatment of the same condition in the nondiabetic ought to be employed. Yet any possible interference with the management of the diabetes must be avoided and the possible limitations or risk which the diabetes may present must be taken into consideration.

In the case of *peripheral or central angiopathy,* if vascular surgery is considered, cognizance must be taken of the usually great extent of the obstructive vascular lesions which may make bypass surgery and amputations more risky than in the nondiabetic. Likewise, rehabilitation procedures for diabetics with vascular impairment must not overlook the systemic character of the disease and of the complication. The compatibility of antihypertensive diuretic drugs, anticoagulants, and vasodilators with the drug management of diabetes must be evaluated carefully.

With regard to *diabetic nephropathy*, particularly the specific intercapillary glomerulosclerosis, the outlook is still very poor. Dialysis may be life prolonging here as in all other types of renal failure. But frequently diabetic nephropathy is precipitated or aggravated by ascending pyelonephritis. Early and vigorous treatment of urinary tract infections and instructions concerning proper hygiene may be successful preventive measures.

Most gratifying progress has been made in *management of diabetic retinopathy*. Photocoagulation and vitrectomy have proved to be most successful in maintaining or restoring vision in instances of advanced proliferative lesions. These procedures are now under consideration for early diabetic retinitis, although it should be remembered that in its early stages the condition may arrest or revert spontaneously. Pituitary ablation, which was more risky and less predictable, has largely been replaced by these procedures. Improvements in microsurgery of the eye, in cataract extraction, and in the prevention and treatment of glaucoma have done much to better the care of diabetics with impaired vision.

The protean picture of the *diabetic neuropathies* still presents innumerable problems in management. No specific treatment is available for the large group of the usually symmetric peripheral neuropathies with or without muscular (amyotrophic) or joint (arthropathic, Charcot joint) involvement, which are responsible for a large sector of chronic morbidity in diabetes. Neither can more than symptomatic relief be offered for the neurovisceropathies secondary to involvement of the autonomic nervous system, such as gastric paresis with its persistent gastric dilatation and diarrhea, bladder atony with urinary stasis and the risk of ascending infections, most disturbing orthostatic hypotension, or impotence. In contrast, it is comforting that some of the diabetic mononeuropathies, particularly those involving the cranial nerves controlling the extraocular muscles, are self-limiting and resolve spontaneously after several weeks. Since such lesions may have a variety of causes, such as toxic, neoplastic, or vascular, the differential diagnosis must be established carefully before the patient can be assured that his lesion is one of the least serious of all the chronic complications of diabetes.

DIABETES MELLITUS IN CHILDHOOD AND ADOLESCENCE

method of
ROBERT B. SCHULTZ, M.D.
Hollywood, Florida

Introduction

The physician responsible for the care of youngsters with diabetes is generally occupied with the prevention of acute catastrophic events such as acute hypoglycemia or diabetic ketoacidosis, as opposed to his counterpart in internal medicine who is generally concerned with the management of chronic complications such as vascular diseases, retinopathy, neuropathy, and nephropathy. In the light of recent studies, however, the pediatrician must now recognize that his role is perhaps more significant in that the care he renders and the attitudes which he generates may ultimately affect the outcome of the longstanding diabetic patient with respect to modification of the aforementioned chronic complications. This article will concentrate, however, on some of the more contemporary methods of treatment of the acute problems with which the pediatrician or pediatric diabetologist is faced.

MANAGEMENT OF EMERGENCIES IN THE DIABETIC CHILD

Diabetic Ketoacidosis

Clinical Presentation. Although severe diabetic ketoacidosis proceeding to coma is a much less common presenting manifestation of the disease today, the reader should nevertheless remain familiar with the classic manifestations. The striking polyuria, polydipsia, polyphagia, and weight loss are rarely misdiagnosed. The clinical features may be manifest over an extended period of days or weeks, or they may appear abruptly when the disease is ushered in by a precipitating illness. When presented with a youngster in ketoacidosis, the physician must not only carefully plan his approach to this primary problem, but must scrupulously search for a possible precipitating illness. Clinical features of the child in ketoacidosis (whether newly diagnosed or an established case) may often be misleading. The finding of leukocytosis *in the absence of fever* is a feature commonly observed at the onset of ketoacidosis. The presence of fever should alert the examiner to the presence of an infectious process. Abdominal findings such as tenderness or diminished bowel sounds (perhaps related to the ileus observed in acidosis or hypokalemia) may raise the question of an acute surgical emergency. Indeed, some youngsters may undergo exploratory laparotomy because of such findings. Acute pancreatitis must repeatedly be mentioned as an initial precipitating cause of childhood diabetes, and the clinician should include a serum amylase or urinary diastase among the tests required from the laboratory. So profound is the effect of acidosis on the gastrointestinal tract that in some 10 per cent of cases, youngsters may present with transient hematemesis. Before proceeding with specific therapy, the clinician should proceed with the following laboratory analyses and procedures:

1. Blood glucose (by customary laboratory methods or estimated by Dextrostix).
2. Serum acetone. This may be tested by use of the Acetest tablet, and, if desired, serial dilutions may be made to quantitate the degree of acetonemia. Since the Acetest tablet does not detect the presence of beta-hydroxybutyric acid, the quantitation of serum acetone may be misleading for those patients in whom this ketone body is excessive.
3. Serum electrolytes: sodium, potassium, chloride, CO_2, blood urea nitrogen (BUN), *serum phosphorus*.
4. Arterial or arterialized blood for blood gases, including pH. These values may be extremely important in subsequent hours as one attempts to assess the success or failure in correcting the acidosis.
5. Serum osmolarity:

$$\text{mOsm./L} = (\text{serum sodium mEq./L.} \times 2) + (\text{blood or serum glucose} \div 18)$$

$$\text{Normal osmolarity} = 286 = 140 \times 2 + 100/18$$

6. Passage of urinary catheter. The sterile introduction of a catheter will provide a specimen for culture and will permit continual evaluation of urine flow.
7. *Passage of a nasogastric tube* in patients who are severely obtunded and have presented with emesis or hematemesis. This will not only help avoid a subsequent aspiration, but will also permit a brief gastric lavage with iced saline, which is all that is usually necessary for stopping the hematemesis of diabetic ketoacidosis.
8. Additional studies such as blood culture, sedimentation rate, febrile agglutinins, and any other appropriate data may be necessary in the search for a precipitating disease process.

Fluid and Electrolyte Therapy. The deficit of water and salts in the youngster presenting with diabetic ketoacidosis is usually quite severe. Balance studies have suggested the following deficits:

Water—100 to 125 ml. per kg.
Sodium—6 to 12 mEq. per kg.
Chloride—4 to 9 mEq. per kg.
Potassium—2 to 8 mEq. per kg.
Phosphate—parallels K^+ depletion.

Repair of the fluid and electrolyte deficit in this disorder demands that the physician have familiarity with the average losses noted and that he familiarize himself with one of the many therapeutic regimens described in the pediatric literature. There is no one universally accepted plan of approach that is best. The following is based on a scheme of therapy which I have found helpful and which has undergone some modifications in the light of new information regarding depletion syndromes described in the literature.

Initial Hydration. The initial hydrating solutions commonly employed are either 0.9 per cent saline or Ringer's lactate solution. The purpose of the initial hydrating solution is to acutely expand the intravascular space, overcome the contracted intravascular volume, and improve renal flow and urine output. A volume of 20 ml. per kg. administered over 1 hour is usually sufficient. If urine flow does not take place, this may be repeated during a second hour. If shock is severe, consider the use of 15 ml. whole blood per kg. as an initial hydrating solution.

Replacement of Deficits. The average youngster presenting in diabetic ketoacidosis has approximately a 10 per cent dehydration. The general plan is to calculate the approximate deficit at the outset and to plan on replacing two thirds of this deficit within the first 12 hours.

Maintenance Requirements. The average maintenance fluids for the patient should be taken into consideration when calculating the fluid requirements for each 24 hour period. Maintenance

TABLE 1. **Average Maintenance Fluid Requirement—1500 to 2000 ml. per m.² per 24 Hours**

WEIGHT (KG.)	SURFACE AREA (SQUARE METERS)
1.0	0.2
3.0	0.2
7.5	0.4
10.5	0.5
13.5	0.6
15.5	0.7
19.5	0.8
23.0	0.9
26.0	1.0
34.0	1.2
38.0	1.3
45.0	1.4
50.0	1.5
55.0	1.6
65.0	1.7

Average maintenance fluid estimates based on body weight alone, noted below, may give slightly higher estimates of fluid needs.

BODY WEIGHT	VOLUME
First 10 kg.	150 ml./kg.
Next 10 kg.	75 ml./kg.
Above 20 kg.	30 ml./kg.

requirements may be calculated by using either of the methods shown in Table 1.

An appropriate maintenance solution contains approximately 30 mEq. per liter of Na and Cl with K added at a concentration no greater than 30 mEq. per liter.

The following is an example of fluid calculations using the aforementioned method. Assume a child of 26 kg. body weight (or 1 square meter of surface area).

1. 10 per cent dehydration in a 26 kg. child gives a deficit of 2600 ml.
2. Maintenance = 2000 ml./M² = 2000 ml.
3. Total = 4600 ml.
4. Initial hydration: 20 ml. per kg. of Ringer's lactate in the first hour = 520 ml. (If no voiding, repeat for a second hour.)
5. Thereafter provide fluids for repair of deficit and provision of maintenance so as to provide two thirds within the next 12 hours: 4600 × ⅔ = 3066 ml. This reduces to a rate of 255 ml. per hour. This volume may be provided by use of 0.3 or 0.45 per cent saline solution.

Although some clinicians recommend the use of glucose-containing solutions from the outset in order to prevent hypoglycemia, the method of insulin administration to be discussed below seldom results in this problem. Consequently, I prefer the use of glucose-free solutions until blood tests have given evidence of a reduction in blood sugar to levels of approximately 200 mg. per 100 ml. At that time 0.3 or 0.45 per cent saline in 5 per cent glucose may be substituted.

POTASSIUM THERAPY. The initial serum K^+ levels do not reflect accurately the profound potassium losses which take place during ketoacidosis. As soon as urine flow is established, K^+ should be added to the intravenous fluids at a rate of 30 mEq. per liter and continued during the period of intravenous therapy. Potassium-containing beverages such as tomato or orange juice may be used once oral intake has begun.

Phosphate Depletion Syndrome. During recent years, considerable interest has been given to the issue of phosphate depletion which takes place during both the development and treatment of diabetic ketoacidosis. Clinically, severe phosphate depletion may be manifest by (1) prolonged stupor long after systemic acidosis is corrected; (2) acute hemolytic anemia; (3) hemorrhage with impaired platelet function; (4) central nervous system (CNS) dysfunction with paresthesias, anorexia, malaise, weakness, convulsions, confusion, and coma; (5) heart failure; (6) generalized myalgia and arthralgia; or (7) hepatic hypoxia.

For these reasons, I strongly recommend the use of phosphate as a potassium phosphate salt to be added to the intravenous solutions in the concentrations noted above in calculating K^+ deficit—i.e., no more than 30 mEq. per liter of K^+ as potassium phosphate.

Alkali Therapy. The use of sodium bicarbonate therapy has become somewhat traditional over the years. However, current thinking suggests that alkali therapy should not be used in *all* cases, and that strict criteria should be employed for its use. In cases of severe acidosis (with pH less than 7.0 or 7.1) or dangerously low serum bicarbonate (5 mEq. per liter or less) bicarbonate therapy may be given slowly intravenously over a 4 to 6 hour period and never as a bolus. The dose should be calculated to raise the serum bicarbonate to approximately 15 mEq. per liter, assuming a 50 per cent distribution of bicarbonate in the body. Calculate as follows: Body weight (26 kg.) × 50 per cent (distribution of HCO_3) × 10 mEq. per liter, the increment desired from 5 mEq. per liter to 15 mEq. per liter = 130 mEq. total. If bicarbonate therapy is used, electrolytes and pH should be carefully monitored, because influences of bicarbonate may worsen the hypokalemia and the hypophosphatemia. For each 0.1 unit increase in pH, serum K usually falls from 0.6 to 1.0 mEq. per liter.

I have witnessed a number of complications of bicarbonate therapy and now prefer to withhold the use of alkali except in those situations noted above.

Parenteral Vitamins. Although there is no good evidence that parenteral vitamins are necessary, their use will not complicate therapy and on theoretical grounds might actually be indicated. Their use should be left to the discretion of the physician.

Insulin Therapy. In the newly diagnosed diabetic patient, schedules of insulin therapy have been recommended as follows:

INTERMITTENT DOSE THERAPY. 1. Give an initial dose of 1 to 2 units per kg. of body weight, administering half intravenously and half subcutaneously. In the presence of shock and circulatory collapse, administer the entire amount intravenously.

2. Measure blood sugar and serum acetone in 2 to 4 hours. If there is no decline in blood sugar, repeat the aforementioned dose.

3. Be certain to have a glucose-containing parenteral fluid in use as blood glucose levels begin to fall to levels of 200 to 250 mg. per 100 ml.

4. Once blood glucose values reach levels of approximately 200 mg. per 100 ml., avoid administering additional insulin.

5. Serum acetone values usually persist for several hours. There is no need to administer additional insulin to correct this ketosis, as long as the blood sugar level shows evidence of returning toward normal.

6. Intermediate acting insulin such as NPH or Lente at a dose of 0.5 unit per kg. may be administered at the outset of therapy or may be withheld until the following morning. If the latter method is chosen, supplements of regular insulin should be continued at 0.5 to 1.0 unit per kg. every 4 to 6 hours, with careful monitoring of blood sugar.

7. If monitoring serum as well as urinary acetone, remember that urinary acetone normally persists long after serum acetone has cleared because of renal concentration of this substance.

8. Carefully monitor sodium, potassium, chloride, blood urea nitrogen (BUN), CO_2, and phosphorus, remembering that *serum potassium* and *serum phosphorus* often decrease markedly during insulin administration.

CONTINUOUS LOW DOSE INFUSION. This method allows a more physiologic delivery of insulin to the patient over a prolonged period of time, is easier to monitor, especially in hospitals where house officers are not present, and permits a more even decline of blood sugar and serum acetone. It has become the method of preference for me and for many clinicians around the country.

1. All the methods for care and monitoring of the patient previously applied are continued.

2. Administer an initial dose of regular insulin of 0.1 unit per kg. intravenously.

3. Then begin an infusion of regular insulin at a rate of 0.1 unit per kg. per hour; technically this is accomplished by placing 50 units of regular insulin in a 250 ml. bottle of 0.9 per cent saline to which has been added 2 to 3 ml. of 25 per cent salt-poor albumin to prevent adherence of insulin to the glass or plastic tubing. Some investigators feel that the addition of albumin is not mandatory. This mixture gives a concentration of 0.2 unit per ml. solution. In the case of the 26 kg. patient given as an example earlier, one would administer 2.6 units per hour = 13 ml. per hour. The careful rate of infusion may be monitored with the use of an IVAC pump. The insulin infusion is attached in "piggy back" fashion to the intravenous fluid line.

4. Fresh insulin solutions should be prepared every 6 to 8 hours.

5. Once the blood sugar level has fallen to levels of approximately 200 mg. per 100 ml. *in the absence of serum acetone,* the infusion may be discontinued. If serum acetone persists, reduce the rate of infusion to deliver approximately 0.05 unit per kg. per hour.

6. Remember, slow *overinsulinization* may take place by either method, resulting in persistent or increasing serum acetone levels in the face of declining blood glucose. The treatment for this is administration of glucose either orally or intravenously and discontinuation of insulin administration.

The methods outlined for treatment of diabetic ketoacidosis apply equally to the newly diagnosed patient as well as to the established patient, with some exceptions. The established patient customarily needs less insulin, and an initial starting dose of regular insulin equal to about 10 per cent of the usual daily dose will suffice. This same dose level may be repeated at 4 to 6 hour intervals as necessary. The continuous infusion technique should be initiated at an insulin dose level of 0.1 unit per kg. per hour but may have to be reduced more rapidly.

Insulin Hypoglycemia

This unfortunate consequence of insulin therapy cannot always be avoided. During the early phase of treatment of diabetic ketoacidosis, it is usually iatrogenic in nature and is corrected simply by (1) increasing the rate of glucose administration, (2) administering 50 per cent glucose intravenously at a dose of 1 to 2 ml. per kg., or (3) administering glucagon at a dose of 0.05 mg. per kg. subcutaneously, intramuscularly, or intravenously, not to exceed 1.0 mg. During the chronic phase of treatment, the occurrence of hypoglycemia is usually the result of excessive insulin dosage, either intentional or accidental, skipping meals or neglect of dietary recommendations, or excessive exercise in the face of inadequate food intake. The symptoms of hypoglycemia should be familiar to all members of the household, friends, and teachers likely to encounter an episode at school. Brochures describing diabetes mellitus are available for school personnel and may be obtained from the American Diabetes Association, 1 West 48th Street, New York, New York 10020. The clinical manifestations are extremely varied but are most commonly characterized by sudden changes in disposition. Often, hypoglycemic episodes occur during the night and awaken the child. I have personally observed youngsters with "night terrors" and nocturnal hypoglycemia, in whom a diagnosis of a true convulsive disorder was subsequently made. Apparently, a sudden decline in blood sugar during the night, although not necessarily to hypoglycemic levels, was sufficient to trigger an epileptogenic focus. Home remedies for the treatment of the irritable hypoglycemic youngster may include candy or sweetened beverages. If the child is physically unable to ingest these substances, then honey or Instant Glucose, which may be purchased from the Diabetes Association of Cleveland, 10205 Carnegia Avenue, Cleveland, Ohio 44106, may be placed inside the child's cheek where rapid absorption takes place. I generally prescribe and demonstrate the use of glucagon to be kept at the child's home. Individual plastic boxes containing single dose vials are available from pharmacies.

Insulin Administration in the Surgical Patient

The youngster scheduled for morning elective surgery may be conservatively managed by administering half the usual dose of intermediate acting insulin at approximately 7 A.M. An intravenous solution of 10 per cent dextrose in 0.45 per cent saline may be used as a peripheral infusion line to provide glucose during the intra- and postoperative periods. Fastidious calculations of glucose-insulin ratios are generally not necessary, but in general 2 to 3 grams of glucose per unit of insulin will avoid hypoglycemia. If an unusually long or complicated operative procedure is planned, the physician would do well to advise the anesthesiologist or his assistant to monitor the patient with frequent determinations of blood glucose, using Dextrostix, with instructions to sample blood from a site distant from the infusion site. Emergency surgical procedures usually take place at some time after the patient has received his customary daily injection of insulin. In this case, the same infusion may be used and supplement of regular insulin administered postoperatively according to levels of blood glucose. A dose of 0.1 unit per kg. may be used as an estimated initial dose and thereafter raised or lowered according to need.

LONG-TERM MANAGEMENT OF THE DIABETIC YOUNGSTER

Insulin Therapy

The posthospital management of the diabetic patient requires frequent communication between the physician and the family. The selection of an appropriate dose of insulin for the patient must be carefully tailored to the individual needs of the youngster, based on his or her daily exercise pattern and dietary needs. Rarely does the activity or dietary intake remain constant, and one must recognize that the selection of an insulin dose, too, is often imprecise. All too often, the parents assume a great deal of guilt because of their inability to precisely control the child's insulin needs. In fairness to the family and the child, the physician must educate and re-educate the family in methods of assessing the degree of glucosuria and insulin dose selection. Immediately upon discharge from the hospital, the patient may be managed on a single morning dose of NPH or Lente U-100 insulin. It is rarely necessary to have to use protamine zinc insulin (PZI) or Ultralente in the growing child. One must emphasize to the family the importance of accurate urine testing during the period immediately following hospital discharge. At some period within the first few months after discharge, most children demonstrate very little need for insulin. This period has been variously described as the "honeymoon" or "recuperative" period. It may actually be necessary to withhold insulin administration until the patient once again demonstrates glycosuria and ketonuria. This "honeymoon" phase may actually last for several months, although more commonly there is simply a brief period of decline in insulin requirement. The decision is the physician's to make, based on his assessment of the child's and the family's ability to cope with this "off-again–on-again" therapy. Precise insulin dosages cannot be legislated. The needs of most children can be fulfilled by a dose ranging from 0.4 to 1.0 unit per kg. per day. As mentioned above, a single morning dose of NPH or Lente usually suffices. If marked glycosuria, associated with thirst and polyuria, occurs during the morning period between breakfast and lunch, then regular insulin may be added to the NPH. Begin by adding an amount of regular insulin equal to approximately 25 per cent of the total NPH dose and re-evaluate the patient's response. In those patients demonstrating nocturnal enuresis with glycosuria and nocturnal thirst, as well as morning glycosuria and acetonuria, there is a clear need for an evening dose of NPH or Lente. This may be initiated by the addition of an evening dose equal to about one third of the morning dose. I prefer to obtain *block urine* testing from my patients (to be described below) prior to the addition of a second dose of insulin. The need for supplemental doses of insulin during intercurrent illnesses should be monitored by the physician, with the family reporting the results of urine tests frequently. Supplements of regular insulin may be needed and can be initiated with a dose equal to approximately 10 per cent of the usual total daily insulin requirement. At times when vomiting and fever coexist during an illness, the physician may find need for use of rectally administered antiemetics, in addition to clear liquids such as Gatorade, Coca-Cola, or ginger ale.

Available Insulin. At present, U-100 insulin is the only commercially available insulin manufactured in this country. It is a purer insulin, called "single peak" insulin, that has replaced the previously used U-40 and U-80 preparations.

Injection Sites. The commonly used injection sites are upper arms, upper outer thighs, lower quadrants of the abdomen, and upper outer quadrants of the buttocks. Injections may be given *perpendicularly* into the subcutaneous tissue of any of these sites. A problem which I commonly encounter in youngsters administering their own insulin is that of hypertrophy and hypesthesia of the injection site (usually the thighs). The diminished sensitivity, once it develops, often results in overuse of these sites, followed by erratic urine results in glucose response. It is presumed that at these hypertrophied sites there is less than optimal insulin absorption and therefore an erratic response to the administered dose. The treatment is simply avoidance of these sites.

Dietary Recommendations

It should be clearly explained to the family and the patient (when age permits) that the dietary needs of the diabetic child are exactly those of any other child of comparable age. The punitive methods of dietary discipline so common in the past should be abandoned. A diet should be carefully planned by the dietitian in accordance with the physician's prescription. The traditional diets recommended in the past have included carbohydrate, 45 per cent; fat, 40 per cent; and protein, 15 per cent. Studies over the past few years, however, have indicated that diets in carbohydrate derived from starch have no adverse effect on postprandial blood sugar or on insulin requirements. The area of greatest concern now centers on the dietary content of cholesterol and saturated fats. Consequently, I agree with recommendations recently made which advocate the following dietary schedule:

Carbohydrate, 55 per cent, with 70 per cent derived from starch and 3 per cent from lactose, sucrose, and fructose; *fat, 30 per cent* and *protein, 15 per cent.*

1. Polyunsaturated : saturated fat ratio of 1.2 to 1.0.
2. Cholesterol limited to 250 mg. per day.
3. Use of lean meats such as lean beef, veal, chicken, turkey, and fish.

The total daily food allowance should be distributed so as to allow for major meals and snacks appropriately spaced to conform to the patient's activity schedule and insulin responsiveness. One of the most important factors to emphasize is consistency in time of eating from day to day so as to minimize the likelihood of hypoglycemia. Appropriate weight gain and normal growth are the best indicators of appropriate caloric intake and insulin dosage. The physician would do well to monitor the patient's blood level of cholesterol and blood lipids every 3 to 6 months.

Exercise

The need for daily exercise cannot be overemphasized. This is a natural part of the child's day, and parents soon learn the wisdom of providing appropriate after-school snacks before children go outdoors to play with friends. Vigorous exercise programs at school, which take place on certain days only, may require a lesser dose of insulin or greater food intake on that particular day. This should be discussed with the parent and the patient so that appropriate precautions may be taken prior to the exercise.

Urine Testing

Ideally, three or four urine tests should be made daily—prior to each meal and at bedtime. The method of second void testing should be taught and recommended to the parent. At present the Clinitest two-drop method is most often recommended for testing. Variations in family and school schedules may require less than the optimal number of daily urine tests, and the physician should attempt to work within the confines of the family's schedule to avoid imposing undue guilt on the parent or child for failing to adhere to a *rigid* schedule. It is desirable to keep most urine tests at a level of 1 per cent when possible. Not infrequently, youngsters show rather erratic urine patterns with frequent urine tests of 3 per cent throughout the day but without polyuria or polydipsia. If the physician is in doubt about the degree of glucosuria in his patient, he may suggest a 24 hour urine collection or block urines at 6 hour intervals—e.g., quantitative collections from 6 A.M. to noon, noon to 6 P.M., 6 P.M. to midnight, and midnight to 6 A.M. Block urine collection permits one to assess those periods when insulin seems to be most or least effective. The quantitation of a 24 hour urine simply requires the measurement of a total volume and then performance of a Clinitest on an aliquot of this urine. One should attempt to keep the number of grams of urinary glucose at a level of less than 10 per cent of total ingested carbohydrate. The latter can be calculated from the diet as total available glucose: (1) 100 per cent of dietary carbohydrate, (2) 58 per cent of dietary protein, and (3) 10 per cent of dietary fat.

Example:

Total daily calories–2000 calories

Carbohydrate:	55% =	1100 calories =	275 grams
Fat:	30% =	600 calories =	66 grams
Protein:	15% =	300 calories =	75 grams

Total available glucose may then be calculated:

Carbohydrate:	275 grams × 100% =	275 grams
Fat:	66 grams × 58% =	38 grams
Protein:	75 grams × 10% =	7.5 grams
Total available glucose		320.5 grams

The 24 hour urine should therefore contain less than 32.0 grams of glucose.

UNIQUE PROBLEMS OF THE CHILD WITH DIABETES MELLITUS

The Somogyi Phenomenon

This phenomenon is perhaps one of the most common manifestations of gradual excessive insulin administration. It describes a situation in which sudden falls in blood sugar are followed by rebound hyperglycemia. This sequence may occur repeatedly throughout the day, but most commonly occurs in late afternoon or in the early morning hours before awakening. The fall in blood sugar which initiates the cycle does not necessarily have to result in true hypoglycemic levels. In fact, more commonly one observes that a precipitous fall from high to even normal levels of blood sugar may be sufficient to induce symptoms of hypoglycemia and initiate the Somogyi phenomenon. The clinician is alerted to this peculiar series of events when parents report symptoms suggesting hypoglycemia with urine tests showing frequent glycosuria. A very subtle manifestation of excessive insulin dosage occurs in the child found to be consistently irritable and grouchy upon awakening, with the morning urines found to contain ketones but free of sugar. This urine pattern must be taught to parents very carefully, for it seems to be the earliest clue to the phenomenon of "overinsulinization," and when recognized may help avoid a subsequent and severe insulin reaction. Occasionally the Somogyi phenomenon may be suspected, but the clinician is not absolutely certain. He may elect to hospitalize the child and obtain absolute blood sugar levels at 3 to 4 hour intervals around the clock, or, more practically, may suggest a 10 per cent reduction in insulin dose with careful monitoring of the urine sugar and acetone over the next 3 to 4 days. This decrease seems safe, and in my experience it has never resulted in an episode of frank ketoacidosis.

Chronic Underinsulinization

The phenomena resulting from less than optimal dosages of insulin may be subtle or overt. The subtle form commonly seen in the adolescent results in continuing polyuria, polydipsia, hyperlipidemia, and surprisingly elevated blood glucose levels. Such patients may claim to feel well while maintaining blood sugars in the 300 to 400 mg. per 100 ml. range. In its most blatant form, chronic underinsulinization manifests itself as diabetic dwarfism or Mauriac's syndrome. This is characterized by short stature, obesity, hepatomegaly, polyuria, polydipsia, hyperlipidemia, and hyperglycemia. Careful reinstitution of an appropriate insulin dose will reverse all the abnormalities.

Autoimmune Endocrine Disorders Associated with Diabetes Mellitus

The association of juvenile diabetes mellitus with autoimmune endocrinopathies such as thyroiditis and/or Addison's disease has been well established. The association with hypothyroidism secondary to thyroiditis is sufficiently common to warrant careful evaluation of the size of the patient's thyroid gland, growth as plotted on a standard grid, and, as recommended by some, annual determination of the presence or absence of thyroid antibodies (microsomal). A sudden unexplained decrease in insulin requirement, associated with weight loss, salt craving, and increased pigmentations, should alert the physician to consider the onset of early Addison's disease.

Emotional Disorders of the Diabetic Child

The physician caring for a youngster with diabetes often finds himself rendering counseling services to the remainder of the family. The many restrictions commonly placed on the diabetic youngster invariably have profound effects on the entire family unit. There is hardly any other disorder which imposes such heavy responsibility on the parent(s) for such things as meal planning, urine testing, and therapeutic decisions regarding daily insulin administration. The metabolic effects of emotional disturbances on the diabetic child are profound, and the physician ignoring this fact will have considerable difficulty in management of his patients. The team approach to total care of the affected youngster and his or her family is often not available in a given community, thus making it necessary to request the assistance of a specialized team from a nearby university.

GOUT

method of
IRVING H. FOX, M.D.,
and WILLIAM N. KELLEY, M.D.
Ann Arbor, Michigan

Gout is a term representing a heterogeneous group of diseases which in full development are manifest by (1) an increase in the serum urate concentration; (2) recurrent attacks of a characteristic type of acute arthritis, in which crystals of monosodium urate monohydrate are demonstrable in leukocytes of synovial fluid; (3) aggregated deposits of monosodium urate monohydrate (tophi), occurring chiefly in and around the joints of the extremities and sometimes leading to severe crippling and deformity; (4) renal disease of uncertain cause which involves glomeruli, tubules, interstitial tissues, and blood vessels; and (5) uric acid urolithiasis. These manifestations can occur in different combinations.

The goals in the therapy of this disease include (1) rapid termination of the acute attack; (2) prevention of future attacks of gout; (3) lowering the serum uric acid to prevent its accumulation in body tissues; (4) prevention of the formation of uric acid stones; and (5) treatment of disorders accompanying hyperuricemia, such as obesity, hypertriglyceridemia, and excess ethanol ingestion.

Treatment of the Acute Attack

Acute gouty arthritis can be effectively treated in most instances with colchicine, indomethacin, phenylbutazone, or oxyphenbutazone. In other patients naproxen or intra-articular corticosteroids may be utilized.

Colchicine. When used within the first 24 to 48 hours of an attack of acute gouty arthritis, intravenous colchicine is highly effective. When 2 mg. is diluted in 20 ml. of isotonic saline solution and infused slowly and carefully into a vein, the patient should receive relief in no more than 6 to 12 hours. If a dramatic response is not observed within 6 hours, 1 mg. may be repeated every 6 hours up to a total dose of 4 mg. during one treatment period. Care should be taken not to infiltrate the colchicine solution, as extravasation can lead to inflammation and necrosis. Gastrointestinal side effects of the drug, which include nausea, vomiting, diarrhea, and abdominal pain, do not occur with intravenous colchicine if the oral colchicine is stopped prior to institution of the intravenous regimen. Leukopenia is a serious potential complication in the patient on prior maintenance colchicine or the patient with hepatic or renal diseases. Accordingly, if a patient has been taking prophylactic colchicine on a long-term basis, no more than 2 mg. should be given intravenously at the time of the acute attack. Intravenous colchicine is contraindicated in the patient with leukopenia or significant hepatic or renal disease.

Oral colchicine may be used in a 0.6 mg. dosage at hourly intervals until joint symptoms ease, gastrointestinal symptoms develop, or the patient has had 12 tablets. However, because of the frequent occurrence of nausea, vomiting, and diarrhea, this form of therapy is recommended only in those patients in whom the diagnosis of gout is not established with certainty. A response to oral colchicine may be of some diagnostic value in this setting.

Indomethacin. Indomethacin may be given in doses of 50 mg. every 6 hours for the first 2 days of an acute attack. Subsequently, 25 mg. four times a day is given until all evidence of acute gout has disappeared. The drug is usually effective, and within 24 hours there is considerable relief of the acute pain, although the swelling and redness may take a few days to disappear. The most common complications include headaches, abdominal pain, and other gastrointestinal complaints. Hematopoietic and central nervous system reactions have been described.

Phenylbutazone. Phenylbutazone is given orally in a dosage of 200 mg. three times each day during the first 1 to 2 days of an acute attack. The drug can then be tapered to 100 mg. four times a day for the subsequent 2 days and then stopped. In no case should it be used for longer than 1 week. Oxyphenbutazone can be given in the same dosage. One of the disadvantages of these two drugs is related to their uricosuric properties; the lowering of serum uric acid and the increase in the renal clearance of uric acid observed with these agents may temporarily interfere with the subsequent diagnostic value of the serum and urine uric acid determinations. Nausea, vomiting, epigastric discomfort, and skin rashes are the most commonly reported side effects. Serious side effects, including bone marrow toxicity and salt and water retention, have been described.

Naproxen. Naproxen may be given in an initial dosage of 500 mg., followed by 250 mg. every 8 hours for up to 48 hours, by which time most patients have responded (this use of naproxen is not listed in the manufacturer's official directive).

Intra-articular Corticosteroids. The aspiration and injection of a crystalline form of corticosteroid into a joint in a dosage of 10 to 40 mg. of prednisone or the equivalent can give relief from the acute attack within 12 hours.

Prevention of Acute Gouty Arthritis

Acute gouty arthritis may develop in any patient with prolonged hyperuricemia. This may occur during the first few months of antihyperuricemic therapy or even longer when large tophaceous deposits are present. Thus prophylactic therapy using low dose oral colchicine, 0.6 mg. twice per day, may be helpful. In a substantial number of patients who cannot tolerate colchicine, indomethacin, 25 mg. twice per day, appears to be effective. Prophylactic therapy may be discontinued 6 to 12 months after the last attack, assuming that the serum urate has been in the normal range and all visible urate deposits have disappeared with antihyperuricemic therapy. In spite of this treatment, patients may still develop an occasional episode of acute gout. Therefore it is useful to supply the patient with appropriate medication and instruction on how to treat the acute attacks.

Antihyperuricemic Therapy

Several available drugs are capable of reducing the serum urate concentration. These antihyperuricemic agents may be divided into those drugs which decrease the synthesis of uric acid and those which increase the renal excretion of uric acid.

Decreased Synthesis of Uric Acid (Allopurinol). Allopurinol diminishes the serum uric acid by inhibiting xanthine oxidase, the enzyme which catalyzes the oxidation of hypoxanthine to xanthine and xanthine to uric acid. The usual daily dosage is 300 mg. Occasionally in particularly resistant cases, 600 to 800 mg. may be necessary. In the few patients with renal insufficiency who require antihyperuricemic therapy, the lowest dosage required to maintain the serum urate below 6.0 mg. per deciliter should be given. Allopurinol may be taken in a single daily dose because of the prolonged half-life of oxypurinol, the active metabolite.

The serum urate begins to decrease within 1 to 2 days and reaches a minimum value within 7 to 14 days. After 3 to 6 months of normouricemia, reduction in the frequency of gouty attacks may be expected to occur. Urinary uric acid is also reduced, thus reducing the formation of uric acid calculi and possibly the progression of gouty nephropathy. Apparent failure of allopurinol to adequately reduce the serum urate to the desired level is usually related to lack of patient compliance.

The most common side effect of allopurinol therapy is the precipitation of acute gouty arthritis. Other reactions include skin rash, fever, leukopenia, thrombocytopenia, hepatitis, vasculitis, or interstitial nephritis. Xanthine crystalluria or lithiasis is rare, having been recorded only in patients with the Lesch-Nyhan syndrome or in patients who have received massive cytolytic tumor therapy. Side effects are most common in patients with renal insufficiency. There are several important drug interactions of allopurinol. The best known is potentiation of the toxicity of 6-mercaptopurine and azathioprine. Allopurinol also increases incidence of bone marrow suppression during cancer chemotherapy with other cytotoxic compounds such as cyclophosphamide.

Increased Excretion of Uric Acid—Uricosuric Drugs. Most uricosuric drugs are weak organic acids which appear to increase the renal clearance of uric acid by inhibiting the renal tubular reabsorption of uric acid. Therapy with uricosuric drugs should be started at a low dose to minimize the increased risk of renal calculi associated with the transient increase in uric acid excretion. The maintenance of adequate urine flow and alkalinization of the urine with oral sodium bicarbonate (2 to 6 grams per day) or sodium citrate (Shohl's solution, 20 to 60 ml. per day) will further reduce the likelihood of uric acid stone formation. Probenecid is administered initially in dosages of 750 mg., increasing to 1.5 to 3.0 grams per day in three or four divided doses over a period of 2 to 4 weeks. Sulfinpyrazone is administered initially at a dose of 150 mg., increasing to 300 to 800 mg. in three or four equally divided doses. Benzbromarone, a newer drug (investigational in the United States of America), can be administered in a single daily dose ranging from 40 to 120 mg. Failure with these drugs has occurred as a result of drug intolerance, concomitant salicylate ingestion, or impaired renal function. Salicylate ingestion at any dose blocks the uricosuric effect of probenecid and sulfinpyrazone and modestly reduces the action of benzbromarone. When the glomerular filtration rate falls to 20 to 30 ml. per minute, uricosuric drugs are ineffective, although benzbromarone may have some antihyperuricemic activity in patients with impaired renal function.

The major side effects of the uricosuric drugs include gastrointestinal symptoms, rash and hypersensitivity, precipitation of acute gouty arthritis, and uric acid stone formation. Uricosuric drugs alter the transport of other organic acids across cell membranes, resulting in numerous drug interactions. The renal excretion of penicillin and ampicillin, for example, is decreased by probenecid, and thus the half-life of these antibiotics is prolonged. Many other drugs with diverse chemical and pharmacologic properties are also uricosuric.

Choice of Drug. The choice of an antihyperuricemic drug should have a rational basis, because the treatment of hyperuricemia in gout is ordinarily carried on indefinitely. Although allopurinol has gained a dominant use in the treatment of hyperuricemia, there remains a place for uricosuric compounds. In general the candidate for a uricosuric drug is the gouty patient without tophi under age 60 with normal renal function who is a normoexcretor of uric acid and has no history of renal calculi.

The indications for allopurinol therapy are as follows: (1) tophaceous gout, (2) gout complicated by renal insufficiency, (3) uric acid excretion greater than 1000 mg. per day, (4) history of renal calculi, (5) hypoxanthine-guanine phosphoribosyltransferase deficiency, (6) secondary hyperuricemia with overproduction of uric acid, (7) prior to the use of cytotoxic agents, (8) allergy to uricosurics, (9) uricosurics ineffective or poorly tolerated, or (10) patient not dependable.

Because the sudden decrease of the serum urate may actually precipitate acute gout, initiation of antihyperuricemic therapy is usually deferred until after the acute episode of gouty arthritis is over. Two to 4 weeks following initiation of antihyperuricemic therapy, it is necessary to check the serum uric acid to ensure a reduction of this value to below 6.4 mg. per deciliter, the concentration at which uric acid saturates extracellular fluid. In the event that the serum urate is not reduced below 6.4 mg. per deciliter and the patient is taking the drug as directed, either an increase in the dose of the medication or combination therapy with a uricosuric drug and allopurinol may be utilized. The latter is rarely necessary, but may be required in patients with extensive tophaceous deposits.

Treatment of Associated Disorders

About 50 per cent of gouty patients have hypertriglyceridemia, about 50 per cent are hypertensive, a large proportion are obese, and a substantial number imbibe excessive quantities of alcoholic beverages. These disorders must be managed with appropriate therapy. A reduction of body weight has been found to lower the serum uric acid. Although a purine-free diet will lower the serum uric acid as well, the availability of potent antihyperuricemic drugs makes this inconvenient and unnecessary for most patients.

Treatment of Hyperuricemia Without Gout

Only a minority of patients with hyperuricemia without gout require therapy. A patient with hyperuricemia and an unequivocal history of a renal calculus should receive allopurinol therapy. Similar therapy should be considered in the asymptomatic hyperuricemic person when the urine uric acid exceeds 700 mg. per 24 hours. Hyperuricemia in malignant disease is usually treated with allopurinol, especially prior to cytolytic therapy. This is an effective method for preventing the occurrence of acute uric acid nephropathy. In the latter instance when a large tumor mass is to be rapidly treated, care should be taken to give 2 to 3 liters of fluid per day and to alkalinize the urine to pH 6.0 to 6.5. The treatment of asymptomatic primary hyperuricemia with a normal 24 hour urinary uric acid excretion remains controversial. There is no evidence to suggest that this form of hyperuricemia leads to progressive impairment of renal function.

THE HYPERLIPOPROTEINEMIAS

method of
JEAN DAVIGNON, M.D.
Montreal, Quebec, Canada

There are three major reasons for wanting to lower plasma lipid levels. The first is to prevent acute abdominal pain and pancreatitis in severe hypertriglyceridemia, a relatively rare occurrence. The second is to reduce the size of unsightly or annoying skin or tendon xanthomas. The third is to prevent, retard, and ideally reverse the atherosclerotic process, especially in the coronary arteries.

In the first two instances, the expected benefit from treatment may be readily appreciated within a relatively short period of time (weeks or months). In the third situation, although much direct and indirect evidence has accumulated to indicate that some atherosclerotic lesions may regress, the benefit is much less tangible for both the patient and the physician, is difficult to objectify, and is likely to be significant on a long-term basis only (years).

The Significance of Elevated Plasma Lipids

Hyperlipidemia is not a diagnosis per se but a biologic sign which should be interpreted in context, taking into account the many variables likely to affect plasma lipid levels. The physician must establish whether diet, alcohol, drugs, hormones (especially contraceptives), toxic substances, physiologic conditions, or specific diseases are responsible for the plasma lipid abnormality. He must sort out the influence of heredity from that of ecologic factors, and must be aware of the situations which may mask a plasma lipid elevation (e.g., recent surgery, weight loss, lipid-lowering drugs, thyrotoxicosis, hepatitis).

Before making the diagnosis of one of the primary types of hyperlipidemia, one must exclude the many causes of secondary hyperlipidemias and seek out the aggravating factors. In practice special attention should be given to obesity, diabetes, hypothyroidism, alcoholism, use of oral contraceptives, pregnancy, nephrotic syndrome, pancreatitis, and biliary obstruction as the more frequently involved causes. One must always remember that primary and secondary hyperlipidemias often coexist in the same individual. For secondary hyperlipidemias, the treatment should be addressed to the underlying condition.

Too often one may conclude erroneously that hyperlipidemia is present on the basis of a single plasma lipid determination in uncontrolled conditions. To avoid being misled by a technical laboratory error, a nonfasting sample, an unduly prolonged venostasis during a difficult venipuncture, or a transient hyperlipidemia, several determinations of plasma cholesterol and triglycerides (preferably three to five) should be obtained over a period of several weeks. Blood must be drawn after a 12 hour fast and preferably on a standard North American diet (i.e., deriving 40 per cent of its calories from fats, mostly saturated). The baseline values thus secured will not only give an idea of the stability of the hyperlipidemia but will also be invaluable later on to assess the response to treatment.

The cutoff points delimiting "hypercholesterolemia" and "hypertriglyceridemia" are arbitrary by definition. If a preventive goal is sought, using two standard deviations above the mean for each age group may be risky, because the "normal population" is rather abnormal from the standpoint of coronary heart disease (CHD) incidence, the large consumption of saturated fats and carbohydrates in North America raising the means much above those of populations with a lower incidence of CHD, such as the Japanese and the Italian. In our laboratory, we tend to adopt the reasoning of Stamler and use a cutoff point of 240 mg. per dl. (100 ml.) for cholesterol and 150 mg. per dl. for triglycerides for an adult of any age in order to include as many persons at risk as possible. Since the risk of developing CHD is a continuous function of plasma cholesterol and since atherosclerosis may develop and progress in the absence of hyperlipidemia, being under the cutoff points does not confer an immunity against atherosclerotic vascular complications. The difficulty in establishing useful "normal limits" is compounded by the fact that plasma lipid values may differ by as much as 20 per cent on the same sample, depending on the methods used.

A large increase in total plasma cholesterol in the presence of normal triglycerides usually reflects an increase in the cholesterol fraction transported by the beta-lipoproteins (low density lipoproteins [LDL]). Indeed, the cholesterol of the alpha-lipoprotein fraction (high density lipoproteins [HDL]), which is higher in premenopausal women than in men, usually contributes less than 45 mg. per dl. to total plasma cholesterol, whereas the cholesterol of the prebeta-lipoprotein fraction (very low density lipoproteins [VLDL]) is less than 35 mg. per dl. when plasma triglycerides are within the normal range. A practical upper limit of normal for LDL-cholesterol is 190 mg. per dl. LDL appear to be the most atherogenic of the plasma lipoproteins, whereas HDL would have a protective role against atherosclerosis.

A rise in plasma triglycerides may reflect an increase in chylomicrons (transporting mainly alimentary fat); an increase in the prebeta-lipoprotein fraction, which is the main carrier of endogenous triglycerides; or an increase in intermediate density lipoproteins (IDL or "remnant lipoproteins"), which normally are readily catabolized into LDL and are present in very small amounts in plasma. Since chylomicrons contain little cholesterol, a mild elevation or a normal plasma cholesterol in the presence of large amounts of triglycerides (e.g., 190 mg. per dl. vs. 1800 mg. per dl., respectively) is likely to be caused by hyperchylomicronemia. Since VLDL contain about 20 per cent of cholesterol, the ratio of cholesterol to triglycerides is greater in hyperprebetalipoproteinemia (e.g., 400 vs. 1800 mg. per dl.). When both cholesterol and triglycerides are high with a ratio close to one (400 and 450 mg. per dl., for instance), the presence of an excess IDL, a lipoprotein usually rich in both cholesteryl esters and triglycerides, may be suspected. Above 300 mg. per dl., triglycerides impart turbidity to plasma. When the plasma sample is set to stand in the cold for several hours, chylomicrons will cause creaming at the top, whereas the smaller VLDL particles will be responsible for a diffuse turbidity throughout the sample.

Classification and Phenotyping

The hereditary hyperlipidemias include several distinct disease entities which must be identified in order to apply the most appropriate treatment. A useful classification of primary hyperlipidemias was proposed in 1965 by Fredrickson and Lees. It was based on both lipoprotein patterns and clinical features, and it was suggested that all patients with increased plasma lipids fell into five distinct phenotypes or categories. With the passage of time, this classification was refined and eventually adopted with slight modifications by the World Health Organization. The qualitative use of paper electrophoresis according to the technique of Lees and Hatch, coupled with the measurement of plasma cholesterol and triglycerides, taught the physician to think in terms of excess exogenous triglycerides (hyperchylomicronemia, type I), excess endogenous triglycerides (hyperprebetalipoproteinemia, type IV), or both (type V), and to recognize the importance of elevated cholesterol in the beta-lipoprotein fraction (type II). Thanks to the efforts of the proponents of this classification, the broad-beta disease (type III, dysbetalipoproteinemia) was singled out as a distinct clinical entity, and it became easier to distinguish the rare familial deficiency in lipoprotein lipase (type I) from the other categories of hyperlipidemia. In many laboratories, lipoprotein electrophoresis became a routine technique, the original paper method being replaced in some by agarose gel or polyacrylamide gel electrophoresis. Unfortunately, some drawbacks to this classification became apparent, and the worthiness of the procedure of lipoprotein phenotyping was challenged. Many physicians found that their patients differed markedly from the highly selected population of patients with xanthomatosis and pronounced elevation of plasma lipids which formed the basis of the original phenotyping system. They realized that most often they were confronted with only mildly abnormal lipids and few physical findings which could help them in diagnosis. In many cases, the lipoprotein pattern did not allow a distinction between type IV (increased prebeta-lipoproteins) and type IIb (increased beta-lipoproteins with a prebeta band). The presence of a sinking prebeta-lipoprotein or Lp(a) which migrates ahead of the beta-lipoproteins could mimic an increase in prebeta-lipoproteins. A broad beta-band turned out not to be necessarily present in type III. Drugs and diet could easily alter the phenotype, and it became evident that a single genetic disease could express itself with different phenotypes in the same family.

The genetic studies of Goldstein and coworkers have helped resolve some of these difficulties. This group performed lipid analyses on 500 survivors of acute myocardial infarction and found 164 to be hyperlipidemic. They tested all available family members of the latter group and found that 54 per cent of the 164 patients had inherited one of three types of familial hyperlipidemia conforming to single-gene transmission (monogenic). In 10 per cent, the classic familial hypercholesterolemia (type II) was recognized with its high penetrance (complete expression in affected children), high plasma cholesterol levels (mean of 350 mg. per dl.), and the presence of tendon xanthomas in several members. The cholesterol : triglyceride ratio was almost always greater than 2, suggesting a high proportion of patients with a type IIa pattern. In 14 per cent, there was an elevation of triglycerides alone with a type IV pattern (hyperprebetalipoproteinemia); in this group, only about 12 per cent of the relatives at risk manifested the lipid defect in childhood (prior to age 20). On the other hand, 30 per cent had a different and previously unreported disease which was termed *familial combined hyperlipidemia.* In this syndrome, plasma lipids tended to show a lesser degree of elevation than in either one of the other two monogenic diseases. Affected individuals rarely manifested an elevation in cholesterol in childhood. Affected members of the same family characteristically showed both hypercholesterolemia and hypertriglyceridemia, but often an affected relative manifested either hypercholesterolemia alone or hypertriglyceridemia alone. Thus in a single family, patterns of type IIb, IIa, or IV (and even type V) could be found simultaneously. In the same study, 15 per cent of the patients could not be classified genetically because of the lack of sufficient relatives. Another 17 per cent had a *sporadic hypertriglyceridemia,* in which an elevation in triglycerides presumably reflected exogenous factors. A last group of 14 per cent, designated *polygenic hypercholesterolemia,* had an elevation of plasma cholesterol, presumably reflecting complex genetic-environmental influences.

Until more is known about the basic genetic defect(s) responsible for the various plasma lipid abnormalities, any classification of primary hyperlipidemias will be subject to revision. In the meantime the physician must adopt a practical and useful classification which will allow him to identify distinct disease entities, recognize their consequences, and apply the most appropriate treatment available. Such a working classification, which takes into account some recent gains in knowledge, is presented in Table 1. There is no need at present to reject the phenotyping system, but its advantages and drawbacks should be recognized. Lipoprotein electrophoresis remains a useful adjunct in diagnosis (especially for types I, III, and V) and helpful during the follow-up period to assess the consequences of treatment. It remains most useful when it is combined with ultracentrifugal analysis and measurements of cholesterol in the various lipoprotein fractions. Unfortunately these techniques are presently available only in specialized centers. In practice, the lipoprotein phenotype may often be inferred from plasma cholesterol and triglyceride concentrations alone, and nomograms have been devised for this purpose.

Controlling the Risk Factors

It is commendable for the physician to make all possible efforts to lower the hyperlipidemia of a patient with ischemic heart disease. However, such efforts may be futile if the other risk factors for coronary heart disease are not recognized and controlled simultaneously. Among these, hypertension, cigarette smoking, and obesity should be amenable to correction in the hope of delaying the onset of atherosclerotic complications.

It is good practice in the routine follow-up of a hyperlipidemic patient to include a blood pressure reading whether he has hypertension or not. These subjects are likely candidates for the development of atherosclerosis. The appearance of hypertension in a previously normotensive subject might be the first indication of the atheromatous involvement of a renal artery. If the patient is hypertensive, the cause of the hypertension

TABLE 1. **Classification of Primary Hyperlipoproteinemias**

NOMENCLATURE	PHENO-TYPE	LIPIDS	POSSIBLE DISTINCTIVE FEATURES	PRESUMPTIVE DEFECT
1. Familial hyperchylomicronemia (fat-induced hyperlipemia) (type I)	I (V)	↑↑TG	Onset in childhood Eruptive xanthomas Abdominal pain Hepatosplenomegaly	Lipoprotein lipase deficiency or deficiency of apo C-II (LPL activator) (Recessive)
2. Familial hypercholesterolemia (familial hyperbetalipoproteinemia) (type II) a. Heterozygous	IIa, IIb	↑↑CHOL N or ↑TG	Tendon xanthomas Premature atherosclerosis Expression in childhood	Impaired β-lipoprotein (LDL) removal Inadequate number of cellular LDL receptors (Dominant)
b. Homozygous	IIa, IIb	↑↑↑CHOL N or ↑TG	Both parents affected Extensive xanthomatosis Thick planar xanthomas Aortic stenosis Early death (<25 years) Resistant to treatment	Absent or very limited number of cellular LDL receptors
c. Pseudohomozygous	IIa, IIb	↑↑↑CHOL N or ↑TG	Same as (b), but only one or no parents affected Responsive to treatment	Unknown Probably represents a distinct disease entity
3. Familial combined hyperlipidemia	IIb, IIa, IV (V)	↑CHOL ↑TG ↑CHOL-↑TG	Lower lipid levels than (2) No expression in childhood Few signs of lipid impregnation Mixed phenotypes in family	Unknown (Dominant)
4. Dysbetalipoproteinemia (broad-beta disease, floating-beta disease) (type III)	III (IIb, IV)	↑↑CHOL ↑↑TG	Planar xanthoma or orange pigmentation of palmar creases Tuberoeruptive xanthomas Punctate xanthomas Glucose intolerance Presence of a "floating β-lipoprotein" (or β migrating VLDL)	Faulty conversion of prebeta-lipoprotein to beta-lipoprotein Accumulation of a cholesterol-rich "remnant" (Recessive or dominant form)
5. Familial hyperprebetalipoproteinemia (carbohydrate-accentuated hypertriglyceridemia) (type IV)	IV (V)	↑↑TG	Arcus corneae, xanthelasma Glucose intolerance Overweight Middle age or late atherosclerosis	Impaired removal of prebeta-lipoproteins (Dominant)
6. Familial mixed hyperlipoproteinemia (type V)	V	↑↑TG	Glucose intolerance Hyperuricemia Abdominal pain, pancreatitis Eruptive xanthomas ↑TG induced by fat as well as sugar	Impaired removal of chylomicrons and prebeta-lipoproteins
7. Familial hyperalphalipoproteinemia	N(↑αLP)	N or ↑CHOL	CHD is rare	Unknown (Dominant)

Abbreviations: TG = triglycerides; CHOL = cholesterol; N = normal; LDL = low density lipoproteins; VLDL = very low density lipoproteins.

should be sought and a systematic and sustained treatment undertaken.

Obesity is often associated with diabetes, hypertension, hypertriglyceridemia, and hyperuricemia. Obese people are often sedentary. All these elements predispose to coronary heart disease. Weight loss and regular exercise will alone improve several of these parameters. In many obese patients with a mild type IV or type V hyperlipoproteinemia, weight control will suffice to maintain the triglycerides within the normal range.

Diabetes is an important risk factor for atherosclerotic cardiovascular diseases. Diabetes may be accompanied by a secondary hyperlipidemia, and conversely many hyperlipidemic patients have glucose intolerance or overt diabetes. To ascertain whether the hyperlipidemia is primary or secondary when it is associated with diabetes, response of lipid concentrations to insulin and a family survey are needed. In the first instance, control of the diabetes should be expected to correct the elevated plasma lipids, and other cases of diabetes may be found in the family without associated hyperlipidemia. In the second instance, a family survey will usually reveal several relatives affected with hypertriglyceridemia, some of them with normal glucose tolerance. In practice, it is academic whether one is secondary to the other or whether both coexist in the same patient (residual hyperlipidemia after control of diabetes and vice versa). The treatment is the same and should be addressed to both problems. Unfortunately, there is yet no evidence to support the view that control of the hyperglycemia will prevent the atherosclerotic complications associated with diabetes.

There is evidence that emotional or physical stress will promote the development of hyperlipidemia and atherosclerosis. In the occasional patient, a reduction in emotional stress will be accompanied by a lowering of plasma lipid concentrations. This aspect should be taken into consideration especially in the high-strung coronary patient in whom a coronary thrombosis might be precipitated by a period of overexertion or emotional stress.

Dietary Management

General Principles. After having recognized the presence of other risk factors and undertaken measures to correct them, while obtaining baseline values for plasma lipids, the next logical step is to put the patient on an appropriate dietary regimen. The dietary management of the hyperlipidemic subject should be guided by the type of lipoprotein abnormality. Exogenous fat will contribute to chylomicron formation and should be restricted in patients with an excess of these particles in circulation (types I and V). High saturated fat and cholesterol intake tend to elevate the cholesterol fraction transported by beta-lipoproteins and should be reduced in hyperbetalipoproteinemia (types IIa and IIb). An excessive intake of simple sugars will usually enhance the endogenous hypertriglyceridemia present in types IIb, III, IV, and V; these patients should thus be encouraged to curb their consumption of refined sugars. The dietary management should also take into account the nutritional habits, the level of physical activity, the degree of overweight or obesity, and the intake of alcohol of the patient. Whether or not the patient eats his meals at home or away from home should be taken into account. The level of caloric intake; the proportion of sugar, fat, protein, and alcohol consumed; the distribution of calories among the various meals; the socioeconomic setting; and the personality of the patient are important variables. Alcohol intake might be responsible in a given patient for a large part of the hypertriglyceridemia observed, or it can account for unexpected fluctuations in the triglyceride levels. *For the obese patient with hypertriglyceridemia, caloric restriction and weight loss should always be the first approach to treatment.* Usually, elevated plasma triglycerides are very responsive to weight loss, whereas beta-lipoprotein cholesterol is little affected.

The dietary management of hyperlipidemia is a great challenge to the patience and perseverance of the physician. He should take all possible measures to motivate the patient and ensure adherence to the dietary regimen. The help of a dietitian is necessary to review the patient's usual dietary habits, to indicate how to bring about the prescribed modifications, to point out the various brands of permissible foods (skim milk cheeses, substitute foods, margarines), to advise on recipes to make the diet more appealing, to consider the economic aspect, and to help reinforce the patient's motivation. The person who prepares the family meals should be present to receive the instructions; no intermediary should be accepted. Giving the instructions to a patient who does not care about cooking is doomed to failure. Even if no other member of a family is affected, it is important to point out that many of the recommended measures might be beneficial to the entire family, as the higher mean plasma cholesterol in the North American population is also associated with a higher rate of coronary heart disease. It is nearly impossible to serve two different menus at every meal at home for any sustained period of time, and temptation for the affected family member might rapidly become irresistible. Follow-up visits should not be too far apart, so that the motivation can be periodically reinforced. The physician must point out from the beginning that the radical change prescribed in dietary habits is definitive and should be pursued for the rest of the patient's life to be of significant preventive value.

Diet and Specific Disease Entity. A summary of the dietary measures applicable to the treatment of specific primary hyperlipoproteinemias is given in Table 2. In *familial hyperchylomicronemia* (type I), any fat intake, whether saturated or unsatured, will contribute to the excess plasma chylomicrons. Medium chain triglycerides (MCT) are an exception to this rule; being absorbed and transported to the liver through the portal system, they will not increase chylomicron formation, but they might contribute to a mild endogenous hypertriglyceridemia. A low fat diet (25 to 35 grams per day), supplemented with MCT to render the diet more acceptable, and the avoidance of any alcohol intake which may precipitate an attack of pancreatitis are the major features of the treatment. The goal is to maintain plasma triglycerides at levels which are not accompanied by abdominal pain, pancreatitis, or eruptive xanthomas and

TABLE 2. **General Guidelines for the Treatment of Hyperlipoproteinemias**

DISEASE ENTITY	DIETARY MANAGEMENT	DRUG THERAPY*
A. Familial hyperchylomicronemia (type I)	1. Low fat intake (25–35 grams/day) 2. MCT supplement 3. No alcohol	No drug effective at present
B. Familial hypercholesterolemia a. Heterozygous type IIa	1. Low cholesterol intake (<300 mg./day) 2. Low saturated fat 3. Increased polyunsaturated fat	1. Cholestyramine (Questran), 16–24 grams/day 2. Clofibrate (Atromid S),† 2 grams/day 3. Nicotinic acid, 3 grams/day 4. Probucol (Lorelco), 1 gram/day 5. Selective combinations of above drugs 6. Addition of second-line drugs (DT_4, β-ST, NEO, PAS) 7. Consider ileal bypass
b. Heterozygous type IIb	1. Reduction to ideal body weight 2. Low cholesterol intake (<300 mg./day) 3. Low saturated fat 4. Increased polyunsaturated fat 5. Control excess intake of refined sugars	Same as above (B,a) except for clofibrate
c. Homozygous type II	Same as for heterozygous type II	1. Nicotinic acid, 3–4 grams/day 2. Cholestyramine (Questran), 24–32 grams/day 3. Clofibrate (Atromid S),† 3 grams/day 4. DT_4 (Choloxin), 8 mg./day 5. Combination of above drugs 6. Addition of second-line drugs 7. Consider portacaval shunt
C. Familial combined hyperlipidemia	1. Reduction to ideal body weight 2. Treat according to type (see Ba, Bb, E) 3. Restrictions may be less stringent than those for familial hypercholesterolemia	1. Treat according to type 2. Use clofibrate cholestyramine probucol dextrothyroxine
D. Dysbetalipoproteinemia (type III)	1. Reduction to ideal body weight 2. Low cholesterol intake 3. Avoid excess of refined sugars 4. Replace saturated fat with polyunsaturated fat	1. Clofibrate (Atromid S), 2 grams/day 2. Use other drugs only if resistance or intolerance to clofibrate occurs: DT_4 or nicotinic acid
E. Familial hyperprebetalipoproteinemia (type IV)	1. Reduction to ideal body weight 2. Cholesterol intake 300–400 mg./day 3. Carbohydrate restricted to 40% of calories 4. Restrict alcohol intake 5. Avoid excess of refined sugars 6. Replace some of the saturated fat with polyunsaturated fat	1. Clofibrate (Atromid S),† 2 grams/day 2. Nicotinic acid, 3 grams/day 3. DT_4 (Choloxin), 4–8 mg./day
F. Familial mixed hyperlipoproteinemia (type V)	1. Reduction to ideal body weight 2. Reduction of fat to 30% of calories 3. No alcohol 4. Reduction of refined carbohydrates 5. Increased protein intake 6. MCT to replace part of fat calories if large excess of chylomicrons 7. If only traces of chylomicrons or mild transient elevation, treat as type IV (E)	1. Nicotinic acid, 3 grams/day 2. Norethindrone acetate (Norlutate), 5 mg. per day; effective in females (investigational) 3. Oxandrolone (Anavar), 2.5 mg. t.i.d. (investigational)
G. Familial hyperalphalipoproteinemia	None needed	None needed

*First steps of treatment are control of risk factors, control of excess body weight, and dietary management. Drugs are added only if dietary approach fails.

†Discontinue clofibrate if total cholesterol (or LDL cholesterol) is increased or shows only a slight decrease (<8%) in type II, or reaches upper limit of normal in type IV.

Abbreviations: DT_4 = dextrothyroxine; β-ST = beta-sitosterol; NEO = neomycin; PAS = para-aminosalicylic acid.

which will reduce the hepatosplenomegaly when present. The ambulatory patient on such a regimen will usually maintain his triglycerides between 500 and 1500 mg. per dl. and stay free of symptoms. In childhood, a 20 to 30 gram MCT supplement will help maintain normal growth and development. Fat-soluble vitamins should also be given.

In *familial hypercholesterolemia with normal triglycerides* (type IIa) a strict low saturated fat (less than 10 per cent of calories), low cholesterol (less than 300 mg. per day) diet with polyunsaturated fat supplementation forms the basis of treatment. Since a single egg yolk contains about 250 mg. of cholesterol, this strict regimen does not allow the use of eggs. The accent should be on lean meats, especially veal, poultry, and fish; the elimination of all dairy products except skim milk; and the liberal use of polyunsaturated oil (corn oil, safflower oil, soybean oil, sunflower seed oil) in cooking, frying, and salads so as to achieve a P/S ratio of at least 1.5. A polyunsaturated margarine should replace butter. The instructions to the patient should be positive, stress the use of fruits and vegetables, and provide him with written guidelines and appealing recipes. A 10 to 15 per cent fall in plasma cholesterol might be expected with this regimen, but it is practically never sufficient to return the cholesterol level to normal. In *familial hypercholesterolemia with some elevation of plasma triglycerides* (type IIb), it is often necessary to add a restriction in refined carbohydrates to cope with the mild associated endogenous hypertriglyceridemia. In our experience, the body weight is higher in these patients than it is in those with type IIa. In some instances it is necessary to control the excess body weight to successfully reduce the elevated plasma triglycerides. In other cases, the hypertriglyceridemia may be the manifestation of an associated diabetes. Some type IIa patients on a strict regimen might at times increase their sugar consumption to the point of raising their plasma endogenous triglyceride concentration.

In the *familial combined* variety of hyperlipidemia, in which a type II as well as a type IV pattern is found, and in which plasma cholesterol levels are not usually as high as in the xanthomatous form, a less stringent low saturated fat–low cholesterol–low refined carbohydrate diet with polyunsaturated fat supplementation should first be attempted as a lipid lowering measure. A "fat-controlled" diet of this type with no carbohydrate restriction has been promoted by the American Heart Association and has met with some success in several types of hyperlipidemia. The dietary management should be guided both by the phenotype and by the response of the plasma lipids to the dietary manipulations.

In *familial hyperprebetalipoproteinemia* (type IV), the calories derived from carbohydrate should not exceed 40 per cent of the total calories. Attention should be given to the excessive intake of refined sugar and concentrated sweets, which should be replaced by complex carbohydrates, proteins, and polyunsaturated fats. The mitigated restrictions in saturated fat and cholesterol (Table 2) are added preventive measures in patients at risk even if plasma cholesterol is not high at the beginning, because in many cases the lowering of plasma VLDL by any means tends to increase LDL-cholesterol. The type IV diet will allow three egg yolks a week and lean meats (beef, pork) with the fat trimmed, while restricting sucrose and concentrated sweets (candy, syrups, jams) as much as possible and encouraging the use of sugar substitutes. In some patients with an important endogenous hypertriglyceridemia, chylomicrons (or very large endogenous particles) might be present intermittently, giving a type V phenotype. In practice, these patients are essentially treated as type IV. The dietary treatment of *familial dysbetalipoproteinemia* has many similarities with the treatment of type IV (Table 2).

The hypertriglyceridemia of the rarer *familial mixed hyperlipoproteinemia* (type V) might be very sensitive to weight loss and control of alcohol intake. In an occasional lean patient with this lipid disturbance, dietary management might be very difficult, with sugars enhancing the hyperprebetalipoproteinemia and small amounts of fat increasing the hyperchylomicronemia. Such patients must be treated with a combination of total fat restriction and sugar restriction with an increased protein intake. MCT supplementation may be used. This diet is difficult to implement, and the patient may maintain his plasma lipids in the 1500 mg. per 100 ml. range from values of 5000 mg. per 100 ml. or more.

In *multifactorial hyperlipidemia,* in which a disease entity may not be singled out to account for the lipid abnormality, an atherogenic, hypercaloric diet is often found to be responsible. Control of body weight, dietary excess, and risk factors is usually strikingly effective in correcting the hyperlipidemia. The phenotype might be helpful in selecting the most appropriate dietary regimen.

Treatment with Drugs

General Principles. The use of drugs constitutes the second line of lipid-lowering measures applicable to the treatment of primary hyperlipidemias (Table 2). Once the physician is satisfied that the diet has been well understood and adhered to, he must decide, after 3 to 6 months, whether lipid-lowering drugs must be added. His decision should be based on the degree of response obtained in the first phase of treatment (lowering of plasma lipids, regression of xanthomas), and on the type of hyperlipidemia and its severity (as judged by its consequence in both the patient and his affected relatives). The drugs should be added to and not substituted for the diet, because the effects of the drugs are usually additive to those of the diet.

In familial hyperchylomicronemia, the use of drugs has been uniformly disappointing and there is no other alternative to dietary management at present. In familial xanthomatous hypercholesterolemia, dietary management is rarely sufficient to achieve good control of the very high plasma cholesterol levels, and drugs must be added in most cases. This is especially true for the homozygous form of this disease, which is highly resistant to therapy. It must be remembered, however, that on occasion a regression of skin lesions might precede by several years the lowering of plasma lipid levels. In familial combined hyperlipidemia as well as in dysbetalipoproteinemia (type III) and familial hyperprebetalipoproteinemia, it is not unusual to obtain a satisfactory response to dietary treatment alone. In many patients, especially in type IV, the physician will have to turn to drugs to reduce the significant residual hypertriglyceridemia which persists in spite of dietary treatment. In familial mixed hyperlipoproteinemia (type V) associated with a decreased lipoprotein lipase activity, some drugs might specifically help control the plasma lipid disturbance.

The list of lipid-lowering substances developed over the past 20 years is overwhelmingly large and bears witness to the fact that the ideal medication has not yet been discovered. There are only a few drugs which have met with some popularity because of their effectiveness, but they all have some drawbacks. When selecting a drug for the treatment of primary hyperlipidemias, one must think in terms of an indefinite period of administration and must choose the most potent agent with the least side effects or potential health hazards.

Specific Drugs. CLOFIBRATE (ATROMID S), 500 MG. CAPSULE. This drug interferes with the synthesis and/or release of VLDL by the liver and increases the biliary excretion of cholesterol. It is most effective in reducing endogenous hypertriglyceridemia. It is mainly excreted by the kidney and has a biologic half-life of about 12 hours, so that preferably it should be administered on a twice a day schedule. The starting dose should be 1 gram twice a day. It may be reduced in an occasional patient who is very sensitive to its lipid-lowering effect. Increasing the dose over 2 grams per day is rarely met by a further decrease in plasma lipids. The effect is rapid and is usually maximal after 3 to 4 weeks of administration.

Indications: Clofibrate is the drug of choice in broad-beta disease (type III) and in familial hyperprebetalipoproteinemia (type IV). In our experience, it has been effective in a good proportion of familial hypercholesterolemia type IIa, in which it will reduce LDL-cholesterol by 20 per cent. It is rarely effective in reducing plasma cholesterol in type IIb, although it does decrease plasma triglycerides. In a large proportion of type IIb and in a small proportion of type IIa, it might even increase LDL-cholesterol, an effect which commands discontinuation of the drug. It will tend to increase LDL-cholesterol in type IV also, occasionally exceeding the upper limit of normal. The same remarks apply to familial combined hyperlipidemia. It is rarely effective in familial mixed hyperlipoproteinemia (type V) when the chylomicrons are in excess. Clofibrate is often used in combination with cholestyramine.

Side effects: These are usually rare and benign, often transient. Gastric irritation, nausea, headaches, and tiredness are among the most frequent. A loss of libido, breast tenderness and enlargement, an increase in appetite, an increased incidence of gallstones, and a transient elevation in liver transaminase have been reported. In rare instances a severe reversible myalgic syndrome may develop, with leg cramps, muscle stiffness, and elevated plasma creatine phosphokinase activity. It may be more frequent and intense when plasma albumin which transports clofibrate is low, as in nephrosis.

Precautions: The lipid-lowering effect is opposed by certain contraceptive drugs. Clofibrate potentiates the effect of coumarin anticoagulants, warfarin (Coumadin); when they are used together, the prothrombin time should be closely monitored and the dose of anticoagulant adjusted downward as indicated. If clofibrate is started in a patient already on warfarin, the dose of anticoagulant should initially be cut by half. In type II, clofibrate should be discontinued if total plasma cholesterol is rising or is decreased by less than 8 per cent. Patients who have previously suffered a myocardial infarction may be at an increased risk of developing an arrhythmia or angina pectoris.

CHOLESTYRAMINE (QUESTRAN), INSOLUBLE POWDER. This is a nonabsorbable, bile acid–binding resin which interferes with the enterohepatic circulation of bile salts. Its hypocholesterolemic effect is linked to the enhanced transformation of cholesterol to bile acids which are lost in the feces and to an increased LDL catabolism. It does not lower plasma triglycerides and may at times raise their concentration in plasma. A daily amount of 12 to 24 grams may be given in two to four divided doses, preferably 30 minutes before a meal. The amount given should be increased gradually to the limit of tolerance or to the point at which adequate cholesterol control is achieved. It must be taken suspended in water, fruit juices, or other liquids. A 20 to 25 per cent decrease of cholesterol beyond the effect of diet alone should be expected.

Indications: Cholestyramine is the drug of choice in familial hypercholesterolemia (types IIa and IIb). It may be used whenever there is an excess of LDL-cholesterol which is not reducible by diet alone. It also reduces the hypercholesterolemia of primary biliary cirrhosis, in which it has been used for the relief of pruritus.

Side effects: Constipation, bloating, gastrointestinal irritation, nausea, vomiting, abdominal cramps and distention, and an occasional fecal impaction in older patients have been reported. Cholestyramine may exacerbate the symptoms of a duodenal ulcer and may aggravate previously asymptomatic hemorrhoids. Steatorrhea may develop with very large doses (>32 grams per day).

Precautions: Cholestyramine may interfere with the absorption of several acidic drugs such as digoxin, coumarin anticoagulants, thyroxine, thiazides, and phenylbutazone. It is necessary to administer these agents 1 to 2 hours prior to taking cholestyramine to avoid such interactions.

NICOTINIC ACID (NIACIN), 100 MG. OR 500 MG. TABLETS. This drug inhibits adipose tissue lipolysis, thus reducing the amount of nonesterified fatty acids transported to the liver for triglyceride synthesis. As a consequence, it decreases the production of VLDL and of their end-product, plasma LDL. It may also interfere with both cholesterol synthesis and catabolism, as well as chylomicrons and VLDL removal. The lipid-lowering doses of this vitamin (2 to 4 grams per day) far exceed the minimum daily requirement (15 mg.) or the therapeutic range for niacin deficiency (500 mg. per day). Because of its many side effects, which may be poorly tolerated, it is best to work up gradually from small doses (100 mg. three to four times daily) over several weeks until the therapeutic range is reached. Giving the drug during a meal or a snack will minimize the side effects. Both triglycerides and cholesterol may be lowered by 20 per cent or more. The effect on triglycerides precedes the effect on cholesterol.

Indications: Because of its many side effects, nicotinic acid is not recommended as a first drug, with the exception perhaps of the homozygous form of familial hypercholesterolemia. It should be used when clofibrate or cholestyramine has failed, has been inadequate, or has had to be discontinued because of some untoward reaction or intolerance. It may be combined with these drugs when they have been only partly effective.

Side effects: Cutaneous flushing of the face or upper part of the body is the most frequent side effect. Other skin manifestations include pruritus, urticaria, ichthyosis, and acanthosis nigricans. Nausea, diarrhea, abdominal pain, dizziness, increased urinary frequency, and dysuria are not uncommon. Hyperuricemia, hyperglycemia, and abnormal liver function tests are often reported. Nicotinic acid may aggravate a peptic ulcer or diabetes, precipitate an attack of gout, or induce gastritis.

Precautions: The use of nicotinic acid is discouraged in overt diabetes mellitus, pre-existing liver disease, active peptic ulcer, and gouty arthritis. The hypotensive effect of ganglionic blockers are potentiated by nicotinic acid, and they should be given together with great caution. Serum enzymes (SGOT, SGPT, LDH, alkaline phosphatase), bilirubin, glucose, and uric acid should be monitored in the course of treatment with nicotinic acid.

DEXTROTHYROXINE (CHOLOXIN), 2 MG. AND 4 MG. TABLETS. The D-isomer of the natural thyroid hormone enhances LDL removal and cholesterol catabolism. Although it has fewer metabolic side effects than levothyroxine, dextrothyroxine retains some at the lipid-lowering doses and may be responsible for increased angina, induction of arrhythmias, and clinical symptoms of hypermetabolism. It must be given with caution in gradually increasing doses (1 mg. daily, with increments of 1 mg. per month) until an effective level is reached (4 to 8 mg. per day) or intolerance supervenes. It may be given as a single daily dose, preferably in the morning. The side effects may be minimized with the concurrent administration of propranolol.

Indications: This drug is a second line choice for the treatment of hyperbetalipoproteinemia. It is also useful in some patients with endogenous hypertriglyceridemia. It may be used in combination with other lipid-lowering drugs to achieve maximum effect.

Side effects: Hypermetabolic effects, exacerbation of anginal symptoms, development of arrhythmias, precipitation of a second myocardial infarction, or aggravation of diabetes mellitus may occur.

Precautions: This agent is contraindicated in patients who have had a myocardial infarction or in patients who are presenting with or have a history of a cardiac arrhythmia of any kind. It should be discouraged in patients with symptomatic ischemic heart disease even without arrhythmia and previous infarction unless they are very closely monitored. Dextrothyroxine tends to potentiate digitalis-like agents and anticoagulants of the coumarin type. It is best to limit the use of dextrothyroxine to young asymptomatic patients without known coronary heart disease and only when diet and other drugs have failed to satisfactorily lower plasma lipids.

OTHER DRUGS. Colestipol, 15 to 25 grams per day in 5 gram doses, another anionic exchange resin, has virtually the same indications, potency and side effects as cholestyramine.

Probucol (Lorelco), 250 mg. tablets, is a newer hypocholesterolemic agent with very few side effects (mainly loose stools or diarrhea). Administration of 1 gram per day in two divided doses will lower plasma cholesterol an average of 12 per cent over the effect of the diet in familial hypercholesterolemia. Although it reduces plasma cholesterol and LDL-cholesterol, it has practically no triglyceride-lowering effect. It is more readily absorbed when given with a meal and tends to accumulate in adipose tissue.

Beta-sitosterol (Cytellin), stable emulsion, 12 to 18 grams per day in divided doses, is a minor cholesterol-lowering agent which interferes with cholesterol absorption. It is a safe drug, virtually free of side effects, to be used in combination in the treatment of familial hypercholesterolemia.

Among the drugs which have not been approved by the Food and Drug Administration for the treatment of hyperlipidemias, but which are useful in certain situations, the following should be mentioned:

Neomycin, 1 to 2 grams per day in three to four divided doses, increases the intestinal loss of cholesterol and is a useful adjunct in the treatment of familial hypercholesterolemia. It has often been used in combination with clofibrate and/or cholestyramine. Side effects are rare, although interference with normal intestinal flora could become a problem. Since nephro- or ototoxicity could develop if the drug were absorbed, it should not be given in ulcerative disease of the bowel or in combination with potentially nephrotoxic or ototoxic agents (streptomycin, kanamycin, gentamicin) or with diuretics such as furosemide and ethacrynic acid.

Norethindrone acetate (Norlutate), 5 mg. per day, a progestational agent, and oxandrolone (Anavar), 2.5 mg. three times a day, were found to stimulate the activity of lipoprotein lipase and are used in the treatment of familial mixed hyperlipoproteinemia (type V) in females and males, respectively. Hormonal side effects may be troublesome, and liver toxicity has been reported.

Para-aminosalicylic acid, 6 to 8 grams per day in one to two doses, 500 mg. tablets, is a potent cholesterol- and triglyceride-lowering agent with frequent side effects such as nausea, vomiting, diarrhea, and an occasional hypersensitivity reaction. It may induce a goiter (a rare occurrence) and should not be used in the presence of renal or hepatic insufficiency or gastric ulcer. A newer purified preparation, PAS-C, has fewer gastrointestinal side effects.

Surgical Approach

Partial Ileal Bypass. This surgical approach was developed by Henry Buchwald at the University of Minnesota primarily for the treatment of familial hypercholesterolemia. The small intestine is measured from the angle of Treitz to the ileocecal valve and is sectioned at the junction of the proximal two thirds and the distal third, or at 200 cm. from the ileocecal valve, whichever is longest. The distal end is sutured, and the segment thus formed is affixed to the anterior tenia of the cecum so as to avoid intussusception. The proximal end is anastomosed end-to-side to the cecum. Since normally most of the bile acids excreted into the bile are reabsorbed in the distal third of the ileum, this operation acts the same way as cholestyramine on plasma cholesterol by interfering with the enterohepatic circulation of bile salts. This form of treatment has several drawbacks which must be weighed against potential benefits. The patient is exposed to the inherent risk of abdominal surgery and anesthesia, which might not be negligible in patients affected with severe coronary or cerebral atherosclerosis. Vitamin B_{12} absorption is impaired, and lifelong injections of this vitamin will be needed to prevent the development of anemia (1000 micrograms every 3 months). Diarrhea usually follows surgery (5 to 20 watery stools per day) and may in some patients be accompanied by weight loss. It is related to the large influx of bile acids into the colon and possibly to some degree of fat malabsorption. In most cases it tends to subside over several months and can be controlled with drugs such as diphenoxylate HCl (Lomotil) or a constipating diet low in residues. In an occasional patient, it might become troublesome enough to warrant restoration of intestinal continuity. The long-range effects are still unknown, although the follow-up of many patients over 10 years has disclosed few complications.

Partial ileal bypass is regarded as the most effective cholesterol-lowering measure. A mean plasma cholesterol decrease of about 40 per cent has been reported in familial type II patients submitting to this type of surgery. The effect is sustained and may allow some relaxation of the dietary restrictions. In view of the numerous effective dietary and drug regimens available for the treatment of other categories of hyperlipidemia, we have restricted its use in our own series to familial hypercholesterolemia (type II). The young adult male with early signs of coronary atherosclerosis and tendon xanthomas, who is from a family with a high incidence of premature ischemic heart disease and coronary deaths and who is unresponsive to the medical management of his hyperbetalipoproteinemia, constitutes a likely candidate for the ileal bypass operation. If some decrease in plasma cholesterol was obtained with cholestyramine, an even better response might be elicited with ileal bypass surgery. It is currently being applied to test the lipid hypothesis in the patient at high risk who has suffered a first myocardial infarction.

Portacaval Anastomosis. For the subject with homozygous hypercholesterolemia (type II), combined therapy with nicotinic acid and cholestyramine is often unrewarding. Partial ileal bypass has not been shown to be very effective. Thomas Starzl in Denver has been successful in correcting the hyperlipidemia and reducing the size of the xanthomas in one such patient with portacaval shunt. Correction of hyperlipidemia in other patients operated upon since then has not been as successful, and serious side effects have been reported. Until more is known of the mechanism of action of this procedure, it remains a strictly experimental and last-resort undertaking. Repeated plasmaphereses and extracorporeal removal of plasma lipoproteins by affinity binding to heparin-agarose are additional treatments which have met with some success in this condition, but are still in the investigational stage.

REACTIVE HYPOGLYCEMIA

method of
JOHN W. ENSINCK, M.D.
Seattle, Washington

Clues to Diagnosis

Hypoglycemia is defined as an abnormal depression of extracellular glucose concentration. The affected patient may display a characteristic symptom complex because of glucose deprivation by the brain. Symptoms resulting from excessive catecholamine release or variable degress of brain dysfunction are elicited with rapid rates of descent of blood glucose levels and/or inordinately low plasma glucose concentrations. Symptomatic hypoglycemia usually occurs when plasma glucose levels fall below 50 mg. per dl. (100 ml.) (blood glucose levels less than 45 mg. per dl.); however, approximately 25 per cent of otherwise normal subjects may have plasma glucose levels less than 50 mg. per dl. after an oral glucose tolerance test (OGTT). In adults the causes of spontaneous (nonpharmacogenetic) hypoglycemic disorders can be segregated into two general categories based upon food intake—those associated with fed or with fasting states. Pathologic glucopenia during short- or long-term fasting (greater than 6 hours) primarily reflects abnormalities in homeostatic mechanisms for de novo glucose production from the liver. In contrast, reactive hypoglycemias are temporally related to nutrient ingestion, and symptoms usually occur within 2 to 5 hours postprandially, depending upon the rate of descent and nadir achieved by plasma glucose. Since glucopenia occurs during the interval between assimilation of sugar and the induction of compensatory increased endogenous glucose production, reactive hypoglycemias comprise abnormalities in the regulatory mechanisms involved in the transition between the fed and fasted states. In comparison with the frequently severe cerebral manifestations ascribable to low plasma glucose levels in fasting hypoglycemia, symptoms associated with reactive hypoglycemia are usually mildly to moderately discomforting owing to triggering of the adrenergic nervous system by the rapid descent of plasma glucose. The patient most frequently complains of faintness, tremulousness, sweating, hunger, palpitation, or mood changes. Chronic fatigue, sustained anxiety, or complaints of mental dullness or lethargy usually do not accompany bona fide hypoglycemia, and the unwary physician should not misattribute these symptoms to hypoglycemia. In patients with reactive hypoglycemia, minor impairment of cerebral cortical function, such as confusion, may occasionally be experienced when plasma glucose levels fall below 35 to 40 mg. per dl. Nevertheless, amnesia, unconsciousness, or seizures rarely ever occur, because counter-regulatory signals rapidly readjust glucose levels, primarily by enhanced hepatic glycogenolysis.

The reactive hypoglycemias are causally related to one or more dietary constituents and can be classified, based on their induction, by (1) glucose, (2) galactose, (3) fructose, or (4) leucine. The glucopenic syndromes caused by ingestion of galactose, fructose, and leucine are genetically transmitted and first appear in infancy and childhood, whereas those induced by glucose occur most frequently in adults. With the exception of patients with insulin-producing tumors who occasionally have reactive hypoglycemia, subjects with glucose-induced hypoglycemia are characterized by normal or slightly elevated fasting plasma glucose levels, and within 5 hours after food intake they sustain an abrupt decline in circulating glucose with symptoms resulting from hyperepinephrinemia usually subsiding within 15 to 20 minutes. The glucose-induced hypoglycemias are usually attributed to (1) excessive secretion of insulin and/or (2) hypersensitivity of peripheral tissues to insulin. These syndromes can often be differentiated solely on the basis of the configuration of the plasma glucose profile and the temporal onset of hypoglycemia in the ensuing period after ingestion of 75 to 100 grams of glucose. Since reactive hypoglycemia can be readily produced in normal subjects deprived of carbohydrates, for correct assessment of glucose homeostasis in such patients it is mandatory that they be tested in standard fashion, which includes 3 days of preparation with 300 grams of oral dietary carbohydrate daily. The test should be performed after an overnight fast with the patient supine. Since, in general, the diagnosis can be established with the postabsorptive glucose profile alone, coincident measurements of insulin levels are not necessary.

Reactive Hypoglycemia Due to Accelerated Glucose Absorption

Symptomatic hypoglycemia occurs most frequently within 90 to 180 minutes after ingestion of a large carbohydrate meal in approximately 5 to 20 per cent of patients who have undergone partial or total gastrectomy, gastrojejunostomy, or pyloroplasty with or without vagotomy. The glucopenic symptoms are usually distinguishable from those caused by "dumping," which are experienced within 1 hour after eating and are related to osmotic distention of the bowel. Characteristically, these patients have a peak plasma glucose exceeding 200 mg. per dl. within 90 minutes after an OGTT, frequently accompanied by exaggerated insulin responses, leading to abrupt descent of plasma glucose to hypoglycemia ranges. There is a rapid transit of glucose with increased delivery of hypertonic sugar into the duodenum, a consequence of the elimination of the gastric reservoir or impaired pyloric sphincter. Insulinotropic substances from the gut plus glucose are thought to evoke an excessive insulin release. Hypoglycemia has also been described in some subjects who have not had gastrointestinal surgery; this has been attributed to a cellular defect with rapid glucose absorption and perhaps enhanced release of insulinotropic enteric factors. Early reactive hypoglycemia with blood glucose nadir around 3 hours also occurs in 20 to 60 per cent of patients with peptic ulcers. Rarely do they have hypoglycemic symptoms.

Therapy. The primary means of treatment for this as for other reactive hypoglycemias is modification of dietary intake in which nutrient content and frequency of ingestion are adjusted so as to minimize the load of carbohydrate absorbed. The approach to dietary maneuvers should be individualized to accomplish abatement of symptoms in the face of convenience of food intake and cost of specific food items. The overall principle is directed to reducing the dietary carbohydrate content especially refined sugars, as well as the total bulk of each meal. In order to maintain isocaloric intake and provide satiety, the meals should be interspersed at regular intervals throughout the waking hours with the least inconvenience. In practical terms, if a weight maintenance diet consists of 35 calories per kg., approximately 12 calories per kg. should be in the form of complex carbohydrates, i.e., starches, 7 to 8 calories per kg. in protein and the remainder in fat. If feasible, intake should be six to eight feedings throughout the waking hours. The rationale of frequency of intake should be carefully explained and re-emphasized to the patient, with the option to adapt the program according to the response and convenience. Increasing fiber content—e.g., gual, a food additive, and pectin from citrus fruit or boiled bran (12 to 15 grams)—may diminish glucose absorption and mitigate symptoms. In virtually all patients, adherence to a dietary regimen has proved effective. In those who for some reason are unable to comply with a dietary program, an anticholinergic drug which inhibits gastric motility and thereby glucose transit time may be effective. Propantheline, 7.5 to 15 mg. by mouth three times daily, is often helpful. Beta-adrenergic blockers such as propranolol, 5 to 10 mg. orally before each meal, have been reported to ameliorate glucopenic symptoms in a few patients. (This use of propranolol is not listed in the manufacturer's official directive.)

Reactive Hypoglycemia Associated with Diabetes Mellitus

Not infrequently spontaneous attacks of hypoglycemia occurring 3 to 5 hours after meals are experienced by patients with mild diabetes who have normal or slightly elevated fasting plasma glucose levels. Diagnosis is established by the presence of hyperglycemia within the first 2 hours of an OGTT, followed by the glucopenic phase. These patients tend to have a higher incidence of obesity and family history of diabetes than do subjects with idiopathic reactive hypoglycemia. The proposed mechanism is a defect in beta cell responses to glucose with a delayed release of insulin, leading to a discordance in the normal insulin-glucose relationships. With time these patients may progress into a more advanced stage of diabetes mellitus and the hypoglycemic manifestations may disappear.

Therapy. If the patient is overweight, a hypocaloric diet frequently leads to abatement of symptoms, and as in other reactive hypoglycemias dietary manipulation forms the basis of treatment (see above). Sulfonylureas have been reported to ameliorate symptoms by tending to "normalize" the release of insulin, leading to partial correction of the aberrant glucose tolerance. Short-term use of one of these agents may be tried on those patients who fail to adhere to diets. Because of the controversial and unresolved results of the University Group Diabetes Program (UGDP) study implicating an adverse effect from tolbutamide, in my judgment long-term use of these drugs for reactive hypoglycemia should be discouraged.

Idiopathic Reactive Hypoglycemia

The most common hypoglycemic syndrome (70 to 80 per cent) occurs in otherwise healthy young adults without previous gastric surgery or history of diabetes mellitus, who have low plasma sugar levels between 2 and 4 hours after food ingestion. Characteristically, these patients tend to be thin, tense, anxious, and compulsive in personality. Symptomatic manifestations of a hyperactive autonomic nervous system are also reflected by gastric hypermotility, nausea, vomiting, and an irritable colon. Although excessive vagal release of insulin has been proposed as a mechanism for the postprandial glucopenia, neither hyperinsulinism nor hyperglycemia is characteristically found in these emotionally labile subjects; hence they have been classified as idiopathic. A small number of such patients may also be obese. Since the cause of hypoglycemia in this heterogeneous group is obscure, claims that some patients in this category may eventually become diabetic are not surprising.

Therapy. As in patients with accelerated glucose absorption and in early onset diabetes mellitus, a modification of dietary intake is the primary treatment. If the patients are within 10 per cent of ideal body weight, a low carbohydrate, high protein, isocaloric diet with increased fiber content and frequent feedings should be prescribed. In those persons who are obese, weight reduction should be encouraged with a diet low in calories and refined carbohydrate, with frequent feedings as described above. Anticholinergics are occasionally beneficial if diet therapy is unsatisfactory. In all patients reassurance and counseling should be stressed, and frequently a tranquilizer such as diazepam, 2.5 to 5 mg. three times daily, is helpful. In more emotionally disturbed patients, psychiatric consultation may be necessary.

Reactive Hypoglycemia Associated with Galactose, Fructose, and Leucine

Hypoglycemia is part of the clinical syndrome following ingestion of galactose (galactosemia), fructose (hereditary fructose intolerance), or amino acids (leucine hypersensitivity). Since these are rare inherited disorders, they usually first appear in infancy and are frequently associated with severe organ dysfunction and mental deterioration. Early diagnosis is mandatory.

Therapy. In galactosemia and hereditary fructose intolerance, enzymatic defects in utilization of these sugars have been characterized. The elimination of galactose and fructose from the diet will prevent the clinical manifestations in these disorders. In patients with leucine sensitivity, the release of insulin is inordinate and the patients may have islet cell hyperplasia. Although not clearly established, restriction of leucine content in the diet may be beneficial. Glucocorticoids such as prednisone in doses of 5 to 10 mg. daily usually cause amelioration of hypoglycemia; however, adverse effects, particularly growth retardation may preclude the use of steroids. Diazoxide in oral doses of 10 to 15 mg. per kg. of body weight may also be effective in control of the hypoglycemic attacks.

OBESITY

method of
LESTER B. SALANS, M.D.
Hanover, New Hampshire

Introduction

Obesity is one of the most prevalent health problems of our society. The obese person suffers more from a variety of illnesses than does the nonobese; abnormalities of carbohydrate and lipid metabolism are more frequent, aggravation of diabetes mellitus, heart disease, joint disease, and gallbladder disease are common, and obesity carries with it significant social, psychological, and economic disadvantages.

Clearly, then, the prevention and correction of obesity are desirable. Most obese patients recognize or can be educated to these facts, and often they begin a weight reduction program with considerable motivation and enthusiasm. Yet, meaningful weight loss is difficult to achieve, particularly when one considers that the goal of any reducing program is not merely to lose weight, but to keep it off. The results of treatment programs for obesity have, almost without exception, been uniformly unsatisfactory; clearly our current therapeutic approach is inadequate. This situation is likely to prevail until a more fundamental understanding of the regulation of eating behavior and body weight is achieved and, as a result, specific therapy can be directed at these processes. Within these limits, the degree of success in the management of the obese patient will depend upon a realistic definition of the goals of treatment and a rational approach to altering the balance between caloric intake and output.

The following paragraphs describe one such approach to the obese individual, based on the concept that the diagnosis of obesity and formulation of a therapeutic plan are the responsibility of the physician, but implementation of this program, while under physician guidance, is conducted by nonphysician resources of the community.

Patient Evaluation

Is Weight Reduction Indicated? The physician must first determine whether reduction in a given patient is justified. To do this a physician must first determine whether the patient is obese; he must be able to distinguish between overweight and obesity, and to identify those who have abnormal patterns of fat distribution but who are not obese. The severity of the obesity must be defined in terms of its degree and the extent to which it impairs the physical, emotional, and economic health of the individual. The coexistence of other health risk factors, such as hypertension, atherosclerosis, and diabetes mellitus which are clear-cut indications for weight loss, and the presence of conditions such as pregnancy and certain acute illnesses which mitigate against weight reduction, must be identified.

Although the diagnosis of obesity depends, in the strictest terms, upon the demonstration of an excessive adipose tissue mass, a practical and reliable clinical method for measuring the amount of adipose tissue in the body is not yet available; thus various indirect methods are employed for assessing body fatness. The most practical approach currently available involves the use of standard tables of weight based on height. Table 1 shows one of the most frequently used tables, adapted from the Metropolitan Life Insurance Company. It must be recognized that this and other indirect methods of assessing obesity are not ideal; they are particularly limited in their ability to identify mild degrees of obesity. In most cases the diagnosis of obesity is obvious from visual inspection and body weight; an individual weighing more than 20 per cent above the upper range for height is obese. The problem is with milder degrees of obesity. Furthermore, such tables alone may fail to distinguish the person who is overweight because of increased muscle mass rather than adipose tissue from the overweight patient with an expanded adipose tissue. Yet, until a practical method for accurate assessment of body fat is available, this appears to be the most reasonable approach. Finally, it must be recognized that some patients, women in particular, may present with normal amounts but abnormal distribution of body fat; these patients are not obese, and weight reduction is not indicated.

Is There a Definable Cause of Obesity? In some instances a specific cause of obesity can be defined; under such circumstances treatment of the underlying cause will usually result in significant and permanent weight reduction. Thus it is important to consider whether a patient is obese because of hypothyroidism, Cushing's syndrome, or one of several other definable but rare causes of obesity. These disorders, however, account for only an exceedingly small fraction of human obesity, and rarely are they responsible for massive obesity. Furthermore, the presence of one of these

TABLE 1. **Fogarty International Center Conference on Obesity Recommended Weight in Relation to Height***

HEIGHT		MEN		WOMEN	
Feet	*Inches*	*Average*	*Range*	*Average*	*Range*
4	10	...	...	102	92–119
4	11	...	...	104	94–122
5	0	...	...	107	96–125
5	1	...	...	110	99–128
5	2	123	112–141	113	102–131
5	3	127	115–144	116	105–134
5	4	130	118–148	120	108–138
5	5	133	121–152	123	111–142
5	6	136	124–156	128	114–146
5	7	140	128–161	132	118–150
5	8	145	132–166	136	122–154
5	9	149	136–170	140	126–158
5	10	153	140–174	144	130–163
5	11	158	144–179	148	134–168
6	0	162	148–184	152	138–173
6	1	166	152–189	...	...
6	2	171	156–194	...	...
6	3	176	160–199	...	...
6	4	181	164–204	...	...

*Height without shoes, weight without clothes. Adapted from the table of the Metropolitan Life Insurance Company.

diseases in an obese patient does not necessarily establish it as the sole cause of the obesity; specific treatment may cause weight loss but not restore the patient to normal body weight. Such improvement is, however, highly desirable, and in every obese patient a specific cause should be sought.

Classification of Obesity. In the overwhelming majority of obese patients a specific cause cannot be discerned; classification of their obesity according to age of onset and severity may, however, be of considerable practical importance, as it may afford some indication of prognosis, and thus better define the objective of treatment and the therapeutic approach to be taken.

Obesity of onset at an early age, particularly within the first few years of life or at puberty, and massive degrees of obesity are the most resistant to medical therapy; weight reduction in these patients is difficult at best, and almost inevitably is followed by regain of weight and restoration of the original state of adiposity. Frequently in this pattern of weight loss, weight gain is repetitive as the obese patient goes from one weight reduction program to another. Such experiences are not only very frustrating to both patient and physician, but are associated with considerable emotional and financial cost. Furthermore, cyclic fasting and refeeding associated with weight loss and regain of weight may be potentially harmful in that this may enhance atherogenic risk factors such as hyperlipidemia. Thus not only is weight reduction in this type of obese patient difficult to achieve and maintain, but the inadequacy of current medical therapy may be associated with serious risk factors. On the other hand, milder degrees of obesity, particularly of onset in adult life, are more amenable to treatment; fortunately this is the most common type of obesity. Classification of an individual's obesity on the basis of age of onset and severity may, then, be of considerable practical importance in determining the therapeutic approach.

Therapeutic Approach

Failure of the current medical approach to early onset, severe obesity has led to the introduction of more drastic measures of treatment. Included among these are various surgical procedures of which gastrointestinal bypass, and specifically jejunal-ileal bypass, is most widely and successfully used. Although this procedure appears to be an effective means of achieving and maintaining weight loss, it may be associated with significant and serious problems for the patient. The mortality rate associated with this procedure may be as high as 5 per cent, and postoperative morbidity may be substantial; persistent diarrhea, fluid and electrolyte disturbances, severe liver disease, and hepatic failure (particularly when postoperative dietary protein intake is inadequate) are but a few of the more serious short-term operative problems. Since jejunal-ileal bypass has been employed in the treatment of obesity for only a relatively short period of time, its long-term consequences are not known. In view of its potential short- and long-term hazards, gastrointestinal bypass remains, in my view, an experimental form of therapy for obesity, which, like any good experiment, should be strictly limited to patients with clear-cut, pressing medical need, and conducted in a setting in which its short- and long-term effects can be very carefully monitored. A less drastic approach to the early onset, massively obese patient may be more appropriate in the usual situation: supportive therapy. In this approach less emphasis is placed on weight reduction, and more on minimization of additional weight gain; symptomatic attention is directed toward associated medical disorders, and to the emotional and socioeconomic capacity and function of the individual. The objectives of this approach are severely limited, to be sure, and the basic problem of obesity is largely ignored; yet in my opinion it offers a reasonable alternative to the inadequacies, frustrations, and risks of other current modes of therapy, at least until our basic understanding of this disorder improves.

Fortunately, the most common type of obesity, adult onset, mild to moderate obesity, is more responsive to medical management. Successful medical management of this type of obesity requires the formulation of a therapeutic plan by the physician, and its implementation through a concentrated and continuous effort on the part of various community resources aimed at quality medical care, emotional support, patient education, and modification of eating habits and physical activity.

Diet. The basis of treatment is dietary, and specifically caloric restriction. Although the optimal diet for weight reduction has yet to be defined, theoretically it is one which contains the least number of calories yet provides total or near total preservation of body nitrogen, minerals, vitamins, and other essential factors. A large number of diets have been introduced in the quest for "optimal." Many of these diets are based on manipulations of the composition of their calories: the ratio of carbohydrate to fat to protein. Too often, however, the proponents of such diets fail to recognize or communicate to the patient the critical importance of total caloric restriction. At this writing no firm evidence exists which militates against the concept that weight loss depends upon caloric deficit and, in turn, that caloric deficit itself depends upon the total number, not the kind, of calories consumed relative to calories expended.

The extent to which calories should be restricted in a given patient depends upon age, body size, sex, and physical activity. Restriction to 800 to 1200 calories per day is generally appropriate for a moderately active woman; 1000 to 1400 calories per day may be more appropriate for a man of similar activity. Obviously, these values need to be adjusted according to the activity, size, and age of the patient. A more precise calculation of desired caloric intake may be achieved based on the fact that 1 lb. of body fat is roughly equivalent to 3500 calories. The patient's daily caloric requirements for weight maintenance may be estimated from standard tables relating caloric needs to body size and physical activity, and recommended calorie intake is based on the desired weekly rate of weight loss. For example, from Table 2 it can be estimated that a 30 year old woman living a "typical" American life style requires approximately 16 calories per pound of desirable weight. If her desired weight is 125 lbs., she will require 2000 calories per day for weight maintenance. Daily intake of 1000 calories will produce a daily deficit of 1000 calories, a weekly deficit of 7000 calories, and thus a predicted weight loss of approximately 2 lbs. per week. Obviously, adjustments must be made for marked variations in physical activity.

Generally two phases of weight loss are observed; an initial period of rapid loss, primarily reflecting loss of body fluid, is followed by a slower rate of weight reduction that predominantly reflects fat catabolism. Frequently, patients become discouraged during this slower, second phase of weight loss, particularly with time and the monotony of a given diet. It is at this time that the introduction of other modalities of therapy to be discussed may be particularly helpful. In addition I have found that the intermittent use of liquid formula diets may be quite useful at this time.

TABLE 2. **Estimated Average Caloric Requirements***

AGE	CALORIES/POUND DESIRABLE WEIGHT†	
1–3	46	
4–6	41	
7–10	36	
	Males	*Females*
11–14	29	25
15–18	22	18
19–22	18	16
23–50	18	16
50	16	14

*Adapted from the Food and Nutrition Board of the National Academy of Sciences-National Research Council Recommended Dietary Allowances, 1974.

†Based on usual physical activity under usual environmental stresses.

These hypocaloric, weight reduction diets should be divided into three or more meals per day, the exact number and pattern of caloric distribution depending upon the individual's eating and activity habits.

Total starvation diets have generated considerable interest and popularity in the treatment of obesity. The rationale for this approach apparently lies in the rapid rate of initial weight loss compared to caloric restriction. This benefit, however, is short lasting; weight loss over the long run is similar for the two methods. Moreover, prolonged starvation may actually be undesirable for several reasons. Lean body mass is lost to a significantly greater degree during total starvation than during caloric restriction. In addition, severe ketosis and mild acidosis may accompany prolonged starvation; the effects of these alterations on cellular function, particularly the cells of the central nervous system and the skeleton, are not fully appreciated. For these reasons, calorie restricted diets seem preferable to total starvation. Certainly, prolonged fasting should not be undertaken in the absence of close medical supervision, and it is contraindicated in certain patients such as those with diabetes mellitus.

The composition of the caloric restricted diet has, as indicated, received wide attention in the management of obesity. The "low carbohydrate diet" (0, or less than 50 grams of carbohydrate per day) has been most popular. When this diet is successful, it is most likely attributable to anorexia induced by severe ketosis, along with lack of palatability, and thus to a reduction in total caloric intake. As discussed above, since the long-term effects of severe ketosis are not yet known, this approach should be employed with caution; it should not be used in the patient with insulin dependent diabetes mellitus, renal disease, or other acidotic states. Even in situations in which attention to dietary composition would seem indicated, as in some of the hyperlipoproteinemias, caloric restriction and weight loss, irrespective of dietary composition, are usually sufficient. If this approach is inadequate, or if the patient is unsuccessful at weight loss, attention to specific alterations in the lipid and carbohydrate content of the diet is then indicated. More recently, attention has focused on low calorie diets composed only of protein, 1.5 grams per kg. of body weight to be exact, fully supplemented with fluid, electrolytes, minerals, and vitamins. With such a regimen it has been possible to nearly restore nitrogen balance after a period of 2 to 3 weeks, and ketosis is reported to be less than with total starvation and low carbohydrate diets. Significant weight loss with a high degree of satiety and preservation of body nitrogen has been reported in patients ingesting this diet. Initial experience, however, indicates certain hazards of this regimen; the levels of uric acid, triglyceride, and cholesterol in the plasma of many of these patients rise substantially. Furthermore, there is no experience with this diet in children and adolescents, and since these periods of active growth and development are exquisitely dependent upon adequate supplies of a broad spectrum of nutrients, it should not be used to achieve weight reduction in obese children until its effects on these processes are defined.

In my view, there is at present no evidence to support the idea that any particular "fad" diet has an inherent advantage over a calorie restricted, balanced "normal" diet in achieving weight reduction; in fact, such "fad" diets may be disadvantageous as discussed above. On the other hand, these diets do provide alternative approaches to weight reduction; a given individual may prefer one type of calorie restricted diet to another for reasons of taste, eating habits, and socioeconomic or other factors, and thus be more likely to adhere to it. If taken under proper supervision, such diets may indeed be of value for certain persons. The basis for recommending any hypocaloric weight reduction diet for an individual patient, and the pattern in which it is to be administered, lies in recognizing its potential hazards and in defining the eating habits of that person, i.e., food tastes, pattern of hunger and satiety, activity and leisure time patterns, and familial, psychological, and economic background. The effectiveness of any hypocaloric dietary regimen will depend upon patient motivation, the ability of the patient to understand the diet and what is expected, and the concomitant use of other therapeutic modalities.

Patient Education. A major factor in determining the effectiveness of weight loss is the motivation of the patient. The obese patient must be made aware of the potential harmful effects of obesity on physical, emotional, and socioeconomic health, and of the advantages of being lean. Satisfaction and reward must be derived as the patient moves from the obese to nonobese state.

The patient must be able to feel that he or she understands and has some control over the recommended treatment program. Thus when a given diet is prescribed, sufficient specific information should be given so that the patient can understand why and how it should be taken. The patient must know that calories do count and understand what constitutes good eating habits, and must be educated to the caloric content of food and the meaning of "the average serving." All of this requires considerable time and effort on the part of the dietitian or nutrition expert, and frequent reinforcement throughout the course of therapy.

Exercise. Several real and potential benefits of a daily exercise program make this an important adjunct to the treatment of obesity. Included among these benefits are (1) an increased expenditure of energy, and therefore a greater caloric deficit than that achieved with dietary restriction alone; (2) a shift in body composition in the direction of increasing lean body mass at the expense of adipose tissue; (3) improvement in cardiac function; (4) improvement in glucose metabolism; and (5) psychological benefit, particularly with respect to improved self-esteem. For these and other reasons, a daily exercise program, carefully planned and tailored to the patient's abilities and physical condition, is an important part of the long-term weight reduction program. Exercise alone, however, is not an effective means of weight reduction; reduced calorie intake is essential. It appears that optimal effects on food intake and body weight are achieved by relatively constant, low levels of aerobic physical activity such as walking, swimming, and bicycling. Table 3 lists examples of specific activities and the levels to be undertaken to achieve a desirable level of physical fitness, based on a program developed by Cooper.

Behavior Modification. Behavior modification is an approach currently receiving considerable attention as a useful adjunct to caloric restriction and exercise in the treatment of human obesity. This approach is aimed at modifying the eating habits and physical activity of the obese patient and thus helping the patient to regulate body weight. Although this may well offer the most promising of the psychological approaches to the management of obesity, its long-term effectiveness remains to be demonstrated. Many obese patients derive considerable benefit from self-help groups, of which Weight Watchers and Tops are perhaps the best known; these groups may be of considerable help in the modification of eating behavior and physical activity, in addition to bolstering motivation.

TABLE 3. **Equivalent Units of Exercise***

Walking: 3 miles in 36 to 43½ minutes
Running: 1½ miles in 12 to 15 minutes
Stationary running: 70 to 80 steps/minute for 20 minutes
Swimming: 700 yards, overhand crawl, in 11:40 to 17:30 minutes
Bicycling: 6 miles in 18 to 24 minutes
Golf: 36 holes
Handball, squash, or basketball, for 40 minutes
Tennis: singles, 4 sets
Skiing: 60 minutes

*The point value of each of these exercise units is 6. A desirable level of physical fitness is achieved by a cumulative score of 30 points weekly.

Psychotherapy. Obesity is very frequently associated with a variety of emotional disturbances. The relationship of these disturbances to obesity has, however, not been fully identified; although psychological factors may enter into the production of obesity, not all persons are obese as a result of these factors. Thus psychological disturbances can contribute to the development and perpetuation of obesity, or they may be the result of obesity. If psychological factors are found to play a role in the cause and maintenance of obesity in a patient, then psychotherapeutic intervention would clearly be indicated. Usually, however, it is difficult to identify cause-and-effect relationships in an obese patient. The decision of whether or not psychotherapy should be initiated in a given patient, then, depends upon an assessment of the nature and magnitude of the disturbance. When psychological factors are clearly a cause, individual or group therapy may be of considerable benefit to the obese patient. On the other hand, even if the causal relationship cannot be established, psychotherapy may be a beneficial adjunct to caloric restriction and exercise. Psychotherapy is also indicated when emotional disturbance is of such magnitude that it significantly interferes with the functional capacity of the patient. In the majority of obese patients, however, psychotherapy appears to add little to caloric restriction and exercise, at least in terms of weight reduction; general emotional support by the physician during the course of weight reduction is usually sufficient.

Pharmacologic Therapy. The role of drug therapy in the treatment of obesity remains to be defined; at present it is the subject of considerable controversy. Not only is there a question of whether the various pharmacologic agents available significantly influence food intake and body weight over the long term, but there is also the problem of addiction and abuse with certain of these drugs. Abuse of the amphetamines is well established. Fenfluramine does not have the central nervous system stimulatory effects of the amphetamines and has a Bureau of Narcotics and Dangerous Drugs (BNDD) classification of IV, but may produce significant drowsiness, depression, and diarrhea. Mazindol is a tricyclic agent with a BNDD classification of III and side effects similar to those of the amphetamine derivatives. Chlorphentermine, diethylpropion, and phendimetrazine share the untoward amphetamine-like effects on the central nervous system, and are classified as III in the BNDD schedule. After analyzing the available evidence on the use of the appetite-suppressant drugs in the treatment of obesity, the editorial board of the Fogarty International Center Conference on Obesity, held in 1973, made the following recommendations:

1. Before deciding to use a drug for weight reduction it is important to evaluate the nature of the derangement which led to the obesity in the first place.
2. There would seem to be little indication for the use of appetite-suppressing drugs or other medications in obesity unless the patient is clinically obese, has obvious medical need, and/or is motivated to lose weight.
3. An appetite-suppressant drug should be used only as part of the treatment, never as the sole therapy, and only with adequate efforts to modify diet and exercise.
4. Since the available data do not indicate that one drug is more effective than another, those drugs with less potential for addiction or abuse would appear to be the preferable agents.
5. There are no presently available criteria (except history) by which one can detect patients who may become psychologically or physically dependent upon these drugs. Therapy should not be prolonged if weight loss cannot be achieved or continued.
6. An appetite suppressant should never be prescribed or dispensed without a careful explanation of the potential side effects and an indication that its use is purely for symptomatic purposes.
7. Injectable forms of these drugs have no place in the treatment of obesity.

A variety of other drugs, including human chorionic gonadotropin, digitalis, diuretics, and thyroid hormone, have been widely used in the treatment of obesity. In my opinion, there is no role for chorionic gonadotropin in the treatment of obesity. Digitalis, diuretics, and thyroid hormone should be employed only when specific indications exist—congestive heart failure, edema, hypertension, and stasis ulcers for digitalis and the diuretics, and clinical and laboratory-demonstrable hypothyroidism in the case of thyroid hormone.

PELLAGRA

method of
WILLIAM B. BEAN, M.D.
Galveston, Texas

Pellagra, first described by Casal in Spain, nearly 250 years ago, with a few elements resembling kwashiorkor, is likely to slip by most alert physicians and medical teams in this country today. Certainly the doctor in his office misses it because he has never seen it and has not been taught about it. The name "pellagra," *pelle agra,* means rough skin. It has nothing to do with photosensitivity. No photochemical reaction is required, although exposure to sunlight is the most common cause of nonspecific damage which determines its cutaneous localization. Most people who suffer from nicotinic acid deficiency have suffered a long time from a reduction of calories and protein of good biologic value. They develop pellagra as but one of a cluster of deficiencies. Absolutely pure nicotinic acid deficiency exists only among bacteria or in laboratory animals.

Pellagra has been a characteristic deficiency where maize, corn, has been the staple energy food. One of the mysteries which developed after it was known that nicotinic acid would correct black tongue in dogs and correct or prevent the manifestations of pellagra was that there was no sharp relationship—sometimes not a close one—between the level of reduction of nicotinic acid in the diet and the probability of getting pellagra. It turned out that tryptophan could be converted into nicotinic acid, although the reverse process does not occur in nature. Because nicotinic acid is a component of two coenzymes, NAD^+ and $NADP^+$, which are concerned with tissue respiration, fat synthesis, and glycolysis, it is not surprising that the energy output is connected with the development of clinical manifestations. We do not know whether North and South American Indians, who used much maize, had pellagra. Where maize was the only or main source of calories, they must have had pellagra.

In many cases, vitamin deficiency diseases are related to that recurring combination of poverty and ignorance. In most practice in the United States, pellagra is secondary to some disease, or process, which reduces the intake and assimilation of a balanced diet or greatly increases need. A diet dependent upon corn for energy not only lacks nicotinic acid but is not rich in tryptophan, which by way of kynurenine and hydroxyanthranilic acid becomes nicotinic acid, although it is not a simple relationship. About 60 mg. of tryptophan may be needed to make 1 mg. of nicotinic acid.

Pellagra used to be recognized by the four D's: dermatitis, diarrhea, dementia, and death. This brings back memories of days when brain tumors were diagnosed by convulsions, hemiplegia, and advanced destruction of the nervous system, not by the early manifestations. Today, in the United States, wheat and corn flour have had restored a modicum of the things milled out, and this flour or meal is referred to as "enriched." It does, indeed, contain added niacin, thiamine, riboflavin, and some minerals. Few persons on reducing diets develop pellagra, despite their poor choice of what they may eat. Others have malabsorption and do not get value returned for what they take in through the mouth. The person who drinks alcohol to excess may get the rest of his calories from salted crackers, potato chips, pretzels, and other naked calories.

If one looks sharply for the bright red tongue, the strange behavior of the alimentary canal, and mental aberration in hospitals where people with diseases of the alimentary canal, cancer, or other chronic ills of the ailing are, pellagra may be recognized. In old persons, the combination of aging, inertia, and neglect by children and friends leads to depression, which is likely to result in eating habits which almost selectively neglect food of good biologic value, especially meats and protein-rich foods.

Specific Treatment

One does not treat a disease, except accidentally, if it is not recognized. Once the notion that pellagra might exist gets into the mind of a physician, he will immediately do what is necessary. Pellagra occurring in hospital patients or in people who have not been exposed to sunlight is often associated with dermatitis from pressure or irritation. This is often overlooked. Diagnosis by exclusion is the resort of those destitute of ideas, but it is still important to remember that if there is a suspicion of vitamin deficiency, no harm will be done by using what is suspected of being the missing vitamin. Unfortunately with pellagra the sore tongue may make it impossible or difficult to ingest food or pills. Thus it may be necessary to start an attack on identified pellagra by giving a significant amount of parenteral nicotinic acid. Within a few hours the red and irritated tongue may resume its normal color. Its edema disappears. The alimentary canal becomes quiet, although it may not return to normal completely. Usually the mental aberrations are corrected rapidly. Most pellagra seen in hospitals is *secondary,* resulting from disease which increases metabolism, reduces absorption, or diminishes appetite and what is eaten. Thus it is likely to be but part of the manifestation of multiple nutritional deficiency states.

Once niacin has been given, the pellagrous patient may rapidly regain appetite, partly because the painful lesions of the mouth and tongue have begun to heal and partly because of a brighter mental outlook. There is also a surge in a sense of well-being, real but hard to measure.

Therapy for patients with less severe or complicated cases should begin with nicotinamide in doses of 100 to 150 mg. twice a day. Sequential release capsules are supposed to maintain a fairly constant level, but this is quite different from the natural three-meals-a-day sequence and advantages are not clearly known. In addition to specific therapy with nicotinamide, a good, balanced, nutritious diet selected from items a patient can and will eat should be prepared. A search should be made for other vitamin, protein, and mineral deficiencies and these corrected if found. Most patients with pellagra suffer from calorie shortage as well as protein deprivation, and these deficiencies should be corrected.

Supportive Therapy

When the patient has made his initial response, we begin a program of complete correction of dietary inadequacies and the employment of a truly balanced diet with approximately 1 gram of protein for each kg. of body weight to help build up the deficiency in those chronically malnourished. Energy material should be provided to keep dietary protein from being used as fuel. For a 70 kg. person, 70 grams of protein will provide just over 11 grams of nitrogen. About 2250 kilogram calories are needed every day. Most routine hospital diets, if eaten completely, provide at least this much. There may be reason to give supplements between meals or to give a large number of small feedings for a while. Supplementary vitamin capsules containing the recommended daily allowances may be useful, but the sheet anchor of therapy is a judiciously chosen, ample, and balanced diet.

Prevention

Although the restoration to flour of portions of the vitamins and minerals milled out has been called "enrichment," this term suggests wishful and wistful thinking rather than careful evaluation. Its effect has been probably more important in reducing beriberi among chronic alcohol addicts, for most of them will eat at least a sandwich a day with some thiamine in white bread. We know that with intervening disease, poverty, and food fads with outrageously unbalanced diets, many forms of malnutrition will continue. Pellagra, although unusual, can be treated and corrected specifically. This may be lifesaving, and it invariably produces a welcome return or increase in the sense of well-being and a restoration of good health.

RICKETS AND OSTEOMALACIA

method of
GUIDO FANCONI, M.D.,
Zurich, Switzerland
and ANDREAS FANCONI, M.D.
Winterthur, Switzerland

Rickets and osteomalacia are characterized by an insufficient apposition of mineral salts in the osteoid tissue. The activity of the osteoblasts is increased, enhancing the proliferation of the osteoid tissue. The main cause of these alterations is the lack or the inactivity of vitamin D.

In the beginning of our century only one form of rickets was known: nutritional rickets. Since vitamin D preparations have become available, vitamin D deficiency is easily cured and prevented and has become a rare disease. This development made it possible to discover many vitamin D resistant forms of rickets. In 1974 Dent published a table in which he enumerated 34 different etiologic types of rickets and osteomalacia: 17 genetic and 17 acquired types. Only the most important of these diseases will be discussed in this article.

Vitamin D_3 (cholecalciferol), which is commercially available, is formed in the skin by ultraviolet irradiation. Vitamin D_3 is hydroxylated in the liver to 25-OHD_3 and in the kidney to 1,25$(OH)_2$-D_3, which acts as a hormone on intestinal calcium absorption with 1000 times greater efficiency than vitamin D_3 (Fig. 1).

Figure 2 schematizes the pathogenesis of vitamin D deficiency rickets; lack of vitamin D and therefore of the hormone 1,25$(OH)_2$-D_3 reduces the intestinal calcium absorption. In order to maintain a constant serum calcium level, more parathyroid hormone is produced. This secondary hyperparathyroidism is typical for vitamin D deficiency and other types of hypocalcemic rickets,

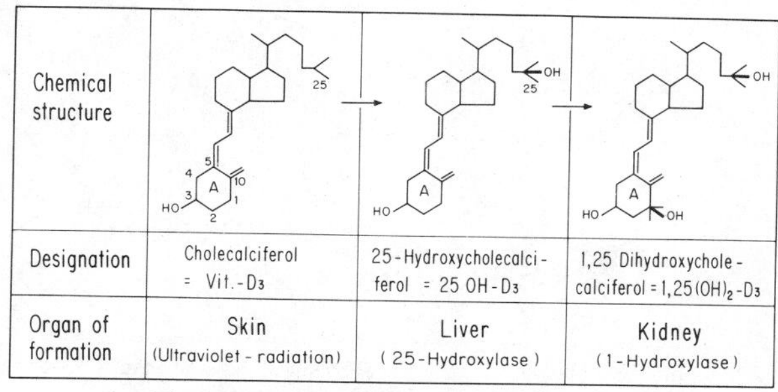

Figure 1. Metabolism of vitamin D_3.

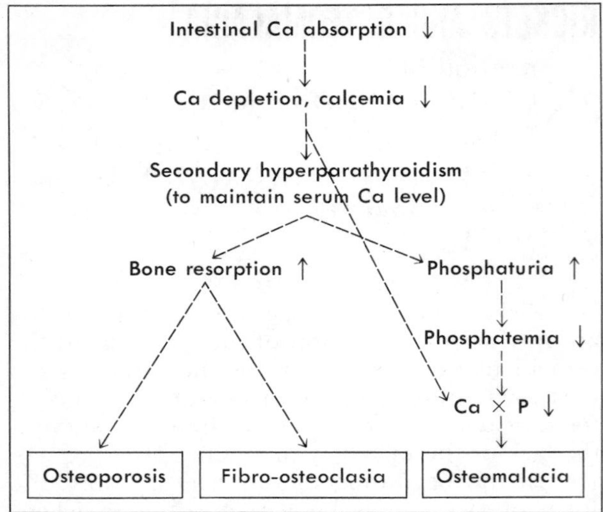

Figure 2. Pathogenesis of vitamin D deficiency rickets.

whereas it is absent in the normocalcemic X-linked hypophosphatemic rickets (phosphate diabetes).

Two etiologic groups of rickets and osteomalacia can be distinguished: (1) *Exogenous causes:* vitamin D deficiency, intestinal malabsorption of vitamin D, and reduced utilization of vitamin D. (2) *Genetic defects,* such as pseudo-vitamin D deficiency and phosphate diabetes. Genetic defects may reduce the efficiency of vitamin D or increase the sensitivity to vitamin D.

However, the limit between the normal variability and a genetic insufficiency is not always clear cut (Fig. 3). The efficacy of vitamin D in normal

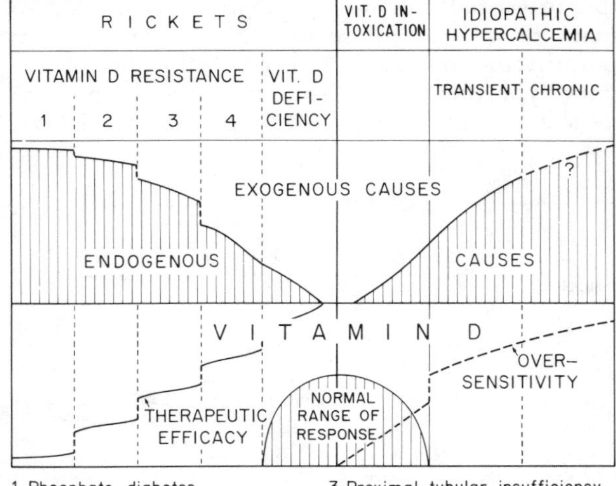

Figure 3.

children varies enormously; children with a tendency to rickets need more vitamin D than other children. On the other hand, some children are constitutionally extremely sensitive to vitamin D. When in England 1000 I.U. of vitamin D per liter was added to the milk, Lightwood noted several cases (about 1 per 1000) of transient hypercalcemia. This disturbance disappeared as soon as the quantity of vitamin D added to the milk was reduced to 400 I.U. per liter. Therefore the daily recommended allowance has been restricted to 400 I.U. of vitamin D for infants, children, and adults.

Vitamin D Deficiency Rickets

Prevention. Every infant (with a very few exceptions, such as those with idiopathic hypercalcemia and untreated hypothyroidism) needs a regular vitamin D supplement in order to prevent rickets. This supplement can be given in the milk preparation; 400 I.U. per liter may be sufficient if the feeding is complete and if this milk is given from the second week of life. If the baby is fed with mother's milk or with a preparation without vitamin D supplement, a vitamin D concentrate in a dose of 400 to 800 I.U. per day is indicated. This applies to full-term as well as premature infants. If one is not sure whether the vitamin is given regularly, e.g., in a primitive population, or if the mother appears to be unreliable, a single massive dose of 200,000 or 300,000 I.U. orally may be given. This excess vitamin is stored in the liver. The dose may be repeated after 3 months in the winter season.

Vitamin D enriched milk has the great advantage of ensuring that all children drinking it, even the poorest and most neglected ones, will be free of rickets. In large "inhuman" cities where the milk is not supplemented with vitamin D, rickets can be frequent among the poor people, whereas among the rich population vitamin D hypervitaminosis can occur because of overdosage. The inconvenience of vitamin D enriched milk is that hypersensitive persons may develop a hypercalciuric intoxication, and we do not know whether arteriosclerosis of older people might be furthered by its use. It is possible that some cases of supravalvular aortic stenosis and peripheral pulmonary stenosis may be due to hypercalcemic intoxication of the fetus.

Treatment. We recommend a daily dose of 5000 to 10,000 I.U. (0.125 to 0.25 mg.) of vitamin D_3 for 3 weeks, corresponding to a total amount of 100,000 to 200,000 I.U. In order to provide enough substrate for the hormonal action in the intestine, a calcium supplement should be added—i.e., 5 to 20 grams of calcium gluconate per day (1 gram contains about 90 mg. Ca^{++}).

There is no need for a special diet. Again, if one doubts that the mother will give the daily treatment, a single oral dose of 200,000 or 300,000 I.U. (5 or 7.5 mg.) may be given by the doctor without danger, as a rachitic infant is not likely to be intoxicated with this amount.

Orthopedic interventions are not necessary in nutritional rickets, as the growing bone will straighten once the metabolic disorder is medically cured.

All the other types of rickets are characterized by an increased need of vitamin D to prevent and/or cure them. They present therefore a certain degree of vitamin D "resistance."

Pseudovitamin D Deficiency Rickets (Vitamin D Dependency)

The genetic transmission is autosomal recessive. The cause is a defect of 1-hydroxylation of the 25-OHD_3 in the kidney. The symptoms are the same as in vitamin D deficiency rickets, but 100 to 1000 times higher daily doses of vitamin D_3 (about 40,000 I.U. [1 mg.]) are necessary for treatment and prevention. However, very small "physiologic" doses (1 or a few micrograms per day) of $1,25(OH)_2$-D_3 or $1\alpha OH$-D_3 are sufficient to produce the same effect. Up to now the administration of vitamin D_3 has been more practical and more economical. The vitamin D supplementation must be given during the patient's entire life.

Familial Hypophosphatemic Rickets

This X-linked hereditary disease was discovered in 1937 by Albright. In 1952, G. Fanconi proposed the name "phosphate diabetes," because the disease is due to a failure of the renal tubular cell to reabsorb phosphate, causing excessive phosphaturia and hypophosphatemia. The serum calcium is normal, and there is no secondary hyperparathyroidism. Owing to the X-linked dominant transmission and the Lyon mechanism, girls (XX) are more frequently but less severely involved than boys (XY). In adults, and particularly in women, hypophosphatemia is often the only sign of the disease. Osteomalacia may reappear when the need for phosphorus is increased, such as during puberty, pregnancy, and lactation.

Treatment consists of phosphate supplements and high doses of vitamin D. In order to raise the serum P level to at least 3 mg. per 100 ml., neutral or slightly acid (pH around 5) sodium phosphate must be given in high and frequent doses regularly distributed over day and night—e.g., 1 to 4 grams dissolved in water given five times daily. The difficulties and the practical limitations of this treatment include the time schedule—i.e., waking the child at night—and the gastrointestinal discomfort, especially osmotic diarrhea. Phosphate treatment alone might decrease the serum calcium and produce secondary hyperparathyroidism. It should be associated with a high dose vitamin D therapy—e.g., 20,000 to 100,000 I.U. (0.5 to 2.5 mg.) per day. The serum calcium level must be regularly controlled to avoid vitamin D intoxication. The risk of hypercalcemia and resultant nephrocalcinosis arises, especially when the patient is immobilized after an orthopedic operation or a disease requiring complete bed rest. In this case the vitamin D treatment must be interrupted, if possible a month before the immobilization. This rule applies to all patients treated with high doses of vitamin D.

If this double treatment is strictly applied and controlled, one might achieve an improvement of skeletal growth and a reduction of bone deformities. However, there is still considerable disagreement concerning its efficacy.

Severe deformities of the legs must be corrected by osteotomies in order to straighten the legs and to prevent arthrosis of badly positioned joints later in adult life.

Hyperazotemic Osteodystrophy

Morphologically this is a combination of rickets with fibro-osteoclasia (caused by secondary hyperparathyroidism) (Fig. 2), osteoporosis, and occasionally osteosclerosis. The pathogenesis is complex, including phosphate retention (by reduced glomerular filtration rate), systemic acidosis, and particularly a depression of the l-hydroxylation of vitamin D in the damaged renal tissue.

Treatment of renal osteodystrophy is very gratifying in patients with severe clinical symptoms (pain, inability to walk, skeletal deformities). Prophylactic treatment should prevent such disturbances. Besides treatment of renal failure, the following three measures should be taken:

1. Aluminium hydroxide given before each meal three times daily to bind alimentary phosphate and therefore to inhibit its intestinal absorption.

2. A supplement of dietary calcium salts (10 to 20 grams of calcium gluconate or lactate per day).

3. Vitamin D_3, 5000 to 40,000 I.U. (0.125 to 1 mg.) per day. This treatment must be carefully controlled by repeated measurements of serum calcium to avoid hypercalcemic vitamin D intoxication and ectopic calcifications. The correct dose of vitamin D must be adjusted for each individual patient. Physiologic amounts (about 1 microgram per day) of $1,25(OH)_2$-D_3 or $1\alpha OH$-D_3 are also effective, but are probably of no advantage for long-term treatment.

In patients with chronic hemodialysis, the treatment and prevention of renal osteodystrophy are similar. However, the calcium concentration of the dialysate (5 to 7 mg. per 100 ml.) adds a new variable. Renal transplantation might reverse the situation or might create new problems with respect to mineral metabolism. Hypercalcemia resulting from continuation of secondary hyperparathyroidism might necessitate partial parathyroidectomy. However, all these problems would be dealt with by transplant nephrologists.

Insufficiency of the Proximal Renal Tubule (Fanconi's Syndrome; de Toni–Debré–Fanconi Syndrome)

This syndrome, discovered in 1936, is in most cases secondary to a genetic disease (e.g., cystinosis, glycogen storage disease, Wilson's disease, tyrosinosis) or to heavy metal (lead, mercury) or drug poisoning (outdated tetracycline). Idiopathic forms are rare and can begin in children as well as in adults. Rickets is caused by renal phosphate loss, renal acidosis, and often an associated intestinal calcium loss. Treatment with vitamin D (20,000 to 40,000 I.U. per day) must be combined with alkali (sodium bicarbonate, sodium citrate, Shohl's solution) and, if necessary, with potassium salts, calcium, and phosphate to compensate for the renal losses of these electrolytes. The serum calcium must be carefully watched to avoid vitamin D intoxication, especially when signs of glomerular failure appear.

Distal Renal Tubular Acidosis

The cause is a failure of the distal renal tubular cells to excrete H ions against a gradient. The disease occurs sporadically or familially, and leads to failure to thrive, growth retardation, rickets, and nephrocalcinosis. Treatment consists of alkali (sodium bicarbonate, 1 to 2 mEq. per kg. per day in divided doses), just enough to correct the acidosis. A low sodium diet is advisable to decrease the solute load. The correction of the acidosis will normalize the growth rate and cure and prevent rickets without vitamin D treatment. However, the nephrocalcinosis, once established, seems to be irreversible.

Similar symptoms appear after ureterosigmoidostomy in patients with exstrophy of the bladder.

Rickets in Intestinal and Hepatic Diseases

In cases of intestinal malabsorption, especially with steatorrhea, the absorption of the fat-soluble vitamin D is inhibited. Therefore osteoporosis and osteomalacia may develop. This might occur after operative reduction of the intestinal tract, in insufficiently treated celiac disease, or in biliary diseases. In liver disease, rickets may be caused by an insufficient hydroxylation of vitamin D_3 to 25-OHD_3. In cases of intestinal or hepatic rickets it is therefore advisable to administer the vitamin D treatment by intramuscular injections—e.g., 300,000 I.U. (7.5 mg.) per month.

If, in underdeveloped countries, malnutrition, infections, parasites, and the like are contributing to cause severe rickets in children under 4 years of age, high doses of vitamin D are necessary to cure the bone disease. After healing, the usual preventive doses are sufficient.

Long-Term Use of Anticonvulsant Agents

Chronic administration of phenobarbital, phenytoin, and other antiepileptic drugs can sometimes produce rickets. These drugs seem to enhance the conversion of vitamin D_3 into more polar inactive metabolites, thus decreasing the availability of substrate for the 25-hydroxylation in the liver. This drug-induced disturbance should be compensated for by an additional vitamin D supply; in fact, this type of rickets can be cured by giving 2000 I.U. of vitamin D_3 orally per day, and can be prevented by giving a smaller prophylactic dose (e.g., 1000 I.U. per day). There is no agreement yet whether all patients on long-term anticonvulsant therapy should receive such preventive therapy.

Tumor Rickets

Some benign mesenchymal tumors have been observed to cause hypophosphatemic rickets or osteomalacia, possibly by producing an unknown vitamin D inhibitor. The bone disease heals quickly and completely after removal of the tumor. If removal is not possible, treatment with pharmacologic doses of vitamin D and phosphate is indicated.

Hypophosphatasia

This genetic bone disease has nothing in common with rickets except a rickets-like appearance of the metaphyses on x-rays. In the malignant neonatal type, the bone lesions are present at birth. It is important to make the diagnosis as early as possible and not to treat these patients with vitamin D, which acts as a poison and produces hypercalcemic intoxication. No treatment is known at present. Complicating hypercalcemia can be reduced by corticosteroids.

Hypercalcemic Intoxication

Vitamin D prevention and treatment of any kind of rickets may cause hypercalcemic intoxication if the dose of the vitamin is too high or if the patient is hypersensitive. It is therefore important that the physician know the first symptoms of hypercalcemia—i.e., apathy, constipation, failure to thrive, polydipsia, and polyuria. Not all the manifestations are present in every case. The control of the serum calcium level and of the urinary calcium excretion is indicated in every suspicious case.

As shown in Figure 3, the *sensitivity to vitamin D* shows considerable individual variations. Some clinical signs might help the physician recognize the degree of sensitivity before he prescribes prophylaxis or treatment: (1) *Tendency to decreased sensitivity:* familial disposition to rickets; familial aminoaciduria; accelerated growth—e.g., in premature infants. (2) *Tendency to increased sensitivity:* retarded growth—e.g., in endocrine disturbances, particularly hypothyroidism; increased density of metaphyseal margins; premature closure of the fontanels or tendency to craniostenosis; advanced bone age in comparison to chronological or height age; or prolonged immobilization.

SCURVY

(Vitamin C Deficiency)

method of
VICTOR HERBERT, M.D.
Brooklyn, New York

Vitamin C

Chemistry. Ascorbic acid is the physiologically active form of vitamin C. Iron and copper salts, alkaline pH, heat, and light facilitate the oxidation of ascorbic acid to dehydroascorbic acid, which remains active as a vitamin. Further oxidation renders the vitamin irreversibly inactive.

Sources. Ascorbic acid is widely distributed, chiefly in plant products, especially vegetables and fruits, whereas grains and cereals contain little. More than 100 mg. per 100 grams is found in broccoli greens, Brussels sprouts, collards, black currants, guava, horseradish, kale, turnip greens, parsley, and sweet peppers. About 50 to 99 mg. per 100 grams occurs in cabbage, cauliflower, chives, kohlrabi, orange pulp, lemon pulp, mustard greens, beet greens, papaya, spinach, strawberries, and watercress. About 30 to 49 mg. per 100 grams is found in asparagus, lima beans, Swiss chard, gooseberries, currants, grapefruit, limes, loganberries, melons (cantaloupe), okra, tangerines, potatoes, and turnips. Potatoes and cabbage may be consumed in large quantities by low-economic groups, and can provide rather large intakes of ascorbic acid.

Absorption. Intestinal absorption of ascorbic acid depends on the amount that is ingested, up to certain limits. If these limits are exceeded, there will be excessive loss of the vitamin in the gastrointestinal tract, with the corresponding osmotic attraction of water and production of diarrhea. Absorbed ascorbic acid is used for metabolic functions and saturation of tissue stores, and excess is largely excreted by the kidneys.

Metabolic Functions. (1) Metabolism of some amino acids. (2) Metabolism of iron and keeping folic acid in the reduced state. (3) Catecholamine metabolism. (4) Connective tissue metabolism via hydroxylation of proline and collagen crosslinking (wound healing). (5) Tooth and bone metabolism. (6) Blood coagulation. (7) Immune response. (8) Electron transport chain. (9) Possibly cholesterol metabolism.

Tissue Stores. Ascorbic acid has been found in large amounts in adrenals, pituitary gland, thymus, and corpus luteum. The saturated body pool of ascorbic acid has been estimated to be 1500 mg., with a daily utilization of 3 per cent (45 mg.). Signs and symptoms of ascorbic acid deficiency appear when tissue stores have been reduced over 80 per cent (body pool below 300 mg.).

Urinary Excretion. Ascorbic acid in excess of metabolic requirements and tissue storage capacity is excreted in the urine. The handling of ascorbic acid is similar to that of glucose. The renal threshold is approximately 1.4 mg. per 100 ml. When larger doses of ascorbic acid are present, the organism adapts by increasing the glomerular filtration rate and catabolism of the vitamin, with urinary excretion of its metabolites. Among these metabolites, one of the best characterized is oxalic acid. The further catabolism of this metabolite differs among individuals, with some persons more susceptible to oxaluria than others after the ingestion of large amounts (above 1 gram) of ascorbic acid.

Requirements

Because a saturated body pool of ascorbic acid is maintained in healthy men by 45 mg. per day, and because 10 mg. or slightly less per day will prevent and even cure clinical scurvy, the National Academy of Sciences recommends a daily dietary allowance (RDA: Recommended Dietary Allowance) of 35 mg. for infants, 40 mg. for children up to age 11 years, 45 mg. for adults, 60 mg. for pregnant women, and 80 mg. for lactating women. These recommendations meet (and actually exceed) the known nutritional needs of essentially all healthy persons. Needs for ascorbic acid may be slightly increased in situations of increased metabolism (e.g., hyperthyroidism), infections, inflammation, drug therapy (estrogens, antacids), smoking, and growth. However, no studies suggest that this increase would exceed the RDA, and alleged "antistress" actions of ascorbic acid have not been confirmed in man. Premature infants seem to do well with 50 mg. per day.

Treatment of Deficiency

Ascorbic acid deficiency is characterized by follicular hyperkeratotic lesions containing fragmented or coiled hairs, perifollicular petechiae, ecchymoses, spongy bleeding gums, poor wound healing, fatigue, swollen joints, muscular aches, and sometimes edema. There may be Sjögren's sicca syndrome or the "neurotic triad" of hysteria, depression, and hypochondriasis.

The only absolute indication for treatment with vitamin C is scurvy. Although as little as 10 mg. per day is enough to treat scurvy, oral doses of 100 mg. three times daily are recommended, and will replenish the body pools within about 5 days. If the patient's mouth is sore, swallowing is difficult, or intestinal absorption is impaired, parenteral administration of 250 to 500 mg. of vitamin C in an isotonic saline solution can be used. With these doses improvement is rapid, and after 1 week the doses should be gradually reduced until the patient is able to achieve a dietary intake of 45 mg. per day. Because malnutrition usually includes deficiencies of other vitamins, the patient should receive, in addition to vitamin C, one multivitamin capsule each day and, as soon as possible, a well-balanced diet. It is safe to continue vitamin supplements for up to 1 month. Doses greater than 100 mg. per day may induce increased catabolism of the vitamin, which continues after the doses have been reduced, and the increased catabolism can produce "rebound scurvy" if doses of 1 gram or more daily are stopped abruptly rather than tapered by about 10 to 20 per cent a day.

Toxic Effects

Although none of the published clinical trials have reported any significant toxicity of ascorbic acid in doses as high as 3 to 6 grams per day for a limited number of days, such large doses should be avoided because of these potential toxic effects: oxalic aciduria and renal stones, uric aciduria, increased urinary calcium, decreased urinary sodium, and hemolytic anemia in patients with glucose-6-phosphate dehydrogenase (G-6-PD) deficiency or sickle cell disease. A case has been reported of acute renal failure and death in a 68 year old man with G-6-PD deficiency who received 80 grams of ascorbic acid intravenously for 2 consecutive days. Large intakes of the vitamin have also been shown to interfere with certain tests for urine or serum vitamin B_{12}, glucose, uric acid, and iron, thus rendering these tests dangerously inaccurate. Destruction of food vitamin B_{12} by megadoses of ascorbate has been reported, but is disputed.

Allegations continue to be made that vitamin C is useful for the prevention and treatment of the common cold. A weak antihistamine effect is alleged. The available evidence, although implying that some slight effects may occur, suggests that any benefit is minimal and that there is no greater value of doses in excess of 200 mg. per day than is achieved by 200 mg. The alleged effects of the vitamin in treatment of cancer are compatible with placebo effect.

VITAMIN K DEFICIENCY

method of
C. THOMAS KISKER, M.D.
Iowa City, Iowa

Introduction

Vitamin K is essential for the synthesis of the vitamin K dependent coagulation factors II, VII, IX, and X. It appears to act in the final conversion of inactive precursor proteins into functional clotting factor molecules. A protein that is similar in structure to prothrombin but lacking activity can be found in animals and in man rendered deficient in vitamin K by the administration of a vitamin K antagonist such as warfarin. This inactive precursor protein can, however, be converted into functional prothrombin in cell free systems with the addition of vitamin K.

In man vitamin K is obtained both from the diet and by synthesis in the intestine. Vitamin K_1 is present in most foods and is particularly abundant in leafy vegetables such as spinach, cabbage, cauliflower, and kale. Animal tissue is a poor source of vitamin K, and breast milk contains only 1.5 micrograms per 100 ml. The adult requirement for vitamin K is approximately 0.03 microgram per kg. of body weight per day. The infant requires significantly more vitamin K, 0.15 to 0.25 microgram per kg. per day. Since the infant diet may consist largely of breast milk, vitamin K deficiency may occur if prophylactic vitamin K is not given.

In addition to dietary intake of vitamin K_1, synthesis of vitamin K_2 by bacteria located in the distal portion of the small intestine and colon provides an additional supply. Both vitamin K_1 and K_2 are fat soluble; thus maintenance of vitamin K nutrition is dependent not only on adequate supply, but also on effective absorption of fat. Patients with fat malabsorption must be considered as candidates for developing vitamin K deficiency and should thus be treated prophylactically.

Prevention

Neonatal. The lowest concentration of vitamin K dependent coagulation factors (II, VII, IX, X) is reached on about the second or third day of postnatal life. After the third day there is a gradual increase in concentration, but adult levels of the clotting factors may not be attained until 6 to 8 weeks of age. There is little storage reserve of vitamin K. The infant diet, particularly breast milk, contains little vitamin K, and the infant has inadequate intestinal bacterial flora for synthesis of the vitamin. Thus significant vitamin K deficiency may occur if additional vitamin K is not provided. One mg. of vitamin K_1 should be given intramuscularly to all full-term newborns at the time of birth. For infants weighing less than 2000 grams, 0.5 mg. of vitamin K_1 intramuscularly is sufficient.

Older Children and Adults. A deficiency of vitamin K can be anticipated in patients with inadequate intake when accompanied by an alteration of the intestinal flora through prolonged broad-spectrum antibiotic therapy. In such patients the prophylactic administration of between 2.5 and 5.0 mg. of water-soluble vitamin K_3 is recommended if the antibiotics are to be continued for more than 14 days in the absence of adequate dietary intake. Vitamin K deficiency can also be anticipated in the older child or adult patient who manifests fat malabsorption as a result of primary intestinal disease or a deficiency of bile salts. Such patients include those with obstructive jaundice, cystic fibrosis, pancreatic carcinoma, small bowel resection, ulcerative colitis, regional enteritis, celiac disease, and sprue. In these patients prophylactic administration of water-soluble vitamin K_3 at a dose of 2.5 to 5 mg. per day, depending upon the age of the patient, will prevent the development of vitamin K deficiency. Should a patient be unable to take the vitamin orally, intramuscular administration of 2.5 to 5 mg. of vitamin K_1 each week is sufficient to prevent vitamin K deficiency.

Treatment

Newborn. Vitamin K deficiency in the newborn is rapidly remedied by the injection of 1 mg. of vitamin K_1 intravenously. When intravenous administration is used, however, the vitamin should be given slowly, as rare reactions, including tachycardia, dyspnea, cyanosis, and anaphylaxis, have been reported. Vitamin K_1 can also be given intramuscularly, providing that the clotting factor deficiencies are not severe enough to cause hematoma formation at the site of injection. Improvement in the prothrombin time will occur within 2 to 4 hours after vitamin K administration and return to normal for age within 48 hours. In most instances this is a rapid enough reversal of the abnormal clotting factor activities that additional therapy is unnecessary. If, however, the infant has a severe or life-threatening hemorrhagic tendency, the administration of 15 ml. of fresh frozen plasma per kg. of body weight should be given in addition to the vitamin K. This amount of plasma will increase the vitamin K dependent clot-

TABLE 1. **Vitamin K Prophylaxis**

PATIENT	PREPARATION	DOSE	ROUTE
Infant			
>2000 grams	K_1 AquaMephyton, Konakion	1 mg. × 1	I.M.
≤2000 grams	K_1 AquaMephyton, Konakion	0.5 mg. × 1	I.M.
Older child, adult			
No restricted intake	K_3 Synkayvite, Hykinone, Menidione	2.5–5 mg. daily	P.O.
Restricted oral intake	K_1 AquaMephyton, Konakion	2.5–5 mg. weekly	I.M.

TABLE 2. **Vitamin K Deficiency Treatment**

PATIENT	PREPARATION	DOSE	ROUTE
Infant			
Mild deficiency	K_1 AquaMephyton, Konakion	1 mg. × 1	I.M.
Severe deficiency	K_1 AquaMephyton	1 mg. × 1	I.V.
Severe deficiency with life-threatening bleed	K_1 AquaMephyton Fresh frozen plasma	1 mg. × 1 15 ml./kg.	I.V. I.V.
Older child and adult			
Mild deficiency	K_1 AquaMephyton, Konakion	2.5–10 mg.	I.M.
Severe deficiency	K_1 AquaMephyton	2.5–10 mg.	I.V.
Severe deficiency with life-threatening bleed	K_1 AquaMephyton Factor IX concentrate (Konyne, Proplex)	2.5–10 mg. 25 units/kg.	I.V. I.V.

ting factor activities sufficiently to allow adequate hemostasis. Currently commercial concentrates of liver dependent factors (Konyne and Proplex) are to be avoided during infancy; at present the use of these concentrates is associated with a high risk for the development of hepatitis. The concentrates also may contain thrombogenic substances which may not be well tolerated by the infant.

Older Child and Adult. Vitamin K deficiency in the older child or adult may be the result of inadequate intake of vitamin K, decreased production by organisms in the gastrointestinal tract, failure of absorption, or interference with the normal function of vitamin K as a result of administration of a vitamin K antagonist such as a coumarin-type drug. Regardless of the cause, correction of vitamin K deficiency in the older child or adult is most rapidly achieved by the intramuscular or intravenous administration of 2.5 to 10 mg. of vitamin K_1. Following administration a significant improvement in the prothrombin time will be apparent within 2 to 4 hours, and complete correction is usual at 24 hours. As previously mentioned, care should be exercised in administration of vitamin K intravenously. The rate of administration should not exceed 1 mg. per minute, with careful observation for signs and symptoms of anaphylaxis.

When bleeding is severe or life-threatening, immediate correction of the clotting factor deficiencies may be indicated. This can be achieved by the administration of prothrombin complex concentrates (Konyne, Proplex). At present, administration of these concentrates is associated with a significant risk for the development of hepatitis. The concentrates also contain variable levels of activated clotting factors, which can cause thrombosis in the recipient. Although these risks may be less with future preparations, currently the concentrates are contraindicated in patients with liver disease and in those with prior thrombotic tendencies. When not contraindicated, the intravenous administration of the concentrate at a dose of 25 units of factor IX per kg. of body weight will immediately correct the clotting factor deficiencies and provide adequate hemostasis until the sustained correction from vitamin K administration has occurred. Fresh frozen plasma, 15 ml. per kg. of body weight given intravenously, will also partially correct the bleeding defect in vitamin K deficiency. Plasma transfusion, however, requires additional time, does not achieve full correction of clotting factor activity, and may result in fluid overload. Fresh frozen plasma transfusion may, nonetheless, be a helpful adjunct to vitamin K administration in patients with severe vitamin K deficiency in whom the prothrombin complex concentrates are contraindicated.

OSTEOPOROSIS

method of
LOUIS V. AVIOLI, M.D.
St. Louis, Missouri

Osteoporosis of the "senile" or "postmenopausal" variety is defined as a skeletal disorder in which the absolute amount of bone is decreased relative to that of younger or menstruating women, although the remaining bone is normal in chemical composition. Symptomatic senile or postmenopausal osteoporosis syndromes are classically considered to result from the universal loss of bone that normally attends senescence in both sexes and begins in the third or fourth decade of life. Although comparable decrements in the functional capacity of the heart, lungs, kidney, and nervous tissue (i.e., nerve conduction time) also attend the aging process, the decrease in bone mass may lead to significant incapacitation and result in fractures and immobilization in the aged person, not only requiring significant hospitalization time but often resulting in relative inactivity.

This is a problem of considerable magnitude; approximately 6.3 million people in the United States are currently suffering from acute problems related to weakened vertebral bones. Perhaps even more significant is the fact that 8 million Americans today have chronic problems related to the spine, compared with 6 million reported in 1963. Moreover, recent epidemiologic surveys indicate that a minimum of 10 per cent of the female population over 50 years of age suffer from bone loss severe enough to cause hip, vertebral, or long bone fractures; surveys performed in homes for the aged and of ambulatory persons 50 to 95 years of age requiring medical care also disclosed symptomatic (i.e., back pain) osteoporosis in 15 and 50 per cent of these populations, respectively.

The consequences of osteoporosis are magnified in the postmenopausal female, resulting in major orthopedic problems in approximately 25 to 30 per cent of postmenopausal women. The incidence of symptomatic osteoporosis appears to be four times greater in women than in men.

Although the total female population in the United States tripled from 31 million in 1900 to 91 million in 1960, the total annual number of vertebral or hip fractures rose from 11,000 to 62,000. The rise in fracture rate was twice as fast as the population gain because of the disproportionate increment in the number of aged females susceptible to fractures of the hip and vertebral column. It should also be emphasized that demographic data indicate that the over-50 age group is the fastest growing minority in the United States and that of the 1 million (approximate) fractures experienced each year by women aged 45 years or older in the United States, about 700,000 are incurred by women with osteoporosis. In 1968, falls were the leading cause of nontransport accidental deaths in all persons and the leading cause of all accidental deaths in elderly white females in the United States. Approximately three quarters of all deaths from falls occur in patients aged 65 and over, with a female : male fracture incidence ratio of 8.1 The rate (per 1000 population per year) of hip fractures in white women resulting from minimal trauma increased from 2.0 at ages 50 to 64, to 5.0 at ages 65 to 74, and to 10 at ages greater than 75 years.

Differential Diagnosis

It appears quite obvious that until the mythological "fountain of youth" is discovered, the physician can only be satisfied with attempting to select those persons at risk of developing vertebral crush fractures or radial and femoral neck fractures with the anticipation of selecting an appropriate *preventive* therapeutic regimen. In this regard, we should not lose sight of the fact that so-called "involutional," "postmenopausal," or "gerontoid" osteoporosis may actually represent a heterogeneity of bone pathology and is often complicated by subtle metabolic or malignant processes. Before embarking on any therapeutic program (which should be considered only *preventive* at this stage of our knowledge), subtle forms of thyrotoxicosis manifested by elevations in T_3 only must be considered, as well as occult forms of multiple myeloma or metastatic carcinoma which may present with diffuse spinal osteopenia and vertebral fracture. Bilateral cortical adrenal nodular hyperplasia without any of the clinical stigmata of Cushing's syndrome may also mimic the "postmenopausal" osteoporotic state presenting with severe cranial osteopenia and vertebral collapse. Adult forms of osteogenesis imperfecta tarda are often missed and not even suspected, because these patients not infrequently lack the classic "blue sclerae" and are unaware (or often uncertain) of familial fracture diathesis. In this regard one should again recall the well documented observations that the incidence of skeletal fractures in osteogenesis imperfecta decreases during the pubescent years, only to occur in females with increasing incidence following ovarian failure. Primary hyperparathyroidism, a metabolic bone disease with a peak incidence in middle-aged females, may also go undetected, especially if the disorder is manifested chemically by intermittent *mild* hypercalcemia and mild elevations in circulating immunoreactive parathyroid hormone (iPTH) beyond the detection of the best of radioimmunoassay techniques. Parenthetically, these women may present with significant hypercalciuria and a rise in serum calcium to abnormal values once estrogen therapy (which is often initiated inappropriately and without careful diagnostic study) is discontinued. Finally, it should be emphasized again that over 20 per cent of aged persons who present with vertebral, femoral, or radial fractures have osteomalacia superimposed on the normal senescent osteopenic process. This skeletal lesion, which is *curable* with vitamin D and supplemental calcium therapy, escapes detection (or, in fact, consideration), because circulating levels of calcium, inorganic phosphate, alkaline phosphatase, iPTH, and vitamin D metabolites may be normal. It is established with certainty only by histologic evaluation of appropriately prepared undecalcified bone biopsy preparations.

Therapy

Once these and a variety of other less common heritable or acquired bone disorders which mimic "osteoporosis" radiographically have been entertained and effectively disposed of, and recognizing that chronic megadose vitamin A therapy, diabetes mellitus, and chronic ethanol abuse also result in an acceleration of the bone loss which attends the aging process, the clinician is then confronted with the therapeutic approach to the "postmenopausal" or "senile" symptomatic or fracture-prone osteoporotic patient. With the exception of the fasting urinary hydroxyproline : creatinine or calcium : creatinine ratios (which are not infrequently elevated in the majority of these subjects) or circulating iPTH values (which may be elevated in 10 to 15 per cent of patients), chemical testing often proves frustrating and unrewarding. Similarly, quantitation of circulating estradiol, estrone, androstenedione, FSH, or LH is of no value diagnostically, because values thus obtained in patients with active "crush fracture" syndromes are no different from those obtained from age-matched females with significantly greater bone mass content and no history of fracture. In some instances, the intestinal malabsorption of calcium is markedly decreased, whereas it is maintained quite well in others. This latter group of patients may respond favorably to dietary supplementation with calcium alone in doses of 1.0 to 1.5 grams per day with rather significant decreases in the annual rate of loss in cortical bone mass. To provide 1.0 gram of elemental calcium, one must administer 5.5 grams of hydrated calcium chloride, 8 grams of calcium lactate, 11 grams of calcium gluconate, 4 grams of calcium acetate, or 2.6 grams of calcium carbonate.

Using metacarpal cortical mass measurements, which are far more sensitive indices of therapeutic responsivity than the routine spinal radiograph, and serial measurements of fasting urinary hydroxyproline : creatinine and calcium : creatinine ratios, it has been demonstrated that some, *but not all*, middle-aged (i.e., 45 to 55 years) females will also benefit from short-term estrogen therapy (e.g., 0.625 to 1.25 mg. of conjugated estrogen preparations daily or cyclically). This approach should be tempered with considerable caution, with routine analysis of the uterine mucosa, because of accumulated evidence of the increased incidence of endometrial carcinoma in patients thus treated.

A variety of other therapeutic regimens have been tried; some (e.g., phosphate supplementation, 1.0 gram per day, or human growth hormone, 0.2 unit per kg. of body weight per day) have proved either deleterious or potentially harmful because of associated therapeutic complications. Advocates of intermittent androgen therapy (e.g., methandrostenolone) cite beneficial effects of long-term therapy (5 mg. per day 3 out of every 4 weeks for 2 years) on total body mineral content as evidence in favor of therapeutic effectiveness. Reports of hepatic toxicity with hepatoma and peliosis hepatis should be acknowledged before adopting this form of therapy chronically, as well as the obvious fact that changes in total body calcium as measured by neutron activation analysis may not necessarily reflect an increase in cortical or trabecular bone mass per se. Histologically, therapeutic regimens consisting of 50,000 units of vitamin D twice weekly and daily calcium supplements of 1.5 to 2.0 grams have also proved effective in suppressing the accelerated bone resorption in osteoporotic patients and the response attributed to suppression of parathyroid hormone release.

Sodium fluoride has also been recommended as a therapeutic aid for the "postmenopausal osteoporotic" patient. Reports of decreased incidence of osteoporosis and collapsed vertebrae in subjects living in areas where the fluoride content of the water supply was greater than 4 ppm., and others citing the potential benefit of sodium fluoride therapy in doses ranging from 10 to 175 mg. per day, are to be contrasted with observations that chronic fluoride administration leads to osteomalacia, an increase in skeletal microfractures, and the exacerbation of arthrosis. Symptomatic improvement has been claimed, however, when fluoride treatment (in doses less than 60 mg. per day) is combined with diets supplemented with calcium in a dosage of 1.0 to 2.0 grams per day. The enthusiasm for this approach must again be tempered by reports of abnormal bone cytology, arthralgia, and joint effusions in patients receiving sodium fluoride for prolonged periods of time, and by others demonstrating decreased mechanical strength of bones of flouride-treated animals in which the bone flouride content approximated that of humans receiving fluoride and supplemental calcium combinations. Rigorous long-term assessment of the effects of chronic fluoride administration on the structural integrity of bone and extraskeletal tissue metabolism and organ function is mandatory before an adequate appraisal of the benefit : risk ratio can be made.

The therapeutic effects reported to occur with calcitonin in Paget's disease of bone have also resulted in limited European trials of this hormone in "osteoporotic" patients. Favorable therapeutic responses to calcitonin for periods ranging from 1 to 29 months judged by symptomatic improvement and decrease in annual fracture rates have been reported when doses ranging from 2 to 100 MRC units per day are given. Although calcitonin is a likely candidate for suppressing the accelerated bone resorption which characterizes the course of an "osteoporotic" patient, long-term calcitonin therapy must presently be considered experimental and *potentially* remedial treatment until more appropriate, well designed double-blind placebo study protocols are developed with quantitative evaluation of the ratios of cortical bone loss, the effect of treatment on parathyroid hormone secretion, and the antibody response to nonhuman calcitonin preparations.

What does the clinician offer his symptomatic "postmenopausal osteoporotic" patient? It would appear appropriate that dietary habits be altered so as to ensure a calcium : phosphate ratio greater than 1.0. This can best be accomplished by supplemental calcium feeding in doses of 1.0 to 2.0 grams per day. As noted earlier, a number of patients will respond to this regimen alone with a gradual decrease in the rate of cortical bone loss. Following an appropriate interval of 6 to 8 months, vitamin D in doses of 50,000 units twice weekly for 1 to 2 months should effectively reverse the osteomalacia of those thus affected and possibly also potentiate the favorable long-term skeletal effect of dietary calcium supplementation. Since estrogen replacement therapy, if initiated more than 6 years following cessation of ovarian activity, is certain to prove ineffective in reversing the progressive fall in bone mass, and since long-term therapy with conjugated estrogens may in fact increase the incidence of endometrial carcinoma, it would appear wise not to arbitrarily subject women in their later postmenopausal years to these agents. Estrogen therapy if initiated should be intermittent (i.e., 3 weeks on and 1 week off) and terminated after 1½ to 2 years.

Conclusion

Despite the therapeutic program selected, the physician should explore sensitive techniques which are readily available to monitor the skeletal response. Routine spinal or pelvic radiographs, or measurements of circulating calcium, phosphate, and alkaline phosphatase, do not presently satisfy this goal. More specific serial quantitation of metacarpal cortical thickness (obtained from routine hand films) and fasting urinary hydroxyproline : creatinine and calcium : creatinine ratios should prove to be much more sensitive indices of the skeletal response in any one patient. Whatever the nature of the therapeutic agent (or agents), skeletal responsivity must be quantitated and the regimen re-evaluated at semiannual intervals. The need to diagnose other potentially remedial metabolic bone disorders must be emphasized, as well as the obvious fact that, once diagnosed, one can only hope to retard the rate of bone loss in a "postmenopausal" or "senile" osteoporotic patient and ideally render symptomatic improvement during the therapeutic interval.

PARENTERAL NUTRITION IN ADULTS

by
CHRISTOF WESTENFELDER, M.D.,
and NEIL A. KURTZMAN, M.D.
Chicago, Illinois

It has been estimated that 3 to 10 per cent of hospitalized patients will require some kind of parenteral nutrition. The aim of such therapy is to maintain normal body composition in the face of decreased oral intake, increased metabolic requirements, and the presence of disorders of the metabolic machinery.

Definitions

Hypocaloric parenteral nutrition is provided when less than 11 kcal. per kg. of body weight per day (as isotonic glucose, amino acids, lipids) is administered. Hyperalimentation exists when total parenteral nutrition is provided. Hyperalimentation is termed hypercaloric when the amount of calories provided exceeds that burned per day. Such parenteral alimentation is required when there are large nutritional deficits to be replaced or prevented. Short-term parenteral nutrition (less than 5 or 6 days) is provided to minimize nitrogen and glycogen losses by the administration of hypocaloric parenteral nutrition. Long-term parenteral nutrition (greater than 5 to 6 days) is designed to allow weight gain, positive nitrogen balance, improved wound healing, and shortened convalescence.

Background (Tables 1 and 2)

A normal adult man weighing 70 kg. has a caloric reserve from fat stores to meet his caloric requirements for 2 months of total starvation (approximately 150,000 kcal.). Caloric reserves from muscle protein (gluconeogenesis) are sufficient for 2 weeks; however, if more than one third to one half of protein stores are catabolized, death usually ensues as a result of respiratory muscle weakness, pulmonary atelectasis, and pneumonia. Carbohydrate reserves present as muscle and liver glycogen and blood glucose are exhausted within 12 hours of the initiation of fasting. Blood glucose concentration is maintained thereafter by gluconeogenesis from endogenous amino acids.

TABLE 1. **Caloric Expenditure During Physiologic Activities and During Disease States**

PHYSIOLOGIC ACTIVITY	EXPENDED KCAL./KG. BODY WEIGHT/24 HOURS	DISEASE STATE
Bed rest	25	Bedridden
Light physical work	30–35	Fever
Moderate physical work	35–40	Sepsis
Heavy physical work	40–50(+)	Extensive burns

Obligatory protein utilization for gluconeogenesis occurs during starvation and is essential because fat cannot be used for the synthesis of glucose. The brain, blood cells, and renal medulla are obligatory consumers of glucose.

During starvation 60 to 70 grams per day of protein is broken down; this amount is equivalent to the loss of 10 to 12 grams of nitrogen in the urine and is associated with the loss of 200 to 300 grams of lean body weight per day. Insulin and glucagon are the primary hormonal regulators of gluconeogenesis and ketogenesis in starvation. Insulin decreases during starvation, resulting in increased lipolysis and increased gluconeogenesis. Glucagon levels also increase during starvation and result in glycogenolysis and increased gluconeogenesis.

Simple administration of 100 grams of glucose per day to a starving patient will reduce urinary losses of nitrogen to 2 to 3 grams per day. After 5 to 6 days of starvation, a striking adaptation to the catabolic state occurs. This adaptation results in a reduction in protein catabolism. The brain, which formerly had been an exclusive glucose user, now uses ketone bodies as fuel. Under this condition of adaptation, 95 per cent of the caloric needs of the body may be met by utilization of fat depots.

In accelerated catabolic states (e.g., sepsis, trauma, burns) the response to starvation is very poorly tolerated and is characterized by accelerated protein catabolism, secondary to an increase in basal metabolic rate, oxygen consumption, and increased energy expenditure. Under these conditions urinary nitrogen losses may exceed 25 grams per day, which is the equivalent of the breakdown of 150 grams of protein, representing the loss of 400 grams of lean body mass. Under conditions of hypercatabolism, the administration of 100 to 400 grams of glucose per day fails to reduce protein

TABLE 2. **Nutrient Requirements**

"NUTRIENT"	KCAL./GRAM	DAILY REQUIREMENT FOR TOTAL PARENTERAL NUTRITION	HOW SUPPLIED
Glucose (dextrose)	4	30–50 kcal./kg. body weight	20–25% solutions
Fat (Intralipid)	9		10% (isotonic)
Nitrogen	4	0.1–0.4 gram/kg. body weight	3–5% solutions of (1) protein hydrolysates (e.g., Amigen, Aminosol); (2) synthetic L-amino acids (1:1.5 ratio essential to nonessential amino acids)
Electrolytes and minerals			
Na		40–120 mEq.	Part of Na can be given as $NaHCO_3$; part of K as $KHCO_3$ or KH_2PO_4
K		40–120 mEq.	
Mg		5–15 mEq.	
Ca		15–30 mEq.	
PO_4		100–300 mEq.	
Trace elements			
Zinc		0.30 μmol./kg. body weight	As their salts
Copper		0.07 μmol./kg. body weight	
Vitamins:			
Water-soluble:			
Thiamine		0.02 mg./kg. body weight	USV parenteral preparation
Riboflavin		0.03 mg./kg. body weight	
Nicotinamide		0.20 mg./kg. body weight	
Pantothenic acid		0.20 mg./kg. body weight	
Biotin		5 μg./kg. body weight	
Ascorbic acid		0.50 mg./kg. body weight	
Pyridoxine		0.03 mg./kg. body weight	
Folate		300 μg./day	
Vitamin B_{12}		30 μg./day	
Fat-soluble:			
Retinol (vitamin A)		10 μg./kg. body weight	
Ergocalciferol or cholecalciferol (vitamin D)		0.04 μg./kg. body weight	
Phytylmenaquinone (vitamin K)		2 μg./kg. body weight	
α-Tocopherol (vitamin E)		15 I.U./day	
Essential fatty acids		(see above: Fat)	Intralipid 10%
Water		30–60 ml./kg. body weight	

catabolism. Protein homeostasis may be maintained in this condition only by the administration of exogenous protein with sufficient calories to meet metabolic demands.

Basic Principles of Total Parenteral Nutrition

The aims of this therapy are to provide all nutrients in a concentrated form in a fashion that does not disrupt fluid and electrolyte homeostasis. Sufficient nonprotein calories should be provided to allow the use of amino acids for protein synthesis. This goal requires the administration of no less than 150 kcal. per gram of nitrogen administered. Hypertonic solutions containing parenteral nutrients must be administered into a large central vein; the usual procedure is to administer these fluids into the superior vena cava. The infused solutions must be given at a constant rate of flow; this procedure avoids fluctuation in blood sugar concentration and facilitates optimal nutrient use. The indications and contraindications for full parenteral nutrition are outlined in Tables 3 and 4.

Parenteral Nutrition Solutions

For short-term hypocaloric parenteral nutrition, the following solution may be used: 1500 ml. 5 per cent dextrose and water to which 40 mEq. KCl has been added, plus 500 ml. 5 per cent dextrose in normal saline. This solution supplies 77 mEq. NaCl and 400 kcal. as glucose. It may be modified according to needs—i.e., if the patient is febrile or has an electrolyte disorder or abnormal cardiovascular, hepatic, or renal function.

A solution for long-term parenteral nutrition is outlined in Table 5. When access to a large central vein is not available, a fat emulsion (Intralipid 10 per cent) may be administered through a peripheral vein. This solution contains 10 per cent soybean oil (54 per cent linoleic, 26 per cent oleic, 9 per cent palmitic, 8 per cent linolenic acids). It also contains 1.2 per cent egg yolk phospholipids and 2.2 per cent glycerin, with pH adjusted with sodium hydroxide to 5.5 to 9.0. The osmolarity of this solution is 280 mOsm. per liter.

For patients with acute renal failure, total parenteral nutrition solutions should be adjusted

TABLE 3. **Indications for Total Parenteral Nutrition**

General
4 to 5 days of starvation and/or >10% loss of lean body weight
Specific
1. Gastrointestinal disorders complicated by:
   a. Enteric or enterocutaneous fistulas
   b. Short bowel syndrome
   c. High alimentary tract obstruction
   d. Malabsorption with normal bowel length, secondary to sprue or ulcerative colitis
2. Functional gastrointestinal disorders
   a. Esophageal dyskinesia post–cardiovascular accident
   b. Hyperemesis gravidarum
   c. Psychogenic vomiting
3. Obtunded sensorium secondary to metabolic or neurologic disorders
4. Excessive metabolic requirements secondary to severe trauma, extensive burns, sepsis, major fractures
5. Preoperatively in patients who suffer from progressive malnutrition
6. Postoperatively if oral intake cannot be resumed within 5 to 7 days and for promotion of anabolism
7. Adjunctive therapy in some cancer patients (improved tolerance of anticancer therapy)
8. Acute renal failure

so that they contain 1.8 per cent essential amino acids and 20 per cent glucose and deliver less than 20 mEq. per day of sodium. Patients with severe cardiovascular or hepatic disease who are retaining salt should also have salt concentration appropriately reduced in their parenteral solutions.

Technical Approach

Ideally the team responsible for the administration of parenteral nutrition should consist of a physician with a strong background in nutrition, a total parenteral nutrition nurse, a surgeon, a pharmacist, and an infectious disease specialist functioning as a consultant.

The preparation of these solutions is performed by the pharmacist. Strict attention to aseptic technique is essential. It is desirable that a laminar flow filtered air hood be employed. Commercial hyperalimentation sets consist of a 1 liter bottle half filled with 50 per cent dextrose under vacuum and a second 0.5 liter bottle containing 5 to 10 per

TABLE 4. **Contraindications for Total Parenteral Nutrition**

Total parenteral nutrition is contraindicated when:
1. The patient is in good nutritional status and only short-term parenteral nutrition is required or anticipated
2. Oral nutrition is feasible
3. Cardiovascular and metabolic derangements are uncorrected
4. Patient is unsalvageable or inevitably dying

TABLE 5. **Composition of Typical Parenteral Nutrition Solutions (Amount per Liter)**

Dextrose (grams)	250
Nitrogen (grams)	4.2*
Na (mEq.)	24
K (mEq.)	40
Mg (mEq.)	10
Ca (mEq.)	1.6
Cl (mEq.)	35
Acetate (mEq.)	52
Phosphate (mg.)	113
Zinc sulfate (mg.)	5
Kcal.	900

Phosphate content of amino acid preparations:

1. Synthetic crystalline amino acids are free of PO_4 (e.g., Cutter, FreAmine)
2. Protein hydrolysates contain the following amounts of PO_4:

a. Amigen (casein)	30 mEq./liter
b. CPH	14 mEq./liter
c. Hyprotigen	25 mEq./liter
d. Aminosol	0 mEq./liter

*Crystalline amino acid preparation (e.g., FreAmine).

cent amino acids. There is a transfer set for aseptic mixing of the two parts of the solution and a separate set for administration to the patient.

The right subclavian vein via an infraclavicular approach (or cutdown) is cannulated (using aseptic technique). The catheter tip is advanced into the superior vena cava above the right atrium. A chest x-ray is obtained to verify correct placement of the catheter. The catheter is fixed by suturing it to the skin; the wound is coated with antibiotic ointment, and a nonocclusive dressing is put in place. This dressing is changed three times per week. The line for fluid administration should contain a filter of 0.22 to 0.45 μ pore size (use of 0.22 μ filter requires the use of a peristaltic pump). The filter should be changed daily. The intravenous tubing should be changed with each bottle of solution. When solutions are changed, the infusion lines should be clamped to avoid air embolization. Blood, albumin, and drugs should *not* be given via the total parenteral nutrition catheter. The catheter should also *not* be used for measurement of central venous blood pressure.

As a rough rule, the fluid should be administered at a sufficient rate to deliver 1 liter the first day, 2 liters the second day, and 3 liters per day thereafter as maintenance. Care should be taken to maintain constant infusion speed. In order to avoid severe hypoglycemia, when the decision to terminate parenteral nutrition is made, fluid administration should be tapered off over 48 hours or 5 per cent dextrose and water or oral feedings begun. The parameters outlined in Table 6 should be monitored.

TABLE 6. **Parameters to Be Monitored**

PARAMETERS	FREQUENCY
1. Body weight, vital signs	Daily
2. Volume of parenteral intake	Daily
3. Oral intake (if any)	Daily
4. Urinary output	Daily total and each voiding
5. Extrarenal losses	Daily
6. Blood measurements	
Electrolytes, BUN	Daily (initial phase)†
Blood sugar	Daily (initial phase)
Osmolality*	Daily (initial phase)
Total Ca, Mg and PO_4	3× weekly
Liver enzymes, bilirubin	3× weekly
Serum proteins	2× weekly
Complete blood count	Weekly
Blood NH_3	2× weekly
7. Urine measurements: glucose, osmolality, acetone	4 to 6× daily (initial phase)
8. Screening for infection	
Clinical observation, status of patient, temperature	Daily
White blood count and differential	As indicated
Blood cultures and culture of infusate and filter	As indicated
9. Fecal and 24 hour urine nitrogen (if diarrhea) in order to assess nitrogen balance	Optional

*May be calculated as follows: $\text{mOsm./kg. } H_2O = 2(Na + K) + \frac{\text{Glucose (mg./dl.)}}{18} + \frac{\text{BUN (mg./dl.)}}{2.8}$. (BUN does not contribute to tonicity.)

†Initial phase: usually the first 3 to 4 days.

Complications

1. Sepsis occurs in 10 to 25 per cent of all patients receiving total parenteral nutrition. Fungus infections are particularly common *(Candida albicans)*. Predisposition for infection may be the result of prior antibiotic therapy or the result of microorganisms in the parenteral alimentation solution itself. This latter fact emphasizes the need for strict aseptic preparation and administration of these fluids. The incidence of infection is significantly reduced by the placement of a 0.22 μ pore membrane filter in the infusion line. If sepsis develops, the parenteral nutrition solution should be discontinued and cultured. The catheter must be removed and also cultured if no other source of infection has been identified.

2. Nonseptic complications related to the catheter include the development of a pneumothorax when the bottle is changed. Also encountered are hemothorax and puncture of the subclavian artery, occasionally accompanied by arteriovenous fistula development; there may be injury to the brachial plexus, cardiac tamponade, cavitating pulmonary infarction from catheter embolus, and thrombosis of the subclavian vein and superior vena cava.

3. Fluid overload, which manifests itself as either hypertension or congestion, may be the result of too rapid infusion of the solution. Careful attention to cardiovascular and renal status prevent the development of this complication. The proper management of this complication consists of reduction of the rate of infusion of the parenteral alimentation solution.

4. Hypertonicity and electrolyte imbalance may likewise result from the administration of parenteral alimentation solutions. Careful surveillance of blood electrolytes and osmolality will allow early identification of this complication and prevent it from becoming clinically significant. If a tendency toward hypertonicity is noted, water should be administered and, if necessary, the amount of hyperalimentation solution infused should be decreased. Both hypo- and hypernatremia may result and are effectively managed by proper attention to water administration. Similarly, hypo- and hyperkalemia may develop and are appropriately treated by the infusion of potassium or the reduction of the amount of potassium in the hyperalimentation solution.

5. Hyperglycemia exceeding 200 mg. per dl. (100 ml.) is rare in the presence of normal pancreatic function. In diabetic patients receiving

hyperalimentation, severe hyperglycemia may develop, which in turn may precipitate the syndrome of nonketotic hyperosmolar coma. The manifestations of this disorder include azotemia, obtundation, and seizures. It is prevented by monitoring both urine and blood glucose levels and by administering regular insulin, 10 to 20 units, when the blood sugar exceeds 200 mg. per dl. and is accompanied by glycosuria. The management of this complication consists of the administration of both regular insulin and hypotonic fluid. It may be necessary to temporarily discontinue infusion of the parenteral alimentation solution.

6. Postinfusion hypoglycemia may occur as a result of inadvertent dislodgment of the catheter or because of interruption of infusion of the hyperalimentation solution. This is especially likely to occur if insulin is being administered concomitantly with the hyperalimentation solution. Management is the infusion of glucose.

7. Hypophosphatemia may occur if the total parenteral nutritional solution does not contain phosphate and is given for more than 7 to 10 days. Under this circumstance serum phosphate may be less than 1 mg. per dl. Severe hypophosphatemia results from the shift of phosphate into muscle and liver cells and not as a consequence of urinary loss. As a result of hypophosphatemia, there may be increased oxygen affinity of red blood cells (because of 2,3-diphosphoglycerate depletion). Other manifestations of hypophosphatemia include paresthesias, hyperventilation, obtundation, seizures, and coma. The disorder is prevented by monitoring the serum phosphate concentration and administering phosphate when required.

8. Hyperchloremic metabolic acidosis may occur with the administration of synthetic amino acid preparations which, when metabolized, result in the delivery of hydrochloric acid to the extracellular fluid compartment. This complication is not seen when protein hydrolysates are administered. It is prevented by monitoring acid-base status and giving $NaHCO_3$ when required.

9. Hyperammonemia may occur in patients with liver disease who are unable to convert ammonia to urea. The ammonia is derived from the metabolism of protein hydrolysates, which contain, in addition, high levels of preformed ammonia. The prevention is to monitor blood ammonia and to give synthetic amino acids to patients with liver disease.

Other, less common complications are outlined in Table 7.

TABLE 7. **Other Complications of Prolonged Total Parenteral Nutrition**

DISORDER	SYMPTOMS AND SIGNS	CAUSE	TREATMENT
Hyperaminoacidemia	Obtundation	Excessive amino acid administration	Glucose, reduce amino acid administration
Hyperphosphatemia	Tetany, paresthesia	Secondary to casein hydrolysates, poor renal function	Synthetic amino acids, correction of volume contraction and Intralipid 10% I.V.
Essential fatty acid deficiency	Dermatitis, poor healing, weakness, thrombocytopenia	Linoleic acid deficiency	Intralipid 10% I.V.
Hypocalcemia	Tetany, paresthesias	Insufficient Ca intake	Calcium salts
Hypomagnesemia	Tetany	Inadequate intake, especially secondary to casein hydrolysate	Mg salts
Anemia	Weakness	Iron, folic acid, vitamin B_{12}, K, copper, zinc deficiency, bleeding	Supplements of deficient compounds, blood transfusion as indicated
Liver enzyme elevation	Hepatomegaly, abdominal pain in right upper quadrant	Excessive fat and glycogen deposition	Reduce amount of total parenteral nutrition

PARENTERAL FLUID THERAPY IN CHILDREN

method of
WILLIAM E. SEGAR, M.D.
Madison, Wisconsin

Parenteral fluids are administered to the child who is unable to consume an adequate intake of water and electrolytes in order to (1) meet the daily normal or physiologic losses of water and electrolytes, (2) replace pre-existing body fluid deficits, and (3) replace abnormal continuing losses of water and electrolytes. Parenteral fluids must be given intravenously. Adequate, safe therapy cannot be provided through the use of fluids administered subcutaneously. Fluid therapy should always be calculated as the amount needed by the child per 24 hours, and the fluids usually should be administered at a constant rate during the entire 24 hour period.

Maintenance Therapy

Every patient, each day, normally loses fairly predictable quantities of water, electrolytes, and calories. Fluid therapy designed to replace these normal losses is usually called maintenance therapy. If the patient in whom fluid therapy is begun is in an adequate state of hydration and if he has not lost excessive amounts of fluid or electrolytes, maintenance therapy will meet his entire needs.

Many systems are advocated for the calculation of maintenance water requirement. It has been shown that the daily physiologic water losses are proportionate to caloric expenditure. It follows therefore that maintenance water requirements are also proportionate to caloric expenditure and that, under most circumstances, water requirement is constant from one patient to the next, when expressed as water needed per unit of caloric expenditure. A convenient unit of reference in calculating maintenance fluid requirements is 100 kcal. For the average hospitalized child, the approximate calorie expenditure in kilocalories can be estimated from one of the following formulas: (1) For the child who weighs up to 10 kg., caloric expenditure is 100 × kg. (2) For the child who weighs 10 to 20 kg., caloric expenditure is 1000 + (kg. − 10)50. (3) For the child who weighs more than 20 kg., caloric expenditure is 1500 + (kg. −20)20. The caloric expenditure per day of three children weighing 5 kg., 15 kg., and 25 kg. would be estimated as 500 kcal., 1250 kcal., and 1600 kcal., respectively.

The maintenance water requirement is the sum of the insensible and renal water losses. When the environmental temperature and humidity are normal, insensible water loss is approximately 50 ml. of water per 100 kcal. per day. Renal water loss varies with the amount of solute that must be excreted and with the concentration at which the solute is excreted, that is, the solute concentration of the urine. If we assume that a normal solute load will vary from 10 to 40 mOsm. of solute per 100 kcal., then 67 ml. of water per 100 kcal. will permit this solute load to be excreted at a urinary solute concentration of 150 to 600 mOsm. per liter. This range of urinary solute concentration can be achieved by any child who does not have severe renal disease. The total maintenance water requirement is the sum of the insensible losses plus renal requirement or 50 ml. + 67 ml. = 117 ml. per kcal. per day. Of this we can assume that 17 ml. will be obtained from water of oxidation. The amount to be given by parenteral administration is therefore 117 ml. − 17 ml. = 100 ml. per 100 kcal. per day.

Maintenance water requirements must be increased when either insensible or renal water losses are greater than normal. Insensible losses may be increased if the child is in a hot environment, has a persistent fever, or has significant hyperventilation. Extra water, usually 25 to 50 ml. per 100 kcal. per day, should be given in these circumstances. Renal water requirement should be increased if the child is undergoing an osmotic diuresis, as in the diabetic with hyperglycemia, or if he is unable to concentrate urine normally. The child with a fixed urine osmolality caused by renal disease and the child with nephrogenic diabetes insipidus are representative examples. In these patients the renal water allotment must be increased from 50 to 250 per cent, and this can be done properly only by monitoring the serum sodium concentration and the weight of the patient. If the level of serum sodium decreases and the body weight increases, less water should be given; if the sodium concentration increases and body weight decreases, more water is needed.

Insensible losses may be decreased if the patient is in a cool environment, is hypothermic, or is breathing air saturated or supersaturated with water vapor. In these instances, less water should be given to meet insensible needs. This is particularly important if the patient cannot excrete dilute urine owing to renal disease or to the presence of appreciable concentrations of circulating antidiuretic hormone (ADH).

Less water is needed to meet renal water requirement if the patient can produce only a concentrated urine (caused by high blood levels of antidiuretic hormone) or if the patient is oliguric. Stress, shock, and recovery from surgery often produce high blood levels of ADH, and since these patients cannot excrete excess water they often cannot tolerate a total water intake of more than 60 to 75 ml. per 100 kcal. per day. Overhydration and hyponatremia do occur in these circumstances, and the patients should be weighed daily and have frequent determinations of their serum sodium concentrations. The anuric patient needs no water except that necessary to replace insensible loss. Thus his water intake is 50 ml. − 17 ml. = 33 ml. per 100 kcal. per day. Even this amount is frequently excessive, and a total water requirement of 20 ml. per 100 kcal. per day is usually more appropriate. Overhydration is a real danger, and the anuric child should be weighed daily. Ideally, his weight should decrease about 0.5 per cent per day if overhydration is to be avoided.

Children require maintenance electrolyte therapy to replace the normal urinary, fecal, and skin losses of sodium, potassium, and chloride. These requirements can also be calculated on the basis of caloric expenditure. As average figures, one can assume that the child needs 3 mEq. of sodium, 2 mEq. of chloride, and 2 mEq. of potassium per 100 kcal. per day to meet his electrolyte maintenance requirements. These are generous figures and usually do not need to be varied when maintenance is varied. This quantity of sodium should not be given to patients with heart failure or liver disease or when a low sodium intake is needed. Potassium is omitted if the child is oliguric, in shock, or suspected of having adrenal insufficiency.

Glucose also must be provided to prevent acidosis and ketosis and to spare the body protein. Not less than 5 grams of glucose per 100 kcal. per day should be given. If less than 100 ml. of water is ordered per 100 kcal. per day, the glucose concentration in the infusate must be increased to more than 5 per cent.

To summarize maintenance therapy, the usual patient needs 100 ml. of water, 3 mEq. of sodium, 2 mEq. of chloride, 2 mEq. of potassium, and 5 grams of carbohydrate per 100 kcal. of energy expenditure per day. In addition to the exceptions previously noted, 60 to 80 per cent of the usual maintenance therapy should be given to premature infants and to full-term newborns during the first few days of life. The glucose concentration in these solutions should usually be greater than 5 grams per 100 ml. of infusate.

Deficit Therapy

Many children have suffered loss of body fluids as a result of pre-existing illnesses at the time parenteral therapy is initiated. Deficits of both water and the electrolyte contained in that water exist. If, in the course of illness, the amount of electrolyte lost with water is proportionate to the concentration of that electrolyte in body fluids, no change in body fluid tonicity results and the child has an isotonic dehydration. If proportionately more water than electrolyte is lost, the concentration of serum sodium and the serum osmolality are increased, producing a hypertonic dehydration. If electrolyte losses are proportionately greater, the serum sodium level and the serum osmolality are less than normal, resulting in a hypotonic dehydration. Experience has shown that of 100 children with dehydration, about 80 will have normal serum tonicity.

Isotonic Dehydration. When body fluids are lost, a portion of that loss originates in the extracellular compartment (approximately 60 per cent); the remainder represents a loss of intracellular fluid (40 per cent). By definition, the loss of 1 liter of extracellular fluid (ECF) (in the patient with isotonic dehydration) includes 140 mEq. of sodium and 100 mEq. of chloride, whereas approximately 150 mEq. of potassium is lost in association with the loss of 1 liter of intracellular fluid (ICF). Deficit therapy consists, simply, of returning to the patient the amount of ECF and ICF that one estimates has been lost. If the estimate were that a child has lost 1 liter of ECF and 500 ml. of ICF, therapy would consist of 1000 ml. of 5 per cent glucose in water containing 140 mEq. of sodium and 100 mEq. of chloride plus 500 ml. of 5 per cent glucose in water containing 75 mEq. of potassium.

There are no laboratory tests that can aid the physician in his attempt to estimate the magnitude of the body fluid deficit. Only the patient's history and the results of physical examination are useful. Certain physical findings correlate in a general way with the degree of fluid deficit. A mild deficit of body fluid represents the loss of 20 to 40 ml. of fluid per kilogram of body weight, or a quantity of fluid equal to 2 to 4 per cent of the body weight. Such a deficit may be characterized by thirst and dry mucous membranes but by little else. A child with a moderate deficit (5 to 7 per cent) has, in addition to the findings previously noted, obvious loss of fluid from around the eyes and, occasionally, minimal changes in tissue turgor. The skin may "tent" owing to loss of elasticity. A depressed fontanelle will be noted in infants. A severe deficit (8 to 12 per cent) presents with obvious changes in skin turgor, depression of the fontanelle, tachycardia, and oliguria. As the deficit approaches 120 ml. per kg. (12 per cent), marked oliguria and evidence of shock will be noted.

Under most circumstances, we assume that about 60 per cent of the body fluid deficit represents loss of extracellular fluid and 40 per cent loss of intracellular fluid. If the illness has been of brief duration (less than 48 hours), we assume that proportionally less intracellular fluid has been lost and that the total fluid loss is somewhat less than might be estimated from the physical findings. If, however, the illness is protracted (more than 7 days), we assume a proportionately greater loss of intracellular fluid and recognize that, based on the physical examination, we may underestimate the magnitude of dehydration. In every instance we estimate the deficit as best we can and return that fluid to the patient, along with his maintenance fluid requirement.

Three examples may clarify the manner in which this is done.

EXAMPLE 1. A 10 kg. infant, ill 3 days, has the physical findings associated with severe (10 per cent) dehydration. The assumptions are that (1) normal maintenance therapy for a child with a caloric expenditure of 1000 kcal. is needed, (2) the child's total body fluid deficit of 1000 ml. (10 kg. × 10 per cent) represents the loss of 600 ml. of ECF (60 per cent of 1000 ml.) and 400 ml. of ICF (40 per cent of 1000 ml.), and (3) the 600 ml. of ECF should contain 600 ÷ 1000 × 140 = 84 mEq. of sodium and 600 ÷ 1000 × 100 = 60 mEq. of chloride, whereas the 400 ml. of ICF should contain 400 ÷ 1000 × 150 = 60 mEq. of potassium. The requirements are shown in Table 1. The child needs 2000 ml. of 5 per cent glucose, to which 80 mEq. of potassium chloride and 114 mEq. of sodium lactate or sodium bicarbonate have been added.

EXAMPLE 2. A 20 kg. child, ill 2 days, has the physical findings of mild dehydration. We assume that (1) maintenance therapy should be based on a caloric expenditure of 1500 kcal. per day, (2) total-body fluid deficits are 600 ml. (20 kg. × 3 per cent), of which approximately 400 ml. represents the loss of ECF and 200 ml. the loss of ICF, and (3) electrolyte losses are proportionate. The requirements are shown in Table 2. Since our assumptions involve errors of greater than 5 per cent, we would probably give this child 2000 ml. of 5 per cent glucose, to which 70 mEq. of potassium chloride and 100 mEq. of sodium lactate had been added.

TABLE 1. **Deficit Therapy Requirements for 10 Kg. Infant with Severe Isotonic Dehydration**

	WATER (ML.)	ELECTROLYTE, MEQ.		
		Na	*K*	*Cl*
Maintenance	1000	30	20	20
ECF deficit	600	84		60
ICF deficit	400		60	
Total	2000	114	80	80

TABLE 2. **Deficit Therapy Requirements for 20 Kg. Child with Mild Isotonic Dehydration**

	WATER (ML.)	ELECTROLYTE, MEQ.		
		Na	*K*	*Cl*
Maintenance	1500	45	30	30
ECF deficit	400	56		40
ICF deficit	200		30	
Total	2100	101	60	70

EXAMPLE 3. A 10 kg. child has been ill 18 hours. He has dry mucous membranes, sunken eyes, and minimal changes in tissue turgor. We assume that (1) the maintenance requirements are normal, (2) since the child has suffered rapid dehydration, the total deficit is only 5 per cent, or less than indicated by examination, and (3) of the fluid lost (500 ml.), more than 60 per cent, perhaps 80 per cent (400 ml.), was extracellular and only 20 per cent (100 ml.) was intracellular. The requirements are shown in Table 3. We would give 1500 ml. of 5 per cent glucose in water, to which 35 mEq. of potassium chloride, 25 mEq. of sodium chloride, and 60 mEq. of sodium lactate had been added.

Hypertonic Dehydration. Hypernatremia (a serum sodium concentration greater than 155 mEq. per liter) is an important complication of dehydration, not only because it is associated with a significant increase in mortality rate, but also because many children who survive an episode of hypernatremic dehydration are left with permanent damage to their central nervous system. Hypernatremia may be produced by the excessive administration of sodium either orally or parenterally to children with diarrheal dehydration and, as such, is frequently the result of mismanagement of a relatively benign illness. Therapy must be designed to lower the serum sodium concentration slowly to prevent the occurrence of cerebral edema. To do this, the usual requirement for maintenance therapy is determined. The deficit is

TABLE 3. **Deficit Therapy Requirements for 10 Kg. Child with Rapid Isotonic Dehydration**

	WATER (ML.)	ELECTROLYTE, MEQ.		
		Na	*K*	*Cl*
Maintenance	1000	30	20	20
ECF deficit	400	56		40
ICF deficit	100		15	
Total	1500	86	35	60

always great, and deficit therapy of 100 ml. per kg. (10 per cent) is usually required, of which one third to one half is given as 5 per cent glucose in water and the remainder is provided by the usual isotonic deficit therapy as previously described. Such therapy will lower the serum sodium concentration by 10 to 12.5 mEq. per day.

EXAMPLE 4. A 10 kg. infant with severe dehydration is seen. The serum sodium concentration is 170 mEq. per liter. The assumptions are that (1) normal maintenance therapy is required, (2) total-body fluid deficit is 1000 ml., of which one third (350 ml.) will be given as 5 per cent glucose in water (this portion of the deficit therapy should not contain electrolyte), and (3) 60 per cent (approximately 400 ml.) of the remaining deficit should be replaced with ECF and 40 per cent (approximately 250 ml.) with ICF. The requirements are shown in Table 4.

Hypotonic Dehydration. Hyponatremia (serum sodium concentration of less than 130 mEq. per liter) is occasionally seen in association with dehydration and is treated by the administration of extra salt. Care must be taken to ensure that the hyponatremic child does not have dilutional hyponatremia and overhydration, in which case extra salt must be given with great care and water restriction may be more appropriate therapy. Treatment of the child with dehydration and hyponatremia consists of maintenance therapy plus the usual deficit therapy plus additional NaCl in an amount sufficient to bring the serum sodium concentration to normal (135 mEq. per liter). Since 0.6 mEq. of sodium per kilogram of body weight will increase the sodium concentration by 1 mEq. per liter, the use of the formula (135 − the observed sodium) × 0.6 × weight in kilograms permits an estimate of the extra NaCl required.

EXAMPLE 5. A 5 kg. infant has a 5 per cent dehydration. The serum sodium concentration is 120 mEq. per liter. The assumptions are that (1) the child needs normal maintenance and deficit therapy, (2) the sodium concentration should be increased 15 mEq. (135 − 120), so 15 × 0.6 × 5 = 45 additional mEq. of NaCl are required, and (3) if the child has convulsions or stupor, this added salt may be given rapidly (15 to 60 minutes) as a hypertonic solution; otherwise it should be added to the parenteral fluids. The requirements are shown in Table 5.

TABLE 4. **Fluid Therapy Requirements for 10 Kg. Infant with Severe Hypertonic Dehydration**

	WATER (ML.)	ELECTROLYTE, MEQ.		
		Na	*K*	*Cl*
Maintenance	1000	30	20	20
Deficit (water only)	350			
ECF deficit	400	56		40
ICF deficit	250		40	
Total	2000	86	60	60

TABLE 5. **Fluid Therapy Requirements for 5 Kg. Infant with Hypotonic Dehydration**

	WATER (ML.)	ELECTROLYTE, MEQ.		
		Na	*K*	*Cl*
Maintenance	500	15	10	10
ECF deficit	150	21		15
ICF deficit	100		15	
Additional NaCl		45		45
Total	750	81	25	70

Shock. Shock caused by dehydration, as may occur with severe diarrhea, is due to the loss of large quantities of extracellular fluid. Similarly, shock caused by burns or crushing injuries or, for example, by retroperitoneal or abdominal surgery is the result of transudation of ECF into the injured tissue. As such, shock should be treated by the rapid infusion of Ringer's lactate solution, 20 to 40 ml. per kg. per hour, until a stable clinical state is obtained. As the injury heals, gradual resorption of the Ringer's solution will occur, leading to a saline diuresis. If plasma or blood is used, hypervolemia and cardiopulmonary overload may result, because these substances cannot be rapidly removed from the vascular system.

Replacement of Abnormal Losses

Maintenance therapy replaces normal water and electrolyte losses. Deficit therapy replaces pre-existing body fluid deficits. An occasional patient will have abnormally large unremitting body fluid losses. These losses may be of upper or lower gastrointestinal fluids, as would occur with continuous gastric or duodenal aspiration or with persistent vomiting or diarrhea. Drainage from a fistula or from a colostomy represents an abnormal loss, as does severe polyuria, persistent sweating, or prolonged hyperventilation. In each instance both the quantity and composition of the fluid must be measured (or estimated) and replaced (volume for volume) by a parenteral solution that has a comparable electrolyte composition. Commercial solutions with the electrolyte composition of "average" upper and lower gastrointestinal secretions are available and should be used for replacement. Large sweat losses can be replaced with additional maintenance fluids, whereas respiratory losses should be replaced by the use of 5 per cent glucose in water. If persistent polyuria occurs, the electrolyte composition of the urine should be determined, and the appropriate replacement therapy can then be determined.

Fluids designed to replace abnormal losses must be given in addition to the usual maintenance therapy and, should a deficit exist, to deficit therapy as well. When replacement fluids are added to a running intravenous infusion, the flow rate must be increased so that all necessary fluids are given in 24 hours.

EXAMPLE 6. A 10 kg. infant receiving gastric suction has evidence of a 5 per cent dehydration. During the past 12 hours, 500 ml. of gastric juice has been removed. The assumptions are that (1) the child needs normal maintenance and deficit therapy, and (2) during the next 24 hours he will need an additional 1000 ml. of fluid that has the electrolyte composition of gastric juice. These requirements can be seen in Table 6. The patient requires 2500 ml. of 5 per cent glucose in water plus 135 mEq. of NaCl and 65 mEq. of KCl during the subsequent 24 hours.

TABLE 6. **Fluid Therapy Replacement for Abnormal Water and Electrolyte Losses in 10 Kg. Child**

	WATER (ML.)	ELECTROLYTE, MEQ.		
		Na	*K*	*Cl*
Maintenance	1000	30	20	20
ECF deficit	300	42		30
ICF deficit	200		30	
Replacement	1000	63	17	150
Total	2500	135	67	200

The total serum CO_2 content and pH determinations are not required for planning appropriate parenteral fluid therapy. Many patients requiring parenteral fluid therapy will have a metabolic acidosis. However, if glucose is provided and body fluid deficits are corrected, the acidosis will be corrected by homeostatic mechanisms, and "titration" of the serum CO_2 with $NaHCO_3$ or Na lactate is not necessary and, indeed, is potentially dangerous.

It is also true that, except for fluids designed to replace abnormal continuing losses, the use of polyionic electrolyte solutions is not recommended. Rather, the total water and electrolyte requirement of the child should be calculated, and the necessary amounts of Na, K, and Cl which are commercially available as concentrated solutions should be added to the appropriate volume of 5 per cent glucose in water, thereby providing each child with fluid therapy designed specifically for him.

SECTION 7

The Endocrine System

ACROMEGALY

method of
RAYMOND V. RANDALL, M.D.
Rochester, Minnesota

Acromegaly is a condition caused by excessive and inappropriate secretion of growth hormone by a tumor of the anterior pituitary or, in rare instances, by an ectopic growth hormone–producing tumor, particularly carcinoid of the lung. Despite the literature of a number of decades ago, it is not clear whether acromegaly can result from hyperplasia of the eosinophilic cells (growth hormone–producing cells) of the anterior pituitary. Although it was previously thought that untreated acromegaly in some instances would become quiescent, so-called "burned out acromegaly," it is now evident that acromegaly, if not treated, continues to be an active process for many decades and may result in death from cardiovascular-renal complications or, less commonly, from expansion of the growth hormone–producing tumor of the pituitary.

Treatment

The objective of treatment in acromegaly is to remove or destroy the pituitary tumor in its earliest stages, thereby (1) stopping or reversing the changes caused by excessive production of growth hormone, (2) preserving or restoring normal pituitary function, and (3) preventing, stopping, or reversing local damage caused by an expanding, space-occupying tumor.

The various modalities of treatment used in treating the pituitary tumors responsible for acromegaly are shown in Table 1.

Studies Prior to Treatment

Before undertaking treatment of the pituitary tumor the clinician should evaluate (1) the extent of the pituitary tumor, (2) the function of the anterior pituitary gland, and (3) the possibility of coexisting endocrine diseases such as primary hyperparathyroidism, insulin-producing tumor(s) of the islet cells of the pancreas and pheochromocytoma(s).

TABLE 1. **Treatment of Pituitary Tumors Associated with Acromegaly**

- Surgery
  - Transfrontal approach
  - Transsphenoidal approach
    - Conventional surgery
    - Cryosurgery
    - Radiofrequency surgery (thermocoagulation)
    - Direct ultrasonic irradiation
- Combination of transfrontal and transsphenoidal approaches
- Radiation
  - Conventional radiation
    - Orthovoltage (high-voltage) x-rays
    - ^{60}Co
    - Linear accelerator
  - Intrasellar implantation of radioactive isotopes
    - ^{90}Y
    - ^{198}Au
    - Other isotopes
  - Heavy particle radiation (cyclotron)
    - Alpha particles
    - Protons
    - Other particles
- Chemotherapy
  - Estrogens
  - Androgens
  - Progesterone
  - Chlorpromazine
  - Somatostatin
  - Bromocriptine
  - Metergoline
- Combination therapy
  - Surgery plus radiation and/or chemotherapy

The various studies which may be used to determine the extent of the pituitary tumor are standard x-ray views of the head; anteroposterior and lateral polytomographic views of the sella, with cuts taken every 2 to 3 mm.; plotting the visual fields; computerized tomography (CT) scan of the head with contrast medium, paying particular attention to the suprasellar and parasellar areas; bilateral carotid angiography with magnification and subtraction views; cavernous sinograms (used in some institutions to detect lateral extension of the pituitary tumor); and measurement of growth hormone in the cerebrospinal fluid (increased when there is suprasellar extension of the growth hormone–producing pituitary tumor). Function of the anterior pituitary is determined by measuring the function of the end-organ endocrine glands—namely, the thyroid, adrenals, and gonads—by measuring the blood values for thyroxine, corticosteroids (cortisol), testosterone, or estrogens, and urinary excretion of 17-ketosteroids and 17-hydroxycorticosteroids (or 17-ketogenic steroids), and by measuring pituitary gonadotropins. Serum prolactin should be measured, because approximately 30 to 50 per cent of growth hormone–producing tumors also produce excessive amounts of prolactin. Under such circumstances, measurement of prolactin, as well as growth hormone, can be used in the post-treatment period to evaluate the effectiveness of treatment.

The possible presence of hyperparathyroidism, pheochromocytoma, and insulin-producing islet cell tumor(s) of the pancreas is determined by the usual tests for these conditions.

Surgical Treatment

Currently we feel that surgical removal of the pituitary tumor is the treatment of choice for hormonally active acromegaly. When successful, this will stop excessive production of growth hormone and also remove the threat of an expanding, space-occupying tumor. Transfrontal approach to the pituitary tumor has long been the time-honored surgical method of treating such tumors, but in the past several years the transsphenoidal approach has become more widely used and, in our opinion, is the method of choice. We do not hesitate to advise this approach even though there may be significant field defects secondary to impingement of the pituitary tumor upon the optic apparatus. When there is significant suprasellar extension of the tumor or lateral extension into one or both cavernous sinuses, we then use a combination of transfrontal plus transsphenoidal surgery.

Transsphenoidal cryosurgery and radiofrequency thermocoagulation surgery were popular a few years ago, but have not proved to be as effective as conventional surgery by the transsphenoidal approach.

Ultrasonic destruction of the pituitary tumor by the transsphenoidal route, although popular in some European countries, has not been widely used in this country, and, in our opinion, has not proved to be as effective as conventional transsphenoidal surgery.

Radiation Therapy

Radiation therapy is available in the United States in the form of conventional high voltage (orthovoltage) x-ray therapy, cobalt-60 and linear accelerator, and the intrasellar implantation of radioactive isotopes, usually radioactive yttrium (^{90}Y) or radioactive gold (^{198}Au), as well as heavy particle radiation using the cyclotron.

We have used radiation therapy as the only means of treatment rather extensively in the past, but it became evident to us as to others, once measurement of growth hormone became available, that in many instances conventional radiation therapy with high voltage x-rays or cobalt-60 was not effective in stopping either excessive production of growth hormone or growth of the pituitary tumor. The intrasellar implantation of radioactive isotopes enjoyed widespread use a few years ago; but this, too, has proved unsuccessful in many instances, and may result in cerebrospinal rhinorrhea or optic nerve or extraocular motor nerve defects more frequently than does conventional transsphenoidal surgery. At this time it is safe to predict that the intrasellar implantation of radioactive isotopes will continue to become less widely used unless more satisfactory techniques for implanting isotopes are developed.

We feel that in selected cases the most effective form of radiation therapy is by heavy particle radiation with the cyclotron, using alpha particles or protons. The main drawback of this type of treatment is that it cannot be used when there is suprasellar extension of the tumor because of potential radiation damage to the optic apparatus. The other disadvantages are that the excessive production of growth hormone may not fall to normal for 6 to 12 months or longer following radiation therapy. Also there may ultimately be a loss of some of the hormonal functions of the normal pituitary. Nonetheless, we feel that this is the treatment of choice in selected patients and have referred a number of patients to Dr. Raymond A. Kjellberg and colleagues at Massachusetts General Hospital, Boston, and Dr. John H. Lawrence and colleagues at the Donner Laboratories, University of California, Berkeley.

Chemotherapy

Ideal treatment of acromegaly would consist of a chemotherapeutic agent which would be easy to administer and nontoxic, would inhibit or reverse tumor growth, and would halt the excessive production of growth hormone by the tumor. Numerous forms of chemotherapy have been tried in an attempt to achieve these objectives, but as yet none has been successful.

Large doses of estrogenic substances, for example, diethylstilbestrol in doses of 5 to 25 mg. orally each day, or androgens, such as testosterone enanthate or testosterone cyprionate in doses of 200 mg. intramuscularly two to three times a week, will negate many of the effects of excessive growth hormone, but can neither permanently stop the excessive production of growth hormone nor stop growth of the pituitary tumor. Similar effects have been noted from the use of medroxyprogesterone, 10 mg. orally every 6 hours, or chlorpromazine, 20 to 25 mg. orally three times a day. Interestingly enough, the hypothalamic hormone, somatostatin (growth hormone–inhibiting hormone) will suppress growth hormone production not only by the normal pituitary but also by growth hormone–producing tumors of the pituitary. However, this material must be given intravenously or intramuscularly (as a short-acting protamine zinc preparation), and hence is not suitable for long-term use. (This use of the aforementioned agents is not listed in the manufacturer's official directive.)

At present the most promising agents seems to be bromocriptine (2-Br-alpha-ergocryptine), a dopaminergic agent, and metergoline, an antiserotonin agent, both of which can be given orally and are effective in many cases of acromegaly in reducing the excessive production of growth hormone to normal. It is not clear at this time what effect these agents have on tumor growth; nor have they been approved for clinical use in the United States. However, these compounds and yet-to-be-discovered related compounds hold great promise for the future in the treatment of acromegaly as well as other hyperfunctioning tumors of the pituitary.

Treatment of Choice

Our current approach to treating patients with active acromegaly is to remove the tumor transsphenoidally, and if the levels of serum growth hormone do not return to normal following operation, or if the surgeon does not think he has removed all of the tumor, to give 4500 to 5000 rads of radiation therapy by linear accelerator to the region of the pituitary. Although it is true that some patients will respond favorably to conventional radiation therapy alone, we are currently unable to separate those patients who will respond from those who will not; hence we do not feel that radiation therapy alone is the treatment of choice, except for selected patients to whom cyclotron therapy is given.

The great appeal of transsphenoidal surgery is that when it is successful the excessive production of growth hormone ceases at once, whereas radiation therapy, if successful, will take up to 6 months or longer before the excessive production of growth hormone ceases. This becomes of great importance in patients with early acromegaly in whom there have been only reversible soft tissue changes rather than the nonreversible disfiguring changes secondary to overgrowth of the affected bony parts. This is particularly important to females, in whom permanent disfigurement is often mentally devastating. When and if effective chemotherapy with dopaminergic, antiserotonin, or similar agents becomes available in this country, it would seem appropriate to administer one of these agents to stop excessive production of growth hormone and, at the same time, give a course of radiation therapy with the thought that if radiation therapy is not ultimately successful in controlling the excessive production of growth hormone and growth of the pituitary tumor, then surgical removal of the tumor could be undertaken. Also, such agents could be advantageously employed in those patients in whom a combination of surgery and radiotherapy has failed to halt the acromegalic process.

Associated Endocrine Diseases

Occasionally, acromegaly may be part of the syndrome of multiple endocrine neoplasias (MEN syndrome), also known as multiple endocrine adenomatosis (MEA syndrome) or Wermer's syndrome, type I, and be associated with coexisting primary hyperparathyroidism and/or insulin-producing tumor(s) of the islet cells of the pancreas. Parathyroid surgery to correct the hyperparathyroidism should be undertaken before operating upon the pituitary tumor when the serum calcium is above 11.0 mg. per dl. (100 ml.). Likewise, surgical correction of islet cell tumor(s) of the pancreas should be performed before operating upon the pituitary tumor if the patient is having moderate or severe hypoglycemic symptoms.

At times acromegaly may be accompanied by coexisting pheochromocytoma(s), and this situation should be corrected surgically before the pituitary tumor is operated upon.

Treatment of Pituitary Failure

Pituitary failure—i.e., secondary failure of the thyroid, adrenals, and gonads—should be looked for by appropriate tests prior to treatment of the pituitary tumor. In general, it has been our experience that pituitary failure present prior to surgical removal of the pituitary tumor will continue to be present following removal of the tumor and/or radiation treatment of the tumor. However, there are enough exceptions to this general rule that we prefer to investigate pituitary function thoroughly following surgery before instituting a course of lifelong endocrine replacement therapy. As the patient with pituitary failure is apt to get into difficulty from secondary adrenal insufficiency rather than from thyroid or gonadal failure in the few months following operation, we measure adrenal function in the immediate postoperative period; if there is definite or questionable adrenal failure, we treat the patient with 25 to 30 mg. of hydrocortisone or cortisone in two to three divided doses daily until thorough endocrine evaluation is undertaken approximately 3 months following treatment of the pituitary tumor. At that time adrenal function is reassessed, along with function of the thyroid and gonads. Subsequently, indicated hormonal replacement therapy is given.

Pitfalls in Dealing with Acromegaly

There are several potential problems in dealing with patients who have acromegaly. The most common is to assume that a pituitary tumor does not exist when the standard x-ray views of the head reveal what appears to be a normal sella. Polytomographic anteroposterior and lateral views with cuts taken every 2 to 3 mm. will often reveal minor changes in the sella contours, diagnostic of a pituitary tumor, which cannot be appreciated on standard x-ray views of the head. Even when polytomographic views of the sella seem to be normal, a pituitary tumor can be present; if we find that hormonally active acromegaly is present, we will then do bilateral carotid angiography with magnification and subtraction views, as this procedure may reveal small pituitary tumors not otherwise demonstrated.

In rare instances acromegaly has been associated with an extrapituitary neoplasm producing excessive amounts of growth hormone. Carcinoid of the lung has been the most common such tumor, and should be excluded when a pituitary tumor cannot be demonstrated. At this time it is not clear whether or not eosinophilic hyperplasia of the pituitary can result in excessive production of growth hormone, but such a possibility must be kept in mind.

Another pitfall is failure to appreciate the fact that hormonally active acromegaly can be present even though the values for growth hormone in the blood are within normal limits. The reason for this is not entirely clear, but we assume that the tumor is producing a growth hormone which is not structurally identical to normally occurring growth hormone, although biologically active, and which is not completely detected by the assay for growth hormone which has been designed to detect normal growth hormone. In such instances we have depended upon other clinical and biochemical indices* to establish the diagnosis of hormonally active acromegaly; when these have been present, we have directed treatment to the pituitary tumor and reversed the hormonally active process.

*Randall, R. V.: Acromegaly. *In* Current Diagnosis–5, H. F. Conn and R. B. Conn (eds.). Philadelphia, W. B. Saunders Company, 1977.

ADRENAL INSUFFICIENCY

method of
JAMES C. MELBY, M.D.
Boston, Massachusetts

Adrenocortical insufficiency is either *primary*, caused by bilateral destruction of the adrenal cortex, or *secondary* (Addison's disease). It may also result from ACTH deficiency, which occurs in hypopituitarism and after prolonged suppression of the hypothalamic-pituitary-adrenal axis by exogenous corticosteroid administration for the therapy of nonendocrine disorders. In primary adrenocortical insufficiency all adrenocortical hormonal steroids are lacking, resulting in the manifestations of both cortisol and aldosterone deficiency. In secondary adrenal insufficiency, aldosterone secretion continues adequately, because it is dependent upon the reninangiotensin system for activation, and all manifestations are due solely to cortisol deficiency.

Treatment

Acute Adrenocortical Insufficiency. Serious suspicion of the presence of acute adrenal insufficiency requires that replacement therapy be given immediately. It is often necessary to treat the patient without a confirmed diagnosis. Prompt administration of cortisol (hydrocortisone), or equipotent doses of its synthetic analogue, is the hallmark of therapy in acute adrenal insufficiency regardless of cause. A bolus of 100 mg. of cortisol as a phosphate or succinate ester should be given intravenously, and an infusion of cortisol phosphate or succinate should be continued at a rate that will deliver 15 mg. per hour for the first 24 hours, with isotonic saline solution as the vehicle. Concomitant administration of isotonic saline solution with or without dextrose, depending upon the presence of hypoglycemia, is usually necessary in the treatment of addisonian crisis. Restoration of the blood pressure may be apparent within minutes and should be established by 1 hour. Volume replacement should be brisk in the first hour (1 to 2 liters of isotonic saline) and judicious after restoration of blood pressure. Volume replacement must *not* be accomplished by the administration of nonobligated water (e.g., dextrose in water) or solutions containing potassium. In the early stages of therapy, provocation of water intoxication by the administration of nonobligated water can occur and lead to a fatal outcome. Synthetic mineralocorticoid administration should not be begun until the patient has recovered from the acute phase of his illness.

In acute secondary adrenocortical insufficiency, treatment with cortisol is identical to that in acute primary adrenocortical insufficiency. Replacement of volume is much less critical in this form of adrenal insufficiency. Isotonic saline solution or dextrose in saline for fluid replacement may be given only with the same prohibition of administration of nonobligated water.

Chronic Adrenocortical Insufficiency. Chronic primary adrenocortical insufficiency (Addison's disease) usually requires replacement with cortisol (hydrocortisone), between 10 and 30 mg. by mouth daily, in doses adequate to abolish postural hypotension, which is the best single index of therapeutic adequacy. Aldosterone replacement may be in the form of 9α-fluorocortisol (fludrocortisone) doses from as low as 50 micrograms every other day to as high as 100 micrograms daily. Addisonians are frequently overtreated with synthetic mineralocorticoids, resulting in edema and hypertension. Female patients may require no mineralocorticoid replacement, except during heat stress in the summer months. Treatment of chronic secondary adrenocortical insufficiency is, almost by definition, limited to patients with hypopituitarism, as patients recovering from hypothalamic-pituitary-adrenal suppression following withdrawal of corticosteroid therapy cannot do so if placed on chronic replacement therapy. Cortisol (hydrocortisone), in doses of 10 to 20 mg. a day, usually suffices. Mineralocorticoid replacement should not be given. In patients who require divided doses of cortisol through the day, it is important to give the majority of the dose in the morning and smaller doses in the mid- or late afternoon. Nocturnal administration of cortisol may lead to insomnia and enhances the possibility of the signs and symptoms of hypercortisonism (iatrogenic Cushing's syndrome).

CUSHING'S SYNDROME

method of
DOROTHY KRIEGER, M.D.
New York, New York

Cushing's syndrome refers to the clinical condition characterized by manifestations of adrenocortical hyperfunction. Such manifestations may be secondary to an excessive production of glucocorticoids alone, or may be associated with an increase in adrenal androgen secretion, or, occasionally in males, with signs of feminization. The cause of such adrenal hyperfunction may reside within the adrenal gland (e.g., adrenal adenoma or carcinoma) with autonomous production of cortisol and suppression of pituitary synthesis and release of ACTH; within the pituitary gland (e.g., basophil or chromophobe adenoma) or the hypothalamus (in both of these instances, associated with increased pituitary ACTH secretion and adrenocortical hyperplasia); or in ectopic tumor production of ACTH (with suppression of pituitary ACTH and stimulation of the adrenal by tumor ACTH). Appropriate therapy can be instituted only after laboratory and roentgen diagnosis have determined the cause of the adrenocortical hyperfunction. Therapy for hyperfunction of all causes is designed to normalize corticosteroid levels.

Adrenal Adenoma

Localization of an adrenal adenoma prior to surgical intervention may be accomplished either by adrenal venography or by iodocholesterol scanning. Ultrasonography and computerized axial tomography may also demonstrate such tumors, although sufficient information is not yet available to determine whether these can replace the aforementioned procedures and what their relative discrimination is with regard to size. Venography may demonstrate tumors as small as 0.5 to 1.0 cm., whereas the smallest tumor localized by scanning was 3.0 cm. It should be noted that thus far there is no diagnostic hallmark that can differentiate conclusively between an adrenal carcinoma and adenoma on venography, although the adrenal carcinomas are usually larger tumors. Lack of uptake of iodocholesterol by adrenal carcinomas has been reported in contrast to the localized uptake seen with adrenal adenomas. Surgical removal of the adenoma is curative. It should be remembered that the contralateral adrenal gland in these patients is atrophic and that adequate corticosteroid supportive therapy is required during operation and in the postoperative state. Patients should receive 100 mg. of hydrocortisone acetate intramuscularly preoperatively and 100 mg. intravenously over each 8 hour period on the day of surgery. This dose is usually tapered, patients receiving 200 mg. of hydrocortisone acetate on the first postoperative day and 100 mg. on the second postoperative day, with further gradual reduction to maintenance levels—usually 37.5 mg. of cortisone acetate daily administered in divided doses of 25 mg. in the morning and 12.5 mg. in the late afternoon. It should be realized that recovery of the function of the contralateral adrenal and of the CNS-pituitary-adrenal axis may take many months. After the patient has been stabilized postoperatively, treatment may be reduced to the 25 mg. morning dose, gradually progressing to alternating this with a 12.5 mg. morning dose and, finally, to a dose of 12.5 mg. on alternate days. At this point adrenal responsiveness to ACTH may be determined. If this is present, further testing may be performed (i.e., pituitary responsiveness either to metyrapone or to vasopressin, as well as to insulin-induced hypoglycemia) to determine adequate function of the CNS-pituitary-adrenal axis, so as to evaluate the patient's ability to respond to stressful situations. When such tests indicate normal responsiveness, all corticosteroid therapy can be withdrawn.

Adrenal Carcinoma

Surgery is the treatment of choice in nonmetastatic disease. If there is evidence of metastatic disease, medical therapy alone is indicated. Such metastases are frequently local, involving adjacent structures such as the kidney, retroperitoneal space, and regional lymph nodes. Distant metastases are most frequent to lung and liver; metastasis to bone or brain is unusual. There is no clear evidence that x-ray therapy is effective in the treatment of an inoperable adrenal carcinoma.

Ortho-para'DDD. The most effective medical therapy appears to be ortho-para'DDD (mitotane [Lysodren]). This interferes with adrenal steroidogenesis, as well as having a direct adrenocortical-cytotoxic effect. Treatment is usually started with 1 to 6 grams per day administered in divided doses. Side effects consist of nausea, vomiting, weakness, and central nervous system symptoms, primarily vertigo, blurred vision, and decreased auditory acuity. With gradual increase in dosage, most of these adverse reactions can be minimized. The maintenance dose may vary from 5 to 20 grams daily. Decreased steroid excretion may occur as soon as 2 to 3 weeks after initiation of therapy, and objective evidence of tumor regression may be seen within 4 weeks. Patients should be followed with determination of either urinary free cortisol or plasma cortisol concentrations; the drug affects the extra-adrenal metabolism of cortisol, so that urinary 17-OHCS measurements are not of value in following such therapy. Available reports indicate both palliation and prolongation of survival.

Aminoglutethimide (Elipten, Cytadrene). This is currently available only for investigational purposes. It inhibits steroidogenesis by blocking the conversion of cholesterol to pregnenolone; it is not cytotoxic. Since the function of adrenal carcinoma is autonomous, there is no resulting compensatory increase of steroidogenesis secondary to any increase in ACTH concentrations that might be induced by the fall in corticosteroids resulting from treatment. It would therefore be expected that such a decrease in corticosteroid secretion would be maintained. The dose employed varies from 1 to 2 grams daily, usually administered in four divided doses. Potential side effects are skin rash, goiter, and sedation. Since this drug also interferes with extraglandular metabolism of corticosteroids, therapy should be monitored by following either urinary cortisol or plasma cortisol concentrations.

Metyrapone (Metopirone). This is another type of drug which acts by suppressing adrenal steroidogenesis, mainly by inhibiting 11-β-hydroxylase and thereby blocking conversion of 11-deoxycortisol to cortisol. Additionally, it also blocks synthesis of cholesterol to pregnenolone. Its efficacy in the treatment of adrenal carcinoma is based on the same considerations as noted for aminoglutethimide. In addition to its side effects of gastrointestinal irritation, both hypertension and hypokalemia may be seen as a result of the increased levels of deoxycorticosterone, which occur as a consequence of 11-β-hydroxylase block. It has no cytotoxic effect on the adrenal. Because of these considerations, it is considered less efficacious than either of the two foregoing modes of therapy.

Surgery. Should there be no evidence of metastatic spread, surgical excision of an adrenal carcinoma is obviously the treatment of choice. Should blood vessel invasion be demonstrated at the time of exploration, medical treatment with Lysodren may be instituted. Since the contralateral adrenal gland may be suppressed, patients should also be maintained on 0.75 to 1.0 mg. dexamethasone daily, and effectiveness of therapy monitored by following urinary free cortisol concentrations. Lower doses of Lysodren may be used than those suggested for metastatic adrenal carcinoma.

Pituitary Tumors

It has been estimated that there is evidence of sellar enlargement, utilizing conventional roentgen techniques, in 10 per cent of patients with Cushing's disease at the time of their initial presentation. The incidence of microadenomas of the pituitary in such patients is not known, although it has been reported that at postmortem approximately 65 per cent of patients with Cushing's disease have pituitary tumors, size unspecified. A recent report, however, describes a more frequent occurrence of ACTH cell hyperplasia rather than adenomas in patients presenting without evidence of sellar enlargement. The microadenomas that have been reported have not necessarily been visualized on polytomography of the sella turcica. There are insufficient data on the results of such microadenectomy, although several cases of cure have been reported without apparent disruption of the function of remaining pituitary tissue. Prolonged follow-up studies are not yet available. With regard to grossly visible pituitary tumors at the time of presentation, remissions have been reported following conventional (cobalt, 4500 R) radiotherapy. How many of the responses to such therapy in Cushing's disease (see below) treated by such a modality represent the response of microadenomatous tissue to such irradiation is unknown.

Ectopic ACTH Syndrome

The most frequent cause of the ectopic ACTH syndrome is a bronchogenic carcinoma, which is usually metastatic at the time of diagnosis, or a pancreatic carcinoma, to which similar considerations apply. Occasionally, the syndrome may be seen with benign tumors, such as bronchial carcinoid tumors or other localized tumors, in which case excision is the treatment of choice. Should excision not be feasible, radiation or chemotherapy of the tumor and its metastases and treatment of the hypercortisolism in addition may improve the patient's condition and remove those symptoms and signs that are secondary to the hypercortisolemia, such as myopathy, psychic effects, evidence of increased catabolism, increased capillary fragility, and hypokalemia. Although not approved by the Food and Drug Administration for this use, either Lysodren or Cytadrene may be employed for this purpose, as discussed under Adrenal Carcinoma. Those pancreatic tumors that are carcinoid in nature may respond to streptozotocin therapy.

Cushing's Disease (Bilateral Adrenocortical Hyperplasia)

The cause of Cushing's disease is at present unknown. It has been suggested that the primary defect is localized to the pituitary gland or, alternatively, to the hypothalamic regulation of ACTH secretion and release. Therapy therefore is directed at eliminating the hypercortisolism present in these patients. The nature of the therapy is in part dependent upon the severity of the disease and the rapidity with which control is indicated. In those patients with severe disease as characterized by markedly elevated blood pressure levels, psychosis, or rapidly progressive osteoporosis, surgical removal of the adrenal glands or, less frequently, of the pituitary may be necessary. Although these therapies are sometimes considered for the mild to moderate forms of the disease (see below), the therapeutic modalities available for these patients are those of some form of pituitary irradiation (other means of pituitary destruction have not been used frequently enough as to evaluate their efficacy), bilateral adrenalectomy, or medical treatment—the last of these designed to remove the abnormal central nervous system drive that has been postulated to be present in some of these patients.

Pituitary irradiation utilizing 4500 R cobalt^{60} is associated with total or almost complete remission in approximately 60 per cent of these patients. An even higher remission rate has been reported in young children with Cushing's disease with no apparent adverse effect on any other modalities of pituitary function. Such remission may not be apparent until 6 to 18 months following completion of pituitary irradiation. It has been suggested that in this interval therapy with agents such as Lysodren or cyproheptadine (see below) might be instituted until the effect of irradiation may be visible. Such a remission consists of reversal of the clinical symptoms of disease and normalization or marked lowering (if not completely to the normal range) of the previously enhanced adrenal corticosteroid secretion. It does not reverse the abnormalities of circadian variation and dexamethasone suppressibility seen in such patients. A higher cure rate is seen following proton beam radiation, but with the risk of producing other pituitary hormone deficiencies. Such therapy is currently available in only two locations (Boston, Massachusetts, and Berkeley, California).

Bilateral adrenalectomy will remove the source of the enhanced cortisol production in such patients (it should be recognized that in some patients residual or aberrant adrenal tissue may remain and eventually hypertrophy to the point of being associated with normal or even enhanced adrenal corticosteroid production). Subtotal adrenalectomy is not effective. Only patients who understand the hazards of adrenal insufficiency and the necessity for permanent maintenance therapy and regulation of such therapy during periods of stress and infection are suitable candidates for such a procedure. Additionally, approximately 15 per cent of such patients will develop evidence of pituitary enlargement and hyperpigmentation (Nelson's syndrome) at an interval of 1 to as long as 16 years following bilateral adrenalectomy. Such pituitary tumors, when they occur, are more aggressive in local extension and more subject to intratumor bleeding with resultant "pituitary apoplexy" than are chromophobe adenomas. It had been previously thought that prior pituitary irradiation at the time of adrenalectomy would prevent the occurrence of such pituitary tumors. There are ample observations at present to show that this is not the case. Since the reported results of pituitary irradiation appear to be so favorable, many clinicians now believe that adrenalectomy should be reserved for those patients in whom such irradiation has failed; repeat irradiation is contraindicated because of the high total dose of irradiation that would have to be delivered.

As bilateral adrenocortical hyperplasia is pituitary dependent, inhibition of adrenal corticosteroidogenesis with either metyrapone or aminoglutethimide will result in enhanced ACTH secretion and hence eventual escape from the metabolic block produced by these agents. Such escape may be overcome by supplemental dexamethasone therapy, but in actuality such treatment is cumbersome and usually not effective. The long-term use of smaller doses of Lysodren (3 to 6 grams daily in divided doses over a 4 to 6 month period, with smaller maintenance doses being continued for as long as 5 years) has also been reported to effect a cure. Again, remission may not be apparent until 4 to 6 months after initiation of therapy. In some patients adrenal insufficiency has occurred, requiring maintenance corticosteroid therapy.

Another form of medical therapy, which is still investigational, is that of the use of antiserotoninergic agents. Reports of efficacy of both cyproheptadine (Periactin) and metergoline, which is a more specific antiserotoninergic agent, have been reported. Such therapy is based upon experimental evidence of a stimulatory role of serotonin on corticotropin releasing factor (CRF) or ACTH release, as well as upon evidence of altered central nervous system function in patients with Cushing's disease (as manifested by abnormalities in sleep electroencephalograms and periodicity of several pituitary hormones such as prolactin and growth hormones) in both the untreated state and when such patients are in remission following pituitary irradiation. The suggested dose is 24 mg. daily in divided doses, although occasionally 32 mg. daily is required. Side effects are increased appetite and occasional somnolence; both of these usually disappear with continued treatment. Studies to date indicate that cyproheptadine is effective in producing a remission in approximately 60 per cent of patients with Cushing's disease (although it may be less effective in the childhood form of the disease) and also in lowering elevated ACTH levels and decreasing the pigmentation seen in patients with Nelson's syndrome. Continuous medication is necessary, as relapses occur on discontinuance. The existence of a subgroup of patients who do not respond raises the question that there may be at least two types of Cushing's disease—one dependent on abnormal CNS drive, and the other of primary pituitary origin.

DIABETES INSIPIDUS

method of
MALCOLM COX, M.D.
Philadelphia, Pennsylvania

Diabetes insipidus (DI) results from a failure in water conservation by the kidneys and is characterized clinically by polyuria, polydipsia, and a urine that is inappropriately dilute relative to plasma tonicity. The evaluation of the polyuric patient should begin with the characterization of the urinary composition with regard to both its solute and water composition. If solute excretion is high, an obligatory water loss (osmotic diuresis) will occur and a primary defect in renal water conservation need not be invoked. An osmotic diuresis is seen in association with poorly controlled diabetes mellitus, in certain patients with chronic interstitial nephritis, and in the polyuric states associated with relief of the obstructed kidney, the recovery phase of acute tubular necrosis, and the transplanted kidney in the immediate postoperative period. In these situations excessive amounts of glucose, sodium, or urea are excreted in the urine and obligate the excretion of large amounts of water (and electrolytes). In such situations therapy should be directed at the correction of the underlying disease process and replacement of fluid and electrolyte losses.

In a pure water diuresis the urine osmolality is lower than the isotonicity usually seen during an osmotic diuresis, and pathologic amounts of glucose, sodium, or urea are absent from the urine. A water diuresis may be due to excessive water intake, such as occurs in patients with psychogenic polydipsia, or to an abnormality in renal water handling per se. The latter may result either from a deficiency of the antidiuretic hormone arginine vasopressin (AVP) (central DI) or from an inability of the kidney to respond appropriately to AVP (nephrogenic DI).

Central DI may be secondary to either an absolute (complete central DI) or relative (partial central DI) lack of circulating AVP. Defects may exist in one or more of the following: (1) the osmoreceptor mechanism, (2) the supraoptic nuclei of the hypothalamus that are responsible for the synthesis of AVP, (3) the axons of these nuclei that are responsible for transporting AVP to the neurohypophysis, and (4) the storage site of AVP in the neurohypophysis. Elevations in the osmotic threshold for AVP release are extremely uncommon, but when combined (as they frequently are) with a loss in thirst sensation, they can result in profound degrees of dehydration and hypertonicity (so called "essential hypernatremia"). Pathologic destruction or degeneration of the supraoptic neurons results in reduction or absence of the capacity to synthesize AVP, and this is presumed to be the mechanism by which central DI results from tumors (e.g., craniopharyngiomas, pinealomas, gliomas, pituitary adenomas), granulomatous processes (e.g., sarcoidosis), and head trauma. Loss of the neurohypophysis by surgical excision or disease does not cause persistent central DI unless the pituitary stalk is sectioned or destroyed far above the posterior lobe (i.e., unless concomitant degeneration of the supraoptic neurons occurs). An intact pituitary stalk is able to release AVP adequately in response to physiologic stimuli. Although potentially remediable causes of central DI should always be carefully sought, the majority of cases remain idiopathic.

Nephrogenic DI results from partial or complete loss of the antidiuretic action of AVP on the collecting tubule. It is useful to exclude from this category disorders caused by defects in the formation and/or maintenance of a maximally hypertonic medullary interstitium, and to restrict the term nephrogenic DI to those disorders in which the impairment of AVP action is due to specific abnormalities intrinsic to the collecting tubule cell. In the former case medullary hypertonicity can be reduced by (1) inadequate delivery of urea to the kidney (e.g., severe malnutrition) and (2) inadequate tubular or vasa recta transport systems (e.g., in chronic interstitial nephritis of any cause, or in association with the use of diuretics such as furosemide, ethacrynic acid, or the organomercurials, all of which inhibit NaCl transport out of the thick ascending limb of Henle's loop). In these situations urinary concentrating ability is only moderately impaired, and at worst the urine is isotonic rather than hypotonic. Clinically significant defects in the intrinsic cellular response to AVP occur in association with electrolyte disorders (hypercalcemia, potassium depletion), in association with the use of certain drugs (lithium, demeclocycline, methoxyflurane), and in patients with hereditary nephrogenic DI. The inference that end-organ unresponsiveness is responsible for the polyuria in the latter disorder has been confirmed by the demonstration of high circulating levels of AVP.

Central Diabetes Insipidus

Once the diagnosis of central DI has been established and a careful search for potentially remediable causes has been made, therapy can be instituted. The mainstay of the therapy of central DI is the administration of some form of antidiuretic hormone, but several nonhormonal modes of therapy are also available.

1. *Aqueous vasopressin (Pitressin)* is a water-soluble posterior pituitary extract containing a mixture of arginine and lysine vasopressin at a concentration of 20 units per ml. The usual dose is 5 to 10 units administered subcutaneously or intramuscularly, with an onset of action within 30 to 60 minutes and a duration of action of 4 to 6 hours. Intravenous use remains investigational. Although aqueous vasopressin is useful diagnostically and in the treatment of acute central DI, it has little use in the chronic treatment of this disorder.

2. *Vasopressin (Pitressin) tannate* in oil is a mixture of arginine and lysine vasopressin and is a long-acting preparation of the antidiuretic hormone principle. It is supplied in a concentration of 5 units per ml. and can be administered subcutaneously or intramuscularly. The usual dose is 2 to 5 units; antidiuresis begins within 2 to 4 hours, and relief of symptoms continues for 24 to 72 hours. This preparation should never be used intravenously. When the ampule is examined, a brown precipitate will be noted; this is the hormone. Before use the ampule must be vigorously shaken and warmed in order to suspend the hormone in the form of an emulsion. Failure to observe these simple precautions is the most common cause of therapeutic failure.

Complications of Pitressin therapy are uncommon. In order to prevent excessive water retention and dilutional hyponatremia, each dose of Pitressin should be repeated only after symptoms of polyuria begin to recur. Local and systemic allergic reactions are very uncommon; should they occur, they can be treated by desensitization. Since vasopressin is a potent vasoconstrictor, patients suffering from vascular disease, especially coronary artery disease, should be treated with caution. Hypertension and coronary insufficiency are unusual with the recommended doses, however. Pitressin may cause abdominal cramps and nausea resulting from stimulation of intestinal smooth muscle contractility. Women may also experience menstrual-like cramps owing to stimulation of uterine contractility.

3. *Synthetic lysine vasopressin (Diapid)* is more stable in solution than synthetic arginine vasopressin and has about two thirds the antidiuretic potency of the latter. It is available as a nonirritating nasal spray containing 50 units per ml. and is sprayed deeply into the nasal passages, 1 to 2 sprays in each nostril. Its major disadvantage is a short duration of action; it must be administered every 4 to 6 hours. However, it does obviate the need for injections in some patients, may be used as an adjunct to parenteral therapy in others, and may be all that is needed in patients with mild degrees of incomplete central DI. This preparation has completely replaced the use of posterior pituitary powder ("pituitary snuff"), which is irritating to the nasal mucosa and has also been associated with allergic pulmonary complications.

4. *DDAVP (1-desamino-8-d-arginine vasopressin)* is a new synthetic analogue of arginine vasopressin with both increased antidiuretic and substantially decreased pressor activity. Extensive therapeutic trials in Europe and more limited investigational studies in this country have shown its efficacy in the treatment of central DI with minimal side effects. It is available as a nasal spray. Since it has a relatively prolonged antidiuretic action (12 to 24 hours), it can be administered in doses of 10 to 20 micrograms once or twice daily. Once it is approved by the Food and Drug Administration, it is likely to become the hormone preparation of choice in the treatment of central DI.

5. *Nonhormonal therapy* of central DI includes such agents as the thiazide diuretics, chlorpropamide, clofibrate, and carbamazepine. (This use of these agents is not mentioned in the manufacturer's official directive.) The use of one or more of these agents, especially when combined with dietary restriction of protein and sodium (to reduce urinary solute and hence obligatory water excretion), can markedly reduce the degree of polyuria and can therefore be a useful adjunct to hormone-replacement therapy. The thiazide diuretics can be employed in patients with complete or incomplete central DI, whereas the other agents are effective only in patients who have some residual capacity to secrete AVP (incomplete central DI).

The *thiazide* diuretics cause a reduction in polyuria by virtue of their ability to decrease extracellular fluid volume and glomerular filtration rate. This results in an increased resorption of fluid in the proximal convoluted tubule and a resultant decrease in urine volume. Since this effect is dependent on maintaining a state of sodium depletion, an excessive intake of sodium will reduce the effectiveness of thiazide therapy. Potent nonthiazide diuretics (such as furosemide) are also effective, but can lead to severe electrolyte disturbances and should not be used. Conventional doses of hydrochlorothiazide (HydroDIURIL, 50 to 100 mg. daily) or its equivalent are effective, and side effects other than hypokalemia are uncommon. (This use of hydrochlorothiazide is not listed in the manufacturer's official directive.)

Chlorpropamide (Diabinese), an oral hypoglycemic agent of the sulfonylurea class, is capable of reducing the degree of polyuria in one third to one half of the patients with incomplete central DI. The initial dose should be 250 mg. daily; this can then be increased in increments of 250 mg. every 3 to 4 days to a maximum of 750 mg. daily until a satisfactory antidiuretic response is achieved. (This use of chlorpropamide is not listed in the manufacturer's official directive.) The magnitude of the response is dose related, but doses in excess of 500 to 750 mg. daily are associated with a significant incidence of hypoglycemia. This limits the usefulness of chlorpropamide therapy in some patients and is a substantial problem in patients with panhypopituitarism in whom antidiuretic doses of chlorpropamide tend to lower the plasma glucose concentration excessively. Despite these drawbacks, chlorpropamide should be tried in most patients with incomplete central DI; especially when combined with a thiazide diuretic, it may be sufficient to control symptoms. Chlorpropamide acts by potentiating the effect of low circulating levels of AVP on the collecting tubule. It has also been suggested that chlorpropamide may increase the release of AVP from the neurohypophysis. Consequently it is ineffective in complete central DI and nephrogenic DI. Other sulfonylureas are either ineffective or less effective than chlorpropamide and should not be employed.

Clofibrate (Atromid-S) is an oral hypolipemic agent which in conventional doses (1 to 2 grams daily) has an antidiuretic action in patients with incomplete central DI. It is somewhat less potent than chlorpropamide. Since it has a short duration of action (6 to 8 hours), it has to be given four times daily, whereas chlorpropamide can be administered as a single daily dose. (This use of clofibrate is not listed in the manufacturer's official directive.) Clofibrate is also associated with a variety of side effects, including gastrointestinal symptoms, myositis, and abnormalities of liver function. Since its only advantage over chlorpropamide is freedom from hypoglycemic reactions, it should not be used as the initial agent in the treatment of incomplete central DI. Clofibrate appears to act by increasing the release of residual AVP from the neurohypophysis, and it is therefore ineffective in complete central DI and nephrogenic DI. Its action is additive with that of the thiazide diuretics and chlorpropamide. Combination therapy may be useful to avert the side effects of large doses of a single agent.

Carbamazepine (Tegretol) is used as an anticonvulsant and in the treatment of tic douloureux; it is also effective in reducing polyuria in patients with partial central DI. It appears to act in a similar fashion to clofibrate, but since it has few advantages over clofibrate, it is not recommended for the routine therapy of incomplete central DI.

Nephrogenic Diabetes Insipidus

The therapy of reversible forms of nephrogenic DI consists of treatment of the underlying electrolyte disorder or discontinuance of the offending drug. Once a definitive diagnosis of hereditary nephrogenic DI has been made, therapy for this rare disorder can be considered. Since these patients are refractory to the action of AVP, therapy is limited to the thiazide diuretics and dietary solute restriction, as discussed previously.

SIMPLE (NONTOXIC) GOITER

method of
GILBERT H. DANIELS, M.D.
Boston, Massachusetts

There is nothing simple about "simple" goiter. The pathogenesis is unknown. There is no iodine deficiency goiter in the United States, contrary to still widely held opinion. Although TSH (thyroid stimulating hormone, thyrotropin) overstimulation was long thought to produce these goiters, the overwhelming majority of patients with nontoxic goiters have normal TSH concentrations.

The presence of thyroid gland enlargement, clinical euthyroidism, and a normal serum thyroxine concentration are generally accepted criteria for simple goiter. However, these criteria are too broad and must be refined to optimize therapy. The presence of an elevated TSH concentration with a diffusely enlarged gland suggests Hashimoto's thyroiditis rather than simple goiter, even in the absence of antithyroid antibodies. A markedly elevated TSH concentration with a nodular goiter suggests the possibility of a biosynthetic defect in thyroid hormone production. In these situations, the TSH elevation probably represents subclinical hypothyroidism, despite the normal thyroxine concentration, and mandates replacement therapy with thyroid hormone. In predisposed persons iodine *excess* or lithium therapy can produce "euthyroid simple goiter" with elevated TSH concentration, and will respond to removal of the offending agent or thyroid hormone therapy.

Hyperthyroidism may develop in persons with nodular nontoxic goiters despite normal thyroxine and free thyroxine concentrations. Early hyperthyroidism in this setting may be mediated by T_3 (triiodothyronine), so called T_3-toxicosis, diagnosed by measuring the total T_3 (not the T_3 resin) concentration. This disorder may be quite subtle, particularly in elderly persons.

A trial of suppressive therapy is often indicated in nodular goiters (see below). However, autonomous foci may develop in such glands, leading to nonsuppressibility. When thyroid hormone is administered in this situation, hyperthyroidism may result. For elderly patients, in whom suppressive therapy is potentially hazardous, the use of TRH (thyrotropin releasing hormone) may be helpful. The inability of a bolus of TRH (200 to 500 micrograms intravenously) to produce a rise in the serum TSH concentration of an untreated patient indicates a nonsuppressible gland and contradicts suppressive therapy. Patients with autonomous foci are prone to develop hyperthyroidism if exposed to excess inorganic (e.g., saturated solution of potassium iodide) or organic (e.g., gallbladder or intravenous pyelogram dyes) iodine-containing compounds.

The thyroid scan can help confirm the presence of multiple nodules when only one or none is clinically apparent in an enlarged thyroid gland. The majority of true simple goiters are nodular rather than diffusely enlarged. The presence of multiple nodules generally means that surgery can be avoided, with the exceptions noted below. The therapy of isolated thyroid nodules will not be considered here. Although the thyroid scan may be helpful in establishing the nature of a substernal mass, the movement of such a mass with swallowing (under fluoroscopic observation) confirms that this is a substernal thyroid.

Suppressive Therapy

Although TSH is not present in excess, suppression of pituitary TSH release by thyroid hormone will cause a decrease in goiter size in about 50 per cent of patients. It will prevent further goiter growth in an undetermined number, as well. Suppressive therapy is usually recommended in younger patients without a history of cardiac disease. Levothyroxine is the agent of choice, providing uniform potency, slow onset of action, and normal levels of serum thyroxine in patients appropriately treated. Initial therapy can begin with 0.1 to 0.15 mg. orally per day. If there is no decrease in the goiter size in 6 to 8 weeks, the dosage can be increased by 0.05 mg., provided the patient remains clinically euthyroid. Final dosages exceeding 0.25 mg. per day are rarely required, and the majority of patients are adequately treated with 0.15 to 0.2 mg. per day. The end-point of therapy is goiter reduction or TSH suppression, whichever comes first. TSH suppression can be determined by an undetectable TSH concentration (provided the assay is sensitive to less than 1 microunit per ml.) or failure of TSH to rise in response to TRH injection. If the goiter does not change in size on suppressive therapy and TSH is fully suppressed, therapy may be continued, provided the gland does not contain autonomous foci. Gland autonomy can be excluded by demonstrating a normal serum thyroxine or a suppressed (less than 5 per cent) 24 hour radioactive iodine uptake while on therapy. There is no need to stop therapy, once initiated, unless hyperthyroidism develops.

With suppression therapy, the nodules often do not change, much of the shrinkage occurring in the paranodular tissue. Occasionally new nodules seem to appear with the onset of therapy, a situation often predicted by prior thyroid scanning. The shrinkage of the normal tissue has allowed the nodules to become more apparent. Extremely large nodular goiters rarely shrink significantly, but perhaps further growth can be prevented.

Simple goiter rarely requires therapy other than careful observation or suppressive therapy with levothyroxine. Pharmacologic dosages of iodides should be assiduously avoided for the reasons mentioned above. Indications for surgery are uncommon, but must be appreciated.

Surgical Indications

A relatively high incidence of malignancy accompanies nodular goiters in small children and nodular goiters which appear after x-ray therapy directed toward the tonsils, adenoids, thymus gland, or facial acne, even after a 20 to 30 year time lapse. Similarly, the presence of suspicious local adenopathy, vocal cord paralysis, or other indications of malignancy dictates surgical therapy. If a large dominant cold nodule is present, a needle biopsy can be performed, or surgical excision should be considered. If continuous growth of a goiter or a nodule within a goiter occurs during suppressive therapy, surgery is recommended.

If a goiter represents a cosmetic burden to the patient, it is best removed, the patient's wishes dictating the therapy in this instance. Minor local symptoms of dysphagia or a sense of pressure will often be relieved by suppressive therapy. However, if tracheal compression is marked or if respiratory embarrassment has occurred, surgery is best considered early. Other local symptoms which do not yield to suppressive therapy can be relieved with surgery. A substernal goiter may cause compressive symptoms only when the hands are raised above the head (Pemberton's maneuver); if such symptoms are noted, surgery is indicated.

HYPER- AND HYPOPARATHYROIDISM

method of
FREDERICK R. SINGER, M.D.
Los Angeles, California

Primary Hyperparathyroidism

Primary hyperparathyroidism is second to malignancies as a cause of hypercalcemia. The development of sensitive radioimmunoassays for the measurement of parathyroid hormone has greatly improved the clinician's ability to diagnose this condition. The use of routine screening tests of serum chemistries has altered the clinical presentation of the disease. In the past patients primarily presented with symptoms of hypercalcemia, bone disease, and renal stones. More recently a significant number of patients have been discovered with asymptomatic hypercalcemia. The definitive treatment of the disease remains surgical; but in view of the necessity of at least partially correcting severe hypercalcemia prior to operation, the medical treatment of symptomatic hypercalcemia will be discussed first.

Medical Management of Hyperparathyroidism. DIET. Since excessive gastrointestinal absorption of calcium may contribute to the hypercalcemia, a low calcium diet (restriction of dairy products) is indicated.

HYDRATION AND DIURESIS. Vomiting, anorexia, and polyuria all may contribute to the development of dehydration. The intravenous administration of 0.9 per cent sodium chloride serves two purposes: it corrects dehydration and induces renal calcium diuresis by inhibiting renal tubular reabsorption of calcium. From 4 to 10 liters per day may be required. After rehydration and establishment of vigorous urinary output, furosemide, 40 to 80 mg., or ethacrynic acid, 50 mg., may be administered intermittently to further increase urinary calcium excretion. It is preferable to carry out this therapeutic regimen within an intensive care unit, as careful monitoring of central venous pressure and urinary output and electrolytes are necessary to minimize the possibility of the patient's developing congestive heart failure, hypokalemia, and hypomagnesemia. Full replacement of the potassium and magnesium losses should be accomplished. If adequate diuresis is achieved, serum calcium concentrations near normal usually can be attained within 24 to 72 hours. Other modes of treatment should then be considered, as this regimen is expensive, requires considerable physician time, and is fatiguing to the patient. Contraindications to its use are the presence of congestive heart failure and anuria.

ORAL AND INTRAVENOUS PHOSPHATE. In patients with low or low-normal serum phosphate concentration, phosphate treatment is highly effective in controlling hypercalcemia. Oral treatment should be instituted with 250 mg. of elemental phosphorus administered four times a day. It is important to administer the last dose at bedtime to avoid a prolonged period between doses. The dose may be increased by 500 mg. increments per day if the desired effects are not attained after 2 or 3 days on a given dose. The maximum tolerated dose is usually 3 grams daily. The serum phosphate concentration should be monitored daily to avoid hyperphosphatemia. Diarrhea may occur at higher doses and usually subsides after reducing the dose. Available commercial preparations are listed in Table 1.

Patients who cannot tolerate oral medication may receive intravenous phosphate as either a sodium or potassium salt in a dosage of 1 gram daily. This should be administered over at least a 6 to 8 hour period to avoid hyperphosphatemia. This regimen has proved safe, but if higher doses are administered over shorter periods of time, a patient may develop hypocalcemia and hypotension and expire.

Phosphate may be used for years in patients who refuse surgery or who have had unsuccessful surgery. The serum calcium will be suppressed in most patients, but there is no evidence to indicate that this treatment prevents the continuing deleterious effects of parathyroid hormone on the skeleton.

TABLE 1. **Some Commercial Preparations of Phosphate**

PREPARATION	1 GRAM OF ELEMENTAL PHOSPHORUS IN:
Oral	
pHos-pHaid	8 0.5 gram tablets
Phospho-Soda	1½ teaspoons
Hyper-Phos K	6 tablets
K-Phos	8 tablets
Intravenous	
Potassium phosphate	30 ml., 1.1 M solution

The use of phosphate is contraindicated in the presence of hyperphosphatemia. If renal function is impaired, the starting dose should be reduced. Potassium phosphate can be used in patients who are in congestive heart failure.

MITHRAMYCIN. Mithramycin is a cytotoxic antibiotic which has been used in the management of certain malignancies such as embryonal cell carcinoma of the testes. It is a potent hypocalcemic agent through its inhibitory effect on bone resorption. It is administered intravenously over a 10 minute period or longer in a dose of 25 to 50 micrograms per kg. The hypocalcemic effect is usually observed within hours, but the maximal effect is often noted after several days. This drug has considerable toxicity. Platelet depression leading to hemorrhage is the most dangerous complication. Impaired renal function and transient rises in hepatic enzymes may also develop. Nausea and vomiting are common side effects which may require treatment. It is preferable to use this drug only if other measures fail. Close monitoring of the toxic effects should be carried out. Repeat injections should be kept to a minimum and should not be administered without knowledge of the platelet count and renal function.

ESTROGENS. Primary hyperparathyroidism is most commonly diagnosed in postmenopausal females. If physiologic doses of estrogens are given to such patients, a decrease in serum calcium concentration of up to 1 mg. per 100 ml. may result. Ethinyl estradiol, 50 micrograms daily, or conjugated estrogens, 0.3 to 1.25 mg. daily, for 3 out of every 4 weeks have proved effective doses. The effects on serum calcium concentration may persist more than 1 year on treatment.

CALCITONIN. Calcitonin is a peptide hormone which has been successfully used in the treatment of Paget's disease of bone. It is a natural antagonist of parathyroid hormone and should be an ideal agent in the management of primary hyperparathyroidism. It does acutely lower serum calcium concentration, but this effect is usually not sustained on repeated treatment. Salmon calcitonin is the form available for use, but it has not been approved for this purpose by the Food and Drug Administration. A dose of 50 to 100 MRC units given parenterally will induce a transient hypocalcemic response.

DIALYSIS. In an occasional patient in whom certain drugs are contraindicated or have proved ineffective, peritoneal or hemodialysis utilizing a calcium-free dialysate may be required to temporarily manage hypercalcemia. Such a patient may have associated complications such as chronic renal failure or congestive heart failure.

The aforementioned treatments may also be useful in managing other diseases which result in hypercalcemia. It should be kept in mind that adrenal corticosteroids are quite ineffective in patients with primary hyperparathyroidism but very efficacious in managing the hypercalcemia of sarcoidosis and various malignancies.

Surgical Management of Hyperparathyroidism. The definitive treatment of primary hyperparathyroidism is surgical. In more than 80 per cent of patients this involves the removal of a single parathyroid adenoma. Because approximately 15 per cent of patients have hyperplasia of all four glands and because abnormal glands may be located in unusual sites such as the mediastinum, it is important that the surgery be undertaken by a surgeon experienced in parathyroidectomy. The following principles should be kept in mind:

PREOPERATIVE PREPARATION. Severe hypercalcemia may lead to dehydration, hypokalemia, and hypomagnesemia. These abnormalities should be corrected prior to surgery.

SELECTIVE VENOUS CATHETERIZATION. In patients who have had previous unsuccessful parathyroid surgery or when a nonparathyroid neoplasm is suspected to be secreting parathyroid hormone, blood samples can be obtained from veins draining the parathyroid glands and other sites. Assay of the samples for parathyroid hormone will frequently point to the most likely site of the excessive hormone secretion. This information can greatly aid the surgeon but is probably unnecessary as a routine procedure owing to its expense and the likelihood that an experienced surgeon has an excellent success rate in previously unoperated patients.

SURGICAL STRATEGY. The decision to operate on a patient with primary hyperparathyroidism should be based on the presence of symptoms, the detection of complications, the age of the patient, and the presence of other disorders which might influence the operative risk. The elderly asymptomatic patient can be followed with or without medical treatment and may never require surgical intervention. Younger patients who are asymptomatic may also be followed; but if the serum calcium concentration is consistently above 12 mg. per 100 ml., surgery is probably advisable. The symptomatic patient, at any age, should be strongly considered as a surgical candidate.

Knowledge of the pathology of primary hyperparathyroidism is important in the surgical management. If on initial exploration of one side of the neck an enlarged gland is found, this should be removed and sent to the pathology laboratory for frozen sections to be made. Further exploration should be carried out to find the other gland on that side. The second gland should be biopsied or even removed for pathologic evaluation. If the large gland is consistent with a parathyroid adenoma histologically and the second gland is normal, the exploration can be terminated, because the incidence of multiple adenomas is very small. If both glands are abnormal, the presence of hyperplasia is likely and the opposite side of the neck should be dissected until the other two glands are found. If hyperplasia is present in all the glands, a subtotal parathyroidectomy, including three glands and a fraction of the fourth gland, should be done. An estimated 100 mg. of parathyroid tissue should remain. A metal clip can be placed as a marker to allow future surgery should hypercalcemia recur because of further enlargement of the remaining gland. The presence of hyperplasia should be suspected in any patient with associated endocrine neoplasia or with a family history of endocrine neoplasia. Should no abnormal glands be found in the neck, the surgeon frequently can explore the superior mediastinum through the neck incision and locate a mediastinal tumor. If none is found, the incision should be closed. Mediastinal exploration through a sternal split should be done at a later time. Selective venous catheterization can be done prior to this procedure.

POSTOPERATIVE MANAGEMENT. Serum calcium concentration begins to decrease within hours after successful surgery. In most patients the concentration will return to normal or slightly below normal levels. In patients with significant bone disease as manifested by increased serum alkaline phosphatase concentration and abnormal x-rays, the "hungry bone syndrome" may develop. Hypocalcemia occurs within several days after surgery and may persist for months if untreated. This state can be distinguished from iatrogenic hypoparathyroidism by measurement of the serum parathyroid hormone concentration. Postoperative magnesium deficiency may also cause hypocalcemia and can usually be diagnosed by measurement of the serum magnesium concentration. If magnesium deficiency is ruled out, the treatment should be a high calcium and phosphate intake, 1 to 2 quarts of milk daily, and pharmacologic doses of vitamin D_2 or dihydrotachysterol. The dose of these agents should be adjusted to maintain serum calcium concentration in the low normal range. A dose of 50,000 units of vitamin D_2 or 0.2 mg. or more of dihydrotachysterol daily may be necessary. As the serum alkaline phosphatase concentration falls with healing of the bone, the dose can be reduced.

Secondary Hyperparathyroidism

Secondary hyperparathyroidism develops as a physiologic response to a state of resistance to the effects of parathyroid hormone. Severe hyperplasia of the parathyroid glands develops most commonly in patients with chronic renal failure and hypocalcemia. Other disorders commonly associated with parathyroid hyperplasia are osteomalacia, rickets, and pseudohypoparathyroidism. The key to treatment is to increase the serum calcium concentration with the judicious use of vitamin D or an analogue and calcium supplementation. A prolonged state of normocalcemia will decrease parathyroid hormone secretion and thereby protect the skeleton against the deleterious effects of the hormone. In patients with chronic renal failure particular care must be taken to normalize the serum phosphate concentration to avoid metastatic calcification. This can be achieved by the use of aluminum hydroxide, 2 tablespoons given four times daily. Large doses of vitamin D_2, 50,000 units or more daily, or dihydrotachysterol, 0.2 mg. or more daily, with 1 to 2 grams of elemental calcium (calcium lactate, 7.7 to 15.4 grams, or calcium carbonate, 2.5 to 5 grams) are often required to correct hypocalcemia. Frequent monitoring of blood chemistries is absolutely imperative in these patients. In patients who are resistant to this treatment, symptomatic bone disease or severe pruritus may be an indication for subtotal parathyroidectomy. This may now be successfully accomplished by removing all parathyroid tissue from the neck and autotransplanting 100 mg. of parathyroid tissue in a forearm muscle. If continuing parathyroid hyperplasia occurs, reoperation can be done under local anesthesia.

Hypoparathyroidism

Hypoparathyroidism may arise as a complication of thyroid surgery, as a rare idiopathic disorder associated with other endocrine deficiencies such as Addison's disease and hypothyroidism, and, not uncommonly, as a reversible complication of severe magnesium deficiency. Tetany may be manifested early in the course of hypocalcemia and can be treated with a short infusion of 10 ml. of 10 per cent calcium gluconate. All patients found to be hypocalcemic should have a serum magnesium concentration determined. If magnesium deficiency is suspected because of alcoholism, malabsorption, or long-term parenteral therapy, magnesium sulfate, 4 ml. of a 50 per cent solution, can be administered parenterally while awaiting the result. If hypomagnesemia is found, treatment should be continued for at least 5 days with 12 ml. of 50 per cent magnesium sulfate to obtain a maximal increase in serum calcium concentration. The drug is best tolerated by intravenous infusion over 12 to 24 hours. Vitamin D or calcium supplementation is not necessary.

The management of chronic hypocalcemia caused by iatrogenic or idiopathic hypoparathyroidism is most easily achieved by the use of high doses of vitamin D_2, average dose 50,000 units daily, or dihydrotachysterol, average dose 0.2 mg. daily, and 1 gram of elemental calcium. The calcium may be obtained from a quart of milk daily, but in some patients persistent hyperphosphatemia will force discontinuation of the milk. In these patients calcium carbonate, 2.5 grams, or calcium lactate, 7.7 grams, will provide 1 gram of elemental calcium. The dose of these agents should be adjusted to maintain the serum calcium concentration at no greater than 9 mg. per 100 ml. in order to avoid hypercalciuria. After changing the dose of vitamin D_2, a change in serum calcium concentration will not occur until at least 2 weeks have passed. Careful monitoring of this test is necessary to avoid hypercalcemia. If hypercalcemia does occur, rapid reversal of this complication can be achieved by inducing a diuresis with intravenous isotonic saline solution and by instituting adrenal corticosteroids in high doses (prednisone, 30 mg. daily).

HYPOPITUITARISM

method of
LUIS F. OSPINA, M.D.,
and JOHN M. LEONARD, M.D.
Seattle, Washington

Introduction

Hypopituitarism most commonly results from a pathologic condition (tumor, infarction, surgical ablation, or infiltrative disease) which directly impairs the synthesis and secretion of hormones by the anterior pituitary gland. Less commonly an abnormality in the production, release, or transport of hypothalamic releasing factors is the cause of pituitary insufficiency. Irrespective of the underlying disorder, hypopituitarism may be partial or total (panhypopituitarism). Prior to initiating lifelong therapy, not only must the extent of pituitary insufficiency be completely defined by appropriate testing; the cause must also be established. If the pathologic process impairing pituitary function is progressive in nature, then partial deficiency may be followed in time by the development of total hypopituitarism.

Releasing Factors

Currently releasing factors are useful in diagnostic testing and not as therapeutic agents.

Growth Hormone Deficiency

Since the absence of growth hormone (GH) in adults does not cause significant clinical problems, therapy with GH is unnecessary. However, in children GH deficiency results in impaired linear growth and dwarfism. In most of these patients, treatment with GH will stimulate linear growth. Persons with constitutional short stature or those in whom growth failure is due to resistance to GH action will not benefit from this form of therapy. Similarly, once epiphyseal closure has occurred, treatment with GH is ineffective.

Once the diagnosis of GH deficiency is firmly established and prior to initiating therapy, the rate of growth should be carefully monitored over a period of 6 to 12 months. Generally the growth rate in these patients is less than 0.25 cm. per month before therapy and will increase to 0.65 cm. or more per month during GH administration. Ideally therapy should be begun at an early age, because each year lost represents height that will have to be recovered later. The greatest increase in growth is usually observed in the first 1 to 2 years of treatment. The response in subsequent years may be diminished.

Variable treatment schedules have been employed. We recommend beginning with 2 I.U. of GH intramuscularly three times each week. If the rate of growth is not increased over a 6 month period, the dose may be increased to 4 I.U. three times per week. Therapeutic response is followed by careful height measurement every 2 to 3 months and bone age determined at 6 month intervals. Treatment is continued until a satisfactory height has been achieved or until epiphyseal closure occurs. Since the majority of patients respond to GH, treatment failure may reflect an inhibiting influence by other factors which affect growth. These include unrecognized hypothyroidism, the concomitant administration of excessive amounts of glucocorticoids, and advanced bone age. Although antibodies to exogenous growth hormone commonly develop, only rarely are they neutralizing. Gonadal steroids (testosterone or estrogen) accelerate epiphyseal closure and therefore may diminish the ultimate response to GH. Initiation of replacement therapy with gonadal steroids should be deferred if possible until a satisfactory height has been achieved.

Growth hormone employed in treatment is obtained by extraction and purification methods from human pituitary glands. The supply of GH is limited. It is available at clinical research centers on an investigational basis and, recently, from a commercial source (Asellacrin, Calbio Pharmaceuticals).

Gonadotropin Deficiency in the Male

Persons with the onset of gonadotropin deficiency prior to adulthood will present with incomplete or absent secondary sexual characteristics. Sexual maturation can be induced with either human chorionic gonadotropin (HCG) or a long-acting ester of testosterone. HCG (APL) has a pituitary LH-like effect in stimulating testosterone production by the interstitial cells of the testes. HCG is administered in a dose of 3000 to 4000 U.S.P. units three times per week for 6 to 9 months. During this period progressive sexual development will become evident, and then the dose may be decreased to 2000 units three times per week. Response is followed clinically and by serum testosterone determinations. The necessity for frequent injections and the expense of HCG are limiting factors to be considered in its application for long-term treatment. We prefer inducing and maintaining secondary sexual characteristics with a long-acting ester of testosterone such as testosterone enanthate (Delatestryl) or cypionate (Depo-Testosterone). Therapy with either testosterone or HCG may result in accelerated bone maturation and epiphyseal closure. Hence it is important not to initiate treatment until satisfactory linear growth has been achieved. In many patients this will mean that androgen therapy is not instituted until age 16 to 18. Occasionally peer problems related to sexual immaturity are such that treatment is begun earlier. When treatment is initiated prior to epiphyseal closure, we begin with a relatively low dose of testosterone (75 to 150 mg.) every 2 to 3 weeks. If epiphyseal closure has occurred, a higher dose of testosterone (100 to 200 mg.) every 10 to 14 days may be employed for more rapid induction of secondary sexual characteristics. In adults testosterone, 200 mg. intramuscularly every 2 to 3 weeks, is satisfactory for long-term replacement. The esters of testosterone are free of serious adverse effects. Occasionally fluid retention or acne necessitates a reduction in dosage. Gynecomastia which may be observed early in the course of treatment with either HCG or testosterone usually subsides without any change in the medication schedule. In elderly patients symptoms of bladder neck obstruction secondary to prostatic hypertrophy may develop or exacerbate during treatment with testosterone. For this reason we employ a short-acting ester of testosterone such as testosterone propionate, 25 to 50 mg. intramuscularly three times per week for 4 to 6 weeks. If no problems are encountered during this time, a long-acting ester of testosterone may be administered.

Gonadotropin Deficiency in Females

In the female gonadotropin deficiency prior to adulthood will result in failure of the development of secondary sexual characteristics and amenorrhea. To induce puberty we use a combination type oral contraceptive containing 50 micrograms of ethinyl estradiol. Once full sexual maturation has been reached, in 2 or 3 years, maintenance therapy with a lower estrogen-containing preparation is satisfactory. As with androgen therapy in boys, administration of estrogen before linear growth is satisfactory may result in accelerated epiphyseal closure with a lessening of adult height.

When fertility becomes a goal, estrogen therapy is discontinued. Ovulation may be induced by the sequential administration of human postmenopausal gonadotropin (Pergonal) and HCG. This therapy is not without risk and therefore should be attempted only in centers experienced with its use and where facilities for daily estrogen determinations exist. The general aim is to induce follicular maturation followed by the induction of ovulation. This is accomplished by administering Pergonal, 75 to 150 I.U. intramuscularly daily for 9 to 12 days. Serum estradiol levels are measured daily to monitor follicular maturation; when the level is greater than 500 picograms per ml., ovulation is induced with 10,000 units HCG intramuscularly. As mentioned previously, treatment with human menopausal gonadotropin should be undertaken only by physicians familiar with its use.

ACTH Deficiency

Although ACTH preparations are available, the requirement for parenteral administration largely limits their use to diagnostic testing. For long-term management of secondary adrenal insufficiency, glucocorticoid hormones are used.

Day to Day Management. Patient education concerning the illness and its potential life-threatening nature is the foundation of successful management. Patients should wear an identifying tag* indicating their immediate need for hydrocortisone. The patient and a household member should be instructed in the technique of administering hydrocortisone hemisuccinate (Solu-Cortef), 100 mg. intramuscularly, in case of emergency when medical assistance is delayed. Adults require between 15 and 30 mg. of hydrocortisone (5 to 7.5 mg. of prednisone or prednisolone) per day. This can be administered by giving two thirds of the dose in the morning on awakening and one third in the evening. If signs of excess glucocorticoid effects are noted, the dose should be reduced.

*Medic Alert Foundation International, Turlock, California.

Management of Stress. Patients must be informed regarding the need for an increase in glucocorticoid requirement during periods of stress. For minor illnesses, such as an upper respiratory tract infection, we instruct our patients to double their maintenance dose until the illness has resolved and they have felt well for at least 2 days. The usual dose is then resumed.

Management of Vomiting. When oral intake is not tolerated, the parenteral administration of glucocorticoids is then indicated. The patient should receive hydrocortisone hemisuccinate, 100 mg. intramuscularly, and contact a physician or be taken to an emergency room for subsequent evaluation.

Management of Acute Adrenal Insufficiency. Treatment of acute adrenal insufficiency must be instituted without delay. In addition to correcting the hormone deficiency and volume depletion, the precipitating cause should be identified and treated. Hydrocortisone hemisuccinate, 100 mg. bolus, is given intravenously immediately, and isotonic saline in 5 per cent dextrose is infused rapidly. Until the patient is stable, 100 mg. of hydrocortisone hemisuccinate intravenously is administered every 6 hours. When the precipitating event has resolved, the dose of hydrocortisone may be reduced over a 4 to 5 day period. Temporary overtreatment with glucocorticoids is preferable to premature reduction in dose.

Management of Elective Surgery. In the evening prior to surgery, a long-acting steroid preparation (100 mg. of cortisone acetate) is administered intramuscularly. On the day of surgery 30 minutes prior to induction of anesthesia, 100 mg. of hydrocortisone hemisuccinate is given intravenously. If the surgical procedure continues beyond 4 hours, an additional 100 mg. of hydrocortisone hemisuccinate is administered intravenously. Post-operatively this dose is repeated every 6 hours for the first 24 hours. On subsequent days the amount of hydrocortisone is reduced by 50 per cent each day until maintenance dose is reached. If post-operative complications develop, hydrocortisone hemisuccinate, 100 mg. intravenously every 6 hours, is resumed until the complication is controlled. Oral administration is instituted when the patient is able to tolerate oral feedings.

Thyroid-Stimulating Hormone (TSH) Deficiency

Isolated loss of TSH is uncommon, and deficiency of this hormone usually is associated with impaired secretion of other trophic hormones. Identification of associated ACTH failure is extremely important, because institution of thyroid replacement before glucocorticoid deficiency has been corrected may result in acute adrenal insufficiency. Treatment of hypothyroidism secondary to TSH deficiency is accomplished by the daily administration of sodium levothyroxine (Letter, Synthroid), 0.1 to 0.2 mg. In patients who are markedly hypothyroid or elderly, the initiation of therapy must be cautious. Begin with thyroxine (T_4), 0.025 mg. per day, and increase by 0.025 mg. approximately every 3 to 4 weeks. If symptoms of coronary insufficiency develop at any point, the dose should be reduced and a more gradual increment may be attempted later. Occasional patients are unable to tolerate usual replacement therapy without exacerbation of underlying cardiac disease, and therefore a lower maintenance dose may be employed. Response to therapy is followed clinically. If serum T_4 levels are measured, errors in interpretation owing to alteration in thyroid binding proteins should be avoided. For obvious reasons, TSH determinations, currently the most accurate laboratory method of following the therapeutic response in primary hypothyroidism, are of no value in the management of these patients. Triiodothyronine (Cytomel), with its rapid onset of action and short half-life, is not recommended for long-term maintenance therapy. In addition, laboratory assessment of adequate replacement is difficult when triiodothyronine (T_3) is used. Combinations of T_3 and T_4 are available; but there is no evidence that they provide any significant advantage, and, because of fixed T_3:T_4 ratios, adjustment of dosage may be less easily accomplished than with levothyroxine. Since preparations of desiccated thyroid may vary in biologic potency, they are less satisfactory for long-term replacement therapy. If desiccated thyroid is employed, the usual maintenance dose is 1½ to 3 grains (90 to 180 mg.) per day.

HYPERTHYROIDISM *

method of
SAMUEL Z. BAVLI, M.D.,
and P. REED LARSEN, M.D.
Boston, Massachusetts

Introduction

Hyperthyroidism is the syndrome produced by the presence in the body of excessive quantities of thyroid hormones. The most frequent causes of this syndrome are (1) Graves' disease, (2) toxic multinodular goiter, and (3) toxic adenoma of the thyroid. This article will deal with the treatment of these forms of hyperthyroidism. Hyperthyroidism resulting from subacute thyroiditis, thyrotoxicosis factitia, and rare causes of hyperthyroidism (e.g., ectopic thyroid tissue, thyroid-stimulating hormone [TSH] secreting tumor, hydatidiform mole) will not be discussed; these diagnoses should be eliminated from consideration before treatment is begun.

*Supported by NIH Grant AM 18616.

General Aspects of Treatment

Patient Education. Because weight loss is usually a prominent feature of their illness, many hyperthyroid patients are worried that they may have cancer. The physician's initial responsibility is to allay such fears. The nature of the disease should be discussed and therapeutic goals explained. One point that should be stressed is that although hyperthyroidism is treatable, it may be weeks to months before the disease is completely under control.

Diet. Many people gain weight excessively once their hypermetabolic states are relieved. The physician should warn the patient of this possibility from the start and advise that conscious control of food intake be exercised as the desired weight is approached.

Anorexia in hyperthyroidism often responds to rest and avoidance of stress. Vitamin supplementation, especially the B vitamins, may be indicated for a few weeks.

Bed Rest. Bed rest is a valuable adjunct in the treatment of severely hyperthyroid patients.

Specific Therapy

Thioamide Drugs. The two drugs of this class that are in current use in the United States are propylthiouracil (PTU) (tablets, 50 mg.) and methimazole (MMI, Tapazole) (tablets, 5 and 10 mg.). Both these drugs inhibit the biosynthesis of thyroid hormones by interfering with the organification of iodine and the coupling of iodotyrosines in the thyroid gland; but only the former one blocks extrathyroidal conversion of thyroxine (T_4) to triiodothyronine (T_3). For this reason we prefer PTU to methimazole.

INDICATIONS. Thioamides are used (1) as the principal therapy in Graves' disease in children and young adults, (2) in severely hyperthyroid patients to control the disease in anticipation of definitive treatment with radioactive iodine (see below), or (3) in preparation for surgery (see below).

Untreated Graves' disease is characterized by spontaneous exacerbations and remissions. Therefore the rationale for definitive treatment of Graves' disease with thioamides is to control the disorder until remission occurs. After a 1 to 2 year course of therapy, permanent remission was found in about 50 per cent of patients in the older literature; however, in recent years the remission rate seems to have fallen to under 15 per cent, perhaps because of an increased content of iodine in our diet. Because of the decreased remission rate, many thyroidologists are now dispensing with a trial of thioamide as definitive therapy.

Patients whose thyroid glands are more than three times normal size seem to have a lower remission rate than do other Graves' disease patients.

DOSAGE. Treatment can be initiated with propylthiouracil (PTU), 150 to 250 mg. every 8 hours, or methimazole, 10 to 20 mg. every 8 hours. (The per mg. efficacy of methimazole is generally stated to be 10 times that of PTU, but in the experience of most thyroid specialists this ratio is probably closer to 15:1.) Improvement in symptoms should begin about 2 weeks after starting treatment. Once improvement has begun, it is generally possible to reduce the dose somewhat. When a euthyroid state has been achieved, it can be maintained in most patients with about 100 mg. of PTU every 8 hours or 10 mg. of methimazole every 8 to 12 hours. In some patients a once-daily dosage schedule of PTU or methimazole may be possible.

DURATION OF THERAPY. When a thioamide is given in Graves' disease with the anticipation of a permanent remission, the drug is continued at a maintenance dose for 1 to 2 years. The choice of this duration of thioamide treatment is arbitrary, and recent preliminary evidence suggests that the likelihood of a permanent remission may be almost as good if the antithyroid drug is stopped as soon as the patient has become euthyroid (an average of 4 months of treatment). When relapse occurs after stopping thioamide administration, it generally does so within a few weeks or months. However, relapse can occur many months or years after discontinuing thioamide treatment. When relapse occurs, either the T_3 or the T_4 or both may be elevated.

EVALUATION OF THE PATIENT DURING THIOAMIDE THERAPY. Symptomatic improvement generally begins about 2 weeks after starting thioamide treatment. Thereafter there should be a progressive gain in weight, as well as a decrease in serum T_4 and T_3 concentrations. The heart rate should return to normal. The patient should be seen about once a month until euthyroid, and then every 3 to 4 months. Serum T_4 and T_3 concentrations should be measured at each visit. After the T_4 and T_3 have fallen to normal, the serum TSH concentration should be measured to determine that the dose of thioamide is not excessive.

Decrease in the size of the thyroid may be an indication that remission has occurred. On the other hand, increase in gland size may indicate either exacerbation of the underlying disease or excessive dosage of the drug. The latter cause of thyroid enlargement may be accompanied by signs and symptoms of hypothyroidism and a rising serum TSH concentration.

Failure of hyperthyroidism to respond to thioamide treatment is generally due to either an insufficient dose or incomplete compliance with the drug regimen.

ADVERSE EFFECTS. Adverse effects occur in about 5 per cent of patients taking long-term thioamides. The most common side effects of thioamides are rash and pruritus. The rash may be mild and disappear spontaneously without discontinuing the drug, or it may take the form of massive urticaria. If drug treatment has to be stopped because of allergic reaction, a different thioamide can be used, as cross-sensitivity rarely occurs. The allergic manifestations should be allowed to disappear before beginning the alternative drug, because otherwise allergy to the alternative drug may be masked. Allergy may also take the form of drug fever.

The most serious side effect of thioamide drugs is agranulocytosis. Agranulocytosis seems to be an idiosyncratic reaction and occurs in at most 0.2 per cent of patients. This event usually occurs during the first few months of treatment, although it may occur at any time. Granulocytopenia occasionally may herald the onset of agranulocytosis, but most cases of agranulocytosis occur precipitously. Thus periodic white blood cell counts are of little value in predicting the advent of agranulocytosis. Furthermore, mild to moderate granulocytopenia is often a manifestation of Graves' disease itself.

Patients taking thioamide drugs should be instructed repeatedly to discontinue the drug at the first sign of a sore throat or fever, and then call the physician. The drug can be resumed if the white blood cell count is not significantly below the pretreatment value. Recovery is the rule if the drug is stopped promptly when agranulocytosis occurs and proper treatment is given. The patient should be placed in isolation and appropriate antibiotics given as needed.

Rare complications of thioamide administration include arthralgias, myalgias, thrombocytopenia, hepatitis, cholestasis, neuritis, periarteritis, lymphadenopathy, loss of hair, change in pigmentation of hair, skin pigmentation, headache, enlargement of salivary glands, edema, and toxic psychosis. Nausea, vomiting, and epigastric distress are occasional side effects of thioamides.

Radioactive Iodine. INDICATIONS AND CONTRAINDICATIONS. ^{131}I is a simple and effective treatment that can be used safely for the treatment of Graves' disease, solitary toxic nodule, or toxic multinodular goiter in almost all patients past the childbearing age. Initially there was fear that radioactive iodine treatment might increase the incidence of leukemia or of thyroid neoplasms, but to date (after more than 30 years of use) studies have been unable to substantiate this fear. For this reason some physicians feel that ^{131}I should be used even in children. However, because of the theoretical long-term risk of carcinogenesis and of recessive mutations (which may not become apparent for two or three generations), the more conservative approach is to limit this form of treatment to patients whose procreative years are past.

Patients who have retrosternal goiters with resulting tracheal compression or obstruction of jugular venous return should not be treated with radioactive iodine, because even the small increase in goiter size which may result from radiation thyroiditis could be hazardous.

Patients who are severely hyperthyroid should be pretreated with a thioamide drug before radioactive iodine is given (see below).

Pretreatment with Thioamide. During the 2 days following administration of a therapeutic dose of ^{131}I, there may be a small increase in the serum T_4 and T_3 concentrations. In severely hyperthyroid patients or in patients with heart disease, even a small increase may be dangerous. Therefore it is wise to treat such patients with a thioamide (using a dose such as described previously) until the serum T_4 and T_3 levels fall to normal. Between 3 and 5 days after stopping the drug the 24-hour radioactive iodine uptake should be measured; ^{131}I treatment should be given immediately thereafter.

Dose. Many schemes have been devised for calculating the dose of ^{131}I. For Graves' disease we administer orally that dose which is calculated (on the basis of the 24 hour RAI uptake) to deliver 5 millicuries to the thyroid gland. In the majority of patients a single dose suffices. If the patient is still hyperthyroid after 4 to 6 months, a second dose can be given. For toxic multinodular goiter or solitary toxic nodule, twice as much ^{131}I should be given per dose.

Response. Except for occasional instances of mild sialadenitis or mild radiation thyroiditis, patients should notice no effects of ^{131}I for about 2 weeks. Thyroid function should then decrease gradually for about 2 to 3 months.

Some physicians treat selected patients with a thioamide for 2 to 4 weeks after the administration of ^{131}I. If post-treatment thioamide is to be given, the drug should not be started earlier than 3 to 4 days after ^{131}I administration, because the thioamide would interfere with organification of the radioactive iodine and hence with the effectiveness of ^{131}I treatment. One disadvantage to post-treatment with thioamide is that it obscures the therapeutic effect of radioiodine and thus prolongs the time needed to evaluate the adequacy of the ^{131}I dose. We do not post-treat with thioamide. Alternatively, post-treatment with iodide can be used (see below).

Long-Term Side Effects. During the first year after ^{131}I therapy for Graves' disease, from 20 to 50 per cent of all patients become hypothyroid. Thereafter about 2 to 5 per cent will become hypothyroid each year. By 20 years after ^{131}I treatment, over 90 per cent of patients are hypothyroid. If a lower dose of ^{131}I is given, the incidence of hypothyroidism during the first year can be reduced to about 10 per cent, but a larger fraction of patients remain hyperthyroid than with the higher dose. Furthermore, the prevalence of hypothyroidism after low dose ^{131}I eventually seems to approach that which occurs after the higher dose. In part, the occurrence of late hypothyroidism may be a feature of Graves' disease per se.

Before radioactive iodine treatment is given, the patient must be told that hypothyroidism will probably develop eventually. The doctor should explain the symptoms of hypothyroidism and instruct the patient to watch for them. If hypothyroidism does occur, lifelong thyroid hormone replacement will be necessary (see pp. 491 to 494).

Surgery. Indications. Subtotal thyroidectomy is indicated for Graves' disease in patients of childbearing age who have failed to have a permanent remission after thioamide treatment, for some cases of hyperthyroidism during pregnancy (see below), for older patients who refuse radioactive iodine, for solitary toxic nodules in patients of childbearing age, and for patients who have large retrosternal goiters producing tracheal compression or obstruction of jugular venous return.

Premedication. Because operating on a patient with active hyperthyroidism entails the risk of postoperative thyroid storm, a thioamide drug should be administered until the patient is clinically and biochemically euthyroid. The thioamide should then be continued at a maintenance level until the day of surgery; iodide, e.g., in the form of a saturated solution of potassium iodide (SSKI), 5 drops orally twice daily, should be added for the last 10 days prior to surgery.

Risks. The risk of mortality with thyroid surgery is essentially the risk of anesthesia, and in young people this should be practically negligible. Postoperative permanent vocal cord paralysis and permanent hypoparathyroidism should occur in no more than 1 per cent in the hands of a skilled surgeon. Transient hypocalcemia in the immediate postoperative period is quite common but usually requires no treatment. The incidence of recurrent hyperthyroidism after a subtotal thyroidectomy for Graves' disease is a function of how much thyroid tissue the surgeon leaves in place; recurrence generally is found in about 10 per cent of patients. Hypothyroidism occurs in 2 to 5 per cent of patients during the immediate postoperative period; but, as with ^{131}I, the prevalence of hypothyroidism increases gradually over a period of years. Ten or 15 years postoperatively hypothyroidism is present in about 30 per cent of patients with Graves' disease. The true prevalence, however, is difficult to estimate, as reported prevalences vary widely, from 6 to almost 50 per cent. The frequency of postoperative hypothyroidism seems to be increased in the presence of high titers of antibodies to thyroid antigens. Hypothyroidism should not occur after removal of a solitary toxic nodule if the other lobe is left intact.

Adjunctive Treatment. IODIDE. Administration of a large quantity of iodide to a patient with Graves' disease results in a decrease in organification of iodine and hence in decreased thyroid hormone synthesis. More importantly, though, there is an immediate inhibition of release of stored hormone from the thyroid gland. This latter effect can be used to hasten the fall of serum T_4 and T_3 concentrations (especially T_3) in severely hyperthyroid patients who are starting a course of a thioamide drug. We use a saturated solution of potassium iodide (SSKI), 5 drops orally once or twice daily. Iodide should be discontinued after 1 to 2 weeks.

Iodide can also be used in selected patients after ^{131}I treatment. If iodide is to be given, it can be administered in a dose such as that mentioned above, and continued for 2 to 4 weeks following ^{131}I treatment, but it should not be started until at least 48 hours after radioactive iodine administration.

The use of iodide preparation for surgery has been discussed (see Surgery, above).

Pruritus, skin rashes, and sialadenitis are occasional complications of iodide administration.

PROPRANOLOL. Propranolol is a β-adrenergic antagonist that can be used for symptomatic relief of many of the symptoms of hyperthyroidism. However, it probably has no effect on the underlying disease. The drug seems not to affect tissue oxygen consumption, but it does decrease heart rate and cardiac output. Thus one of the basic metabolic abnormalities has not changed, but the mechanism for delivering oxygen to the cells has been impaired. Propranolol is indicated in the treatment of thyroid storm and may be useful as an adjunct to decrease the heart rate in patients with tachyrhythmias caused by hyperthyroidism. It should be used with caution, if at all, in patients who have myocardial failure. The dose of propranolol is 20 to 40 mg. orally four times daily. Propranolol is contraindicated in patients with asthma, nonarrhythmia-related congestive heart failure, or history of hypersensitivity to this drug.

Special Situations

Pregnancy. Although authorities are of divided opinions on whether a thioamide drug or surgery is the treatment of choice for hyperthyroidism during pregnancy, all agree that radioactive iodine should not be used in this situation, because radioactive iodine crosses the placenta, and ablation of the fetal thyroid would result.

Most opinions favor the use of thioamide drugs for control of hyperthyroidism during pregnancy. Since these drugs do cross the placenta to some extent, the total daily dose should be limited to at most 150 mg. of propylthiouracil (PTU) or 10 mg. of methimazole. Larger doses continued past mid-gestation risk the occurrence of a large goiter in the baby, with consequent tracheal compression. Fortunately, in some women pregnancy tends to ameliorate hyperthyroidism and hence to decrease the dose of drug required to control the disease. A few cases of aplasia cutis have been reported in the offspring of women who received methimazole, but not PTU, during pregnancy. Therefore at present PTU seems the safer drug to use.

Surgery is an acceptable alternative to drug treatment, with the one provision that surgery not be undertaken during the third trimester, as it may precipitate labor.

Iodide should not be used in pregnant patients, except briefly in preparation for surgery. Chronic administration of iodide during pregnancy frequently results in a large goiter in the neonate. The safety of propranolol with respect to fetal development is unproved, and therefore it should not be given routinely to the pregnant patient.

Thyroid Storm. Thyroid storm, or thyrotoxic crisis, is an exaggerated form of severe hyperthyroidism, generally of abrupt onset, and characterized by hyperpyrexia, extreme tachycardia (often accompanied by congestive heart failure), and altered mental state (usually obtundation or delirium). It usually occurs in patients who have a prior history of hyperthyroidism in whom acute psychologic or physiologic stress has occurred, most commonly infection or surgery. The dividing line between thyroid storm and severe hyperthyroidism is hard to define.

Untreated thyroid storm is almost universally fatal, but with proper treatment a reduction in mortality rate to 20 per cent can be achieved.

General Support. The most immediate need is to reduce the body temperature and heart rate. External cooling should be used as needed, as well as acetaminophen (Tylenol, Spectra, and other brands), 325 to 650 mg. every 4 to 6 hours. Acetaminophen is preferable to aspirin, because the latter drug displaces T_4 and T_3 from thyroxine binding globulin, thus leading to an increase in free thyroid hormones. Oxygen should be administered in order to improve tissue oxygenation to meet the high metabolic demand.

Intravenous dextrose-containing solutions, with or without electrolytes as indicated, should be given in order to replete liver glycogen stores, which are decreased in the hyperthyroid patient. Glucose administration also exerts a nitrogen-sparing effect. Vitamins, especially B vitamins, should be given.

Specific Antithyroid Measures. PTU, 400 mg. orally every 6 hours (by nasogastric tube if necessary), should be given to block the synthesis of thyroid hormones and to decrease peripheral conversion of T_4 to T_3. Alternatively, methimazole, 30 mg. orally every 6 hours, can be used; however, as mentioned previously, this drug lacks the peripheral effect of PTU. One hour after PTU is started, iodide should be given to prevent release of stored T_4 and T_3 from the thyroid gland. (The reason for the 1 hour wait is to allow time for the onset of action of PTU and thus prevent the iodide load from providing substrate for further hormone synthesis.) The iodide can be given as a saturated solution of potassium iodide (SSKI), 5 drops orally every 6 hours, or as intravenous sodium iodide, 1 gram by continuous infusion over 24 hours.

Dexamethasone may be given at a dose of 1 mg. every 6 hours (orally or intravenously) in order to decrease the extrathyroidal conversion of T_4 to T_3 and to cover the possibility of relative adrenal insufficiency.

Blockade of Peripheral Effects of Thyroid Hormones. Propranolol may be used to decrease the heart rate and control many of the features of hyperthyroidism. This drug should be given orally, 20 to 40 mg. every 4 to 6 hours; if oral administration is impracticable, propranolol can be given by slow intravenous infusion (at 1 mg. per minute), 2 to 4 mg. every 4 to 6 hours. The use of propranolol should not alter the use of digitalis glycosides or diuretics when appropriate for atrial fibrillation and congestive heart failure. If propranolol is contraindicated—e.g., in patients with asthma or nonarrhythmia-related congestive heart failure—guanethidine (Ismelin) may be used at a dose of 20 to 50 mg. orally every 8 hours. Alternatively, reserpine, 1 to 3 mg. intramuscularly every 8 hours, can be used. It should be borne in mind that an acute surgical abdomen often is a consideration in patients with thyroid storm, and depletion of catecholamines brought about by guanethidine or reserpine may complicate surgical intervention.

Ophthalmopathy. Mild exophthalmos is common in Graves' disease and usually requires no specific treatment. When symptoms are present in mild to moderate ophthalmopathy, simple measures generally suffice. Burning and itching of eyes can be alleviated by the instillation of 1 per cent methylcellulose eye drops. Photophobia can be relieved by wearing dark glasses, and shielded glasses are useful for wind sensitivity. If the lids cannot be closed completely, they may have to be taped shut at night in order to prevent corneal desiccation. Orbital edema can be decreased by elevating the head at night. If orbital edema is severe, salt restriction and a diuretic may be used. Chemosis may be treated with corticosteroid eyedrops, but such treatment should not be used for mild chemosis, as corticosteroid administration may decrease resistance to herpes simplex conjunctivitis. Diplopia can be dealt with temporarily by using an eyepatch. In most cases diplopia will resolve spontaneously.

When ophthalmopathy is severe, more aggressive methods may be necessary. If infiltrative ophthalmopathy is progressive, with loss of visual acuity, and if the measures mentioned above are ineffective, a trial of prednisone should be instituted, at a dose of 40 to 120 mg. orally daily in divided doses. Antacids may be given together with prednisone in order to decrease gastric irritation, particularly if there is a history of peptic ulcer or gastritis. As soon as the ophthalmopathy comes under control, the dose of prednisone should be decreased gradually to the lowest effective dose, usually about 20 mg. daily. Eventually prednisone administration should be shifted to an every-other-day schedule. After 4 to 6 months the dose should be tapered and discontinued. Systemic corticosteroids should not be used for Graves' ophthalmopathy unless an immediate threat to visual acuity or a visual field defect is present.

When medical therapy fails to relieve severe ophthalmopathy, surgical orbital decompression (removal of part of the bony orbit) should be performed. Alternatively, x-ray treatment directed at the retro-orbital tissues sometimes is effective.

The course of Graves' ophthalmopathy is unpredictable and does not necessarily mimic that of the hyperthyroidism. However, it is the clinical impression of many that the ophthalmopathy tends to be aggravated if the patient is allowed to become hypothyroid.

HYPOTHYROIDISM

method of
MERVILLE C. MARSHALL, JR., M.D.,
and BRUCE D. WEINTRAUB, M.D.
Bethesda, Maryland

Deficient circulating levels of L-thyroxine (T_4) and L-triiodothyronine (T_3), or impairment of their actions, results in the clinical and biochemical features of hypothyroidism. There are a variety of causes of hypothyroidism which can be characterized as primary (thyroidal), secondary (pituitary), or tertiary (hypothalamic). The current concept of the hypothalamic-pituitary-thyroid axis is that the thyroid synthesizes and secretes thyroid hormones under the stimulative influence of thyrotropin (TSH) released by the pituitary gland. The pituitary gland, in turn, is stimulated to release TSH by thyrotropin-releasing hormone (TRH), but is inhibited by the thyroid hormones via a negative feedback regulatory circuit.

In primary diseases of the thyroid causing hypothyroidism, serum thyroid hormones are low, leading to an elevation of serum TSH. Secondary hypothyroidism is defined as a disorder of the pituitary gland resulting in low TSH levels and consequent low T_3 and T_4. Tertiary hypothyroidism, in which disease at the level of the hypothalamus presumably results in inadequate secretion of TRH, also exhibits low TSH and thyroid hormone levels. Endogenous TRH levels in man cannot be readily measured; however, the TSH response to exogenous TRH provides an additional useful diagnostic test.

When 500 micrograms of TRH (Protilerin) is given as a single intravenous bolus injection to normal subjects, the serum TSH rises from a basal value of 0.5 to 4 microunits per ml. to a peak value of 10 to 25 microunits per ml. in 20 to 30 minutes, and gradually returns to normal over the next 60 to 90 minutes. In primary hypothyroidism, basal TSH is elevated, and there is an increased response to TRH. Although an elevated basal TSH level is sufficient for the diagnosis of primary hypothyroidism, in mild cases the exaggerated response to TRH may be helpful in confirming the diagnosis. In secondary hypothyroidism, there is no rise in serum TSH in response to TRH; in tertiary hypothyroidism, there is a definite response to TRH, which is often delayed, with TSH reaching peak levels at approximately 45 to 90 minutes. Recent evidence suggests, however, that the results of TRH testing may not always be a reliable guide to the anatomic location of central nervous system disease.

Treatment

The preferred treatment of hypothyroidism of any cause is replacement of thyroid hormones, although certain cases of congenital abnormalities of iodine metabolism by the thyroid and, outside the United States, endemic iodine deficiency can be treated with chronic iodine administration. Over the course of several decades, a variety of regimens have been employed, and most of them have been successful. There are no long-term, controlled studies to definitively indicate which regimen is the best. Our recommendations are based upon current knowledge of thyroid physiology and pertinent clinical and experimental data.

Thyroid hormones are available as preparations derived from animal glands, or as the pure synthetic hormones. Thyroid, U.S.P. (Thyrar, Thyrocrine) is a powder of defatted porcine thyroid glands. It is specified to have an iodine content of 0.17 to 0.23 per cent; however, the iodine is in the form of T_4, T_3, and iodoproteins in varying proportions, with consequent variable potency. Thyroid Strong tablets are also prepared from defatted, desiccated thyroid glands, and contain 0.3 per cent iodine. One tablet of Thyroid Strong is equivalent to 1½ grains of thyroid, U.S.P. Thyroglobulin, N.F. (Proloid) is a purified extract of porcine thyroid gland that is subjected to bioassay, and hence has a more constant biopotency. It is also standardized to give a T_4:T_3 ratio of approximately 2.5:1. Pork thyroid "liquid" capsules, U.S.P. (S-P-T) are likewise standardized to give the same T_4:T_3 ratio as thyroglobulin, N.F. Levothyroxine, U.S.P. (Synthroid, Letter, Cytolen, Levoid) is the synthetic sodium salt of T_4. Tablets of different strengths are available for several brand names; however, it should be noted that the color code of the tablets differs for each brand name. Switching from one brand to another could lead to confusion and inadvertent over- or underdosage by the patient, unless forewarned. Levothyroxine is also available in a parenteral preparation. Liothyronine, U.S.P. (Cytomel) is the synthetic sodium salt of T_3. Only tablets for oral use are marketed; however, preparations for parenteral use are available from the manufacturer. Liotrix (Euthroid, Thyrolar) is a mixture of synthetic T_4 and T_3 in a 4:1 ratio. Euthroid tablets contain 0.06 mg. T_4 and 15 micrograms T_3; Thyrolar tablets contain 0.05 mg. T_4 and 12.5 micrograms T_3. The relative potencies of these preparations are as follows: 0.1 mg. of T_4 = 50 micrograms of T_3 = 60 mg. of thyroid U.S.P. or thyroglobulin approximately = 1 tablet of liotrix. Whereas 25 micrograms of T_3 was once considered the equivalent of 0.1 mg. of T_4, it has recently been shown that 50 micrograms of T_3 is required to achieve the same degree of TSH suppression as 0.1 mg. T_4 (see below).

Approximately 40 per cent of both endogenous and exogenous T_4 is converted to T_3, and the proportion of circulating T_3 that is derived from monodeiodination of T_4 has been calculated as 40 to 90 per cent. Also, although T_3 is more metabolically active than T_4, there is evidence that T_4 per se has hormonal activity independent of its conversion to T_3. In addition, oral T_4 given once daily produces stable serum levels of both T_4 and T_3 that can be readily monitored, wheras oral T_3 produces wide swings in serum T_3 levels after each dose, and no change in T_4 levels. For these reasons, we believe that T_4 is the therapeutic agent of choice for hypothyroidism. It most closely mimics normal physiology; it does not include T_3 and thereby avoids acute changes in serum T_3; and it has a reliable, standardized potency. Thyroid, U.S.P. is the least expensive of the thyroid preparations, but suffers from its potentially inconstant potency. Thyroglobulin, U.S.P. is only slightly less expensive than T_4. All the T_3-containing agents are much more expensive; and, although the wide swings in serum T_3 levels caused by each of these agents have not been proved detrimental, such variations in thyroid hormone level are certainly nonphysiologic. If T_3 is prescribed, it should be given in divided doses to minimize the acute changes in serum T_3 levels.

The advent of sensitive radioimmunoassays for TSH and TRH testing has made possible a more precise definition of euthyroidism. As discussed above, primary hypothyroidism is characterized by elevated basal TSH levels and an exaggerated response to TRH. Recent studies have shown that 0.1 to 0.2 mg. of T_4 daily will render most patients euthyroid as judged by normal serum T_4, T_3, and TSH levels and a normal TSH response to TRH. Patients with mild disease, by both clinical and laboratory criteria, often are adequately replaced with only 0.1 mg. T_4 daily, whereas patients with more severe disease generally require 0.15 to 0.2 mg. T_4 daily. Progression of the disease process may necessitate changes in the replacement dose of T_4. If T_3 is used in the treatment of hypothyroidism, 75 to 100 micrograms is required to normalize serum TSH.

Serum TSH assays are widely available and provide the most convenient means of determining efficacy of treatment. When the T_3, T_4, and TSH values are normal, a patient may still have subclinical hypo- or hyperthyroidism which would be revealed by an abnormal TRH test. However, the need to adjust therapy to such fine control by means of TRH tests has not been demonstrated. In the absence of TSH assays, normalization of *both* T_4 and T_3 should be the goal of therapy. *Normal* T_4 with *subnormal* T_3, as well as *normal* T_3 with *low* T_4, is often associated with elevated TSH levels.

In secondary or tertiary hypothyroidism, basal TSH levels are not helpful, although TRH tests could be followed in tertiary hypothyroidism. Thyroid hormone levels and clinical status are therefore important to follow. Conditions that raise thyroxine-binding globulin (TBG) (e.g., pregnancy, birth control pills, genetic defects) or lower TBG (e.g., steroids, androgens, nephrosis, cirrhosis, genetic defects) will cause parallel changes in serum T_4 and T_3 levels. Free T_4 or free T_4 index measurements are unaffected by TBG concentration.

Young patients can be started on full maintenance dose immediately. Patients over 50 years of age and patients with coronary artery disease are more safely started on low doses, 0.025 to 0.050 mg. per day, and gradually increased to full maintenance dose with increments of 0.025 to 0.050 mg. at monthly intervals. Theoretically, the shorter half-time of disappearance of T_3 (1 to 2 days) versus T_4 (6 to 8 days) may favor use of the former in patients with heart disease, who are prone to develop worsening angina during therapy. However, the acute rise in serum T_3 levels after oral T_3 administration may pose an added risk for these patients, which may overshadow its theoretical advantage.

If patient adherence to a daily drug regimen is not reliable, it is possible to give the total weekly dose of T_4 once per week with effective replacement and no toxic symptoms. The daily dose of T_4 can also be administered as daily subcutaneous injections. The most important factors in maintaining euthyroidism are convincing the patient of the necessity of lifelong replacement and intermittent clinical and laboratory evaluation. It should also be noted that these recommendations are for *replacement* therapy and do not pertain to *suppressive* therapy for other thyroid disorders.

Myxedema Coma

Myxedema coma is readily recognized in the patient with the characteristics of severe hypothyroidism: edematous facies, large tongue, loss of eyebrows, alopecia, and slow reflexes. Mentation ranges from stupor to frank coma. Often, the patient has a history of gradual deterioration that becomes precipitous upon exposure to stress or cold, or with the onset of infection.

The following features are of particular interest: (1) *Hypotension* is resistant to vasopressors unless thyroid hormone is given. (2) *Hyponatremia* is attributed to a combination of the decreased glomerular filtration rate seen in hypothyroidism and inappropriate antidiuretic hormone (ADH) in the case of primary hypothyroidism, but is generally a result of adrenal insufficiency in the case of secondary hypothyroidism. Glucocorticoids are required for the treatment of the latter; water restriction is advocated, and overhydration must be prevented in either case. (3) *Hypoglycemia* of uncertain cause should be treated with intravenous glucose. (4) *CO_2 narcosis* may require assisted ventilation. (5) *Hypothermia,* often considered the hallmark of impending coma, is treated only with blankets; active reheating is deleterious. (6) *Occult gastrointestinal hemmorrhage* is often associated with fecal impaction. (7) *Pericardial effusion* is common, but tamponade is quite rare.

Myxedema coma has a mortality of up to 40 per cent, even with modern modes of therapy. Rapid clinical assessment and initiation of therapy prior to laboratory confirmation are critical. Baseline serum T_3, T_4, TSH, and plasma cortisol levels should be obtained for later documentation of thyroid and adrenal status. Recent data support the following regimen: a loading dose of 0.4 to 0.5 mg. of T_4 intravenously, followed by 0.1 mg. T_4 intravenously daily until the patient can take oral medications. Improvement of vital signs can be seen within 6 to 12 hours, and return of consciousness can occur in 24 to 36 hours. A significant decline in TSH also occurs within the first 24 hours of treatment. Intravenous T_3, 25 to 50 micrograms daily, has been used with success; however, parenteral T_3 must be specially prepared from kits obtained only directly from the manufacturer. T_3 has also been given orally, 12.5 micrograms every 6 hours, but with the attendant risks of nasogastric intubation and the uncertainty of drug absorption in the presence of coma. The use of T_3 in the treatment of myxedema coma has not been reassessed, and the optimal dose of T_3 has not been established. Moreover, these doses of oral T_3, based upon early studies, differ significantly from current recommendations for the use of oral T_3 in urgent therapy as outlined below.

Glucocorticoids are probably a valuable adjunct to thyroid hormone therapy for two reasons: (1) the possibility of hypopituitarism with adrenal insufficiency cannot be immediately excluded; and (2) it is possible that the return to normal metabolism could cause increased clearance of serum cortisol and consequent relative adrenal insufficiency, even in the absence of hypopituitarism. Hydrocortisone, 200 to 300 mg., is given intravenously the first day and tapered over the next few days.

The patient should be carefully examined for a source of occult infection, even in the absence of leukocytosis, fever, and tachycardia. Other causes of coma—e.g., cerebrovascular accidents, drug overdose—should not be overlooked. Occasionally, anemia is severe enough to warrant transfusion.

Urgent Therapy

Except in the case of myxedema coma, rapid thyroid replacement is rarely necessary. Occasionally, when surgery is imminent in the face of the unexpected discovery of hypothyroidism, urgent therapy may be warranted. In such instances, the T_4 regimen described above can be employed, or 75 to 100 micrograms of T_3 orally per day can effect rapid replacement. The risks of such therapy in patients with possible cardiac disease should be carefully considered.

Pregnancy

Untreated maternal hypothyroidism is associated with a high incidence of fetal morbidity and mortality, and maternal hypothyroidism should therefore be promptly treated. During normal pregnancy, there is an increase in serum total T_4 level concomitant with a rise in thyroxine-binding globulin (TBG) secondary to elevated estrogen production. Free T_4 and TSH levels are normal. In hypothyroidism, total T_4 may be in the normal range, but still low for pregnancy. Free T_4 is low, and in the case of primary hypothyroidism TSH is elevated. There are no recent studies on replacement therapy for hypothyroidism in pregnancy; in general, a regimen similar to that for nonpregnant patients is recommended—i.e., 0.15 to 0.2 mg. T_4, or its equivalent, per day. It must be noted, however, that adequate replacement should return total T_4 to the normally high basal levels of pregnancy, and, in the presence of elevated TBG, larger doses of T_4 may be needed initially to correct the deficiency. A normal free T_4 level is a useful indicator of adequacy of replacement therapy. It should also be remembered that thyroid hormones appear in the milk of nursing mothers; if thyroid supplements are properly administered, this should pose no danger to the infant.

Cretinism and Pediatric Hypothyroidism

The prevailing concept of fetal-neonatal thyroid hormone physiology is as follows: (1) there is little if any exchange of thyroid hormones and TSH between maternal and fetal circulations; (2) reverse T_3 is found in high concentrations in fetal serum and amniotic fluid; (3) at the time of birth, there is an abrupt rise in neonatal serum TSH levels, declining to baseline over the next 2 to 3 days. T_4 and T_3 also rise post partum.

It is pertinent to mention new advances in neonatal screening for hypothyroidism. Three methods have had preliminary clinical trials: (1) measurement of T_4 on filter paper spotted with blood at 2 to 3 days of age (as in the procedure used for routine phenylketonuria screening); (2) measurement of T_4 in umbilical cord blood; and (3) measurement of TSH in cord blood. The first two methods are the simplest, and will detect a significant number of cases of clinically inapparent hypothyroidism. On the basis of the preliminary trials, the American Thyroid Association now recommends initial screening for congenital hypothyroidism, using either filter paper T_4 or cord blood T_4 assays (depending upon availability), and TSH testing of suspicious samples. An incidence of congenital hypothyroidism of 1 in 5000 to 6000 has been found with these screening methods.

Congenital hypothyroidism may be due to athyreotic cretinism, usually resulting from a defect in embryogenesis of the thyroid gland, or goitrous cretinism, resulting from inborn errors of thyroid metabolism, iodine deficiency, or maternal ingestion of goitrogens, which, in contrast to thyroid hormones, readily cross the placenta. Inadvertent administration of radioactive iodine to a pregnant woman can cause fetal thyroid destruction. Juvenile hypothyroidism—i.e., hypothyroidism acquired during childhood or adolescence—is most commonly caused by Hashimoto's thyroiditis.

It is known that treatment of congenital hypothyroidism prior to age 3 months yields a 78 per cent chance of subsequent mental development into "normal" range (IQ greater than 85). The clinical signs of congenital hypothyroidism often are meager immediately post partum, causing delay in diagnosis. Undoubtedly, neonatal screening provides the best means of early diagnosis. A history of siblings with cretinism, and/or a history of maternal thyroid abnormality should raise the index of suspicion for a given neonate.

The treatment of hypothyroidism in children, as in adults, has been reassessed. Several studies show that a mean oral dose of 2.8 to 4.4 micrograms per kg. of T_4 per day will normalize thyroid function tests, including TSH levels, in children aged 1 to 16 years. Neonates require higher replacement doses of T_4, averaging 10 micrograms per kg. Again, T_4 is the therapeutic agent of choice. The use of desiccated thyroid in children has been reported to cause symptomatic hypertriiodothyroninemia. Thyroid hormone and TSH levels should be followed, but the ultimate criterion of adequate therapy is restoration of normal growth and development. Normalization of serum alkaline phosphatase can serve as a parameter of adequate replacement; bone age also correlates with thyroid status, but this response is slow. Overtreatment can cause acceleration of bone maturation and premature craniosynostosis. Intrauterine diagnosis and treatment of fetuses at risk for hypothyroidism are still experimental.

"Subclinical Hypothyroidism"

Patients who are clinically euthyroid but have elevated TSH with normal T_4 and T_3 levels are generally considered to have "compensated" thyroid failure. Opinion is divided upon whether to treat such patients with thyroid hormone in order to normalize serum TSH. In any case, when "subclinical hypothyroidism" is discovered, close follow-up of the patient is important for early detection of frank hypothyroidism.

Thyroid Hormone Side Effects and Drug Interactions

Thyroxine itself has essentially no side effects at correct dosage. Early symptoms of overdosage include palpitations, nervousness, diaphoresis, heat intolerance, headaches, and insomnia.

Recently, a study purporting to show an association between thyroid hormone therapy and the prevalence of breast cancer has been widely publicized. Criticism of this report has been detailed in a statement released by the American Thyroid Association. An association between primary thyroidal disease and breast cancer has been suspected, but numerous studies to date have reported conflicting results. An association between breast cancer and thyroid hormone treatment per se has not been demonstrated.

Absorption of oral T_4 is variable and ranges from 30 to 90 per cent, whereas T_3 absorption is generally complete. Absorption of T_4 is decreased in the presence of cholestyramine, and ingestion of the two drugs should occur at least 5 hours apart.

Thyroid hormone will potentiate the actions of oral anticoagulants, adrenergic agonists such as epinephrine (Adrenalin), ephedrine, isoproterenol, and tricyclic antidepressants. Dosage adjustment of these agents may be necessary. Thyroxine will also decrease glucose tolerance in diabetic patients, and may necessitate an increase in the dosage of oral hypoglycemic agents or insulin. As previously mentioned, any patient taking steroids may be at risk for developing relative adrenal insufficiency when thyroid hormone is started; hence steroid requirement should be closely monitored.

THYROID GLAND MALIGNANCIES

method of
ANDRE J. VAN HERLE, M.D.
Los Angeles, California

The proper therapeutic approach to the treatment of thyroid cancer is highly controversial. Part of this controversy is due to certain recognizable elements which make evaluation of therapy uncertain. These include (1) the difficulty in certain instances of arriving at an accurate pathologic diagnosis; (2) the age of the patient at the time the tumor is discovered; (3) the experience of the surgeon performing the thyroid surgery; and (4) the varying degrees of involvement of the different histologic tumor types. Each of these factors may contribute to the outcome of the therapy administered to a patient with thyroid cancer, making it nearly impossible to formulate a uniform therapeutic approach.

It is generally accepted that a surgical approach is indicated once the malignant nature of a thyroid lesion is highly suspected or proved by external biopsy or cytologic evaluation of a thyroid aspirate. Although this viewpoint is challenged by a minority of thyroidologists, who claim that suppressive therapy with thyroid hormone may be sufficient to control differentiated thyroid tumors, we believe that a patient should not be denied surgical resection of a malignant thyroidal tumor.

It is difficult to determine the type of surgical approach advisable for a subject with thyroid cancer, because the procedure frequently depends on the presentation of the lesion at the time of surgery. Some guidelines, however, can be proposed. The type of surgical resection to be applied depends on several factors, one of which is the histologic type of the tumor. We will first discuss tumors of relatively rare incidence—namely, medullary and anaplastic carcinomas—and follow this with a discussion of the more common differentiated thyroid tumors.

The type of surgical approach we recommend in patients with medullary carcinoma is a near total thyroidectomy. This operative procedure involves the removal of both thyroid lobes and the isthmus of the thyroid gland, leaving a small rim of thyroid tissue at the upper pole of both thyroid lobes in the tracheoesophageal groove in order to preserve parathyroid function. A modified neck dissection is indicated if lymph node involvement is obvious during the intervention. This operation preserves the sternocleidomastoid muscle as well as the spinal accessory nerve and the internal jugular vein and prevents a number of cosmetic deformities which may follow the sacrifice of these structures. The rationale for such an aggressive approach with this type of tumor is based on two observations: (1) this tumor is mostly multicentric within the lobes of the thyroid gland; and (2) surgery is the only therapeutic intervention that can reduce the tumor mass, because it is composed of C-cells which are not amenable to treatment with radioactive iodine. The measurement of thyrocalcitonin in the circulation of such patients not only is a good marker for the presence of such tumors prior to surgery (especially in conjunction with stimulatory tests) but also indicates the existence of residual tumor tissue after surgery or the development of metastases.

The diagnosis of an anaplastic carcinoma should always be confirmed by means of a biopsy, and a surgical consultation should not be denied the patient. Frequently, surgical resection of the tumor is impossible and will usually not affect the final outcome in patients with this notoriously malignant tumor. Therapy is consequently palliative; tracheostomy is frequently performed to prevent suffocation, and external radiation therapy is attempted. Certain authors feel there is a difference in the outcome of poorly differentiated carcinomas, the small cell carcinoma being more responsive to surgical treatment followed by irradiation therapy than anaplastic carcinomas, the latter being more malignant.

Differentiated thyroid tumors are slightly less malignant than medullary carcinomas of the thyroid. These include papillary, follicular, or mixed papillary-follicular carcinomas and represent roughly 90 per cent of all malignant thyroid tumors. Follicular carcinomas of the thyroid are in general more malignant than the papillary carcinomas. The latter type tends to metastasize to lymph nodes, in contrast with the former which tends to spread via a hematogenous route.

The surgical approach for differentiated carcinomas is essentially similar to that described for medullary carcinomas of the thyroid. A near total thyroidectomy is recommended with a modified neck dissection if lymph node involvement is present. The rationale for this approach can be summarized as follows: (1) The incidence of intraglandular and extraglandular spread exceeds 80 per cent in patients with thyroid malignancies. (2) The resection of all glandular tissue prevents monopolization of ^{131}I by normal glandular tissue, and its removal facilitates subsequent radioisotope therapy directed toward residual tumor tissue if this is indicated.

The reported incidence of degeneration of differentiated tumors to undifferentiated tumors should also be taken into account. The exact histologic nature of a thyroid lesion is sometimes not provided at the time of surgery, as frozen sections could be interpreted as being benign, yet permanent sections reveal the malignant nature of the lesion. In those circumstances a reintervention is mandatory to remove the residual thyroid tissue. In a number of instances additional tumor tissue is found in the remaining resected lobe.

No matter how skilled the surgeon and how thorough his attempt to remove all thyroid tissue, a total thyroidectomy is rarely achieved. Therefore ablation with ^{131}I radioactive iodine is frequently necessary following near total thyroidectomy to eradicate residual thyroid tissue and to maximize the chances of discovery of thyroid metastases or regrowth at a later stage with total body scans. A dose of 30 millicuries of ^{131}I is appropriate initially, although more than one dose may be required to achieve this goal. This initial ablative dose can be administered shortly after surgery before starting supplementation therapy with thyroid hormone (±3 weeks) or could be administered at a later date (2 to 3 months) if the patient is too debilitated after surgery to tolerate an episode of hypothyroidism. The administration of thyroid hormone in suppressive doses (0.2 mg. of L-thyroxine [Synthroid] per day) is indicated following surgery. This dose of thyroid hormone will not only suppress thyroid-stimulating hormone (TSH) levels in most of the patients, a goal to be reached because of the presumed TSH dependence of most of these lesions, but will also maintain a euthyroid state. The evaluation of serum TSH levels in these patients will help assess whether acceptable suppression is achieved. The therapy with thyroid hormone should be instituted for the patient's lifetime, to be interrupted only for total body scanning or therapeutic administration of ^{131}I.

The patient should not take any form of thyroid hormone supplementation for approximately 1 month prior to any scanning or ablative procedures in order to obtain an adequate level of thyroid-stimulating hormone (TSH). An alternative approach is to discontinue therapy with L-thyroxine (L-T_4) 1 month prior to the date of the planned total body scan and start the patient on T_3 therapy, 75 micrograms per day for a period of 2 weeks. The T_3 therapy should be stopped 2 weeks prior to the planned scanning. This schedule then prevents the discomfort of hypothyroidism in these patients. The circulating TSH level achieved under these conditions is usually as high as the levels achieved after the intramuscular administration of exogenous bovine TSH, and makes the latter superfluous. Additionally, the administration of exogenous bovine TSH may lead to severe allergic reactions and to the development of antibodies which may inactivate TSH.

The late follow-up in patients with differentiated thyroid carcinoma following a surgical procedure should include all the following studies:

1. Clinical evaluation, with special attention to the recurrence of a nodule or masses in the neck area, the development of lymph nodes, the development of hoarseness, dysphagia, or dyspnea, or a tenderness in bony areas.
2. Chest x-rays, which may reveal the unsuspected presence of metastases.
3. A total body scan on a yearly basis for a period of 3 years, and every 3 years thereafter, always while the patient is off suppressive therapy. If no uptake is demonstrated in total body scan, the patient should immediately resume suppressive therapy with L-thyroxine (200 micrograms per day).
4. The measurement of serum thyroglobulin, a specific protein of the thyroid, which is released by most differentiated thyroid tumors and their metastatic lesions in the circulation. This measurement should be considered the counterpart of thyrocalcitonin measurements in medullary carcinomas of the thyroid to discover metastatic disease of this tumor.

Patients should be evaluated by the aforementioned screening tests (with exception made for the total body scan) at least once a year after their surgical procedure or after ablation with ^{131}I to ascertain if they are still clinically free of disease. In the evaluation of the adequacy of thyroid hormone supplementation, T_4 and TSH levels are of importance. Serum calcium and phosphorus levels should be assessed to determine whether or not normal calcium balance is maintained in subjects who experienced hypoparathyroidism after surgery, or to detect new cases of hypoparathyroidism which sometimes occur late after surgery. The use of doxorubicin and bleomycin as therapeutic agents should still be considered investigational at present.

PHEOCHROMOCYTOMA

method of
GABRIEL SPERGEL, M.D.
Brooklyn, New York

The rarity of pheochromoctyoma is due primarily to the failure to look for this tumor and not to its true prevalence. Approximately 0.5 per cent of all hypertensive patients harbor a pheochromocytoma. Although a rare cause of sudden death, pheochromocytomas contribute to the vast morbidity and mortality caused by hypertension. The management of this disorder is now well established and routinized, and physicians should be familiar with a treatment protocol.

Diagnostic Features Relating to Therapy

The diagnosis of pheochromocytoma is based on the finding of significantly elevated plasma or urinary concentrations of catecholamines or their degradation products. We discourage the use of retroperitoneal CO_2 insufflation studies and retrograde selective adrenal vein catheterization, because they are dangerous and may precipitate a hypertensive crisis even in the well-prepared patient. The preoperative preparation requires a chest x-ray, including a lateral view to look for "posterior" mediastinal masses; an intravenous pyelogram with nephrotomography to see the course of the ureters and evaluate the suprarenal areas for masses; and a neck x-ray to look for calcifications that might suggest the presence of medullary thyroid carcinoma. We do not perform stimulatory tests (glucagon or tyramine) or blocking tests (phentolamine) unless clinically indicated in a patient with borderline laboratory results or one with a convincing history and physical findings and with negative catecholamine assays. Some patients with pheochromocytoma will have a low blood volume, and this is of importance as it must be corrected prior to surgery. Serum calcium and phosphorus values should be obtained, because a significant number of these patients may have the multiple endocrinomatosis (MEA) syndrome (Type II), which usually includes hyperparathyroidism. If available, an assay of thyrocalcitonin is of value in determining the presence of medullary thyroid carcinoma, even in the asymptomatic relative of a patient with the Type II MEA syndrome. In addition to the knowledge that family members of a patient with the MEA syndrome may be similarly affected, the presence of the syndrome means that the surgeon has to look for bilateral and multiple pheochromocytomas which are present in a majority of these family members.

Preoperative Management

It has been our policy to treat all patients with a combination of long-acting α-adrenergic blocking agents (phenoxybenzamine HCl) and β-adrenergic blockers (propranolol). If one uses only the α blockers, one may unmask β activity, and then bouts of tachycardia may ensue. When the β blockers are used alone, they may precipitate hypertensive crises. Operations are to await the successful control of blood pressure and heart rate and rhythm. Surgery under other than ideal conditions leads to a mortality rate in excess of 50 per cent. We have seen no deaths during elective surgery for a pheochromocytoma in over 30 patients.

Therapy with blocking agents is begun with phenoxybenzamine (Dibenzyline), 10 mg. orally twice daily, and propranolol (Inderal), 10 mg. orally three times daily; the latter is not to be used in patients with a history of bronchial asthma. The rapid acting α blocker, phentolamine (Regitine) is of little use because of a short half-life. The phenoxybenzamine (Dibenzyline) may be increased by 10 mg. every 2 to 3 days until the paroxysms and/or the hypertension is controlled. The largest dose we have used is 80 mg., but much larger doses may be necessary. Side effects are usually minimal but include a stuffy nose, anorexia, abdominal cramps, and postural hypotension. The propranolol is effective not only because of its β-adrenergic blockading activity but also because of its antirenin properties, and patients with pheochromocytoma have very high renin values owing to catecholamine stimulation. The dose of propranolol is increased every 2 to 3 days by 10 to 20 mg. until tachycardia and catecholamine-induced arrhythmias are abolished. The usual dose required is 40 mg. daily, but we have used as much as 400 mg. daily in a single patient. Side effects include bloating, fluid retention, unmasking of asthma, and significant and symptomatic bradycardia.

The selected doses of these oral agents is continued up to the evening prior to surgery. There are reports in the literature that sudden cessation of the β blockers can lead to arrhythmias, myocardial infarction, and death—especially if the doses of the agents used are large and if the patient has ischemic heart disease. The anesthesiologist must also be aware that these α and β drugs will potentiate the hypotensive effect of preoperative medications as well as the hypotensive properties of anesthetic agents.

Because of the intense vasoconstrictive effects of the catecholamines, some patients with pheochromocytoma may have constricted blood volumes. As sympathetic blockade is achieved, the blood volume may fall further. This should be corrected by replacement with whole blood prior to and during the initial moments of surgery. It is our custom to stay 2 to 3 units of blood ahead of the intraoperative blood loss.

Additional problems such as the presence of hypercalcemia from concomitant hyperparathyroidism (Sipple's syndrome—multiple endocrinomatosis, Type II) must be treated with intravenous fluids and Fleet's Phospho-Soda or other forms of hypocalcemic therapy. It is a mistake for the surgeon to attempt parathyroidectomy prior to removal of the pheochromocytoma. Obviously, the patient is to be in the best possible condition, and electrolyte imbalance, infection, and hyperglycemia are all to be well controlled prior to attempting surgery.

Intraoperative Management

A team approach is the only way to manage these patients during surgery. The head of the team should be the endocrinologist or cardiologist with the most experience in dealing with arrhythmias and hypertensive emergencies. The anesthesiologist must be aware of the possible adverse effects the agents he uses may have on this patient who has partial α- and β-adrenergic blockade. The surgeon must be aware of all the unusual places the pheochromocytoma may be hidden and must be prepared to cease operating at any time at the request of the internist.

Prior to administration of preoperative sedation, an arterial line must be cannulated so that direct and continuous monitoring of blood pressure measurements can be made. Electrocardiographic (ECG) leads should be placed so that the cardiac rate and rhythm can be simultaneously monitored. We have found it convenient to have all these parameters displayed on a single console. Central venous pressure should also be monitored prior to surgery and intraoperatively. At least two intravenous lines should be open to permit administration of drugs, fluids, and blood as needed. The central venous line may be so used if necessary. No fluids other than isotonic saline solution should be used with the intra-arterial line, as dextrose solutions can cause thrombosis with subsequent distal gangrene. All solutions that may be necessary and all drugs should be prepared and ready for use. We have found it convenient to have syringes filled with 5 mg. phentolamine on the ready, as well as a bottle of 500 ml. 5 per cent glucose in water containing 50 mg. phentolamine. Similarly, a 500 ml. bottle of 5 per cent glucose in water containing 5 ampules of norepinephrine (Levophed) should be available. It is our policy not to hang up the latter on an intravenous (IV) pole to prevent accidental use of the bottle when not indicated. Syringes with intravenous digoxin (Lanoxin), propranolol, lidocaine, and hydrocortisone should be available.

In our institution, induction of anesthesia is begun with short-acting barbiturates such as secobarbital. Using scopolamine and pancuronium (Pavulon) or d-tubocurarine, intubation is accomplished. Methoxyflurane (Penthrane) or enflurane (Ethrane) is the anesthetic agent of choice, because neither one sensitizes the myocardium to catecholamines and less arrhythmias are expected. As soon as the skin is incised, we begin the administration of whole blood, and it is our custom to stay 2 units ahead of blood loss to prevent the "flabby heart" syndrome, which is an irreversible complication of a catechole-depleted myocardium attempting to contract in a volume-depleted patient. Curare, succinylcholine, and gallamine are not used by us. Diethyl ether, cyclopropane, and halothane are to be avoided. Some of the worst arrhythmias occur during intubation, perhaps secondary to hypoxia or direct stimulation of pharyngeal and tracheal nerve plexuses. These bursts of myocardial activity are usually short lived and spontaneously cease when the anesthesia begins.

It is suggested that the surgeon use an anterior abdominal incision rather than approach through the flank, as it must be remembered that pheochromocytoma may be multiple, bilateral, and found almost anywhere in the abdomen and sometimes in the chest. Exploration should proceed cautiously, with the surgeon stopping all activity when hypertensive crises or arrhythmias are thought to be due to his touching the tumor or its blood supply. It is our custom to have the internist instruct the surgeon when to stop or start and to have him administer the appropriate antihypertensive or antiarrhythmic agent. When the tumor is located, the venous drainage should be ligated before the arterial supply is interrupted. On occasion, this may mean a large amount of blood may be trapped within the tumor. If the tumor is intra-adrenal, the entire adrenal is sacrificed. All adherent tissue, including the kidney, may similarly have to be sacrificed in an en bloc dissection. Once the blood supply to and from the tumor is interrupted, the blood pressure should fall to or toward normal. If it does not, another tumor is to be expected and the surgeon should be urged to continue exploration. If the blood pressure falls to shock levels, infusions of norepinephrine should be started. If adrenalectomy is done, hydrocortisone infusion should be started.

Hypertensive crises—we have seen blood pressure values as high as 380/240 mm. Hg—should be treated with bolus injections of 1 to 5 mg. of phentolamine (Regitine) or by infusion of the previously prepared Regitine in dextrose and water solution. A tachyrhythmia, usually sinus, will most often respond to lowering of the blood pressure; if not, propranolol in 1 mg. boluses may be used. Ventricular irritability usually responds to lowering of the blood pressure; if not, we give lidocaine in doses of 50 to 100 mg. intravenously by bolus infusion.

Postoperative Management

Patients are usually kept in the recovery room or intensive care unit for up to 48 hours, with monitoring of the blood pressure and electrocardiogram (ECG) continuing throughout. After the pulse and pressure are stable, the arterial line is removed and the patient is returned to his room. Recovery may be simple, or the patient may require adrenal steroids and antihypertensive medications. The latter is usually due to continued hypertension from irreversible small vessel disease and/or renal ischemia and rarely is due to a missed tumor. Therapy with alpha-methyldopa and propranolol may be successful. About 10 days after surgery, urinary metanephrine or vanillylmandelic acid (VMA) values can be studied again, as prior measurement may reflect only release of stores of catecholamines rather than new synthesis. If the catecholamine measurements are elevated, treatment with α- and β-adrenergic blockers or α-methyl-para-tyrosine should be started.

Medical Therapy

If the patient refuses surgery, is not a candidate for an operation, has had surgery and still has elevated catecholamine levels, or has a metastatic functioning pheochromocytoma, medical treatment is required. This consists of using appropriate doses of α- and β-adrenergic blocking agents, just as was described for preparation of the patient for surgery. This is usually sufficient, even in patients with functioning metastases. Signs and symptoms may ameliorate or disappear despite the fact that plasma and urinary levels of catecholamines and their metabolites are high. If control is not achieved and paroxysms or continued levels of unacceptable blood pressure remain, α-methyl-para-tyrosine, a false precursor in the synthesis of epinephrine and norepinephrine (investigational) may be used. A 50 to 90 per cent reduction in pressure and urinary values of catecholamines may ensue with improvement in the patient.

Other members of the patient's family should have 24 hour urines examined for catecholamines. If hypercalcemia was a part of the patient's syndrome, this, too, should be looked for in the relatives, along with evidence for medullary thyroid carcinoma.

Medical therapy may continue indefinitely. Metastases usually occur to lung, brain, and bone. Bone lesions may respond to cobalt radiation. In our hands, the other metastases respond to nothing and are soon fatal. Symptoms and signs directly relating to action of the catecholamines can usually be relieved completely or at least in part.

The pregnant patient with a pheochromocytoma is a rare and special case. It is necessary to remove the tumor as soon as possible, and the risk to the fetus must be taken. Best survival for mother and child is said to occur when surgery is attempted in the second trimester. This makes sense, but experience with this condition is limited.

THYROIDITIS

method of
ROBERT L. PEAKE, M.D.
Galveston, Texas

Suppurative Thyroiditis

Acute bacterial infection of the thyroid (with local abscess formation) is rare since the advent of antibiotics. It is usually the result of generalized sepsis or direct extension from infection in adjacent structures in the neck. Symptoms include severe pain, tenderness, and localized swelling and heat in the thyroid. Systemic symptoms of infection and sepsis are present. The organisms most commonly associated are streptococci, staphylococci, pneumococci, and coliforms. Treatment includes appropriate antibiotics (depending on the most likely organism) until cultures and sensitivities are available. With abscess formation, incision and drainage are necessary. Complete recovery is the rule.

Granulomatous Thyroiditis (Subacute, Acute-Nonsuppurative, de Quervain's Thyroiditis)

Granulomatous thyroiditis presents with "sore throat" (pain and tenderness in thyroid), recent thyroid enlargement, pain on swallowing radiating to the jaw and ears, fever to 104°F. (40°C.), and generalized malaise. In addition, the patient often has symptoms of hyperthyroidism with increased nervousness, tremulousness, palpitations, and increased sweating. Circulating thyroid hormones are elevated. Differential diagnosis depends on the tenderness of the thyroid, elevated erythrocyte sedimentation rate (>60 mm. per hour), and a very low 24 hour ^{131}I uptake (most often <2 per cent per 24 hours). This disorder is considered to be a viral infection. It often develops acutely; symptoms increase for 3 to 5 days and persist for 1 to 3 weeks. Severity of symptoms is variable, and there may be recurrences over the subsequent 2 years.

Therapy Directed at Thyroiditis. The disease process is self-limited, but symptomatic relief and reassurance are required. Initial therapy should consist of 0.6 to 0.9 gram (10 to 15 grains) of aspirin every 4 to 6 hours, combined with rest, local heat to thyroid, and sedation. Rarely are narcotics required for pain relief. Aspirin dosage should be maintained for 2 weeks and then tapered gradually over the next 2 to 3 months.

Adrenal steroids may be employed if symptoms are very severe, or if the patient fails to respond to aspirin in 48 to 72 hours. Prednisone or equivalent is given at a dose of 10 to 15 mg. every 6 hours for the first 2 weeks, and then is gradually decreased over the next 6 weeks. Failure to respond to both salicylates and steroids should make one review the diagnosis. It has been found that the acute symptoms can recur as one decreases or discontinues either salicylates or steroids; in such a case, repetition of the aforementioned regimen is required. Recurrences may be more common in patients in whom steroids have been employed, or this may merely reflect the fact that the inflammatory process was more severe.

If thyroid enlargement persists after inflammation and hyperthyroidism have resolved, or in patients with two or more recurrences of the acute syndrome, thyroid hormone in full replacement doses (0.2 mg. of thyroxine or 200 mg. [3 grains] of thyroid extract) should be employed to decrease thyroid size and requirement for function.

Therapy for Associated Hyperthyroidism. Since this is often mild and transient, therapy with sedation (15 to 60 mg. of phenobarbital every 6 to 8 hours) may be all that is required. When hyperthyroidism is more severe, propranolol (Inderal) in doses of 20 to 40 mg. every 6 hours may be used. (This use of propranolol is not listed in the manufacturer's official directive.) Symptoms usually resolve in 2 to 3 weeks even without therapy.

The disease process usually resolves completely (but with the possibility of recurrences for up to 2 years). Transient hypothyroidism may occur, but it is seldom permanent. Rarely, there will be residual scarring and resulting nodularity in the gland, which may be confused with nodular goiter and/or carcinoma.

Chronic Lymphocytic Thyroiditis (Hashimoto's Thyroiditis, Struma Lymphomatosa or Autoimmune Thyroiditis)

This disorder is very common and presents usually as a painless thyroid enlargement. The gland is often asymmetrically enlarged, increased in firmness and lobular (varies from "pebbly" feeling to frank nodularity). This disorder probably accounts for most diffuse goiters in the United States and for at least two thirds of goiters in children and adolescents.

This disorder is familial and autoimmune in pathogenesis, and abnormalities of cell-mediated and humoral immunity have been demonstrated. The use of radioimmunoassay for antithyroglobulin antibodies has demonstrated their presence in 75 to 90 per cent of patients with diffuse goiter. (Tanned red cell and complement-fixing tests are considerably less sensitive.) The patient is usually euthyroid, and thyroid function tests are normal or at the low range of normal. Since this disorder is one of progressive thyroid destruction with resulting fibrosis and scarring, patients may present with hypothyroidism, and this disorder is considered to account for virtually all patients with "idiopathic" or primary hypothyroidism. Transient or mild hyperthyroidism also may be the presenting picture for this disorder (see Silent or Painless Thyroiditis, below).

Although it has been common practice to observe and reassure patients with small diffuse goiter, there is reason to treat all diffuse goiters with thyroid hormone in sufficient doses to suppress thyroid-stimulating hormone (TSH). Minimal degrees of thyroid enlargement (one and a half to three times normal size) can be expected to return to normal size with this treatment. Larger and firmer glands almost always decrease in size but may not return completely to normal. Slow and gradual increase in size, increasing firmness, and increasing nodularity can be expected without treatment. The earlier one treats diffuse goiter, the more complete and satisfactory the response.

Preferred treatment is with L-thyroxine in eventual doses of 0.2 to 0.3 mg. per day (0.15 to 0.2 mg. is usually sufficient to suppress TSH to normal levels). In euthyroid patients, begin at 0.1 mg. for 1 week, then increase to 0.2 mg. for 1 week, and then 0.3 mg. alternating with 0.2 mg., or 0.3 mg. daily. In patients who are hypothyroid or myxedematous, start at 0.025 or 0.05 mg. and increase at 2 to 3 week intervals. Thyroid extract may be used instead, with a final dose of 200 mg. (3 grains) per day. Maximal decrease in the gland usually occurs between 3 and 6 months. With small goiters, one may wish to discontinue therapy after 6 to 12 months to see if thyroid enlargement recurs. If recurrence is seen and in larger glands, thyroid hormone in full replacement doses is continued for life.

Surgery is rarely indicated in diffuse goiter. Indications can be a predominant nodular area which does not concentrate radioiodine, cosmetic concerns, or obstructive symptoms with very large glands. Carcinoma may coexist with lymphocytic thyroiditis, and thus the presence of positive antithyroid antibodies does not exclude carcinoma.

It is also important to remember that multiple areas of decreased or absent uptake are common in thyroid scans in this disorder, and careful correlation of palpable nodules with the appearance of the scan should be made. Before considering surgery for cosmetic or obstructive reasons, one should obtain maximal decrease in gland size with 6 to 12 months of thyroid hormone treatment. It is absolutely essential that all patients treated with subtotal resection of the thyroid be on thyroid hormone in replacement doses for life, because the remaining tissue will again increase in size, and/or the patient will have increased likelihood of hypothyroidism.

Iodide therapy in this disorder, or when used to treat chronic obstructive pulmonary disease, will often cause increasing thyroid size and/or hypothyroidism by blocking thyroid hormone secretion (lithium salts produce a similar effect). Development of hyperthyroidism has also been reported during iodide therapy. For these reasons and the fact that iodine deficiency is very rare in this country, iodide therapy for diffuse goiters is to be discouraged.

Graves' disease may coexist with chronic lymphocytic thyroiditis, and these disorders probably share some elements of autoimmune pathogenesis. This combination probably accounts for patients with exophthalmos without hyperthyroidism (euthyroid Graves' disease) and for the high incidence of hypothyroidism after ^{131}I therapy for Graves' disease.

Silent or Painless Thyroiditis

A newly described syndrome with diffuse goiter and mild and transient hyperthyroidism (lasting only a few weeks) is silent or painless thyroiditis. Patients with mild hyperthyroidism but without goiter have also been described. Except for no history of inflammation and pain in the thyroid, this disorder resembles granulomatous thyroiditis with transient hyperthyroidism, and iodine uptake is very low (<5 per cent). Biopsies to date have revealed chronic lymphocytic thyroiditis, and antithyroglobulin antibodies by radioimmunoassay are positive.

It would appear that this syndrome is another combination of Graves' disease and chronic lymphocytic thyroiditis. Since hyperthyroidism is transient, treatment should consist of sedation (phenobarbital), propranolol (see Granulomatous Thyroiditis, above, for doses) and antithyroid drugs—not ^{131}I therapy. (This use of propranolol is not listed in the manufacturer's official directive.) The main importance is distinguishing this syndrome from Graves' disease.

Riedel's Thyroiditis (Chronic Sclerosing Thyroiditis)

This is a rare disorder associated frequently with chronic sclerosing mediastinitis, retroperitoneal fibrosis, or chronic sclerosing cholangitis. There is progressive destruction and replacement of the thyroid with fibrous tissue. The gland is hard and attached to surrounding tissues with associated involvement of nerves and vessels in the neck or mediastinum. Treatment consists of surgical biopsy and sectioning or removal of the isthmus. More extensive resection is usually impossible and dangerous because of involvement of adjacent structures in the neck. High dose adrenal steroids have also been employed in severe cases and have been beneficial in symptomatic relief. Thyroid function is usually preserved until late in the disease when the patient can become hypothyroid.

Radiation Thyroiditis

Therapeutic doses of ^{131}I for hyperthyroidism often are accompanied with local pain, tenderness, and exacerbation of hyperthyroidism. The clinical picture is identical to that of granulomatous thyroiditis, varying in severity. Treatment consists of aspirin or, rarely, corticosteroids as discussed above. This disorder begins 5 to 10 days after treatment and runs a course of a few days to 1 to 3 weeks.

MALIGNANT CARCINOID SYNDROME

method of
HAROLD BROWN, M.D.
Houston, Texas

The dramatic symptomatology of the classic malignant carcinoid syndrome is usually a late manifestation of the disease, and the physician will be confronted with a long-term management problem. The syndrome is characterized by episodes of flushing, particularly of the upper part of the body, with cyanosis and venous telangiectasia; intestinal hyperperistalsis with abdominal cramps, borborygmi, and diarrhea; a peculiar valvular heart disease with collagenous deposits on the endocardium, particularly of the right side of the heart, resulting in pulmonic stenosis and tricuspid regurgitation and stenosis; and bronchial constriction, which is the least frequent component of the syndrome.

In most subjects with the syndrome the tumor arises from the ileum and there are extensive deposits in the liver, but the origin may be from any portion of the gastrointestinal tract, including the pancreas and gallbladder, the lung, ovary, testis, thyroid, and thymus.

At first the symptomatology was attributed to the elaboration of serotonin, but it is now appreciated that these tumors may secrete other substances, including 5-hydroxytryptophan, histamine, prostaglandins, kallikreins—which form bradykinin—catecholamines, ACTH, melanocyte-stimulating hormone (MSH), insulin, calcitonin, gastrin, antidiuretic hormone (ADH), glucagon, and vasoactive intestinal peptide.

Since patients with the syndrome are usually not surgical candidates, except in specific instances to be detailed, symptomatic therapy is usually employed.

Surgery

Occasionally, the syndrome may arise from carcinoids in the lung, ovary, or testis, and resection may be curative. In most patients there will be extensive hepatic metastases that preclude surgery. Rarely some palliation may be achieved by resection of a large mass of tumor in the liver or omentum. The anesthesiologist should be aware of the tendency of these subjects to develop hypotension, particularly with the administration of sympathomimetic compounds.

Flushing

In some patients the attacks may be precipitated by specific foods, alcohol, or large meals, and avoidance of these factors will diminish attacks. The bouts of flushing may be brought on by emotional upsets, and sedation with tranquilizers such as chlorpromazine (Thorazine) may be effective. The phenothiazines are also mild alpha-adrenergic blocking agents that tend to inhibit kinin formation. Phenoxybenzamine (Dibenzyline), an alpha-receptor blocker, may also be tried, beginning with a dose of 10 to 20 mg. per day and increasing to 60 mg. if necessary. (This use of phenoxybenzamine is not listed in the manufacturer's official directive.)

Corticosteroids in pharmacologic doses have been effective in alleviating the prolonged and incapacitating flushing attacks in patients with bronchial carcinoids.

Gastrointestinal Symptoms

There is considerable evidence that serotonin is involved in the gastrointestinal manifestations, and antiserotonin agents usually give relief. Methysergide (Sansert), a potent antiserotonin agent, can be tried in doses of 2 to 4 mg. as often as every 4 hours, with most of the medication being taken during the period when symptoms are maximal. (This use of methysergide is not listed in the manufacturer's official directive.) One should omit therapy for several weeks every 6 months after gradually decreasing the dose to reduce risk of producing retroperitoneal or other organ fibrosis, which is, however, reversible. Cyproheptadine (Periactin) has also been effective in doses of 4 to 8 mg. two or three times per day. The diarrhea will also respond to traditional antidiarrhea medication such as paregoric or diphenoxylate with atropine (Lomotil).

Heart Disease

The manifestations of heart disease are treated in the usual fashion. Patients with valvular heart disease and intractable failure should be considered for a valvular prosthesis.

Antitumor Therapy

Response to radiation and chemotherapy leaves much to be desired, although radiation is useful to treat local deposits in skin or bone.

Various chemotherapeutic agents have been tried with little success and should be employed only on an investigational basis in desperate situations. It is hoped that new and more effective agents or combinations will be forthcoming.

Asthma

Attacks of bronchoconstriction can be relieved by administration of epinephrine or similar agents via nebulizer. The small amount of drug delivered locally to the lung does not appear to cause exacerbation of the flushing attack or to provoke hypotension.

General

The lifespan of these patients may be decades, and they must be encouraged to tolerate minor discomforts. Their symptoms may vary in intensity from time to time for unknown reasons. Some of the attacks are accompanied by hypotension, which usually resolves without specific treatment. If a vasoconstrictive agent is required, the usual sympathomimetic agents—norepinephrine (Levophed), metaraminol (Aramine), or mephentermine (Wyamine)—are avoided, and only the direct acting α-receptor agents, such as phenylephrine (Neo-Synephrine) or methoxamine (Vasoxyl), should be employed after volume replacement if the patient remains symptomatic.

Patients with marginal food intake and those with high 5-HIAA excretion should receive supplements of 50 to 100 mg. of niacin per day as part of their daily multivitamin supplement.

SECTION 8

The Urogenital Tract

BACTERIAL INFECTIONS OF THE URINARY TRACT (MALE)

method of
LYNN H. BANOWSKY, M.D.
San Antonio, Texas

Asymptomatic bacilluria is rare in either pediatric or adult males. Lower urinary tract irritative symptoms (burning, frequency, urgency) are the most common presenting complaints. If the infection is confined to the lower urinary tract and has not gained access to the patient's bloodstream, fever is usually not a prominent part of the symptomatology (less than 38.3°C. [101°F.]). Fever greater than 38.3°C. (101°F.) should alert the physician to the likelihood of urosepsis, the most common portals of entry being the urethra, prostate, and kidney.

A significant number of men with urinary infections will have as a predisposing factor a structural defect in their urinary tract. The most common abnormalities are various congenital anomalies (e.g., ureteropelvic junction obstruction, ureterovesical reflux), bladder outlet obstruction, urethral stricture, urinary stone, urinary tract fistula, or urinary tract neoplasm. Most patients should have an intravenous pyelogram to exclude significant structural abnormalities. If the infection is severe or becomes chronic, a complete urologic evaluation is indicated.

Treatment

Acute Infections. Patients who present with an acute infection but no urosepsis can be started on a variety of effective oral antimicrobial agents. My own preference is nitrofurantoin macrocrystals, 100 mg. three times daily. Other equally effective drugs are penicillin G, 400,000 units orally four times daily; ampicillin, 250 mg. orally four times daily; trimethoprim, 80 mg.–sulfamethoxazole, 400 mg., 2 tablets orally twice daily; or cephalothin, 250 mg. orally four times daily. Treatment should be continued for 10 to 14 days.

The goal in treating urinary infections is the complete eradication of the offending organism from the urine. For this to be determined, follow-up cultures should be obtained during treatment and at appropriate intervals after cessation of therapy. The persistence of even a low colony count of the same organism indicates that therapy has failed and that additional treatment is indicated. Disappearance of the patient's symptoms is not a reliable index of effective antimicrobial therapy.

Urosepsis. The patient who presents acutely ill with urosepsis not only requires prompt and vigorous antibiotic therapy but also needs prompt urologic evaluation to exclude significant underlying causes of the sepsis such as urinary tract stone or residual urine. As the offending organism is usually not known, a combination of antibiotics should be used initially. Ampicillin, 500 mg. to 1 gram, or cephalothin, 500 mg. to 1 gram, intravenously every 6 hours, and gentamicin sulfate, 3 to 5 mg. per kg. per day in three equally divided doses every 8 hours, is an effective combination for most common urinary tract pathogens. Dosage of these drugs must be adjusted according to the patient's level of renal function.

Chronic Bacterial Prostatitis. The prostate is the usual focus of chronic urinary tract infections in the male. Bacteria residing in the prostate infect the urine and result in symptoms. Most antibiotics do not diffuse well into the prostatic tissue, and as a result permanent eradication of the prostatic focus of infection is difficult. Sterilization of the patient's urine, however, results in complete symptomatic relief. Long-term suppression can be accomplished safely with a variety of antibiotics, including nitrofurantoin macrocrystals, trimethoprim-sulfamethazole, tetracycline, and penicillin G. Selection of the specific drug depends on identification of the organism and its sensitivity pattern.

The selected antibiotics can usually be given in a markedly reduced dose and only twice daily—

e.g., nitrofurantoin macrocrystals, 50 mg. twice daily. The last dose (P.M.) should be given after the patient has voided and just before retiring to bed. This allows the medication to stay in his bladder overnight for maximal effectiveness.

Male Patients with Long-Term Indwelling Urethral Catheters. There are no data to support the use of antibiotics to suppress infection in patients who have long-term indwelling urethral catheters. Infection in these patients is inevitable. The use of antibiotics accomplishes only a change in type of organism or a change in sensitivity patterns—usually to a more resistant strain. Antibiotics in these patients should be reserved for clinical infections.

Supportive Care. Some simple advice can often make the patient much more comfortable until the antimicrobials have had an opportunity to control the infection. Forcing fluids mechanically dilutes and lowers the bacterial count in the bladder. Drinks containing alcohol irritate the bladder, intensify the symptoms of vesical irritability, and should therefore be avoided until the patient is asymptomatic. Warm sitz baths as desired, plus an analgesic such as oral codeine, usually provide adequate symptomatic relief.

BACTERIAL INFECTIONS OF THE URINARY TRACT (FEMALE)

method of
WILLIAM T. BOWLES, M.D.
St. Louis, Missouri

One of the most common diseases treated in the urologist's office is acute cystitis in the female patient. The shortness of the female urethra, the proximity of the periurethral glands, which easily become infected, and the anatomic proximity to the vagina are all factors which may contribute to the increased incidence of lower urinary tract infection in females.

In our office, we obtain a catheterized urine specimen for immediate analysis and culture. Voided urine in the female is not reliable unless the physician himself makes sure that, in the process of obtaining the voided specimen, there is no labial or vaginal contamination. If the diagnosis of urinary infection is made, the patient is placed on appropriate medication and instructed to call back in 48 hours for the results of the culture. If there is no relief of symptoms in the intervening period, the culture results should enable the physician to select the drug of choice. Rapid response to the therapy is the rule; if the patient continues to have symptoms, further investigation is mandatory.

Single Episode of Cystitis

A patient who develops acute cystitis without hematuria should be treated for a minimum of 10 days with the drug of choice. If symptoms and urine have cleared completely at the end of this time, no further investigation is warranted. If the patient noted hematuria during the episode of bladder infection, intravenous pyelogram and cystoscopy should be performed once the infection has cleared. Often, a urinary tract tumor will bleed concurrently with the onset of symptoms of urinary infection, and coincident clearing of the hematuria with the administration of therapeutic drugs may give the practitioner a false sense of security.

Repeated Episodes of Cystitis

Recurrent urinary infections in the female in the absence of congenital abnormalities or stones are almost always reinfections. Stamey has shown that bacteriuria is preceded by colonization of the vaginal vestibule by colonic pathogens. Patients with repeated episodes of cystitis in many cases may be managed with low-dose, antimicrobial prophylaxis once the acute infection has been eradicated. In sexually active women, a low dose of a urinary antimicrobial taken at the time of sexual intercourse may suffice in preventing recurrence of infection. Prophylactic, low-dose therapy may be required for months or years.

If the urine fails to clear rapidly with treatment, the physician should suspect urinary tract disease as a cause of the persistent bladder infection. Intravenous pyelograms will yield important information about the status of the kindeys and drainage systems. Chronic pyelonephritis may be apparent on pyelography, and this finding may necessitate long-term antibiotic therapy to clear the urine. Findings of obstruction of the urinary tract may require surgical correction. Stricture of the ureteropelvic junction, calculous disease, ureteral stricture, or neurogenic dysfunction all may contribute to the chronicity of urinary infection. The presence of persistent pyuria with or without hematuria and the absence of bacteriuria should suggest the possibility of tuberculous genitourinary infection, and appropriate cultures should be obtained.

In addition to intravenous urography, cystography may add important information. It may demonstrate the presence of vesicoureteral regurgitation or reflux which, together with infection, may lead to pyelonephritis and renal destruction. Reflux may be secondary to congenital dysfunction of the ureterovesical valve mechanism or may be secondary to actual or functional obstruction of the vesical outlet. When persistent ureterovesical reflux is noted, surgical correction of the ureterovesical junction may be considered.

Cystoscopy may reveal other causes of recurrent infection such as foreign body in the bladder, bladder diverticulum, or a significant residual urine. The finding of a large residual urine without evidence of bladder outlet obstruction may suggest neurogenic dysfunction of the bladder and require a neurologic evaluation to rule out such diseases as multiple sclerosis, spinal cord tumor, tabes dorsalis, and bladder dysfunction secondary to herniated intervertebral disc.

Persistent Bacteriuria in Older Females

Many septuagenarian and octogenarian females will be discovered to have apyuric bacteriuria without symptoms of bladder infection. The bacteriuria will usually clear rapidly with treatment but will rapidly recur after cessation of therapy. In the presence of normal renal function, it is questionable whether anything is to be gained by treating these asymptomatic patients; however, long-term suppression with antimicrobials will usually maintain urine sterility.

Choice of Drugs (in Order of My Preference)

Sulfonamides. The great majority of initial episodes of cystitis are caused by *Escherichia coli* organisms, which are sensitive to sulfonamides. A good choice would be sulfamethoxazole (Gantanol). An initial dose of 2.0 grams is followed by 1 gram twice daily. The patient should be instructed to maintain an adequate urinary output during sulfonamide therapy.

Nitrofurantoin (Furadantin, Macrodantin). This drug is effective against a wide variety of gram-negative organisms and has the added advantage of not producing resistant colonic bacteria. Severe nausea is occasionally seen and would require the substitution of another agent. Nitrofurantoin is extremely useful in long-term prophylaxis. Doses as low as 50 mg. per day are effective in preventing recurrences.

Sulfamethoxazole-Trimethoprim Combination (Septra, Bactrim). This new drug combination utilizing 400 mg. of sulfamethoxazole and 80 mg. of trimethoprim in a single tablet is quite effective in rapid clearing of bacteriuria. Trimethoprim has the added advantage of preventing vaginal colonization by its properties of diffusion in the vaginal fluid at bactericidal concentrations, and thus is an excellent choice for prophylaxis at low dosage. One-half tablet daily will usually prevent recurrent infections. The usual dosage in the adult for an acute infection is 2 tablets twice daily. It is hoped that trimethoprim alone may become available for use in patients exhibiting allergy to sulfa compounds.

Penicillin. Although not usually indicated by disc sensitivity testing, penicillin G, being rapidly excreted in high dosage in the urine, is often effective against many forms of *E. coli.* Its chief advantage is its low cost. It is also effective against certain strains of *Proteus mirabilis* and is useful in patients with history of struvite stones secondary to the presence of urea-splitting organisms such as *Proteus mirabilis*. The usual dosage would be 500 mg. four times daily.

Nalidixic Acid (NegGram). This agent is effective against a wide range of gram-negative bacteria, including Proteus and Pseudomonas in some patients. It is well tolerated and should be administered in a dose of 1 gram four times daily. Occasional photosensitivity reactions occur, and patients should be warned to avoid direct exposure to sunlight while taking the drug.

Chloramphenicol (Chloromycetin). This drug is used much less frequently than formerly because of the recognition of severe and often fatal blood dyscrasias which may develop secondary to its administration. In severe infections, however, it may be lifesaving, and it is very efficacious in the treatment of certain gram-negative infections. Certainly, it should be utilized only after appropriate sensitivity studies have been performed and the patient has been made aware of the possible hazard.

Methenamine. One of the first agents available for the treatment of urinary tract infections, this drug is still occasionally useful in modern therapeutics. It should be remembered that the drug is excreted in an inactive form and becomes active only when hydrolyzed to formaldehyde in an acid urine. This process takes several hours, and in the presence of frequency of urination the drug is usually eliminated in the inactive form. Administration should be accompanied by periodic testing of the urinary pH to make sure that an acid urine is maintained. The drug is available combined with mandelic acid for acidification as Mandelamine and is usually administered in the dose of 1 gram four times daily. This drug should not be utilized for the treatment of an acute urinary tract infection.

Other Drugs. In resistant infections, sensitivity tests may show that injectable drugs are necessary for proper treatment of the infection. Such treatment should properly be given in the hospital. A wide variety of injectable drugs such as cephalothin, kanamycin, streptomycin, colistin, gentamicin, tobramycin (Nebcin), and amikacin sulfate (Amikin) are available for hospital use.

There are several other oral compounds available, such as cephalexin, carbenicillin, and ampicillin, that are equally effective in urinary tract infections. Because of their high cost, I use these drugs only after appropriate culture and sensitivity testing.

BACTERIAL INFECTIONS OF THE URINARY TRACT (FEMALE CHILDREN)

method of
GEORGE W. KAPLAN, M.D.
San Diego, California

Urinary infections in girls are quite common, as infections of the urinary tract are second in frequency only to infections of the upper respiratory tract in childhood. Significant bacteriuria occurs in approximately 1 per cent of all newborn infants; interestingly, in this age group, there is a male preponderance of infections. However, after the first month of life the sex incidence of urinary tract infection changes and females will predominate. Approximately 1 per cent of schoolgirls will be found to have significant bacteriuria at any given time, and 5 per cent of all girls will have a urinary infection at sometime during their childhood.

The mode of presentation can be quite different from that usually seen in adult females. Although typical lower urinary tract symptoms can occur in children, the usual symptoms of urinary tract infection are nonspecific and include abdominal pain, fever, failure to thrive, gastrointestinal complaints, and foul-smelling urine. Many children are completely asymptomatic. Hence, it is necessary to have a high index of suspicion so that urinary infections will be discovered promptly, thereby, ideally, minimizing morbidity and sequelae.

Urinary infections in girls are among the most underdiagnosed, as well as the most overdiagnosed, problems of childhood. This apparent paradox derives from several different factors. First, in many prepubertal girls, voided urine passes first into the vaginal vault prior to exiting from the introitus; any urine collected by voiding (even by the "clean-catch" method) may be a mixture of bladder urine and vaginal content, resulting in a high incidence of overdiagnosis. Additionally, there is a "sham syndrome" in which lower tract symptoms are present without infection. On the other hand, because the symptom complex is often not characteristic, urinary infections are not sought, and consequently are often underdiagnosed. Children tend to void more frequently than adults, so that infection may be present even though bacterial counts in the urine are less than 10^5 organisms, another frequent source of underdiagnosis.

Urinary infection is not, in and of itself, a final diagnosis, much as anemia is not considered a final diagnosis. There should be an attempt to define the mechanism by which the child became infected to best minimize recurrence of infection. In addition, an attempt at localization of the infection is important, because the long-term implications of pyelonephritis, as opposed to cystitis, may be quite different.

The standard method of urine collection in infants—i.e., the use of a bag applied to the perineum—and voided specimens in older girls are of value only if normal urinalyses and urine cultures are obtained. When there is question about the diagnosis or when one must immediately institute therapy after obtaining a specimen, a more reliable means of obtaining specimens (either suprapubic aspiration or urethral catheterization) should be employed. Many urinary infections in children have the potential to result in renal scarring. Consequently, it is felt that every girl should be studied radiographically with both intravenous urography and voiding cystourethrography following her first documented urinary infection. To avoid subjecting children to unnecessary x-ray exposure and their parents to unwarranted cost, it is quite important that initial diagnosis be as accurate as possible.

The first therapeutic decision that must be made is whether the child with the infection can be safely managed as an outpatient or whether hospitalization is necessary. Many children with upper urinary tract infection will become dehydrated because of inability or unwillingness to drink adequate amounts of fluid. Large urine volumes are an adjunct to therapy, and acidosis from dehydration can complicate management. Hence, high fever, prostration, vomiting, or diarrhea might indicate that in-hospital treatment is preferable. The child ill enough to require hospitalization is probably best managed with intravenous fluids and parenteral antibiotics. Although antibiotic therapy is dictated by the results of urine cultures and sensitivity studies, it is not necessary to wait for the results of these studies prior to initiating therapy. A urine culture is obtained by a reliable method, and therapy is instituted pending the results. Broad-spectrum antibiotics that yield high tissue and urine levels are preferred for initial management. Antibacterial agents have no place in the initial management of serious urinary infections.

Ampicillin can be utilized in doses of 50 to 100 mg. per kg. per day intravenously. When there is known to be a high incidence of ampicillin-resistant organisms or when patients are allergic to penicillin, cephalothin (50 to 100 mg. per kg. per day) or cefazolin (25 to 50 mg. per kg. per day) is a good alternative. For patients suspected of or proved to have organisms resistant to the aforementioned drugs, gentamicin (3 to 5 mg. per kg. per day), kanamycin (15 mg. per kg. per day), colistimethate (2.5 mg. per kg. per day), or carbenicillin (50 to 100 mg. per kg. per day), can be utilized. Tobramycin and amikacin are usually reserved for instances of proved resistance to the aforementioned drugs. Doses of all antibiotics may have to be reduced, depending on the child's level of renal function. If after 48 hours the child is not responding to treatment or if a repeat urine culture is not sterile, therapy should be changed in accord with culture and sensitivity results.

Some children with urinary infections are either unable or unwilling to empty their bladder completely. Residual urine may interfere with the effectiveness of therapy. Consequently, an indwelling catheter is occasionally of benefit as a therapeutic adjunct. This is especially so in the child with vesicoureteral reflux or with lower tract obstruction. Antipyretics are administered to decrease the child's metabolic needs and fluid requirements, and antiemetics are utilized to combat vomiting, when present.

In the child who has a milder infection and is not so seriously ill, outpatient therapy is completely appropriate. If it is thought that the infection is most likely pyelonephritis, oral broad-spectrum antibiotics such as ampicillin (50 to 100 mg. per kg. per day) or cephalexin (50 to 100 mg. per kg. per day) are used. Tetracycline is not utilized in children, because it tends to stain the teeth. Chloramphenicol is not used because of a high incidence of aplastic anemia. If the infection is thought to be in the lower tract only, an agent such as sulfisoxazole (150 mg. per kg. per day), nitrofurantoin (5 to 7 mg. per kg. per day), nalidixic acid (50 mg. per kg. per day), or trimethoprim-sulfamethoxazole suspension is utilized.

For the child who has moderate dysuria, warm sitz baths several times daily are often beneficial in promoting bladder emptying. Phenazopyridine, by and large, is not much help. Because many children develop incontinence with urinary infections, this drug has the disadvantage of permanently staining underclothing and bed sheets. In addition, its dose form is not easily decreased, and methemoglobinemia is a definite hazard of excessive dosage.

Once the initial infection has been treated, obstructive lesions should be sought radiographically and, when present, corrected. The indications for surgical intervention are beyond the scope of this discussion. Therapy of 10 to 14 days is felt adequate for first infections, although there is some evidence that 5 days of therapy may be sufficient. The reinfection rate is quite high, and approximately 80 per cent of girls having one infection will experience a second infection within 2 years of initial diagnosis.

Problems such as infrequent voiding, detergent (bubble bath) use, pinworm infestation, and chronic constipation should be sought and corrected when possible. Urethral dilation has not been shown to be efficacious in eradicating infection in controlled studies, although many uncontrolled studies purport to demonstrate utility. Internal urethrotomy carries some risk of morbidity and probably should not be used in children.

Children with frequent recurrences of infection, especially those proved to have cystitis follicularis or vesicoureteral reflux (when nonoperative management has been elected), are best treated with long-term suppressive antibacterial therapy to prevent reinfection. Because it is largely excreted in the urinary tract and does not alter bowel flora, nitrofurantoin, 25 to 50 mg. once or twice daily, is ideal for this purpose. However, many children cannot tolerate this medication because of gastrointestinal upset. Trimethoprim–sulfamethoxazole has the theoretical advantage of obliterating pathogenic organisms from the vulva; inasmuch as this is the usual reservoir of organisms entering the urinary tract, this drug is also efficacious when administered once a day at bedtime. Other alternatives are sulfisoxazole, methenamine mandelate, and menthenamine hippurate given once or twice daily. When long-term suppressive therapy is utilized, it should continue for a minimum of 6 months in those children with cystitis follicularis or until vesicoureteral reflux has resolved in patients with that problem. All children with proved urinary infections should be followed with periodic urine cultures for a minimum of 1 year following withdrawal of medication.

CHILDHOOD ENURESIS

method of
DOMENICO J. MANZONE, M.D.,
and LOWELL R. KING, M.D.
Chicago, Illinois

Definition

Enuresis is the involuntary voiding of urine at an age by which bladder control should be present. At 2 years of age approximately 40 per cent of children will wet the bed, and at age 5 only 10 per cent of children are still enuretic. It is generally agreed that by 36 months most children will have acquired the necessary inhibitory and facilitating higher cortical centers needed to control voiding, with diurnal preceding nocturnal control.

Etiology

Many theories regarding the etiology of enuresis have been proposed. However, since bed-wetting is a symptom, not a disease, no single explanation will suffice for all cases. The most supported theory cites a delay in the maturation of the inhibitory control mechanisms over bladder functions as the cause of enuresis. The lack of inhibition is consistent with the reduced bladder capacity found in the majority of enuretics, which is functional and accompanied by slight daytime frequency. About one half of enuretics will have cystometrograms similar to those of infants, with elevated intravesical pressure and spike-like detrusor contractions during filling. There is considerable evidence from sleep research to implicate sleep disturbance with altered arousal mechanisms as a major factor in bed-wetting. In the nonenuretic child bladder contractions occur only in REM sleep, and these contractions often result in normal awakening to void. In enuretics uninhibited spike-like detrusor contractions occur in non-REM sleep. The enuretic episode generally starts in stage 4 nondreaming, non-REM sleep, and as sleep lightens to stage 1 or 2, voiding occurs. The belief that it is more difficult to awaken enuretics may be valid, but such a situation could be related to the depth of sleep at the time of enuresis.

Genetic factors play a role in enuresis. Monozygotic twins are concordant for bed-wetting twice as often as dizygotic twins. When both parents have a history of enuresis, 77 per cent of the children will be symptomatic, whereas when one parent has been enuretic, 44 per cent of the offspring will be enuretic. The vast majority of enuretics do not have an underlying psychoneurosis. The cure of enuresis by a variety of nonpsychiatric modalities does not result in symptom substitution by the patient. Of course, psychopathology and enuresis can coexist, and in some situations enuresis and encopresis are behavioral responses in emotionally disturbed children. Environmental factors may be responsible for enuresis or may cause relapse of bed-wetting after a period of control. This is frequently observed in broken homes, after the arrival of a new sibling, or after traumatic separation of mother and child.

Food allergies have recently been found to cause reduced bladder capacity with increased vesical irritability in a small minority of enuretics. Diet therapy with the elimination of offending foods has been successful. Unfortunately IgE levels have not been helpful in identifying these children with food intolerances.

We find a number of enuretics who have pinworm infestation and are cured when the pinworm is eradicated. In the patient with a suspected infestation, we use the Scotch Tape technique to identify the characteristic eggs found on the perineum, and treat the entire family with pyrantel pamoate.

Treatment

Enuresis is "normal" in the younger child, and we feel that it is not proper or worthwhile to treat enuresis in children 3 or 4 years old. Early therapy is less successful, and can be harmful to the developing psyche by underlining the inadequacy of the child. In view of the low incidence of organic lesions (1 to 6 per cent), a full urologic work-up is not necessary in primary enuresis. Prior to commencement of therapy a careful history and physical examination will identify those patients requiring further study. A normal abdominal, spinal, and genital examination and normal urinary stream, in addition to intact perineal sensation, anal sphincter tone, and bulbocavernosus reflex, point to anatomic and neurologic integrity of the child. A normal urinalysis and specific gravity rule out significant renal disease. A negative urine culture excludes undetected bacteria. A higher index of suspicion for organic lesions should be maintained in the adolescent enuretic and in the child with recurrent enuresis. When enuresis is accompanied by a poor urinary stream, abnormal physical findings, or daytime urgency incontinence and dribbling, investigation for underlying organic disease should be undertaken. For this group of patients a urologic work-up should include a voiding cystourethrogram along with excretory urography, and cystoscopy when these radiographic studies are abnormal or questionable. Urodynamic studies, including intravesical pressure, urethral flow, and pelvic floor–external sphincter electromyography, may identify specific voiding dysfunctions in the older persistent enuretic. When enuresis is concomitant with infection, the enuresis will usually stop when infection is eliminated and further infection prevented. After bladder irritation subsides, the child may still have to learn the techniques of normal urinary control.

No single therapeutic plan has proved effective in every patient with enuresis, and a combined approach is often most effective.

Responsibility-reinforcement is based on active participation of the child and includes a progress record kept by the patient with rewards, such as a star on the calendar, for each dry night. A dialogue with the physician takes place in the course of several interviews, and is part of the step-by-step reinforcement. Improvement takes longer than it does in conditioning or drug programs, but the relapse rate is lower. These techniques can be effectively incorporated in other modes of therapy.

Conditioning therapy is based on an electrolytically triggered alarm which evokes two responses: awakening and micturitional reflex inhibition. Ultimately the child will awaken before voiding. The alarm system is cumbersome, needs supervision, and requires a mean period of 16 to 17 weeks to achieve dryness.

Bladder training involves a daily log of voided volumes, forcing fluids, and extending the intervals between voiding. This overtraining by fluid stress eventually improves bladder capacity and ultimately urinary control.

Drug therapy in combination with active participation of the child is most successful in our hands. The basic assumption is that the child himself must wish to change his behavior pattern. We ask the child to stop drinking 1½ hours before bedtime. This is something the cooperative child who wants to stay dry can do, whereas he may not be able to stop wetting the bed. If the child does not restrict fluid voluntarily, he is signaling that he is rebelling, and that there is another problem. If enuresis persists despite fluid restriction, we add imipramine hydrochloride (Tofranil), 25 mg. at bedtime for children 5 to 8 years old, and imipramine pamoate (Tofranil-PM),* 75 mg. for older children; or propantheline bromide (Pro-Banthine),* 7.5 mg. for children aged 5 to 7 and 15 mg. for older children before retiring; or ephedrine sulfate plus atropine sulfate (Enuretrol), 1 tablet for 5 to 10 year old children and 2 tablets for 11 to 15 year old children. These medications, especially imipramine, should be dispensed in childproof packages. The drug and fluid restriction program is continued for 2 to 4 months; if the regimen is successful, we find relapse relatively unusual when the child is weaned from the drug. When imipramine is effective, a measurable increase in functional bladder capacity occurs. Use of imipramine to compensate for a state of immaturity provides an opportunity to control the symptomatic event until further development allows for spontaneous remission. Often imipramine will help interrupt the pattern-habit of enuresis, leaving the child dry when the drug is discontinued.

*See manufacturer's official directive before prescribing Tofranil, Tofranil-PM and Pro-Banthine for enuresis in children.

EPIDIDYMITIS

method of
JEROME P. RICHIE, M.D.
Boston, Massachusetts

Acute epididymitis, or epididymo-orchitis, represents a significant cause of morbidity in males, especially in those between the ages of 20 and 50 years, and results in a high loss of job productivity. This entity is responsible for more time loss in the military than is any other urologic disease. Promptness in establishment of the diagnosis and institution of therapy is essential in order to reduce morbidity and job-related time loss.

Acute epididymitis is an inflammatory process, usually originating in the globus minor at the lower pole of the testicle. The inflammation may spread and involve the remainder of the epididymis, the testicle, and, in severe cases, the surrounding scrotal skin (fixation) or spermatic cord (funiculitis). The onset is usually gradual, with increasing swelling and tenderness of the epididymis; associated irritative symptoms may be present. In the early stages of the disease, the inflamed epididymis may be palpated as a discrete tender area posterior to and separated from the testicle; in such patients the diagnosis is straightforward. In more advanced stages, however, the induration involves the entire testicle, making differentiation from tumor, torsion of the spermatic cord or testicular appendages, hernia, and hydrocele virtually impossible. The Doppler examination may be helpful in distinguishing testicular torsion from epididymitis.

Treatment

1. Absolute bed rest. This may be accomplished on an outpatient basis unless sepsis requiring intravenous antibiotics intervenes.

2. Elevation of the scrotum. The preferred method is by the Bellevue bridge, which consists of placement of wide pieces of tape on the anteromedial thighs to effect scrotal elevation. Other, less satisfactory methods include placement of a rolled towel between the legs and scrotal support.

3. Pain alleviation. Local injection of the spermatic cord at the pubic tubercle with 5 to 10 ml. of 0.5 per cent bupivacaine (Marcaine) will most often result in immediate and dramatic relief of pain. The desired effects tend to persist far longer than the duration of the anesthetic and may be attributed to the relief of spasm. One injection usually will suffice and need not be repeated. Local application of ice packs will also help minimize pain. Oral analgesia with aspirin or propoxyphene

napsylate (Darvocet-N), 100 mg. every 4 hours, may be needed for moderate pain, and aspirin with codeine every 4 hours for severe pain.

4. Systemic antibiotics. Oral or parenteral antibiotics are indicated only in patients with urinary infection (dysuria, pyuria, and frequency), marked tenderness of the prostate on rectal examination, or signs of sepsis. A broad-spectrum antibiotic is preferred, such as tetracycline, 250 mg. four times daily, or cephalexin (Keflex), 250 mg. four times daily. Only a small minority of patients are truly infected and thus require antibiotics.

5. Steroids. These drugs are indicated in every noninfected patient to reduce inflammation, decrease morbidity, and shorten the course of the disease. Prednisone, 80 mg. every other day, is given for a total of five doses, and then discontinued. No adverse effects have been noted with this dosage for this time period.

6. Anti-inflammatory agents. Oxyphenbutazone is not recommended in the therapy of epididymitis. The potential serious or fatal side effects, such as aplastic anemia or leukemia, are too severe to justify use of this agent for benign disease.

7. Surgical intervention. Epididymectomy should be considered in recurrent epididymitis, in a protracted course of epididymitis, and in elderly persons. Epididymo-orchiectomy may be required in patients with marked skin fixation and abscess formation.

Bed rest should be continued until the patient is free of pain. Limited ambulation is then instituted, with gradual return to full function. Scrotal support is generally helpful during the recuperative period.

Induration of the epididymis may take several months to resolve completely, although relief of pain should be obtained in the first several days. Careful follow-up with repeated examination of the scrotal contents is mandatory to ensure complete resolution. Any residual masses may require surgical exploration to exclude malignancy.

BALANITIS AND BALANOPOSTHITIS

method of
ROBERT T. PLUMB, M.D.
San Diego, California

Balanitis is inflammation of the glans penis and posthitis is inflammation of the prepuce. These seldom occur separately, and so the word balanoposthitis is the commonly accepted terminology.

It occurs in local conditions such as phimosis, redundant prepuce, growths on the prepuce or glans, or retention of secretions (smegma) or urine. Precipitating causes are a wide spectrum of bacteria or chronic fungus or yeast, chiefly *Candida albicans* infections.

Management

Simple hygienic procedures are adequate in most patients. These consist of retraction of the foreskin and mild soap and water cleansing with careful drying by patting. The prepuce should not be left retracted because of the fear of paraphimosis. Wet compresses in the more acute inflammatory phase are indicated. Use of a butterfly (gauze with hole cut in it) and Burow's solution, 30 ml. (1 oz.) to 500 ml. (1 pint) of cold water, or Domeboro tablets (aluminum subacetate) to make a solution as directed on the package is mild and effective. The wet compresses are used for 1 hour three to four times per day. In the interval between wet dressings a bland cream is used. This same approach is acceptable in the treatment of infants. Creams or preparations using a gel base, such as betamethasone benzoate (Benisone, Flurobate), betamethasone valerate (Valisone), fluocinolone acetonide (Synalar), or halcinonide (Halog), are more desirable than ointments to prevent maceration in these warm, moist areas. Oral antibiotics are seldom indicated.

Antibiotic creams are also used, but their use should be preceded by smear, culture, or KOH preparation to rule out the presence of a fungal or yeast infection.

Those patients with proved fungal or yeast infection may use one of the following antifungal creams:

For *Candida albicans* infection: amphotericin (Fungizone) or triamcinolone acetonide, nystatin, neomycin sulfate, and gramicidin (Mycolog).

For fungal infections: tolnaftate (Tinactin).

Effective against both yeast and fungi: clotrimazole (Lotrimin), haloprogin (Halotex), or miconazole (Micatin).

For bacterial infections: flurandrenolide with neomycin sulfate (Cordran) or neomycin sulfate and triamcinolone acetonide (Neo-Synalar).

Surgery

Local conservative therapy is usually successful; however, if the foreskin cannot be retracted, a dorsal slit should be done, using 3-0 catgut for hemostasis. A dorsal slit is also advisable if the patient has fever or inguinal lymphadenitis. A careful examination of the glans should be made.

Dark-field examination or biopsy should be done on all lesions. The meatus should be inspected for the presence of a meatal stricture.

A circumcision is the ultimate in cure and should be carried out after acute and subacute lesions have subsided. This eliminates the warm bacterial culture area provided by the foreskin. In the elderly a dorsal slit may be adequate.

Diabetes

Balanitis may be the presenting complaint in patients with undiagnosed diabetes. Studies to rule out diabetes are indicated. Diabetic males are more prone to this problem, and circumcision is recommended.

GLOMERULAR DISORDERS

method of
GEORGE B. THEIL, M.D.
Milwaukee, Wisconsin

Acute glomerular injury may occur through a variety of mechanisms, among which the most well recognized or established are immunologic, toxic, and vascular. A number of specific diseases which produce their effects through one or another of these pathways may be conveniently characterized in outline form by utilizing the format of Table 1, in which the example is that of the glomerulonephritis of systemic lupus erythematosus.

The immunologic basis for damage and glomerular insufficiency has been recognized in a growing number of specific systemic, neoplastic, and infectious diseases in which the antigen, antibody, and its resultant complexes have been at least partially deciphered. Circulating antibody may also be directed toward normal or possibly altered glomerular basement membrane, as in Goodpasture's syndrome or rapidly progressive proliferative glomerulonephritis (RPGN). An immunologic mechanism is probable in several other recognized forms of renal damage in which the antigen or potential antigen and its evoked antibody have not been as well defined—e.g., membranous glomerulopathy and the Schönlein-Henoch syndrome. The evidence for these being immunologically mediated is the frequent demonstration on immunofluorescent staining of kidney biopsy specimens of deposits containing complement and/or other immunoglobulin components. There remains a pool of idiopathic disorders principally under the heading of the idiopathic or minimal lesion nephrotic syndrome, in which "immunologically oriented" therapy (a glucocorticoid and/or an immunosuppressive compound) is effective, although there is no conventional evidence that an immunologic mechanism is operative. Toxic glomerular nephropathy, although a complex phenomenon, is most probably caused by direct chemical injury to either tubular or glomerular components or both. Classically, the aminoglycoside antibiotics (most recently, gentamicin and amikacin) are the offending agents. Other toxic nephritides such as that produced by methicillin probably work through a hypersensitivity mechanism to effect their damage in addition to direct interstitial and glomerular injury. Although the precise mechanisms have not been unequivocally worked out, the functional effect is that of impairment of glomerular filtration. A vascular basis for glomerular disorders can be obstructive owing to disseminated intravascular clotting or clotting in the kidney per se, or may fall under the heading of vasculitis, associated either with fibrinoid necrosis alone or with actual cellular infiltration of arterioles or medium-sized arteries. Glomerular insufficiency is related to accelerated or malignant hypertension; Shwartzman or Shwartzman-like reactions, including the hemolytic-uremic syndrome; and diseases of unknown cause, such as polyarteritis nodosa. The last-named condition may prove ultimately to relate to a somewhat different mechanism through a hepatitis-associated antigen. It is therefore obvious that there may exist an overlapping of causal factors. This is best exemplified by the Shwartzman reactions and polyarteritis nodosa, in which all three of the basic mechanisms may participate.

The spectrum of potentially injurious agents thus presents a diagnostic and then a therapeutic challenge to the clinician and emphasizes the need for a careful differential diagnosis when a patient has the history, physical signs, and laboratory data compatible with acute glomerular involvement. In general, the more profound and chronic the disease process, the greater the clinical and biochemical dislocations will be (Table 2). None of the values in any of the columns are proposed to be absolute, but are tabulated for ready refer-

TABLE 1. **Levels of Sophistication in the Description of Glomerular Disorders***

A. Mechanism of disease
   Immunologic
B. Etiology
   Deposition of complement-linked DNA–anti DNA complexes in the subendothelial and other regions of the renal glomeruli
C. Other mediators of glomerular damage
   Polymorphonuclear rhexis, protease and lysozyme liberation, kinin release, activation of the complement cascade and of the clotting mechanism
D. Functional assessment
   See Table 2
E. Pathogenesis
   Frequently progressive glomerular compromise unless therapy is instituted with glucocorticoids, immunosuppressive agents, or both
F. Clinical syndrome
   Systemic illness with pleuropericarditis, hematologic abnormalities, arthritis, other multisystem manifestations, and/or the nephrotic syndrome
G. Therapeutic response
   Generally good

*Example given is for the glomerulonephritis associated with systemic lupus erythematosus.

TABLE 2. **Functional Assessment of Renal Glomerular Insufficiency**

DEGREE OF SEVERITY	CLINICAL SYMPTOMS*	BLOOD UREA NITROGEN (MG./DL.)	CREATININE CLEARANCE (ML./MIN.)	BLOOD PRESSURE (MM. HG)	HEMOGLOBIN (GRAMS/DL.)	TOTAL SERUM BICARBONATE (MEQ./LITER)
0	None	15	100	130/80	14	25
1+	None	25	50	150/90	12	20
2+	Rare	50	25	160/100	10	15
3+	Occasional	100	10	170/110	8	10
4+	Usually	200	5	180/120	6	5

*Obviously influenced by the systemic manifestations of the disease associated with the renal problem.

ence to approximate the clinical and laboratory findings which can be expected. The physician must appreciate that occasionally there might be a deviation or exaggeration of one of these abnormalities. However, in general, as the glomerular filtration rate decreases, anemia, hypertension, and azotemia parallel each other in degrees of severity. In addition, when such a patient has oliguric renal insufficiency with salt and water retention, electrolyte abnormalities, and acidosis, it may be difficult to immediately differentiate an acute or rapidly progressive glomerular disorder from other sudden and primarily nonglomerular renal insults such as bilateral renal artery occlusion, obstructive uropathy, or even acute tubular necrosis. The possibility of the latter diagnosis should alert the clinician to consider early in the course a complete urologic work-up. The physician must also be aware of the consequences of the renal functional compromise, including the acquired susceptibility to lower doses of many therapeutic agents which are potentially toxic. It should also be emphasized that the usual case presenting with chronic persistent and/or progressive glomerular deterioration is not readily classifiable, and thus the tabulations under many of the headings in Table 1 will be essentially blank and not as nicely illustrated as in the example given of systemic lupus erythematosus with glomerulonephritis.

The hallmark of significant glomerular disease, in addition to proteinuria, is the measurement of glomerular filtration which can be approximated clinically by the creatinine clearance. Clinicians are frequently at a loss to assess with confidence the trend of glomerular filtration. This observation is of critical importance relative to when therapy should be started or stopped or to evaluate the effects of therapy or changes caused by the disease. The following formula provides an approach to a reasonably precise estimation of significant changes of glomerular filtration:

$$td = \frac{\overline{X}^1 - \overline{X}^2}{W^1 + W^2}$$

$\overline{X}^1$ and $\overline{X}^2$ are the mean of 4 hour creatinine clearances done on 3 successive days during the initial or basal examination ($\overline{X}^1$) and any other follow-up examination ($\overline{X}^2$). W^1 and W^2 represent the respective difference between the high and the low 4 hour creatinine clearance on these same 3 successive days during the two periods to be compared, W^1 being the initial and W^2 being the follow-up difference. A value exceeding 0.5 is indicative of a significant change in glomerular filtration rate. The renal biopsy remains an important adjunctive tool which can provide the clinician with either a definitive answer or appropriate clues regarding the nature of the glomerular insult or other renal lesions which suppress normal glomerular filtration.

General Treatment Measures of Glomerular Disorders

Experience for most of the general measures is derived from patients with the classic immunologic disorder, acute post-streptococcal glomerulonephritis, or from patients with acute reversible renal insufficiency (acute tubular necrosis).

Bed Rest. Whether or not strict bed rest is employed is dictated by the severity of the clinical symptoms and should obviously be enforced most diligently when cardiovascular complications are present. Confinement to bed is generally limited to the period of any associated acute cardiovascular involvement, and physical activity is then gradually increased as tolerated, regardless of persistent hematuria and proteinuria. There is no evidence that prolonged bed rest or restrictions of normal tolerated physical activity influence the subsequent course of these diseases.

Diet. When the patient is first seen, oral intake should be limited to approximately 1 liter of relatively potassium- and sodium-free liquids containing sufficient calories (400 or more) in the form of carbohydrate to alleviate ketosis and lessen endogenous protein catabolism. This regimen permits evaluation of the degree of renal functional restriction, oral tolerance, and the clinical status while appropriate electrolytes, acid-base parameters, and nonprotein nitrogenous constituents are measured. This is of particular importance when the disease is acute, symptomatic, and associated with suppression of renal function. In patients with the least severe disease, a general diet with liquids ad libitum and modest dietary sodium restrictions (4 grams of sodium chloride daily which contains approximately 70 mEq. of sodium) is prescribed. In more severe disease, sodium restriction to 2 grams of sodium chloride (35 mEq. of sodium) and protein to 0.5 gram per kg. of body weight per day is indicated, together with some restriction of the amount of total fluid intake. With oral intolerance or in the severely oliguric patient, parenteral replacement and maintenance are used in the form of 10 to 20 per cent dextrose in water. This allows appropriate restriction of the volume of fluid intake (500 to 800 ml. daily) to make up for the average insensible fluid loss plus an amount equivalent to the urine output for the previous 24 hours.

Nausea. Nausea can be decreased by chlorpromazine (Thorazine), 10 to 25 mg. intramuscularly, or other comparable antinausea agents. Promethazine hydrochloride (Phenergan), administered intramuscularly (12.5 to 25 mg.), may be an effective sedative. If possible, avoid the use of sedatives or other drugs which depend principally on renal excretion for their route of elimination from the body, particularly when renal functional impairment is evident. Meperidine (Demerol) may be used for pain.

Antibiotics. The use of antibiotics should be dictated by the nature of any accompanying or precipitating infection, administering a loading dose and adjusting the maintenance doses to the metabolism of the antibiotic and to the degree of impairment of kidney function. Routine urine cultures should also be done, because some acute and even chronic renal glomerular disorders may have accompanying genitourinary infections.

Treatment of Complications

In addition to the general measures outlined above, a number of complications resulting from renal decompensation are quite common and may need treatment. Some of the complications may be prevented, and the patient should be evaluated continuously with this thought in mind.

Congestive Heart Failure. Attention should be directed to the treatment of the increased volume expansion so common to heart failure in this setting. A trial of diuretics such as furosemide (Lasix) is useful and may be successful by inducing a prompt and adequate diuresis. Digitalization can be accomplished by one of the conventional programs. The dose schedule is dictated by the rapidity with which digitalization is desired and must be modified for the degree of renal insufficiency present. If oliguria is present to any appreciable degree or if the patient has bradycardia, digitalization and digitalis maintenance become more difficult. Electrolyte abnormalities, particularly hyperkalemia or hypokalemia or rapid changes from high serum potassium to relatively low serum potassium values, make the digitalized patient extremely vulnerable to digitalis toxicity and potentially serious arrhythmias.

Hypertension. Mild hypertension will not require definitive therapy and may actually be prevented from becoming a serious threat by careful attention to salt and water balance (volume control). Occasionally a more vigorous approach than bed rest and sodium and water restriction may be required. Antihypertensive drugs, in general, can adversely affect the glomerular filtration rate, and, if moderately severe nitrogen retention is present (plasma or serum urea nitrogen greater than 100 mg. per dl.), caution must be exercised to avoid further impairment of renal function with sudden dropping of systemic arterial pressure. This is usually a more important consideration, however, in the long-term management in chronic renal insufficiency. Hydralazine, diazoxide, and/or nitroprusside can support the patient during a hypertensive crisis. Other agents are rarely necessary if attention is given to fluid overload as outlined in the preceding discussions of general management and congestive heart failure.

Electrolyte Disturbances. In addition to usually mild obligatory renal sodium wastage, potassium loss and hypokalemia may occur and may be accentuated by the use of diuretic agents. Oral replacement in doses of 2 to 4 grams potassium chloride (30 to 70 mEq. K) daily are then indicated. Hypokalemic nephropathy is an avoidable added insult. If hyperkalemia is a problem, glucose and insulin, calcium, oral sorbitol or lactulose, potassium-binding resins, or dialysis may be used, together with absolute potassium restriction. Hyperkalemia is potentially life threatening and must be treated immediately and expertly.

Acidosis. For symptomatic acidosis, additional sodium in the form of bicarbonate, citrate, or a flavored lactate solution is employed orally, together with protein restriction to 0.5 gram per kg. per day or less to reduce the fixed acid load. Shohl's solution (140 grams of citric acid and 98 grams of sodium citrate in 1 liter of water), 10 to 20 ml. four times daily (40 to 80 mEq. Na^+), may also be employed.

Anemia. Anemia will not require treatment if the patient is asymptomatic or if the packed cell volume is above 25 per cent. Symptomatic anemia is best treated by the cautious use of packed red cells, 1 unit daily for 3 successive days.

Metabolic Bone Disease. Hyperparathyroidism is a problem only in the chronically acidotic or hyperphosphatemic patient. The effects of hyperparathyroidism may be suppressed by prescribing appropriate doses of oral calcium and vitamin D and instituting dietary phosphate restriction and oral gel therapy directed at decreasing gastrointestinal phosphate absorption.

The general measures outlined above address the treatment of the abnormalities which arise as a result of glomerular disease, which itself may present with a variable degree of severity and may also vary in the individual rate of progression. There are more certitude and hard data available in treating these sequelae of glomerular disorders than in treating the underlying "cause" of the disease. The most obvious exceptions are the toxic disorders, in which the offending agent can be discontinued if it is part of therapy, or immunologic glomerular disease associated with certain malignancies, in which their removal will generally reverse the kidney disease. The same is true for treating the glomerular disorders associated with infections such as bacterial endocarditis or infected ventriculoatrial shunts. There are also case reports in the literature describing impressive successes with glucocorticoids, immunosuppressive drugs, heparin or sodium warfarin anticoagulation, acetylsalicylic acid, dipyridamole, and indomethacin; the latter five drugs are directed at protecting the glomeruli from reactions which follow the hosts' response to immune complexes or cytotoxic antibodies. It is important to emphasize that the results in careful studies (in which the glomerulopathy is reasonably well defined and a format such as Table 1 is employed) are usually *less* optimistic and *more* conservative than in the wealth of isolated and many times empiric uncontrolled observations. Table 3 attempts to list the additional diseases or disease settings in which treatment is accepted to be of value or probable value in the resolution of the *acute* or profound glomerular disorder. The term "immunosuppressive agents" refers to cyclophosphamide or azathioprine. Prednisone is the oral glucocorticoid generally used, and hydrocortisone is the preferential drug for parenteral therapy. A word of caution must be injected at this point. The physician is required to consult the accepted indications for a given drug as compiled in periodicals such as the Physicians' Desk Reference and particularly the inserts in the drug package which outline the accepted indications. They must be specifically stated or the patient informed regarding the exceptions to drug use.

A Special Manifestation of Glomerular Involvement

The *nephrotic syndrome* may be caused by any of a number of factors producing glomerular damage with increased permeability and massive proteinuria. In general, it is characterized by proteinuria exceeding 3 grams daily, hypoalbuminemia, hypercholesterolemia, hyperlipidemia, double refractile lipoid bodies in the urinary sediment, sodium retention, and anasarca. Other manifestations include an increased susceptibility to infections and occasion-

TABLE 3. **Treatment of Glomerular Disorders**

GROUPING	SPECIFIC THERAPY OF ACCEPTED OR PROBABLE VALUE
Immunologic	
Bacterial endocarditis	Appropriate antibiotics
Infected arteriovenous shunts	Appropriate antibiotics
Other infections	Appropriate antibiotics
Glomerulopathy with neoplasia	Treat the underlying malignancy
Systemic lupus erythematosus	Glucocorticoids, immunosuppressive agents
Idiopathic membranous glomerulopathy	Glucocorticoids
Schönlein-Henoch purpura	Glucocorticoids, immunosuppressive agents
Goodpasture's syndrome	Bilateral nephrectomy?, plasmapheresis?, glucocorticoids
RPGN	Glucocorticoids, immunosuppressive agents
Toxic	
Drug-induced neuropathy	Discontinue medication; see recommendations under specific drug nephrotoxicity
Vascular	
Hemolytic-uremic syndrome	Antihypertensive agents Glucocorticoids? Treat any associated infection
Other	
Minimal-lesion nephrotic syndrome	Glucocorticoids, cyclophosphamide
Wegener's granulomatosis	Glucocorticoids, immunosuppressive agents
Shwartzman reaction with disseminated intravascular clotting	Glucocorticoids, heparin Treat any associated infection

ally significant hypovolemia or even hypovolemic shock. A variable degree of glomerular insufficiency can accompany the nephrotic syndrome.

The list of recognized disease processes and toxic agents that may provoke this syndrome is large indeed, and any of the agents discussed previously can be responsible. The prognosis and the type of treatment employed are functions of the precipitating disease, which emphasizes again the need for a complete diagnostic work-up. A renal biopsy should be done in virtually every patient with the nephrotic syndrome. The most successful outcome is to be expected in the minimal-lesion nephrotic syndrome. The glucocorticoids are the main therapeutic agents employed in most patients. It is not within the province of this therapeutic outline to debate the merits of the individual hormones that have been employed. Steroidal dosages may be calculated according to their anti-inflammatory equivalents with respect to cortisone or hydrocortisone. The major considerations are the induction of diuresis and reversal of proteinuria, a program of maintenance, and, finally, the withdrawal of steroids. When therapy is entirely successful, all urinary, biochemical, and clinical findings of "nephrosis" revert to normal. Prognosis should be somewhat guarded, as late relapses may occur; fortunately, they are frequently responsive to treatment with steroids. Cyclophosphamide is an important alkylating agent which may be used in conjunction with prednisone to treat such relapses or corticosteroid-resistant minimal-lesion nephrotic syndrome. (This use of cyclophosphamide is not listed in the manufacturer's official directive.) The dose employed is approximately 2 mg. per kg. of body weight as a single daily dose. The physician must consult the appropriate literature to assess the type and success of therapy in the individual patient (cause of the nephrotic syndrome), as many systemic diseases, among other agents, may cause a nephrotic syndrome.

General Management

Diet. The diet should be low in sodium, containing at least initially from 0.5 to 1 gram of sodium chloride (10 to 20 mEq. Na) per day and should contain at least 1 gram of protein per kg. of body weight. Because of problems with the palatability of very low sodium diets, consultation with the hospital dietitian should be sought.

Induction of Diuresis. Prednisone is given in a dosage of 1 mg. per kg. of estimated dry weight for 6 to 8 weeks, although in minimal-lesion nephrotic syndrome usually no more than 4 weeks of prednisone is required. If this trial is unsuccessful, a repeat course may be indicated following a rest period of 5 to 7 days without steroids. Profuse diuresis may begin in the drug-free interval. If more than one intensive course is necessary, the steroid may be started at a higher level or another steroid may be selected and started in equivalent high doses. Cyclophosphamide, as outlined above, may be used when indicated.

Maintenance Therapy. Maintenance prednisone should be continued after the onset of diuresis. However, the steroid dose is now given 3 days per week (approximately every other day). The program may have to be continued for 1 year, although clinical judgment and the nature of the case may be such that withdrawal of maintenance steroids can be accomplished at a much earlier date. We should obviously guard against the tendency toward continuing pharmacologic doses of glucocorticoids when the patient's disease is proved refractory.

Steroid Withdrawal. The maintenance dose is decreased by 25 per cent every week, and then the hormone therapy may be discontinued if the patient's urine remains protein free or there is minimal proteinuria.

Additional Considerations. 1. The systemic use of chlorothiazide or furosemide is of value in patients who are edematous, and should be given in conjunction with the steroid. Other diuretics, either alone or in combinations, should also be used when indicated.

2. As a rule, potassium supplementation is not necessary and need not be used routinely prior to the onset of diuresis. Once diuresis has been established, the plasma level provides an adequate index of body need in this situation. If the level is borderline low (3 mEq. per liter or less), a daily dose of 2 to 4 grams of potassium chloride (30 to 70 mEq. K) may be administered orally.

3. Thoracentesis and abdominal paracentesis for the removal of small amounts of fluid are justified for respiratory embarrassment or physical comfort, and have been reported to be associated occasionally with the onset of significant diuresis.

4. Parenteral salt-poor serum albumin, 1 unit (25 grams) on 3 successive days, can be a valuable therapeutic adjunct in effecting diuresis.

5. Evidence of nitrogen retention, hyperglycemia, or an elevated blood pressure is not a contraindication to glucocorticoid therapy, but must be approached and treated knowledgeably. The same admonition applies to the awareness of any of the potential hazards when intensive steroid or immunosuppressive therapy is used.

6. Spironolactone in doses of up to 50 mg. four times daily may be a useful diuretic in nephrotic states, in which there is usually excess aldosterone excretion.

PYELONEPHRITIS

method of
C. RITCHIE SPENCE, M.D.
Fort Sam Houston, Texas

Introductory Remarks

Acute pyelonephritis refers to a focal inflammatory reaction to the renal parenchyma and/or collecting system. It is usually caused by gram-negative organisms which originate from the intestinal flora. *Escherichia coli* is the most common organism (75 per cent), followed by Klebsiella, Enterobacter, *Proteus mirabilis,* Pseudomonas, and *Streptococcus faecalis.*

Several pathways by which bacteria may reach the kidney have been suggested, including the lymphatic, hematogenous, and, most importantly, ascending pathways. As women are affected more often than men by a wide margin, it necessarily follows that the ascending route is most favored owing to the shorter urethra in the female. Pyelonephritis in the male is most uncommon and probably results from an established focus of infection in the prostate or the presence of obstructive uropathy.

Treatment

Supportive Measures. 1. *Activity:* The patient is placed at bed rest.

2. *Fluids:* Fluids are administered, preferably via the parenteral route, for first 24 to 48 hours until such time as the clinical status of the patient can be ascertained with confidence. Two thousand to 3000 ml. is optimal intake whether intravenously or by mouth.

3. *Diet:* Clear liquids are given if the patient's clinical condition permits; otherwise, nothing by mouth.

4. *Fever:* If the patient's temperature is greater than 101°F. (38.3°C.), consider acetylsalicylic acid every 4 hours, either by mouth (650 mg. [10 grains]) or by rectal suppository (1300 mg. [20 grains]). Consider *cooling measures* for a temperature greater than 103°F. (39.4°C.).

5. *Pain:* Codeine sulfate (30 to 60 mg.) or meperidine hydrochloride (50 to 75 mg.) intramuscularly every 4 hours may be necessary for relief.

Antibiotics. General Considerations. If the patient has no prior history of urinary infections and a nosocomial cause is unlikely, *Escherichia coli* will most often be the causative organism. Therapy should be initiated as soon as possible and directed against *Escherichia coli* until such time as the urine culture can verify the choice of antibiotic.

A history of recurrent pyelonephritis or a nosocomial (i.e., instrumentative) cause should alert one to the possibility of other, more resistant organisms such as Proteus, Klebsiella, and Pseudomonas. If the culture reveals Proteus, a careful search for urinary stone should be initiated.

It should be emphasized that the parenteral route is preferred during the initial phases of therapy. This ensures optimal blood levels of antibiotics and avoids gastrointestinal intolerance caused by an oral antibiotic or that associated with the pyelonephritis. It is suggested, then, that an antibiotic be chosen which is available in both parenteral and oral forms. If, after 48 to 72 hours, the clinical condition has improved significantly, the oral form may be substituted, provided sensitivity studies confirm the suitability of the medication.

Pregnancy will limit the choice of antibiotics. It has been suggested that sulfonamides be avoided during the last trimester because of the possible development of hyperbilirubinemia and kernicterus. Other authors hold that the risk is theoretical at best and use sulfonamides during all phases of pregnancy without reported difficulty. Tetracycline should be avoided without question during pregnancy owing to its potential for causing discoloration of deciduous teeth in the fetus and producing fatal hepatotoxicity in the mother.

Chloramphenicol should be avoided in all patients unless sensitivity studies specifically permit no other medication.

Specific Antimicrobials. The following drugs which have a parenteral and oral form are recommended:

1. *Ampicillin,* 1 to 2 grams intravenously over a 30 minute period every 6 hours. Oral dose is 250 to 500 mg. every 6 hours.

2. *Cephalothin,* 1 to 2 grams intravenously over a 30 minute period every 6 hours. Oral dose is 250 to 500 mg. every 6 hours.

3. *Carbenicillin,* 2 to 5 grams intravenously over a 1 hour period every 4 hours. Carbenicillin should not be used alone because of the rapid development of resistance, but, instead, with another drug (e.g., gentamicin) for serious infections caused by Pseudomonas, Enterobacter, and indole-positive Proteus. Oral dose is 2 tablets every 6 hours.

The following drugs are available in parenteral form only:

1. *Gentamicin sulfate,* 3 mg. per kg. of body weight (total daily dose) given in divided doses intramuscularly every 8 hours for 5 to 7 days.

2. *Kanamycin,* 1 gram intramuscularly immediately, followed by 500 mg. intramuscularly every 12 hours for 5 to 7 days.

3. *Tobramycin,* 1 to 1.5 mg. per kg. of body weight (total daily dose) given in divided doses every 8 hours intramuscularly. This drug may be more effective against Pseudomonas than is gentamicin.

The following antimicrobials are available in oral form for long-term management after parenteral therapy has been concluded:

1. *Nitrofurantoin macrocrystals (Macrodantin),* 50 to 100 mg. by mouth every 6 hours.

2. *Sulfonamides:* Sulfisoxazole (Gantrisin), 1 gram every 6 hours, or sulfamethoxazole and trimethoprim combination (Septra or Bactrim), 2 tablets twice daily.

3. *Nalidixic acid (NegGram),* 1 gram every 6 hours.

4. *Tetracycline,* 250 to 500 mg. every 6 hours, or one of the newer synthetic tetracyclines, such as doxycycline (Vibramycin), 100 mg. daily, which, unlike any other tetracycline, has the added advantage of being useful in patients with impaired renal function.

Duration of Therapy

The controversy regarding length of therapy still persists. For initial, uncomplicated pyelonephritis, I prefer 14 to 21 days of total therapy (parenteral and oral). If the episodes are recurrent and the culture demonstrates the same organism, then my preference is for 6 weeks of total therapy. The occasional patient may require a long-term low-dose regimen (e.g., nitrofurantoin macrocrystals [Macrodantin] once or twice a day) for control.

Follow-up

After treatment the patient should have follow-up cultures at 2 weeks, at monthly intervals for 3 months, and then every 3 months up to 1 year. All patients with a history of pyelonephritis should have a complete urologic evaluation to include excretory urography, voiding cystourethrography, and cystoscopy.

TRAUMA OF THE GENITOURINARY SYSTEM

method of
NORMAN R. ZINNER, M.D.,
and NAND S. DATTA, M.D.
Los Angeles, California

Introduction

The presence of hematuria—whether gross or microscopic—in an injured patient must always raise the suspicion of injury to the genitourinary system. The converse is not true. The absence of hematuria in an injured patient does *not* eliminate the possibility of severe damage. The physician must be aware of the possibility of urinary tract injury from the nature of the incident and retain an index of suspicion whenever a question exists.

To illustrate, complete avulsion or transection of the renal pedicle from an automobile accident or gunshot wound may result in a normal urinalysis. Similarly, the urine in patients with unilateral ureteral transection from external trauma or by ligation during pelvic surgery will be clear in about half the cases.

The general management of the patient with genitourinary system injury begins in the emergency room when the patient is first seen and the injury suspected. The management of the specific lesion follows afterward.

In presenting our approaches to management, we take the reader to the emergency room where the patient first appears and trace the steps to be taken in the sequence required.

General Approach to Genitourinary Injuries

Abdominal Trauma Which Appears to Spare the Bladder. These types of injuries fall into two categories: penetrating injuries, such as gunshot or stab wounds to the mid or upper abdomen; and blunt trauma which involves the abdomen without fracture of the bony pelvis but may be associated with fracture of lower ribs or transverse processes of lumbar vertebrae. Renal and ureteral injuries should be considered in patients with injuries in either category. Since virtually all the patients with penetrating abdominal wounds will be explored surgically (because of the high incidence of abdominal visceral damage), the kidneys and possibly the ureters can be examined directly. Nonetheless, preoperative tests can be most important, because an injury may be missed or the extent not well appreciated. At the least, besides a urinalysis, the intravenous pyelogram (IVP) is most revealing. By contrast, patients sustaining blunt trauma are sometimes managed by expectant observation, and tests are even more vital here. The urologic considerations for observation will be discussed later.

The initial general management depends largely upon the patient's condition, the effectiveness of resuscitative therapy, and the facilities available at the time. All such patients will require intravenous fluids, airway maintenance, and some x-ray studies. Accordingly, the approach to the genitourinary system can begin at the time the patient arrives in the emergency room and the intravenous infusion is started.

1. Inject 50 to 100 ml. of suitable urologic

contrast material into the intravenous line directly or hang 150 ml. of isotonic saline solution with 150 ml. of contrast material onto the intravenous system by piggyback technique. This will permit later excretory urography (IVP) without extending the preoperative time period.

2. Catheterize the patient and examine the urine.

3. Monitor urine output.

4. Evaluate renal function, assess renal or ureteral damage, and study for urinary extravasation when the usual kidney-ureter-bladder film (KUB) is made.

If the patient is rushed to the operating room without radiologic examination in the emergency room, intraoperative roentgenograms can then be made to at least establish the presence of a functional contralateral kidney should nephrectomy be required for the injured kidney.

Abdominal Trauma Which Appears to Involve the Bladder. Injuries to the bladder from penetrating wounds are variable but should be considered if the wound of entry or exit is in the lower abdomen or when clinical signs suggest the possibility of bladder involvement. Bladder injury should be suspected in blunt trauma which has produced fractures of the bony pelvis. It will be found in 25 per cent of such patients. It should also be suspected in alcoholic patients who come to the emergency room after having fallen while inebriated and with a full bladder.

When bladder involvement is suspected, a cystogram should precede the excretory urogram. The following cystographic sequence is performed:

1. Catheterize the patient and examine the urine. Remember the urine may be normal even if bladder rupture is massive.

2. Obtain a cystogram with a rapid four film sequence as follows:

Film No. 1—KUB with patient supine. (This also provides any other information needed from the KUB.)

Film No. 2—Let 100 ml. of suitable contrast medium run into the bladder under gravity. If extravasation is seen, empty the bladder and conclude the study at this point.

Film No. 3—If there is no extravasation in Film No. 2, continue from a height of about 30 cm. above the bladder. This is done most simply by attaching an Asepto syringe without its bulb to the catheter which is extended vertically. Do not force the fluid in. The purpose of the low volume film is to avoid continued bladder filling if there is massive extravasation, as shock can be worsened if large quantities of the hypertonic contrast material enter the peritoneal cavity. In the high volume film, this can be suspected if the fluid suddenly starts running much faster than it did at the start.

Film No. 4—Drain the bladder and rinse it with saline. Any extravasation which was previously obscured by the contrast-filled bladder will now be evident, as it will not be washed out by the saline irrigation and the bladder is empty.

This entire sequence requires 5 or 10 minutes, and the patient can be otherwise attended. He need not be turned from side to side. Fluoroscopic control will substitute for Films 2 and 3 if available.

3. Now inject 50 to 100 ml. of a suitable intravenous contrast material as in Step 1 for abdominal trauma which appears to spare the bladder.

4. Monitor urine output.

5. Expose the intravenous pyelogram (IVP) films when appropriate.

By performing the cystogram before the IVP, the diagnosis of urinary extravasation from the bladder is not confused with extravasation of contrast material from an injured lower ureter. Furthermore, if the IVP is done first, contrast material will squirt continually into the bladder from the ureter. Even with continuous catheter drainage, it is very difficult to keep the bladder completely empty, and the small amount of contrast agent within the bladder may mimic extravasation after the postwashout (fourth) film.

Pelvic and Genital Trauma Involving the Male Urethra. Clinical management focuses here on the distinction between urethral injuries *above* the urogenital diaphragm (external urethral sphincter) and those *below* the urogenital diaphragm. The approach to treatment is entirely different for the two, and misunderstanding can lead to severe consequences. Fortunately, the clinical distinction is not difficult.

Lacerations and avulsions above the diaphragm occur in blunt trauma to the pelvis and are usually associated with bony pelvic fractures. There is no bleeding from the urethral meatus, because blood is trapped proximal to the external sphincter. On rectal examination, the prostate may be palpated high in the pelvis, having been dislocated from its normal low lying position.

Lacerations and crush injuries below the diaphragm occur in straddle accidents such as those which occur when a man slips on a stepladder and crushes his perineum from below. There is usually bleeding from the meatus, because the urethral injury is distal to the sphincter. Initial management of possible urethral injuries differs radically from the others described.

1. *Do not ask the patient to urinate.* If the patient urinates and there is a laceration or transection of the urethra, this urine may extravasate into the

periurethral areas. Often the injury itself is not initially associated with extravasation, and this act of voiding in the emergency room may be the first time extravasation occurs.

2. *Do not pass a catheter.* Blind insertion of the relatively stiff urethral catheter may convert a partial urethral separation to a complete one.

3. Instead, first obtain a retrograde urethrogram. If there is no extravasation and the urethra is intact, a catheter may then be passed, if desired or necessary. If the urethra is in continuity but a small area of extravasation is noted, a small soft catheter can often be guided gently into the bladder if care is taken to avoid further urethral injury.

4. The cystogram and excretory urogram can then follow as indicated.

Genitosacral Injury Not Involving the Urethra. 1. Initiate the usual general resuscitative and supportive measures.

2. Assess the integrity of the urinary system as outlined.

3. Evaluate the scrotum and its contents for rupture of the testicles and integrity of the vascular supply. The vascular phase of a scrotal scan, using sodium pertechnetate, will demonstrate this rather well if there is uncertainty.

4. Evaluate the penis for laceration of the corpora. Perform corpora cavernosogram if laceration or rupture is suspected. This is done by inserting an 18 gauge needle into either corpora and injecting 10 ml. of contrast material while exposing an x-ray film. Laceration of the corpora is indicated by extravasation of the contrast medium.

Specific Treatment for Genitourinary Tract Injuries

Penetrating Renal Injuries. Most peacetime penetrating renal injuries result from low velocity handgun missiles and knife wounds. Nearly all require abdominal exploration as mentioned. If celiotomy is performed and the renal injury diagnosed in advance, the kidney should be managed at the same time. Essentials of treatment are as follows:

1. First, control the vascular pedicle. This can be approached through the base of the mesentery by an incision over the aorta in the midline or by reflecting the right or left colon medially. The artery should be isolated and secured with umbilical tape or a vascular clamp. Back bleeding can be prevented by then securing the vein. Gerota's fascia should be left intact until the vessels are secured to maintain any tamponade which has developed.

2. Now, incise Gerota's fascia and mobilize the kidney. Visualize the entire kidney and explore it thoroughly.

3. Debride all devitalized tissues and ligate or reanastomose branch vessels within the renal hilus. Major vascular injury can be repaired with proper exposure, using usual vascular techniques. One should be aware of the possibility of thrombus formation or arterial obstruction from intimal avulsions within the main renal artery.

4. Scrupulously suture ligate bleeding parenchymal vessels.

5. Suture the renal collecting system with 4- or 5-0 absorbable atraumatic interrupted sutures.

6. Reapproximate open parenchyma when possible, using No. 2 chromic catgut. Vertical mattress sutures placed over bolsters made from multiple strands of the No. 2 gut provide good hemostasis and closure for the ruptured portion of the kidney.

7. Oversew the renal capsule when possible with continuous 4-0 absorbable sutures.

8. If reapproximation of injured kidney sections is not possible, oversew the opened area with any available renal capsule or a patch of peritoneum, viable omentum, or fat.

9. Drain the kidney through the retroperitoneum. Allow the drain to remain in place until urine drainage ceases. This may be 7 to 14 days or longer. Cessation of urinary leakage from the kidney in the the postoperative period should be confirmed by an IVP before removing the drains.

10. Obtain follow-up films in several months and again about a year later. If, during the repair, ischemia time is expected to be prolonged, the kidney should be cooled.

Postoperatively, one should caution the patient about delayed bleeding, which can occur up to 3 months afterward. Subcapsular hematoma may produce a Page kidney in certain circumstances, and follow-up should include observation for hypertension. In fact, all renal injuries should be followed for hypertension for at least a period of 1 year.

Nonpenetrating Renal Injuries. The principal decision in nonpenetrating injuries is to determine if renal exploration is required. Renal contusions are decided easily—no exploration is needed and the patient is managed by bed rest, forced fluids, observation, and serial urograms. Hematuria will clear, and healing is usually uneventful.

At the other end of the scale, major injuries with massive destruction and a completely shattered kidney are also rather straightforward. Both categories mentioned comprise approximately 85 per cent of all blunt renal injuries. The remaining 15 per cent are the most difficult to manage, because decisions regarding surgical exploration or whether to salvage a damaged kidney are less certain. The approach is as follows:

1. Follow the measures outlined under Abdominal Trauma Which Appears to Spare the Bladder (p. 517).

2. Type and cross-match 4 to 6 units of whole blood and transfuse as necessary.

3. Administer intravenous fluids as required.

4. Administer broad-spectrum antibiotics intravenously.

5. If the patient was in shock, the likelihood of acute tubular necrosis may be decreased by the administration of 40 mg. of furosemide (Lasix) intravenously.

6. Reinject the patient with 100 ml. of contrast material administered rapidly and obtain a nephrotomogram within 15 to 30 seconds after completion of the injection. This set of films will delineate renal parenchyma in most cases and reveal lacerations. Later films made in sequence will better demonstrate the extent of extravasation.

7. If now necessary, perform renal arteriography. This is most important in patients in whom there is no renal function on one side and thrombosis or complete avulsion of the pedicle is suspected. A sodium pertechnetate renal scan may also be helpful in ascertaining arterial supply to the kidney and can also be used for delineation of the renal parenchyma and for diagnosis of urinary extravasation.

8. If a segmental vessel is found to be bleeding during selective arteriography, autologous clot or shredded absorbable gelatin sponge (Gelfoam) can be injected into that particular vessel to stop the bleeding.

9. If the lacerations deeply involve the collecting system or the extravasation is severe, exploration and repair are required. A flank or subcostal (Lyons) approach may be easier than a transabdominal incision, but the incision will depend upon the nature of the injury, the experience of the surgeon, and the repair required. The subcostal approach allows easy access to the anterior and posterior surfaces of the kidney and its major vessels while remaining behind the peritoneum. The intra-abdominal contents can be explored through this incision if necessary.

From this point on, management of the kidney itself is the same as that for penetrating injuries. Renal and upper ureteral injuries associated with significant pancreatic injury raise the possibility of postoperative pancreatic fistula or digestion of the repaired kidney by pancreatic juices. Unless an excellent barrier can be constructed to separate kidney from pancreas, the kidney should probably be removed if the pancreas is also injured.

Ureteral Injuries. Most ureteral injuries are iatrogenic and are reported to occur in 3 to 5 per cent of pelvic operative procedures. The majority of such injuries accompany gynecologic operations. Violent trauma accounts for a small fraction of ureteral injuries but should not be overlooked, because unsuspected ureteral laceration or transection can lead to urinoma and abscess formation. Late ureteral obstruction can also develop.

Ureteral Injuries Produced by External Trauma. The general approach to ureteral trauma is the same as that indicated under Abdominal Trauma Which Appears to Spare the Bladder (p. 517). About 90 per cent of ureteral injuries which result from penetrating trauma will be associated with other major visceral injuries, and all must be explored and repaired. Preoperative urograms will provide the diagnosis in over 80 per cent of cases by demonstrating the extravasation. A negative urinalysis can be especially deceptive in these cases. Careful exploration of the retroperitoneum is required during celiotomy when ureteral damage is considered possible.

If the injury is near the renal pelvis, ureteropyeloplasty by any well described technique is the safest and simplest approach. Nephrostomy with stent can be performed, although primary closure without any foreign body within the urinary system is also acceptable. In all cases, broad-spectrum antibiotic coverage and generous retroperitoneal drainage are required.

Injuries to the mid-ureter can normally be managed in the following fashion:

1. Debridement.
2. Spatulation of both ends.
3. Watertight, end-to-end anastomosis with six to eight separate 4- or 5-0 absorbable sutures or with an interlocking continuous mattress suture.
4. A 1 to 2 cm. ureterotomy is made about 5 cm. proximal to the anastomosis. This serves as a diversion and puts the anastomosis to rest. Alternatively, primary closure without stent or vent can be used and generally leads to good results. T-tube ureteral drainage is not desirable. Alternative means of inserting stents are unreliable, and diverting nephrostomy is generally not required.

Distal ureteral injuries are best handled by ureteroneocystostomy by any of the many well-described techniques. The bladder can be brought to the ureter by psoas hitch or a bladder flap. If a ureteroneocystostomy is performed, a suprapubic cystostomy should be performed.

In all cases, ureteral anastomoses should be made without tension. If there is difficulty, alternative possibilities include the following:

1. Transureteroureterostomy.
2. Autotransplantation of the kidney into the pelvis with ureteroneocystostomy.
3. Cutaneous ureterostomy with secondary repair later.
4. Ureteral ligation with nephrostomy and secondary repair later.
5. Interposition of ileum between the proxi-

mal ureter and the bladder. This may be considered in very extensive ureteral loss. A preliminary nephrostomy usually tides over the acute phase, and this procedure is done at a second stage.

IATROGENIC URETERAL INJURIES. Ureteral injuries after pelvic surgery result from transection, ligation, or devascularization and comprise the majority in this category. In most instances, the primary problem for which the injury-producing operation was performed will influence the decision in therapy of the injured ureter.

Transections recognized at the time of the initial operation can be repaired by ureteroneocystostomy. Those that are recognized later require immediate exploration, drainage, and either ureteroneocystostomy or transureteroureterostomy. At times, the induration, inflammation, and even frank abscess make repair difficult. If there is sufficient length to the good section of proximal ureter, transureteroureterostomy may still be possible, but one should bear in mind the potential of infecting the uninvolved side. If some primary repair is not feasible, drainage with nephrostomy or temporary cutaneous ureterostomy can be done to salvage the kidney.

Ligation discovered at the time of the initial operation can be undone. If there is a question regarding the viability of the ligated section, it is best to resect the section and reimplant the ureter. Ligation that is recognized afterward can be treated by ureteral reimplantation. Occasionally, a ureteral catheter can be inserted to bypass the obstructing location, but this is generally only helpful for the short term.

Ureterovaginal fistulas can be treated expectantly or by the passage of a ureteral catheter if there is no abscess or urinoma. Some will heal spontaneously, but many will require later repair. In these circumstances, repair by ureteroneocystostomy can be performed after 3 to 6 months. This allows time for the inflammatory process to subside, and the procedure can be done with greater security. Alternatively, a transureteroureterostomy can be performed at the time the injury is discovered, but the ultimate outcome is less secure. If there is ureterovaginal fistula with urinoma and abscess formation, or if there is significant obstruction to the distal ureter, a diverting nephrostomy may allow the area to heal and prevent later complications from developing. A repair can then be performed in 3 to 6 months.

Urinary Bladder Injuries. The ruptured urinary bladder should be repaired surgically as soon as possible. The abdomen is explored through a midline vertical incision which can be extended superiorly if needed to manage associated injury to intra-abdominal organs. If the rupture is intraperitoneal, the peritoneum is opened and the intraperitoneal organs inspected. If the rupture is extraperitoneal and injury to other intra-abdominal organs is not suspected, the peritoneum is not entered. In either case, the bladder is opened and inspected for the number, location, and extent of lacerations. Wound edges are debrided and the bladder is closed in two layers, using running sutures of 3-0 plain catgut for the muscularis and mucosa and interrupted sutures of 2-0 chromic catgut for the muscular and serosal layers. The closure is watertight. One or more Penrose drains are used. Before the bladder is repaired, any bony fragments from a fractured pelvis are removed. In the male, the bladder is drained by a suprapubic tube rather than a urethral Foley catheter, as the latter can result in urethritis, prostatitis, epididymitis, and—later on—urethral stricture formation. In the female, a large indwelling urethral catheter may be satisfactory.

Prostatomembranous Urethral Injury. Injury to the posterior urethra may present as partial or complete avulsion, usually at the level of the prostatic apex. The distinction is important. In incomplete avulsion the prostate will be at its normal location and rectal examination may not be helpful. The retrograde urethrogram may reveal a streak of contrast medium going into the prostatic urethra, but one should also see localized extravasation. In complete avulsion the prostate is displaced cephalad and the retrograde urethrogram shows unmistakable evidence of the lesion. If the lesion is incomplete, a small catheter (14 or 16 F.) may be introduced *gently* into the bladder. The catheter should be left indwelling for 2 to 3 weeks. If resistance is met when the catheter is inserted, it should be withdrawn, no further attempt made, and suprapubic cystostomy performed.

If the avulsion is complete, an entirely more serious set of considerations exists. This injury can result in severe and prolonged disability. Mortality rates exceeding 40 per cent have been reported, although death is usually from the associated injuries. The specific urinary tract lesion often results in sexual impotence, urethral stricture, and/or urinary incontinence. The sexual impotence may be due to the injury itself or may result from surgical trauma at the time of initial management.

The difficulties in managing these patients acutely, combined with the high complication rate, have led to increasing acceptance of simple suprapubic cystostomy with drainage of the perivesical space. This is the safest approach for the immediate problem in most situations, and secondary repair is done later. However, when the patient is stable, the exposure adequate, and the surgeon experienced in this problem, a primary repair can then be the best solution.

In primary repair, an attempt should be made

to realign the urethra without further local damage, after careful debridement of frayed edges. The mucosa tends to be pulled from within the more bulky periurethral tissues, and this redundant mucosa is cut flush with the rest of the urethra on either end.

Realignment is accomplished by the following method. The bladder is opened and a Robinson catheter is passed from the bladder through the urethra. This is seen to exit from the proximal end of the avulsed urethra. A Foley catheter is then passed through the external urethral meatus. This is seen to exit from the distal end of the avulsed urethra. These two catheters are then sutured together, and the Foley catheter is guided into the bladder. The proximal and distal ends of the urethra are then sutured with full thickness interrupted 4-0 chromic catgut. The Foley balloon is inflated and the catheter left in place. A cystostomy is also placed and a seton from the Foley is brought through the cystostomy opening to guide later passage of a urethral catheter if there is some problem.

Primary repair of the urethra may be considered under the following circumstances:

1. The surgeon has enough experience.
2. The patient's general condition permits a prolonged delicate repair.
3. A large hematoma or continuous oozing of blood is not obscuring the field of repair.
4. Torn ends of the urethra are easily identified.
5. Torn ends of the urethra are not badly ecchymosed or edematous, making the primary repair impossible.

Penile Injuries. In all significant penile injuries, integrity of the urethra as well as that of corpus cavernosa should be determined by a retrograde urethrogram and a corpus cavernosogram in order to determine the location and the extent of the injury. Urethral injuries should be handled as discussed later on.

Injury to the Corpus Cavernosum. This type of injury is treated by evacuation of the hematoma, debridement of the edges of tunica albuginea, and reapproximation with running sutures of 2-0 chromic catgut. The basic problem in the "fractured penis" is a tear in the tunica albuginea of the corpus cavernosum with hemorrhage, hematoma formation, and distortion of the organ. We do not believe in managing these patients conservatively, because a number of these patients develop penile contracture subsequently. Surgical repair of the tear in tunica albuginea should be done as soon as possible.

Penile Amputation. Treatment consists of primary reanastomosis whenever possible. As the preparations are being made for surgery, the severed penile part should be treated in iced Ringer's lactate solution containing 1000 U.S.P. units of heparin per 100 ml. and a broad-spectrum antibiotic. A tourniquet should be applied to the base of the penis in the emergency room. The ends of the penile stump and the severed part are debrided and anastomosed with 2-0 absorbable suture material. An end-to-end urethral anastomosis is performed in an elliptical fashion over a urethral Foley catheter, using interrupted sutures of 4-0 chromic catgut, excluding the urethral epithelium. The skin of the distal segment is removed up to the very base of the glans, and the denuded penis can be buried in scrotum or beneath the mons pubis, allowing the glans to be exposed. The penile shaft is later freed and skin cover borrowed from these areas, making sure that the graft is not too bulky. If the severed part of the penis is not available in the first place, local reshaping measures are done. They consist of ligation of subcutaneous blood vessels, oversewing of corpora, and performance of meatoplasty in a fashion similar to the one used for conventional partial penectomy for carcinoma. Significant penile amputation may subsequently be treated by staged plastic reconstruction by the use of a tubed pedicle graft. Self-inflicted penile injuries are best treated jointly by the urologist, plastic surgeon, and psychiatrist.

Avulsion of Penile Skin. The object in initial management of the patient with degloving injuries of the penis consists of saving as much skin as possible to allow for subsequent coverage of the penis. Small wounds may fill in by the growth of the surrounding skin without contracture. Large dermal defects can be covered by scrotal skin. Extensive loss of penile shaft skin can be treated initially by burying the penis in the scrotum, followed by subsequent full-thickness skin grafting from this area. If the patient is uncircumcised and the prepuce is still intact, its mobilization and pulling over the penis in a fashion similar to glove over a finger can provide cover for practically the whole pendulous part of the penis. Thermal injuries of the penis can be treated initially by the usual methods for burns. Final treatment would depend upon the extent of the loss of skin, and is based upon the general principles outlined above.

Scrotal Injuries. Scrotal skin is quite redundant. Accordingly, there is seldom a problem in providing sufficient cover for the intrascrotal organs. If enough skin is available to cover the testes, the initial treatment consists of generous debridement, thorough irrigation with an antibiotic solution, and primary closure of the wound with drainage and a compression dressing. It is very important to sustain hemostasis before the wound is closed.

Some patients may appear to have very little

available scrotal skin. However, adequate mobilization of the skin at the time of surgery may result in sufficient cover. If not, the wound may be allowed to heal by secondary intention, using wet to dry dressings. Subsequently, it may be possible to mobilize the skin further to cover the testes, but the danger of infection should be considered. When there is total skin loss, the testes should be buried subcutaneously within the thigh. They should remain above the fascia to preserve the cool temperature environment needed for their proper function.

Testicular Injuries. *Testicular contusions* are treated conservatively by cold packs, scrotal support, and analgesics.

Open testicular wounds will be treated by open surgical exploration. The exact repair depends upon the extent of the injury. *Laceration* of the tunica albuginea is debrided and closed primarily with running sutures of 3-0 absorbable material. The part of the testis that cannot be covered with tunica albuginea should be removed (partial orchiectomy), hemostasis restored, and the tunica albuginea then closed.

The badly shattered testis should be removed. However, every attempt should be made to salvage any viable part of the testis for possible hormone production.

Transection of the vas deferens is treated by immediate reanastomosis.

Anterior Urethral Injury. Injury to the anterior urethra should be suspected if there is blood at the external urinary meatus and perineal swelling and ecchymosis. The diagnosis of the location and the extent of the injury is made by a retrograde urethrogram. In some patients, in addition to a urethrogram, urethroscopy may be required to completely evaluate the extent of the injury. A minor tear in the anterior urethra can be managed by letting it heal over a small (14 or 16 F.) Foley catheter, which is left indwelling for 10 to 14 days. Major urethral injury is managed surgically, either by primary closure or by secondary closure preceded by preliminary suprapubic cystostomy. Primary closure is done in patients with localized injury and in the absence of urinary extravasation and/or local infection. Sufficient length of corpus spongiosum is mobilized proximal and distal to the area of the injury. The devitalized tissues are adequately debrided and urethral ends are reanastomosed without tension in an elliptical fashion, using interrupted sutures of 4-0 chromic catgut, excluding the urethral epithelium. A small (14 or 16 F.) Foley catheter is left indwelling for 10 to 14 days. Patients with extensive tissue damage with marked perineal hematoma and/or extravasation of urine, with or without local infection, are better treated by preliminary proximal urinary diversion by suprapubic cystostomy. Perineal hematoma may be managed conservatively by cold compresses, broad-spectrum antibiotics, and analgesics. Urinary extravasation and local infection are managed by adequate drainage and subsequent wound care. Three or 4 months after the perineal wounds heal, definitive repair of the urethral problem is undertaken, after re-evaluation by retrograde urethrogram and urethroscopy.

BENIGN PROSTATIC HYPERPLASIA

method of
EVERETT D. HENDRICKS, M.D.
Prescott, Arizona

Evaluation of the Patient

Benign prostatic hyperplasia produces a progressive enlargement of the prostate which results in an obstruction to the outflow of urine from the bladder. The patient with this condition may have symptoms of frequency, urgency, and nocturia; he may have a slow starting urinary stream with poor force; or he may have any combination of these symptoms. The patient may be found to have secondary effects of his prostatic obstruction such as residual urine, vesical cellules or diverticula, hydronephrosis, or azotemia. These are late findings, however; proper and timely treatment of prostatic obstruction will result in their prevention.

If symptoms of nocturia and frequency with a slow, hesitant, or interrupted stream and a feeling of not emptying his bladder are severe enough to make a patient desire relief, he should be considered for surgery whether or not residual urine is present. In many ways the bladder can be considered as analogous to the heart. Both are muscular organs. In both, hypertrophy and thickening of the wall may occur when an increased load is placed upon them owing to stenosis of the orifice through which their contents must be expelled. When this obstruction is too great and too prolonged, both undergo decompensation by dilatation, loss of tone, and inability to empty efficiently. Just as the cardiologist aims to prevent the development of cardiac decompensation and congestive failure in the patient with valvular heart disease, so the urologist strives to prevent decompensation of the urinary bladder with resultant vesical dilatation, residual urine, and often some degree of permanent loss of vesical and renal function. When, however, the secondary effects of vesical neck obstruction have occurred—namely, residual urine, vesical cellules or diverticula, hydronephrosis, or azotemia—clear-cut indications for prostatic surgery are present.

Although symptoms and secondary findings are usually well correlated with the size of the prostate, exceptions to this rule are frequent. Many times a patient with a huge prostate will void freely with no secondary effects. Likewise, severe symptoms and signs of prolonged obstruction may be found in the patient with a small prostate. Thus whether or not a patient should receive treatment for prostatism is dependent not upon the size of his prostate but upon the severity of his symptoms and presence of undesirable secondary effects from the obstruction.

Usually the evaluation of the patient with these signs or symptoms is not difficult. Occasionally, however, a patient's symptoms and findings do not correlate well with his prostatic size, his age, or his past history. In this patient the urologist may suspect an abnormality of sensory or motor innervation of the bladder producing a neurogenic vesical dysfunction. Adequate urodynamic studies should then be done prior to any surgery. In this way those patients may be identified whose problems are not primarily prostatic and for whom prostatic surgery might be inappropriate.

Nearly all patients with benign prostatic hyperplasia (BPH) will need surgery if complete retention develops. One should always determine, however, whether or not a recently administered medication may have caused the retention. Frequently atropine-like drugs, antispasmodics, bronchodilators, antihistamines, muscle relaxants, and tranquilizers, whether prescribed by a physician or purchased over the counter, are guilty of causing urinary retention. Eliminating these medications can at times eliminate the patient's difficulty in voiding without surgery.

When a patient experiences complete urinary retention and requires catheterization, one should always insert an indwelling Foley catheter. Emptying the bladder once with a catheter and then allowing the patient to go without a catheter is almost surely to be followed by repeated retention. Then, however, the vesical distention is frequently complicated by infection with absorption of bacteria into the systemic circulation via the defects in the urinary mucosa produced by the initial catheterization. By placing a Foley catheter initially, repeated distention of the bladder is avoided and the bacteriuria that may result is not associated with the severe complications that may occur with a distended bladder. The catheter is connected to a drainage apparatus to keep the bladder empty at all times until corrective surgery can be planned.

For the patient with significant symptoms and signs of benign prostatic enlargement, surgery is the only effective and satisfactory treatment. Some patients with this condition have concurrent urinary infection, and will improve after treatment of this infection. A few may have chronic congestive prostatitis with a boggy prostate and copious prostatic secretion; they may benefit from massage. Some patients may also have urethral strictures that may be dilated effectively with sounds. Most patients, however, have pure benign prostatic hypertrophy (or hyperplasia), and their problem is a mechanical one; the prostate has enlarged in such a manner as to obstruct the urethra at the outlet of the bladder. Nothing other than mechanical removal of the obstruction is of help. Medication, massage, and sounds all have no real effect on their symptoms. Medical treatment of benign prostatic hyperplasia is in the experimental phase at present and may well be very effective at some time in the future. At present, hormones, antibiotics, antihistamines, steroids, and the like have no practical value. After appropriate evaluation, the prostate should be removed by the type of surgical procedure best suited to that patient. If the patient's health will not permit surgery, urinary drainage is usually necessary. This should be provided by an indwelling urethral catheter, or a suprapubic cystostomy if the urethral tube is not well tolerated, either permanently or until the patient's condition improves sufficiently to allow prostatic surgery.

History and physical examination supplemented by chest x-ray, blood chemistries, blood counts, urinalysis, electrocardiogram, and excretory urogram are usually sufficient to properly evaluate the patient for surgery. The excretory urogram is essential. It reveals important information regarding the condition of the kidneys, ureters, and bladder. It helps estimate prostatic size and thus aids in selection of the proper operation. It reveals the amount of residual urine without catheterization. The present or previous use of steroids by the patient is information of prime importance. The presence of a stable hemostatic mechanism is usually adequately established by the absence of a history of bleeding tendencies, the nonuse of anticoagulants, and an adequate supply of platelets as noted by the differential leukocyte count.

Types of Surgery

The obstructing prostatic tissue is either removed through the urethra with a resectoscope or excised or enucleated through a surgical incision. The operation used is the one which the surgeon feels will provide the patient with the most benefit, the least morbidity, and the least risk.

Transurethral Approach. For many years

urologists used this procedure to do a partial resection of the prostate. Although many patients benefited, this was fraught with undesirable complications such as secondary bleeding, persistent urinary infection, and recurrent obstruction. In recent years, with both the improved electroresectoscopes and the cold-cutting punch resectoscope, which I prefer, urologists are endeavoring to remove all obstructing tissue. When this is done, postoperative hemorrhage and recurrent obstruction occur almost as rarely after transurethral surgery as after the open operations. Because the transurethral operation carries a significantly reduced mortality, less pain, earlier ambulation, a shorter hospital stay, and a shorter period of postoperative disability, I prefer this operation to any other when it can be used. Since larger glands cannot easily be resected in a reasonable time, I do not perform transurethral resection when I anticipate that the prostate will be larger than 60 grams. In addition, one cannot perform transurethral resection when severe ankylosis of the hips prevents the patient from getting into a lithotomy position, or when the urethra is too small or strictured to accept the instrument, even after internal urethrotomy or external perineal urethrostomy. The use of isotonic irrigating solutions to prevent intravascular hemolysis and acute renal tubular necrosis and the reduction of urethral strictures by the use of the Otis urethrotome have made transurethral removal of the prostate a safer and better operation.

Vesicocapsular Prostatectomy. When the prostate gland is too large to be completely removed with the resectoscope, an incisional approach is used. Likewise, when there are stones in the bladder that are too large to be crushed with a lithotrite and removed through the urethra or if diverticula of the bladder are to be removed, an open operation through an incision is preferred.

I prefer an operation called the vesicocapsular prostatectomy. This is done through a lower abdominal incision, either midline or transverse. The bladder and prostate are approached extraperitoneally, and a vertical incision is made in the bladder through the anterior vesical neck extending into the prostatic capsule. The urethral orifices are identified, and the vesical mucosa is incised around the enlarged prostate, which is then removed by sharp and blunt dissection. The urethra is severed with the scissors at the apex of the prostate. Good visual and operative access to both the prostatic fossa and the bladder is obtained, and any ancillary surgery to the bladder or vesical neck is done while a hemostatic pack is in the prostatic fossa. Bleeding areas are identified and fulgurated or suture-ligated. Suture ligatures are placed in the vesical neck at 5 and 7 o'clock to secure the large arteries to the prostate. If it seems appropriate, a wedge can be resected from the vesical neck at this time and the vesical mucosa sutured over this area to the floor of the prostatic capsule. A No. 24 F. Foley catheter is left in the urethra and with enough water in the bag to keep it out of the prostatic fossa. Occasionally, when bleeding is more marked than usual, a No. 24 Foley catheter is left as a cystostomy tube. The bladder and prostatic fossa are closed tightly. Catheters are usually removed by the fifth or sixth day, and the patient is usually home by the seventh or eighth day. In my opinion this operation combines the best features of the retropubic and the transvesical (suprapubic) prostatectomies.

Retropubic Prostatectomy. This operation is done by an abdominal approach, but the prostate is removed through a transverse incision in the prostatic capsule. This gives excellent vision of the prostatic fossa for control of bleeding, and these patients may have less postoperative discomfort from spasm, because the bladder has not been opened. The surgeon is somewhat handicapped, however, by poorer access to the bladder, both for inspection and for carrying out other procedures on the bladder. It has become a favorite with many urologists, and its good results and low mortality make it worthy of continued use.

Transvesical (Suprapubic) Prostatectomy. This operation is also done through a lower abdominal incision. A small longitudinal anterior incision is made in the bladder and the prostate enucleated through this incision. Bleeding is controlled by spontaneous capsular contraction aided by pressure of the Foley catheter bag. Some urologic surgeons have preferred to place a temporary pursestring suture around the vesical neck after removing the prostate. By thus temporarily separating the prostatic fossa from the bladder, clot tamponade is utilized to stop bleeding from the prostatic bed and clots are prevented from plugging the catheter.

Perineal Prostatectomy. This operation is done through an incision in the perineum, either just above or just below the external rectal sphincter. The prostatic capsule is incised posteriorly and the enlarged gland enucleated. It is an operation that has been extensively utilized and in many cases has had good results. Postoperative impotency and incontinence are probably greater with this operation than with the other approaches, however. Markedly enlarged glands are difficult to remove with perineal approach. Rectal injury, although uncommon, is a serious complication when it does occur. Mortality is low, and poor-risk patients tolerate this procedure well. In my experience, however, this poor-risk patient with the small to medium-sized gland is better treated with a transurethral operation, because I believe that the risk of complications is less.

Complications

Cardiovascular Complications. In any substantial series of patients with benign prostatic hyperplasia, a considerable number of elderly and poor-risk patients are included. Even these patients tolerate careful prostatic surgery well. Despite precaution, myocardial infarction, cerebrovascular complications, and thrombophlebitis with emboli do occur. The death rate in all patients having surgery for benign prostatic hyperplasia is less than 2 per cent and is considerably less than 1 per cent for transurethral operations. Any significant reduction of this complication rate could be accomplished only by denying the benefits of prostatic surgery to high-risk elderly patients, many of whom may need it the most.

Urethral Stricture. Urethral strictures can occur in any patient who has had a catheter or an instrument in the urethra. Thus this condition is more common after the transurethral procedure but can occur with any type of prostatic surgery. Adequate meatotomy, use of an internal urethrotomy or perineal urethrostomy, nonreactive catheters, and early removal of catheters have markedly reduced the incidence of this annoying complication.

Vesical Neck Contracture. Contracture at the vesical neck results from excess formation of scar tissue with a diaphragm-like constriction at the vesical outlet. The cause is not precisely known. I have found that leaving the mucous membrane undisturbed at the vesical neck as much as possible helps reduce the incidence of contracture of the vesical neck. The milder forms need no treatment or merely an occasional dilatation with urethral sounds; more severe forms require incision with Colling's knife or excision with the resectoscope.

Infections. It is the reduction of sepsis that has been most responsible for reducing the mortality rate of prostatic surgery from the 20 to 30 per cent of a few decades ago to the present low figure of 1 to 2 per cent. Improved surgical techniques, improved patient status, chemical and nutritional advances, blood transfusions, bacteriologic studies, and antibiotics have nearly eliminated serious infection as a complication of prostatectomy. Renal infections are very rare. Epididymitis is nearly nonexistent if the vasa deferentia are tied or crushed. During the vesicocapsular prostatectomy I ligate each vas deferens inside the pelvis just where the vas turns medially after traversing the internal ring, lateral to the bladder. This is done while a pack is in the prostatic fossa. During transurethral resections, I have found vasopaxy or vas ligation equally effective in preventing epididymitis and it takes only a few minutes. Osteitis pubis, a potential complication in any retropubic operation, has occurred only once in many years, and this after a retropubic prostatectomy.

Hemorrhage. Most prostatic operations are completed without serious blood loss, primary or delayed, and most patients do not require transfusion. However, profuse bleeding can occur at any such operation and, particularly in the poor-risk patient, requires replacement with whole blood or the appropriate fractionated products of whole blood. Despite allegations against it, I am never averse to a "1-unit transfusion," when the need for 1 unit clearly exists and, after its administration, there is no need for a second unit.

By control of specific points of bleeding, however, serious bleeding can usually be controlled at surgery. Bleeding in the first several postoperative hours is usually due to the patient's reaction to pain after the anesthetic wears off. The resultant straining and spasm of the bladder open new bleeding areas. This can be avoided and treated by adequate analgesia in the postoperative period.

Delayed bleeding, occurring 1 to 3 weeks postoperatively, is common but usually not serious. It often occurs because patients have exerted undue tension with the abdominal muscles and thus increased the pressure on their bladder, either by exercise or by straining to defecate. I caution patients against any exercise more vigorous than walking for 3 or 4 weeks postoperatively and urge them to take whatever laxatives, either dietary or medicinal, necessary to prevent straining. Sexual activity is interdicted for 1 month after surgery. Despite these precautions, however, occasionally a patient will have sufficient secondary bleeding about 2 weeks postoperatively to require catheter evacuation and, rarely, cystoscopy and electrocoagulation of bleeders and transfusion. If adequately treated, there are no serious sequelae.

Vesical Hypotonia. The dilated hypotonic bladder in the patient who has delayed surgery too long and carried a large residual urine for a long time will often regain much of its normal tone after removal of the obstructive prostate. Occasionally, however, the loss of tone is not completely reversible and the patient is unable to empty the bladder completely, even after complete elimination of the mechanical obstruction. (This is seen particularly in patients who have previously had an abdominoperineal operation.) This patient then continues to carry some residual urine and is susceptible to recurrent urinary infection. Parasympathomimetic drugs—e.g., bethanechol chloride (Urecholine), in doses of from 5 to 25 mg. three times a day—are at times helpful and well tolerated in the usual patient. Double voidings—

i.e., going back to void a few minutes after the first attempt—and Credé's abdominal expression are often useful in this type of patient. Occasionally, some type of continuous prophylactic drug therapy such as a sulfonamide, a nitrofurantoin, or a methenamine preparation aids in prevention of infections in these patients.

Extravasation. When veins and venous sinuses are opened during transurethral surgery, irrigating solutions enter the vascular spaces and are added to the intravascular fluids. When an isotonic solution (I use 3.3 per cent sorbitol) is used, intravascular hemolysis is minimal and the acute tubular necrosis that previously was a threat when water was the irrigant no longer occurs. Since hypervolemia and secondary hyponatremia can be significant complications of intravascular absorption of irrigating solutions, even if isotonic, one should take steps to avoid these phenomena. By keeping the head of pressure of the irrigating fluid as low as is consistent with visibility, recognizing and controlling venous bleeding as it occurs, and judiciously limiting the length of resection, one can keep venous absorption and its complications to a minimum.

Extravasation of irrigating fluid through the thin prostatic capsule or a perforated bladder need not result in serious consequences if it is promptly recognized. The procedure should be terminated, a catheter placed for good drainage of the bladder, and Penrose drains immediately placed down to the area of extravasation through a small suprapubic incision. By far the most important factor is being alert to this possibility, so that the condition is recognized quickly.

Incontinence. Incontinence after surgery for benign prostatic obstruction is fortunately extremely rare today. Many patients have urgency control problems in the first several hours or few days immediately after the catheter is removed, but I have seen very few persistent control problems of significance. When these occur, they have occurred in patients who had pre-existing longstanding extensive urethral and prostatic infection with scarring and prostatic calculi. I am certain that in these patients the ravages of previous infection had destroyed the elastic character of the membranous and bulbous urethra so essential to urinary continence. One should be alert to this possibility in weighing the indications for surgery in these patients with extensive and longstanding pre-existing infection of the prostate and posterior urethral strictures.

Impotency. Sexual potency is not affected by the transurethral and abdominal operations. I tell these patients before surgery that their sexual potency after surgery will be neither impaired nor enhanced by the operation. It is important to warn them that, after prostatic surgery, the seminal fluid ejaculates backward into the bladder during orgasm; otherwise they are often puzzled and occasionally troubled by orgasm without normal ejaculation of fluid. Reduced or absent potency probably does occur in a significant number of patients after the perineal prostatectomy. This is, I feel, a contraindication to the perineal operation in the sexually active male.

PROSTATITIS

method of
GEORGE W. DRACH, M.D.
Tucson, Arizona

Prostatitis represents one of the most difficult treatment problems to face the medical practitioner. Its causation is often uncertain, its cure is often temporary, and recurrence is common. Do we have any practical methods to treat prostatitis? I believe we do. "Prostatitis," however, refers to a series of diseases of differing causes. Before any significant therapeutic plan can be initiated, it is first necessary to attempt to decide the most likely cause of the patient's prostatic complaints.

A treatise on diagnosis of prostatitis is beyond the purpose of this article. Let us assume that the basic evaluation of prostatitis (which includes divided urinary and prostatic specimens for analysis and culture; examination of the bladder, prostate, and urethra; and urinary flow studies) has been accomplished. Patients may then be assigned to one of several categories of prostatitis: bacterial, mycotic, inflammatory, or prostatodynia. Each of these may be further divided into acute or chronic, and so forth. An additional pain syndrome may sometimes be confused with prostatitis: the postoperative perineal causalgia or neuralgia of patients who have had prostatic surgery with resultant electrical or surgical injury to branches of the pudendal or obturator nerves. These patients should be referred to specialists in treatment of such diseases.

Bacterial Prostatitis

Patients with bacterial prostatitis constitute the smallest group, in my experience, of those with prostatitis-like symptoms. In these patients, the causative organisms are consistently recovered from prostatic fluid cultures. These patients often have relapsing urinary infection caused by their prostatic organisms. In general, the most serious such infections are due to gram-negative bacteria, with *Escherichia coli,* Proteus species, or Klebsiella being most common. Gram-positive organisms may also cause prostatitis; Enterococcus represents one especially difficult organism to treat when it becomes established in the prostate. A Staphylococcus (either *S. epidermidis* or *aureus*) may also cause prostatitis, but their causative roles must be carefully confirmed by quantitative bacterial cultures. The Staphylococcus is also one of the most common contaminants of the urethra, so that recovery of small numbers from prostatic fluid may represent contamination only. Almost any other bacterial species known has been implicated as a cause of prostatitis, and most mycotic organisms, including tuberculosis, have also been demonstrated to cause prostatitis in humans.

Inflammatory Prostatitis

Some patients with complaints of perineal pain, urinary urgency and frequency, and "poor voiding" go through complete evaluations and have no evidence of bacterial or mycotic cause for the prostatic symptoms. Their only persistent finding is a tender, edematous prostate with prostatic fluid which contains significant numbers of white blood cells, mucus, and other evidence of chronic inflammation. This inflammatory prostatitis indicates some chronic irritative activity in the prostate, but by our present techniques we are not able to designate some specific causative agent. Perhaps Trichomonas infestation had occurred, or perhaps the causative agent is Mycoplasma or Chlamydia. These agents cannot be easily demonstrated, so the presumptive diagnosis is made on the basis of a high index of suspicion, such as knowledge of occurrence of trichomoniasis in the patient's wife. Or perhaps the inflammatory process is created by autoimmune disease or allergic phenomena. Nevertheless, the end result is prostatic inflammation without demonstration of a specific bacteriologic cause.

Prostatodynia

Lastly, we have the generally younger patient who has complaints of prostatic difficulty but in whom we find no bacterial cause, no evidence of prostatic inflammation, and normal urinary anatomy. Most such patients demonstrate only prostatic tenderness upon examination and also show mild to moderate decrease in voiding flow rate. If urethral pressure profiles are done on these patients, they show remarkable irritability and spasm of the prostatic urethra. (Patients with bacterial or inflammatory prostatitis may also have these urodynamic abnormalities.) I prefer to call this process prostatodynia and avoid the terms prostatitis or prostatosis.

Let us now proceed to develop the plan for treatment of bacterial or inflammatory prostatitis or prostatodynia according to the category into which we have placed our patient.

Treatment of Bacterial Prostatitis

Acute bacterial prostatitis is a potentially serious process which can result in septicemia or abscess formation. Patients are often afflicted with high fever, chills, nausea, and vomiting, so hospitalization is often necessary in order to administer intravenous antibiotics and other medications. The antibiotic selected should be based on knowledge of the organism most likely to be causing the disease. If the patient has had previous urinary infections, it is best to select initial therapy which would be specific to his most recent urinary infection.

Most physicians now know of the diffusion barrier that prohibits passage of many standard antibiotics into the prostate. For this reason, only certain drugs such as sulfamethoxazole-trimethoprim, erythromycin, doxycycline, minocycline, and a few others are generally recommended for treatment of prostatitis. In acute prostatitis, however, the barrier to drug diffusion into the prostate is not as prominent, so that one may select any antibiotic to which the causative organism is sensitive and expect a favorable effect.

Other supportive measures may be necessary. Urinary retention, caused by prostatic edema, may require urethral or suprapubic catheter drainage of the bladder. Bed rest should be advised during the first days of therapy in an attempt to further decrease prostatic edema. The patient should have gentle rectal examinations performed on several occasions to detect possible prostatic abscess. If such an abscess forms, it must be drained surgically, usually by the transurethral or perineal route.

Chronic bacterial prostatitis is much more commonly encountered than acute prostatitis. These patients have an intact barrier to perfusion of many antibiotics into the prostatic tissue or fluid, so physicians must select for administration those drugs mentioned above which both penetrate the prostate and are effective in killing the bacteria that are causing the prostatitis. Typical treatment regimens for chronic prostatitis involve much longer courses of therapy than 10 day regimens for urinary infection. The minimum duration of therapy of prostatitis in my hands is 6 weeks. I have had patients on antibiotic therapy for as long as 6 months before we have achieved control of their disease—and even then some of these patients will relapse again after several months of being free of disease. The cure rate for bacterial prostatitis is about 30 to 40 per cent, and those who cannot be cured are placed on continuous antibiotic suppression to avoid complications of urinary infection return, possible sepsis, and chronic debilitation.

If the prostatic organism is shown to be sensitive to one of the following medications, the dosages used are as follows: sulfamethoxazole-trimethoprim: 2 standard tablets or 1 double strength tablet twice daily; erythromycin, 500 mg. every 6 to 8 hours; doxycycline or minocycline, 100 mg. twice daily; or chloramphenicol (Chloromycetin), 500 mg. every 6 hours. Precautions regarding use of these drugs, as indicated in their product literature, must be followed. Injectable drugs such as kanamycin, streptomycin, gentamicin, or tobramycin have been reported to result in cure of chronic prostatitis when given in usual dosages for periods of 10 days to 2 weeks.

Patients with chronic draining prostatic sinuses, infected prostatic calculi, or badly scarred prostates may not respond to the aforementioned therapy and may require surgical correction of the prostatic abnormality. This may be accomplished by the transurethral route when feasible, but some patients are finally cured only after they have undergone total perineal or retropubic prostatectomy. In other instances, diseases which predispose the patient to chronic prostatitis, such as meatal stenosis or urethral stricture, must be corrected before one can expect cure of prostatitis by antibiotics. All such surgical procedures carry inherent risks such as impotence which must be thoroughly understood by patient and physician.

If all else fails and the patient is placed on therapy to suppress urinary infections which result from chronic prostatitis, several drugs are useful. These include methenamine mandelate, 1 gram four times daily; methenamine hippurate, 1 gram twice daily; nitrofurantoin, 50 mg. four times daily; or sulfa preparations, 500 mg. four times daily.

Treatment of Inflammatory Prostatitis

On the assumption that at least some of those patients with inflammatory prostatitis have an infection with some type of microorganism, most are first placed on a trial of treatment with one of the drugs I have found most useful: doxycycline or minocycline, 100 mg. twice daily for 2 weeks. If the patient responds to this trial, therapy is continued for a full 6 weeks. These drugs of the tetracycline series are known to penetrate the prostate and are selected for this trial because they are also most likely to affect the unusual microorganisms which may cause prostatitis, such as Chlamydia, Mycoplasma, or others.

When suspicion exists for presence of Trichomonas, or when these parasites are seen in prostatic fluid, metronidazole is usually effective therapy. It is given in dosages of 250 mg. three times daily for 7 to 10 days to both the patient and any sexual partner.

If there is no response to these forms of therapy and the inflammatory process continues, one of three drugs may be useful in decreasing the patient's symptoms, although I have seldom seen cures result. An antihistamine such as diphenhydramine, 25 to 50 mg. three or four times daily, or promethazine hydrochloride, 12.5 to 25 mg. three times daily, sometimes provides relief when symptoms are especially bad; or oxyphenbutazone, 100 mg. three times daily, may control the inflammatory process and associated symptoms.

Over the years, a few of my patients with this inflammatory type of prostatitis have ultimately developed prostatic carcinoma, so that I now watch carefully for carcinoma in these patients. It seems to me that those patients who develop carcinoma get almost no relief from any of the foregoing medications or any other therapy of prostatitis, but they are markedly relieved when the correct diagnosis is ultimately made and specific therapy for carcinoma (such as estrogenic hormones) is begun.

Treatment of Prostatodynia

This syndrome, as mentioned previously, involves the occurrence of symptoms similar to prostatitis in a patient with no evidence of bacterial or inflammatory disease of the prostate. Most such patients are less than 50 years of age. Their major problem is inappropriate function of the prostate and prostatic urethra, with both voiding and sexual abnormalities.

Several types of medications must often be tried in an attempt to control the symptoms in these patients. I often begin with low doses of diazepam, 2 mg. three or four times daily. The drug is used more for its smooth-muscle relaxing effect than for tranquilization. Antispasmodic agents may also help. Flavoxate, 100 mg. four times daily, or hyoscyamine, 0.15 mg. four times daily, will sometimes decrease intensity of symptoms in these patients. Most "miracle" cures I have seen in patients in this category have occurred after treatment with phenoxybenzamine, which is used for its alpha-blocking effects on the prostatic urethral musculature. (This use of phenoxybenzamine is not listed in the manufacturer's official directive.) Patients respond to dosages ranging from 10 mg. daily to 10 mg. three times per day. They must be warned of the side effects of dizziness, hypotension, and loss of ejaculation. In fact, occurrence of these side effects has prohibited use of this drug in a number of patients. But when the drug can be tolerated successfully, significant improvement can occur. Interestingly, patients who respond favorably to this drug also show objective improvement in urinary flow rates and velocity. Perhaps it will eventually be possible to treat prostatodynia with alpha-blocking drugs which do not have such potent side effects on vascular functions.

Nonspecific Aspects of Treatment

Most patients with these chronic diseases of the prostate feel threatened and confused by their problem. They are often rendered more anxious by our apparent inability to effectively treat their prostatic affliction. Reading the previous paragraphs indicates that much of the therapy recommended is based on trials of this or that. It is inevitable, then, that part of the therapy provided by the physician must include an understanding that for most cases of prostatitis or prostatodynia there is no instant cure, and that any cure achieved will require lengthy communication and cooperation between patient and physician. Psychologic support of the patient's anxieties during this treatment period can be one of the most important aspects of the therapy rendered.

Sitz baths for 30 minutes once or twice daily may help relieve prostatic discomfort. Prostatic massages can be of use if the patient has inspissated secretions in the prostatic ducts, but their routine use in the treatment of prostatitis is of no proved value. Some authors have recommended that prostatic massages, if done, be performed no more often than every 5 days.

As our knowledge of various causes of these prostatic diseases improves, so too should our treatment continue to improve. It is hoped that we will soon be able to relieve all patients with "man's hidden disease," prostatitis.

ACUTE RENAL FAILURE

method of
WILLIAM D. MATTERN, M.D.
Chapel Hill, North Carolina

Acute renal failure results from an abrupt reduction in glomerular filtration rate (GFR); if sustained, this loss of function leads to profound and ultimately fatal alterations in the volume and composition of the extracellular fluid. Traditionally, the onset is heralded by a dramatic fall in urinary output (oliguria if output is less than 400 ml. per day, and anuria if less than 50 ml. per day), but nonoliguric acute renal failure is being recognized more frequently now that blood urea nitrogen (BUN) and serum creatinine concentration are monitored routinely in hospitalized patients.

The many causes of acute renal failure can be grouped for clinical convenience into three categories: (1) prerenal, (2) renal, and (3) postrenal. The prerenal causes include hypotension, dehydration, congestive heart failure, and, less commonly, an acute interruption of renal arterial flow or venous drainage. The postrenal cause is obstruction, most commonly resulting from prostatic enlargement in older men. The renal parenchymal causes are numerous, but by far the most common is acute tubular necrosis (ATN).

Strictly speaking, ATN is a pathologic designation that has been applied to a clinical syndrome. It occurs in two general settings. The first is following surgery, trauma, or sepsis in association with a temporary reduction in blood pressure. The second is after exposure to a nephrotoxin. The major categories of nephrotoxins include drugs, radiographic contrast agents, anesthetics, and pigments (hemoglobin and myoglobin).

Initial Measures

It is often impossible at the outset to know whether an abrupt decline in urinary output represents the onset of ATN or is the consequence of a reversible nonrenal condition such as dehydration or obstruction. This is particularly true in the settings associated with hypotension. Although the oliguria may indicate the onset of ATN, it may also reflect the normal physiologic response of the kidney to a reduction in perfusion pressure below the level at which intrarenal autoregulation can maintain a normal GFR. It is critical in the initial approach to treatment that every effort be made to distinguish and correct any reversible nonrenal conditions.

Evaluation of the Urine. Appropriate analysis and interpretation of urinary changes remains the most useful method of distinguishing a reversible reduction in GFR from the established reduction of ATN. It is essential that a sample of urine be obtained at the outset, before treatment is initiated, particularly with agents such as mannitol or furosemide (Lasix).

In prerenal conditions such as hypotension, dehydration, and congestive heart failure, the urine sediment is unremarkable. The urine sodium concentration is less than 20 mEq. per liter, and often less than 10 mEq. per liter. The urine specific gravity is usually above 1.015, and the urine osmolality is greater than 400 mOsm. per kg. The urine to plasma (U/P) osmolality ratio is greater than 1.3, and the U/P creatinine ratio is greater than 20.

In ATN the urine sediment contains pigmented casts and renal tubular cells in 80 per cent of cases. The urine sodium concentration is usually greater than 20 mEq. per liter. The urine specific gravity is "fixed" at about 1.010, and the osmolality is close to 300 mOsm. per kg. The U/P osmolality ratio is usually less than 1.2, and the U/P creatinine ratio is less than 20, and often less than 10. The typical changes in urine composition cannot be interpreted as evidence for ATN in the patient with pre-existing chronic renal disease, and prerenal conditions must carefully be excluded by other means.

The findings of red cells and red cell casts suggests acute glomerulonephritis, whereas the finding of many white cells suggests the possibility of papillary necrosis. If the dipstick test of the urine is positive for blood (the orthotolidine reaction) and no red cells are seen, hemoglobinuria or myoglobinuria should be suspected.

Correction of Reversible Nonrenal Conditions. Dehydration is suggested by decreased skin turgor, orthostatic hypotension, and a low central venous pressure. After the urine sample is obtained, treatment is initiated with isotonic saline solution, given intravenously, at a rate of about 200 ml. per hour. Congestive heart failure is indicated by the usual constellation of findings, including cardiac enlargement, an S_3 gallop, rales, an elevated pulmonary capillary wedge pressure, peripheral edema, hepatic enlargement, distended neck veins, or an elevated central venous pressure. After the urine sample is obtained, treatment is initiated with diuretics and digitalis. Obstruction is suspected when an enlarged prostate and distended bladder are noted. In this situation a single in-and-out catheterization of the bladder is indicated to determine postvoid residual volume.

In the patient with hypotension and oliguria, an indwelling urinary catheter may be indicated for the first few hours of treatment so that changes in urine flow can be observed in relation to changes in perfusion pressure, or until a diagnosis of ATN is established. Immediate efforts are made to correct the hypotension. Deficits in extracellular or intravascular fluid volume are replaced with isotonic saline solution, albumin, plasma, or blood, as indicated by the nature of the deficit, while central venous pressure is monitored. A volume challenge may also be indicated in the hypotensive patient who does not have a demonstrable deficit, but care should be exercised to avoid fluid overload, especially if cardiac reserve is limited.

The Use of Mannitol and Furosemide. Controversy continues about the use of these agents in acute renal failure. The administration of mannitol generally is favored in selected situations of high risk for ATN, preferably before the insult or immediately afterward. Two such situations are (1) during surgery which involves the abdominal aorta, and (2) following a hemolytic transfusion reaction. In the former situation, an intravenous infusion of 50 ml. of a 25 per cent solution of mannitol can be given over 5 minutes before the aorta is cross-clamped. An intravenous infusion of a 15 per cent solution of mannitol at a rate of 2 ml. per minute can then be continued for the next hour. The same protocol can be used after a hemolytic transfusion reaction combined with the intravenous administration of saline at a rate of 200 ml. per hour. Both infusions should be discontinued if oliguria supervenes. Mannitol administration may also be considered in the patient who has become oliguric after the onset of hypotension following surgery, trauma, or sepsis—once again, after the urine sample has been obtained for evaluation. While treatment is being initiated to correct the hypotension, 50 ml. of a 25 per cent solution of mannitol is infused intravenously over 5 minutes and repeated once after 15 minutes. Further administration is to be avoided. If the oliguria persists, the retained mannitol, which is slowly metabolized, may cause an osmotic shift of water into the extracellular fluid, aggravating fluid overload or precipitating heart failure.

The evidence suggesting that furosemide may prevent ATN is not convincing. Too frequently, a transient increase in urine output after its administration is interpreted as indicating that ATN has not occurred. As a consequence, appropriate management is delayed and serious fluid overload may develop in the interval.

Established Acute Tubular Necrosis (ATN)

The oliguric phase of ATN typically lasts 10 to 14 days, but not infrequently persists for 3 to 4 weeks and occasionally even longer.

Fluids and Electrolytes. Salt and water intake should be limited in the normally hydrated patient to allow for the 0.5 to 1.5 pound daily weight loss anticipated under these conditions. Observed renal and gastrointestinal water losses are replaced, plus estimated insensible loss (400 to 600 ml. per day in the afebrile patient). Water intake is subsequently adjusted according to the serum sodium concentration. If hyponatremia develops, intake is further restricted.

Sodium and chloride are provided only in amounts adequate to replace measured nonrenal losses. In many patients extracellular fluid volume is significantly expanded at the outset of management because of prior saline administration, as evidenced by edema or a frankly elevated central venous pressure. In this setting treatment with large doses of furosemide has been advocated, to increase renal salt and water excretion. Furosemide is given by intravenous injection at a rate of 100 mg. per 5 minutes, starting with 100 mg. and increasing at 12 hour intervals by 100 mg. per dose until a total daily dose of 1000 mg. is reached (this dose is higher than that listed in the manufacturer's official directive) or an adequate change in urine output is achieved. Such treatment does not alter the GFR or shorten the period of established ATN. If other indications are present, dialysis usually provides a more rapid and predictable means for restoring extracellular fluid volume to normal.

Potassium losses are not replaced and intake is restricted as much as possible, the main constraint being the extent to which protein intake is restricted (i.e., a 20 gram protein diet contains about 40 mEq. of potassium). Despite maximal restriction, the serum potassium concentration usually rises. Treatment is related to the rate of rise, the absolute levels, and associated changes on the electrocardiogram (ECG).

If potassium accumulation is gradual and other indications for dialysis are absent, the cation exchange resin, sodium polystyrene sulfonate (Kayexalate) is given. It is commonly prepared as a suspension in a solution containing sorbitol, such that each 60 ml. contains 15 grams of Kayexalate and 20 grams of sorbitol. This suspension is given in doses of 60 to 100 ml., by mouth or by retention enema, at about 3 to 4 hour intervals. For each gram of Kayexalate administered, about 1 mEq. of potassium is exchanged for 2 mEq. of sodium. For this reason, its use may be contraindicated in the presence of fluid overload or when cardiac reserve is limited.

The potassium concentration may rise rapidly, particularly when ATN is associated with tissue injury, sepsis, internal bleeding, or severe acidosis. Bascially, a rapidly rising potassium concentration is an indication for hemodialysis, as relatively large amounts of potassium (200 mEq. or more) can be removed within 6 hours. Peritoneal dialysis may remove a similar amount, but only 4 to 6 mEq. is removed with each exchange and the total treatment time spans 36 hours.

If the potassium concentration is between 6.5 and 8.0 mEq. per liter and the ECG shows peaking of the T waves, 50 ml. of a 7.5 per cent solution of sodium bicarbonate (45 mEq.) is injected intravenously over 5 minutes and repeated after 10 and 15 minutes in order to shift potassium into cells temporarily until total body stores can be reduced by dialysis or Kayexalate therapy. If the potassium concentration is above 8.0 mEq. per liter or more severe ECG changes are noted (diminished P waves or broadening of the QRS complex), 5 to 10 ml. of 10 per cent solution of calcium gluconate is injected intravenously over 2 minutes, while continuously monitoring the ECG, and repeated once after 5 minutes, in order to stabilize membrane potentials and thereby directly antagonize the cardiac effects of the hyperkalemia.

In uncomplicated ATN, metabolic acidosis develops gradually and plasma bicarbonate concentration falls by about 2 mEq. per day. If respiratory compensation is normal; treatment can be withheld until the bicarbonate concentration falls below 15 mEq. per liter. Alkali is then given, usually as Shohl's solution, a combination of citric acid and sodium citrate which contains 1 mEq. of alkali and 1 mEq. of sodium in each ml. of the solution. The average daily dose required to maintain plasma bicarbonate at 15 mEq. per liter is 45 ml. If acidosis is more severe, the accompanying sodium load with larger doses may be prohibitive and correction by dialysis is indicated.

Diet. The goals of dietary therapy in acute renal failure are to minimize the rate of catabolism and reduce the accumulation of the end-products of nitrogen metabolism. These goals are best achieved by a diet which provides a caloric intake in the range of 2500 and a protein intake of 20 grams, using proteins which have a high content of essential amino acids, such as eggs. In the less alert patient whose gastrointestinal tract remains intact, oral hyperalimentation by nasogastric feeding tube can be undertaken using Amin-Aid. Each pack contains 6.6 grams of essential amino acids, 0.8 gram of nitrogen, 654 nonprotein calories, and less than 2 mEq. of sodium and potassium. When mixed with 250 ml. of water, the final volume is 340 ml. and the osmolality is 1125 mOsm. per kg. The average dose is 3 packs a day. To avoid osmotic diarrhea, the amount of water is increased as much as possible and the mixture is given in small aliquots or by continuous drip. In the patient whose gastrointestinal tract is not functional, parenteral hyperalimentation, using a mixture of hypertonic glucose and essential amino acids, has been advocated recently as an alternative to the more traditional daily infusion of the "nitrogen sparing" 100 grams of carbohydrate (1000 ml. of 10 per cent dextrose in water). The administration of the hypertonic glucose and amino acid solution requires a central venous catheter. Scrupulous attention to the catheter skin site is necessary to avoid infection, preferably by specialized hyperalimentation teams; unless such personnel are available, the infection risk may outweigh the potential benefit in nutrition.

Dialysis. When the established period of ATN is relatively short, and particularly in the nonoliguric patient whose general condition is good, careful management of diet, fluids, and electrolytes may obviate the need for dialysis. In the majority of patients, however, dialysis is usually indicated to correct fluid overload, restore the chemical composition of the extracellular fluid toward normal, or reverse symptoms of uremia.

Peritoneal dialysis is the method of choice in uncomplicated cases. Blood chemical values shift gradually toward normal, minimizing the risk of the dialysis dysequilibrium syndrome; large volumes of excess salt and water can be removed, with a minimum risk of sudden hypotension resulting from disproportionate depletion of intravascular volume; and the need for a vascular access and the exposure to heparin which are required before hemodialysis can be avoided. Peritoneal dialysis may not be possible (1) after recent abdominal surgery, particularly if abdominal drains are present; (2) if assisted ventilation is required, as distention of the peritoneal cavity with dialysate may elevate the diaphragms and further impair ventilation; or (3) in the catabolic patient, if the BUN and serum potassium concentration are rising rapidly.

A major goal of hemodialysis is to maintain the predialysis BUN below 125 mg. per 100 ml., and preferably below 100 mg. per 100 ml. After trauma, or in the severely catabolic patient, even daily treatment may fail to achieve this degree of chemical control. Conventional access to the circulation is by a Scribner shunt which is left in place at the wrist or ankle throughout the period of established ATN. The two problems with this access are infection and clotting. The latter problem is most likely to occur in the patient whose blood pressure is unstable. A recent alternative method of vascular access in acute renal failure involves repetitive, percutaneous placement of a catheter in one of the femoral veins. "Single needle" dialysis is done via the catheter, which is removed at the end of each treatment. Excellent flows are obtained, even in the hypotensive patient who may be receiving pressor agents during the dialysis. By alternating from one femoral vein to the other with successive treatments, as many as ten or more treatments can be done.

Complications

Infectious. Infection is the leading cause of death. The most common sources are the urinary tract, wounds, and the lung. Indwelling urinary catheters are not necessary to monitor urine output. Once ATN is established and outlet obstruction has been excluded, catheters should be removed. In the unresponsive male patient, urine may be collected subsequently by condom catheter drainage. The skin sites of intravenous catheters and Scribner shunts should receive scrupulous care, and the intravenous sites should be changed every few days. Peritonitis remains a risk with peritoneal dialysis, particularly with the bottle-hanging method in general use. Strict sterile technique in catheter placement and repositioning is essential. Special attention by nursing personnel is also required when injecting additives into the bottles and in placing the drain line so as to prevent backflow of effluent.

Cardiovascular. Fluid overload, volume-dependent hypertension, and anemia all predispose to congestive heart failure. Prior to dialysis, acute pulmonary edema was the most common cause of death. Pericarditis may develop as a complication of acute uremia and is an indication for dialysis. It is frequently associated with atrial arrhythmias and pericardial effusions, but the latter seldom lead to tamponade in this setting. Rapid changes in the serum potassium concentration and hypokalemia should be avoided in patients receiving digitalis. Peritoneal dialysate contains no potassium, and hemodialysate contains potassium at a concentration of 2.0 mEq. per liter. Potassium, as KCl, may be added to either type of dialysate, as indicated.

Hematologic. Anemia is to be expected, and all efforts should be made to avoid blood transfusions unless (1) they are necessary to maintain intravascular volume and blood pressure, (2) hematocrit-related angina develops in a patient with pre-existing coronary heart disease, or (3) the hematocrit falls below 15 per cent. Frozen red cells are the preferred blood product, because they carry the least risk of hepatitis and sensitization to HLA antigens. If frozen blood is not available, washed packed red cells should be used. Iron loss invariably complicates the anemia, and folate deficiency develops as a consequence of loss during dialysis. Oral iron supplements should be given when possible, but parenteral iron should not be administered. Folate is replaced in the amount of 1 mg. per day.

Neurologic. Confusion, lethargy, and obtundation in the acutely ill patient may, or may not, be manifestations of uremic encephalopathy. Dialysis is indicated if the BUN is greater than 100 mg. per 100 ml. Persistence of the symptoms then indicates the need for further evaluation. Seizures occur in severe acute uremia as a manifestation of encephalopathy, and also following rapid correction of blood chemical values as a manifestation of the dialysis dysequilibrium syndrome. They are often precipitated, during hemodialysis, by a transient drop in blood pressure. Treatment is given with intravenous diazepam (Valium), and 5 to 10 mg. is injected at a rate no greater than 5 mg.

per minute. The dose may be repeated after 10 minutes and again after 20 minutes. Blood pressure, respiratory rate, and mental status are monitored closely to avoid hypotension, respiratory depression, and obtundation. Further treatment is rarely required, and phenytoin has not been demonstrated to have a definite protective effect for the seizures which occur in this setting.

Gastrointestinal. When anorexia, nausea, and vomiting develop as manifestations of acute uremia, they are relieved by dialysis. In the past, bleeding stress ulcers were a frequent complication, especially in patients presenting with ATN after severe trauma or major surgery. Frequent hemodialysis in this setting appears to have reduced the incidence of this complication. Ileus remains a frequent complication in the common settings of ATN, and inactive intestinal peristalsis may retard the outflow of dialysate. Bowel perforation continues to occur as a complication of trocar placement for peritoneal dialysis, with an incidence of about 1 per cent. It may present with feculent return or as glucose-positive, watery diarrhea. The trocar is left in place and surgical consultation is obtained.

Drugs. The removal of drugs by glomerular filtration or by diffusion across the peritoneal or hemodialysis membrane is determined by (1) the plasma concentration, (2) the molecular weight, (3) the degree of binding to plasma proteins, and (4) the volume of distribution. Major modifications of drug dosage and intervals of administration may be necessary when GFR is sharply reduced, and further adjustments may be required in connection with peritoneal or hemodialysis. New information about pharmacokinetics in renal failure is accumulating rapidly now that methods for determining individual drug levels are being applied more widely. Standard references should be consulted when selecting initial drug dosage (Bennett et al.: JAMA, *230*:1544, 1974); whenever possible, blood levels should be obtained as a guide to subsequent therapy.

Antibiotics are the most commonly used group of drugs in acute renal failure. Some antibiotics, such as the aminoglycosides, have significant dose-related nephrotoxic potential, and careful regulation of blood levels during therapy is essential. Intraperitoneal instillation of antibiotics is recommended in treating the peritonitis which complicates peritoneal dialysis. By adding the antibiotic to the dialysate, the drug is delivered directly to the site of infection; after a single systemic loading dose, therapeutic blood levels can thus be maintained.

Digitalis is not removed by dialysis.

The Diuretic Phase

The diuretic phase is initiated by a rather predictable stepwise increase in urine output over 7 to 10 days, from oliguric levels to 2 to 3 liters per day. Clearance initially remains low, and then gradually rises. The BUN and serum creatinine concentration continue to rise for the first few days, gradually plateau over the next several days, and then slowly begin to decline toward normal after the diuresis is well established. Medical management is continued for the first week, and dialysis may be required. The diuresis is characterized by an obligatory loss of water, salt, and potassium. Appropriate upward adjustments in intake are required to prevent dehydration, volume contraction, and hypokalemia. By the third to fourth week, renal function is approaching normal and the renal regulation of water and electrolyte excretion is restored.

Prognosis. The mortality in ATN remains high, mainly because of the serious nature of the underlying conditions with which it is associated. In uncomplicated cases, a recovery rate of 80 per cent or better has been documented. Radionuclide imaging using iodohippurate sodium (Hippuran), the Hippuran renal scan, has provided an extremely accurate, noninvasive method for predicting the potential for recovery during the period of oliguria. Serial scans which continue to show some uptake of Hippuran correlate, in over 90 per cent of cases, with subsequent recovery of function. Long-term studies in patients who have recovered indicate that many will continue to demonstrate mild impairment of function 5 to 10 years after the episode.

Prevention

The likelihood of ATN in a surgical setting may be reduced by (1) avoiding dehydration prior to surgery, (2) scrupulous attention to volume replacement during surgery, and (3) careful maintenance of blood pressure in the immediate postoperative period. In medical and surgical settings, careful initial assessment of renal function and regular monitoring during the administration of potentially nephrotoxic drugs are essential. This latter point is particularly important in the elderly. With aging there is a gradual reduction in GFR. There is a parallel reduction in muscle mass and decrease in the rate of creatinine production. Thus a serum creatinine concentration of 1.0 mg. per 100 ml. in a 65 year old patient may reflect a GFR that is 50 per cent below normal. Several recent articles provide methods of correcting for age when estimating GFR from the serum creatinine concentration (Gault and Cockcroft: Nephron, *16*:31, 1976).

CHRONIC RENAL FAILURE

method of
CARL M. KJELLSTRAND, M.D.,
Minneapolis, Minnesota
and T. L. JOHNSON, M.D.
Duluth, Minnesota

Principles

The exact cause of most chronic renal diseases is unknown, although they are generally incurable and are relentlessly progressive. The most common cause of renal failure is chronic glomerulonephritis, which is immunologically mediated and of varied causes. Because treatment with immunosuppressive drugs may retard or even halt destruction of the kidney (see pp. 511 to 515), careful clinical and histologic assessment of patients with chronic kidney disease is mandatory.

Curable forms of renal disease are interstitial nephritis secondary to analgesic abuse, hypercalcemic nephropathy, nephritis of subacute bacterial endocarditis, nephrosclerosis secondary to hypertension, and obstructive uropathy. Unfortunately, because the cause of the disease is usually unclear, treatment can only be directed toward the symptoms. This symptomatic treatment falls into four main categories: (1) retarding the progression of the disease by treating the aggravating complications; (2) maintenance of homeostasis by manipulating diet, electrolytes, and fluid; (3) treating organ-specific problems and arranging a logical, long-term follow-up; and (4) anticipation of the eventual need for chronic dialysis or transplantation, or both, before irreversible or life-threatening complications occur.

Slowing Down the Progression of Disease

Natural Progression. Most chronic renal diseases progress at a constant rate. The level of serum creatinine is the most convenient clinical yardstick of kidney function. Creatinine, excreted mainly by glomerular filtration, is produced at a relatively constant rate in most persons. The percentage of residual renal function can be estimated by dividing 100 by the serum creatinine level. Therefore at a serum creatinine level of 1 mg. per 100 ml., the renal function is approximately 100 per cent, whereas a serum creatinine of 5 mg. per 100 ml. reflects 20 per cent residual function. It may be useful to plot the percentage of renal function against time, because the decline in renal function usually follows a straight line. Deviations from this straight decline suggest an acute exacerbation.

The slope of the line (rapidity of deterioration) varies considerably between patients. Kidneys may be totally destroyed in only a few weeks, as in the case of rapidly progressive glomerulonephritis, although progression usually takes place over many years. For example, diabetic nephrosclerosis progresses relatively rapidly, whereas pyelonephritis and congenital diseases (hypoplasia-dysplasia, and polycystic kidneys) progress slowly. The progression of the bulk of kidney diseases, including chronic glomerulonephritis and nephrosclerosis, falls in between.

Some renal diseases are curable or at least amenable to the halting of their progression. Notable among these is analgesic nephropathy. If a patient can discontinue the intake of drugs containing analgesics (particularly phenacetin), progressive failure can be halted, and function is often improved. By controlling hypertension the course of nephrosclerosis can be altered. Also, the relief of any urinary tract obstructions will ameliorate the functional deterioration associated with the obstruction. Detection and treatment of hypercalcemia can halt the progressive renal failure associated with hypercalcemia nephropathy. The chronic nephritis associated with bacterial endocarditis or chronic bacteremia, such as "shunt nephritis," can be cured by eradication of the underlying focus of infection.

The blood urea nitrogen (BUN) may be used to follow kidney function, but is less suitable because, unlike creatinine, which is produced at a constant rate, the production of BUN is heavily influenced by dietary protein consumption. A patient with serious kidney disease may have a normal BUN during restriction of protein, whereas high BUN levels may be found during only moderate renal insufficiency if the protein consumption is high.

Renal insufficiency can be divided into three clinical stages. The first is the early asymptomatic stage. Usually there are no symptoms of uremia below a creatinine of 3 mg. per 100 ml., although edema formation and hypertension may be troublesome. The second stage is moderate renal insufficiency, with a creatinine level from 3 to 8 mg. per 100 ml. During this time, there are usually signs of increasing fatigability, anemia may become a problem, and the patient's working capability declines. The final clinical stage is severe renal insufficiency, with a creatinine level over 8 mg. per 100 ml. Problems with weakness, lethargy, nausea, and vomiting become more frequent, and symptoms and signs of overhydration, pericarditis, and neuropathy may appear.

Deviations from these patterns indicate the need to re-evaluate the patient, and particularly to consider iatrogenic problems, which are discussed later.

Hypertension. Renal disease is frequently complicated by hypertension. This hastens the progression of the disease by adding nephrosclerosis. Thiazide diuretics are appropriate for initial treatment of hypertension during the early stages of renal failure. Agents such as chlorthalidone (100 mg. once or twice per day) or hydrochlorothiazide (50 to 100 mg. once or twice per day) are suitable. When the serum creatinine level reaches 3 to 4 mg. per 100 ml., it is best to substitute furosemide (40 mg. one to three times per day) for the less potent diuretic agents. A second choice is propranolol in a starting dose of 10 mg. four times per day, up to 120 mg. four times per day. If this regimen is not sufficient or if side effects occur, hydralazine (10 to 100 mg. two to four times per day) or prazosin (1 to 5 mg. two to four times per day) may be used. Control of blood pressure by twice daily medication regimens will improve patient compliance. Alpha-methyldopa or clonidine is used as a fourth-line drug. Their side effects of fatigue and lethargy are frequently added to that of uremia. Guanethidine and reserpine should be avoided because they may decrease renal function. The patient can cooperate by checking his or her own blood pressure at home.

Hypertensive crises are best dealt with through the use of a constant infusion of nitroprusside supplemented by intramuscular hydralazine injections. Diazoxide combined with furosemide is also an effective treatment for hypertensive crises (see pp. 206 to 223).

Urinary Tract Infections. Urinary tract infection is a frequent complication of other forms of renal disease and aggravates the renal insufficiency already present. Symptoms, such as fever or back pain, should be investigated by taking cultures of the urine and sensitivity determinations, followed by appropriate therapy. Many antimicrobial agents are both nephrotoxic and excreted by glomerular filtration; therefore their doses must be modified (see Drugs, below).

Drugs. Iatrogenic complications are common in the care of uremic patients, and may either hasten renal failure or aggravate the symptoms of uremia. Alphamethyldopa may cause lethargy and fatigue that are indistinguishable from the symptoms of uremia. Because many drugs are both nephrotoxic and excreted by the kidneys, toxic levels are both more common and more dangerous in the patient with pre-existing renal insufficiency. The most commonly used nephrotoxic drugs are the aminoglycoside antibiotics (gentamicin, tobramycin, kanamycin, and amikacin), methoxyflurane anesthetic agents, tetracyclines, and phenacetin-containing analgesics.

Many other drugs require modified dosage when renal insufficiency is present. There are two articles that are addressed in particular to this problem: "A guide to drug therapy in renal failure" (JAMA, *230*:1544, 1974); and Anderson et al.: Clinical Use of Drugs in Renal Insufficiency (Springfield, Ill., Charles C Thomas, 1976).

Obstruction. Obstruction may be a contributing factor in the patient with deteriorating renal function. Prostatic hypertrophy and kidney stone disease are two common examples, both of which are also frequently complicated by urinary tract infection. Sloughing papillae may also obstruct, and are most frequently seen in patients with diabetic nephropathy or chronic pyelonephritis or who have a history of abusing analgesics. Infusion pyelography and urologic evaluation are important tools in the treatment of the patient with chronic renal failure.

Acute Exacerbation of Renal Failure. Hypertensive crisis, urinary tract infection, drug intoxication, and obstruction may acutely exacerbate chronic, slowly progressive renal failure. The most common cause, however, is *sudden dehydration,* usually precipitated by gastroenteritis, overuse of diuretics, or inappropriately instituted sodium restriction. Vigorous intravenous rehydration should be instituted with a goal of 50 per cent replacement within the first 12 hours. The serum electrolytes, BUN, and creatinine should be monitored every 12 hours. Repeated physical examinations, monitoring of central venous pressure, and a daily roentgenogram of the chest will aid in assessing volume repletion and preventing fluid overload with pulmonary edema.

During acute exacerbation, three life-threatening situations may occur: hyperkalemia, acidosis, or fluid overload. The treatment of these complications is dealt with on pages 530 to 534.

Special Problems. OPERATIONS. A series of problems may be encountered when it is necessary to perform operations on patients with chronic renal failure. The operation itself may impose an acute, usually transient, exacerbation of renal failure. Particularly dangerous is the indiscriminate preoperative habit of restricting the patient's fluid intake, and the patient should go to the operating room well hydrated. In patients with serum creatinine levels above 3 to 4 mg. per 100 ml., the kidneys can be protected through the use of mannitol-furosemide infusion. Mannitol (20 per cent) can be infused at 20 ml. per hour, starting 2 to 3 hours before operation, continuing through it, and then tapered and discontinued over the next 6 to 12 hours. Furosemide, in a dose roughly corresponding to 100 mg. for each mg. per 100 ml. of serum creatinine, is added to 500 ml. mannitol. Thus the patient with a serum creatinine level of 3 mg. per 100 ml. has 300 mg. of furosemide added to the mannitol solution. A patient with a serum creatinine of 7 mg. per 100 ml. has 700 mg. added. To avoid dehydration, replace urine with half isotonic or isotonic saline solution to which 20 to 60 mEq. of potassium chloride has been added per liter solution.

In the patient with severe renal insufficiency with a serum creatinine level of approximately 8 mg. per 100 ml., or a BUN level above 100 mg. per 100 ml., preoperative dialysis will correct the bleeding abnormality of uremia.

PREGNANCY. Patients with serum creatinine levels over 3 mg. per 100 ml. are usually sterile. If pregnancy occurs, there is an increased incidence of spontaneous abortion. There is little evidence to support the contention that pregnancy may aggravate renal failure. An exception to this may be active lupus nephritis in which marked kidney deterioration has been reported during or shortly after pregnancy. Aggravation of the nephrotic syndrome is frequently observed during a pregnancy. A major problem encountered during pregnancy is exacerbation of hypertension, and a patient with severe hypertension should therefore be advised against planned pregnancy. Birth control pills, however, frequently aggravate hypertension.

Maintenance of Homeostasis

As the renal disease progresses, the kidneys' ability to maintain homeostasis is curtailed. Each patient may demonstrate a number of physiologic aberrations, but all patients with severe renal insufficiency are unable to meet any extreme situation. Thus a patient with severe chronic renal failure can tolerate neither a large sodium load nor a sudden sodium restriction. Although there is considerable individual variation, progressive loss of nephrons thus results in a diminished ability to regulate electrolyte and water balance.

Uremia. Some of the symptoms of chronic renal failure, such as fatigue, pruritus, and particularly nausea, vomiting, and hiccups, seem to be caused by the accumulation of urea and toxins that are end-products of protein metabolism. Both the BUN levels and such symptoms can therefore be reduced by protein restriction. The high biologic-value protein-reduced diets are unpalatable, and should be reserved for specific situations. If the patient does not notice any improvement, the diet will not be followed. The gastrointestinal symptoms are the main indication for a trial with diet. Even some patients with BUN levels over 100 mg. per 100 ml., with no obvious symptoms, report a definite improvement after a protein-restricted diet is used. The protein intake should be tailored to the stage of renal failure, and may be estimated by performing a creatinine clearance and using the following levels of restriction. Patients with creatinine clearances greater than 30 ml. per minute usually do not require protein restriction. Those with a creatinine clearance of from 20 to 30 ml. per minute are given 0.7 gram of protein per kg. of body weight; from 5 to 20 ml. per minute, 0.4 gram per kg.; and less than 5 ml. per minute, 0.3 gram per kg. (high quality protein Giordano-Giovanetti diet). Caloric intake must be maintained at 30 to 50 calories per kg. of body weight to avoid catabolism.

When the diet is reduced below 70 grams of protein per day, iron and vitamin supplements should be used. It is unnecessary to treat the hyperuricemia of uremia, unless the patient develops gout (see Bone and Joints, p. 538).

Sodium-Water Edema. Avoid unnecessary sodium restrictions in patients with chronic renal failure. Sodium restriction should be instituted when severe hypertension is present, because sodium-fluid overload makes hypertension almost impossible to control. Other indications are heart failure and edema.

There is no reason to restrict fluids unless oliguria is present, because patients usually drink enough to maintain a normal serum sodium concentration. Patients with diabetic nephropathy have a unique liability to develop sodium and fluid overload.

Severe incapacitating edema can develop in nephrotic patients. In the early stages of renal insufficiency, this can usually be dealt with by dietary sodium restriction and the use of thiazide diuretics, such as chlorthalidone, 100 to 200 mg. per day, or hydrochlorothiazide, 50 to 100 mg. twice daily. During moderate and severe renal insufficiency, however, this therapy is frequently not sufficient. The second drug to be added to the thiazides is spironolactone, 25 mg. two to four times a day. If diuresis does not result, furosemide should be gradually added to the thiazide-spironolactone combination. It may be necessary to use doses up to 1 to 2 grams per day. (This dose of furosemide is not listed in the manufacturer's official directive.) After a patient's edema is controlled, this dose can usually be reduced considerably. In most instances, it is inadvisable and dangerous to completely resolve the edema, because the resulting intravascular hypovolemia may exacerbate the renal failure. Complications of the therapy are hypovolemia, orthostatic hypotension, hypokalemia, and sometimes gout. It takes a good patient-doctor relationship to balance the side effects of this drug therapy against the side effects of the edema.

In extreme cases of edema, the infusion of 50 to 200 ml. per day of 25 per cent salt-poor albumin over several days may be necessary. This increases plasma oncotic pressure and mobilizes the edema so that diuresis can result. The nephrotic syndrome of chronic glomerulonephritis frequently improves as renal function deteriorates.

Acidosis. Severe renal failure is invariably associated with some degree of acidosis. However, bicarbonate levels above 16 to 18 mEq. per liter need not be treated. Moderate acidosis will improve with the use of oral calcium carbonate as described below for Calcium and Phosphorus. Patients with more severe failure require sodium bicarbonate in a dose of 15 to 60 mEq. per day. Oral sodium bicarbonate is sometimes complicated by gastric bloating, and in these instances Shohl's solution (14 grams of citric acid, 9 grams of sodium citrate in 100 ml. of water) can be prescribed. One gram of sodium bicarbonate supplies 12 mEq. of bicarbonate; 10 ml. of Shohl's solution supplies 10 mEq. of bicarbonate.

Potassium. The potassium balance of a patient with renal failure is usually self-regulated until the disease reaches its end-stage. Therefore potassium problems are usually encountered only during an acute exacerbation. In those few patients who develop hyperkalemia without an acute exacerbation, dietary potassium restriction and oral sodium polystyrene sulfonate (Kayexalate), 15 to 30 grams per day, may be necessary. Hypokalemia is a common complication of diuretic therapy and must be detected and corrected, because it can lead to acute exacerbation of the uremia.

Calcium and Phosphorus. Malabsorption of calcium and deficient excretion of phosphorus are invariable concomitants of moderate renal insufficiency. Both the high serum phosphorus and decreased calcium absorption give rise to secondary hyperparathyroidism, which leads to bone disease. During moderate renal insufficiency (creatinine over 3 mg. per 100 ml.), the patient should be started on phosphorus-binding agents. Aluminum hydroxide, most conveniently supplied in capsules (Alu-Caps or Dialume), is given in doses of 0.5 to 2 grams two to four times a day, depending on the serum phosphorus level, which should be maintained within the normal range. Antacids that contain magnesium should not be used in these patients because of the risk of magnesium intoxication. Calcium carbonate should also be given to patients in moderate renal insufficiency in doses of 1 to 2 teaspoons of powder two to four times a day, in order to keep the serum calcium above 8 mg. per 100 ml. (see also Bone and Joints, below).

Organ-Specific Symptoms and Follow-up

General. As the renal disease progresses, weakness, lethargy, and decreasing physical capacity ensue. These symptoms are usually not encountered until the patient enters moderately severe renal failure, with a serum creatinine level greater than 5 to 6 mg. per 100 ml. If the symptoms occur earlier, drug intoxication may be the cause. When the patient approaches severe renal failure, decreased libido, impotency, and amenorrhea ensue. There is no known treatment for these symptoms.

Gastrointestinal Problems. With the progression to severe renal failure, the symptoms originating from the gastrointestinal tract become disturbing to the patient. The patient may complain of a bad taste in the mouth, and fetor uremia may be noted. This can be controlled by careful dental hygiene, with frequent mouthwashings and toothbrushing. Nausea and vomiting occur with increasing frequency as the disease progresses. These symptoms usually occur with BUN levels greater than 100 mg. per 100 ml. and may be expected to resolve with the institution of protein-restricted diets (see Uremia, p. 537).

In the patient with more severe uremia, trimethobenzamide (Tigan), 250 mg. capsules a half hour before meals, or suppositories (200 mg.) when needed may help. Phenothiazine derivatives (Thorazine, Compazine), however, may induce neurologic symptoms and contribute to fatigue, and should not be used.

Patients with severe uremia are also more prone to develop gastroduodenal ulcers, pancreatitis, and either diarrhea or constipation. The treatment for these conditions is no different from that in the patient with normal renal function. Drug modifications may be necessary because of decreased renal clearance (see Drugs, p. 536).

Bone and Joints. Some degree of bone disease is present in all patients with moderate to severe uremia. Impaired absorption of calcium and deficient excretion of phosphorus lead to moderate hypocalcemia and hyperphosphatemia. Hypocalcemia stimulates parathyroid gland activity and causes secondary hyperparathyroidism. Metabolic acidosis may also contribute to bone disease. There may be no clinical manifestations of bone disease, although some uremic patients may develop bone pain, spontaneous fractures, or periarthritis. (Treatment is outlined under Calcium and Phosphorus, above.) If bone pain occurs in spite of aggressive treatment, the patient should be referred to a nephrology center for a trial with one of the new vitamin D metabolites. Regular vitamin D should not be used because of its long half-life and the possibility of prolonged toxicity.

Some patients also develop pain in their joints. If gout is present, colchicine or phenylbutazone may be used for short-term treatment, if the doses are reduced to one-half to one-third when there is moderate renal insufficiency. If hyperuricemia is associated, allopurinol should be used in the smallest effective dose. Probenecid is inefficient against the serum uric acids and provides no benefit to the patient with moderately severe renal failure.

Skin. Pruritus can be a disabling symptom of uremia. It may occur when hyperphosphatemia is present, and in some instances it is alleviated with the use of aluminum hydroxide gels. High levels of parathyroid hormone and calcium can also induce pruritus. It is also possible that some uremic toxins cause pruritus, because improvements have been noted when protein-restricted diets were used. Uremic patients seem to have less than normal sebum and sweat formation, and their skin is usually dry; therefore moisturizers and skin creams are useful. Symptomatic treatment with antihistamines, such as diphenhydramine (Benadryl), 25 mg. two to three times a day, or hydroxyzine pamoate (Vistaril) 50 mg. every 6 hours as necessary, may be needed.

Hematologic. All patients with progressive renal failure become anemic. The anemia develops slowly; therefore a sudden decrease in a patient's hemoglobin level indicates bleeding. Other causes may be deficiencies (folic acid, vitamin B_{12}, and iron), particularly if the patient is on a restricted diet. Results of the serum iron and iron binding capacity tests may be misleading in uremic patients, and evaluation of the bone marrow may provide a more accurate assessment of iron storage. Vitamin and iron supplements should be prescribed when appropriate. When the patient enters severe renal insufficiency and has incapacitating anemia, a trial with testosterone derivatives (nandrolone decanoate [Deca-Durabolin], 100 mg. per week intramuscularly) may stimulate erythropoiesis, although the masculinizing side effects can be particularly disturbing to some women patients.

Patients with advanced renal failure should not be given blood transfusions unless hemorrhage or life-threatening anemia occurs. Transfusions decrease the patients' bone marrow activity, pose a hazard of hepatitis, and may make later transplantation impossible because of presensitization to white blood cell antigens.

Coagulation. As the patient becomes severely uremic, the coagulation process becomes increasingly abnormal, primarily as the result of altered platelet function. These patients usually do not bleed spontaneously, but there is an increased risk of bleeding during operations. Platelet transfusions are not of value, because transfused platelets do not function normally in a uremic patient. If the patient bleeds, all medications known to impair platelet function (i.e., analgesics, antihistamines) must be discontinued. There is no known cure for the bleeding diathesis other than dialysis, which will rapidly improve platelet function.

Cardiovascular System. If cardiac failure develops, it is usually caused by sodium-fluid overload with hypertension, and this should be the target of therapy. Large doses of furosemide may be needed with severe renal insufficiency, at times requiring up to 1 to 2 grams orally in divided doses daily. (This dose is higher than that listed in the manufacturer's official directive.) Rapid infusion of high-dose furosemide may cause deafness, which is usually transient. Digitalis is rarely needed. Digoxin is the preferred preparation, and the maintenance dose must be reduced by 50 per cent for patients with severe uremia.

Pericarditis is a specific complication of severe uremia. Although some patients may respond to dietary treatment, pericarditis almost always requires dialysis.

Pulmonary System. Although there is no apparent specific pulmonary disease present in uremic patients, an incipient pulmonary edema (frequently appearing as a "butterfly pattern" on roentgenograms) is a consequence of fluid overload. Patients with moderate fluid overload sometimes develop pulmonary edema rapidly after seemingly minor upper respiratory tract infections. High doses of furosemide may save the patient's life (see Cardiovascular System, above). Fluid overload can also be treated through the induction of diarrhea. A 70 per cent sorbitol solution in a dose of 2 ml. per kg. may be used orally, or 10 to 15 ml. per kg. of a 20 per cent sorbitol solution can be given rectally. Patients with functioning gastrointestinal tracts usually lose between 2 and 4 kg. of body weight in 12 to 24 hours by this method.

Neuromuscular System. Lethargy and an inability to concentrate are common occurrences during severe renal failure. If these symptoms occur before the serum creatinine is 7 to 8 mg. per 100 ml., iatrogenic (drug intoxication) or electrolyte problems may be the cause. Asterixis, confusion, and psychosis may occur when the uremia is extreme. Dialysis is the only effective treatment for these problems. Tetany and convulsions are usually related to electrolyte abnormalities, particularly hyponatremia and hypocalcemia, but they may also be triggered by hypertension.

All patients with moderate uremia will have clinical evidence of peripheral neuropathy with decreased nerve conduction velocity. Symptoms of paresthesias or pain in the feet or legs may herald an abrupt worsening of their disease. Physical signs include decreased vibratory sensation and absent deep tendon reflexes. Progressive neuropathy is another indication for the initiation of dialysis.

Follow-up

Chronic renal failure is a disease that takes many years to develop, and close cooperation between physician and patient is necessary to successfully deal with all of the symptoms associated with it.

During the *early asymptomatic stage*, only twice yearly visits that include a physical examination, blood pressure, serum creatinine level, urinary protein determination, and urine cultures are necessary. The patient must be examined more often as edema and hypertension occur.

As the patient enters into *moderate and severe renal failure*, more frequent contact is necessary. When the serum creatinine reaches the level of 6 to 8 mg. per 100 ml., the patient should be seen not less frequently than every other month.

At this stage, the physical examination should include particular attention to blood pressure and the secondary complications of hypertension, as well as signs of pericarditis and neuropathy. Determinations of BUN, creatinine, electrolytes including bicarbonate, calcium, phosphorus, and alkaline phosphatase should be made. If symptoms are present, urine cultures should be performed. The hematocrit should be measured. If the anemia is out of proportion to the renal failure, evaluation for bleeding or iron or vitamin deficiencies should be undertaken.

The patient should keep a weekly chart of his or her weight. If the patient is hypertensive, blood pressure readings, taken both sitting and standing, should be recorded two or three times a week.

As the stage of moderate renal failure is entered, treatment with oral calcium and aluminum hydroxide gel should be started to retard the developing bone disease. When special diets are used, vitamin and iron supplements are added. Sodium bicarbonate is prescribed as acidosis progresses, and antihypertensive medications and diuretics are used as necessary. Protein restriction is used increasingly during the late stages of kidney failure. Testosterone may be tried for anemia, and one must be alert to the signs and symptoms of pericarditis and neuropathy.

Both the physician and the patient must be aware of the gradual onset of symptoms and also of the patient's individual tolerance. For the same degree of uremia, patients with polycystic kidneys seem to tolerate uremia well and have fewer symptoms than the patient with glomerulonephritis. Diabetic patients, on the other hand, frequently develop uremic symptoms and complications much earlier than others. Sudden deterioration is frequently iatrogenic in origin or is caused by dehydration.

Definitive Therapy

Several options are available for patients with chronic renal failure; both dialysis and transplantation are successful procedures. The 8 or 9 year cumulative survival in middle-aged patients with a related donor kidney transplant is approximately 85 to 90 per cent, and in chronic dialysis and cadaver transplantation the 9 year cumulative survival at the most successful centers is 60 to 70 per cent. Children as young as 1 year, and adults older than 60, have had successful transplants. Diabetic patients are now regular transplant recipients. Therefore almost all patients with severe uremia should be evaluated by a dialysis-transplant team.

The first contact should be made during early renal failure so that the patient is familiarized with the dialysis-transplant team. The patient should be seen by a nephrologist before the serum creatinine is 8 mg. per 100 ml. Diabetic patients should be seen when the serum creatinine is about 5 mg. per 100 ml. At this time, a pretransplant work-up should be initiated, and an arteriovenous fistula for future dialysis should be created. Failure to refer patients before reaching end-stage renal disease may severely complicate dialysis treatment later. Almost all patients, including those who would like to undergo transplantation, require a period of hemodialysis.

The patient should be started on dialysis as definitive therapy or as a preparation for his or her transplant no later than when the creatinine level reaches 12 to 13 mg. per 100 ml., or 8 to 9 mg. per 100 ml. for diabetic patients. Although some patients may feel relatively well at these levels, life-threatening or disabling complications occur frequently. The risks of continued conservative management at this level of renal function are unacceptable in view of the present success of dialysis and transplantation.

GENITOURINARY TUBERCULOSIS

method of
RICHARD J. BOXER, M.D.,
and RICHARD M. EHRLICH, M.D.
Los Angeles, California

The diagnosis of genitourinary tuberculosis must be confirmed prior to initiating chemotherapy. The diagnosis should be based on the identification of *Mycobacterium tuberculosis* in culture and the finding of acid-fast bacilli in the stained urinary smear or, less commonly, tissue biopsy. Guinea pig inoculation has been abandoned by most laboratories, but is still worthy of consideration if the clinical index of suspicion is high despite prior negative cultures. The urine specimen should be the first voided morning urine; collections on 3 separate days are necessary to be certain the diagnosis is not missed through patient or laboratory error. It is important to have the patient off antibiotics at the time of urine collection. Tetracycline has some tuberculostatic effect and can interfere with culture and diagnosis.

If the urinary smear or culture is positive, prompt initiation of chemotherapy is indicated. If radiologic changes are highly suspicious for tuberculosis, then consideration should be given to starting chemotherapy prior to laboratory confirmation, as cultures take at least 6 weeks.

Isolation in a hospital or sanatorium is no longer necessary unless concomitant active pulmonary lesions are demonstrated. Since *M. tuberculosis* is spread by inhalation, proper disposal of the urine is necessary and all patients should sit when voiding. General measures include good dietary intake, a multivitamin supplement, and exercise. However, it is recommended that the patient refrain from strenuous exercise for a period lasting at least 6 months.

Family members and close contacts must be screened for pulmonary tuberculosis by skin tests and chest roentgenograms. An adult who manifests a newly positive skin test must be followed with chest roentgenograms every 3 to 6 months, although specific chemotherapy is not indicated. On the other hand, a child with a positive skin test should be considered a recent converter and should undergo isoniazid (INH) therapy for 1 year, during which time chest x-rays should be performed every 3 to 6 months.

Gow (J. Urol., *115*:707, 1976) reappraised the traditional 2 years of medical therapy. He suggested that 6 months of rifampin, ethambutol, and INH were sufficient to eliminate tuberculosis from the urinary tract. In addition, 63 per cent of his patients had major surgery. The short course is experimental, and until much more data and follow-up are presented, we will continue to recommend 2 years of chemotherapy.

The cornerstone of therapy is the proper use and combination of medicines for 2 years. The patient must understand the importance of taking the medication and the possible untoward effects as manifested by fever, skin rash, decrease in color perception or visual field, tinnitus, hearing loss, vertigo, peripheral neuritis, or gastrointestinal distress. In addition, general malaise and jaundice are important signs of drug-induced hepatitis.

Surgery is indicated for intractable pain, fever, persistently positive cultures, ureteral stricture, a persistently nonfunctioning kidney, or caseating epididymitis. Surgical intervention may be an important adjunct to medical therapy.

Specific Chemotherapy

The value of employing multiple drugs in the therapy is to decrease the number of resistant organisms. The following treatment is used at the University of California, Los Angeles (UCLA) Hospital:

1. Isoniazid (INH), 300 mg. per day by mouth.
2. Ethambutol, 15 mg. per kg. once per day taken by mouth.
3. Cycloserine, 250 mg. twice daily by mouth.
4. Pyridoxine (Vitamin B_6), 100 mg. daily by mouth.

Streptomycin has been replaced in all but special instances. If cultures indicate that the *M. tuberculosis* is susceptible only to streptomycin, the drug is used. Ototoxicity, vestibular toxicity, and the pain and inconvenience of intramuscular injections, as well as the demonstration that the drugs listed above are a highly effective combination, have caused us to avoid streptomycin; however, if it is used, a baseline audiogram is recommended.

The toxicity of *isoniazid* (INH) specifically involves the central or peripheral nervous system and the liver. The former toxicity is well known and can be largely prevented by the daily use of pyridoxine, 100 mg. Attention has recently been focused on INH-induced hepatitis. The Center for Disease Control (CDC), in a joint communiqué with the American Thoracic and American Lung Societies (Morbidity and Mortality Weekly Report, February 22, 1975), states that "monitoring by routine laboratory tests (e.g., serum glutamic oxaloacetic transaminase [SGOT], serum glutamic pyruvic transaminiase [SGPT], serum bilirubin, and alkaline phosphatase) is not useful in predicting hepatic disease in INH recipients and therefore is not recommended. However, in evaluating signs and symptoms, such tests are mandatory." If the SGOT level does not exceed three times normal and no signs or symptoms exist, "INH may be continued with caution and careful observation," the CDC states.

Gastrointestinal distress is the primary untoward effect of *para-aminosalicylic acid* (PAS), but sodium PAS is usually better tolerated with less bloating and diarrhea; nonetheless, some patients experience episodes of gas and loose stools throughout the period of treatment. Thus we have replaced PAS with ethambutol as a primary drug because patient compliance is significantly better and thus further ensures continuation of the multiple drug regimen.

Ethambutol is equally effective as PAS yet avoids annoying gastrointestinal distress. Retrobulbar neuritis that produces loss of visual acuity, inability to distinguish the color green, and impairment of peripheral vision are a few untoward effects occasionally observed when ethambutol is taken. Hyperuricemia may also follow prolonged administration in rare instances. Half of this medication is excreted in unchanged form in the urine; thus smaller doses should be used in those patients with azotemia. The dosage is 25 mg. per kg. of body weight during the first 2 weeks, and then 15 mg. per kg. taken by mouth daily.

Cycloserine is well tolerated and the toxicity is low when the dosage is 250 mg. twice daily. The toxicity is usually seen in the central or peripheral nervous system and can be controlled by pyridoxine. Skin rash and hepatic toxicity have been noted but not frequently.

Ethionamide, chemically similar to INH, is an alternative drug that is reserved for resistant organisms and otherwise rarely used. It is highly toxic, and liver function tests must be monitored. The dosage is 250 mg. three times daily by mouth.

Rifampin is a new bactericidal drug that is proving highly effective against *M. tuberculosis.* Although it is now used almost exclusively for retreatment, it may eventually become a primary drug. Because of hepatotoxicity, liver function tests should be monitored. It has been reported that the intermittent use of rifampin commonly results in allergic reactions such as urticaria, dyspnea, bronchospasm, thrombocytopenia, and renal failure. A "flu" syndrome is the most common untoward effect. Therefore the intermittent use of rifampin is not recommended. Cohn (JAMA, *228*:828, 1974) has noted the decreased effectiveness of oral contraceptives as well as menstrual irregularities with rifampin administration.

Three of the commonly used drugs (INH, cycloserine, and ethionamide) have shown some ability to irritate the central nervous system; therefore excessive stimulants such as amphetamine sulfate (Benzedrine) or coffee should be avoided. Anticonvulsant medication may be necessary.

Surgical Therapy

Surgical therapy is an important adjunct to chemotherapy. Although it is rarely necessary, nephrectomy is indicated for intractable pain, hematuria, persistent fever, bacterial infection behind stenosed calyces, hypertension secondary to a tuberculous kidney, ureteral stricture not amenable to dilatation, drug intolerance, or failure of prolonged medical therapy. Obstructing cicatricial lesions of calcyes can cause renal destruction, and partial nephrectomy, usually of the upper pole, may preserve the remaining kidney. When a solitary kidney is affected, partial nephrectomy may be extremely important. Although we have not found it necessary, some surgeons advocate cavernostomy (speleostomy) for obstruction of a calyceal neck.

Ureteral reimplantation for distal ureteral cicatricial obstructions can save the kidney. If the lesion is situated in the middle or proximal third of the ureter, interposition of the intestine (ileal ureter) can be successfully employed.

Bladder contracture, a frequent problem, can cause severe symptoms which can be alleviated by cystoplasty, using cecum if the ureterovesical junctions are intact. However, if there is vesicoureteral reflux, an ileocecocystoplasty is the preferred procedure. This effectively eliminates reflux by interposing the ileocecal valve.

Epididymectomy is indicated for patients with caseation of the epididymis.

Follow-up Care

Danger exists in the event of recurrence, resistance, or cicatricial obstruction. A routine urinalysis should be performed every 4 to 8 weeks; if pyuria increases, the physician is alerted to possible recurrence or resistance, and urine concentrates for acid-fast bacilli or cultures should be promptly initiated. Routine culture for bacteria every 2 months is also indicated to detect secondary infections.

An intravenous urogram (IVP) should be done every 3 months during the first year, every 6 months in the second year, and every 2 years thereafter. Ureteral obstruction can frequently be prevented by calibration. Thus using a No. 6 F. catheter, ureteral calibration should be done every 4 months during treatment and every 6 months thereafter for 5 years. During cystoscopy, if bladder ulcerations are seen, a solution of neomycin sulfate (500 mg.), bacitracin (10,000 units), and 2 per cent procaine hydrochloride is instilled.

Renal function should be monitored frequently by measuring serum creatinine and blood urea nitrogen. Serial blood pressures should also be done.

Genitourinary tuberculosis can be effectively controlled if diagnosed early in its course. It is important to note that the disease can affect all ages and should be considered in the differential diagnosis when dealing with unexplained cases of fever, urinary tract infection, hematuria, pyelonephritis, papillary necrosis, or ureteral stricture. Finally, because tuberculosis is spread by the hematogenous route, it is a systemic disease capable of affecting both kidneys.

Acknowledgment

The authors thank Barbara J. Kahn, M.P.A., for her help in writing this manuscript.

TUMORS OF THE GENITOURINARY TRACT

method of
HARRY GRABSTALD, M.D.
New York, New York

Prostate

Benign Tumors. Symptomatic benign prostatic hypertrophy and, very rarely, the benign leiomyoma should be removed by prostatectomy by any one of four techniques: transurethral, suprapubic, retropubic, or perineal.

Malignant Tumors. By far the most important malignant tumor of the prostate is the adenocarcinoma. There are 55,000 new cases seen each year. Therapy depends upon grade and stage of the disease. For practical purposes, four stages of the disease will be considered.

STAGE 1. Incidental cancer is the form discovered upon removal of the specimen for presumed benign disease. It is conceivable that a simple prostatectomy may have removed all malignant tissue. My personal preference is not to follow simple prostatectomy with radical total prostatectomy. Factors to be considered include the patient's age and condition, and the grade and stage of tumors—i.e., percentage of prostate removed which is involved by cancer. For high grade cancers occupying a large portion of the gland, external therapy may be suggested. If the patient is young—50 to 60 years of age—then total (radical) prostatectomy may be done if the patient is willing to assume the risk of 100 per cent impotence and 5 to 20 per cent or more incontinence.

My choice of treatment is to follow with rectal examinations to see if there is an increase in size and degree of induration and then to use external radiation therapy. Lymphangiography may give a clue regarding node status. If proper therapy is predicated on proper diagnosis, i.e., accurate staging, then lymph node involvement should be documented. Repeat biopsy may be indicated.

STAGE 2. Early operable prostatic cancer is manifest by an asymptomatic small isolated nodule in the prostate and should be treated by total prostatectomy, including prostate and capsule and seminal vesicles. Preliminary biopsy is mandatory, as 50 per cent of "hard prostates" are benign. When total prostatectomy is performed by the retropubic approach, lymphadenectomy may be accomplished, although the value of this procedure is not known. A second and perhaps equally good method of treatment is radiation therapy by external or interstitial means. We favor the latter technique, using ^{125}I which has a lower morbidity.

STAGE 3. Approximately 35 to 50 per cent of patients are seen in this stage. This consists of locally advanced disease with involvement of most of one or both lobes and possibly seminal vesicles. External radiation therapy for larger glands and interstitial or external radiation is the suggested therapy. Estrogenic hormones—e.g., stilbestrol, 3 mg. daily—or bilateral orchiectomy may be used, although I have generally saved these methods for patients with metastases. Transurethral resection may be required when there are obstructive symptoms.

STAGE 4. Locally extensive cancer with distant metastases is managed by means of hormone therapy or castration and transurethral resection if necessary. In many instances, response to hormone therapy is favorable and transurethral resection may be obviated. The superiority of one form of estrogenic hormone over another has never been demonstrated, and, in fact, the dosage of estrogenic hormones has not been standardized. Three mg. daily is generally adequate.

Perhaps the most challenging prostatic cancer patients are in relapse—i.e., those who have once responded to hormone therapy but are now in failure. Cortisone, adrenalectomy, and hypophysectomy are all procedures of limited merit. There is no cancer chemotherapeutic agent that has been found to be consistently useful in the management of patients with prostatic cancer who are in relapse. Cytoxan and 5-fluorouracil (5-FU) are occasionally useful.

Sarcoma of the Prostate. The most common forms of sarcoma of the prostate are the round cell, spindle cell, leiomyosarcoma, and rhabdomyosarcoma. Except for lymphosarcoma, these sarcomas are generally quite radioresistant. Total prostatectomy as a part of an anterior exenteration is indicated.

Penis

Benign Tumors. CONDYLOMATA ACUMINATA. Methods of therapy are topical and surgical.

Topical: Application of podophyllin is often effective but time consuming. The medication may prove irritating, especially to glans and scrotal wall. The use of 5-fluorouracil cream or solution (Efudex) has recently been found to be effective and is probably the topical agent of choice.

Surgical: Simple electrofulguration under local anesthesia is easily performed and effective, and may, when the lesions are neither too large nor numerous, be carried out as an office procedure.

The surgical method of choice is circumcision, with removal of as many condylomas with the prepuce as possible. Simple fulguration of the remaining lesions is effective. Circumcision is the only means by which recurrence can often be prevented.

A malignant variant is known (Buschke-Loewenstein tumor), but the lesion is not considered premalignant.

MISCELLANEOUS, RARE BENIGN TUMORS. These include parameatal cyst, lipoma, fibroma, glomus tumor, hemangioma, and lymphangioma. Treatment consists of simple complete surgical excision with verification of the benign nature of the tumor. Attention to other areas, if the disease is a part of a systemic or more diffuse process, such as hemangioma, is advised.

Prominent cutaneous papillae occurring on the coronal margin of the glans may resemble papillomas but should not be confused with condylomata acuminata. Excisional biopsy, for proof of benignity of the lesion, and circumcision comprise the treatment of choice, although if not prominent or bothersome, the lesions may be left untreated.

Penile horns represent extreme forms of keratosis. They may develop on a wart or acanthoma, and many grow to extreme size, up to 9 cm. in length. These should be excised, for they tend to undergo malignant change over a long period of time.

Premalignant Tumors. Among the so-called premalignant or preinvasive tumors are included erythroplasia of Queyrat, carcinoma in situ (Bowen's disease), and leukoplakia.

Complete local excision of the tumor with close follow-up examination is the treatment of choice for each of these lesions, especially when circumcision has not previously been performed. The incidence of cancer in patients with erythroplasia of Queyrat is high. Actually, the term erythroplasia of Queyrat is a synonym for in situ cancer.

Occasionally local partial amputation or radiation therapy is required because of the extensive nature of the lesions, despite their microscopic appearance.

Malignant Tumors (Primary). By far the most common and important tumor of the penis is the epidermoid or squamous cell carcinoma. The treatment is as follows:

1. Adequate and prompt biopsy of all penile ulcers which do not heal quickly is mandatory. This is especially true in the uncircumcised or in those circumcised after childhood.

2. Simple partial penile amputation with a 2 cm. margin proximal to the tumor is generally adequate. A period of approximately 2 weeks is allowed to elapse in order to theoretically permit whatever tumor is in the lymphatics between penis and inguinofemoral nodes to reach these areas and to allow secondary inflammation of these nodes to subside, as 50 per cent of enlarged nodes are inflammatory. Penis cancers which are noninfiltrating and less than 2.5 cm. in size may be treated by supervoltage external radiation therapy. Even if there is residual or recurrent disease, surgery can still be accomplished.

3. Bilateral superficial and deep groin and pelvic node dissection, including femoral, external, internal and common iliacs, is advocated when nodes are palpable. Neither preoperative nor postoperative radiation therapy is recommended to groins.

More extensive tumors involving a great portion of the shaft of the penis may require radical penectomy with permanent perineal urethrostomy.

Miscellaneous malignant tumors include sarcoma and malignant endothelioma. The treatment of choice is partial or total amputation of the penis, depending upon the margin obtainable.

Malignant Tumors (Secondary). Secondary tumors of the penis are not uncommon; they are mostly of prostatic, bladder, or rectal origin. Extensive surgery is generally not indicated, for the prognosis is poor. Simple penile amputation may be necessary to control pain, bleeding, or infection.

Both primary and metastatic melanomas of the penis are rare. For the primary tumor, partial amputation of the penis, if possible, is carried out along with superficial and deep groin dissection in continuity. When the disease is metastatic, the nature and extent of the generalized melanomatosis would dictate to a great extent the therapy of the penile metastasis. Local excision for control of pain may be required.

Testis

All testicular tumors should be considered malignant. Therapy includes treatment of the primary tumor, regional lymphatics, and distant metastases.

The Primary Tumor. Simple orchiectomy with ligation of the spermatic cord at the level of the internal ring should be performed as soon as the diagnosis of tumor is suspected.

Aspiration or open biopsies should not be performed under any circumstances, for local tumor spillage may markedly alter the course and prognosis.

Early orchiectomy affords the earliest and simplest means of making a histologic diagnosis, which information, in turn, is vital to planning further therapy.

Regional Lymphatics. The testis drains to the retroperitoneal periaortic and pericaval nodes. Radical retroperitoneal lymphadenectomy is recommended in patients with embryonal carcinoma and teratocarcinoma. This applies whether or not there is proof of existence of tumor-containing nodes, as evidenced by ureteral deviation on pyelography, physical findings, or lymphangiography. External radiation therapy may also be used for those who refuse node dissection. There is no proof of the superiority of surgery over radiation therapy. The reliability of markers (alpha-fetoprotein, CEA, and β-subunit gonadotropin) may someday make it feasible to eliminate the need for node dissections in some patients.

Node dissection is not recommended for seminoma because of the radiosensitivity of the tumor and the excellent results obtained with radiation.

Patients with seminoma should be treated by simple orchiectomy followed by supervoltage radiation therapy, utilizing a tumor dosage of 2000 to 3000 R in 2 to 4 weeks.

The cancer chemotherapy to be described may be considered in the management of patients with extensive retroperitoneal node disease which is inoperable or nonresectable.

Following chemotherapy with the newer combinations of agents, re-exploration or second-look procedures are often warranted. External radiation therapy may be used for such nodal disease, although masive involvement is generally radioresistant.

Distant Metastases. Progress in the treatment of metastatic testicular cancer has been most gratifying. By utilizing drug combinations and by treating properly and to toxicity, high response rates are noted. The present agents of choice include vinblastine, actinomycin D, bleomycin, cisplatinum, cyclophosphamide, doxorubicin, and chlorambucil in various carefully monitored combinations. These agents are effective but toxic, and great care should be taken in their use.

Adrenal

The treatment for almost all tumors of the adrenal gland, whether cortical or medullary, whether hormonal or nonhormonal, consists of total removal of adrenal and tumor.

When adrenalectomy is performed for pheochromocytoma, a drop in blood pressure must be anticipated and carefully treated by having the anesthesia team prepared to use agents to raise blood pressure, such as phentolamine (Regitine), when the tumor is removed.

Total surgical excision of a neuroblastoma is the preferred treatment, although this tumor is particularly often inoperable because of local invasion of vital structures.

When primary aldosteronism is secondary to adrenal tumor, simple removal of the cortical adenoma is the treatment of choice.

When adrenalectomy is to be performed for Cushing's syndrome secondary to an adrenal cortical tumor, the patient should be prepared preoperatively by steroids, which should be continued postoperatively. Adrenal cortical carcinomas, hormonal or nonhormonal, are best treated by total adrenalectomy. The treatment of choice for metastatic adrenal carcinoma is o,p′-DDD. No other agent appears useful.

Scrotum

Benign Tumors. Scrotal sebaceous cysts are common. They may be treated by simple surgical excision when symptomatic. Other benign tumors include dermoid cysts, angiomas, hemangiomas, lipomas, and fibromas—all of which may be excised surgically for diagnostic as well as for cosmetic or symptomatic purposes.

Malignant Tumors. Epithelioma or cancer of the scrotum is fortunately rare today. The treatment is wide surgical excision. Although little information is available relative to the value of superficial and deep groin dissection in the management of these patients, it should be carried out after a period of 2 to 3 weeks following scrotal surgery if nodes are palpable.

Kidney

Benign Tumors. Benign tumors of the kidney are rare unless one includes simple benign cortical cysts as tumors. Although one may suspect either tumor or cyst, in any one given patient with a renal mass and a filling defect on pyelograms, only further studies or exploration will yield the definitive diagnosis. For this reason, all renal masses should be evaluated with CT (computerized tomograms) and arteriography.

Simple cortical adenomas, usually incidental

autopsy findings, are very rarely of a size sufficient to be clinically manifest.

Malignant Tumors. The three most important and common tumors of the kidney are renal cell adenocarcinoma (hypernephroma), nephroblastoma (Wilms' tumor), and tumors of the renal pelvis (transitional cell).

RENAL CELL CANCER WITHOUT METASTASES. Total nephrectomy is the treatment of choice for renal cell adenocarcinoma without metastases. An incision appropriate to remove kidney, perirenal fat and fascia, and adjacent lymph nodes and to facilitate early pedicle ligation is preferable. The incidence of direct extension to the perirenal fascia is high, and a radical nephrectomy should therefore include removal of all surrounding perirenal fat, fascia, and nodes. I prefer a transabdominal approach. Renal infarction via the renal artery may help decrease blood loss at nephrectomy.

Routine preoperative irradiation is not recommended, and the value of postoperative irradiation is uncertain.

RENAL CELL CARCINOMA WITH METASTASES. Nephrectomy in the presence of metastases may be considered (1) as a part of a planned therapeutic approach in which both the primary renal tumor and metastatic disease are to be removed, (2) with the faint hope that metastases might regress after nephrectomy, and (3) for the purpose of palliation of local or systemic symptoms. In instances when surgery may be contraindicated, radiation therapy is of occasional value, especially in the palliation of hematuria.

Although there are scattered reports of response of renal cell adenocarcinoma to chemotherapy, results with the chemotherapy of this tumor have been generally very poor. The natural history of the tumor may be responsible for some of the "favorable" reports to date.

NEPHROBLASTOMA (WILMS' TUMOR). The treatment of choice for Wilms' tumor is nephrectomy as soon as possible by the transperitoneal approach. Postoperative irradiation therapy is recommended with an accepted dose range of 3000 to 4000 R over 3 to 4 weeks, beginning on the day of or following surgery. As a rule, however, nephrectomy in children is not difficult regardless of tumor size.

Postoperative radiation is not recommended when the child is under 1 year of age, or when the tumor is encapsulated, has not crossed the midline, and has not been spilled in its removal.

Cure rates with Wilms' tumor are much higher over the past few years since the advent of prophylactic cyclic chemotherapy utilizing actinomycin D and vincristine.

TUMORS OF THE RENAL PELVIS. The treatment of choice for transitional cell carcinoma of the renal pelvis is total nephroureterectomy with resection of a cuff of bladder so as to ensure complete removal of the intravesical portion of the ureter. The patient should be followed by cystoscopy and urine cytology.

Ureter

All ureteral tumors should be considered malignant. The treatment of choice is total nephroureterectomy with resection of a bladder cuff.

Urinary Bladder

Proper therapy is predicated upon accurate staging and upon an understanding of the behavior and pathology of bladder tumors.

Benign Papillomas. Transurethral resection with electrocoagulation is the treatment of choice and yields excellent results. Repeat cystoscopy every 3 months during the first year, every 4 to 6 months during the second year, and annually thereafter should be carried out. Open surgical treatment of benign papillomas should be avoided when possible. Even repeated transurethral resection, when tumors are multiple, is to be preferred to open surgery.

True papillomatosis, in which the bladder wall mucosa is virtually replaced by papillomas and in which relatively little normal mucosa is seen, may occasionally require total cystectomy and urinary diversion. Even in such patients, however, a trial of conservative therapy may sometimes yield surprisingly good results. Intravesical thiotepa may occasionally decrease the frequency with which transurethral surgery may be required.

Malignant Epidermoid Cancer. SUPERFICIALLY INFILTRATING LOW-GRADE TUMORS. The initial treatment of choice for superficially infiltrating tumors of low grade is transurethral resection when the tumor is cystoscopically accessible. When the tumor may not be completely resected transurethrally because of location, segmental resection is utilized. Unfortunately, most bladder tumors do not occur in the dome or in areas where adequate segmental resection is possible. Urine cytology is a mandatory part of follow-up after transurethral resections.

Under certain circumstances, total cystectomy is the treatment of choice even when the tumor is superficially infiltrating. For example, when there is rapid recurrence or evidence of residual tumor after conservative surgery, when tumors are multiple, or when ureteral orifices or bladder neck may be compromised by lesser procedures, cystectomy may be required.

DEEPLY INFILTRATING HIGH-GRADE TUMORS. When tumors are of deep stage and high grade, transurethral techniques are generally of little value. The treatment of choice is segmental bladder resection when a single tumor is found in the dome of the bladder or in an area permitting resection with a 4 cm. margin of healthy bladder wall.

Anterior exenteration (radical total cystectomy) includes removal of bladder, pelvic fascia, peritoneum and lymphatics, prostate, and seminal vesicles in men or uterus, tubes, ovaries, and upper vagina in women; it should be considered when lesser sugical procedures cannot be utilized. Whether segmental resection or radical cystectomy is performed, the procedures should be preceded by external radiation therapy. The most commonly utilized is cobalt. The dosage is either 200 R in 5 days or 4000 R over 4 weeks.

External irradiation as the sole therapeutic modality may be utilized in patients with infiltrating tumors when surgical excision is not feasible because of age or general conditions. Supervoltage irradiation with a dosage of 6000 R tumor dose is advocated. Urinary diversion by ileal conduit may be combined with irradiation therapy and is indicated when urinary symptoms are severe and when there are progressive hydronephrosis and danger of impending renal failure. Postoperative irradiation is generally of little palliative value and of no curative value when bladder tumors are inoperable because of extensive local disease or because of nodal involvement. Radiation will not prevent recurrences.

Urethra

Male Urethral Tumors (Benign). Condylomata acuminata, although they more often involve the penile skin, may also involve the distal urethra and should be treated by excisional biopsy (to rule out cancer) and transurethral fulguration. Other benign tumors include urethral polyps, adenomas, and papillomas. These are best managed by excisional biopsy and electrofulguration. Urethroscopy and urethrography are mandatory to rule out those tumors which cannot be seen by simple inspection of the meatus. Intraurethral topical fluorouracil (Efudex) may be tried.

Male Urethral Tumors (Malignant). The most common malignant tumor of the male urethra is the squamous cell (epidermoid) cancer. Others include columnar cancers, adenocarcinomas, transitional cell carcinomas, and melanomas.

The treatment of choice depends upon tumor size, location, and extent of disease. Simple partial penile amputation should be carried out for cancers of the distal urethra. Most urethral tumors occur in the bulbous portion of the urethra and are generally very extensive invaders of local structures. Radical total cystectomy, prostatectomy, and penectomy with simultaneous lymphadenectomy is the treatment of choice. Urinary diversion by ileal conduit is the diversionary procedure of choice. Most patients have extensive perineal masses and fistulas, and simple excision is impossible. Interstitial irradiation techniques and external irradiation may be utilized when the tumor is inoperable or when the age or general condition of the patient precludes radical surgery. Radiation techniques, regardless of the mode of administration, are not curative. Radiation therapy may be combined with simple suprapubic cystotomy, although the latter diversionary procedure is not always satisfactory because urethral leakage of urine via the perineum and/or the fistulas or urethra often continues. After ablative surgery is accomplished and after a 3 to 4 week delay, during which time antibiotics may be used, radical groin dissections should be carried out if there are inguinal nodes involved.

Female Urethral Tumors (Benign). Benign tumors of the female urethra include papillomas, fibromas, and angiomas, and are treated by simple excisional biopsy and fulguration. Cancer must be ruled out. When urethral caruncles are symptomatic, excisional biopsy and fulguration is mandatory.

Adequate excision of distal urethral tumors in the female may be aided by insertion of a Foley catheter, distention of the balloon, and traction so as to facilitate adequate examination of the urethra, which may then be inspected by eversion of the meatus.

Female Urethral Tumors (Malignant). Cancer of the female urethra may offer an extreme therapeutic challenge, because local excision is rarely possible. Total cystectomy, urethrectomy with lymphadenectomy, and urinary diversion by ileal conduit is the treatment of choice unless only the distal third is involved and local excision is possible.

Interstitial implantation techniques utilizing iridium and other radioactive materials are now being utilized with increasing frequency for distal third tumors, and the results, in some hands, are equal to those obtained by radical surgical means. In those patients in whom radical surgery may not be feasible, interstitial and external radiation therapy is the treatment of choice. I prefer anterior exenteration preceded by external radiation therapy.

URETHRAL STRICTURES

method of
SHLOMO RAZ, M.D.
Los Angeles, California

Female Urethral Stricture

Etiology. The cause of female urethral stricture may be chronic urethritis, atrophic vaginitis resulting from estrogen deficiency, or a congenital or functional abnormality (an example of the latter would be external sphincter spasticity).

Treatment. Treatment of urethral stricture in the female will depend on the cause of her condition. When atrophic vaginitis is suspected as a reason for the narrowing, a high dosage of local estrogen cream is helpful. When chronic urethritis is present with recurrent urinary tract infection, urethral dilatations can be used, but the results of these procedures are unpredictable. Pharmacologic treatments are aimed at relaxing the bladder neck and urethra, and mainly consist of alpha-adrenergic blocking drugs, such as phenoxybenzamine hydrochloride (Dibenzyline). Surgical procedures such as internal urethrotomy are sometimes indicated, but there is a risk of developing urinary incontinence after the procedure.

Male Urinary Tract Strictures

Etiology. The cause can be inflammatory in nature, such as gonorrhea, or congenital, owing to abnormal development of the urethra. Strictures may follow trauma, which can be iatrogenic or due to straddle trauma to the perineum. Surgical trauma can stem from endoscopy, catheterization, or transurethral surgery of the urethra.

Treatment. Treatment of urethral stricture in the male is usually not pharmacologic; it consists chiefly of urethral dilatations, which can be done progressively with small filiforms and followers when the urethra is very narrow, or by utilizing metallic sounds. Internal urethrotomy is very useful as a surgical treatment, with endoscopic incision of the area of narrowing and the use of an indwelling catheter for various periods of time to allow healing around the catheter for the widened urethra. Plastic operations on the urethra can be done, using skin grafts freed from penile skin or pediculated grafts from scrotal skin. These procedures can be done as a single or two stage operation. For short strictures end-to-end anastomosis after excision of the urethra and wide dissection of the proximal and distal aspects of the urethra can be used.

NONGONOCOCCAL URETHRITIS

method of
DAVID ORIEL, M.D.
London, England

Definition and Diagnosis

Urethritis is characterized clinically by dysuria and urethral discharge (although asymptomatic infections are possible), and in the laboratory by an excess of polymorphonuclear leukocytes (PMN) on a Gram-stained smear of urethral exudate and the presence of pyuria. Urethritis is either gonococcal or nongonococcal. Clinical differentiation between gonorrhea and nongonococcal urethritis (NGU) is unreliable, and therefore some laboratory investigation is necessary. Except in special circumstances, it is bad practice to treat men for urethritis without determining its type.

The following specimens are collected: (1) a smear of urethral exudate for Gram staining, (2) a second urethral specimen for culture for *N. gonorrhoeae,* and (3) the first 10 ml. of voided urine, to be examined in the laboratory for the presence of pyuria. Microscopy for gram-negative intracellular diplococci is quick, simple, and at least 90 per cent accurate for the diagnosis of gonorrhea in men, but should always be supplemented by culture. Men with NGU show an excess of PMN (at least 20 per high power field) on the Gram-stained urethral smear and laboratory evidence of pyuria, but no intracellular diplococci on microscopy and negative cultures for *N. gonorrhoeae.*

About 50 per cent of infections of NGU are caused by *Chlamydia trachomatis.* The cause of the remainder is uncertain, but some may be caused by *Ureaplasma urealyticum* ("T-strain" mycoplasma). Facilities for culturing these organisms are not generally available at present. Postgonococcal urethritis (PGU) occurs when a patient treated for gonorrhea has persistent urethritis despite the elimination of *N. gonorrhoeae.* It is thought to be due to an original mixed infection with gonorrhea and NGU, and the management of NGU and PGU is identical.

Antimicrobial Therapy

The penicillins, spectinomycin, and metronidazole are all ineffective in the therapy of NGU and should not be prescribed. The drugs of choice are the tetracyclines, with erythromycin as second choice. The following regimens are effective:

1. Tetracycline or oxytetracycline, 250 mg. four times daily for 2 weeks. The medication should be taken either 1 hour before or 2 hours after meals. Since tetracyclines chelate with calcium, milk and milk products are prohibited during therapy; for similar reasons, antacids containing aluminum or magnesium should also be avoided.

2. Minocycline, 100 mg. twice daily for 2 weeks. This drug provides high serum and tissue concentration, dietary restrictions are unnecessary, and patient compliance is better with twice daily dosage. However, it should be mentioned that some patients experience vestibular side effects with this antibiotic.

3. Erythromycin stearate, 250 mg. four times daily for 2 weeks, is a satisfactory alternative for patients unable to take tetracyclines.

The ideal duration of antimicrobial therapy for NGU is unknown, but a course of less than 2 weeks is probably suboptimal.

General Measures

Nongonococcal urethritis is sexually transmissible, and patients should refrain from intercourse until they are judged cured. If such restraint is impossible, a condom should be used. Alcohol is traditionally prohibited during therapy. The value of this measure is uncertain, but clinical experience indicates that alcohol does aggravate urethritis in some patients, and it seems sensible to avoid or reduce its consumption during therapy.

Monitoring Response to Treatment

After completing treatment, the patient will need re-examination two or three times during the following month, the initial diagnostic tests being used to confirm that he no longer has significant urethritis. If at the end of this time he is symptom free, with no laboratory evidence of urethritis, he may be regarded as cured. Men who are progressing favorably may normally resume intercourse 2 or 3 weeks after starting therapy.

Management of Female Contacts

Some physicians do not advise examination or treatment of female contacts of men with NGU. However, NGU is a sexually transmitted disease, and many of these women have been shown to be infected by *C. trachomatis* and other pathogens. *C. trachomatis* causes cervicitis and may be involved in the pathogenesis of salpingitis; it causes many cases of ophthalmia neonatorum. Untreated female contacts of men with NGU can certainly reinfect their partners or infect new ones. There are therefore good reasons why these women should be examined and treated. Because of the difficulty of deciding clinically whether a woman has a nongonococcal genital infection, many authorities recommend epidemiologic treatment with a tetracycline or erythromycin after associated infections have been excluded.

Management of Relapsing Nongonococcal Urethritis (NGU)

Treatment of the kind outlined will cure about 80 per cent of men with NGU, but unfortunately the remainder either will have persistent symptoms and signs of urethritis after therapy or will relapse subsequently. In a few patients this relapsing NGU persists for months or even years and may cause much distress.

Although the causes of relapsing NGU are not fully understood, the clinician may usefully ask himself the following questions:

1. Has the patient taken his medication according to instructions? Should a change of antimicrobial be considered?
2. Have regular sexual contacts received epidemiologic treatment? Is there any possibility of reinfection from a new source?
3. Is the patient perpetuating the urethritis himself by trauma ("squeezing" or "stripping")?
4. Has he developed prostatitis?
5. Has he any rare cause of urethritis, unresponsive to tetracycline or erythromycin, such as trichomonal, candidal, or herpetic urethritis?
6. Has he developed a urethral stricture or other urologic disease?

Each of these points will require consideration. If, after 2 or 3 months, the cause of repeated relapse cannot be identified, urologic investigation for prostatitis, stricture, or other urogenital disease is certainly advisable.

Emergency Situations

There may be occasions when a patient develops acute urethritis under circumstances in which even limited laboratory investigation to ascertain the cause is not possible. What should be prescribed? The drug of choice is tetracycline or oxytetracycline, 500 mg. four times a day for a week. This treatment will cure most infections of gonorrhea and is adequate for NGU. Careful follow-up examination should be performed as soon as laboratory facilities are available.

Conclusion

NGU is one of the most common sexually transmitted diseases, with an estimated 2 million cases a year in the United States alone. Because it causes discomfort and anxiety, with the possibility of complications either in the men or in their female partners, thorough and effective treatment is highly desirable.

RENAL CALCULI

method of
LYNWOOD H. SMITH, M.D.
Rochester, Minnesota

Stone formation within the urinary tract is a common complication caused by a variety of metabolic disorders. A classification of these disorders would be as follows: (1) the renal tubular disorders, including renal tubular acidosis and cystinuria; (2) inborn errors of metabolism, including primary hyperoxaluria and xanthinuria; (3) the hypercalcemic states, with primary hyperparathyroidism being most common; (4) uric acid lithiasis; (5) urolithiasis associated with gastrointestinal disorders; (6) idiopathic urolithiasis; and (7) secondary urolithiasis with infection and obstruction. Prior to a discussion of the diagnosis and treatment of each of these disorders, it is important to review the general considerations of the medical evaluation and treatment that apply to all patients forming calculi within the urinary tract.

A number of features in the clinical history are important in the evaluation of a patient with renal calculi. The age of onset or detection of urolithiasis may suggest specific disorders and may also provide a clue concerning the question of whether or not the stone formation will be recurrent. The younger the age of onset, the greater the chance that the patient will have recurring stone formation if not treated. Common problems in adults, such as idiopathic urolithiasis, hyperparathyroidism, and uric acid lithiasis, are rare in children. Rare causes of urolithiasis in adults, including renal tubular acidosis, cystinuria, and primary hyperoxaluria, are more common causes of calculus formation in children. Idiopathic urolithiasis and uric acid lithiasis occur more frequently in males; primary hyperparathyroidism is more common in females. A family history of urolithiasis may suggest an inherited metabolic disorder. Medications such as vitamin D, carbonic anhydrase inhibitors, and absorbable antacids may promote calculus formation. Dietary excesses of calcium, oxalate, and purines, especially when combined with a low fluid intake, may increase the supersaturation of the urine and the tendency for crystal formation and growth. History of residence in a known stone-stress area, such as the southeastern United States, may affect the tendency to produce calculi. The appearance and composition of any stone passed may be helpful; patients may have old stones available, and, if so, these should be obtained and analyzed. The frequencies of colic, stone or gravel passage, hematuria, and infections are important in the overall evaluation. The need for and the type of surgery should be recorded. Often, particularly helpful information concerning the natural history of the calculus formation can be obtained from previous roentgenograms.

The laboratory evaluation of patients with urolithiasis is outlined in Table 1. Additional tests that may be needed or helpful in the diagnosis of specific metabolic disorders will be reviewed subsequently as they apply to these disorders. The extent of the laboratory evaluation will vary with individual patients. In a 60 year old male with several renal calculi that have not changed over the past 5 years, a serum calcium, uric acid, and creatinine; a urine culture; and roentgenograms of the urinary tract would suffice. A young patient or a patient with calculi that are obviously recurrent would require a complete laboratory evaluation.

An important aspect of the medical evaluation of a patient with renal calculi is the assessment of metabolic activity or recurrent nature of the stone formation. This not only determines need for specific therapy, but also provides a means to evaluate effectiveness of that therapy. Criteria to assess metabolic activity, in use in our stone clinic since 1965, are as follows: "Surgically active urolithiasis" is present when there is colic, obstruction, or infection associated with a stone. This in no way implies metabolic activity, because the stone causing symptoms may have been present for many years without change. "Metabolically active urolithiasis" is considered present when one or more of the following criteria are met: (1) new stone formation by roentgenograms within the past year, (2) stone growth by roentgenograms within the past year, and (3) the passage of documented gravel within the past year. Metabolic activity cannot be assessed in the presence of the secondary conditions of infection and obstruction. These must first be treated and eliminated. If none of these criteria are present and previous roentgenograms are adequate, the patient is said to have "metabolically inactive urolithiasis," and he is followed at yearly intervals on an adequate fluid intake. If previous roentgenograms are not

TABLE 1. **Laboratory Evaluation of Patients with Renal Calculi**

Serum
Calcium × 3
Phosphorus
Uric acid
Creatinine/BUN
Alkaline phosphatase
Protein electrophoresis
Urine
Urinalysis
Urine culture and antibiotic sensitivity
Urinary pH (fasting state)
Urine chemistry (24 hour collection—normal diet)
Calcium
Phosphorus
Uric acid
Oxalate
Cystine
Creatinine
Renal function
Creatinine clearance
Roentgenograms
Excretory urograms
KUB with tomograms
Stone analysis (if available)

available or are inadequate, the metabolic activity is classified as "indeterminate" and the patient is followed at regular intervals on a high fluid intake with dietary restriction when necessary.

In a series of 101 consecutive patients with indeterminate metabolic activity, 64 (63 per cent) were subsequently found to have inactive disease. Had they been treated without establishing its need, approximately two thirds of the patients would have been committed to a lifetime of therapy that may have been unnecessary.

The final general considerations relate to therapy. First, all patients with renal calculi should be carefully instructed in fluid intake. Ideally, a 240 ml. (8 oz.) glass of fluid hourly while awake, plus 240 to 480 ml. (8 to 16 oz.) of fluid, if up during the night, should be the goal, with at least half of the fluid as water. If dietary excesses in terms of calcium, oxalate, or purines are present, they should be eliminated. This program with patient compliance will control calculus formation in 60 per cent or more of the patients and is the cornerstone of preventive therapy of urolithiasis. Specific therapy is added and does not replace the need for the high fluid intake. Second, most disorders associated with urolithiasis are chronic; continued follow-up is required to ensure adequate control of the calculus formation, reassess the treatment program and patient compliance, and review treatment results and future plans with the patient. Only with regular follow-up of patients with urolithiasis can effective treatment be accomplished.

METABOLIC DISORDERS COMPLICATED BY RENAL CALCULI

Renal Tubular Acidosis (RTA)

Definition. Type I RTA (distal RTA) may be inherited or acquired and is characterized by an inability of the distal nephron to generate or maintain steep lumen-peritubular hydrogen ion gradients. Ammonia production and bicarbonate conservation are usually normal. Hyperchloremia, hypokalemia, systemic acidosis, and urinary wasting of sodium, potassium, calcium, and phosphorus occur. Nephrolithiasis, urolithiasis, osteomalacia, and muscle weakness may occur.

Diagnosis. Urine pH will be greater than 5.5 (usually 6.0) in the presence of systemic acidosis (plasma bicarbonate less than 20 mEq. per liter) without evidence of bicarbonate wasting in the urine. Urine pH should not be evaluated in the presence of bacteriuria, as bacterial metabolism may alter the results.

Special Test. Ammonium chloride load: A solution of NH_4Cl to provide 100 mg. per kg. per 24 hours is given. Urine and systemic pH are monitored. When plasma bicarbonate falls below 20 mEq. per liter and urine pH is above 5.5 (usually above 6.0) without bicarbonate wastage in the urine, the diagnosis is confirmed.

Treatment. Metabolic replacement is given, including sodium, potassium, and bicarbonate (90 to 150 mEq. of base per 24 hours in divided doses). Neutral orthophosphate has been added in a few patients in whom stone formation has not been controlled by metabolic replacement.

Cystinuria

Definition. Cystinuria is an inherited disorder of amino acid metabolism in which there is abnormal transport of cystine, ornithine, lysine, and arginine in the kidney and intestinal tract. Because of the limited solubility of cystine in urine, cystine stones may form in the urinary tract. No other recognized clinical abnormalities occur.

Diagnosis. Diagnosis is confirmed by increased urinary excretion of cystine (greater than 400 mg. per 24 hours), ornithine, lysine, and arginine; cystine stone by analysis; and the presence of cystine crystalluria in the morning fasting urine.

Treatment. 1. Urine volume is maintained above 3 liters per 24 hours. The patient is instructed to get up during the night, by alarm clock if necessary, to drink 480 ml. (16 oz.) of water.

2. Alkalinization of urine to pH above 7.0 is achieved with citrate solution (Polycitra, 15 mEq. base per 15 ml.) as 15 ml. four times daily or $NaHCO_3$. Titrate treatment by measuring urine pH with nitrazine paper.

3. D-Penicillamine, 250 to 500 mg. four times daily, is given 30 minutes before meals and at bedtime. *Note:* This is a potentially toxic drug; it should be used for stone dissolution when cystine should be reduced to 200 mg. per 24 hours or less, and for those patients whose disease cannot be controlled with hydration and alkalinization alone. Here dosage can be adjusted to maintain cystine in the range of 400 to 500 mg. per 24 hours.

Primary Hyperoxaluria

Definition. Primary hyperoxaluria is a rare inherited disorder of glyoxalate metabolism associated with increased urinary excretion of oxalate. Type I hyperoxaluria, glycolic aciduria, is the most common form and is due to a deficiency of soluble 2-oxalglutaric:glyoxalate carboligase having increased excretion of oxalic and glycolic acids. Type II hyperoxaluria, L-glyceric aciduria, is due to a deficiency of D glyceric dehydrogenase and is associated with increased excretion of oxalate and

L-glyceric acids. Onset is commonly in childhood, with recurrent calculi and nephrocalcinosis progressing to renal failure and early death if not treated. Extrarenal oxalate deposits, termed oxalosis, occur when renal failure is present.

Diagnosis. Diagnosis is confirmed by hyperoxaluria (100 to 300 mg. per 24 hours) in the absence of secondary causes such as gastrointestinal disorders.

Treatment. Pyridoxine, 50 mg. three times daily, will reduce oxalate excretion in 20 to 50 per cent of these patients. Neutral orthophosphate (NeutraPhos—100 mg. elemental phosphorus per 30 ml. [1 oz.] or K-Phos Neutral—250 mg. elemental phosphorus per tablet) may be given as 2 grams of elemental phosphorus per 24 hours in four divided doses. Orthophosphate cannot be used if glomerular filtration rate is less than 30 ml. per minute.

Xanthinuria

Definition. Xanthinuria is an extremely rare disorder of purine metabolism associated with a deficiency of xanthine oxidase. Xanthine calculi have occurred in approximately 50 per cent of the reported cases.

Diagnosis. Diagnosis is confirmed by xanthinuria with low serum and urinary uric acid, and by presence of a xanthinine stone. Therapy with xanthinine oxidase inhibitors must be ruled out.

Treatment. Maintain a high urine volume with dietary restriction of purines.

Hypercalcemic States

Definition. Any cause of hypercalcemia may cause renal calculi, but the most common are primary hyperparathyroidism and immobilization. Although malignancy is the most common cause of hypercalcemia, calculus formation resulting from the hypercalcemia and hypercalciuria of malignancy is rare.

Diagnosis. Diagnosis is confirmed by hypercalcemia, usually with hypercalciuria. Diagnostic studies are directed toward defining the cause of hypercalcemia.

Special Test. Serum immunoreactive parathyroid hormone assay.

Treatment. Therapy is determined by the primary cause of the hypercalcemia.

Uric Acid Lithiasis

Definition. GOUT. Approximately 25 per cent of the patients with gout form uric acid stones. The frequency of this complication increases when uricosuric agents are used without increasing fluid intake and alkalinization of the urine.

IDIOPATHIC URIC ACID LITHIASIS. The cause remains unknown. Serum and urine uric acid are normal. Typically, these patients excrete a persistently acid urine.

MYELOPROLIFERATIVE DISORDERS. With active disease and during therapy, there is increased metabolism of purines with overproduction of uric acid.

LOW URINE OUTPUT STATES. These are most commonly seen in elderly males with prostatism in whom fluid intake is self-restricted, and in patients with ileostomies. In both situations urine volume is low and pH is acid with normal uric acid excretion.

Diagnosis. Diagnosis is confirmed by uric acid stone by analysis, demonstration of abnormal uric acid metabolism with hyperuricemia and hyperuricosuria, and a radiolucent stone on roentgenograms.

Treatment. 1. High fluid intake.

2. Alkalinization of urine to pH 6.5 following urine pH with nitrazine paper. This increases the solubility of uric acid ten-fold.

3. Allopurinol, 300 mg. daily. If the kidney is not obstructed, uric acid stones can be dissolved with 3 to 6 months of treatment. Allopurinol can then be stopped unless the patient has gout, a myeloproliferative disorder, or an ileostomy, for which continuation may be required.

Urolithiasis Associated with Gastrointestinal Disorders

Definition. URIC ACID LITHIASIS. As previously discussed, patients with ileostomy and excessive diarrhea lose water and bicarbonate from the gastrointestinal tract, resulting in a low urine volume with acid pH. In this setting uric acid is poorly soluble and uric acid lithiasis may occur. The diagnosis and treatment have already been discussed.

ENTERIC HYPEROXALURIA. In conditions of malabsorption, including small bowel disease, small bowel resection, chronic pancreatitis, cirrhosis, and conditions of bacterial overgrowth of the small bowel, there may be increased absorption of dietary oxalate by the colon, producing hyperoxaluria without increase in L-glyceric or glycolic acids in the urine. Steatorrhea with the coprecipitation of calcium with fatty acids leaves increased amounts of oxalate in solution and available for absorption. (1) *Diagnosis:* Demonstration of hyperoxaluria without increased excretion of L-glyceric and glycolic acids in the urine in the presence of gastrointestinal disease. (2) *Treatment:* Dietary restriction of oxalate and fat with calcium supplement if urinary excretion of calcium is low. Cholestyramine, 4 grams three to four times per day, is given to patients with bile acid diarrhea.

This may increase water absorption and urine volume; at the same time it nonspecifically binds oxalate in the colon, decreasing its absorption.

Idiopathic Urolithiasis

Definition. Idiopathic urolithiasis, including idiopathic hypercalciuria, is the diagnosis currently made in 70 to 80 per cent of patients with renal calculi. It is a syndrome that includes several as yet ill-defined diseases. The diagnosis is one of exclusion after known causes of urolithiasis have been ruled out. From 50 to 75 per cent of these patients will have hypercalciuria. In the majority of these patients the hypercalciuria is due to increased calcium absorption from the diet. Recent observations suggest that this may be related to a disturbance in vitamin D metabolism with increased production of $1,25(OH)_2D_3$. A much smaller group may have a primary renal leak of calcium with modest secondary hyperparathyroidism. Other abnormalities that have been reported in these patients include (1) decreased crystal growth inhibitors, including citrate; (2) modest increased urinary excretion of oxalate with calcium oxalate stone formation; (3) excretion of persistently alkaline urine with calcium phosphate calculi but with a normal capacity to acidify the urine; and (4) hyperuricosuria with calcium oxalate calculi, thought to be related to heterogeneous nucleation (epitaxial crystal growth).

Diagnosis. Again, this is a diagnosis of exclusion made after other causes of calculus formation have been ruled out. The urinary excretion of calcium should be measured initially on the patient's normal diet, with more than 300 mg. per 24 hours considered hypercalciuria. If dietary calcium is low, increased calcium intake (as 1 liter [quart] of milk per day; approximately 800 mg. of calcium) can be given for 3 days with repeat measurement of urinary excretion of calcium.

Special Tests. To separate patients with absorptive hypercalciuria from those with a renal leak of calcium, measurement of the 2 hour excretion of calcium after an overnight fast of at least 14 hours is helpful. An excretion of less than 20 mg. during the 2 hour collection is considered a normal response; it is seen in healthy subjects and in patients with absorptive hypercalciuria. More recently, comparison of the state of saturation with inhibitor activity for the calcium crystal systems has been used to assess the tendency to form calculi and the effects of specific forms of therapy.

Treatment. Initially metabolic activity must be assessed in these patients to determine need of therapy. Once this need has been established, several effective treatment programs are available.

1. Thiazides, such as hydrochlorothiazide, 50 mg. twice daily, or trichlormethiazide, 2 mg. twice daily, are particularly effective when significant hypercalciuria is present, as these agents will decrease the urinary excretion of calcium by approximately 50 per cent. A high sodium intake can overcome this effect; therefore moderate sodium restriction may be necessary. Approximately 80 per cent of these patients will stop calculus formation.

2. Orthophosphate is usually given as the neutral salt to provide 1.5 to 2.0 grams of elemental phosphorus per 24 hours in three or four divided doses. The dosage is critical and may have to be increased to control stone formation if a lower dose was initially used. Approximately 40 per cent of the patients treated with orthophosphate will lose old stones, usually during the first 3 to 6 months of therapy. This is the treatment of choice in patients with normocalciuria, but it is equally effective in patients with hypercalciuria. More than 90 per cent of the patients will have complete cessation of calculus formation. It should not be used if glomerular filtration is less than 30 ml. per minute. Recent studies suggest that the alkaline salt of phosphate may be more effective, but this is currently being used only in those patients whose stone formation is not adequately controlled with the neutral salt. This treatment decreases urine calcium and increases inhibitor activity.

3. Allopurinol, 300 mg. per day. In patients with hyperuricosuria and calcium oxalate calculi, reduction of the urinary excretion of uric acid has been reported to effectively stop stone formation that is thought to be due to heterogeneous nucleation.

Secondary Urolithiasis

Definition. Calculus formation associated with infection and obstruction should be considered secondary, requiring careful metabolic evaluation in patients with this condition. Both infection and obstruction occur commonly without calculus formation; therefore it is reasonable to assume the stone formation is in part related to a primary metabolic abnormality that is complicated by urolithiasis. Stones produced in this setting often take on a staghorn configuration and are moderately radiopaque with laminations. The crystal composition is typically struvite (magnesium-ammonium-phosphate), related to the alkalinity of the urine from bacterial metabolism of urea (urease-producing bacteria; most commonly Proteus sp.).

Diagnosis. Diagnosis is made by demonstration of bacteriuria with urease-producing bacteria and alkaline urine (pH often greater than 7.5), and by stone analysis showing struvite. A complete metabolic work-up should be done to diagnose primary stone disorders. Metabolic activity can be assessed only after secondary problems have been eliminated.

Treatment. Therapy leading to cure is frequently possible in these patients but must include careful attention to each of the following elements:

1. Identification and treatment of infection with bactericidal therapy starting 48 hours before surgery. Total time of treatment is 10 to 14 days.
2. Surgical removal of all infected calculi, with restoration of urinary tract anatomy when possible.
3. Careful metabolic evaluation, with treatment of specific metabolic abnormalities (i.e., hyperparathyroidism, cystinuria) when indicated.
4. Long-term follow-up with suppressive antibacterial therapy and acidification (usually 6 to 12 months). Urine should be cultured monthly for 3 months, then at 3 month intervals for 1 year, and then annually. Re-evaluation of stone formation should be undertaken at 3 month intervals for 1 year and then annually. Adequate follow-up is critical to successful treatment of these patients.

Summary

For patients with all forms of renal calculi, effective preventive therapy is potentially available. Treatment is based on a careful definition of the underlying metabolic abnormalities and secondary conditions, as well as on the assessment of metabolic activity. Critical to success is the continued long-term follow-up of these patients.

SECTION 9

The Venereal Diseases

CHANCROID

method of
THOMAS E. CARSON, M.D.
New Orleans, Louisiana

Chancroid is a sexually transmitted disease caused by *Hemophilus ducreyi*. The infection is uncommon in temperate zones but may become very significant in tropical climates. The clinical disease is rare in women.

The incubation period of chancroid is short, ranging from 3 to 5 days. The disease characteristically presents with multiple tender purulent ulcerations on the penis, mainly in the uncircumcised under the foreskin and in the sulcus. There is usually associated bilateral, tender inguinal lymphadenopathy.

Although primarily clinical, the diagnosis of chancroid may be aided by the finding of characteristic clusters or "school of fish" arrangements of pleomorphic, gram-negative coccobacilli on Gram's stain of exudate from the lesions.

Treatment

1. After concurrent syphilis has been ruled out by dark-field examination, the treatment for chancroid is oral tetracycline or sulfisoxazole. At least 2 weeks of therapy are required for cure, but often therapy must be extended to over 1 month.

Therapy with tetracycline is preferred and is given in a dosage of 500 mg. four times a day. This is continued until complete clearing of the lesions is noted and tenderness in the lymph nodes has subsided. If syphilis has been missed, this dosage of tetracycline for 2 weeks or more is curative. Allergic reactions are fewer with tetracycline than with sulfonamides.

Sulfisoxazole is adequate in the treatment of chancroid. A loading dose of 4 grams should be given, followed by 1 gram four times a day until clinical cure is accomplished. Sulfa drugs do not interfere with incubating syphilis, and serologic tests for syphilis should be obtained 2, 4, and 6 months following treatment to ensure that syphilis has not been missed.

2. Topical therapy is a frequently neglected and very important adjunct in the treatment of chancroid. The duration of antibiotic therapy may be decreased as much as half with intensive topical therapy.

Frequent compresses with a washcloth or gauze, sopping wet with plain cool water, are recommended for simplicity. These should be applied three to six times a day for 10 to 20 minutes. The lesions should then be adequately dried and a shake lotion containing 3 per cent iodochlorhydroxyquin applied. Formulation of a suggested shake lotion is as follows:

Iodochlorhydroxyquin	3.0
Zinc oxide	20.0
Talc	20.0
Glycerin	10.0
Water q.s. ad.	100.0

This preparation promotes drying. The patient should be instructed not to remove the caking that will develop after frequent applications to the lesions.

3. Fluctuant lymph nodes may occur in untreated or neglected cases. Resolution of the buboes will be hastened by aspiration through an 18 gauge needle and local heat applications.

Simple pyoderma is a frequent infection of the genitalia and is clinically difficult to distinguish from chancroid. The usual findings on Gram's stain are mixtures of gram-negative rods and gram-positive cocci. Treatment is the same as for chancroid; a differential characteristic is more rapid clinical clearing in pyoderma—usually within 7 to 10 days.

On the rare occasion when oral tetracycline and intensive topical therapy as previously outlined fail to result in clinical cure, kanamycin, 500 mg. intramuscularly twice daily for 6 to 14 days, is recommended.

GONORRHEA

method of
SUMNER E. THOMPSON, III, M.D.,
and PETER L. PERINE, M.D.
Atlanta, Georgia

The treatment of gonorrhea should be based on a proper diagnosis by Gram stain or culture for *Neisseria gonorrhoeae*; a test-of-cure culture should be made 3 to 14 days after therapy. The Gram stain is highly sensitive and specific only for the diagnosis of gonococcal urethritis and conjunctivitis. Infection of other sites, the endocervix, vagina, anal canal, and oropharynx, should be confirmed by culture, as the Gram stain is much less sensitive and specific for *N. gonorrhoeae*.

The following regimens are recommended for treating uncomplicated gonococcal urethritis in men and asymptomatic endocervical, vaginal, and/or rectal infection in women: (1) Aqueous procaine penicillin G, 4.8 million units intramuscularly (2.4 million units in each buttock), simultaneously with 1.0 gram of probenecid by mouth. (2) Ampicillin, 3.5 grams, or amoxicillin, 3 grams by mouth, together with 1 gram of probenecid by mouth administered simultaneously.

Patients who are allergic to penicillin or probenecid can be treated with either of the following agents: (1) Tetracycline hydrochloride, 1.5 grams by mouth as a loading dose, followed by 0.5 gram four times per day for 4 days (total dose of 9.5 grams). The drug should be taken on an empty stomach and without milk to prevent binding of the drug in the gastrointestinal tract. (2) Spectinomycin hydrochloride, 2.0 grams in a single intramuscular injection.

Since lack of patient compliance contributes to treatment failure, a single dose regimen is preferred over multiple dose regimens.

Patients may fail treatment for gonorrhea if the infecting gonococci are resistant to the drug given for treatment. Of considerable importance is the recent appearance of penicillinase-producing *N. gonorrhoeae* (PPNG) in many parts of the world, including the United States. The PPNG have acquired an R-factor plasmid that codes for the production of beta-lactamase enzymes which destroy penicillin, ampicillin, amoxicillin, and some of the cephalosporin group of antibiotics. PPNG are highly prevalent in certain areas of the Far East, and many of the PPNG infections reported in the United States have occurred in merchant seamen, tourists, and military personnel returning from that area of the world. The prevalence of PPNG in the United States (approximately 150 cases from more than 20 different states from September 1976 through April 1977) is too low to warrant changes in the recommendation for penicillin or ampicillin as the drug of choice for initial treatment of uncomplicated gonorrhea, unless the patient is a sexual contact to a patient with proved PPNG infection. Since PPNG do not produce unique clinical signs of infection, the following procedures are recommended: (1) All patients who fail treatment of gonorrhea should have a culture for *N. gonorrhoeae* done. (2) Patients who fail treatment and patients with recent sexual exposure in the Far East should be treated with spectinomycin hydrochloride, 2.0 grams intramuscularly. (3) All positive test-of-cure cultures of *N. gonorrhoeae* should be tested for penicillinase production. All state laboratories are equipped to perform tests to confirm penicillinase production by *N. gonorrhoeae.* (4) Patients with PPNG infection should be reported to local public health authorities, who will initiate investigations of the patients' sexual contacts. (5) Spectinomycin hydrochloride is the only drug of proved efficacy for PPNG infections. Patients with PPNG infection who fail treatment with spectinomycin may be cured by treatment with sulfamethoxazole-trimethoprim, 9 tablets daily in a single dose by mouth for 3 days. (This use and dose of sulfamethoxazole-trimethoprim are not listed in the manufacturer's official directive.)

The incidence of complications after PPNG infections appears to be the same as that after the usual gonococcal infection. Treatment of complicated PPNG infection should include an aminoglycoside antibiotic such as kanamycin, 2 grams intramuscularly daily (this dose of kanamycin may be higher than that listed in the manufacturer's official directive), or parenteral gentamicin in a dose of 3 mg. per kg. per day until the infection is cured, together with the procedures outlined below.

In small series of men with anorectal gonococcal infection, treatment with the single dose penicillin or ampicillin regimens recommended for uncomplicated urethritis resulted in treatment failures in 10 to 30 per cent of cases. Some authorities feel that multiple day therapy with an antibiotic is required to eradicate this infection. Tetracycline hydrochloride, 0.5 gram by mouth four times per day for a total dosage of 9.5 grams, may be effective.

Men treated for gonococcal urethritis may have a persistent urethral discharge that is both Gram-stain and culture negative for *N. gonorrhoeae*. Such postgonococcal urethritis may result from coincident infection with *Chlamydia trachomatis* or Mycoplasma species which are not affected by penicillin and its congeners. The recommended treatment for postgonococcal urethritis is tetracycline, 0.5 gram four times a day by mouth for at least 7 days.

Disseminated Gonococcal Infections (DGI)

Gonococcal bacteremia produces a disease spectrum ranging from the relatively benign tenosynovitis-dermatitis syndrome to subacute progressive endocarditis. Those with the tenosynovitis-dermatitis syndrome frequently do not require hospitalization. However, patients with true septic arthritis, meningitis, or endocarditis should be treated in the hospital. Other categories of patients requiring hospitalization are those in whom the initial diagnosis is not clear; those in whom a dramatic response to therapy is not observed within 24 hours (continued fever or progression of joint symptoms); and those in whom compliance with therapy is doubtful. Short-term therapy for gonococcal bacteremia is feasible, because gonococci causing DGI are almost uniformly sensitive to penicillin and tend to be quite sensitive to the other commonly used antigonococcal antibiotics as well.

Recommended Treatment for the Tenosynovitis-Dermatitis Syndrome. (1) First choice: Aqueous procaine penicillin G with probenecid by mouth as in uncomplicated gonorrhea. This is to be followed by 0.5 gram of ampicillin or amoxicillin four times daily by mouth for 4 to 7 days. (2) Alternatives: ampicillin, 3.5 grams, or amoxicillin, 3 grams, by mouth in a single dose with 1 gram of probenecid, followed by 0.5 gram of ampicillin or amoxicillin four times a day for 5 to 7 days.

Penicillin-allergic patients can be treated as follows: (1) Tetracycline hydrochloride, 1.5 grams initially, followed by 0.5 gram of tetracycline by mouth four times a day for 5 to 7 days on an empty stomach. Superior efficacy of minocycline or doxycycline over generic tetracycline has not been established for gonorrhea. (2) Erythromycin in any of its forms, 0.5 gram four times a day by mouth for 5 to 7 days. All forms except the estolate should be taken while fasting. Estolate has the advantage of being well absorbed after feeding, and therefore has less gastrointestinal toxicity.

Recommended Treatment for Septic Arthritis. Aqueous crystalline penicillin G, 8 to 10 million units a day intravenously for a minimum of 3 days. Dramatic improvement usually occurs within 2 days. The regimen may be extended for additional days with ampicillin or amoxicillin, 0.5 gram every 6 hours by mouth.

Penicillin-allergic patients can be treated in the following fashion:

In our hands, the oral erythromycin regimen outlined above has proved as efficacious as penicillin. Repeated aspiration of the fluid from the inflamed joint through a large-bore needle may also be beneficial. Open surgical drainage of the joint or instillation of intra-articular antibiotics is unnecessary, and may delay healing. Intra-articular antibiotics may cause a chemical synovitis not easily distinguished from continuing infection.

Recommended Treatment for Gonococcal Meningitis and Endocarditis. Gonococcal meningitis should be treated with 20 million units of aqueous crystalline penicillin G intravenously daily for a minimum of 10 days. The same daily dose of penicillin for 4 weeks is used for endocarditis.

Every effort should be made to adequately document penicillin allergy before using an alternative regimen, as none of the alternatives have been adequately assessed in these conditions. A high-dose cephalosporin (e.g., cephalothin, 6 to 12 grams per day intravenously) can be used for 4 weeks in treating endocarditis, but cannot be used in meningitis. Alternative regimens for treating meningitis are chloramphenicol, 2 to 4 grams a day initially given intravenously, or tetracycline hydrochloride, 0.5 gram intravenously every 6 hours for 10 days.

Salpingitis, Pelvic Inflammatory Disease (PID)

Gonococci may be cultured from the endocervix of women with their first episode of salpingitis in 50 to 80 per cent of cases. Culture of a culdocentesis sample reveals this pathogen less frequently, and often shows a polymicrobial flora containing anaerobes. A purely anaerobic flora is most likely to occur late in the disease course—in repeated attacks of salpingitis, or in chronic disease. Because gonococci are associated with acute salpingitis, the initial management should be at least adequate for gonococci. Most anaerobic organisms are also sensitive to penicillin, *Bacteroides fragilis* being the exception.

After PID is diagnosed, a decision must be made about hospitalization. Six indications for hospital admission are (1) a questionable diagnosis (e.g., inability to rule out appendicitis, ectopic pregnancy, or torsion of an ovarian cyst); (2) nausea and vomiting such that oral medications cannot be used; (3) presence of an adnexal mass; (4) evidence of generalized peritonitis; (5) poor response to an outpatient antibiotic regimen; and (6) pregnancy.

Patients who are hospitalized usually need the supportive treatment of intravenous fluids, bed rest, and analgesics, as well as the following drug therapy: (1) Aqueous crystalline penicillin G, 20 million units per day intravenously until there is definite clinical improvement, followed by ampicillin or amoxicillin, 0.5 gram four times a day by mouth, to complete 10 days of therapy. (2) Nonpregnant women with no evidence of renal failure who are allergic to penicillin may be treated with tetracycline hydrochloride, 0.5 gram intravenously every 6 hours, switching to the same dosage by mouth as soon as possible, to complete a minimum of 10 days of treatment.

Combined penicillin-aminoglycoside therapy is widely used for inpatient therapy. This combination may be unnecessary, because, in our experience, enteric aerobic gram-negative rods are rarely the cause of salpingitis. In patients with multiple recurrences of salpingitis, or relapsing chronic disease, and antibiotic directed specifically against *B. fragilis* may be combined with the penicillin therapy. Clindamycin, 0.25 to 0.5 gram intravenously every 6 hours, switching when possible to the same dose orally, or chloramphenicol, 0.5 to 1 gram four times a day intravenously or by mouth, may be used. Every effort to establish the presence of *B. fragilis* should be attempted before these potentially toxic drugs are used.

There is a definite place for surgery in managing PID. The indications for surgical intervention are (1) failure of clinical improvement after an adequate trial of antibiotic therapy; (2) the presence of a pelvic abscess which does not disappear after medical management; (3) suspected leakage or rupture of a pelvic abscess; and (4) serious doubts concerning the actual diagnosis. The timing of the surgical management of PID must be individualized.

Outpatients should be treated with either the aqueous procaine penicillin G or ampicillin/amoxicillin regimen used for uncomplicated gonorrhea. Both regimens should then be followed by 2 grams per day of oral ampicillin or amoxicillin for at least 10 days. Alternatively, tetracycline hydrochloride, 0.5 gram by mouth four times a day for at least 10 days, may be used.

Pharyngeal Infection

Pharyngeal gonococcal infections are difficult to treat, as gonococcal pharyngeal infections do not respond either to ampicillin or its congeners or to spectinomycin. The regimens of choice are aqueous procaine penicillin G plus the probenecid regimen or the tetracycline regimen given for uncomplicated gonorrhea. Sulfamethoxazole-trimethoprim tablets, 6 a day by mouth for 3 days, have also been successful in eradicating gonococci from the throat. (This use of sulfamethoxazole-trimethoprim is not specifically listed in the manufacturer's official directive.)

The major difficulty in treating gonococcal pharyngeal infection is establishing the diagnosis. Patients frequently have no symptoms and a normal-appearing pharynx. Care must be taken to obtain adequate culture specimens; both tonsils should be swabbed vigorously to ensure express of material from the crypts. Because other Neisseria organisms normally reside in the oropharynx, Gram stains should not be used for diagnosis. Organisms which grow on Thayer-Martin medium must be confirmed as *N. gonorrhoeae* by sugar fermentation patterns.

Gonococcal Infection in Infants and Adolescents

Infants may be infected with gonorrhea during passage through the birth canal of an infected mother. The most common site of neonatal infection is the conjunctivae (ophthalmia neonatorum), characterized by a profound mucopurulent conjunctivitis affecting both eyes, with onset within 1 week after birth. The infants should be hospitalized and treated with (1) aqueous crystalline penicillin G intravenously, 75,000 to 100,000 units per kg. per day in four doses, or aqueous procaine penicillin G intramuscularly, 75,000 to 100,000 units per kg. per day in two doses, for 7 days; plus (2) saline irrigations and instillation of penicillin, tetracycline, or chloramphenicol eyedrops every 2 hours. Bacitracin is not effective, and antibiotic eyedrops alone are not indicated.

Uncomplicated vulvovaginitis and urethritis do not require hospitalization. Both may be treated at one visit with aqueous procaine penicillin G, 75,000 to 100,000 units per kg. intramuscularly, and probenecid, 25 mg. per kg. by mouth. Follow-up test of cure should be obtained in all patients, and the source of infection should be identified, examined, and treated. Adolescents with infection complicated by peritonitis or arthritis should be hospitalized and treated with penicillin as recommended for ophthalmia neonatorum.

Children under 6 years of age with allergy to penicillin should be treated with erythromycin, 40 mg. per kg. per day in four doses by mouth for 7 days for uncomplicated disease. Complicated disease should be treated with cephalothin, 60 to 80 mg. per kg. per day. in four doses intravenously for 7 days. Children older than 6 may be treated with an oral regimen of tetracycline, 25 mg. per kg. per day in four doses for 7 days (see manufacturer's official directive before using in young children), or an intravenous regimen of tetracycline, 15 to 20 mg. per kg. per day in four doses for 7 days.

Epidemiologic Treatment

The sexual partners of patients with gonorrhea should receive treatment for gonorrhea at the first visit. It is of interest that a high percentage of male sexual contacts of infected women may have asymptomatic infection, and their urethral exudate is often falsely Gram stain negative for gonococci.

Test of Cure

In general, follow-up urethral culture and cultures from other appropriate sites in men and cervical, anal, and other site cultures in women should be obtained 3 to 14 days after completion of therapy.

Most persisting or recurrent gonorrhea occurring after adequate therapy is reinfection. In addition, none of the recommended drug schedules are 100 per cent effective. There is about a 4 per cent failure with aqueous procaine penicillin G and probenecid, a similar rate for tetracycline, and an 8 to 10 per cent failure with ampicillin and probenecid. In addition, failure rates increase correspondingly with increased gonococcal resistance to antibiotics, and gonococci resistant to one antibiotic tend to be more resistant to others. The exception to this is spectinomycin; thus, since failures to spectinomycin do not increase as the organism becomes more resistant to penicillin, ampicillin, and tetracycline, spectinomycin is the drug of choice for patients failing treatment with other antibiotics.

GRANULOMA INGUINALE

method of
THOMAS A. CHAPEL, M.D.
Detroit, Michigan

Granuloma inguinale is a specific chronic granulomatous disease caused by *Calymmatobacterium granulomatis*. This condition is traditionally classified as a venereal disease, although its sexual transmission is controversial.

Therapy

1. Tetracycline, 500 mg. orally four times daily, is often effective over 2 to 3 weeks. It is advisable to continue therapy for 2 weeks after clinical healing.

2. Streptomycin, 0.5 to 1.0 gram intramuscularly twice daily, is usually effective within 14 to 21 days.

3. Gentamicin, 40 mg. twice daily intramuscularly, *or:*

4. Chloramphenicol, 0.5 gram every 8 hours orally, cures most lesions within 3 weeks.

A diagnosis of granuloma inguinale should be established by crush preparation or biopsy before treatment is begun. If an antibiotic is effective, a clinical response is usually evident within 7 days and healing within 3 to 5 weeks. Strains of *C. granulomatis* have occasionally become resistant to tetracycline and/or streptomycin. If resistance develops to both tetracycline and streptomycin, gentamicin or chloramphenicol should then be used. Prolonged follow-up is recommended, because relapse can occur several months after treatment of the primary lesion.

LYMPHOGRANULOMA VENEREUM

method of
THOMAS A. CHAPEL, M.D.
Detroit, Michigan

Lymphogranuloma venereum (LGV) is a systemic, sexually transmitted disease caused by members of the genus Chlamydia. The disease is characterized by a small, transient initial lesion usually located on the genitalia or perineum. This is followed by regional lymphadenitis and/or chronic inflammation in the adjacent connective tissue of the infected areas.

Success of therapy can usually be monitored by resolution of clinical signs. It is recommended that lymphogranuloma venereum complement fixation titers (LGV-CF) be ascertained before treatment and every 3 to 4 months for 1 year after apparent cure to detect relapse or reinfection. The patient should be re-treated if any evidence of reactivation appears. Re-treatment is also recommended for patients who have not shown a two tube fall in LGV-CF titer 6 weeks after initial treatment.

Therapy

1. Tetracycline, 0.5 gram four times daily for at least 3 weeks.

2. Sulfisoxazole, 4.0 grams orally, followed by 1.0 gram four times a day for at least 3 weeks.

Fluctuant lymph nodes should be aspirated with a large bore needle and a syringe. Rectal stricture sometimes seen with LGV should be managed by dilatation at 2 week intervals. Refractory cases may require surgery.

SYPHILIS

CDC RECOMMENDED TREATMENT SCHEDULES, 1976

U.S. Department of Health, Education, and Welfare/Public Health Service

The following recommendations were established by the Venereal Disease Control Advisory Committee* after deliberation with therapy experts.†

Few data have been published on the treatment of syphilis since CDC revised these recommendations in 1968. Penicillin continues to be the drug of choice for all stages of syphilis. Every effort should be made to document penicillin allergy before choosing other antibiotics, because these antibiotics have been studied less extensively than penicillin. Physicians are cautioned to use no less than the recommended dosages of antibiotics.

Early Syphilis (Primary, Secondary, Latent Syphilis of Less Than 1 Year's Duration)

1. Benzathine penicillin G, 2.4 million units total by intramuscular injection at a single session. *Benzathine penicillin G is the drug of choice because it provides effective treatment in a single visit.*‡ OR

2. Aqueous procaine penicillin G, 4.8 million units total: 600,000 units by intramuscular injection daily for 8 days. OR

3. Procaine penicillin G in oil with 2 per cent aluminum monostearate (PAM), 4.8 million units total by intramuscular injection: 2.4 million units at first visit, and 1.2 million units at each of two subsequent visits 3 days apart. *Although PAM is used in other countries, it is no longer available in the United States.*

Patients Who Are Allergic to Penicillin. 1. Tetracycline hydrochloride,* 500 mg. four times a day by mouth for 15 days. OR

2. Erythromycin (stearate, ethylsuccinate, or base), 500 mg. four times a day by mouth for 15 days.

These antibiotics appear to be effective but have been evaluated less extensively than penicillin.

Syphilis of More Than 1 Year's Duration (Latent Syphilis of Indeterminate or More Than 1 Year's Duration, Cardiovascular, Late Benign, Neurosyphilis)

1. Benzathine penicillin G, 7.2 million units total: 2.4 million units by intramuscular injection weekly for 3 successive weeks. OR

2. Aqueous procaine penicillin G, 9.0 million units total: 600,000 units by intramuscular injection daily for 15 days.

The optimal treatment schedules for syphilis of greater than 1 year's duration have been less well established than schedules for early syphilis. In general, syphilis of longer duration requires higher-dose therapy. Although therapy is recommended for established cardiovascular syphilis, there is little evidence that antibiotics reverse the pathology associated with this disease.

Cerebrospinal fluid (CSF) examination is mandatory in patients with suspected, symptomatic neurosyphilis. This examination is also desirable in other patients with syphilis of greater than 1 year's duration to exclude asymptomatic neurosyphilis.

Published studies show that a total dose of 6.0 to 9.0 million units of penicillin G results in a satisfactory clinical response in approximately 90 per cent of patients with neurosyphilis. There is more published clinical experience with short-acting penicillin preparations than with benzathine penicillin G. Some clinicians prefer to hospitalize patients with neurosyphilis, particularly if the patient is symptomatic or has not responded to initial therapy. In these instances they treat patients with 12 to 24 million units of aqueous crystalline penicillin G given intravenously each day (2 to 4 million units every 4 hours) for 10 days.

Patients Who Are Allergic to Penicillin. 1. Tetracycline hydrochloride, 500 mg. four times a day by mouth for 30 days. OR

2. Erythromycin (stearate, ethylsuccinate, or base), 500 mg. four times a day by mouth for 30 days.

---

*R. H. Henderson, M.D., Chairman, Venereal Disease Control Division, Bureau of State Services, Center for Disease Control, Atlanta, Ga.; J. H. Miller, Executive Secretary, Venereal Disease Control Division, Bureau of State Services, CDC; D. Fouser, WNET-TV, New York, N.Y.; H. Hamilton, Editor, *Urban Health*, Atlanta, Ga.; G. H. Handy, M.D., Department of Health and Social Services, Madison, Wis.; B. Krohn, Barbara Krohn, and Associates, Seattle, Wash.; S. Nixon, M.D., Floresville, Tex.; M. O. Shinn, EOC of Imperial County (Cal.), Inc., El Centro, Cal.

†V. Cave, M.D., Brooklyn, N.Y.; P. E. Dans, M.D., University of Colorado Medical School, Denver, Colo.; N. J. Fiumara, M.D., State Department of Public Health, Boston, Mass.; A. R. Hinman, M.D., State Department of Public Health, Nashville, Tenn.; R. H. Kampmeier, M.D., Central State Hospital, Nashville, Tenn.; L. Klein, M.D., Grady Memorial Hospital, Atlanta, Ga.; W. Ledger, M.D., University of Southern California Medical Center, Los Angeles, Cal.; W. McCormack, M.D., Boston City Hospital, Boston, Mass.; G. McCracken, M.D., University of Texas Medical Center, Dallas, Tex.; N. B. Nichols, M.D., University of Oklahoma Health Sciences Center, Oklahoma City, Okla.; P. L. Perine, M.D., Virginia Mason Clinic, Seattle, Wash.; M. F. Rein, M.D., University of Virginia, Charlottesville, Va.; J. P. Sanford, M.D., Uniformed Services University of the Health Sciences, Bethesda, Md.; A. L. Schroeter, M.D., Mayo Clinic, Rochester, Minn.; P. F. Sparling, M.D., University of North Carolina, Chapel Hill, N.C.; L. Taber, M.D., Baylor College of Medicine, Houston, Tex.; E. C. Tramont, M.D., Lt. Col., M. C., Walter Reed Army Medical Center, Washington, D.C.

‡Italics indicate commentary.

*Food and some dairy products interfere with absorption. Oral forms of tetracycline should be given 1 hour before or 2 hours after meals.

There are NO published clinical data which adequately document the efficacy of drugs other than penicillin for syphilis of more than 1 year's duration. Cerebrospinal fluid examinations are highly recommended before therapy with these regimens.

Syphilis in Pregnancy

Evaluation of Pregnant Women. *All pregnant women should have a nontreponemal serologic test for syphilis, such as the VDRL or RPR test, at the time of the first prenatal visit. The treponemal tests such as the FTA-ABS test should not be used for routine screening. In women suspected of being at high risk for syphilis, a second nontreponemal test should be performed during the third trimester. Seroreactive patients should be expeditiously evaluated. This evaluation should include a history and physical examination, as well as a quantitative nontreponemal test and a confirmatory treponemal test.*

If the FTA-ABS test is nonreactive and there is no clinical evidence of syphilis, treatment may be withheld. Both the quantitative nontreponemal test and the confirmatory test should be repeated within 4 weeks. If there is clinical or serologic evidence of syphilis or if the diagnosis of syphilis cannot be excluded with reasonable certainty, the patient should be treated as outlined below.

Patients for whom there is documentation of adequate treatment for syphilis in the past need not be re-treated unless there is clinical or serologic evidence of reinfection such as darkfield-positive lesions or a four-fold titer rise of a quantitative nontreponemal test.

1. Patients at All Stages of Pregnancy Who Are Not Allergic to Penicillin. Penicillin is given in dosage schedules appropriate for the stage of syphilis, as recommended for the treatment of nonpregnant patients.

2. Patients at All Stages of Pregnancy Who Are Allergic to Penicillin. Erythromycin (stearate, ethylsuccinate, or base) is given in dosage schedules appropriate for the stage of syphilis, as recommended for the treatment of nonpregnant patients. Although these erythromycin schedules appear safe for mother and fetus, their efficacy is not well established. Therefore the documentation of penicillin allergy is particularly important before treating a pregnant woman with erythromycin. *Erythromycin estolate and tetracycline are not recommended for syphilitic infections in pregnant women because of potential adverse effects on mother and fetus.*

Follow-up. Pregnant women who have been treated for syphilis should have monthly quantitative nontreponemal serologic tests for the remainder of the current pregnancy. Women who show a four-fold rise in titer should be re-treated. After delivery, follow-up is as outlined for nonpregnant patients.

Congenital Syphilis

Congenital syphilis may occur if the mother has syphilis during pregnancy. If the mother has received adequate penicillin treatment during pregnancy, the risk to the infant is minimal. However, all infants should be examined carefully at birth and at frequent intervals thereafter until nontreponemal serologic tests are negative.

Infected infants are frequently asymptomatic at birth and may be seronegative if the maternal infection occurred late in gestation. Infants should be treated at birth if maternal treatment was inadequate, unknown, or with drugs other than penicillin, or if adequate follow-up of the infant cannot be ensured.

Infants with congenital syphilis should have a CSF examination before treatment.

Infants with Abnormal CSF. 1. Aqueous crystalline penicillin G, 50,000 units per kg. intramuscularly or intravenously daily in two divided doses for a minimum of 10 days. OR

2. Aqueous procaine penicillin G, 50,000 units per kg. intramuscularly daily for a minimum of 10 days.

Infants with Normal CSF. *Benzathine penicillin G, 50,000 units per kg. intramuscularly in a single dose. Although benzathine penicillin has been previously recommended and widely used, published clinical data on its efficacy in congenital neurosyphilis are lacking. If neurosyphilis cannot be excluded, the procaine or aqueous penicillin regimens are recommended. Since cerebrospinal fluid concentrations of penicillin achieved after benzathine penicillin are minimal to nonexistent, these revised recommendations seem more conservative and appropriate until clinical data on the efficacy of benzathine penicillin can be accumulated. Other antibiotics are not recommended for neonatal congenital syphilis.* Penicillin therapy for congenital syphilis after the neonatal period should be with the same dosages used for neonatal congenital syphilis. For larger children the total dose of penicillin need not exceed the dosage used in adult syphilis of more than 1 year's duration. After the neonatal period, the dosage of erythromycin and tetracycline for congenital syphilitics who are allergic to penicillin should be individualized but need not exceed dosages used in adult syphilis of more than 1 year's duration. Tetracycline should not be given to children less than 8 years of age.

Follow-up and Re-treatment

All patients with early syphilis and congenital syphilis should be encouraged to return for repeat quantitative nontreponemal tests 3, 6, and 12 months after treatment. Patients with syphilis of more than 1 year's duration should also have a repeat serologic test 24 months after treatment. Careful follow-up serologic testing is particularly important in patients treated with antibiotics other than penicillin. Examination of CSF should be planned as part of the last follow-up visit after treatment with alternative antibiotics.

All patients with neurosyphilis must be carefully followed with serologic testing for at least 3 years. In addition, follow-up of these patients should include clinical re-evaluation at 6 month intervals and repeat CSF examinations, particularly in patients treated with alternative antibiotics.

The possibility of reinfection should always be considered when re-treating patients with early syphilis. A CSF examination should be performed before re-treatment unless reinfection and a diagnosis of early syphilis can be established.

Re-treatment should be considered when (1) clinical signs or symptoms of syphilis persist or recur; (2) there is a sustained four-fold increase in the titer of a nontreponemal test; or (3) an initially high-titer nontreponemal test fails to show a four-fold decrease within a year.

Patients should be re-treated with the schedules recommended for syphilis of more than 1 year's duration. In general, only one re-treatment course is indicated because patients may maintain stable, low titers of nontreponemal tests or have irreversible anatomic damage.

Epidemiologic Treatment

Patients who have been exposed to infectious syphilis within the preceding 3 months and other patients who on epidemiologic grounds are at high risk for syphilis should be treated as for early syphilis. Every effort should be made to establish a diagnosis in these cases.

Reported by Venereal Disease Control Division, Bureau of State Services, CDC.

SECTION 10

Diseases of Allergy

ANAPHYLAXIS AND SERUM SICKNESS

method of
JAMES I. TENNENBAUM, M.D.
Columbus, Ohio

Definitions

Anaphylaxis may be one of the most dramatic and extreme of medical emergencies. Often it occurs suddenly when least expected and is therefore more dangerous. It is an immunologically mediated reaction following the introduction of a specific antigen (allergen) into any suitably sensitized individual. This antigen-antibody reaction results in the explosive release of pharmacologically active chemical mediators, such as histamine, slow-reacting substance of anaphylaxis (SRS-A), and eosinophilic chemotactic factor of anaphylaxis (ECF-A) from mast cells and basophils. These mediators have profound effects on smooth muscle, capillaries, and mucus glands and are responsible for the signs and symptoms that affect four major organ systems: skin, respiratory, gastrointestinal, and cardiovascular. The effect to which each system is involved is variable in individual patients and presents as follows:

Skin: urticaria, angioedema, erythema, pruritus.

Respiratory: wheezing, dyspnea, choking, laryngeal stridor, cyanosis.

Gastrointestinal: nausea, vomiting, abdominal cramps, diarrhea (occasionally bloody).

Cardiovascular: vascular collapse with shock, ischemic changes on electrocardiogram (ECG), cardiac arrhythmias.

The severity is variable, ranging from a mild skin rash to death, depending on the extent of involvement of each organ system.

Antigens which commonly induce anaphylaxis are drugs such as penicillin and heterologous antiserum, stinging insect venoms, pollen extracts, and, rarely, certain foods. Some agents, such as iodinated contrast media and aspirin, produce identical reactions by some undefined nonimmunologic release of chemical mediators. These idiosyncratic reactions have been called *anaphylactoid* reactions. The clinical appearance and management are the same, however.

Serum sickness classically is an allergic reaction that develops in many patients following the therapeutic administration of foreign (usually equine) serum. It is manifested clinically by fever, skin eruptions, joint symptoms, lymphadenopathy, and occasionally neuritis. The symptoms are caused by toxic circulating antigen-antibody complexes. The symptoms usually appear 7 to 12 days following initial exposure to the antigen but may occur sooner (accelerated serum sickness) in patients who have antibodies from previous exposure. Today the serum sickness syndrome is more commonly induced by drugs, particularly penicillin, because of the use of human serum, especially human antitetanus serum.

Management

Prevention. The best way to manage anaphylaxis is to avoid it if at all possible. Many reactions follow unnecessary use of drugs. The following steps will decrease the risk of severe reactions.

1. Take a careful allergy history from every new patient. Especially noted should be any previous adverse reactions to any injected or ingested substance.

2. Warn the patient to avoid exposure to any substance to which he is known to be sensitive. The patient should wear an identity bracelet or pendant indicating a known allergy. These can be obtained from the Medic Alert Foundation, Turlock, California 95380.

3. Prescribe drugs, only when absolutely indicated, by mouth rather than by injection whenever appropriate.

4. A Hymenoptera insect–sensitive patient or family member should be taught emergency care following a sting to include epinephrine (Adrenalin) administration and ingestion of an antihistamine preparation and ephedrine. Stinging insect emergency medical kits are commercially available. After self-treatment, the patient should proceed to the nearest medical facility for further treatment as indicated. Immunotherapy (hyposensitization) with Hymenoptera extract

should be given to such patients in an attempt to minimize reactions to future stings.

5. Allergenic extracts administered to hay fever and asthma patients should be given only when a physician is on the premises and according to carefully prescribed schedules. A patient should wait in the physician's office for at least 20 minutes following the injection so that any adverse reaction may be treated promptly.

6. All patients should be current in their immunization with tetanus toxoid to eliminate the need for horse serum antitoxin. Immune sera of human origin should be used whenever possible, to avoid induction of serum sickness.

7. Patients known to be sensitive to foods, drugs, or food additives must read labels of all packaged or prescribed products. Aspirin-sensitive patients should be given a list of all drugs and foods known to contain salicylates.

8. Topical application of certain drugs, such as antibiotics, antihistamines, and local anesthetics, should be avoided, as such application carries a high risk of sensitization.

Treatment. Treatment should be individualized according to severity and the system involved. Immediate treatment is mandatory.

1. The most important agent regardless of the cause is epinephrine. Once anaphylaxis has been diagnosed, 0.3 to 0.5 ml. of epinephrine (1:1,000) should be given subcutaneously. If the inciting agent was an injectant, another 0.2 ml. should be given in the injection site. This may be repeated in 15 to 30 minutes if needed. Proportionately smaller doses should be used in children.

2. A tourniquet should be applied proximal to the site of a drug injection or insect sting whenever possible.

3. Administer diphenhydramine hydrochloride (Benadryl), 50 to 100 mg. intramuscularly.

4. Oxygen should be administered by any means available, should cyanosis or severe dyspnea be present.

5. If wheezing is present without hypotension, 500 mg. of aminophylline should be given intravenously over 20 to 30 minutes.

6. The patient should be hospitalized, if he does not respond promptly to the aforementioned measures.

7. A patent airway must be maintained by endotracheal intubation or tracheostomy.

8. If the initial hypotension does not respond quickly to subcutaneous epinephrine, an intravenous infusion of isotonic saline should be started and a vasopressor such as levarterenol or metaraminol administered in sufficient quantities in this infusion to maintain adequate blood pressure.

9. Corticosteroids are not useful in the immediate treatment of anaphylaxis, as they have a slow onset of action. In patients with severe respiratory distress or hypotension unresponsive to other measures, corticosteroids should be used. One hundred mg. of hydrocortisone by intravenous push should be given immediately, followed by 300 mg. in divided doses for 24 to 48 hours.

10. Should cardiac arrhythmias or cardiac arrest occur, immediate appropriate cardiopulmonary treatment, as indicated by ECG and central venous pressures, should be instituted.

11. Antihistamines (Benadryl, 50 mg. every 6 hours) are most useful for the management of the urticaria and angioedema associated with serum sickness. In addition, ephedrine, 25 mg. every 6 hours, may afford relief when used concomitantly with antihistamines. Aspirin is effective for the relief of fever and joint symptoms. In severely affected patients, steroids in high doses, 40 to 60 mg. of prednisone initially, followed by gradual tapering and withdrawal over 7 to 10 days, are extremely effective. Occasionally, a clinical relapse may occur when therapy is discontinued, requiring another short course of treatment.

ASTHMA IN ADULTS

method of
JOHN A. ARKINS, M.D.
Milwaukee, Wisconsin

The diagnosis of asthma is usually not difficult. It can be broadly defined as reversible obstructive airway disease which may or may not be allergic in nature. The disease is characterized by intermittent episodes of wheezing, coughing, and dyspnea with mucoid sputum production.

In general, treatment can be subdivided into two major categories: specific therapy and symptomatic therapy.

1. *Specific therapy:* (a) Avoidance. If the patient is clinically sensitive to environmental antigens such as danders, pollens, molds, or foods, he can either totally avoid these substances or at least reduce exposure. Before removing or avoiding these substances, there must be good clinical evidence of sensitivity as demonstrated by history, skin test, radioallergosorbent test (RAST), or challenge. (b) Hyposensitization. This method is valuable only in the atopic (IgE mediated) diseases in which inhalant sensitivity has been demonstrated by one of the techniques listed in (a).

2. *Symptomatic therapy:* This is therapy directed at (a) relieving bronchial smooth muscle contraction, (b) relieving edema of the mucosa and (c) reducing the production of mucoid sputum. Other factors playing a role, such as hypoxia, dyspnea, anxiety, and hyperventilation, will respond, when (a), (b), and (c) are relieved.

To approach the problem of treatment specifically, asthma will be considered under the following headings: mild, moderate, and severe (status asthmaticus).

Mild Asthma

This form of asthma is usually seasonal, IgE mediated, and easily controlled with a minimum of medication on an intermittent basis.

Specific therapy is important here and may result in complete relief of the disease. There may be important precipitating factors such as exercise, cold air, and anxiety. Specific therapy may require only that sympathomimetic amines such as ephedrine sulfate, 25 mg., terbutaline, 5 mg., or metaproterenol, 20 mg., be given. Combination drugs containing theophylline offer no advantage. Inhaled sympathomimetic amines are dramatic in their effect, but patients tend to overuse them so they are generally not recommended. Isoproterenol is a major offender in this regard. Infrequent use of isoetharine (Bronkosol) or metaproterenol (Alupent, Metaprel) is safer. Refills of these agents must be regulated to ensure that the patient is not overusing them.

Moderate Asthma

This form of asthma is a more severe form of seasonal asthma or may occur on a perennial basis. It may or may not be IgE mediated. It is often precipitated by upper respiratory infections.

Specific therapy is also important in these patients; however, symptomatic therapy is of utmost importance. These patients are frequent visitors to the emergency room unless their asthma is controlled. An organized approach to these patients is as follows:

Theophylline Preparations. Numerous preparations are on the market. The active ingredient is anhydrous theophylline. A starting dose of 3 mg. per kg. (usually 200 mg. in the average adult) every 6 hours orally is used. Because of marked individual variation in metabolism of this drug, each patient will require different dosages, ranging from 800 to 1600 mg. daily. Theophylline blood value measurements are available at many institutions. A level of between 10 and 20 micrograms per ml. is ideal. Toxic reaction occurs in most patients at levels above 20 micrograms per ml. The blood should be drawn 5 to 6 hours after the last dose.

Sympathomimetic Amines. Oral drugs in this category are almost on a par with theophylline. These drugs, ephedrine, 25 mg., terbutaline, 5 mg., or metaproterenol, 20 mg., must be taken on a regular basis around the clock at 4 to 6 hour intervals. Many combination drugs containing theophylline are available: e.g., hydroxyzine, barbiturates, and glyceryl guaiacolate. These offer no advantage over the single drugs. The aerosol drugs are also in this category, and the statement regarding their use in mild asthma also applies here.

Mediator Inhibitors. There is currently only one drug in this category. It is cromolyn (Aarane, Intal). It is not a bronchodilator but does inhibit mediator release from mast cells. It is useful in atopic (IgE mediated) asthmatics. It is administered by inhalation in a Spinhaler in a dosage of 1 capsule (20 mg.) four times daily. This drug may reduce the requirements for sympathomimetic amines and lessen the need for corticosteroids.

Corticosteroids. If the aforementioned methods are unsuccessful in controlling asthma, corticosteroids are indicated. A starting dose of prednisone, 40 to 60 mg. per day, is usually satisfactory. This dose is maintained until there is a definite clinical response, and then is tapered to the minimal tolerated daily dose or, better yet, alternate day dosages. Other forms of corticosteroids may be used; however, prednisone is effective in the majority of patients. There is no need for parenteral steroids or ACTH.

An aerosol corticosteroid is also available. It is beclomethasone (Vanceril). This has the definite advantage of not being systemically absorbed, so that the production of a Cushing-like syndrome is not a problem. The usual starting dosage is 2 or 3 inhalations four times daily. After the patient responds, the dosage can be reduced.

Expectorants. Fluids are probably the best expectorants; however, potassium iodide, 10 drops four times daily, and glyceryl guaiacolate, 200 mg. four times daily, are commonly used and may be helpful in some patients. A good mucolytic agent is acetylcysteine (Mucomyst), but it should be given in a 10 per cent solution with a bronchodilator, as it may aggravate the asthma if used in a higher concentration.

Antibiotics. As most respiratory infections are of viral cause, the indiscriminate use of antibiotics should be avoided. If the signs of bacterial infection are present—i.e., purulent sputum with many polymorphonuclear cells and bacteria, fever, chills, and leukocytosis—then antibiotics should be administered after a culture is taken. If the patient is not penicillin sensitive, ampicillin, 1 gram per day for 10 days, is used. Tetracycline, 1 gram per day for 10 days, would be a good alternative.

Toxicity. With all these drugs there is toxicity:

Theophylline: gastrointestinal upset, arrhythmias, convulsion.

Sympathomimetic amines: cardiac stimulation, adrenergic stimulation.

Cromolyn: very few—local irritation, dermatitis.

Corticosteroids: all the effects of hypercortisolism.

Beclomethasone: monilia overgrowth.

Severe Asthma (Status Asthmaticus)

This is the most severe form of asthma and is life threatening. The patient must be hospitalized. A team approach is advisable, including the primary physician, allergist, pulmonary specialist, and anesthesiologist.

All the approaches listed under symptomatic therapy for moderate asthma are applicable here. Initial therapy must be guided by the physiologic status of the patient. Serial blood gases must be used to monitor direction. Usually a low P_{CO_2} and elevated pH are seen initially, reflecting hyperventilation. If the P_{CO_2} rises above normal, reflecting acidosis, the patient is becoming worse and will need more aggressive therapy.

Initially the bronchodilators are started as follows:

1. Epinephrine 1:1000, 0.4 to 0.5 ml. subcutaneously, repeated every 30 minutes for four to five times.
2. Theophylline: If the patient has had no prior therapy, give a loading dose of 5.6 mg. per kg. of theophylline ethylenediamine (aminophylline) intravenously, followed after 20 to 30 minutes by a maintenance dose of 250 to 500 mg. intravenously every 6 hours. Blood levels are extremely useful here. If the patient has been given theophylline, then maintenance should be instituted.
3. Ephedrine sulfate, 25 mg., or other beta-stimulator, every 4 to 6 hours.
4. Corticosteroid: hydrocortisone, 4 mg. per kg. every 2 to 4 hours until definite clinical improvement is apparent for 24 hours; then the dosage is reduced.

Further measures include the following:

1. Oxygen therapy to correct the hypoxia.
2. Hydration: 5 per cent dextrose in ½ isotonic saline solution should be used.
3. Antibiotic therapy if a bacterial infection is suspected.
4. If there is no response in 24 hours and the patient is developing acidosis, then intubation and mechanical assistance should be provided. Volume respirators are the best.
5. Miscellaneous: (a) Mucolytic agent such as acetylcysteine by nebulization or sodium iodide, 1 gram in the intravenous solution daily. (b) Avoid alkaloids unless the patient is on full assisted respiration. (c) Sodium bicarbonate, 90 mEq. intravenously over 10 minutes, followed by 44 mEq. increments if pH is below 7.3.

In summary, status asthmaticus represents a medical emergency. The key to successful management is an adequate understanding of the underlying pathophysiologic principles and the institution of immediate and aggressive therapy. Bronchodilators around the clock, hydration and expectoration, corticosteroids, and oxygen therapy with careful monitoring are the initial measures. Antibiotics, if indicated, sodium bicarbonate, and mechanical respirators with or without intubation of the patient may be instituted if the initial therapy is not adequate. Treatment should be continued for 24 to 48 hours following marked improvement to ensure that a recurrence will not develop. Following discharge, these patients must be carefully observed and trained to increase their medications when the asthma increases. Instructions are given in the use of bronchodilators on an around-the-clock basis, using beta-adrenergic stimulators such as ephedrine, terbutaline, or metaproterenol, therapeutic amounts of theophylline, and adequate hydration. In addition, early recognition of infection and the use of expectorants and corticosteroids (when indicated) are necessary. Usually with this regimen and a patient educated by the physician to use medications properly, recurrences can be kept at a minimum.

ASTHMA IN CHILDHOOD

method of
ROBERT H. SCHWARTZ, M.D.
Rochester, New York

Introduction

The clinical spectrum of asthma includes an occasional transient nuisance, episodic disability, chronic disabling disease, life-threatening status asthmaticus, and respiratory failure. The full impact of asthma on the developing child, on the family, on the local community, and on the national economy has yet to be determined. Approximately 100 children die from asthma each year in the United States. However, elimination of this mortality is not the only goal of management. For the child, goals are prevention, relief, and cure. Fortunately, most asthma in childhood is physiologically mild, and with proper comprehensive management children can be helped to "outgrow" both disease and disability. True biological severity as well as the child-parent behavioral responses to the illness must be considered. The major interim goals are to help the child perform at least ordinary daily activities typical for children of that age and to educate both the child and parents to manage the disease within the family's life style.

Definition of Asthma

Minden and Farr have defined allergy as a "broad group of untoward physiologic responses which are mediated by a variety of fundamentally different immunologic mechanisms." It is well known that asthma usually has an allergic basis. However, it is also triggered by nonimmune factors such as exercise, viral and bacterial infection, psychic stimuli, meteorologic changes, cold, and exposure to irritating dusts and chemicals, especially air pollution. These stimuli provoke asthma through neural and neurohumoral pathways. Modern understanding of these pathways, especially the mediators of the asthmatic response, has resulted in far better pharmacologic management than in the past.

Asthma is a condition which results in diffuse but reversible airways obstruction. Reversibility occurs either spontaneously or following appropriate therapy. Whatever the predominant trigger mechanism for the individual patient, a state of bronchial hyperresponsiveness ("twitchy lung") exists, resulting in (1) edema of bronchial mucosa, (2) constriction and hypertrophy of bronchial smooth muscle, and (3) hypersecretion by bronchial mucous glands.

Principles of Management

There are six basic principles in the management of childhood asthma: (1) understanding the biological basis of asthma, (2) prevention (prophylaxis) of allergic disease, (3) identification of and avoidance of pertinent offending allergens, (4) symptomatic and/or prophylactic therapy with drugs, (5) hyposensitization (immunotherapy) with extracts of those common allergens which cause symptoms and which cannot be avoided, and (6) education and rehabilitation of the child-patient and his family. All these principles must be considered and applied to children with chronic, severe, and intractable asthma. All need not be applied to the child with only occasional wheezing. Treatment failures often occur when either drug therapy or hyposensitization is solely relied upon.

The Biologic Basis of Asthma. Asthma is frequently familial and therefore probably has a genetic basis. As with allergies in general, the mode of inheritance is incompletely understood. The family history of allergy can usually be obtained in 40 to 70 per cent of children with asthma. Unilateral and bilateral family histories carry an increasing risk of developing asthma. Atopic dermatitis and hay fever seem to be genetically related to asthma, and a prior history of these is frequently followed by the development of asthma. About 50 per cent of children with ragweed hay fever will subsequently wheeze to some extent. Obviously, many undefined asthma risk factors need to be defined. For the present, it is best to regard allergy and asthma as independent but closely linked tendencies. Allergy is the tendency to develop an immunologic response, usually IgE antibodies, to allergens encountered in the natural environment. These antibodies sensitize the surface of mast cells in the respiratory tract. On re-exposure to the allergens, mast cells release mediators (histamine and others) which act on small blood vessels, mucus-secreting glands, and smooth muscle in airways. Irritant receptors are also stimulated by histamine. Airways are subsequently narrowed by edema, mucus accumulation, and, in the case of asthma, direct and reflex bronchoconstriction. When this reaction occurs in the lungs, asthma ensues. When it occurs in the nose, the entity is allergic rhinitis. What distinguishes the patient with asthma from the patient with only allergic rhinitis is probably an inherited bronchial hyperreactivity ("twitchy lung"). Some argue that the development of hyperreactivity is initially facilitated by the inflammatory effects of infection in early childhood. Pertussis, measles, and, more recently, respiratory viruses (RSV and adenovirus) have been implicated. Inheritance of bronchial hyperreactivity alone (without allergy) can account for the 25 per cent of asthmatic patients in the pediatric population who have "intrinsic" asthma. Severe viral infection can conceivably do the same. It will be difficult to completely define the interrelationships of genetic, environmental, infectious, and neurohumoral risk factors which contribute to the development, chronicity, and severity of asthma. Both the scientist and the patient's physician must arrive at and be able to communicate a working explanation. This may have to change from time to time. In this respect, the science and the art are similar. Methods to safely detect the presence or absence of bronchial hyperreactivity in the young child with allergic rhinitis will certainly be helpful in the anticipatory management of many such children seen by the pediatrician.

Prevention (Prophylaxis) of Allergic Disease. Children of allergic parents are more apt to develop respiratory allergies. It has also been observed that between 50 and 80 per cent of infants who have atopic dermatitis subsequently develop, in later childhood, asthma or allergic rhinitis. Several studies have shown that only 25 per cent of asthmatic children spontaneously outgrow their asthma by adolescence. Where in the course of human development can the physician intervene and attempt to avoid these consequences?

SPECIAL DIET. Potentially allergic newborns are placed on a diet free of cow's milk products, wheat, eggs, and chicken for the first 9 months of life. Milk-substitute soybean preparations (Isomil, Neo-Mull-Soy, ProSobee, Soyalac) contain adequate vitamins and provide adequate nutrients for normal growth. Breast feeding is an admirable alternative. In one study, this prophylactic diet has reduced the incidence of atopic eczema by three fourths as compared to sibling controls. The development of major respiratory allergies in those children who do develop eczema may be reduced by as much as 75 per cent. A significant decrease in the development of bronchial asthma and perennial allergic rhinitis has been accomplished. This approach, as recommended by Glaser and Johnstone, has both its proponents and its critics. Immunologic immaturity of the gastrointestinal tract IgA secretory system with leakage of foreign proteins into the systemic circulation has been cited as the condition of initial sensitization. IgE production is stimulated. Avoidance of foreign proteins, potential antigens, and allergens during this period of IgA secretory maturation prevents early sensitization and possibly the priming effect of further sensitization. After IgA secretory maturation, specific IgA prevents epithelial penetration and systemic sensitization. Studies from England are beginning to support the rationale for this type of diet, which has been used in Rochester, N.Y., for many years. The allergen-avoidance regimen reduced the incidence of eczema during the first year of life. Also, those children had lower serum IgE levels at 6 weeks of age. The approach has yet to be conclusively proved effective. It is reasonable if applied to offspring of allergic parents. It offers some, but not complete, hope for prevention. Its disadvantages are the increased expense and the extra stress which it may impose on the parent-child relationship. The latter occurs primarily because of the specially imposed circumstances. These may encourage parents to regard the healthy infants as ill and can set the stage for future abnormal health behavioral patterns.

HYPOSENSITIZATION (IMMUNOTHERAPY). The value of appropriate specific hyposensitization therapy in the relief of hay fever and asthma has withstood the subjective test of time and is still surviving the objective scrutiny of rigorous laboratory and clinical investigation. Unfortunately, the allergen content of almost all injection material is not standardized, and therefore the details of this procedure vary from physician to physician throughout the country. Nevertheless, the studies of Johnstone (Rochester, N.Y.) have suggested that such therapy may alter the natural history of allergic disease of childhood. When hyposensitization therapy was administered using the highest tolerated dose of allergen mixtures, 78 per cent of children were free of symptoms by their sixteenth birthday. In contrast, only 22 per cent of placebo-treated children "outgrew" their asthma. There is good evidence for the efficacy of immunotherapy with aqueous extracts for the treatment of asthma caused by pollens (ragweed and grasses) and some evidence for house dust and dust mite *(Dermatophagoides pteronyssinus)*. Little objective evidence is available to support the efficacy of mold spore allergen hyposensitization, and control studies have not been reported to show the effectiveness of injections of animal danders. There is scant, if any, objective evidence that injections of stock or autogenous bacterial vaccines are effective in controlling asthma even in children whose symptoms are provoked only by "respiratory infections." Since, in children, these infections are usually viral in cause, the rationale for even undertaking such therapy is difficult to explain. Perhaps a better approach would be the development of effective safe viral vaccines to be used in very early infancy aimed at providing host resistance against the most important respiratory viruses (RSV, parainfluenza, and influenza). These viruses are able to invade and disrupt the surface epithelial structures of airways. They are the common causes of bronchiolitis of infancy and childhood, and when these infections are severe, protracted, or recurrent, they seem to predispose to the future development of asthma.

Identification of and Avoidance of Pertinent Offending Allergens. Identification of offending allergens is made by correlation of history with results of allergy skin tests or RAST (radioallergosorbent tests).

In the first 2 years of life, food allergens (milk, eggs, wheat) are the most common allergenic factors. The trial elimination diet for 7 to 14 days, with stepwise reinstitution of individual foods at 5 to 7 day intervals after symptoms have cleared, is the best way to detect these sensitivities. A careful hypoallergenic diet consists of a milk substitute (some children are sensitive to soybeans), rice cereal, apples, pears, carrots, sweet potatoes, and lamb. Skin tests are not entirely reliable in determining food allergy. A negative test does not indicate a lack of sensitivity; nor does a positive test mean definite clinical sensitivity.

During the second year of life and thereafter, inhalant sensitivities as a cause of respiratory allergies should be suspected. House dust, animal danders, vegetable seeds, molds, and pollens are potential sensitizers.

House dust is a heterogeneous mixture of degenerative plant fibers, animal danders, molds, bacteria, and house dust mites *(Dermatophagoides pteronyssinus* and *D. farinae).*

Animal danders are epidermal (hair and skin) products shed most usually from indoor pets (cat and dog). In rural areas other animals may be implicated. Chicken, duck, and goose feathers are found in pillows, quilts, and upholstered furniture. Vegetable products include kapok (pillows, mattresses, upholstered furniture, life preservers, and toys), and flaxseed (upholstery, wave sets, shampoos, and hair tonics).

Mold spores are important causes of inhalant allergies in children. In the United States, the two most important outdoor molds responsible for seasonal respiratory allergies are Alternaria and Hormodendrum. Symptoms occur between late March and November in most localities. Indoor molds (Penicillium and Aspergillus) are encouraged by dampness and high humidity. Mold growth is also encouraged by both warm and cool mist vaporizers used by parents in the frequently prescribed treatment of respiratory symptoms. Office and home humidifiers are commonly another sorce of mold antigens.

Pollen sensitivities are most easily recognized. If parents (or patient) can determine the exact time that respiratory symptoms begin and when they become less severe or end, the physician can correlate them with the pollination timetable of his locality. Trees, grasses, and weeds pollinate sequentially in many areas of the United States. In some areas of Texas and Florida, grasses pollinate almost throughout the year.

One must remember that as the respiratory epithelium becomes primed by inhalant allergens or respiratory infection, similar respiratory symptoms may be precipitated or compounded by inhalant, nonantigenic irritants such as smoke, odors, and fumes. Wheezing with exercise and postexercise bronchospasm also occur more frequently during periods of allergen-induced symptoms.

Skin testing is the most important diagnostic method. It helps to confirm the historical data, allows general assessment of the degree of tolerance to further injection therapy, and redirects one's attention to the history when unsuspected positive tests are found. When a positive pollen test is found with a negative history, evaluation during subsequent pollen seasons may be rewarding in that early clinical sensitivity may be discovered. Antihistamines should not be taken for 24 hours prior to skin testing. Hydroxyzine (Atarax) should not be taken for 48 to 72 hours prior to skin testing. Sympathomimetics, aminophylline, and phenothiazine tranquilizers also suppress the development of positive immediate skin tests. Cromolyn sodium and corticosteroids (both systemic and inhalable) do not suppress immediate skin tests. Scratch tests with antigenic extracts of the common allergens known to be present in the environment should be performed first. In small children, and frequently in older children, scratch tests may suffice in determining important pollen sensitivities. In order to avoid large and severe reactions, scratch tests should be done prior to intradermal testing. Intradermal testing should be done only with the inhalant allergens to which the child did not react on scratch testing. Do not test any allergens to which the child is thought to be extremely sensitive (those such as peanuts and shellfish which are known to provoke immediate symptoms in the patient). Provocation testing (conjunctival and inhalational) more directly relates the allergen with production of allergic symptoms. However, these tests should be performed only by those experienced in these methods. Inhalation bronchial challenge is of value in asthmatic patients with multiple positive reactions to skin testing. I usually reserve RAST testing for those children whose reaction to the skin testing situation makes it impossible to accomplish this procedure. RAST testing, which detects specific serum antibody, is also useful for detection of specific stinging insect venom hypersensitivity. These antigens are not now commercially available for skin testing.

For the patient with respiratory allergy, avoidance of inhalant allergens and irritants shares equal importance with drug and hyposensitization therapy in reducing the total allergic load and raising the symptomatic threshold. This point cannot be overemphasized. Printed instructions on avoidance of house dust, molds, animal danders, pollens, and specific food allergens can be obtained from textbooks on allergy. As the child spends a good portion of the 24 hour day in his bedroom, major emphasis should be placed on reduction of inhalant allergens in this area. The room can be made attractive with an aim toward simplicity. Wool carpeting, stuffed furniture, and heavy draperies should be avoided. Items containing feathers or hair should be eliminated. Cats, dogs, and other hairy animals should not be allowed in the house. Mattresses and box springs should be completely covered (Allergen-Proof Encasings Inc., 1450 East 363rd Street, Eastlake, Ohio 44094). Avoid insect and other house sprays in the bedroom. Outdoor clothing or household articles should not be stored in the bedroom. A central air filter on the furnace should be replaced monthly. If the home is heated by forced hot air, the outlet to the bedroom should be closed. Electronic air cleaners (either portable or attached to the central heating system) are of considerable value in preventing exposure to allergenic particles. The aim of any mechanical device is to deliver to the patient's bedroom fresh outdoor air filtered free of pollen and mold spores. During the pollen season bedroom windows should be kept closed, especially at night when the concentration of pollen in the outdoor air is usually greatest. Outdoor allergens cannot be avoided; however, certain steps can be taken to minimize exposure, such as remaining indoors on windy days, avoiding participating in grass cutting, and keeping car windows closed when taking a drive. The control of indoor molds is difficult. A dehumidifier in the basement may be helpful. In contrast, proper humidification of the house during the winter months is of value to a patient with respiratory symptoms. When it is feasible for the patient to spend a major part of the pollen season in an area of relatively low pollen concentration, this is desirable.

Obviously, all these restrictions need not be applied to every patient. The severity and chronicity of the allergic and asthmatic problem will determine the extent of intervention.

Symptomatic and/or Prophylactic Treatment with Drugs. General Considerations. Pharmacologic management is a principal modality of asthma therapy. Children should not be regarded as "little adults." Drug doses and dosing intervals cannot be based on adult studies. Absorption, body metabolic compartment distribution, and catabolism are different for children and differ from child to child. The aim of therapy is to provide a drug dosage whose bioavailability is such as to provide a rapid blood level within the effective therapeutic range, yet not exceeding that level which results in toxicity. The interval of dosage must maintain a level within that range.

Because of recent pharmacokinetic studies with xanthines (theophylline and its derivatives) in children, it is now appreciated that the therapeutic range for serum theophylline is 10 to 20 micrograms per ml. Levels greater than 20 micrograms per ml. may be associated with toxic effects which include insomnia, irritability, restlessness, tremors, convulsions, coma, vomiting, hematemesis, dehydration, tachycardia, cardiac arrhythmias, and shock. The method of high-pressure liquid chromatography for serum theophylline determinations should be available in most medical centers. The biologic half-life varies from 1.4 to 7.8 hours in children. This makes it most desirable to obtain serum theophylline levels for those children who do not respond and who require long-term therapy. The determination is also useful in the effective management of status asthmaticus and respiratory failure.

I try to avoid fixed-combination drugs. These usually contain a xanthine (such as aminophylline or theophylline), ephedrine, and a tranquilizer, the last used to counter the excitatory effects of ephedrine (insomnia, tachycardia, tremor, headache, nervousness, irritability, anorexia, nausea, vomiting). Undesirable side effects from ephedrine, hydroxyzine (drowsiness and hallucinations), and phenobarbital (paradoxical excitation in children) may be encountered when increasing the dose of these fixed-combination drugs to achieve therapeutic theophylline levels.

However, sympathomimetics (beta-2 adrenergic agonists) have a synergistic bronchodilator action when used with theophylline. When used initially or in addition to theophylline, they are frequently effective in controlling the asthma attack. When given as separate medications, this procedure will allow independent adjustment of dosage.

Drug dosage, especially now because of the myriad of xanthine and theophylline preparations available, should be calculated on the basis of their anhydrous theophylline content. For reference, some frequently used preparations are listed in Table 1. Also listed are some fixed-combination drugs which may be effective in episodic acute asthma but are not recommended for continuous use in the difficult-to-control chronic asthmatic child. Oral sympathomimetics can be used alone at the initial onset of mild episodic wheezing or along with a pure theophylline drug in chronic or refractory states when theophylline alone is not effective.

The pharmacologic actions of both theophylline and sympathomimetics are to increase intracellular cyclic 3′5′-adenosine monophosphate (AMP). Elevation of AMP levels prevents mediator (histamine and others) release from mast cells and causes bronchial smooth muscle to relax. Theophylline does this by competitively blocking phosphodiesterase, an enzyme which degrades cyclic AMP to 5′-AMP. Sympathomimetics, by virtue of their beta-2-adrenergic action on adenyl cyclase, increase cyclic AMP production from ATP. Sympathomimetics (such as epinephrine) have both beta-2 and beta-1 action in addition to alpha receptor stimulation. Alpha and beta agonists produce undesirable effects (alpha—vasoconstriction, ureterocontraction, uterine contraction, intestinal smooth muscle

TABLE 1. **Selected Oral Xanthines and Xanthine Combination Bronchodilators**

PREPARATION	GENERIC NAME	THEOPHYLLINE (ANHYDROUS) EQUIVALENT	AVAILABLE THEOPHYLLINE (MG.)	OTHER ACTIVE INGREDIENTS
1. Aminophylline	Aminophylline U.S.P.	86%	86 mg. per 100 mg. tablet 172 mg. per 200 mg. tablet	None None
2. Choledyl	Oxtriphylline	64%	64 mg. per 100 mg. per 5 ml. 64 mg. per 100 mg. tablet 128 mg. per 200 mg. tablet	Elixir, 20% alcohol None None
3. Elixophyllin	Theophylline (anhydrous)	100%	27 mg. per 27 mg. per 5 ml. 100 mg. per 100 mg. per 5 ml. 200 mg. per 200 mg. tablet	Elixir, 20% alcohol Suspension, None None
4. Lufyllin	Dyphylline	70%	140 mg. per 200 mg. tablet 280 mg. per 400 mg. tablet	None None
5. Slo-Phyllin	Theophylline (anhydrous)	100%	27 mg. per 27 mg. per 5 ml. 100 mg. per 100 mg. tablet 200 mg. per 200 mg. tablet	Syrup None None
6. Somophyllin	Aminophylline	86%	90 mg. per 105 mg. per 5 ml.	None
7. Theolair	Theophylline (anhydrous)	100%	125 mg. per 125 mg. tablet 250 mg. per 250 mg. tablet	None None
8. Asbron	Theophylline sodium glycinate	50%	50 mg. per 100 mg. per 5 ml. 150 mg. per 300 mg. tablet	Elixir, 15% alcohol Guaifenesin, 33 mg. Guaifenesin, 100 mg.
9. Brondecon	Oxtriphylline	64%	64 mg. per 100 mg. per 5 ml. 128 mg. per 200 mg. tablet	Elixir, 20% alcohol Guaifenesin, 50 mg. Guaifenesin, 100 mg.
10. Duovent	Theophylline (anhydrous)	100%	130 mg. per 130 mg. tablet	Guaifenesin, 100 mg. Ephedrine, 24 mg. Phenobarbital, 8 mg.
11. Marax	Theophylline (anhydrous)	100%	32.5 mg. per 32.5 mg. per 5 ml. 130 mg. per 130 mg. tablet	Syrup, 5% alcohol Ephedrine, 6.25 mg. Hydroxyzine, 2.5 mg. Ephedrine, 25 mg. Hydroxyzine, 10 mg.
12. Quibron	Theophylline (anhydrous)	100%	50 mg. per 50 mg. per 5 ml. 150 mg. per 150 mg. capsule	Elixir, 15% alcohol Guaifenesin, 30 mg. Guaifenesin, 90 mg.
13. Tedral	Theophylline (anhydrous)	100%	32.5 mg. per 32.5 mg. per 5 ml. 65 mg. per 65 mg. per 5 ml. 130 mg. per 130 mg. tablet	Elixir, 15% alcohol Ephedrine, 6 mg. Phenobarbital, 2 mg. Suspension Ephedrine, 12 mg. Phenobarbital, 4 mg. Ephedrine, 24 mg. Phenobarbital, 8 mg.

Notes:

1. Guaifenesin—previously known as glyceryl guaiacolate.
2. Many other brands are available. See Physician's Desk Reference.
3. Dosage for children should be calculated on the basis of available theophylline at 3 to 5 mg. per kg. to be given no more frequently than every 6 hours. "Trough" serum theophylline levels can be obtained 6 hours after the dose (just before the next dose). "Peak" levels can be obtained 1½ to 2 hours after the dose. This will help identify children who eliminate theophylline more slowly or more rapidly. A dosage of 5 mg. per kg. body weight every 6 hours should not be exceeded unless it is possible to monitor serum theophylline levels.

relaxation, anal sphincter contraction; beta-1—cardiac contraction, intestinal smooth muscle relaxation) and do not contribute to bronchodilation.

Sympathomimetics are catecholamines, and, except for ephedrine, the common ones used therapeutically (epinephrine, ethylnorepinephrine, and isoproterenol) are rapidly degraded by catechol-O-methyl transferase. Modern efforts have been aimed at producing (pure) beta-2 agents of longer duration. Metaproterenol and terbutaline are available in the United States. Salbutamol (Albuterol) has been used with success abroad. Only metaproterenol has been approved by the Food and Drug Administration for use in children (less than 12 years of age).

The aforementioned drugs are still the mainstay of asthma therapy. Proper dosage, timing, and duration of therapy, I believe, have reduced childhood disability, number of office visits for epinephrine injections, and hospitalizations over recent years. However, some patients remain difficult to manage. Even this group has been significantly reduced with the use of cromolyn sodium (Intal, Aarane), and beclomethasone (Vanceril). A small group still requires intermittent short courses (3 to 5 days) of oral short-acting steroids (prednisone). A few will require continuous alternate day steroids, and a rare minority will require daily steroid therapy.

Cromolyn sodium is a powder which, if administered by inhalation (special Spinhaler) prior to allergen exposure, prevents the release of histamine and other mediators from specific IgE-sensitized mast cells. It is not an antihistamine; nor is it a bronchodilator. Therefore it is ineffective in the treatment of acute asthma. It is effective in allergen-induced asthma when used regularly (four times per day) and prior to known allergen exposure. Moderate to good control of about half the asthmatic patients has been achieved in several studies. A 1 month trial in children with perennial asthma requiring frequent or continuous bronchodilators should be used. If improvement occurs, it can be continued. During acute asthmatic flare-ups, it should be temporarily discontinued. It is difficult for children less than 5 years of age to self-administer the 20 mg. dose by the special inhaler. (The use of cromolyn sodium in children under 5 years is not recommended in the manufacturer's official directive.)

Exercise-induced bronchospasm and asthma (that following 8 to 10 minutes of strenuous exercise) can frequently be prevented by administration of theophylline, metaproterenol, ephedrine, or cromolyn sodium, ½ to 1 hour prior to exercise.

Adrenal corticosteroids are very effective for the treatment of asthma. Their use is limited by undesirable side effects. Steroids should be reserved for those children with severe intractable asthma who do not respond to other measures in a reasonable amount of time. The dose should be the smallest which satisfactorily controls symptoms, and the duration of treatment should be as short as possible. For acute intermittent therapy, they can be given in tapering doses three times a day over 5 days and stopped abruptly without suppressing the adrenal gland. Prompt treatment with steroids should be undertaken when there is severe exacerbation of asthma in a child who had long-term steroid therapy discontinued within the previous year. Intravenous steroids should be started immediately when the diagnosis of status asthmaticus is made, both because of the seriousness of the situation and because the onset of action is delayed (4 to 6 hours). For long-term therapy, the best schedule is the lowest dosage which will control symptoms, given once every other day before 8:00 A.M. This schedule will result in the least adrenal suppression. Administration of corticosteroids early in the morning mimics the natural diurnal variation of plasma cortisol concentration. When daily therapy is required, attempts should be made to achieve control with the lowest amount of single morning dosage. Short-acting steroids (prednisone, prednisolone, or methylprednisolone) should be used. When steroids are used for more than 5 days, dosage reduction should be gradual over a period of 1 to 2 weeks. Dosage reduction for those children on long-term alternate day therapy should be at a rate not exceeding 2.5 mg. of prednisone reduced every 2 weeks. For those on daily therapy the reduction rate should not exceed 1 mg. per month. After discontinuing steroids, recovery of a normal pituitary-adrenal response to stress may take as long as a year. So throughout that period the life of a child with severe chronic asthma is constantly at risk at times of stress. Steroids should not be used as a substitute for the parameters of management discussed (environmental controls, bronchodilator therapy, and hyposensitization when indicated). Because of their impressive beneficial action, parents may be reluctant to discontinue steroids; therefore, prior to institution of steroid therapy, parents should be advised of the multiple undesirable effects of long-term therapy. Children on long-term steroid therapy should be seen regularly by their physician, even when asymptomatic. These visits allow the opportunity to re-evaluate the patient's clinical status, to attempt to reduce steroid dose, and to anticipate frequent side effects such as growth retardation, hypertension, incipient diabetes mellitus, and posterior subcapsular cataracts.

Topically active corticosteroid aerosols (beclomethasone dipropionate [Vanceril]), now available in the United States, make it possible to administer effective doses of steroids without producing systemic side effects. These should be started in the chronic asthmatic prior to the use of oral steroids. They are also used in the steroid-dependent asthmatic while reducing oral steroids and, ideally, discontinuing them. When attempting systemic steroid reduction, extreme caution must be exercised. It is best to switch to an alternate day schedule, giving twice the daily dose prior to 8:00 A.M. and then very gradually tapering at the rate of 1 mg. of prednisone per month. Acute respiratory infections and severe attacks of asthma should be promptly treated with large doses of prednisone. They can be used in the severe seasonal asthmatic who cannot be controlled with oral theophylline and/or oral beta-2 agents. Cromolyn sodium should be tried before steroid inhalation. With beclomethasone, control is usually achieved in 2 to 3 days of two 50 microgram–metered inhalations four times a day (total daily dose equals 400 micrograms). Little or no adrenal suppression occurs. When more frequent inhalation is necessary to control symptoms, some adrenal suppression can be expected. Success rate in weaning patients from oral steroid use varies from 20 to 90 per cent in reported studies. Success is dose dependent. The development of oropharyngeal candidiasis is also dose dependent. Occasionally, the larynx may become involved. So far, no instances of Candida extending to the bronchi or lungs have been reported. In order to try to avoid oral thrush, I request that patients rinse their mouths with water after each inhalation. Oral thrush is easily controlled with nystatin (Mycostatin) oral suspension (rinse mouth and swallow 4 ml. [400,000 units] four times a day and continue for 2 days after thrush has disappeared). Huskiness of voice and sore throat are other side effects.

Hyposensitization (Immunotherapy). Until other methods are developed, hyposensitization therapy remains an important adjunct in the treatment of respiratory allergies such as asthma. The in vitro system of leukocyte histamine release has been used to measure cellular sensitivity to antigen and levels of blocking (IgG) and reaginic (IgE) antibodies. After many years of empiric use of the method of hyposensitization, an immunologic basis of clinical improvement is beginning to be understood. Several studies have provided evidence to indicate that hyposensitization may result in (1) increased titers of blocking antibody; (2) stabilization of the titers of reaginic antibody during the pollen season; and (3) prolonged and intense hyposensitization, which may result in true desensitization of leukocytes which contain histamine.

These methods are now being applied to assess the value of immunotherapy with extracts of many allergens previously used, to develop and evaluate the effectiveness of purified antigens, and to help determine when hyposensitization should be discontinued.

Antihistamines and decongestants may be tried for one or two seasons in children with hay fever. However, it is strongly recommended that hyposensitization therapy be instituted in children with a history of grass or weed pollinosis and a positive skin test for grass or ragweed, regardless of the severity of their symptoms. This early therapy may be important in preventing the development of seasonal and perennial bronchial asthma. If avoidance of allergens by bronchial asthma patients is impossible (pollens and outdoor mold spores, or unsuccessful indoor mold spores and house dust), hyposensitization should be undertaken. This therapy will increase the likelihood that the child will outgrow his asthma. By and large, animal danders can be avoided. Severe reactions to injections of these allergens can occur. They should be administered only under unusual circumstances and then given cautiously, starting with very dilute solutions.

The process of hyposensitization injections consists of a series of injections of allergenic extracts, beginning with small concentrations and gradually increasing to the maximum tolerated dose (swelling more than 3 to 5 cm. in diameter or marked swelling at the site of injection for over 24 hours). Subcutaneous injections are initially given once or twice weekly, with at least a 3 day interval between doses. When a maintenance dose is achieved, injections may be given at 3 to 4 week intervals. Injections should be continued for at least 1 year after the child is completely free of symptoms and does not require medication. The same dose is given if the interval between injections is 14 to 28 days. Between 28 and 42 days the dose is reduced by 25 per cent. Between 42 and 56 days, the dose is reduced by 50 per cent. During the pollen season, injections may be given once or twice weekly, although dosage may have to be reduced, as larger local reactions can occur at this time. Perennial therapy is the best prospect for lasting protection. It is recommended over coseasonal and preseasonal methods.

Following injections a child should always be kept under medical observation for at least 30 minutes. The size of local reactions should be recorded. Generalized reactions (flushing, itching of palms or throat, hives, angioedema, cough, wheezing) should be treated promptly:

1. Apply tourniquet proximal to the site of injection.
2. Give epinephrine (1:1000), 0.1 ml. subcutaneously into the exact site of injection to slow antigen absorption.
3. Give epinephrine (1:1000) subcutaneously above the tourniquet or into another extremity (enough to make a total dose of 0.01 mg. per kg.).
4. Evaluate the airway. Be prepared to give oxygen if there is cyanosis and to establish an airway if obstruction occurs.
5. If the reaction is severe, give diphenhydramine (Benadryl), 10 to 50 mg. (2 mg. per kg.) intravenously or intramuscularly.
6. Be prepared to administer aminophylline, 6 mg. per kg. at a rate no faster than 1 ml. per minute. Aminophylline is supplied in 10 ml. ampules containing 250 mg. The dose should be administered over a 5 to 10 minute period. After the patient responds, an antihistamine and bronchodilator should be continued for the next 8

hours, as relapse may occur when the action of the initial medication subsides. Epinephrine (Sus-Phrine), 0.005 ml. per kg., usually provides this protection. The patient or parents should report to the physician on arriving home.

Education and Rehabilitation. Comprehensive care not only includes the modes of management already discussed but also includes education of parents as to the mechanisms of allergic reactions, reasons for hyposensitization, and the actions of the several medications that may be prescribed. Similar discussions with the child or adolescent to the best of their comprehension should be undertaken. The mysteries and misconceptions of allergy should be dispelled. Follow-up conferences should include re-emphasis of environmental controls, assessment of the effectiveness of medication, and inquiry as to the development of new problems. Physician contact only during periods of crisis is undesirable, especially with asthmatic patients. These children need to be evaluated during asymptomatic periods. The meaning of asthma to the patient and within the family constellation must be explored. In chronic asthma, psychologic counseling may be indicated. In rare situations when management is unsuccessful, it may be advisable to have the patient re-evaluated and to continue care at a specialized residential treatment center.

Asthmatic children should be encouraged to participate in physical activity.

Exercise-induced bronchospasm and asthma occur in all ages but are more common in children. They are especially prevalent in severe asthmatics, occurring in 85 to 90 per cent of boys and 65 per cent of girls. They may occur in latent asthmatics and even in allergic patients with hay fever. They are best elicited by a free running mode of exercise and least by swimming. Asthmatic children and adolescents avoid sports participation because of the occurrence of exercise-induced bronchospasm. Regular swimming should be encouraged, as it improves posture, physique, muscle tone, and fitness. Other athletic activities, such as track, soccer, and basketball, readily provoke exercise-induced bronchospasm. Sometimes a warm-up period will decrease its occurrence. Exercise-induced bronchospasm can frequently be prevented by the use of an oral theophylline or beta-2 bronchodilator drug 30 to 60 minutes prior to exercise. Inhalation of cromolyn sodium 15 minutes prior to exercise has also met with some success. Combinations of ephedrine and theophylline have additive effects in diminishing exercise-induced bronchospasm when administered 1 hour prior to exercise.

Home, Office, Emergency Room, and Hospital Management

Treatment at Home. Mild asthmatic attacks of slow onset usually respond to simple oral medication with theophylline (see Table 1) or a theophylline-ephedrine bronchodilator combination drug. In patients known to wheeze, I usually instruct parents to start therapy at the onset of upper respiratory symptoms and/or cough, and to continue them on an every 6 hour schedule during the daytime (8:00 A.M., 2:00 P.M., 8:00 P.M.). If symptoms occur at night or wheezing is moderate, then the 6 hour schedule should include a fourth (2:00 A.M.) dose. Other 6 hour schedules can be used according to the family life style. Patients should be encouraged to maintain adequate oral fluid intake. I do not prescribe other so-called mucolytic agents by either oral or inhalation routes. Mild asthmatic attacks can also be treated with oral metaproterenol (Metaprel, Alupent) in the following dosages: for children 6 to 9 years old (less than 60 pounds), 10 mg., 1 teaspoon, or ½ tablet; and for children over 9 years (more than 60 pounds), 20 mg., 2 teaspoons, or 1 tablet. This can be given every 6 hours. I prefer to start theophylline initially, and then, if there is no response, to add metaproterenol to the 6 hour schedule. Medications are continued for 2 to 3 days after symptoms have subsided, as sometimes it takes this long for pulmonary function to subclinically return to normal. This practice may also prevent early recurrence of lower respiratory symptoms. Physical activity should be limited during and for 2 to 3 days following acute flare-ups. Antihistamines for allergic rhinitis can be continued if there is mild wheezing. However, if wheezing is severe or protracted, they should be stopped, as they are thought to dry lower respiratory secretions. In this instance, I prescribe a 2 to 3 day course of long-acting nasal drops such as oxymetazoline hydrochloride (Afrin). The dose for children over 6 years of age is 2 to 3 drops of a 0.05 per cent solution in each nostril every 12 hours. A 0.025 per cent solution can be used for children 3 to 6 years of age. Prolonged and excessive use should be avoided. With mild chronic wheezing, theophylline can be used chronically on a round-the-clock 6 hour schedule. Metaproterenol is added for acute exacerbations. In these cases, serum testing should be done to achieve and assure adequate theophylline dose and serum level. The child should be seen at periodic intervals and followed with interval history, physical examination, and pulmonary function tests. The pulmonary function tests (forced vital capacity [FVC], forced expiratory volume in 1 second [FEV_1], and maximum mid-expiratory flow rate [MMEFR]) before and after exercise and before and after injection of epinephrine (0.01 ml. per kg.—no more than 0.5 ml.) can be used to assess bronchial irritability and degree of airway obstruction. The indications and use of cromolyn sodium, beclomethasone, and oral steroids have been discussed. I make every attempt to avoid the use of Freon-propelled aerosol adrenergic agents in children. However, they frequently give much appreciated, prompt relief. Metaproterenol, isoetharine, and isoproterenol can be given by this method. The disadvantages of hand nebulizers are dependence and habituation, especially by preteenagers and teenagers. Patients using these devices frequently delay seeking physician attention when their asthma gets worse. Parents should be advised about the too frequent use of "nebs" and should become concerned if used more than two breaths every 4 to 6 hours. Parents should control their use. In the rare teenager who benefits from hand nebulizers, I usually do not prescribe refills unless I am sure of that person's self-health care maturity. Overuse of isoproterenol nebulizers has led to undesirable consequences such as paradoxical bronchospasm, cardiac arrhythmias, and sudden death.

Treatment in the Physician's Office. Children with moderate asthmatic attacks of acute onset and those whose asthma is not controlled by home management should be seen promptly at home, in an emergency room, or in the physician's office. The following should be documented: time since onset of attack; treatment with previous drugs, especially aminophylline and steroids; fluids retained in previous 24 hours; presence of fever or vomiting; quality and quantity of any sputum production; respiratory infection in family or contacts; and exposure to known and potential allergens. Special attention on physical examination should be paid to the state of hydration, temperature, pulse rate, respiratory rate, degree of muscular fatigue, and presence or absence of cyanosis. Extent of wheezing should be estimated and pulsus paradoxus measured. Pulsus paradoxus is an abnormal decrease in systolic arterial blood pressure with inspiration. Normally the difference between inspiratory and expiratory systolic pressure does not exceed 5 mm. Hg. During an asthmatic attack the difference often exceeds 10 mm. Hg. A larger paradox indicates severe asthma. Pulse rate, respiratory rate, auscultatory examination of air exchange and wheezing, and pulsus paradoxus should be used to evaluate response to therapy.

Initial therapy is epinephrine 1:1000 (0.01 ml. per kg. —not more than 0.5 ml.) given subcutaneously. Children whose attacks are of short duration usually respond to the first injection within 5 to 10 minutes. If response occurs, epinephrine aqueous suspension (Sus-Phrine) 1:200 (0.005 ml. per kg.) is given subcutaneously. The dose of Sus-Phrine should not exceed 0.3 ml. Sus-Phrine is a long-acting preparation in which 20 per cent of the epinephrine is immediately available and the remainder over about 8 hours. Patients are then requested to remain on their oral bronchodilator therapy at 6 hour intervals for the following 2 to 3 days. In some patients with mild asthma, one can learn that an initial dose of Sus-Phrine is quite satisfactory. In all instances oral hydration is encouraged. Those patients who do not respond to the first injection of epinephrine may be given the same dose two more times, at 20 minute intervals. During this time, oral hydration is encouraged. Also, if the patient has not received oral theophylline in the previous 6 hours, an oral dose of 5 mg. per kg. is given. Any patient who is cyanotic should receive 40 per cent oxygen by Venturi mask. This can also be given to patients in severe distress before, during, and for 10 to 15 minutes after epinephrine (Adrenalin). Oxygen relieves anxiety, corrects the hypoxia of the ventilation-perfusion abnormality in asthma, and reduces the fall in arterial oxygen tension which frequently accompanies acute bronchodilation following use of epinephrine and/or theophylline.

Children who do not respond to these therapies should be sent immediately to an emergency room at the nearest hospital (preferably one with an intensive care unit) for further attention and admission. The admitting diagnosis is status asthmaticus. I believe no more than 90 minutes should elapse in making this decision.

When hospital distance is great and the patient has not received a theophylline derivative, intravenous fluids should be started (5 per cent glucose in one-quarter isotonic saline solution) at a rate of 60 ml. per kg. per 24 hours. Intravenous aminophylline at a dose of 5.6 mg. per kg. diluted in three volumes of intravenous fluid should be given over 15 to 20 minutes. This is a loading dose. Serum theophylline levels can be measured after arrival at the hospital. The first dose of a corticosteroid should also be given. This can be either hydrocortisone sodium succinate (Solu-Cortef), 200 mg., or methylprednisolone sodium succinate (Solu-Medrol), 40 mg., intravenously.

Either will be repeated every 4 to 6 hours during the treatment of status asthmaticus.

Treatment in the Emergency Room. As in the physician's office, severe or prolonged attacks of asthma demand the immediate attention of a physician. Secondary pathophysiologic changes may occur rapidly in children, making reversibility progressively more difficult. Expiratory obstruction produced by the basic abnormal bronchial responses leads to pulmonary hyperinflation, increased dead space, decreased compliance, and increased resistance to air flow. This results in alveolar hypoventilation, uneven ventilation, and increased work of breathing. Retained secretions may contribute to atelectasis. Dehydration, infection, and muscular fatigue increase the severity of these changes. Regional differences in ventilation and perfusion initially result in arterial hypoxemia (decreased Po_2), which later, as more airway obstruction and muscular fatigue occur, may be combined with hypercapnia (increased Pco_2). Especially in children less than 5 years of age, respiratory acidosis resulting from hypercapnia is frequently compounded by a metabolic acidosis (accumulation of lactic acid and ketones) resulting from hypoxemia, increased muscular work or breathing, vomiting, dehydration, and starvation. Acidosis, hypoxemia, and hypercapnia render the bronchial musculature less responsive to bronchodilators, at the same time leading to pulmonary arterial vasoconstriction, pulmonary hypertension, right heart strain, and cardiac failure. Metabolic derangements lead to cardiac arrhythmias and cardiopulmonary arrest. Therapy is aimed at each of these processes with a goal of reversibility and prevention of progression. Careful and frequent assessment of the patient is therefore advisable.

Initial treatment and evaluation in a hospital emergency room should be no different than initial treatment in a physician's office (see above). The decision to admit the child to the hospital and to begin further therapy should not take longer than 90 minutes from the time the patient enters the front door. Pediatric patients who are sick enough to require intravenous fluids and intravenous aminophylline in the emergency room are sick enough to be admitted to a well staffed hospital floor or pulmonary intensive care unit. There is no question that the small child who has been ill more than 1 day with severe wheezing, dehydration, and fatigue should be immediately treated and admitted to the hospital. Any child who did not respond to epinephrine in his physician's office should be immediately treated further and admitted to the hospital. It is also my opinion that the child with chronic asthma and repetitive exacerbations with repeated visits to the emergency room should be admitted to the hospital for more comprehensive care and reevaluation. Parents sometimes do need relief from the chronic stress of caring for their children. Hospitalization alleviates this family morbidity and provides an environment which may be free of home allergens which have been contributing to the child's illness. Hospitalization also provides an opportunity for re-education and social reevaluation which may not have been accomplished on an outpatient basis. A plan for continuity of care can be established or reaffirmed. The success of "breaking" the asthmatic episode frequently becomes only a secondary goal in long-term management. To treat the asthmatic episode, giving the patient some pills without arranging follow-up by a primary physician or specialist, is poor emergency room medicine.

As in office treatment, history and physical examination data should be obtained. Again, other conditions which cause wheezing, such as aspiration of foreign body, should be considered. In those patients who do not respond to initial therapy, complications of asthma, such as pneumomediastinum, pneumothorax, or atelectasis, should be reconsidered. Atelectasis and pneumonia should be considered in those patients who have residual localized rales following relief of wheezing with bronchodilators.

Laboratory studies should include white blood cell count and differential, hematocrit, serum electrolytes, urinalysis, posteroanterior and lateral x-rays of the chest, sputum Gram stain, bacterial and/or viral respiratory cultures, and arterial blood gases (Pao_2, $Paco_2$, pH, and base excess). If the child has been given oral theophylline within the previous 6 hours, a serum theophylline level should be obtained.

Treatment in the Hospital. Most children with acute asthma are apprehensive from dyspnea, a feeling of suffocation, and increased work of breathing. Unresponsiveness of asthma to epinephrine, in addition to its frequently associated effects (tachycardia, tremulousness, and vomiting), contributes to the apprehension, which may progress to a state of terror. Every effort should be made to maintain a calm atmosphere during this time of medical crisis. The physician's self-confidence or lack of confidence is easily perceived by the child-patient as well as by the parents. A systematic approach is reassuring to all concerned.

Initial therapy should be started immediately.

1. Status asthmaticus is the lack of improvement or of sustained improvement of severe

asthma after three subcutaneous injections of epinephrine 1:1000 (0.01 ml. per kg.) given at 20 minute intervals.

2. A rapid systematic history and physical examination will have already been done.

3. If oxygen has not been started, it should be immediately (Venturi mask at FIO_2 = 40 per cent).

4. Intravenous fluids (one-quarter isotonic saline solution in 5 per cent dextrose) should be given at a rate of 60 ml. per kg. per 24 hours.

5. Initial venous blood samples can be obtained at the time of intravenous needle insertion (complete blood count, serum electrolytes, serum theophylline, serum for acute phase viral antibody studies).

6. If theophylline or its derivatives have not been given in the previous 24 hours, then aminophylline, 5.6 mg. per kg., should be diluted in equal parts of intravenous fluid and administered over 20 minutes. If the patient received theophylline at a dose of 5 mg. per kg. or less between 6 and 8 hours ago, a serum theophylline should be drawn, and aminophylline, 3 mg. per kg., should be given over 20 minutes. When the child has received theophylline in therapeutic amounts in the previous 6 hours, an immediate serum theophylline value should be obtained and maintenance aminophylline started at a constant infusion dose of 0.9 mg. per kg. per hour. When in doubt, obtain a serum theophylline level and start the constant infusion. The rate should be regulated with a constant infusion pump.

7. At this point, about 20 to 30 minutes after aminophylline has been infused, beta-adrenergic therapy should again be considered. Epinephrine may now be effective. One dose may be tried. However, I prefer to use an aerosolized bronchodilator (5 drops of isoproterenol 1:200 in 2 ml. of saline or 10 drops of isoetharine in 2 ml. of saline delivered with oxygen). It has been suggested that concomitant use of epinephrine and isoproterenol may increase the risk of cardiac arrhythmias. Therefore it is wise not to administer these drugs within 1 hour of each other.

8. Corticosteroids (Solu-Cortef, 200 mg., or Solu-Medrol, 40 mg.) should now be given intravenously.

9. If blood gases have not been obtained, this should be done. Direct arterial sampling from the radial, dorsalis pedis, or posterior tibial artery can be accomplished using a well heparinized syringe with a 23 gauge needle.

10. A portable posteroanterior and lateral chest x-ray is obtained. Patients should not be sent to the x-ray department unless accompanied by the respiratory care team.

11. Ideally, the child with status asthmaticus should be managed in an intensive care unit with a pediatrician, a nurse, and an inhalation therapist. An anesthesiologist must be available for consultation, should see the child early, and should be prepared for nasotracheal intubation and controlled ventilation if pulmonary failure occurs.

12. If the aforementioned measures took place or were started in the emergency room, the responsible physician should accompany the child to the new location (well-staffed hospital floor or intensive care unit). A physical examination, laboratory data, therapy, vital signs and response flow sheet should be started. Observations should be made frequently and recorded.

13. Several centers have found the clinical asthma scoring method of Wood and Downes to be useful (Table 2). Impending and acute respiratory failure can be anticipated. Along with measurement of pulsus paradoxus, this system can also be used to follow improvement. Through experience, Wood and Downes at Children's Hospital of Philadelphia have found that 75 per cent of children, with $Paco_2$ of 55 torr (mm. Hg) or higher after routine therapy, develop values in excess of 65 torr (mm. Hg). Thus, a $Paco_2$ of 55 torr (mm. Hg) indicates impending failure, and a value of 65 torr (mm. Hg) or greater is indicative of acute respiratory failure.

Further therapy depends upon the clinical

TABLE 2. **Clinical Asthma Score**

CRITERIA	0	1	2
Cyanosis (or Pao_2)	None (70–100)	In air (<70)	In 40% O_2 (<70)
Inspiratory breath sounds	Normal	Unequal	Decreased to absent
Use of accessory muscles	None	Moderate	Maximal
Expiratory wheezing	None	Moderate	Marked
Cerebral function	Normal	Depressed or agitated	Coma

Impending respiratory failure = score ≥5, $Paco_2$ ≥55 torr after routine therapy.
Acute respiratory failure = score ≥7, $Paco_2$ ≥ 65 torr.

Further therapy depends upon the clinical response up to this point, the rapidity of improvement, or the occurrence of deterioration. Efforts are aimed at (1) correction of acute metabolic abnormalities, (2) hydration, (3) bronchodilatation, and (4) preparedness in the event of respiratory failure. The following should be considered and dealt with:

1. Hypoxia: Humidified oxygen should be given in concentration to maintain Pa_{O_2} greater than 60 mm. Hg and preferably between 80 and 100 mm. Hg. Whether given by Venturi mask or oxygen tent, inspired oxygen (F_{IO_2}) should be measured. Nasal cannulas should be avoided, as F_{IO_2} cannot be measured easily and children with severe asthma frequently breathe through their mouths.

2. Acidosis: Children frequently have a mixed respiratory and metabolic acidosis. With severe status asthmaticus, sodium bicarbonate (1 to 2 mEq. per kg.) should be given initially over 10 minutes and then as often as necessary to maintain the blood pH above 7.30. The dose can be calculated on the basis of base deficit (base deficit = − base excess): dose of sodium bicarbonate (mEq.) = (− base excess) × 0.3 × weight (in kg.). Aerosol bronchodilator (isoproterenol or isoetharine) should again be tried at this point, as pH correction may now allow for bronchodilator response.

3. Hydration: Recommendations for hydration and maintenance fluid therapy, based on the concept that hydration helps to liquefy bronchial secretions and to liquefy mucus plug, have ranged from maintenance fluid rates to 2 to 3 times maintenance. High intrathoracic pleural pressures occur throughout both inspiration and expiration in children with severe asthma. This contributes to fluid retention within lung tissue and impaired gas exchange. In addition, renal fluid retention occurs in acidosis and hypoxic states. Patients on mechanical ventilators also retain fluid. Therefore overhydration, especially with hypotonic solutions, should be avoided. Unless dehydration is clinically evident, intravenous fluids should not be initially administered at a rate greater than one and a half times maintenance (50 to 60 ml. per kg. per 24 hours or 1500 ml. per square meter body surface area per 24 hours). Sodium requirement is 3 mEq. per kg. per 24 hours, and potassium is 2 mEq. per kg. per 24 hours. Twenty-four hour fluid and electrolyte requirements should be divided into four 6 hour bottles. The potassium concentration should not exceed 40 mEq. per 1000 ml. of fluid. Fluid intake and output should be recorded, as well as urine specific gravity. The volume of fluid used to deliver intravenous medications should also be recorded. Cumulative blood volumes taken for various tests should be documented.

4. Aminophylline can be given by several different protocols. Whichever is used, theophylline serum levels should be monitored. Two methods have been used with success in Rochester, N.Y.: (a) A loading dose of aminophylline of 5 mg. per kg. given intravenously over 20 minutes and repeated every 6 hours. Theophylline serum levels are obtained 30 minutes after the dose is delivered and just before the next dose. Levels above 10 micrograms per ml. and below 20 micrograms per ml. are therapeutic. Some patients develop symptoms of toxicity between 15 and 20 micrograms per ml. (b) A loading dose of 5.6 mg. per kg., followed by a constant infusion of 0.9 ml. per kg. per hour. In some children the constant infusion rate had to be gradually increased to 1.3 mg. per kg. per hour to achieve serum theophylline levels greater than 10 micrograms per ml.

5. Aerosolized bronchodilators: Isoproterenol 1:200 (5 drops in 2 ml. of saline) or isoetharine (10 drops in 2 ml. of saline) delivered by nebulizer with oxygen should be administered every half hour for the first 2 hours and then every 2 to 4 hours as the clinical course dictates. The child's heart rate should be monitored and inhalation therapy discontinued if the rate exceeds 180 beats per minute or if the rhythm becomes irregular.

6. Steroids are continued every 4 to 6 hours. They may be stopped abruptly if used for less than 5 days in a child who has not received steroids in the previous year.

7. Sedation: Although recommended by some, sedation should not be used unless the patient reaches a point of respiratory failure as outlined above and is supported by controlled ventilation. Relief of bronchospasm and/or hypoxemia is the best "sedative." Excessive amounts of morphine, barbiturates, meperidine, and phenothiazines have been noted as factors contributing to death from asthma. Depression of respiration, increased pulmonary vascular resistance, and release of histamine have been cited as possible mechanisms of such an outcome.

8. Antibiotics: It is not recommended that antibiotics be administered to all children with status asthmaticus. However, some children in status have accompanying bacterial infections. Aids in making a decision to start an antibiotic include history of mucopurulent sputum or nasal discharge prior to the attack, fever (may not be present), elevated leukocyte count (can be elevated after epinephrine), and pneumonic infiltrate on x-ray and Gram's stain of the sputum. Specific etiologic diagnoses should be made by culture and

antibiotic therapy adjusted as appropriate. Inquiry should be made as to a history of penicillin allergy. Many attacks of acute asthma occur with viral infections. Viral respiratory cultures should be obtained, as well as acute and convalescent serum.

9. Postural drainage is useful in helping to mobilize bronchial plugs and secretions. It should not be used in early, severe status asthmaticus with tight wheezing. Head-down positioning, splinting of one side of the chest in the lateral position, breath-holding, dislocation of the oxygen mask, and increased agitation all may contribute to a sudden severe hypoxic episode. When loose rales become evident on chest auscultation, this procedure can be introduced. It is most effective when given immediately after aerosol bronchodilator therapy.

10. Intermittent positive pressure breathing (IPPB) ventilators should be avoided, as they induce bronchoconstriction and may cause pneumomediastinum and pneumothorax.

11. Respiratory failure and controlled ventilation: The physician must check the patient hourly for the first several hours to make sure that the patient is ventilating adequately and that hydration is proceeding on schedule, and to observe and record the response to medication therapy. A single nurse should be assigned to the patient for each shift. If a pulmonary intensive care unit is not available and standard procedure not set up for this type of patient, the physician-in-charge should be present when a different nurse comes on the case. Signs of respiratory failure have been outlined. These should be reviewed and evaluated frequently and made clear to all personnel involved. An anesthesiologist should be notified when each patient with status asthmaticus is admitted to hospital. It is at this time that thoughts of potential dangers should be contemplated; thus if he needs to act, he will have familiarity with the patient. Bronchoscopic aspiration of mucoid secretions is rarely indicated in children. Endotracheal intubation with an inert polyvinyl chloride tube is preferred over tracheostomy in children. Although subglottic stenosis has been reported, these tubes have been left in place for 1 week without serious complications. Intravenous pentobarbital and a short-acting muscle relaxant may facilitate insertion of the endotracheal tube. The patient should be well oxygenated with 100 per cent oxygen prior to endotracheal intubation and immediately afterward. Oxygen concentration is reduced as indicated. Assisted ventilation is initially given by bag and then by mechanical means. Endotracheal aspiration at 15 to 30 minute intervals or as needed, using aseptic technique, should be employed. Care should be taken not to apply suction, as this will remove oxygen as well as secretions from the lungs. Volume-controlled respirators are preferred to pressure-controlled devices. Pressure-controlled devices do not deliver an adequate tidal volume when lung compliance is decreased and airway resistance is decreased. Volume-controlled ventilators deliver the required tidal volume irrespective of the pressure required to deliver that volume. They also have a mechanical alert system to warn of excessive pressure. If excessive pressures are necessary to provide adequate ventilation, succinylcholine, 2 mg. per kg., may be injected intramuscularly. This produces muscle paralysis and apnea in 3 to 4 minutes, preventing coughing against the ventilator and eliminating chest wall spasm. Although curare (d-tubocurarine) releases histamine, many have found it effective because of its prolonged action and rapid reversibility with atropine and prostigmine. Sedation, along with controlled ventilation and muscle paralysis, is advisable. Observe for signs of arterial hypotension, pneumothorax, and tension pneumothorax, as these are complications of mechanical ventilation. The electrocardiogram, in addition to those parameters previously mentioned, should be monitored. Sufficient concentration of oxygen is administered to achieve a Pa_{O_2} between 80 and 100 mm. Hg. Tidal volume is usually begun at 10 ml. per kg. of body weight. Minute ventilation (tidal volume times respiratory rate) should be adjusted so that carbon dioxide levels are reduced slowly and respiratory alkalosis avoided. Appropriate bronchodilators, steroids, and fluid therapy should be continued. Mechanical ventilation may be discontinued when wheezing becomes low-pitched with loose rhonchi, compliance improves, the chest becomes less hyperinflated, and blood gases have returned to normal while on F_{IO_2} of 40 per cent or less. This usually takes 24 to 72 hours.

ALLERGIC RHINITIS DUE TO INHALANT FACTORS

method of
JOHN J. STEVENS, M.D.
La Jolla, California

It is estimated that 10 to 20 per cent of the population suffers from nasal allergy. Rhinitis may be mild and seasonal or chronic and perennial, and may be present from infancy to old age.

Specific Treatment

The primary approach to alleviating the symptoms of inhalant nasal allergy is to eliminate or decrease exposure to the responsible antigens.

Animals. People who are known to be allergic should avoid contact with all animals, and no animals should be allowed in the home, particularly the bedroom. This is important from a prophylactic standpoint, even if the person is not having much clinical difficulty at the time. In warm climates, animals may be kept outside all year, but even this compromise often results in difficulty, as animal hair and dander will stick to clothing and be brought into the home. No stuffed animal trophies should be in the home. All felt rug pads should be removed, as these frequently contain animal hair. No feather pillows are allowed in the home. Dacron pillows should be substituted. No covers are needed for such pillows.

Insecticides. Those which contain pyrethrum should be especially avoided, and all insecticides may act as nonspecific irritants.

Kapok. Furniture stuffed with kapok should be eliminated or covered with dustproof coverings. No kapok stuffed animals are allowed.

House Dust. Chronic and perennial problems are frequently aggravated by house dust sensitivity. The home should be kept as dust-free as possible, especially the bedroom, which should be simply furnished, using washable throw rugs and curtains. The floor should be of a hard surface, and the entire room damp-dusted regularly to remove accumulations of dust. All stuffed animals except those stuffed with nonallergic materials should be eliminated. One or two of the child's favorite stuffed animals may be selected and stuffed with Dacron or foam rubber. There should be few pictures, books, statues, and so forth, all of which tend to accumulate dust. If there is a forced air heating system, the filter should be cleaned or replaced monthly. A foam rubber mattress and covered box springs are advisable, and both should be covered by dustproof coverings, which may be acquired from any large department store or by writing to Allergen-Proof Encasings, 1450 E. 363rd St., Eastlake, Ohio 44094. Emulsified oil compounds such as Allergex (Hollister-Stier Laboratories, Los Angeles, California) help retard dust formation when sprayed into rugs, curtains, and stuffed furniture. Carpets should preferably be of a synthetic type, such as nylon. At times, skin testing with stock house dust produces a minimal response, whereas testing of an extract made from the patient's own house dust will elicit a marked reaction. In these cases, hyposensitization with this autogenous house dust may give better results than with stock dust.

Molds. Warm, damp, moist, musty areas where molds tend to accumulate should be avoided, such as barns, cellars, attics, closets, and garages. In warm, moist climates, the woodwork and walls can be painted with a paint containing a mold inhibitor. Cupboards, woodwork, and bathroom showers may be cleaned with a chlorine solution (Clorox), which helps to eradicate molds. House plants are a major source of mold and should be avoided.

Air Filtration. Efficient air conditioners and electrostatic precipitators are available which remove varying amounts of pollen and dust from the air, and can be recommended as adjuncts. When the patient is building a home, consideration can be given to having an air conditioner with precipitating filters built into the heating unit, as this is the most efficient system. Single room units are less effective and should be checked to ensure that they do not emit significant amounts of irritating ozone.

Pollens. There are few inhabited places on earth where pollens are not found in abundance, at least during certain seasons of the year. It is true that exposure to a certain pollen, such as ragweed during the late summer and fall in the midwest and east, can be avoided by going to the seashore or mountains or taking an ocean voyage. However, it is impractical for many people to vacation during this period, and a move to another part of the country which has a longer growing season will frequently transform the seasonal pollinosis of the east into a chronic and perennial problem of the west. Advising a patient to move because of allergic rhinitis is therefore rarely justified. Since pollens cannot be avoided, a more practical course is specific antigen injection therapy.

Immunotherapy—Hyposensitization. The technique of administering aqueous extracts of pollen, mold, and environmental antigens in an attempt to render the patient less responsive to subsequent exposure to these inhalants has been developed over the past 70 years. The details of hyposensitization procedures are beyond the scope of this presentation, and may be found by referring to A Manual of Clinical Allergy, by Sheldon, Lovell, and Mathews (2nd ed., Philadelphia, W. B. Saunders Co., 1967). In general, the patient's sensitivity is first elicited by skin testing, and the appropriate starting solution is based on this sensitivity. Gradually, the concentration is increased until a maintenance dose is reached. This is continued every 2 to 3 weeks until the patient is asymptomatic and then for 1 or more years. If symptoms return after discontinuance, injections are resumed. It is usually best to give injections in a perennial fashion; however, with a clear-cut seasonal problem, preseasonal treatment can be given beginning several months prior to the anticipated season. The consensus is that approximately 70 to 80 per cent of patients with pure inhalant sensitivity improve with specific hyposensitization.

Aqueous extracts have been the mainstay of treatment. However, in recent years, treatment with alum-precipitated antigens has been introduced. This material is weakly antigenic, and therefore can be given in stronger concentrations at longer intervals. Maintenance is reached more rapidly than with aqueous extracts. Those who use these extracts report them to be as effective as aqueous extracts, but the few well-controlled studies indicate that they may not be as effective as aqueous treatment. For many years, there has been a great deal of interest in developing a safe repository form of therapy with emulsions of extracts in oil. At present, emulsion therapy is considered investigational by the Food and Drug Administration. Autogenous urine injections are not recommended and are potentially harmful.

Complications. Chronic, perennial allergic rhinitis is frequently complicated by nasal polyps and infection of the sinuses. Sinus involvement should be suspected when the patient does not respond to the previously outlined measures. Irrigation of the antra and, at times, antrostomy will be necessary to provide adequate drainage. Appropriate antibiotics following culture of sinus secretions are indicated. Nasal polyps are removed only if mechanical blockage of the airway or sinuses is marked. When repeated infection of the upper air passages occurs, immunization with a stock or autogenous bacterial vaccine may be of benefit. The few well-controlled studies conducted with vaccines have failed to show significant improvement.

Patients with allergic rhinitis may aggravate the situation by the frequent use of vasoconstricting nose drops, resulting in a superimposed chemical rhinitis. Nose drops must be discontinued if the patient is to improve. Frequently, the task of weaning the patient is a difficult one. The patient should be allowed to use nose drops as often as he likes in one nostril, while allowing the other side to recover. When he can breathe through the recovered side, nose drops must be stopped completely. If this fails, corticosteroids will be necessary for 1 to 2 weeks, starting with oral prednisone, 40 mg. in divided doses, and decreasing the dose every 2 days as follows: 40, 20, 15, 10, 5, and 0 mg.

Symptomatic Treatment

Antihistamines. Antihistamines compete with histamine at cell receptor sites. There are many antihistamines available, and several varieties should be tried before they are abandoned. One drug may work well for a particular patient and be ineffective for another. Also, after a period of time, a certain antihistamine may lose its effectiveness, and switching to a different class will again afford relief. If the second antihistamine loses effectiveness, going back to the first may give relief. Long-acting preparations are preferred. Generally, the most effective antihistamines have the most sedative properties. An ephedrine-like vasoconstrictor is added to a number of antihistamines, and these will give additional relief in certain cases. In mild cases, antihistamines may be the only therapy necessary in addition to elimination procedures. If antihistamine is started, 1 to 2 weeks prior to the usual onset of seasonal rhinitis and taken regularly, symptoms frequently are much less that season. If the patient waits and begins antihistamine after the onset of symptoms, it may not be as effective.

Nose Drops. As mentioned previously, nose drops with vasoconstrictors should be avoided because of the possibility of a chemical rhinitis with rebound. Oxymetazoline hydrochloride (Afrin) is reported to be less likely to produce rebound, and the occasional use of this long-acting preparation twice daily for brief periods of 3 to 4 days may be permitted.

Cromolyn Sodium. Solutions of cromolyn sodium (Intal, Aarane), as well as the powder, have been used locally in the nose with reported success. This material is thought to prevent release of chemical mediators from mast cells. Cromolyn is not presently available for nasal use in the United States.

Corticosteroids. Corticosteroids are useful because of their anti-inflammatory properties. However, in view of their well-known serious side effects, they should be avoided if at all possible and used only in the most severe, acute cases of allergic rhinitis, and then for as brief a period of time as possible.

SYSTEMIC. There are many different corticosteroids available, but none of these have any distinct advantage over prednisone. Treatment is initiated with a dose of 40 mg. a day, and decreased by 5 to 10 mg. every 2 days. Improvement is not expected for 12 to 24 hours. Some have advocated the use of long-acting injectable corticosteroids (triamcinolone) for seasonal allergic rhinitis or to interrupt a particularly severe episode of allergic rhinitis. These drugs may suppress adrenocortical function for as long as 2 to 3 months and may occasionally cause menstrual irregularities. ACTH is not advised because of the possibility of developing anaphylactic reactions even to synthetic ACTH.

LOCAL. Some patients will obtain temporary relief when prednisolone (Hydeltra), 0.3 ml., is injected into each inferior turbinate. This can be repeated once or twice at 7 to 10 day intervals. In recent years, the topical application of dexamethasone nasal spray (Decadron Turbinaire) has been introduced. This preparation will give relief to some patients, and nasal polyps may even be reduced. At times, it must be discontinued because of an irritating, burning sensation. It is started with 2 sprays in each nostril three times a day, gradually decreasing the dose until the least number of sprays that gives reasonable control of symptoms is reached. There will be some absorption of this preparation, resulting in the usual side effects of corticosteroids. However, the side effects, such as adrenocortical suppression, will be less than with systemic corticosteroids. Nasal septal perforation has been reported in a few patients after long-term use.

A newer preparation, beclomethasone dipropionate (Beconase), has been used with equal success in Europe. This topical corticosteroid is very poorly absorbed, giving it a significant advantage over Decadron in regard to decreased potential systemic side effects. Beclomethasone is not presently available for nasal use in the United States, but is available for treatment of asthma (Vanceril). Other poorly absorbed topical corticosteroids are being studied (flunisolide, betamethasone-17 valerate, triamcinolone) and are expected to be available in the future.

ADVERSE REACTIONS TO DRUGS: HYPERSENSITIVITY

method of
GUY A. SETTIPANE, M.D.
Providence, Rhode Island

The frequency of adverse reactions to drugs in hospitalized patients is estimated to be 3 per cent. Adverse reactions to drugs may be classified as follows: *side effects* (undesirable pharmacologic effect), *toxicity* (overdosage), *interactions* with other drugs, *idiosyncrasy* (unusual reaction not related to known pharmacologic action), *intolerance* (increased pharmacological effect with small doses), *allergic reactions*, and *pseudoallergic reactions*.

Allergic reactions are defined as an altered response to a drug mediated by an immunologic mechanism. Pseudoallergic responses to a drug are described as adverse reactions that are not mediated by an immunologic mechanism, but are clinically similar to the signs and symptoms of true drug allergy.

Clinically, allergic reactions to drugs may be manifested by urticaria-angioedema, pruritus, erythema, fever, bronchospasm, shock, and death. Immunologically, drug allergy and other hypersensitivity reactions are categorized by the Gell and Coombs classifications (Table 1).

Some drug hypersensitivity reactions, such as penicillin allergy, may manifest symptoms which can be classified as type I, II, III, or IV. For example, penicillin has been known to produce immediate shock and death (type I), hemolysis (type II), serum sickness (type III), and delayed reactions, which may occur up to 2 weeks later (type IV).

Examples of pseudoallergic reactions, which are nonimmunologic, are the urticarial or bronchospastic reactions produced by aspirin and tartrazine. Antibodies to these drugs have not been found in patients who have adverse reactions to them.

Pseudoanaphylactic reactions to penicillin have been reported; they are thought to be due to microembolization to the lungs and brain as well as direct toxicity from the procaine component of aqueous procaine penicillin G after intravenous infusion.

Atopy does not appear to predispose persons to hypersensitivity reactions to drugs, and the frequency of drug allergy appears to be the same in atopic and nonatopic subjects. However, there is evidence that asthmatic patients may have a more severe reaction to a drug than nonatopic persons when a drug hypersensitivity does occur. Also, pseudoallergic reactions to aspirin are found more frequently in asthmatic patients, who may experience severe reactions to this drug and related compounds such as indomethacin, sodium benzoate, mefenamic acid, phenylbutazone, ibuprofen (Motrin), and tartrazine. Therefore it is imperative that drugs be administered cautiously to asthmatic patients to avoid the possibility of adverse reactions.

Another principle of drug allergy is that children may have less drug hypersensitivity reactions than adults. This observation is usually attributed to a decreased exposure to certain drugs. As a child becomes older, his exposure rate to drugs, such as penicillin, is increased through use, and therefore the risk of developing IgE antibodies to a drug becomes greater. Another possibility for a decreased frequency of drug allergy in children may be explained on the basis of an immature immunologic system.

Most drugs are haptens and stimulate the immunologic system by combining with endogenous macromolecules such as proteins, which serve as a hapten carrier. Once antibodies are produced to the hapten-carrier complex, the presence of hapten alone can combine with the specific antibody producing an antibody-antigen reaction with the release of anaphylactic mediators such as histamine, slow-reacting substance of anaphylaxis (SRS-A), chemotactic factors, and prostaglandins. In order to produce these allergic mediators, the hapten must be at least bivalent, because univalent haptens do not cause the release of allergic mediators.

Drugs do not usually react with endogenous macromolecules, but in vivo degradation products of these drugs may react with endogenous proteins, resulting in antigenic stimulation of the immunologic system. These breakdown products of drugs may combine with certain

TABLE 1. **Types of Hypersensitivity (Gell and Coombs)**

TYPES	CLINICAL CLASSIFICATION	ONSET OF REACTION	ANTIBODY OR MEDIATORS
I	Acute anaphylaxis	Several minutes	IgE
II	Cytotoxic or cytolytic reaction	Minutes to hours	IgG or IgM, complement
III	Arthus reaction (immune complex disease)	Usually several days	IgG
IV	Delayed reaction	48 hours	Lymphocytes

proteins or specific internal structures such as the lung or blood, so that the resulting antigen-antibody reaction may be directed chiefly against certain body tissues, resulting in organ-specific pathology. For example, penicillin may be degraded in vivo to benzylpenicillenic acid, which combines with endogenous proteins to form benzylpenicilloyl haptenic groups (the major antigenic determinant of penicillin; the "minor" antigenic breakdown products of penicillin are benzylpenicillin, benzylpenicilloate, benzylpenilloate, and benzylpenicilloylamine). Some of the degraded products of penicillin may combine with protein molecules on red blood cells, thus stimulating the immunologic system to produce antibodies against the complex of breakdown products of penicillin and tissue. The next exposure to penicillin may result in hemolytic anemia (Gell and Coombs type II reaction). If shock or acute anaphylaxis occurs, then a Gell and Coombs type I reaction mediated by IgE antibodies has been activated.

Management of Adverse Reactions—General Principles

1. Stop the offending drug.
2. Administer aqueous epinephrine (1:1000), 0.2 to 0.3 ml. subcutaneously or intramuscularly depending on the severity of the reaction and cardiac status of the patient.
3. Epinephrine may be repeated in 15 to 20 minutes in severe reactions.
4. If the drug-allergen was given intramuscularly, retard absorption from the injection site by local infiltration of 0.1 to 0.2 ml. of 1:1000 epinephrine. If the injection site is on an extremity, apply tourniquet proximally.
5. Maintain airway patency. Insertion of an endotracheal tube or performance of a tracheostomy may be necessary.
6. Intravenous infusion of isotonic saline should be begun in moderate to severe cases.
7. Diphenylhydramine (Benadryl), 10 to 50 mg. by the intramuscular route, may be administered.
8. If epinephrine has not reversed vascular collapse, a drip infusion of norepinephrine (Levophed, 1 ampule [4 ml. of 0.2 per cent solution], added to 1 liter of 5 per cent dextrose solution) may be infused at a rate of up to 2 to 3 ml. per minute as required to maintain blood pressure.
9. If bronchospasm occurs and is not relieved by epinephrine, begin an intravenous infusion of aminophylline (6 mg. per kg. in 250 ml. of intravenous solution).
10. Corticosteroids (equivalent of 200 mg. hydrocortisone every 4 to 6 hours) may be given even though the beneficial effects may be delayed in onset.
11. The patient should be observed closely for 2 to 3 hours after recovery from acute anaphylaxis. If symptoms persist, hospitalization may be necessary.
12. After recovery from acute anaphylaxis, epinephrine (Sus-Phrine), 0.10 ml. subcutaneously, may be given to maintain a symptom-free state.

Desensitization to drugs such as penicillin is not recommended because of the hazards involved, except under extraordinary circumstances. Whenever there is a history of drug allergy, other drugs with similar pharmacologic action should be chosen.

TABLE 2. **Frequency of Adverse Reactions to Aspirin**

CONDITION	FREQUENCY (%)	PREDOMINANT SYMPTOM PRODUCED
Chronic urticaria	23	Angioedema-urticaria
Asthma	4	Bronchospasm
Normal	0.9	Either bronchospasm or angioedema-urticaria

TABLE 3. **Drugs Frequently Implicated in Systemic Reactions**

Penicillin
Sulfonamides
Aspirin
Heterologous serum
Anesthetics
Iodides and radiopaque materials
Insulin
Barbiturates
Tranquilizers
Tetracyclines and other antibiotics

The drug of choice for treatment of type I hypersensitivity reactions is epinephrine, followed by antihistamines and corticosteroids. The drugs of choice for treatment of type IV hypersensitivity are corticosteroids. For treatment of type II and III hypersensitivity reactions, the primary drugs are corticosteroids, which may be supplemented by epinephrine and antihistamines as the clinical situation requires.

It is recommended that persons with definite adverse reactions to drugs should carry with them information about their drug sensitivities at all times.

ALLERGIC REACTIONS TO INSECT STINGS

method of
RICHARD EVANS, M.D.
Washington, D.C.

Between four and eight persons per thousand of the population of the United States are at risk of a severe allergic reaction to the sting of an insect. There is no apparent difference in the incidences of insect sting allergy in the normal population and what is considered the allergic population.

Hypersensitivity reactions to stinging insects are immediate type IgE-mediated reactions and are capable of eliciting serious, even fatal, systemic anaphylactic reactions. Such sting reactions are confined almost entirely to the order of Hymenoptera. Honeybees, yellow hornets, bald-faced hornets, yellow jackets, wasps, and the imported fire ant are members of this order. Until most recently the diagnosis of hypersensitivity to insect stings was left to the history alone. The availability of in vitro tests of immediate hypersensitivity, including antigen-induced leukocyte histamine release and serum specific IgE antibody measurement by the radioallergosorbent test (RAST) procedure, has greatly facilitated the identification of those patients at risk of anaphylaxis. Furthermore, these tests have helped to confirm the validity of skin testing with specific insect venoms in the diagnosis of hypersensitivity in these patients. Such diagnosis is important in order to plan appropriate treatment programs.

A patient who has sustained a recent insect sting and who then develops manifestations of anaphylaxis, such as angioedema, laryngoedema, urticaria, bronchospasm, or hypotension, should be considered to be suffering a medical emergency and provided immediate treatment. This treatment is outlined in Table 1.

Insect sting allergic patients can be protected from subsequent serious reactions by the use of allergen immunotherapy. A protective IgG antibody response is seen in patients who are treated with immunotherapy using specific venom or venom-rich insect body extracts. These materials are expected to be released from investigative restrictions in the very near future. The treatment course is similar to that of standard allergen immunotherapy which employs increasing amounts of injected extract material as tolerated by the patient. The initial immunotherapy dose should be below the threshold of skin reactivity, and the ultimate maintenance dose should be approximately twice the amount of the average insect sting (50 to 100 micrograms for the honeybee; 25 to 50 micrograms for the vespids). Once a patient has reached this maximum dose, he should be maintained on injections of that dose at monthly intervals for an indefinite period of time.

All patients must be instructed in measures of avoiding stinging insects. These include prohibiting walking outdoors barefoot, keeping bees, or attempting to destroy insect nests. Particular caution should also be used in picnicking outdoors in the summer months. All sensitive patients should have an emergency kit containing a syringe preloaded with 1:1000 aqueous epinephrine within reach at all times. These kits can be purchased from the Hollister-Stier Company and from the Nelco Company. Sublingual isoproterenol (Isuprel) is not an adequate substitute for epinephrine. Patients at risk should be identified with a Medic-Alert identification tag.

Unusual reactions to the sting of an insect, such as encephalitis, nephritis, and nephrotic syndrome, are not characteristic of IgE reactions and should not be treated with immunotherapy. Prolonged, painful, local reactions may be treated with diphenhydramine (Benadryl), 1 mg. per kg. up to 50 mg., orally, every 4 to 6 hours, and/or prednisone, 30 mg. daily, for 3 days.

TABLE 1. **Method of Emergency Treatment**

1. The emergency treatment of choice is 1:1000 aqueous epinephrine, 0.01 ml. per kg. to a maximum of 0.3 ml., subcutaneously; this may be repeated every 20 minutes as necessary
2. Diphenhydramine (Benadryl), 1 mg. per kg. up to 50 mg., intramuscularly or intravenously; this may be repeated every 4 to 6 hours
3. Corticosteroids, hydrocortisone equivalent of 5 mg. per kg. up to 500 mg. intravenously, every 4 to 6 hours
4. Maintenance of airway and blood pressure as necessary

SECTION 11

Diseases of the Skin

ACNE VULGARIS

method of
ALAN R. SHALITA, M.D.
Brooklyn, New York

Acne vulgaris is the single most common skin disease. It affects approximately 80 per cent of the teenage population and, contrary to popular belief, may persist well into the third and fourth decades of life. Acne is a disease of the pilosebaceous follicle with a multifactorial cause. The pathogenesis includes an androgen-dependent increase in sebum production, proliferation of the follicular microflora (principally *Propionibacterium acnes*), and alterations in follicular keratinization. This results in the clinical lesions of acne—namely, open comedones (blackheads), closed comedones (whiteheads), papules, pustules, and nodulocystic lesions. Current therapy is directed toward suppression of these lesions and is usually remarkably effective.

Topical Therapy

Many acne patients may be successfully treated with topical therapy alone. For comedonal and mild inflammatory acne, therapy is initiated with tretinoin cream 0.05 per cent daily. The patient should be advised that an initial erythema and exfoliation may occur, that an exacerbation of inflammatory lesions is possible during the first month of therapy, and that an increased sensitivity to sunburn is likely. For the sunburn, judicious exposure combined with a para-aminobenzoic acid (PABA)-containing sunscreen is advisable. Patients with a pronounced seborrhea or those refractory to the 0.05 per cent tretinoin cream may tolerate a 0.1 per cent cream or the 0.05 per cent tretinoin swabs or liquid—all of which have a tendency to produce more pronounced erythema and desquamation. An alternative dosage form is the 0.025 per cent gel, which is particularly useful in treating inflammatory acne. Significant therapeutic improvement does not usually occur before 4 to 6 weeks, and 12 weeks are normally required for optimal therapeutic benefit. Topical tretinoin appears to exert its effect on the keratinizing epithelium of the follicle.

Benzoyl peroxide gels are very good topical antibacterial agents. Therapy is usually initiated with a 5 per cent gel applied daily. Refractory cases may require the 10 per cent concentration or more frequent application. Although little erythema occurs, there may be considerable desquamation.

Many patients benefit from the combined use of topical tretinoin and a benzoyl peroxide gel, one applied in the morning and the other at night. The effects of the two drugs appear to be additive. Some patients, however, will not tolerate the "dryness" produced by this regimen. One may then try therapy with each drug on alternate days.

Topical antibiotic solutions such as those containing erythromycin and clindamycin offer promise as additions to the therapeutic armamentarium. At the time of this writing, however, they are still experimental, and there are few data available on the stability of extemporaneous preparations.

Preparations containing various combinations of sulfur, resorcin, and salicylic acid, particularly in tinted lotions and creams, may be useful when used judiciously. They accelerate the resolution of inflammatory lesions while providing cover.

Systemic Therapy

Broad-spectrum antibiotics remain valuable tools in the treatment of inflammatory acne. Therapy is usually initiated with 500 to 1000 mg. of tetracycline hydrochloride or erythromycin. The dose is decreased at appropriate intervals according to the therapeutic response. Minocycline, 50 mg. daily to three times daily, is occasionally useful in patients who appear to be refractory to the aforementioned agents. An alternative is larger doses of tetracycline. One thousand five hundred to 3000 mg. of tetracycline is effective in patients with severe nodulocystic acne who have not responded to lower doses. The safety of the long-term use of these antibiotics for acne treatment is now well established.

In resistant acne in women, systemic estrogen therapy is beneficial. This can be administered in the form of oral contraceptives. Most useful are those containing 80 to 100 micrograms of ethinyl estradiol or mestranol. Those containing norgestrel as the progestational agent appear to be contraindicated because of their apparent mildly androgenic effect.

Systemic steroids are frequently useful for short periods in recalcitrant nodulocystic acne. Doses of 30 to 40 mg. of prednisone per day may be used if rapidly tapered.

Local Therapy

Intralesional injections of triamcinolone acetonide or triamcinolone hexacetonide (2.5 to 5 mg. per ml.) are most useful in achieving the prompt resolution of inflammatory lesions, particularly those of the nodulocystic variety. No more than 0.5 mg. should be injected into any single lesion of the face in order to minimize local atrophy. The hexacetonide salt should be limited to lesions of the chest and back, because it may produce more pronounced and prolonged atrophy.

Cryotherapy with liquid nitrogen probes, liquid nitrous oxide, or solid CO_2 is also useful in treating large inflammatory lesions. An initial edematous reaction is followed by relatively prolonged resolution of nodulocystic lesions.

The physical removal of comedones with a comedo extractor is frequently of benefit. Incision and drainage of inflammatory lesions rarely accomplishes more than intralesional steroids or cryotherapy.

PSEUDOFOLLICULITIS BARBAE

method of
CHARLES S. THURSTON, M.D.
San Antonio, Texas

Pseudofolliculitis barbae (PB), commonly called "shaving bumps," is a medical problem prevalent among most blacks but very few whites. Men with PB characteristically have stiff and strongly curved beard hair, which, when shaved, tends to "ingrow" 2 or 3 days later. The consequence is a foreign body type of inflammatory papule or pustule, which, in turn, may progress into a large nodule or abscess. The associated itching and pain can be severe, but are quickly relieved when the ingrown hair—foreign body—is spontaneously or manually released.

The PB problem, although genetically predisposed by a characteristic type of beard, is precipitated and severely aggravated by improper shaving techniques such as shaving too closely. Unfortunately, even when very meticulous shaving practices are followed, the genetically prone may occasionally develop PB of varying severity. Milder cases may show fewer than 20 papules or pustules, whereas hundreds of such lesions are noted in moderate and severe cases. Numerous inflammatory nodules and abscesses may also be noted in the more severe cases.

Acute Management

In all but the mildest cases, some medical management is required during the acute phase of PB. The following measures are recommended:

1. Discontinuance of all shaving for a minimum of 3 weeks for mild cases and up to 6 to 12 months for the more severe cases. The beard may be kept neatly trimmed with clippers or scissors to a minimum of ¼ inch.
2. Manual release of all clinically visible ingrown hairs with a sterile needle. The patient should be taught to release, daily, other ingrown hairs as they become visible. He should be cautioned against plucking hairs from the root.
3. Warm tap water compresses.
4. Topical corticosteroid lotions.
5. A 2 week "burst" of systemic corticosteroids, beginning with 30 to 40 mg. per day of prednisone, is valuable in the more severe cases.
6. Systemic antibiotics may also be needed in severe cases when secondary infection has intervened.

Topical and systemic medications are rarely needed for more than 2 weeks. On the other hand, resumption of shaving should be completely avoided until all ingrown hairs have been released and all inflammatory lesions have disappeared.

Control Measures

Education. Education of the patient is an important first step in PB control. The patient should be taught early that there is no guarantee that his PB can be cured unless he is willing to abstain from shaving permanently. He can be reassured, however, that with sincere motivation on his part, he may be able to retard or prevent the development of PB by following well disciplined shaving practices. The physician may play an important role as an instructor in this effort.

Choice of Shaving Methods. Patients with PB may expect varying degrees of successful shaving by using one or more of the following shaving methods: (1) an adjustable razor, (2) a chemical depilatory, or (3) electric clippers. None of these methods is ideal, and therefore the "best" method is the one the physician can most expertly and enthusiastically teach and the patient can enthusiastically accept and diligently follow. It must be emphasized that no matter what method is chosen, shaving should not be resumed until all PB lesions have completely cleared.

Instruction of Shaving Methods. ADJUSTABLE RAZOR. The adjustable razor offers the patient a chance to have a neatly shaven appearance each day. However, this method requires considerable skill as well as motivation; it is outlined as follows:

1. Remove pre-existing beard with electric clippers, leaving $^{1}/_{16}$ inch of stubble.
2. Wash the beard area, using warm water and bath soap on a rough washcloth.
3. Rinse with warm water.
4. Squeeze a modest amount of shaving cream on the fingers and gently massage it on the entire beard area in a circular motion. If lather dries prior to completing shave, reapply.
5. Insert a sharp razor blade into the adjustable razor and adjust the blade angle to the midsetting.
6. Shave the well lathered beard area, using the following precautions: (a) Use gentle, even strokes without pressing the razor against the face or stretching the skin with the other hand. (b) Use as few strokes as possible in an effort to shave every hair. Hard-to-shave areas may require shaving in more than one direction. (c) Do not substitute pressure for a sharp blade. Generally speaking, if more than two strokes are necessary to cut the hair, a new blade is needed. A change of blade is usually necessary after one to three shaves, depending upon "toughness" of the beard.
7. Rinse the face and inspect it for remaining embedded hairs.
8. Release embedded hairs with a toothpick, and trim with small iris or cuticle scissors.
9. Apply after-shave lotion.
10. Repeat the shaving procedure daily at approximately the same hour.

CHEMICAL DEPILATORY. The use of these agents, barium sulfide and calcium thioglycolate, has become more widely accepted since "odor-free" brands have been placed on the market. Nevertheless, the depilatories are potentially irritating, and great care should be taken when they are first used. In fact, the novice should pretest the chemical on a 2 cm. hair-bearing area of the forearm.

The steps in the shaving procedure are as follows:

1. Remove the pre-existing beard with clippers, leaving $^{1}/_{16}$ inch of stubble.
2. Wash the beard area, using warm water and mild bath soap on a rough washcloth.
3. Rinse with warm water.
4. Apply the freshly prepared paste on one half of the bearded area.
5. Remove the paste within 3 to 5 minutes, before it dries, using the edge of a plastic spatula, tongue blade, or table knife.
6. Rinse the area thoroughly with warm water.
7. Repeat steps 4, 5, and 6 on the other half of the beard area.
8. Apply after-shave lotion.
9. Repeat the shave every 3 to 5 days, depending upon the degree of irritation.
10. As beard hairs regrow between shaves, keep their tips free by gentle brushing with a toothbrush.

ELECTRIC CLIPPERS. Of all the shaving methods, the use of electric clippers is technically the least difficult to master. The significant points to be emphasized are as follows:

1. The beard should be trimmed so as to leave a minimum of $^{1}/_{16}$ inch of stubble.
2. Pressing the clippers against the face while attempting to trim beard hairs lying close to the skin surface must be avoided.
3. Close-lying hairs must be kept free from re-entering the skin by daily gentle scrubbing with a rough washcloth and brushing with a toothbrush.
4. Hairs which become embedded should be released daily with a toothpick or sterile sewing needle.
5. The electric clipper shave should normally be repeated every 1 to 2 days.

ALOPECIA

method of
P. E. HUTCHINSON, M.B., M.R.C.P.
Leicester, England

A prerequisite to management of any condition is accurate diagnosis. However, there is generally a lack of familiarity with diseases affecting the hair, and therefore this aspect has been emphasized below. The approach is to categorize hair diseases according to clinical presentation and mechanism of affection of the hair. From a careful history and examination of the scalp, four main clinical patterns emerge as shown in Table 1.

The mechanism of hair involvement is determined by an examination of scalp skin, looking particularly for signs of inflammation or scarring; by an examination of scalp hairs in situ with regard to the distribution of

TABLE 1. Categories of Hair Disorders, Based on Clinical Presentation and Mechanism of Hair Loss

1. Increased rate of hair shedding
    - Loss of telogen hairs (telogen effluvium)
    - Loss of broken hairs (anagen effluvium)
    - Loss of whole anagen hairs (anagen effluvium proper)
2. Diffuse hair thinning
    - Decrease in hair shaft diameter in a proportion of hairs
3. Patchy alopecia
    - Noncicatricial
        - Loss of telogen hairs
        - Loss of broken hairs
        - Loss of whole anagen hairs
        - Decrease in hair shaft diameter
    - Cicatricial
4. Failure to grow long hair
    - Loss of telogen hairs
    - Loss of broken hairs

hair lengths and the form of the distal ends—i.e., whether they are fractured or have fine tapering tips as produced in early anagen; by an examination of shed hairs, evaluating shed hair count per day and examining the morphology of the hair roots; and, finally, by an examination of plucked hairs, in particular evaluating the number of hairs in each of the two main phases of the hair cycle—i.e., anagen and telogen.

Following this preliminary categorization, a final diagnosis is reached by the relevant specific investigation.

INCREASED RATE OF HAIR SHEDDING

The primary complaint is of an excessive loss of scalp hair. Objective evidence of such a complaint is necessary, as this is an area which is a ready target for subjective distortion, particularly by an anxious patient. A degree of objectivity can be gained by a formal hair count. The patient is first asked to wash the hair and then to collect all shed hairs separately for each day over the following 5 days. The average daily count should not exceed 100 hairs per day.

There are three possible pathogenic categories, and these, together with the possible specific causes, are shown in Table 2.

Telogen Effluvium

This is the loss of hairs which have entered telogen prior to shedding—i.e., the follicles have ceased active growth. Usually not more than 30 per cent of the scalp hairs are affected. This might be regarded as an exaggerated and synchronized form of normal physiologic molting. Normal scalp hair follicles undergo successive phases of hair growth, anagen, lasting for approximately 3 to 5 years, followed by quiescence, telogen, lasting for approximately 3 months. At the end of the growth period a terminal club is produced on the hair shaft, which results in the mature telogen hair. The length of the hair cycle and the total number of scalp follicles are such that the expected hair fall per day is approximately 50 hairs. In autumn this count may be higher, as there is evidence of a seasonal molt in man.

TABLE 2. Increased Rate of Hair Shedding—Individual Causes

- Telogen effluvium
    - Systemic disease
        - Infection
            - Following febrile episodes
            - Influenza
            - Gastroenteritis
            - Syphilis
        - Nutrition
            - Severe dieting
        - Endocrine
            - Pregnancy (ca. 3 months following delivery)
        - Neoplasia
            - Systemic malignancy
        - Drugs
            - Anticoagulants, e.g., dextran, heparin
            - Antithyroid drugs, e.g., carbimazole, iodides
            - Estrogens (ca. 3 months following cessation), e.g., contraceptive pill
            - Sodium valproate
        - Environment
            - Air flight (3 months following)
    - Anagen effluvium (broken hairs)
        - Hair disease
            - Alopecia areata
        - Systemic disease
            - Autoaggressive
                - Systemic lupus erythematosus
            - Drugs
                - Alkylating agents, e.g., azathioprine
                - Antimetabolic agents, e.g., methotrexate
                - Mitotic arresting agents, e.g., colchicine
                - Thallium*
                - Vitamin A intoxication*
                - Boric acid*
- Anagen effluvium (whole anagen hairs)
    - Skin disease
        - Tinea amiantacea

*Suspected mechanism for agent listed.

The diagnosis of telogen effluvium is established from (1) the history of an acute shedding episode and increased hair counts, the shed hairs being exclusively telogen hairs, and (2) an increased telogen count in plucked samples. In this second investigation approximately 50 hairs are plucked from a single site on the scalp. The number of hairs in telogen is counted by examination under a hand lens or microscope. The normal telogen count is determined by the relative duration of telogen to the whole cycle, which is approximately 10 per cent. The limits of the telogen count are largely dependent on chance sampling effect in a binomial situation, together with true individual variation. In practice the upper limit of normal is approximately 25 to 30 per cent.

It is evident from Table 2 that most causes are acute self-limiting processes and therefore require no treatment. In fact it is likely that the precipitating factor is no longer in evidence at the time of presentation of the hair problem, as there is a latency of approximately 3 months prior to the shedding period, representing the time telogen hairs remain in the follicle before shedding. However, syphilis and systemic malignancy are also possible causes, and these must be investigated by appropriate clinical and laboratory procedures.

Anagen Effluvium (Broken Hairs)

Anagen effluvium is the loss of hair which was actively growing immediately prior to being shed. In normal use the term refers to the loss of fractured hair. The mechanism for this is an abrupt decrease in the cellular output of the follicle matrix owing to an acute metabolic insult to the proliferating cells. Up to 90 per cent of scalp hairs may be involved.

The most common cause of anagen effluvium is the use of cytotoxic drugs. This would appear to be a general effect of antimitotic drugs, occurring, for example, with alkylating agents such as azathioprine, antimetabolic agents such as methotrexate, and mitotic arresting agents such as colchicine. Similarly thallium, vitamin A intoxication, and systemic poisons such as boric acid may act by such a mechanism.

The hair is shed within a few days following the use of the drugs, and regrowth is prompt if the hairs remain in anagen.

Usually the cause is self-evident—e.g., cytotoxic therapy; but rarely the cause is found only by very detailed drug or occupational history, as exemplified by recent cases of accidental self-poisoning from boric acid contained in mouthwashes and soap powders. Hair may be lost by a similar mechanism in such diseases as systemic lupus erythematosus and alopecia areata, in which the insult is presumably cellular and perhaps immunologic rather than pharmacologic. Diagnosis of these two conditions is not a problem when related to the total clinical picture.

The anagen effluvium of cancer chemotherapy is self-curative, and no treatment is necessary. Attempts at prophylaxis have been made by the use of a tight band around the scalp to restrict scalp blood flow during therapy, but this has met with only mixed success.

Anagen Effluvium (True)

What might be called "true" anagen effluvium is the loss of complete anagen hairs. The mechanism involved is presumably the loss of normal hair anchorage such that relatively small traction forces are able to dislodge hairs from their follicles. The diagnosis is made on the basis of shed hairs being *intact* anagen hairs.

The cause of this is tinea amiantacea. This is basically an eczematous process which involves the outer one third of the follicular outer root sheath. The history is of loss of clumps of hairs with adherent scale. On examination of the scalp there are patches of scale which coat the proximal end of the hairs in an enveloping shroud.

Treatment is simple and effective, comprising 2 per cent sulfur and 2 per cent salicylic acid in aqueous cream, applied to the scalp through multiple partings nightly and shampooed out twice weekly, with a strong detergent shampoo.

DIFFUSE HAIR THINNING

Here the primary complaint is of an apparent decrease in hair count per unit area, not necessarily associated with increased hair fall. The problem is diffuse on the scalp but has a particular impact in the vertical region. In the later stages baldness may result. There is no objective clinical investigation for the evaluation of decreased hair density. Early change must be assessed by eye and compared with the expected density for the appropriate age and sex. Mean hair density decreases with age, starting in the third decade, and more markedly so in males than in females. The word *apparent* has been stressed, as the actual hair count per unit area is not dramatically affected. The predominant change is from normal wide-diameter terminal hair to successively finer hair. Diffuse hair thinning is therefore usually a problem of hair shaft diameter rather than hair count per unit area. In the extreme instance of complete vertical male pattern baldness, normal terminal hair is totally replaced by very fine, barely discernible vellus hair. The causes are listed in Table 3.

Genetic Causes

By far the most common causes are genetic, the male and female pattern alopecias, and there are at least two distinct genetic conditions. For full expression in addition to genetic constitution, androgens are important, and therefore these conditions are more evident in the male.

Male Pattern Alopecia. There are at least two distinct genetic entities. The first is an autosomal dominant trait with a high degree of penetrance and an onset in the third or early fourth decade. The earliest clinical manifestations are caused by a reduction in the duration of anagen, which results in a failure to grow long hair on the vertex and consequent increased shedding rate. Telogen counts of plucked hair samples are markedly elevated, usually greater than 40 per cent. The condition is rapidly progressive, and total vertical baldness can be expected within a few years.

The second condition is again probably inherited as an autosomal dominant trait. The onset, however, is

TABLE 3. **Diffuse Hair Thinning—Individual Causes**

Hair follicle disease
- Genetic
  - Male pattern, autosomal dominant, early onset
  - Male pattern, ? autosomal dominant, late onset
  - Female pattern, ? autosomal dominant, ? polygenetic

Systemic disease
- Nutrition
  - Iron deficiency
- Endocrine
  - Thyroid disease
  - Hyperandrogen states
- Drugs
  - ? Aspirin
  - ? Amphetamines

usually later, in the fourth to sixth decade; telogen counts are somewhat raised but not to the same extent as in the preceding condition, and the disease is far less rapidly progressive.

Female Pattern Alopecia. This is much less common than male pattern alopecia. The genetics of the condition is not fully established, but there is some evidence for an autosomal dominant mode of inheritance. Onset may be as early as the early third decade. In contrast to the male pattern alopecias, the frontal hair line is typically retained and telogen counts are normal or very slightly raised, with a mean of approximately 15 per cent on the vertex. Although there may be a marked decrease in apparent hair density at a young age, the condition is not rapidly progressive, and baldness does not result from this condition until late middle age if at all.

Diagnosis of these conditions is made by the clinical pattern of involvement, by the clinical signs mentioned above, and, particularly in the first male type, by the family history. Possible acquired factors, which are detailed below, should be excluded.

Management in the well-adjusted male is not difficult, with a simple explanation of the disease and reassurance that the hair loss is not an indicator of systemic illness. In the female, however, who usually sees the condition as a potential cosmetic and social disaster, it is necessary to give firm assurance that the condition does not behave as the rapidly progressive male condition and that she can expect, with suitable hair styles, a cosmetically acceptable covering for a good number of years.

Systemic Causes

Only a small number of diffuse alopecias are related to systemic causes, which are listed in Table 3. The relevant diagnostic procedures should be performed.

It is not worthwhile intensively investigating biochemically the androgen status of women with diffuse hair loss unless there is associated hirsutism. The decreased diameter of scalp hair is a far less sensitive indicator of androgen levels than the increase in diameter of the secondary sexual hair of the upper lip, beard, or central chest. This is not to deny, however, a possible critical role of androgen in female pattern baldness, which could result from increased end-organ—namely, scalp follicle—responsiveness.

A small clinical clue to possible hypothyroidism from the scalp hair is a raised telogen count in a plucked sample.

Iron deficiency is a widely recognized cause of diffuse hair loss. There is, however, little hard evidence either of a pathogenetic role for iron deficiency or of improvement of the hair condition following treatment. However, it is prudent to investigate and treat any abnormality in the iron status.

Systemic drugs are probably an insignificant cause of the problem, although recently amphetamines and aspirin have been implicated. Because of its extremely wide use, any implication of the combination contraceptive pill is important. There is no doubt that cessation of the use of the contraceptive pill, as with any estrogen, may produce a telogen effluvium, but a separate question is whether diffuse thinning may occur *during* therapy. The present state of knowledge may be summarized by stating that there is no evidence that the contraceptive pill causes diffuse hair thinning, and there is some evidence that it does not in the majority of persons. A further point is that possible effects of different absolute and relative amounts of the two components have not been investigated. If there were a deleterious effect on hair of either component, the most likely would be progesterone, which may have androgenic activity. Estrogens, however, have antiandrogenic activity. A reasonable course in the female with diffuse hair thinning and who desires to take the contraceptive pill is to suggest a medium estrogen– and low progesterone–containing product.

PATCHY HAIR LOSS

The first diagnostic procedure is to determine whether such a loss is scarring (cicatricial). In scarring alopecia the affected skin is thickened and nonsupple, has limited mobility over the scalp compared to normal tissue, and may even be hard to the touch. Gentle traction on hairs on the margin of the patch has little effect on the affected skin, whereas in noncicatricial loss this may produce elevation of the skin of the affected area.

Noncicatricial

Possible mechanisms of hair loss here cover the same range as for the previous two syndromes; they are listed in Table 4.

The hair loss in syphilis is really diffuse as previously described, but there may be focal accentuation. Hair loss in these areas is not complete.

Alopecia Areata

The hair loss in patches of alopecia areata results from a combination of fracturing and loss of telogen hairs. The affected skin is normal or slightly erythematous, and within the areas there is virtually complete alopecia apart from a sparse short stubble. There may be further patches of alopecia on the body and fine regular pitting of the nails.

The major diagnostic procedure is the demonstration of the exclamation mark hair. This is essentially a short, broken telogen hair, but the most important feature is a diminutive telogen bulb. The short, broken hairs should be plucked from the involved scalp with

TABLE 4. **Patchy Hair Loss—Individual Causes**

Noncicatricial
- Loss of telogen hairs
  - Alopecia areata
  - (Syphilis)
- Loss of broken hairs
  - Alopecia areata
  - Tinea capitis
  - Mechanical trauma
- Loss of anagen hairs
  - Tinea amiantacea
- Decrease in diameter
  - Mechanical, prolonged traction

Cicatricial
- Restricted local scalp disease
  - Severe infection—e.g., fungal
  - Folliculitis decalvans
  - "Hot combing"
  - Irradiation
- Skin disease
  - Lichen planus
  - Discoid lupus erythematosus
  - Morphea
  - Cicatricial pemphigoid
  - Necrobiosis lipoidica
- Systemic disease
  - Lupus vulgaris
  - Tertiary syphilis
  - Sarcoidosis
  - Carcinoma—secondary deposits

epilating forceps and examined with a hand lens or microscopically for this feature. Short, broken hairs with normal-sized telogen bulbs are not diagnostic of alopecia areata and may also be found in extrinsic causes of hair fracturing—e.g., trichotillomania. Further investigations in alopecia areata are a screen for circulating organ-specific autoantibodies, including thyroid, adrenal, and parietal cell, as well as appropriate endocrine studies if these appear clinically indicated. If high titers of autoantibodies are demonstrated together with normal endocrine function, the patient is followed for future possible endocrine disease.

In the majority of adult patients with alopecia areata the disease spontaneously remits within a year. Unfavorable prognostic pointers are childhood onset, the presence of a family history of alopecia areata, a family or personal history of atopy, total body involvement, and duration of the initial patch of alopecia areata lasting greater than 6 months.

Two main forms of therapy have been used: locally injected corticosteroids, including jet injectors, and systemic corticosteroids. Widespread alopecia areata makes the first treatment impractical, but there was initial enthusiasm for its use in more localized alopecia areata. However, any success must be evaluated in the light of the high spontaneous remission rate, and recent studies have not confirmed a significant beneficial effect. Systemic steroids in doses of approximately 40 mg. of prednisolone daily are effective in promoting regrowth even in longstanding alopecia totalis. However, on cessation of therapy there is invariably relapse, and maintenance dosage must be high to continue control. The ratio of beneficial to unwanted effects of systemic steroids in alopecia areata is therefore unfavorable.

Tinea Capitis

The mechanism of hair loss in fungus infection of the scalp is by hair fracturing, resulting from invasion of the hair shaft by fungus. Many different members of the genera Trichophyton and Microsporum are possible causes. Typically the clinical appearance is of patches of short lusterless broken hairs. There is a variable inflammatory response of interfollicular scalp skin, varying from chronic scaling to acute inflammation with pustules. Fluorescence in ultraviolet light occurs in the diseased hairs in the majority of organisms.

Diagnosis of tinea capitis is based on clinical appearance, fluorescence, and potassium hydroxide preparations of involved hair when hyphae are visible within the hair shaft.

The mainstay of treatment is now griseofulvin. The adult dose is 0.5 to 1 gram daily (250 to 500 mg. in children) taken after the main meal of the day. Treatment must be continued until there is complete clinical cure. Side effects of the drug are usually not severe and include drowsiness, nausea, diarrhea and skin eruptions. Discoid lupus erythematosus–like syndromes, transient leukopenias, and exacerbations of porphyria in the predisposed may also occur.

Mechanical Trauma

The mechanical force finally responsible for fracturing is usually the tensile force generated by grooming—e.g., brushing and combing—or by deliberate pulling. Whether a hair breaks as the result of mechanical stress depends upon the balance between the magnitude of the applied forces and the intrinsic strength of the hair shaft. Conditions may be classified according to whether the applied traction forces are of an abnormally high magnitude or whether there is an intrinsic weakness of the hair shaft. Individual causes are listed in Table 5.

Trichotillomania

This is an underdiagnosed condition that is often mistaken for alopecia areata. In only a small percentage of patients is there an underlying incapacitating psychiatric illness. Usually the patients are rather obsessional, introverted, preadolescent children.

The mechanism of fracturing is usually from a plucking action, a lock of hair having been wound around a finger. There is a patchy hypotrichosis, and numerous broken hairs feel like a coarse stubble under the examining finger. There are also multiple, short, newly growing anagen hairs with fine tapering distal

TABLE 5. **Patchy Hair Loss from Mechanical Trauma—Causes**

High tensile forces
  Trichotillomania
  Curly or woolly hair
Fragile hair
  Structural
    Congenital
      Monilethrix
      Pili annulati
    Acquired
      Worn cuticle
  Biochemical
    Congenital
      Pili torti
      Menkes' steely hair disease
    Acquired
      Ultraviolet light damage
      Bleaching
      Permanent waving or straightening

tips, representing regrowth from previous insult. On plucking the short broken hairs, many are in anagen, which distinguishes the condition from alopecia areata. The telogen count of plucked samples is usually very low.

The course of the disease is often quite long, even in the childhood type, with a mean duration of approximately 5 years.

The first step in management is the detection of any serious underlying psychiatric condition and subsequent psychiatric referral. In the average case it is difficult to know whether the patient is fully aware of the action. There seems little point in confronting the patient with the diagnosis, although the parents should be fully informed. The patient may be reassured that there is no serious organic disease of the hair follicles, and that regrowth can be expected when conditions are right.

Curly Hair—"Woolly Hair." Abnormally high tensile forces may be generated by brushing and combing this sort of hair when the comb becomes readily entangled in the curly locks. This may be a major cause of problems in the hair of blacks and in the genetically determined conditions of woolly hair.

Congenital Structural Defects of the Hair Shaft

These include rare conditions such as monilethrix and pili annulati, both of which are inherited as autosomal dominant traits. In monilethrix the hair is beaded and has nodules of relatively normal hair shaft diameter interposed between very narrow segments. Because of the fine diameter of the latter, the hair is vulnerable to minor tensile forces. In pili annulati there are bands of alternating light and dark zones in the hair. The basic pathology is the presence of cavities in the cortex of the abnormal segments which reduce the effective hair shaft diameter.

Acquired Structural Defects

This results from damage to the hair cuticle, the damaging agent again being grooming. The hair shaft might be likened to a bundle of long steel rods (the cortex) bound together by thin binding wire (the cuticle). The strength of the system is along the length or growth axis. Stability against lateral forces is provided by lateral cohesion afforded by the cuticle. If this is worn, the central elements are free to "fray" and may be individually snapped, producing the appearance of trichorrhexis nodosa. Excessive frictional wear may be produced in normal hair by excessive grooming. Particularly harmful is the practice of "back-combing," in which the hair is brushed from the distal ends toward the scalp. This opposes the ratchet effect of the free margins of the cuticle, which point upward like scales on a pine tree. Hair which is excessively vulnerable to frictional damage is again very curly hair.

Congenital Biochemical Defects of the Hair Shaft

There are several different conditions associated with biochemical defects of the hair shaft. All of these seem to share as a final common biochemical defect an increase in free sulfhydryl groups of the hair shaft. There may also be systemic involvement—e.g., mental deficiency. These conditions include Menkes' steely hair disease and pili torti. Menkes' disease is related to abnormal copper metabolism and is associated with mental deficiency, vascular disease, and bone disease in the early months of life and is invariably fatal without treatment. Pili torti are simply twisted hairs, in which there is rapid axial rotation of the hair shaft of 180 degrees without curling. This is not a single entity but may occur in several poorly defined conditions. In some of these there is a biochemical defect, and again there may be associated mental deficiency. A clinical clue to an underlying biochemical defect is a characteristic bleach-blond color to the hair, which may result from complexing of melanin precursors with free thiol groups.

Acquired Biochemical Defects

Ultraviolet Light. Hair is surprisingly vulnerable to ultraviolet light, such that continuous exposure to a full summer season of natural sunlight may produce approximately 50 per cent decrease in stress required for 15 per cent extension. This may in large part be responsible for the sporadic occurrence of hair fragility in otherwise perfectly healthy young adults who indulge in long periods of sunbathing on the beach, punctuated by immersion in the sea and vigorous toweling of the hair.

Cosmetic Procedures

These include oxidation, bleaching, reduction, permanent waving, and hair straightening. In addition to the effect on melanin, bleaching also affects the disulfide bonds of keratin, but bleaching itself is usually not a cause of excessive fragility in normal hair. Chemical permanent waving or hair straightening consists of cleavage of disulfide bonds and realignment by mechanical measures, followed by reoxidation. Problems may arise if the reoxidation is incomplete because of technical incompetence, or if the hair has been previously bleached and disulfides are unable to reform. Bleached hair therefore should not be subjected to permanent waving.

Diagnostic procedures in traumatic alopecias include historical details of cosmetic procedures such as grooming techniques, the use of permanent waving or straightening, bleaching, and sun exposure. The hair shaft should be examined microscopically for structural changes. In children, if hair fragility is associated with a light-bleached color of the hair and pili torti, investigations should include serum copper levels and amino acid chromatography.

Treatment of those conditions caused exclusively by external agents is dependent on an accurate diagnosis and avoidance of the responsible agent. In conditions associated with congenital hair shaft defects and in extrinsically damaged hair, until new growth has occurred, the following advice should be given:

1. Minimize mechanical trauma. (a) Brush and comb with care, pulling out the comb if it should become caught up in the hair. (b) Avoid back-combing. (c) Avoid excessive toweling following bathing. (d) A proprietary conditioner, which covers the hair with a slippery film, may also help.

2. Avoid chemical damage. (a) Shampoo the hair with a shampoo having a neutral pH (keratin is vulnerable to alkali attack). (b) Avoid permanent waving or straightening of the hair. (c) Avoid excessive sun exposure of the hair.

Tinea Amiantacea. This condition has been mentioned above. The impact is in fact usually focal, producing a patchy hair loss. The diagnosis and treatment are as described above.

Prolonged Mechanical Traction. This is a completely different category of mechanical damage from that described above. Certain hairstyles, such as the pony tail or plaiting, and certain cosmetic procedures, such as the application of hair rollers, particularly when worn in bed, produce chronic traction on the hair. The follicular response is a reduction in hair shaft diameter, as is found diffusely in the patterned alopecias.

Diagnosis depends on the clinical suspicion roused by the pattern of involvement, which corresponds to the sites of maximum traction—e.g., the frontal hair line from the pony tail, and the temples and parietal areas above the ears from rollers. Early diagnosis is imperative, as the changes are irreversible.

Cicatricial Alopecia

The mechanism of hair loss here is through replacement of hair follicles with fibrous tissue. The causes are listed in Table 4. The diagnosis of a cicatricial alopecia can usually be made by clinical examination through the features listed above.

Diagnosis of the specific cause is based on scalp biopsy, clinical examination of the whole skin, general physical examination, and appropriate laboratory procedures. In discoid lupus erythematosus and lichen planus the scalp lesions may be solitary, in which case biopsy of the edge of a lesion combined with immunofluorescence will establish the diagnosis.

In general management is directed at the underlying cause. Symptomatic treatment in noninfective, nonmalignant conditions is aimed at any active lesions. Once scarring has occurred, treatment is useless. The patient is told to report if there is progressive growth in an old lesion or if new lesions develop. These may be treated by the intralesional injection of corticosteroids; 0.1 ml. of triamcinalone acetonide (5 to 10 mg. per ml.) is injected intradermally at 1 to 2 cm. intervals, up to a maximum dose of 20 mg. This may be repeated at monthly intervals. The most effective syringe is a dental syringe in which the fine needle screws on to the barrel, thus allowing greater injection pressures.

FAILURE TO GROW LONG HAIR

There are two pathogenic mechanisms which may produce this effect, shortening of the growing period of the hair follicle, with subsequent excessive loss of telogen hair, or diffuse fracturing of the hair shafts.

The first may be an isolated defect, or it may occur in association with other hair or skin diseases—e.g., familial woolly hair and hidrotic ectodermal dysplasia. Diagnosis is established by the presence of fine tapering distal tips of the short hair shafts. No treatment is available.

The causes of hair fracturing which may be associated with a diffuse impact are trichotillomania and the congenital and acquired hair shaft defects. The investigation and management of these are as described for patchy hair loss.

CANCER OF THE SKIN

method of
WILMA F. BERGFELD, M.D.
Cleveland, Ohio

Important skin cancers to recognize and treat are the basal cell carcinoma, squamous cell carcinoma, and malignant melanoma. All these neoplasms appear most frequently on sun-exposed sites and in fair-skinned, blue-eyed persons. Early recognition and treatment offer a good prognosis.

Basal Cell Carcinoma

Basal cell carcinomas are slow-growing neoplasms, which are locally destructive and rarely metastasize. These neoplasms are frequently seen on sun-exposed surfaces of fair-skinned, blue-eyed persons; however, they may also be observed on the unexposed skin surfaces. Clinically the basal cell carcinoma may present as a psoriasiform patch, papule, nodule, and/or scar, with or without superficial or deep ulceration. Basal cell carcinomas with the histologic appearance of a morphea or metatypical basal cell carcinoma are biologically active and will demonstrate local invasion. The metatypical basal cell carcinoma on rare occasions is known to metastasize.

Treatment consists of total removal of the neoplasm. This can be accomplished by electrosurgery with curettage, cryotherapy, surgical excision, radiotherapy, and chemosurgery. Chemosurgery, fixed and fresh tissue techniques, is a histologically controlled excision of the neoplasm. This technique allows for microscopic removal of the entire neoplasm, which diminishes the recurrences. Chemosurgery is recommended for all recurrent basal cell carcinomas, morphea, and metatypical basal cell carcinomas and lesions of the nasal alae and nasal fold.

Squamous Cell Carcinoma

Squamous cell carcinoma is a rapidly growing cutaneous neoplasm which metastasizes frequently. Squamous cell carcinomas are often preceded by premalignant skin conditions such as actinic keratosis, cutaneous horn, Bowen's disease, erythroplasia of Queyrat, leukoplakia, and radiation dermatitis. Those squamous cell carcinomas which develop in actinic keratoses have a better prognosis, metastasizing less frequently, than those that develop de novo.

Squamous cell carcinomas are most frequently seen on sun-exposed skin; however, they may be seen on unexposed skin, especially in patients who have ingested arsenic or have received radiation therapy to the site. Clinically a squamous cell carcinoma may present as a hyperkeratotic papule, nodule, or tumor, with or without ulceration. Those patients with histologically moderately or poorly differentiated squamous cell carcinomas should be evaluated for metastases to local lymph nodes.

Treatment of choice is excision of the squamous cell carcinoma. In small lesions electrosurgery with curettage, cryotherapy, or chemosurgery may be employed. Radiotherapy is ineffective, as these tumors are radioresistant.

It is necessary that the physician recognize and treat all premalignant skin lesions in an attempt to diminish the incidence of squamous cell carcinoma. If these lesions are difficult to remove totally, the patient should be periodically reevaluated for the development of squamous cell carcinoma.

Malignant Melanoma

Malignant melanoma is a melanocytic skin tumor which may present de novo or within a junctional nevus, compound nevus, or melanotic freckle of Hutchinson. The biologic activity of a malignant melanoma may be rapid or may be slow growing for many years, with sudden rapid growth and metastases. Malignant melanomas are considered a highly malignant disorder with poor prognosis. The more superficial malignant melanomas—Clark levels I, II, and III—can be effectively treated with wide excision. The nodular malignant melanoma—Clark levels IV and V—have poor prognosis, and all treatment modalities are limited. Treatment of a nodular malignant melanoma is excision with chemotherapy and/or immunotherapy.

Early recognition and treatment of the superficial malignant melanoma improve the prognosis of these lesions.

Malignant melanomas are also seen more frequently on sun-exposed skin of fair-complexioned persons. Common sites of malignant melanoma are noted to be the head and the lower extremities.

Follow-up

All patients with malignant skin tumors should be followed yearly for 5 years. In the first year they are seen every 4 to 6 months. Recurrences of skin tumors should be confirmed by skin biopsy and the lesions removed by one of the modalities mentioned.

CREEPING ERUPTION

method of
JOHN H. HICKS, M.D.
Miami, Florida

Creeping eruption (sandworm, larva migrans) is apparently a vanishing disease, at least in some parts of the southeastern United States. Whereas 20 years ago many infestations would be treated during summer rainy months, now only an occasional case is seen.

This decreased incidence is thought to be due to the discovery of thiabendazole for therapy and its widespread use in cats and dogs by veterinarians. This disease is caused by the cat and dog hookworms, *Ancylostoma braziliense* and *Ancylostoma caninum.* Infested cats and dogs pass eggs in the feces which, under appropriate conditions of moisture, warmth, and sandy soil, hatch out into infective larvae. Children are most commonly infested while playing in sand piles, and this is often an occupational disease in plumbers.

Systemic Therapy

Thiabendazole (Mintezol) is given in severe infestation when topical therapy is impractical. The medication is used as tablets or suspension at 10 mg. per pound of body weight twice daily for 2 to 3 days (See manufacturer's official directive regarding duration of treatment). Side effects are common, including nausea, dizziness, and stomach distress.

Topical Therapy

When infestation covers limited areas of the body, topical thiabendazole (Mintezol) may be applied directly to the lesion or under Saran Wrap. (Topical use of thiabendazole is not listed in the manufacturer's official directive.) If used without airtight occlusion, it should be washed off and reapplied four to five times daily. It is rubbed in well at the most active end of the sandworm track. The medication is sticky and marshmallow flavored for oral use, but is quite practical for topical therapy.

Course of Disease

When using systemic thiabendazole, usually pruritus ceases within a few days. The tracks begin to show less redness with resolution, and swelling starts to regress. Often patients may develop transient urticaria caused by the dying larvae; in most instances, this is not to be confused as an allergic reaction to the medication.

When topical therapy alone is used, one sees "survival of the fittest" in its truest state. Some larvae die quickly; others are resistant. The length of treatment needed is directly proportional to the number of larvae present and may require 1 to 3 weeks of therapy. Most infestations may be handled adequately with topical therapy alone.

Other Measures

Reassurance and explanation of the disease process are welcomed by mothers, because small children are most commonly involved. They should be told that there is no multiplication of worms in the human body, and that when the involvement is on the buttocks, the worms do not ordinarily parasitize the mucous membrane of the rectum.

Since pruritus is severe, excoriations and secondary bacterial infection are common. The application of a topical antibiotic such as bacitracin or erythromycin gluceptate (Ilotycin) is a valuable local treatment.

Other adjuncts of some value, although they are not anthelmintic, are oral trimeprazine (Temaril) for itching and, occasionally, systemic steroids. The latter alter the inflammatory response considerably and give much relief in severe cases. Ice cold compresses often give relief from itching when other measures fail. Freezing the lesions with Freon, ethyl chloride, or liquid nitrogen is not now recommended. Only about one third can be "blistered out," and this method is somewhat outdated.

DECUBITUS ULCER

method of
JESS R. YOUNG, M.D.
Cleveland, Ohio

Reddened Areas

The major emphasis in any decubitus ulcer care program must be prevention. The skin of all patients, particularly those at high risk for decubitus ulcer development, must be watched constantly. Once any area of skin becomes reddened, pressure on this area must be minimized 100 per cent of the time. The patient should be turned at least every 2 hours while he is awake, and the time of turning should be recorded on a "turning sheet." If this regimen is followed, decubitus ulcers will not develop.

Other measures can be used to aid in the program:

1. A foam rubber mattress template with a silicon gel flotation pad insert works very well, provided that the foam rubber mattress is placed on a regular mattress and is covered by one sheet. The flotation pad is inserted in this foam rubber mattress, encased in a stocking net. The pad should never be covered with a pillow case; nor should Chuxs be used.

2. An air mattress may help if the apparatus is not defective, if the patient does not weigh too much, and if only one sheet is applied over the mattress. If Chuxs are needed, the air mattress does not work well.

3. A sheepskin will offer protection if the patient does not sweat excessively. It is especially good for protecting the heels and elbows. If Chuxs are needed under the buttocks, the sheepskin is not effective.

4. Protective boots help protect the feet and heels.

5. If the patient is old or has dry skin, a skin lotion with a lanolin base (such as Lanolor) should be used instead of soap for his daily bath (soap tends to dry out the skin).

6. The skin can be sprayed with tincture of benzoin to protect it. Cover this sprayed area with powder afterward.

7. Castellani's paint or gentian violet is effective if there is weeping from the reddened areas.

8. A water bed may be effective in minimizing pressure, but some patients suffer fear and insecurity while in such a bed.

9. An inexpensive "water bed" can be devised by filling an ordinary camping air mattress with water, and by using an electric blanket beneath the mattress to keep the water at body temperature.

10. The Stryker Circ-O-Lectric bed may also be effective in minimizing pressure on reddened areas.

Ulcerated Areas

1. All the measures used in the treatment of "reddened areas" are also effective in the treatment of open ulcerations. However, when the ulcer is present, the minimizing of pressure on the area 100 per cent of the time becomes absolutely mandatory.

Any or all of the following measures may be tried, but their effectiveness has been questionable:

1. A heat lamp should be set up about 12 inches from the area, and used for 15 minutes four times daily.

2. Paint the edges of the open areas with tincture of benzoin.

3. After cleansing with hexachlorophene (pHisoHex), Wescodyne or potassium permanganate (1:10,000) soaks can be used several times daily.

4. After cleansing with pHisoHex, a mixture of equal amounts of magnesium–aluminum hydroxide (Maalox) (or milk of magnesia) and granulated sugar is applied to the area. The ulcer is cleansed, and the mixture is changed daily.

5. Fibrinolysin and desoxyribonuclease (Elase) ointment can be used if debridement is a problem. The ulcer in the surrounding area must be watched carefully when this is used because of the danger of sensitization.

6. Spread 10 per cent ichthammol (Ichthyol) in Lassar's paste thickly on a gauze sponge large enough to cover the ulcer and its borders. Press this firmly against the skin. Cover with a large, soft dressing such as an abdominal (ABD) pad. Change the dressing every day. When changing the dressing, any adherent paste can be removed easily with a gauze sponge saturated with mineral oil.

7. Oxygen therapy can be tried for very deep and draining areas. The areas are irrigated with hydrogen peroxide and then washed with hexachlorophene (pHisoHex). A hole is punched in the bottom of a large wax paper container (such as is used at the bedside to hold ice for the patients), and then an oxygen catheter with 100 per cent oxygen running is placed in the bottom of this container. The open mouth of the container is placed against the ulcer for a 15 to 20 minute period daily.

CONTACT DERMATITIS

method of
F. A. THOMAS, M.D.
Kansas City, Missouri

Coping with the many manifestations of contact dermatitis requires an awareness of possible eliciting agents; this knowledge admixed with the distribution (location) of the lesions can usually result in an accurate diagnosis and hence guide successful therapy. Other useful aids would be a history of exposure to new agents, chemicals, working conditions, or personal activities. At times the agent can be an item in the patient's environment that has been used before without incident. Common offenders would include cosmetics, jewelry, Rhus, and the like.

Also helpful in proper treatment is an understanding of two basically distinct types of reactions: allergic contact dermatitis and primary irritant dermatitis. Allergic contact dermatitis is distinguished from primary irritant dermatitis by its ability to occur in sensitized persons. Even a small amount of antigen can elicit an enormous response in sensitized persons. In contradistinction, primary irritant dermatitis does not depend on previous antigen sensitization, but instead occurs from agents that would produce irritation in most persons with sufficient exposure.

Topical Therapy

Topical therapy can be divided into three stages, each with its own particular mode of therapy. At times the stages may overlap, and hence one type of therapy can be used in more than one stage. Most eruptions show this transitional morphology as they improve (i.e., acute eruptions becoming subacute).

Acute Dermatitis. Acute dermatitis consists of vesicular or oozing skin with much edema, burning, or itching. Lesions can be overtly bullous. Wet dressings are the mainstay until the oozing and vesiculation subside.

1. Burow's wet dressing (1 Domeboro tablet per pint of cool water) applied for 10 to 15 minutes two or three times daily.

2. Colloidal oatmeal wet dressing (1 teaspoon of Aveeno colloidal oatmeal powder to 1 quart [liter] of water). For larger extensive areas, a soothing bath in colloidal oatmeal can be used.

3. Sodium chloride (2 teaspoons in a quart [liter] of water yields a 0.9 per cent solution). This can be used as wet compresses or soaks.

4. Potassium permanganate compresses applied 15 minutes three times daily (one 1½ grain tablet [100 mg.] per quart [liter] of water). When used warm, these compresses work well for infected areas.

Subacute Dermatitis. In subacute dermatitis there is generally less oozing and less edema, as well as some subsidence in appearance. The aforementioned preparations can be used, as well as the following lotions:

1. Hydrocortisone with menthol and camphor (Heb-Cort MC), 0.25 per cent. This is very useful as a local antipruritic agent because of its menthol and camphor ingredients. It also has 0.25 per cent hydrocortisone for anti-inflammatory effect. In addition, it works well on Rhus dermatitis.

2. Corticosteroid lotions. These can be used when pure corticosteroid effect is desired. Flurandrenolide (Cordran) lotion and triamcinolone (Kenalog) lotion are both useful. A suitable shake lotion can be made by mixing 90 ml. of sterile distilled water with 15 grams of betamethasone valerate (Valisone) cream. Menthol 0.5 per cent can be added to the shake lotion for added antipruritic effect.

Chronic Dermatitis. Generally dry type lesions with some thickening and scaling are present. The mainstays of therapy are the corticosteroid creams and ointments. In general creams have better cosmetic acceptance and the ointments have better vasoconstrictive effects. Usually the thicker, dried, and lichenified lesions respond better to ointments than to creams.

The fluorinated topical steroids are preferred when maximal effect is desired. I frequently use betamethasone valerate (Valisone) or fluocinonide (Lidex) preparations. Betamethasone valerate has the added advantage of being paraben-free. Other effective topical corticosteroids are flurandrenolide (Cordran), fluocinolone (Synalar), and triamcinolone (Aristocort, Kenalog).

Systemic Therapy

The type and amount of systemic therapy are dependent upon the extent and severity of the dermatitis as well as upon the presence or absence of seondary infection.

Antihistamines. For moderate cases of contact dermatitis the use of antihistamines and antipruritics is helpful in alleviating some discomfort. Commonly used agents are diphenhydramine (Benadryl), hydroxyzine (Atarax), and cyproheptadine (Periactin). Sedation seems least with Atarax. All three preparations are available in syrups or elixirs for accurate pediatric dosage.

Antibiotics. Secondary infection complicating contact dermatitis is an indication for systemic antibiotics. Usually the organism is in the gram-positive spectrum and is susceptible to such antibiotics as erythromycin (Erythrocyn, E-Mycin) or clindamycin (Cleocin). A culture should be done to confirm the organism's sensitivity to specific antibiotics. I prefer to avoid the penicillins in the presence of pre-existing dermatitis unless sensitivity studies show resistance to other agents.

Corticosteroids. The use of corticosteroids should be reserved for severe and extensive cases of acute contact dermatitis, bearing in mind their contraindications and side effects.

Most cases of moderately severe involvement will respond to the following tapered dose of prednisone: 40 mg. daily for 2 days, then decreasing 5 mg. every other day for a total of 2 weeks (i.e., 40, 40, 35, 35, 30, 30, mg.). This schedule may be modified for especially severe cases by starting at 60 mg. of prednisone per day and following the same tapered dose over 3 weeks. For elderly patients, triamcinolone (Kenacort, Aristocort) may be used, because it does not cause water retention. Corticosteroids are pharmacologically more effective if given each morning in one dose: an antacid preparation may be added the first few high dosage days. For children, dexamethasone (Decadron elixir) and betamethasone (Celestone) syrup are useful. They are given in one third to one half the adult dose, depending on the weight of the child.

Persistent Dermatitis

Chronic dermatitis that follows an episode of contact dermatitis must be carefully evaluated. Low-grade contact dermatitis may arise from allergy to various preservatives used in medicaments (e.g., parabens, ethylenediamine, EDTA) or to one of the active ingredients used in medicaments (e.g., neomycin, nitrofurazone). Another possibility to consider is persistence of the dermatitis from the use of ill-advised home remedies. Cross-sensitivities of various medications must be explored, because some systemic preparations cross-react with chemically related topical agents.

Prevention

Prevention is usually possible once the causative agent is identified. In the case of cosmetics, suitable hypoallergenic products are available (Almay, Allercream, Ar-Ex, Marcel). For most industrial allergens, either protective clothing or removal from suffices. For hand eruptions a suitable barrier cream may be worthwhile.

DERMATITIS HERPETIFORMIS
(Duhring's Disease)

method of
HARRY IRVING KATZ, M.D.,
and STEVEN EARL PRAWER, M.D.
Fridley, Minnesota

Introduction

Dermatitis herpetiformis (DH) is a cutaneous disease of unknown cause characterized by chronic pruritus, multiform skin lesions, occult gastrointestinal pathology (gluten-induced enteropathy), and dramatic response to test doses of either sulfones or sulfapyridine. The intensity of the patient's pruritus can lead to deep excoriations, pigmentary changes, and scar formation that obscure the primary grouped (herpetiform) macules, papules, and discrete small tense vesicles distributed in a symmetrical mirror image–like fashion over the scalp, elbows, scapulae, buttocks, and knee regions. Diagnostic confirmation includes light microscopic fibrin and polymorphonuclear subepidermal papillary microabscesses, along with deposits of IgA on direct immunofluorescence found in clinically normal skin.

Treatment

Systemic treatment is necessary because topical measures are disappointing. Long-term maintenance treatment with either one of the sulfones or sulfapyridine, along with certain dietary restrictions is the mainstay of therapy for DH. However, screening tests should be obtained prior to institution of even test doses of these medications. We routinely obtain a complete blood count (CBC), glucose-6-phosphate dehydrogenase (G-6-PD), SMA-12, and urinalysis. A normal G-6-PD level is essential, because the sulfones and sulfapyridine can precipitate a hemolytic crisis in patients with deficient amounts of this enzyme. In addition, frequent clinical and laboratory follow-up is necessary because significant untoward side effects can occur, including headache, neurologic impairment (peripheral neuropathy), gastrointestinal disturbance, methemoglobinemia, thrombocytopenia, hemolytic anemia, leukopenia, agranulocytosis, aplastic anemia, renal damage, hepatitis, toxic epidermal necrolysis, and a variety of other cutaneous eruptions. We obtain a complete blood count and reticulocyte counts every 1 to 2 weeks until the patient is stabilized. Follow-up CBC, SMA-12, and methemoglobin determinations are obtained at 3 to 6 month intervals.

Dapsone (Avlosulfone)* is one of the more commonly used sulfones and is dispensed as either 25 mg. or 100 mg. tablets. Although not mentioned as an official indication, Dapsone is frequently used in DH. We start the patient on dapsone, 25 mg. four times daily. Usually within 24 to 48 hours, the patient has a prompt response, becoming asymptomatic and noting a cessation in the development of new lesions. Although a dosage of dapsone greater than 100 mg. per day occasionally may be necessary, caution must be used, because the incidence of side effects increases. Maintenance dosage of dapsone is determined by the gradual reduction in the amount that is given consistent with the signs and symptoms in a particular patient. The usual daily maintenance dose is 25 to

*This use of dapsone is not listed in the manufacturer's official directive.

100 mg. of dapsone per day. Alternatively, sulfapyridine (0.5 gram tablets) can be used instead of dapsone. After an initial dose of 2 to 6 grams per day in divided dosage, a maintenance level of 0.5 to 2 grams per day may be necessary. However, with sulfapyridine, increased oral intake of water and/or alkalization of urine are necessary to prevent crystallinuria. Follow-up urinalysis with microscopic examination is recommended if sulfapyridine is used.

The adjunctive elimination of iodides, iodine, and gluten from the diets of patients with DH is a measure that may help prevent exacerbations or contribute to the establishment of the lowest maintenance dose of either dapsone or sulfapyridine. A gluten-free diet can be very limiting; however, in a few patients with DH, scrupulous adherence to such a regimen may achieve a complete remission without any medications. Most patients need a combination of dietary restrictions and long-term dapsone or sulfapyridine in order to control their disease.

ATOPIC DERMATITIS

method of
JAMES J. LEYDEN, M.D.
Philadelphia, Pennsylvania

Atopic dermatitis is unquestionably one of the most common dermatologic problems. In general, diagnosis is not difficult except for certain localized forms of the disease. Many highly effective therapeutic agents are available, and yet the overall management of this disorder remains a challenge. Successful therapy, as in all chronic conditions characterized by frequent relapses, involves patient education and compliance.

Patient Education

Patients and/or their parents must be taught that atopic dermatitis represents an inherited tendency for their skin to become irritated, pruritic, and eventually inflamed. Parents often are misinformed that they or their child has an "allergy," and they go from doctor to doctor searching for the cure for this "allergy." Patients must learn that their skin is "different," and that it will itch and become irritated and inflamed by situations and materials which tend not to bother the rest of the population. For example, it has been experimentally demonstrated that atopic dermatitis patients have a lowered threshold for pruritic stimuli which can be set off by such normally harmless factors as wool fibers or exercise. Experimental data have also established that the skin of those with atopic dermatitis is significantly more susceptible to low grade irritants such as soaps and environmental changes. It is also clear that, as is commonly seen in any chronic disease, excessive emotional stress can result in exacerbations of atopic dermatitis.

Patients and parents in particular should know that, despite all attempts to prevent flare-ups, these will periodically occur and that they are not the "fault" of the family. Parents should also be counseled about the potential problem of children's sensing that exacerbations of their eczema symptoms lead to parental guilt feelings and undue secondary gain. Care must be taken to ensure that children with eczema do not become unduly protected and lead special lives.

Prevention of Trouble

1. Keep the infant's nails clipped to prevent undue excoriations.
2. Avoid wool fibers.
3. Bathe with lukewarm water and in the winter months follow with a lubricant such as Eucerin or Vaseline Intensive Care Lotion applied to *damp* skin. Lubricants trap moisture and minimize scaling and cracking of the skin which provoke pruritus and eventually lead to dermatitis.
4. Use mild soaps only, e.g., Dove or Neutrogena, and stress that mildness is only relative and that excessive washing with these soaps can be irritating.
5. Avoid overheated bedrooms and excessive use of covers.
6. Don't be upset if a child itches after playing—overheating stimulates itching. The benefit of playing far outweighs the price of a temporary itch.
7. Avoid physical contact with relatives with active herpes simplex lesions, and avoid smallpox vaccination or contact with those recently vaccinated. Patients with atopic dermatitis are far more susceptible to severe generalized viral infection.

Diet

No evidence exists to clearly implicate dietary factors. Occasionally children will develop hives from certain foods—e.g., albumin—which can then precipitate enough itching and scratching to instigate a full-scale attack of atopic dermatitis. Such situations are uncommon, and the common practice of eliminating one food after another produces frustrated parents and does not benefit the patient. Testing for immediate-type allergy is of little use in the management of atopic dermatitis.

Pruritus

No single truly antipruritic drug exists. Antihistamines are useful. The drug I find most useful is hydroxyzine (Atarax). Children and adults alike with atopic dermatitis often tolerate and require what seem like relatively high doses. The dose should be pushed till benefit or drowsiness occurs, particularly at bedtime. A good dose one half hour before intended sleep will lead to a peaceful night for patient and parent alike.

Management of Acute Flares of Dermatitis

When the skin becomes acutely inflamed and pruritic and is oozing, I employ cool tap water compresses for 5 to 10 minutes four times daily, followed by application of a fluorinated steroid cream or ointment (e.g., Synalar or Valisone). There is now strong evidence to endorse the common practice of adding an antibiotic, either topically if the dermatitis is localized or systemically in the form of erythromycin if the dermatitis is widespread. Nearly every patient who has oozing and crusting of the skin lesions will contain sufficient levels of *Staphylococcus* that the addition of an antibiotic produces significant benefit. Antibiotics are of use only in the first few days to a week. Subsequently, as oozing and crusting subside, antibiotic therapy should be discontinued. Once the acute dermatitis has been controlled, I switch patients to a nonfluorinated steroid such as desonide (Tridesilon) or to a 1 per cent hydrocortisone preparation (Hytone). Once there is no further inflammation, topical steroids are discontinued and hydroxyzine (Atarax) is used as needed. A common mistake made at this point is to fail to make sure that the patient has medicaments on hand at home for the next occasion, which surely will come. Patients tend to have less trouble as they get older, but they never lose the tendency; when and if conditions are correct, an acute attack will result.

For severe, generalized attacks (more than 50 per cent of body surface involved), I employ systemic erythromycin, 250 mg. four times daily, and systemic steroids, 1 to 2 mg. per kg. per day. This is an entirely safe short-term procedure in an otherwise healthy patient and produces rapid clinical improvement. Widespread application of fluorinated steroids is extremely expensive and usually also results in a systemic steroid effect. After 7 to 10 days patients can be quickly weaned from systemic steroid and switched to a topical agent to apply to residual areas of dermatitis. As long as doctor and patient clearly view systemic steroids as a *short-term* modality, the benefit far exceeds the extremely small risk involved.

Localized Frequently Misdiagnosed Atopic Dermatitis

Two localized forms of atopic dermatitis are commonly misdiagnosed by nondermatologists: (1) scalp and (2) foot involvement.

On the scalp atopic dermatitis appears as a severe flaking (dandruff-like) with moderate to severe pruritus. A clinical clue is found in the history in that frequent shampooing does not control the scaling and, in fact, usually intensifies both scaling and pruritus, in contradistinction to the benefit seen in dandruff and seborrheic dermatitis. Another clue is age—dandruff is almost nonexistent in prepubertal children. Just as in atopic dermatitis of the body, the overuse of potential irritants such as detergent shampoos must be minimized. Gentle shampooing two to three times a week at most, with a shampoo such as Johnson's Baby Shampoo is usually sufficient to keep the scalp and hair clean and at the same time to avoid irritation. Application of fluocinolone (Synalar) solution or betamethasone valerate (Valisone) lotion two to three times daily is applied to pruritic areas or any area of frank dermatitis. Once itching and any rash are controlled, topical steroids are discontinued, with instructions to promptly restart if pruritus recurs.

The most frequently misdiagnosed form of atopic dermatitis is the variety localized on the feet. Typically, atopic dermatitis of the feet appears as a dry, scaling, fissuring dermatitis most pronounced on the balls of the feet and the undersurface of the toes. Characteristically, patients describe this condition as worsening in the winter and improving in the summer—similar to the usual course for atopic dermatitis elsewhere on the body. The usual misdiagnosis is that of "athlete's foot," implying a fungus infection. Typically fungus infections are most symptomatic in the summer, not in the winter; with fungus infections, moreover, usually one can find toe web and toenail involvement, which is not seen in atopic dermatitis. The treatment is the same as elsewhere—namely, cessation of all excessive washing and scrubbing, application of topical fluorinated steroids for the acute flare-up, and then nonfluorinated steroids or hydrocortisone until clear. In this form of atopic dermatitis, ointments are superior to creams because of the pronounced fissuring usually present.

NEURODERMATITIS

method of
WESLEY K. GALEN, M.D.
Birmingham, Alabama

Neurodermatitis is a disorder characterized by symptoms of intense itching or burning. Skin signs of this disorder may include scaling, hyperpigmentation or hypopigmentation, erythema, excoriations, erosions, and lichenification (thickening of the skin), frequently to the point of plaque or nodule formation. These changes are the result of chronic scratching or rubbing by the patient. Classically it has been subdivided into localized neurodermatitis or lichen simplex chronicus, and generalized neurodermatitis or atopic dermatitis. The latter disorder is discussed on pages 599 to 600. This discussion will be limited to lichen simplex chronicus and its variants and will not include considerations of other skin signs of neuroses or psychoses such as trichotillomania, neurotic excoriations, delusions of parasitosis, or factitial dermatitis. It will not cover generalized pruritus, which may be caused by any number of conditions from cholinergic urticaria to essential pruritus caused by serious underlying disorders.

Lichen simplex chronicus may develop at any location on the body, but appears most frequently to involve certain areas such as the neck, lower legs, ankles, scalp, vulva, scrotum, or perianal area. Since it is a diagnosis of exclusion, it is most important that underlying or associated dermatoses be searched for and treated. For instance, contact dermatitis to nickel in jewelry may initiate and perpetuate dermatitis on the neck; xerosis or venous stasis may underlie dermatitis of the lower legs or ankles; yeast vaginitis or intertrigo may precipitate intense vulvar or perianal pruritus. Treatment aimed at predisposing problems frequently helps in the treatment of lichen simplex chronicus. Once such factors have been considered, treatment of lichen simplex chronicus may be approached. It is important to remember that whatever the precipitating events, environmental or psychogenic, the patient is now suffering the consequences of a vicious itch-scratch cycle. Thickened and damaged skin is more vulnerable to pruritus than is normal skin; hence, unbearable pruritus may be elicited by numerous environmental and psychogenic stimuli—i.e., intense heat or cold, rough fabrics, or anxiety. Such pruritus demands scratching, so the skin is reinjured and made more and more vulnerable.

Treatment

Explaining these factors to the patient and emphasizing the role of rubbing and scratching in causing lichen simplex chronicus are of paramount importance. Reassurance is helpful. Rarely, psychiatric consultation is necessary.

Antihistamines such as hydroxyzine (Atarax, Vistaril), 25 to 50 mg. every 4 to 6 hours, (Temaril Spansules), every 12 hours, or cyproheptidine (Periactin), 4 mg. every 6 hours, may help by their sedative as well as antihistaminic effects.

Cool compresses with clear water or very dilute Domeboro solution may compete as effectively with itching as does pain, the inevitable consequence of intense scratching.

Topical steroid creams or ointments such as flurandrenolide (Cordran), fluocinonide (Lidex), betamethasone (Diprosone, Valisone, or Fluobate), triamcinolone (Aristocort, Kenalog), or hydrocortisone (Hytone, Nutracort) applied twice daily help significantly. Occasionally it is necessary to use these under occlusion (plastic wrap) to enhance their penetration through very thickened skin. It is important to monitor topical therapy, especially occlusive topical therapy, in order to avoid atrophy, telangiectasia, and stria formation which may develop after chronic use.

Rarely plaques of lichen simplex chronicus will defy these therapeutic attempts and will require the intralesional injection of steroids. Nodular lesions on the legs, known as prurigo nodularis, most frequently require this mode of therapy. Triamcinolone acetonide (Kenalog) diluted with isotonic saline or lidocaine (Xylocaine) to a concentration of 2 to 4 mg. per ml. may be infiltrated into such plaques or nodules. The patient should be advised that transient or permanent localized atrophy may follow this.

It is important to avoid the use of topical anesthetics (the 'caine preparations), topical antihistamines (e.g., diphenhydramine with calamine), and complex mixtures of antibiotics and steroids on these chronic lesions because of their sensitizing abilities. To superimpose a contact dermatitis on such irritated areas could be disastrous.

POISON IVY DERMATITIS

method of
WILLIAM L. EPSTEIN, M.D.
San Francisco, California

Exposure to poison ivy, poison oak, or poison sumac is the most common cause of allergic contact dermatitis in the United States. The result is an acute eczematous eruption, which fortunately heals in 2 to 3 weeks, barring intervention of complications or re-exposure to the offending allergen. No cure exists. Treatment is aimed at reducing morbidity.

The rash of poison ivy is red and itchy when it first appears; it rapidly becomes vesicular or blistery. If treatment is begun in the earliest phase with very potent corticosteroids such as fluocinonide (Topsyn Gel) 0.05 per cent, betamethasone benzoate (Benisone Gel), fluocinolone acetonide (Synalar HP) 0.2 per cent, or betamethasone valerate (Valisone) 0.1 per cent, three times daily, the rash may in some instances be prevented from its full development; certainly the patient is made much more comfortable. Once the blisters have appeared and the area is weeping, these corticosteroids are less effective. Also because of their high potency and tendency for increased absorption, they should not be used for long periods of time or over large areas of the body. If the rash has been present for several days, conventional therapy with cool soaks (Burow's solution 1:40), tepid baths (starch and soda, Aveeno), and shake lotions (calamine lotion without additives) are called for. Avoid overdrying and cracking of the skin. Topical antihistamines in the acute phase may induce contact sensitization. Systemically, aspirin in large doses (0.6 gram [10 grains] every 3 to 4 hours) or antihistamines in sedative doses may reduce pruritus. A hypnotic at bedtime (chloral hydrate, 0.5 to 2.0 grams [7½ to 30 grains]) is required occasionally. If edema becomes noticeable, as often happens when the dermatitis occurs on the face or genitalia, I use systemic corticosteroids (see Severe Dermatitis, below).

In the healing stages, when the skin is dry and scaly, pruritus is best controlled by use of topical corticosteroids.

Severe Dermatitis

The patient suffers agonizing discomfort from oozing, crusting, itching, and smarting. Therapy is active; all the stops are pulled. The patient is instructed to rest at home, compressing or bathing every 2 or 3 hours for 10 to 15 minutes at a time. Aspirin and sedatives are prescribed as needed. Systemic corticosteroids are used routinely unless specifically contraindicated. Best results are obtained with large amounts. I prefer repository corticotropin injection (ACTH Gel), 80 units, given intramuscularly twice daily on the first visit (the patient returns later for the second injection). Repeat single injections of 80 units of ACTH Gel, given on the third and fifth days, often suffice to control the disease, but in each case the dose and frequency of injection depend upon the response. The same degree of control requires an initial dose of 400 to 600 mg. of hydrocortisone or its equivalent (80 mg. of triamcinolone or methylprednisolone [Medrol]). The dose is reduced gradually over 7 to 10 days. Flare-ups occur when withdrawal is too rapid. The value of a very large initial dose cannot be overemphasized; most failures are recorded by physicians loath to administer a therapeutic dose.

Administration of poison ivy extracts is contraindicated in the management of the acute disease. Usually it produces no effect, but occasionally the dermatitis is aggravated by such misguided therapy.

Complications

A major cause for concern is the appearance of a secondary pyoderma. This hazard becomes significant whenever the patient is hospitalized. Complications of corticosteroid therapy always remain a possibility, but they rarely develop in short-term therapy of otherwise healthy persons. Uncommonly, nephrosis or nephritis may follow a bout of poison ivy dermatitis. Rarely granulomatous hypersensitivity follows use of zirconium-containing lotions.

Re-exposure most commonly accounts for a prolonged siege of dermatitis. The patient should be instructed to have potentially contaminated clothing, including shoes, towels, sheets, sleeping bags, and the like, washed or cleaned. The allergenic oleoresins are nonvolatile oils which oxidize very slowly or not at all in the absence of moisture. Fomites, such as children, animals, clothing, rocks or brush, tools, athletic or hiking equipment, furniture, automobiles, or accessories, may transfer the allergen to sensitive persons. Cross-reacting allergens are found in mango rind, cashew nut shell oil, India marking nut, and Japanese lacquer. Instruction in the nature of poison ivy allergens is a vital prophylactic measure. Avoidance of exposure may, however, prove impossible.

Prophylaxis

Many methods and treatments have been devised to destroy the plant or protect the patient. None is wholly effective.

Chemical destruction or physical removal of the plant may temporarily reduce exposure, but permanent eradication of the weed is not feasible; besides, indirect contact from fomites may occur.

Barrier creams, topical detoxicants, and the like give inadequate protection. Thorough washing after exposure does not prevent a severe dermatitis in highly sensitive persons; it may, however, reduce the reaction in those who are less sensitive. Harsh soaps and vigorous scrubbing offer no advantage over simple soaking in cool water.

Immunologic prophylaxis is possible. It is, however, a rigorous procedure demanding supervision by a physician. The danger of untoward effects is considerable. Large amounts of active allergens must be ingested over long periods of time; when therapy is stopped, sensitivity rapidly returns. This form of treatment should be reserved for very sensitive persons who for reasons of work or environment cannot avoid allergenic exposure. Of the experimentally proved agents (crude poison ivy oleoresin, synthetic pentadecyl catechol, and cashew nut shell oil), only the crude oleoresin is commercially available at this time. Many companies supply it in over-the-counter preparations, but these either are wholly inactive or are so dilute as to be valueless for prophylaxis.

A reliable active oleoresin is supplied by Hollister-Stier Laboratories (107 S. Division Street, Spokane, Washington 99202). The standard desensitization set contains 15 ml. each of 1:100, 1:50, and 1:25 dilutions of oleoresin in corn oil (a total of 1050 mg. of allergen). Instruction sheets are enclosed. The important point is to increase the dose of allergen in a dropwise fashion as rapidly as the patient's tolerance allows. Onset of itching means that the increment is too great. When this happens, the dose is reduced by 2 to 5 drops; after pruritus subsides, it is increased again. Other untoward reactions, such as dermatitis, urticaria, or dyshidrosis, may occur if the cardinal symptom of pruritus is ignored or not recognized. This preparation occasionally causes pruritus ani; dividing the dose tends to reduce this complication. The total dose for hyposensitization varies between 2000 and 3000 mg. (After the first set is completed, 1:25 dilutions should be used in doses of 1 to 1.5 ml. daily.) Once hyposensitization therapy is completed and the drug is stopped, sensitivity tends to return within 1 to 3 months so that many patients are required to remain on a maintenance dose all the year round. According to tolerance, this can be 1 to 2 ml. of 1:25 dilution twice a week.

SEBORRHEIC DERMATITIS

method of
JAMES W. BARD, M.D.
Lexington, Kentucky

Seborrheic dermatitis is very common. It is manifested as a red, slightly papular eruption which tends to have a greasy scale. It runs the gamut from a mild scruffy dandruff to acute, exudative, fiery red, and widespread lesions. The cause is not known, but circumstantial evidence implicates sebaceous gland activity. The disease is one of pubertal and postpubertal individuals and of infants still under maternal hormonal influence. Neurologic disease, such as parkinsonism and some seizure states, precipitates or worsens seborrheic dermatitis.

The treatment of seborrheic dermatitis is based on location and severity. In general, treatment is suppressive rather than curative. Patients are often unhappy to find that no simple lasting cure exists.

Scalp (the Most Commonly Affected Area)

For noninflammatory dandruff—i.e., an increase in scalp scaliness with little or no associated erythema—increase the frequency of shampooing. Two or three times a week is a minimum; more commonly, alternate days or even daily. The brand of shampoo is not so important as the frequency of use and instructing the patient to shampoo the scalp and not the hair. Popular over-the-counter shampoos are usually effective.

For more resistant dandruff, use one of the keratolytic, sulfur, or selenium sulfide shampoos. Selenium sulfide shampoos, represented by Selsun or Exsel, should not be used more than twice a week. X-Seb shampoo with and without tar contains 4 per cent salicylic acid. Zincon contains zinc pyrithione and is similar to Head and Shoulders shampoo. Sebulex and Capitrol are also effective. These may all be used daily if necessary.

For dandruff plus erythema and more papular lesions, shampoo as above and add a topical corticosteroid just after shampooing. Triamcinolone acetonide spray (Kenalog), 10 mg. per 150 grams, is used with a long tube to apply the spray to the scalp. Barseb Thera-Spray is similar and contains hydrocortisone. Betamethasone valerate lotion (Valisone 0.1 per cent) and betamethasone benzoate lotion (Flurobate 0.025 per cent) or fluocinolone acetonide solution (Synalar 0.01 per cent) may also be used.

For rather thick and crusty lesions, pretreat with 5 per cent liquor carbonis detergens in Nivea oil for 6 to 8 hours before shampooing, and follow with topical corticosteroids as above. The treatment should be repeated daily until the skin is clear. As the dermatitis improves, instruct the patient to use the minimum treatment necessary to keep the eruption under control.

If the seborrheic dermatitis is complicated by secondary infection from excoriations, use an appropriate systemic antibiotic. Systemic corticosteroids in uncomplicated scalp involvement are seldom or never indicated.

Face (Erythema and Scaling of the Eyebrows and Paranasal Areas)

Extension of seborrheic dermatitis from the paranasal to the malar areas makes a "butterfly" rash, which can be distinguished from the rash of lupus erythematosus by chronicity, morphology, and the presence of other areas of skin involved with typical seborrheic dermatitis.

For mild slightly scaly and red areas, wash the face with mild castile, Neutrogena, or Purpose soap twice daily, using the fingers to massage the lather around. Rinse well and apply hydrocortisone cream ¼ or ½ per cent.

For more red and papular lesions use 1 per cent hydrocortisone lotion or desonide cream (Tridesilon). Avoid using fluorinated topical steroids on the face so as not to cause atrophy and telangiectasia.

If topical steroids fail, switch to 40 per cent sulfur in Aquaphor for a time and then return to topical hydrocortisone.

If the eruption is very red and the scales appear moist, proceed as in the following paragraph.

Intertriginous Areas (Axillae, Chest, Inframammary, Umbilical, and Retroauricular)

Seborrheic dermatitis in these areas tends to follow a course of acute dermatitis with erythema and exudation to chronic dermatitis with epidermal hypertrophy and scaling. In the latter stages the lesions are hard to differentiate from psoriasis. However, the treatment for both diseases is the same.

In the presence of any weeping dermatitis, wet dressings are in order. Domeboro or Bluboro is mixed, 1 packet to 1 pint of water, to make a modified Burow's solution and is applied via a saturated cotton cloth left in place for about 1 hour two to three times a day. The wet pack is followed with topical corticosteroid lotion such as flurandrenolide (Cordran *lotion* 0.05 per cent) or triamcinolone lotion (Kenalog 0.1 per cent).

If the eruption is widespread and acute, a course of a systemic steroid may be indicated. Prednisone is given at a starting dose of 50 mg. and is reduced by 5 mg. each succeeding day.

As the dermatitis subsides, use the *cream* or *ointment* forms of the aforementioned topical steroids.

Intertriginous seborrheic dermatitis is occasionally complicated by secondary opportunistic Candida and bacterial infections manifested as pustules and purulent discharge. Culture will reveal which is present. Topical nystatin is effective for Candida. (Be cautious in using a cream containing the preservative ethylenediamine, as it is a common cause of skin sensitization and contact dermatitis.) Systemic antibiotics are used for bacterial infections. Topical antibiotics are of little help. Since infection in this instance is a secondary phenomenon, treating the primary seborrheic dermatitis should heal both.

Most chronic external otitis is really seborrheic dermatitis and can be treated with a plain corticosteroid solution such as outlined for Dandruff plus Erythema, above.

Crural seborrheic dermatitis occurs most often in infants. Distinguish it from diaper dermatitis by involvement of the creases in the skin. Diaper dermatitis tends to spare the creases, whereas seborrheic dermatitis begins in the crural folds. Gentle washing with soap and application of a dilute hydrocortisone lotion such as ¼ per cent Nutracort lotion should be effective.

STASIS DERMATITIS AND ULCERS

method of
JOHN C. MAIZE, M.D.
Buffalo, New York

Stasis dermatitis and stasis ulceration are due to the increased hydrostatic pressure in the superficial veins of the leg, which occurs when the valves of the deep venous system and calf perforating veins become incompetent. This is commonly the result of destruction of the deep venous valves during recanalization of a thrombus. These valves may also degenerate with age, and poorly understood genetic factors can result in their premature degeneration. When the hydrostatic pressure in the cutaneous capillaries exceeds the colloid osmotic pressure, edema forms, followed by diapedesis of red blood cells and structural changes in the capillaries. Marked venous congestion can result in ischemic necrosis of the epidermis, which is followed by ulceration. Trauma in the presence of marked hypostatic edema may also precipitate ulceration.

Stasis changes are rarely the result of primary lymphedema or lymphedema secondary to lymphatic obstruction by tumor or lymphangitis unless complicated by venous insufficiency. Edema resulting from congestive heart failure, cirrhosis, nephrosis, or hypoproteinemia may complicate venous insufficiency and must be looked for and treated appropriately.

Stasis changes predominantly involve the skin of the lower third of the leg. Edema is the sine qua non of stasis dermatitis. Initially it is soft and pitting, but eventually it becomes brawny. Mottled pigmentation results from deposition of hemosiderin and increased melanin production secondary to inflammation. Erythema, scaling, and fissuring signal the development of stasis dermatitis. This may progress to epidermal erosion, oozing, and crusting. Vesiculation is not seen unless there is superimposed contact dermatitis to medications or impetiginization. Pruritus commonly leads to lichenification by chronic rubbing. Varicose veins are commonly present. Stasis ulcers develop on the medial aspect of the leg, usually over the malleolus or just superior to it.

Topical therapy alone will provide only modest or temporary relief of symptoms. Prolonged improvement can be achieved and maintained only by alleviating the increased pressure in the superficial venous system. Pressure gradient therapy is often effective in reaching this goal. Venous insufficiency is a lifelong disease, and the degree of therapeutic success correlates directly with the patient's insight and cooperation as well as the follow-up control provided by the physician.

Stasis Dermatitis

The involved skin of patients with stasis dermatitis is particularly prone to the development of allergic contact dermatitis. Two classes of medication are the most common offenders. These are the topical 'caine-type anesthetics, which are used for relief of pruritus, and the topical antibiotics, particularly neomycin, which are commonly prescribed for real or suspected infection. The patient should be cautioned not to apply these to his skin; the same holds true for any other products not specifically prescribed by the physician.

Acute Stasis Dermatitis. A short period of bed rest with the affected leg elevated is necessary to reduce edema. The dermatitis will not resolve until the edema is reduced. Pressure therapy ordinarily is not well tolerated during the acute phase.

Open wet dressings should be applied every 4 hours for 15 to 20 minutes, using four to six layers of soft roll gauze (Kerlix) or strips of a clean soft sheet soaked with tepid tap water. Burow's solution diluted 1:20 or 1:40, potassium permanganate 1:8000, or isotonic saline solution may also be used, but these probably add little to the effect of plain water.

After soaking, 1 per cent hydrocortisone cream or a fluorinated steroid cream is applied sparingly to the area. Ointments should be avoided during the acute phase, because they interfere with evaporation and may lead to maceration.

Subacute or Chronic Stasis Dermatitis. Wet dressings should be discontinued, because excessive drying of the skin may produce fissures.

Topical steroids should be continued to be applied four times a day. An ointment or emollient base is often tolerated better than a water-washable cream base.

Secondary Infection. Secondary infection is common in all phases of stasis dermatitis and may present as either impetigo or erysipelas. If there is evidence of secondary infection, a culture should be taken and appropriate systemic antibiotic therapy initiated, depending upon the results of the sensitivity studies. Topical antibiotics are not ordinarily effective, and some may lead to sensitization.

Follow-up Care. After the dermatitis resolves, the topical corticosteroids should be discontinued, because long-term use of fluorinated steroids may produce atrophy. Hydration of the skin can be maintained by the application of an emollient cream such as Eucerin or unscented cold cream.

Stasis Ulcer

If stasis dermatitis is present, the measures outlined above should be used.

Bed rest should be maintained, with the affected leg elevated until gross edema is reduced.

Necrotic tissue and crusts must be removed to encourage the growth of granulation tissue at the ulcer base. Crusts may be removed by using tepid tap water compresses twice daily for 20 minutes to soften them, followed by grattage with dry 4 × 4 gauze pads. This usually suffices also for loose necrotic debris. For more tenacious necrotic material, collagenase (Santyl) is useful. This should be applied to the ulcer bed overnight, followed by wet compresses and gauze grattage in the morning. Burow's solution must not be used, because it will inactivate the enzyme. If available and convenient, daily whirlpool treatments are efficient for debridement and accomplish this with a minimum of discomfort. Thick eschars may sometimes require surgical debridement, but this procedure is painful and adequate local anesthesia is often difficult to obtain when the ulcer is large.

Colonization of the ulcer by mixed flora is the rule rather than the exception and does not require specific therapy. Infection, manifest by a purulent exudate or cellulitis in the skin surrounding the ulcer, should be managed by appropriate systemic antibiotic therapy as determined by culture and sensitivity studies. Pseudomonas infection often responds well to wet compresses of ¼ to ½ per cent acetic acid solution applied for 20 minutes four times daily.

Between compresses the ulcer should be covered with a Telfa dressing secured by paper tape. Packing of the ulcer with such materials as absorbable gelatin or sugar does not hasten healing but does create difficulty in cleaning the ulcer.

For recalcitrant ulcers, excision of the fibrous ulcer bed followed by skin grafting may be necessary.

Management of Venous Insufficiency

Adequate long-term control of stasis dermatitis and stasis ulcers depends upon relieving the increased pressure in the superficial venous system. This can be accomplished and maintained by pressure gradient therapy.

Severe edema and acute stasis dermatitis must be brought under control by bed rest and the methods previously outlined.

When ambulation becomes possible, the extremity should be wrapped with a 3 inch Ace bandage from the forefoot to the knee before the patient arises from bed. Greater pressure is applied to the foot and lower leg than to the upper leg in order to establish a gradient. The patient must be carefully instructed in the proper application. Several Ace bandages should be available so that soiled ones can be laundered.

If the patient is unable to use Ace bandages properly, an Unna's boot (Dome-Paste Bandage, Gelocast) may be applied instead. This should be changed every 4 to 7 days, depending upon the amount of exudate from the ulcer. As in the case of Ace bandages, the Unna's boot should be tighter around the foot and lower leg than the upper leg.

When most of the edema has subsided, the patient's leg should be measured accurately and custom fitted with a Jobst support stocking. This should be put on before arising in the morning and worn for the entire day. Ordinary elastic stockings and support hose are not usually effective. The Jobst stocking must be refitted periodically because of the gradual loss of elasticity.

Other helpful measures include (1) avoidance of long periods of standing; (2) intermittent rest periods during the day, with the legs elevated above the level of the heart; and (3) elevation of the foot of the bed.

Role of Surgery in the Management of Venous Insufficiency

Removal of the superficial venous system cannot be expected to remedy the basic problem, which is incompetency of the deep venous system. Varicosities may be eliminated, but elastic stockings will still be necessary to control edema. If an ulcer persists or recurs over the site of an incompetent perforator, ligation of the incompetent perforator can help prevent further ulceration at that site.

DERMATOMYOSITIS-POLYMYOSITIS

method of
CLARK HUFF, M.D.
Denver, Colorado

Polymyositis is an inflammatory disease of muscle defined by a combination of features: (1) symmetrical weakness of proximal muscles, (2) a characteristic muscle biopsy, (3) compatible electromyographic findings, and (4) elevated levels of skeletal muscle enzymes in the serum. In association with (5) characteristic skin findings, the disease is termed dermatomyositis. Present evidence supports an immunologic pathogenesis. As with other diseases diagnosed by clinical criteria, it is unclear whether cases diagnosed as dermatomyositis-polymyositis represent a homogeneous entity. For instance, the disease in children is somewhat different clinically and prognostically from the adult form. In addition, because of overlapping clinical features, other muscular and connective tissue diseases occasionally may be diagnosed as dermatomyositis-polymyositis. Such difficulties in defining the disease and in excluding other similar diseases have created some uncertainty in interpreting the results of therapeutic studies.

Before attempting any therapy, one should make every effort to verify the diagnosis. If three or four of the five proposed criteria cannot be met, other diagnoses should be seriously considered. If the diagnosis of dermatomyositis-polymyositis is relatively certain, the results of therapy must be closely scrutinized by monitoring the disease activity at weekly intervals. The serum levels of muscle enzymes (serum glutamic oxaloacetic transaminase [SGOT] or creatine phosphokinase [CPK]) and the strength of affected muscle groups are commonly used to gauge the results of therapy.

Treatment

Bed rest and physical therapy are important therapeutic recommendations for the patient acutely ill with marked weakness and muscle tenderness. As these symptoms resolve, activity may be gradually increased. Physical therapy is essential for prevention of permanent musculoskeletal deformities.

Glucocorticoid drugs remain the primary mode of therapy. Most therapists strongly advocate glucocorticoid therapy at high doses early in the course of disease, so that irreversible muscle destruction may be prevented. The earlier the drug is given, the greater the chance of a favorable response. Daily oral doses of prednisone of 1 to 2 mg. per kg. (60 to 120 mg. for an adult), either in divided or single morning doses, are given initially. The higher doses of prednisone and the divided dose schedule are usually reserved for the more severely ill patient. After a therapeutic response to the drug, as demonstrated by increasing muscle strength and decreasing serum levels of muscle enzymes, one should maintain the initially high prednisone dosage for 2 to 8 weeks. Subsequently, the goal is to maintain the response on the lowest possible dose of prednisone, given in a single morning dose. The initial decrease in prednisone dose may be relatively large (20 to 25 per cent of the initial dose); however, subsequent decreases in dosage should be much smaller (5 to 10 per cent of the initial dose every 2 weeks). If the disease exacerbates as the prednisone is withdrawn, the dosage should be increased until a remission is seen. If a moderate daily prednisone dosage is achieved (20 to 30 mg. in an adult), one should attempt to institute an alternate-day regimen in order to minimize the adverse effects of the drug. Glucocorticoid drugs themselves may cause a myopathy. If weakness increases without concomitant elevation of muscle enzymes, a steroid myopathy must be considered, and more rapid tapering of the prednisone or converting to an alternate-day regimen may be warranted. By carefully monitoring the parameters of disease activity, one may individualize the prednisone dosage for each patient. In many patients after months or even several years of therapy, the prednisone can be withdrawn completely.

Cytotoxic or immunosuppressive drugs have been used when 2 to 3 months of high dose glucocorticoid therapy was unsuccessful, or when the dosage of glucocorticoid required for control of the disease was dangerously high. These drugs are used as adjuncts to glucocorticoids; however, even for their "steroid-sparing" effects, they must be considered investigational. Intermittent methotrexate use (0.5 to 0.8 mg. per kg. per week) has been most successful for this purpose. Daily azathioprine (50 to 150 mg.) has also been used.

Since skin involvement in dermatomyositis is largely asymptomatic, topical therapy may be unnecessary. A bland lubricant may be helpful when scaling is a major complaint. Avoidance of ultraviolet light and use of a sun screen are helpful in the patient whose skin lesions are light induced. If the skin lesions are markedly inflammatory, use of a low to medium potency topical steroid drug, such as 1 per cent hydrocortisone, 0.01 per cent fluocinolone, or 0.025 per cent triamcinolone, may be valuable. Chronic use of potent topical steroids should be avoided because of the local cutaneous complications of these agents, such as atrophy and telangiectasia.

Therapy of calcinosis cutis, often the most disabling component of the disease in children, is exceedingly difficult. Both surgery and diphosphonate therapy have been helpful in individual patients.

Although the association of adult-onset dermatomyositis with malignancy appears to be real, the frequency of the association is not clear. Probably no more than 15 to 20 per cent of adults with dermatomyositis have associated malignancy. Response of dermatomyositis to removal of an associated cancer has been reported only rarely. Nevertheless, the adult with dermatomyositis should have a thorough evaluation for an associated neoplasm.

THE ERYTHEMAS

method of
ALAN H. SCHRAGGER, M.D.
Allentown, Pennsylvania

The traditional generic term of *erythemas* collects under one heading a miscellaneous group of diseases that share only a reaction pattern of vasodilation of the small vessels of the subpapillary plexus and dermal papillae. Those that have a known cause seem to represent a hyperactivity to a foreign substance, be it viral, bacterial, physical, or chemical. This commonality is based on morphologic descriptions of the varying patterns of erythemas of the skin—e.g., nodular, annular, marginal, or multiforme; these patterns will be discussed under suitable subheadings.

Erythema Nodosum

Erythema nodosum is important as a reaction pattern of response to immune complexes or sensitized lymphocytes. The reaction damages vessel walls and leads to extravasation with a characteristic bruising appearance. The lesions are primarily on the pretibial area as a diffuse deep red erythema, with induration and tenderness. Multiple nodules may appear and even coalesce. As evolution progresses, the extravasation gives rise to the appearance of a bruise; hence, the name erythema contusiformis. New crops of nodules may appear as old ones fade.

The disease is most common among women in the 20 to 30 year age group. Causes include the reaction to streptococcal infections, tuberculosis, sarcoidosis, viruses, yersiniae, mycoses, drugs, enteropathies, and malignancies. Initial investigation should include chest x-ray, antistreptolysin-O (ASO), skin tests, and an erythrocyte sedimentation rate (ESR) as an initial screen. Chest x-ray findings of bilateral lymphadenopathy, along with fever, a scalene node, and erythema nodosum, compose Löfgren's syndrome, which has been recognized as an entity accompanying sarcoid or of undetermined cause.

Therapy is best directed to the primary cause. If this is undetermined, bed rest and salicylates offer symptomatic relief. Oral steroids, although initially effective, are hard to discontinue because of recrudescences and therefore are to be avoided except in unusually severe cases and when the danger of aggravating an underlying cause—i.e., tuberculosis—has been eliminated.

Erythema Multiforme

Erythema multiforme is by far the most important of this group of diseases. This condition seems to be a step-up in severity of an allergic reaction from urticaria. The body response is more severe and persistent, and may progress to such damage of the lower level of the epidermis that bullae appear. The characteristic lesions of a gradually expanding circle of erythema, which clears in the center and then develops new lesions within, are widely known as iris or bull's eye lesions. These can progress to a more severe manifestation, with widespread bullae involving not only the skin but also the mucous membranes. The eyes, mouth, vulva, and rectum can be affected. Internal organs can have manifestations, with lungs, kidneys, and intestines reacting.

The cause is varied, with reactions attributed to immune response from a virus—in particular, herpes simplex, but also including poliomyelitis, mumps, orf, variola vaccines, and atypical pneumonia. Bacterial infections, mycotic infections, collagen vascular disease, and malignancies, with or without radiation therapy, can also be a cause. Drug reactions are often extremely severe, particularly to hydantoins, phenobarbital, penicillin, salicylates, sulfonamides, and phenolphthalein.

With early signs of only macules and papules, therapy can be expectant with high doses of hydroxyzine (Atarax), 200 to 400 mg. daily. The disease may progress rapidly; if widespread vesicles appear, steroids should be started at a level of 100 mg. of hydrocortisone every 4 hours. After stabilization, oral prednisone, 80 to 100 mg. daily, is indicated initially. Supportive care may be required. If a generalized bullous reaction develops (the Stevens-Johnson syndrome), sterile sheets, reverse isolation, intravenous fluids, and the support of a burn unit can be lifesaving. The most dangerous sequela is eye damage following corneal ulceration or panophthalmitis. An ophthalmologic consultant will usually recommend saline soaks, mydriatics, and topical antibiotics. The mouth may be very painful, with swollen desquamating membranes making swallowing impossible. Lidocaine (Xylocaine Viscous) as a mouthwash can be very helpful. After bullae have stopped appearing, the steroids can be tapered rapidly. Scarring of the skin is unusual, but there may be corneal opacities or synechiae. The usual course is 2 to 6 weeks, with a mortality of 5 to 15 per cent reported.

Other Erythemas

A group of erythemas may be described according to their morphologic appearance.

Erythema annulare centrifugum presents as spreading annular lesions with raised borders and some scaling. The cause is rarely delineated; it is felt to be an immunologic response.

Erythema chronica migrans is seen primarily as a reaction to the bite of a tick of the family Ioxididae. The lesion starts several weeks or months after the tick bite and spreads to enormous proportions. Penicillin or tetracycline is effective treatment.

Erythema gyratum perstans is seen in association with internal malignancies, with bizarre waves of woody-appearing erythema. The erythema may disappear after surgical removal of the primary lesion, only to reappear with the development of metastases.

Erythema marginatum rheumaticum is seen in about 10 per cent of children with rheumatic fever as pale, delicate rings of infiltrated erythema over the abdomen and trunk, usually lasting only a few hours. Recurrent crops are not uncommon.

Erythema ab igne is seen usually over the anterior skin of persons chronically exposed to fierce heat. The skin develops a chronically reticulated appearance with hyperpigmentation, telangectasias, and dryness. In later years, nodules and squamous cell carcinoma may develop. Avoidance of heat and emollients will give symptomatic relief, but the changes are irreversible.

Erythema elevatum diutinum has multiple, annular, firm, flat lesions with an elevated edge, frequently found on the dorsum of the hands of middle-aged persons. Histopathology shows leukocytoclasis and hyalin around capillaries, putting this condition in the allergic vasculitis classification and differentiating it from granuloma annulare. Therapy has given poor results, although dapsone (investigational for this use) has been reported effective.

Erythema induratum of Bazin has had a questionable relationship to the tubercle bacillus. It is seen as multiple, firm nodules, frequently with ulceration, that appear on the back of the lower legs of young women. Antituberculosis therapy has cleared some of these lesions; others clear in warm weather.

Erythema induratum of Whitfield is found in middle-aged women with chronic vascular insufficiency who develop painful nodules on the dorsum of the leg without ulceration and a histopathologic picture resembling that of nodular vasculitis. Therapy requires rest, elevation, diuresis, and treatment of infection if present. Cortisone can be helpful.

SUPERFICIAL FUNGUS INFECTIONS OF THE SKIN

method of
ANDREW H. RUDOLPH, M.D.
Houston, Texas

Superficial fungus infections of the skin can be divided into the superficial mycoses, dermatophytoses, and candidiasis.

SUPERFICIAL MYCOSES

Tinea Versicolor (Pityriasis Versicolor)

Tinea versicolor is a very common superficial fungus infection caused by the organism *Malassezia* (pityrosporon) *furfur*. Lesions usually consist of asymptomatic, scaly patches characteristically located on the upper trunk and neck. The disease may involve large areas of the skin, and a Wood's light examination is often helpful in assessing the extent of involvement. In winter the lesions are usually fawn to brown in color; but in summer, because the presence of the fungus interferes with normal tanning, the lesions will often appear lighter than the surrounding skin. With increased ultraviolet exposure, this color difference becomes more prominent and is often the reason the patient seeks medical help. Although treatment may eradicate the fungus infection, the patient should be advised that it may take many months to resolve this color difference.

Griseofulvin is not effective in the treatment of tinea versicolor, but numerous topical agents have been used with varying success. A satisfactory treatment, especially in those patients with extensive involvement, is the use of selenium sulfide (Selsun) shampoo. Following a bath or shower, the shampoo is applied as a lather to all areas of the skin from the neck down to the waist. The lather is allowed to dry for 30 minutes and is then rinsed off thoroughly. This regimen is repeated at weekly intervals for 2 weeks, and then once a month for 3 months. Between treatments with the selenium sulfide shampoo, a 25 per cent solution of sodium thiosulfate, used alone or in combination with 1 per cent salicylic acid in 10 per cent isopropyl alcohol and propylene glycol (Tinver lotion), should be applied twice daily to all visible scaly areas. Tolnaftate 1 per cent (Tinactin), haloprogin 1 per cent (Halotex), miconazole nitrate 2 per cent (MicaTin), or clotrimazole 1 per cent (Lotrimin) can also be used effectively, but these agents are expensive and for that reason are usually restricted to the treatment of limited infections.

The patient should be reassured that this is a benign disorder, but that recurrences, especially during the hot humid months, are common in susceptible persons. These recurrences usually respond to re-treatment and can be minimized by having the patient use a soap containing salicylic acid and sulfur after the initial therapy.

Tinea Nigra

Tinea nigra is a superficial fungus infection caused by the organism *Cladosporium wernecki.* The asymptomatic black or brownish-black macular lesions of tinea nigra generally occur on the palmar surface of the hand or, less commonly, on the plantar surface of the foot.

Treatment with a mild keralytic fungicide such as Whitfield's ointment is usually successful. Tincture of iodine, 2 per cent salicylic acid and 3 per cent sulfur ointment, or one of the newer topical agents such as clotrimazole 1 per cent (Lotrimin) can also be used. Topical tolnaftate (Tinactin) is reportedly ineffective, as is oral griseofulvin.

DERMATOPHYTOSES

Tinea Capitis

Tinea capitis is a fungus infection of the scalp and hair which usually occurs in children. It is uncommon in adults. Depending upon the degree of inflammation present, tinea capitis may be classified into noninflammatory and inflammatory types. The epidemic, noninflammatory type is most commonly caused by an anthropophilic fungus such as *Microsporum audouini* or *Trichophyton tonsurans* and is characterized by patchy alopecia, broken hairs, mild scaling, and minimal inflammation. Sporadic, inflammatory tinea capitis is usually due to a geophilic (soil) or zoophilic (animal) organism such as *Microsporum gypseum, Microsporum canis,* or *Trichophyton mentagrophytes.* Inflammatory tinea capitis usually presents with hair loss, inflammation, and pustulation of the scalp. In certain patients a painful, elevated, boggy, erythematous mass (kerion) may develop. In severe inflammatory tinea capitis, permanent hair loss may result. The classification of tinea capitis into noninflammatory and inflammatory types is arbitrary, and exceptions are common; for example, *T. tonsurans* can induce either a noninflammatory or an inflammatory response.

Topical therapy alone is not effective in the management of tinea capitis, and griseofulvin is indicated in the treatment of all types. Griseofulvin in the microcrystalline form (Fulvicin-U/F, Grifulvin V, Grisactin) is most commonly used. A dose of 5 mg. of the microcrystalline form of griseofulvin per pound (0.45 kg.) of body weight per day is usually adequate for children. Thus very small children can be treated with 125 mg. of griseofulvin suspension daily; children from 30 to 50 pounds (14 to 23 kg.), with 125 to 250 mg.

daily; and children over 50 pounds (23 kg.), with 250 to 500 mg. daily. A dose of 0.5 to 1 gram daily of griseofulvin microsize is usually adequate in most adult patients. Better gastrointestinal absorption of griseofulvin occurs when it is ingested after meals with a high fat content and when the total daily dosage is divided into two equal doses. Ultramicrosize griseofulvin (Gris-PEG) can also be used in approximately half the total dosage recommended for microcrystalline griseofulvin. However, except for enhanced bioavailability, the ultramicrosize preparation does not seem to offer any significant advantage, increased effectiveness, or added safety over the microsize form. The total dosage of griseofulvin must be individualized, and long periods of treatment may be required. Since incomplete treatment may be accompanied by relapse, it is best to continue the griseofulvin for 2 weeks after all clinical and laboratory examinations are negative. In most cases, the usual course of therapy is 6 to 8 weeks. Post-treatment follow-up should continue for an additional 6 to 8 weeks. Since griseofulvin is fungistatic rather than fungicidal, concomitant topical therapy is often helpful. The application of a mild topical antifungal agent may decrease dissemination of spores and infected particles and hasten resolution. Ointments can be used, but solutions are usually better accepted. Other adjuvant measures, such as clipping the hair around the lesion to facilitate shampooing, removal or restriction of infected fomites, and a search for a source of the infection, are indicated. Siblings should be examined and treated if infected. With modern therapy there is no justification for extensive absences from school.

In inflammatory tinea capitis moist compresses and thorough but gentle daily shampooing are helpful to keep the scalp clean and to promote drainage. Although a kerion looks like a severe bacterial infection, it is not and should be regarded as an allergic inflammatory response of the scalp to the presence of fungi in the hair follicle. Kerions are treated with griseofulvin in the same dosage and duration as noninflammatory tinea capitis. In some patients, systemic steroids for 1 to 2 weeks may be necessary to calm the inflammation. Topical fungicides can be used as previously indicated but are ineffective by themselves.

Tinea Barbae

This is usually an inflammatory fungus infection of the bearded area of the face and neck caused by various species of Trichophyton and Microsporum, but most commonly by *Trichophyton mentagrophytes* or *Trichophyton verrucosum.*

Tinea barbae is managed similarly to tinea capitis of the inflammatory (kerion) type. Wet compresses should be used to remove any crusts or scales. A topical antifungal agent such as clotrimazole 1 per cent (Lotrimin) or miconazole nitrate 2 per cent (MicaTin) can be applied topically, and griseofulvin should be administered orally.

Tinea Corporis

Dermatophyte infections of the glabrous skin can be used by many Microsporum and Trichophyton species or *Epidermophyton floccosum.*

These infections, if limited in area, can usually be managed successfully by topical treatment alone. Miconazole nitrate 2 per cent (MicaTin), clotrimazole 1 per cent (Lotrimin) or haloprogin 1 per cent (Halotex) should be applied twice daily to all involved areas, taking into consideration that the advancing border of the fungal infection may extend up to 6 cm. beyond the margin of the visible lesion. Following topical treatment, pruritus is usually relieved within 1 week, and cures are usually obtained within 3 to 6 weeks. To reduce the possibility of relapse, treatment should be continued for 1 week after all the lesions have cleared. In exceptional cases, prolonged topical treatment may be required.

Extensive cutaneous involvement, lesions at hard-to-reach sites, involvement of the hair follicle, or chronic or recurrent infections may require the addition of oral griseofulvin. Griseofulvin microsize, 250 to 500 mg. twice daily after meals for 1 month, is usually adequate. Incomplete treatment with griseofulvin may be followed by relapse.

Tinea Cruris

Tinea cruris is commonly caused by *Trichophyton rubrum, Trichophyton mentagrophytes,* or *Epidermophyton floccosum.*

The treatment of tinea cruris is dependent upon the history and physical examination. In new, limited infections, a topical antifungal agent such as clotrimazole 1 per cent (Lotrimin) or miconazole nitrate 2 per cent (MicaTin) applied twice daily for 2 to 4 weeks is often sufficient. After clearing, maintenance therapy with one of these agents or dusting the involved area with tolnaftate (Tinactin) powder may help prevent recurrence.

Patients with chronic or recurrent tinea cruris unresponsive to topical therapy, those with extensive lesions, or those with follicular involvement should also be treated with griseofulvin, 0.5 to 1 gram daily for 30 days.

Severe inflammatory tinea cruris or tinea cruris which has become secondarily infected may require treatment with topical or systemic steroids and systemic antibiotics. Since tinea cruris may develop secondary to a dermatophyte infection of the feet, any concomitant tinea pedis should also be treated.

Tinea cruris is prone to recur, and instructing the patient on preventive local measures is important. Tight underclothing or pantyhose which produces sweating and chafing in the groin should be avoided and the wearing of loose-fitting cotton clothing encouraged. The use of powders to decrease sweating and maceration may also be helpful.

Tinea Pedis

Tinea pedis is usually caused by the same fungi that most commonly cause tinea cruris: *Trichophyton rubrum, Trichophyton mentagrophytes,* or *Epidermophyton floccosum.* Tinea pedis may present clinically as a chronic scaling eruption with or without hyperkeratosis, as an interdigital infection, or as a vesiculopustular eruption.

Early, mild tinea pedis can often be treated with a good topical agent such as miconazole nitrate 2 per cent (MicaTin) applied twice daily. However, chronic infections will usually require oral griseofulvin, 0.5 to 1 gram for 30 days, along with a good topical agent. Antifungal therapy is continued until a clinical and laboratory cure is achieved. The dry, scaly, diffuse type of infection of the soles is particularly difficult to cure, and relapse is frequent. Treatment may have to be continued for up to 3 months, and it may be necessary to use a keralytic agent such as 10 per cent salicylic acid in petrolatum along with the topical antifungal agent.

The intertriginous or vesicular variety of tinea pedis is often complicated by a superimposed bacterial infection. This should be treated with bed rest, elevation of the foot, and wet compresses with Burow's solution (1:10 to 1:20) for 15 to 30 minutes three to four times a day. The use of systemic antibiotics is usually necessary, especially if the tissue reaction is severe or lymphangitis is present. If autoeczematization is present, systemic corticosteroids may be required. After resolution of the bacterial infection, appropriate antifungal therapy should be initiated.

Tinea pedis is difficult to cure and control because of the moist, warm environment of the feet. Efforts to keep the feet cool and dry are helpful; these include drying the feet thoroughly after bathing and frequently airing them; avoiding nylon hose or other synthetic fabrics which interfere with the dissipation of moisture, and wearing instead cotton absorbent socks; and avoiding tennis shoes and wearing sandals, perforated shoes, or alternating pairs of shoes to permit their drying. Good foot hygiene is important, and a powder such as tolnaftate (Tinactin) may be used liberally twice daily. Despite these measures, recurrences are common, and some infections persist no matter what therapy is used or what precautions are taken.

Tinea Manuum

The management of the patient with tinea manuum is essentially the same as that recommended for tinea pedis, although environmental factors do not play as critical a role. The infection may remain unilateral for many years, a phenomenon yet unexplained. Tinea manuum is usually accompanied by tinea pedis, and both sites of infection should be treated at the same time. If required, topical treatment may be supplemented by griseofulvin microsize, 0.5 to 1 gram per day for approximately 4 to 8 weeks. The dry, scaly, diffuse type of palmar infection is difficult to cure, and relapse is frequent.

CANDIDIASIS

Cutaneous Candidiasis

Superficial fungus infections of the skin can also be caused by *Candida albicans.* This infection does not respond to griseofulvin, making it very important to draw a clinical distinction between lesions caused by *Candida albicans* and those caused by dermatophytes. Candidiasis is usually made worse by a hot, humid environment and is therefore often limited to areas of increased perspiration or maceration. Frequent sites of involvement are the intertriginous areas such as the groin, gluteal cleft, inframammary areas, and axilla.

Initial therapy of acute intertriginous candidiasis should be similar to that of an acute contact dermatitis. Moist compresses with cool tap water for 15 minutes two or three times a day are both soothing and drying. After each compressing, the area should be allowed to dry thoroughly and then a topical preparation applied. In acute cases, this can be a topical steroid followed by or used in combination with nystatin (Mycostatin) or amphotericin B (Fungizone). A shake lotion containing these ingredients may also be used. Newer agents, such as miconazole nitrate 2 per cent (MicaTin) or clotrimazole 1 per cent (Lotrimin) are also effective. Paraben-free preparations should be used, as this preservative can sensitize an already aggravated site. In this regard, preparations containing ethylenediamine should also be avoided because of their potential sensitizing properties. In less acute cases it is probably best not to use a medication containing a topical steroid but to rely only on the anticandidal agent. Use of harsh soaps and vigorous scrubbing are contraindicated. In axillary candidiasis the patient should be instructed to avoid the use of deodorants and other irritating substances. The patient should be instructed on the role of environmental factors and the necessity of keeping the involved areas cool, dry, and well aerated, both during treatment and after clearing to prevent recurrence. Patients with candidiasis, especially those with recurrent infections, should be thoroughly evaluated to rule out any predisposing factors such as endocrine abnormalities, underlying malignancies, or immunologic defects. Candidiasis in patients receiving long-term broad-spectrum antibiotics, systemic corticosteroids, cytotoxic agents, or immunosuppressive drugs is often severe and resistant to therapy.

DRUG ERUPTIONS

method of
LAFAYETTE G. OWEN, M.D.
Louisville, Kentucky

A rash caused by a drug will usually improve if the offending drug is stopped. Without treatment, however, resolution of the eruption may take several days or even weeks. Until the drug intake is stopped, nothing except emergency management should be considered.

A difficult but very common problem is presented by the patient who is receiving a number of drugs at one time. It is then necessary to discontinue all nonessential drugs. If a certain type of medication is necessary to maintain life, a different class of drugs should be substituted. An example would be the substitution of a nonthiazide diuretic for hydrochlorothiazide (Hydrodiuril).

It has been said that almost any drug can produce almost any rash; diagnosis is not always easy, and standard texts of dermatology should be consulted for lists of common troublemakers among drugs and the type of rash each causes.

Further management of drug rashes depends on the type and severity of the eruption.

Severe Reactions. The most severe skin eruptions that may be caused by drugs are erythema multiforme, involving both skin and mucous membranes (Stevens-Johnson type), and toxic epidermal necrolysis, in which the skin becomes red and then superficially denuded, resembling a scald. Of great interest is the recent appreciation that treatable microbial infections can produce precisely these same rashes. Mycoplasma-caused atypical pneumonia can produce erythema multiforme, and staphylococcal infection can cause the scalded skin picture. Before blaming a drug for either of these rashes, one should consider the possibility of the existence of these treatable infections.

In drug-induced severe erythema multiforme or toxic epidermal necrolysis, the patient should be hospitalized and given usual supportive care. Corticosteroid at the level of 120 mg. prednisone per day is the starting dose we use. Sometimes the starting dose is given as 80 mg. methylprednisolone sodium succinate (Solu-Medrol). As the patient improves, dosage is reduced accordingly. Wet dressings (isotonic saline or Burow's solution 1:40) and local debridement are most helpful in preventing secondary infections. Lidocaine (Xylocaine Viscous) is of help in reducing oral pain. Usually even severely ill patients can be spared the risks of intravenous therapy by drinking liquid formula diets immediately after the mouth is numbed with lidocaine (Xylocaine).

Urticarial Reactions. Severe reactions should be treated with epinephrine (1:1000), starting with 0.2 ml. With severe urticarial reactions, prednisone, 20 to 30 mg. per day, should be given for 5 to 7 days. Antihistamines in high dose usually control less acute rashes. Chlorpheniramine (Chlor-Trimeton), 4 mg. tablets, can be taken two, three, or even four at a time every 4 hours without risk, providing that the patient is kept from driving an automobile or operating machinery. An epinephrine bitartrate inhaler (Medihaler-Epi) is useful for the patient to carry in case of acute distress.

Morbilliform Reactions. These are usually treated symptomatically with antihistamines. In severe cases 15 to 20 mg. of prednisone per day may be given. Aveeno baths (4 tablespoons to a tub of lukewarm water) and an ointment containing the following should be applied four or five times daily:

Menthol ¼ per cent
Phenol ¼ per cent
Valisone Cream 0.1 per cent, 15 grams
Velvachol to make 60 grams

Drug-Induced Photosensitivity. Eruptions on light-exposed areas may be due to drugs taken internally as well as to photosensitizing films left by the newer soaps. In addition to stopping such drugs as sulfonamides, sulfonylureas, phenothiazines, and thiazides, the patient should be treated with antihistamines, Aveeno baths, and the aforementioned ointment. In some cases steroids should be given, starting with 30 mg. prednisone per day. If the light-induced eruption persists for several weeks, an antimalarial drug such as quinacrine, chloroquine, or hydroxychloroquine should be given (1 tablet twice daily for 2 weeks and then 1 daily). (This use of these agents is not mentioned in the manufacturer's official directives.) The patient should be instructed to avoid the sun when possible and to wear a sun protective agent if outdoors (Solbar, PreSun, Pan Ultra, or Maxafil).

Corticosteroid-Induced Acne. Patients taking corticosteroid for control of serious blood dyscrasias or colitis often develop a steroid-induced acne. This can usually be controlled with customary acne treatment without interruption of the required dose of steroid.

HERPES SIMPLEX

method of
MICHAEL JARRATT, M.D.
Houston, Texas

Herpes simplex virus is virtually ubiquitous in man. Eighty to 90 per cent of the normal adult population have circulating antibodies to herpes simplex virus, indicating previous infection. After causing an acute and painful primary infection with a usual duration of 2 to 4 weeks, herpes simplex virus has the unique capacity to ascend sensory nerves and establish latent infection in dorsal root ganglia. At periodic and unpredictable intervals thereafter, the virus reactivates and descends along sensory nerves to the cutaneous surface, where it causes shorter duration (5 to 7 days), self-limited recurrent lesions. Herpes simplex virus also causes recurrent keratoconjunctivitis, Kaposi's varicelliform eruption, disseminated infection of the newborn, and temporal lobe encephalitis. Treatment of each of these clinical presentations of herpetic disease will be discussed individually.

Primary Mucocutaneous Infection

Gingivostomatitis. Primary herpetic gingivostomatitis is a disease of children and young adults. The primary infection is characterized by very painful and widespread erosions in the mouth and pharynx. The pain is frequently severe enough to compromise adequate oral fluid intake. The erosive process heals spontaneously in 2 to 4 weeks.

No specific antiviral therapy is available. Consequently, treatment consists of supportive measures.

1. Sodium bicarbonate in warm tap water. Use as a mouthwash and a gargle four to six times daily.
2. Topical anesthetic agents. Viscous lidocaine (Xylocaine) or dyclonine hydrochloride (Dyclone) may be held in the mouth as frequently as necessary to maintain relief of pain.
3. Oral analgesics. Codeine or even meperidine (Demerol) may be required for adequate pain relief.
4. If the infection is severe and protracted, hospitalization and intravenous fluid and electrolyte maintenance may be required.

Vulvovaginitis. Primary herpetic vulvovaginitis is a venereally transmitted disease of adolescents and young adults. Extensive erosion involving the mons pubis, perineum, labia majora and minora, and vagina is accompanied by intense, marked soft tissue edema and exquisite pain. The infection resolves spontaneously in 2 to 4 weeks.

No specific antiviral therapy is available. Consequently, treatment consists of supportive measures.

1. Warm tap water sitz baths four times daily.
2. Topical anesthetics. Anesthetic sprays containing benzocaine (Americaine) aerosol may afford some relief of pain when applied four times daily after sitz baths. However, there is a rather high incidence of allergic sensitization to "caine" topical anesthetics. Therefore if itching, erythema, or edema should grow worse during the course of the treatment with topical "caines," the topical anesthetic agents should be discontinued immediately.
3. Oral analgesics. Oral codeine or even meperidine (Demerol) may be required for adequate control of pain.
4. Involuntary muscle spasm and intense local edema may interfere with urination. Hospitalization and Foley catheter drainage may be required in some cases.

Recurrent Cutaneous Infection

Herpes Labialis (Fever Blisters, Cold Sores), Herpes Genitalis (Venereal Herpes), Herpetic Whitlow (Recurrent Infection of Fingers and Hands). There is no single therapeutic modality that is fully effective in decreasing the duration or the recurrence rate of cutaneous herpes simplex infection. Consequently, numerous treatment modalities are recommended by many physicians.

ETHER. Ordinary diethyl ether is a topical anesthetic agent and a lipid solvent which dissolves the capsule of the herpesvirus particle. Topical application of diethyl ether three or four times daily to *early* recurrent lesions will provide symptomatic relief and may decrease the duration of the lesions.

THYMOL IN CHLOROFORM. Thymol is an antiviral agent which interferes with herpesvirus protein synthesis. Thymol also is a topical anesthetic agent. Chloroform is a lipid solvent which dissolves the herpesvirus particle capsule. Topical application of 4 per cent thymol in chloroform twice daily at the *earliest sign* of a new recurrent lesion will give symptomatic relief and may decrease the duration of the lesion.

GLUTARALDEHYDE.* Glutaraldehyde 2 per cent, buffered with sodium bicarbonate to pH 7.5, appears to dry lesions effectively, but the solution is unstable in the bottle and precipitates in only 3 to 5 days after mixing. Fresh solution should be applied only to new lesions twice daily.

LIQUID NITROGEN. A light freeze to a *very early* recurrent lesion with liquid nitrogen on a cotton applicator may abort progression of the lesion.

CORTICOSTEROIDS. 1. Topical corticosteroid. *Very early* and very frequent (every 1 to 2 hours) application of a high potency topical corticosteroid cream is reported by some clinicians to abort further progression of recurrent lesions. Although the use of topical corticosteroids is contraindicated in herpetic keratoconjunctivitis, there is no evidence that topical application of corticosteroids to recurrent cutaneous lesions is detrimental.

2. Intralesional corticosteroid. Subcutaneous injection with a 30 gauge needle of triamcinolone acetonide (Kenalog) parenteral suspension, diluted with isotonic saline solution to 3 mg. per ml., may abort the progression of early erythematous plaque stage lesions or enhance the healing of early vesicular lesions.

NUCLEOSIDES. 1. Idoxuridine (IDU). Ophthalmic preparations of 0.1 per cent IDU in solution or ointment base (Stoxil, Herplex, Dendrid), although effective in the treatment of herpetic keratoconjunctivitis, have been shown to be ineffective in recurrent cutaneous disease such as herpes labialis, herpes genitalis, and herpetic whitlow. Recent experience with 5 per cent IDU in dimethylacetamide (DMAC) (investigational) indicates that this preparation will decrease the duration of lesions by 50 per cent, but will not decrease recurrence rates. Early experience with this preparation also indicates that there may be a high incidence of contact allergic sensitization.

2. Vidarabine (Vira-A); adenine arabinoside (Ara-A). Topical vidarabine (Vira-A), like IDU, has been shown to be effective in herpetic keratoconjunctivitis, but to be ineffective in recurrent cutaneous disease such as herpes labialis, herpes genitalis, and herpetic whitlow.

PHOSPHONOACETIC ACID. Phosphonoacetic acid is a new anti-herpesvirus agent which specifically inhibits viral DNA synthetase. It has been shown to be very effective in vitro and in animal model studies. Human studies are currently under way. If the human studies reveal both efficacy and safety, the drug would be released for human use.

IMMUNE STIMULATORS. 1. Repeated smallpox vaccination. Although this has been a rather common approach to therapy for frustrating recurrent disease, and although there are numerous anecdotal reports of its efficacy, double-blind, controlled studies indicate that repeated smallpox vaccinations had no more effect on the course of recurrent herpes infections than did placebo vaccinations. Since there is some risk both to the patient receiving vaccinia virus and to others exposed to the vaccinia virus, this therapeutic modality should be discontinued.

2. Bacille Calmette Guérin (BCG) inoculation. One uncontrolled, open study indicating success with BCG inoculation for treatment of recurrent herpes genitalis in women is published in the obstetrics and gynecology literature. Three subsequent double-blind and controlled clinical studies, however, have shown no effect of BCG inoculation on the course of recurrent herpetic disease, and local abscess formation occurred in up to 25 per cent of patients.

3. Levamisole. Levamisole is a drug with a unique capacity to boost cell-mediated immunity. At present, several open, uncontrolled studies of levamisole in the treatment of recurrent herpes simplex infections indicate that the drug, when administered periodically, may decrease the recurrence rate of frequently recurrent disease. Large, double-blind controlled studies with levamisole in recurrent herpes infections, currently under way, will be completed within the next 12 to 18 months. If these studies indicate efficacy and safety for the drug in the treatment of recurrent herpes infections, it will likely be approved by the Food and Drug Administration for general use. The drug is not currently available for human use in the United States.

DYE-LIGHT PHOTOTHERAPY. Photoactive heterotricyclic dyes are dramatically lethal in the presence of light for herpes simplex virus in vitro. Four years ago, initial studies indicated that the topical application of photoactive dye and visible light to recurrent herpetic lesions would not only enhance healing but also decrease recurrence rate. More recent studies have cast doubt on the efficacy of dye-light therapy. Furthermore, laboratory studies with dye-light disrupted herpesvirus show

*Investigational for this use.

that, although viral infectivity is destroyed by dye-light therapy, the virus particles' mutagenic capacity remains intact. Whether this laboratory finding indicates an oncogenic risk for man is still open to considerable debate. A large double-blind and long-term study of the efficacy and safety of dye-light therapy is now under way. Study results will be forthcoming shortly.

VACCINE. Since patients with frequently recurrent herpes simplex infections have high circulating humoral antibody titers to herpesvirus, there is good reason to suspect that a herpesvirus vaccine might not prove effective in the therapy of recurrent disease. However, there is recent animal model evidence that herpesvirus vaccines and circulating anti-herpesvirus IgG may interact with the cell-mediated system to enhance resistance against herpes simplex virus infection. The only herpesvirus vaccine currently available for human use outside the United States is Lupidon-G. However, neither the safety nor the efficacy of Lupidon-G has been established in properly controlled studies.

Recurrent Keratoconjunctivitis

Recurrent herpetic infection of the eye is a major cause of blindness. The earliest and least severe form of ophthalmologic disease is superficial dendritic keratitis. With multiple recurrences, however, deeper ameboid ulcers develop and sometimes give rise to severe stromal keratitis.

Several treatment modalities are available.

Simple Debridement. Superficial dendritic ulcers are topically anesthetized and debrided, after which the eye is patched during epithelial healing.

Nucleosides. 1. Idoxuridine (IDU), 0.1 per cent solution or ointment (Stoxil, Herplex), is applied to the infected eye every 1 to 2 hours during the day and every 2 to 4 hours during the night.

2. Vidarabine (Vira-A). Topical Vira-A for recurrent herpetic keratoconjunctivitis is as effective as IDU, is relatively nontoxic, and does not cross-react with IDU in allergic patients.

3. 5-Trifluoromethyl-2-deoxyuridine (TF-3). In human studies outside the United States, TF-3 has been shown to be as good as or better than IDU or Ara-A in the treatment of herpetic keratoconjunctivitis. Human studies in the United States, however, are in their early stages, so the drug will probably not be available for use in less than 1 to 2 years.

Corticosteroids. Topical application of corticosteroids is definitely contraindicated in the treatment of dendritic and ameboid herpetic ulcers of the cornea. Some controversy exists as to the usefulness of topical corticosteroids in the treatment of deep stromal keratitis.

Kaposi's Varicelliform Eruption (Eczema Herpeticum)

Eczema herpeticum is a widespread cutaneous infection which occurs in patients with preexisting skin diseases such as atopic eczema, Darier's disease, and the epidermolytic hyperkeratosis form of ichthyosis. The infection usually runs its course and heals spontaneously in 2 to 3 weeks. Secondary infection with staphylococci and streptococci may be a significant complication. At present the mortality rate is less than 10 per cent because of modern techniques of dealing with pyogenic infection and fluid and electrolyte imbalance.

No specific antiviral therapy is yet available. Consequently, the treatment consists of supportive measures.

1. Wrap moist and exudative areas with Kerlix gauze rolls wet with aluminum acetate 1:40 solution (Domeboro, Bluboro). After 20 or 30 minutes remove the Kerlix wraps, and sponge severely involved areas with povidone-iodine (Betadine) in water. Repeat the wet compresses and sponging three or four times daily.

2. If secondary pyogenic infection ensues, treat with appropriate oral or intravenous antibiotics.

3. In the event of high fever and toxicity, hospitalization and appropriate management of fluid and electrolyte imbalances may be necessary.

Disseminated Infection of the Newborn

If a mother has active infectious herpetic cervicitis or herpes genitalis during delivery, the newborn infant is at risk for the development of disseminated herpes simplex virus infection spreading from the skin to the brain and other internal organs. The infection has a very high morbidity and mortality rate. Consequently, rather extraordinary therapeutic measures may be justified.

1. Wet to dry aluminum acetate compresses followed by povidone-iodine washes should be applied as described for Kaposi's varicelliform eruption.

2. If secondary pyogenic infection of the skin ensues, appropriate intravenous antibiotics are indicated.

3. Single volume exchange transfusion from a donor with a history of herpetic infection of the appropriate type (type 1 or type 2) may be helpful. The deficiencies in newborn humoral and cellular immunity may be partially corrected not only by the transfusion of type-specific immune globulin

but also by the administration of donor lymphocytes sensitized to herpes simplex virus.

4. Adenine arabinoside (Ara-A), although not yet available for general use, may prove to be effective when administered intravenously in doses of 10 to 15 mg. per kg. per day.

Encephalitis

Herpes simplex virus encephalitis is a temporal lobe infection with very high morbidity and significant mortality. Intravenous idoxuridine and cytosine arabinoside (Ara-C) have proved to be too toxic for systemic use. Currently human studies with adenine arabinoside (Ara-A), 15 to 20 mg. per kg. per day intravenously, are encouraging. However, Ara-A is not yet approved for human use in the United States.

Other therapeutic approaches consist entirely of supportive care.

HIDRADENITIS SUPPURATIVA

method of
FRED F. CASTROW II, M.D.
Houston, Texas

The lesions of hidradenitis suppurativa are caused by a blockage of the apocrine sweat glands with subsequent secondary infection. The term apocrinitis applies to the acute stage and is characterized by nonsuppurative, tender, nodular lesions. Apocrinitis and hidradenitis occur where there is an abundance of apocrine glands, such as the axillary region, genitocrural region, buttocks, umbilicus, breast, and occasionally aberrant sites. The early nodular lesions are tender, but not of the exquisite nature of a furuncle. The lesions are often misdiagnosed and treated as furunculosis or perirectal abscesses. In the early stage of the disease the lesions are confined principally to the dermis but later dissect toward subcutaneous tissue and form multiple sinus tracts which erupt to the surface. Hypertrophic scars occur frequently. The lesions have the tendency to become very resistant to all types of conservative treatment. In cases of advanced hidradenitis suppurativa, the lesions dissect laterally to form pockets filled with pus and a characteristic gelatinous material. It should be noted that as these lesions advance and spread laterally, they rarely or never break into the deep subcutaneous tissue.

If there are a few isolated lesions only, they can be treated under local anesthesia, but treatment of the more extensive eruption must be performed under a general anesthetic. The steps of the method are as follows:

1. A probe is inserted into each sinus tract, and the superficial tissue is incised so as to effect complete exteriorization. The multiple interconnecting sinus tracts often give the lesion a honeycomb appearance. Any redundant tissue is removed during this stage of the procedure.

2. The multiple cavities containing pus and the sticky gelatinous material are adequately drained, and the lining is thoroughly curetted with a dermal or uterine curette.

3. The entire exteriorized area is extensively coagulated with a bipolar current. The bipolar electrocoagulation serves to stop the bleeding, helps destroy the lining of the cavity, and minimizes postoperative pain by temporarily sealing the nerve endings.

4. Starting on the first postoperative day, hot compresses or sitz baths are utilized three times daily, and antibiotics, such as the combination of neomycin-polymyxin-bacitracin, are applied locally. Immediate postoperative discomfort is negligible and is tolerated better than the preoperative pain inherent in the hidradenitis.

Many patients are cured by the operation; in others, a few new lesions develop. These new abscesses are treated early in the same manner as the original ones. Complete healing in severe cases occurs within 3 weeks to 2 months after the operation. The average time required for complete healing varies from 4 to 6 weeks.

The precursor lesions of hidradenitis, comedones, may be treated with the use of vitamin A acid locally. The vitamin A acid should be applied sparingly and only frequently enough to produce minimal erythema. Systemic antibiotics, especially tetracycline, are of adjunctive benefit to control the secondary bacterial infection but should not be relied upon to bring about complete resolution of the hidradenitis. Superficial x-ray therapy and various other surgical approaches have been used effectively in the treatment of hidradenitis suppurativa, but these methods require either special equipment or specialized surgical skills.

KELOIDS

method of
ARTHUR C. RESSMANN, M.D.,
J. L. PIPKIN, M.D.,
and RONALD J. RESSMANN, M.D.
San Antonio, Texas

There is no one modality that can be considered the treatment of choice in all keloids. Location of the keloid, particularly over or near reproductive organs or over the thyroid; size; age of keloid; and thickness are all factors that affect or dictate the type of therapy. X-ray therapy, surgery, intralesional injection of relatively insoluble corticosteroids, and cryotherapy are the most commonly employed methods. When surgical excision of keloid tissue is performed, it is followed by either x-ray or intralesional corticosteroid therapy, or both.

Early Keloids (1 to 6 Months)

Intralesional Corticosteroid. Triamcinolone acetonide (Kenalog) is used for intralesional therapy. Kenalog parenteral, 10 mg. per ml., is diluted to 5 mg. per ml. with 2 per cent lidocaine (Xylocaine). This combination of local anesthetic with the corticosteroid lessens the discomfort of injection and also reduces the possibility of atrophy if the injection is accidentally placed outside the keloid. Sterile disposable plastic syringes with a 26 gauge needle may be used; however, the needle must be securely placed on the syringe or it will pop off under pressure. Although Luer-Lok syringes will prevent this, the glass syringe may break under pressure. The size of the lesion determines the amount of corticosteroid injected; however, 20 mg. is the maximum amount given at one treatment. The treatment is repeated at 2 week intervals until the keloid begins to regress and show surface crinkling. The treatment may then be given at longer intervals and less corticosteroid used until the desired result is achieved.

The corticosteroid must be injected evenly into the keloid. If this is done, the area being treated will slowly whiten as the corticosteroid is injected. Care must be taken not to inject the corticosteroid outside the keloid, or atrophy of fat and adjacent tissue may occur with an undesirable result.

Cryotherapy: Liquid Nitrogen. Thin, early, slightly pruritic keloids may be treated successfully with liquid nitrogen. Treatment is administered every 2 to 3 weeks. Slight pressure with a cotton swab dipped in liquid nitrogen is applied long enough to produce slight blistering. It is of no help in thick keloids, and its effectiveness is limited.

X-Ray Irradiation. X-ray irradiation is probably the treatment of choice in early keloids. However, possible genetic effects, particularly when keloids are located over reproductive organs and thyroid, increased patient resistance to all forms of irradiation, and lack of x-ray training in dermatology teaching centers is causing this modality to be used less frequently.

The keloid is outlined in ink, leaving a 2 mm. margin of normal skin. Transparent celluloid is placed over the outlined keloid, and the outline is traced in ink on the celluloid.

The celluloid outline is traced on a lead sheet 0.5 mm. thick by means of a Beaver blade point, and the outline on the lead is carefully carried out. The opening in the lead sheet will match exactly the outlined keloid. This is securely held in place with liquid Duo adhesive and tape.

X-ray treatment is administered with the following factors: Maximar 100, KV 100 MA 5, filter 1 mm. aluminum, FSD 30 cm., HVL 1 mm. aluminum. An air dose of 250 R is administered. The same dose is administered in 2 weeks and again in 1 month. Usually three to four treatments are given, with the total being 750 to 1000 R. In thicker keloids the dosage and filtration may be increased.

Old Keloids

The keloid is first surgically excised, suturing normal skin using a running subcuticular No. 4 nylon suture.

X-ray irradiation is first administered at the time of removal of sutures, and the treatment regimen is the same as x-ray irradiation of early keloids.

If x-ray irradiation is not indicated for reasons previously outlined, intralesional corticosteroid may be started or one may defer treatment until it is certain that the keloid will recur.

In old keloids that are not amenable to complete surgical excision, the keloid may be shaved flush with the skin, using a sterilized Gem razor blade, hemostasis being accomplished with pressure or Monsel's solution. This is then followed immediately by the routine for x-ray irradiation or intralesional corticosteroid therapy or a combination of both. This is particularly useful in large ear lobe keloids, surgical excision of which would result in a deformed or no ear lobe.

Effectiveness of Therapy

The most desirable result is nonrecurrence of a keloid following complete surgical removal requiring no follow-up therapy and a line scar. However, in most patients the result is changing a thick, unsightly symptomatic keloid into a flat asymptomatic scar. Patients should be made aware of this before treatment is started.

In early keloids intralesional corticosteroid therapy is gaining favor because of resistance of patients to x-ray irradiation and possible genetic effects.

In old keloids surgical removal followed by a combination of x-ray irradiation and intralesional corticosteroid therapy is probably the most effective treatment.

LICHEN PLANUS

method of
WILLIAM A. CARO, M.D.
Chicago, Illinois

Lichen planus is a chronic inflammatory disease of unknown cause affecting skin and frequently oral mucous membranes. The disease usually occurs in adults, and lesions favor the volar aspects of the wrists and the ankles initially. The lower back, genitalia, and oral mucous membranes also are commonly involved. The disease may take from several weeks to several months for full development. The classic skin lesion is a flat-topped, polygonal, somewhat shiny papule with a characteristic violaceous hue. Over the surface of the lesion one may see small whitish points or delicate white lines (Wickham's striae). Lesions usually arise de novo but also can arise at sites of minor skin trauma such as scratch marks (Koebner phenomenon). On the lower extremities the lesions may be larger, thicker, and rougher in appearance (hypertrophic lichen planus). Most patients with lichen planus have some degree of itching, and this may be severe. When the mouth is affected, the buccal mucosa usually shows a white lacelike pattern, and patients with severe involvement may have mucosal ulcerations. Milder oral involvement usually is asymptomatic, although more severe lesions may be painful and may interfere with eating. Lichen planus also may affect the nails and the scalp with hair loss.

Drugs, including gold, antimalarials, quinidine, antituberculous agents, phenothiazines, and thiazides, may produce lichen planus–like eruptions, and contact with color film developers may produce similar lesions.

Treatment

Because many patients itch and are under stress, mild tranquilizers and sedatives may be of value. Hydroxyzine (Atarax, Vistaril), 10 to 25 mg. three or four times a day, has been helpful. Corticosteroid creams (e.g., Aristocort, Kenalog, Cordran, Synalar, Valisone) should be applied two or three times daily at full strength, although with extensive lesions the cost factor may dictate a more economical concentration. In chronic and resistant lesions such as hypertrophic lesions on the legs, nighttime occlusion with a plastic film such as Saran Wrap will enhance penetration of the topical corticosteroid. Individual recalcitrant lesions also benefit from the intralesional injection of corticosteroid suspensions such as triamcinolone acetonide (Kenalog) suspension, 5 to 10 mg. per ml. Sterile isotonic saline solution may be used as a diluent, and the areas should be injected evenly using small amounts. Ten mg. should be the maximum injected at one time, and injections can be repeated as necessary at 3 to 4 week intervals.

Symptomatic relief may be obtained in extensive lichen planus with the use of colloidal oatmeal baths (1 cup Aveeno colloidal oatmeal powder to a tub of tepid water) or an antipruritic lotion such as 0.25 per cent menthol in a hydrophilic lotion (Shepard's, Nutraderm). When all treatment measures fail and the patient is disabled by the eruption, oral prednisone may be employed at 20 to 30 mg. daily for 3 to 6 weeks, followed by gradual withdrawal over a 3 to 4 week period.

Symptomatic mouth lesions respond poorly to treatment, although diluted mouthwashes, topical anesthetics such as lidocaine (Xylocaine Viscous), and applications of topical corticosteroids (triamcinolone acetonide in emollient dental paste [Kenalog in Orabase]) may be tried. Intralesional injection of corticosteroid suspensions also may be helpful.

The clinician should recognize that the course of lichen planus is quite variable, and the eruption may last many months to a year or longer even with treatment.

PHOTOSENSITIVITY AND SUNBURN

method of
JOHN A. PARRISH, M.D.
Boston, Massachusetts

Introduction

The sun is the energy source of all life on earth and emits a wide range of electromagnetic energy extending from radiowaves, through infrared, visible, and ultraviolet to x-rays. It is the ultraviolet (UV) component (290 to 400 nm.) of sunlight which causes most skin reactions. Because shorter wavelengths are absorbed by atmospheric ozone and longer wavelengths are much less effective, it is the middle ultraviolet (UV-B, 290 to 320 nm.) which primarily causes sunburn, suntan, and skin cancer. However, long wavelength ultraviolet (UV-A, 320 to 400 nm.) may augment these cutaneous reactions, and it is this waveband that is primarily responsible for most drug- or chemical-induced photosensitivity reactions. Sensitivity in certain diseases may extend into the visible portion of sunlight or artificial light.

Photoprotection

Tanning. Melanin, the pigment naturally occurring in skin, is unquestionably the best sunscreen. Genetic factors, however, determine the constitutive (base-line) skin color of a person, as well as the ability to tan in response to UV exposure. Cautious graduated exposures permit progressive tanning without sunburn in all but the poorest responders. Both the ability to tan and its final extent may be increased by PUVA (oral psoralen, e.g., methoxsalen [0.6 mg. per kg.], followed by exposure to artificial or solar UV-A). Great care with exposure times is essential, as severe phototoxicity can result from the steep dose-response curve. Ideally a radiometer should be used to monitor the UV-A dose.

Sun Avoidance. Any measures that reduce exposure of the skin to strong sunlight should be exploited. Outdoor activities should be timed to avoid the peak UV-B times (10:00 A.M. to 2:00 P.M.). Long hair growth helps shade the ears and neck. Broad-brimmed hats and long-sleeved clothing significantly reduce the impact of harmful ultraviolet rays, but it should be remembered that light-textured materials, especially when wet, only partially block the passage of UV-B. Beach umbrellas, although protecting against direct sunlight, may not prevent sunburn from UV-B scattered from the sky or reflected from sand. Windowglass blocks UV-B but not UV-A. This may be relevant in the management of certain photosensitivity states (see below).

Sunscreens. Sunscreens occupy a position in the borderline between medications and cosmetics, and the subject is clouded by misconceptions and folklore. The most common incorrect belief is that certain preparations can promote a tan. Since tanning and sunburn both result from the same ultraviolet waveband, one cannot be promoted independently of the other. Many of the innumerable commercially available preparations that claim to promote tanning provide no protection whatsoever. The most effective and cosmetically acceptable sunscreens are those which contain para-aminobenzoic acid (PABA), PABA esters, benzophenones, and cinnamates (Table 1) in suitable vehicles that promote adherence to the skin. Drug-induced and endogenous photosensitivity reactions (e.g., polymorphic photodermatitis) require screens effective against the longer ultraviolet wavelengths (Solbar, Uval, Piz Buin Exclusive Extrem). In the treatment of certain light-induced pigment disorders (e.g., melasma), opaque sunscreens must be used (Reflecta, Covermark). Ideally, sunscreens should be applied 30 to 60 minutes before the onset of sun exposure and must be reapplied after swimming or excessive sweating.

TABLE 1. **Topical Sunscreens**

ABSORBING AGENT	EXAMPLES
PABA	PreSun, Pabanol
Esters of PABA	Sea & Ski, Pabafilm, Block Out
Benzophenones	Solbar, Uval
Combinations (cinnamates and benzophenones)	Piz Buin

Treatment of Sunburn

1. Cold compresses of isotonic saline or Burow's solution 1:40 or plain tap water.
2. Tepid tub baths with or without nonirritating additives (e.g., bath oils).
3. Topical fluorinated steroids such as triamcinolone cream 0.025 per cent three or four times daily and under compresses. Steroid-induced vasoconstriction may reduce erythema, itching, and general discomfort. However, there is no evidence that corticosteroids diminish cell damage.
4. Severe sunburn or dangerous accidental overexposure may be treated with systemic corticosteroids. In normal, healthy persons a brief course (e.g., oral prednisone, beginning with 40 to 60 mg. and tapering over 4 to 8 days) will abort severe sunburn.

Photosensitivity Disorders

Solar Urticaria. Solar urticaria is a rare disorder, probably of several different pathogenic mechanisms, in which hives appear within minutes of exposure to sunlight. If the threshold is high enough, some patients can be controlled simply by avoiding prolonged unprotected sun exposure. Other very sensitive patients must avoid any daytime exposure. Most patients are not helped by antihistamines. It is possible to slowly build up sun tolerance by using carefully metered, graduated exposure to artificial light which stimulates pigmentation and possibly depletes the UV-induced mediators of urticaria.

Polymorphous Light Eruption. Severe reactions may be managed as outlined for sunburn, but chronic use of systemic corticosteroids is not recommended. If patients anticipate an unavoidable intense or prolonged sun exposure, they may take a short course of hydroxychloroquine sulfate (Plaquenil), 200 mg. once or twice a day beginning 2 or 3 days prior to exposure. (This use of Plaquenil is not listed in the manufacturer's official directive.) A potential adverse effect of long-term use is deposition in the retina and occasionally irreversible retinal damage. Ocular examinations are advisable once or twice a year, depending upon frequency of use.

Long-term management of mild cases can be achieved by simply avoiding midday sun and using sunscreens. Those more photosensitive patients can also be treated by a careful course of PUVA which tans, depletes mediators, or diminishes lymphocyte capabilities. Beta-carotene (120 to 180 mg. orally per day) is occasionally beneficial. Usually no treatment is required in winter.

Porphyria Cutanea Tarda. The precipitating agents, commonly ethanol or estrogens, should be sought and withdrawn. Phlebotomy has proved to be the most useful treatment to date. Remove 300 to 500 ml. of blood every 3 to 4 weeks until urine porphyrins are normal, or until the hematocrit falls to 85 per cent of its original value. Alkalinization of urine and small doses of antimalarials are still experimental, require close supervision, and may be dangerous, but are sometimes effective.

Erythropoietic Protoporphyria. The most impressive symptom is burning pain within minutes of light exposure, followed by edema and itching if the patient remains in the sun. Oral beta-carotene (Solatene), 60 to 240 mg. daily, decreases subjective symptoms dramatically in some patients. It often requires 6 to 8 weeks of therapy before significant symptomatic relief is noticeable.

Lupus Erythematosus. Sunburn or chronic sun exposure may precipitate or aggravate lesions of chronic discoid lupus erythematosus. Moderate sun exposure often is not harmful to uninvolved skin. Sunscreens are suggested, and hydroxychloroquine (Plaquenil) and topical steroids may be used during times of disease activity. Patients with systemic lupus erythematosus should avoid being sunburned.

Drug-Induced Photosensitivity. Many drugs and chemicals can cause phototoxic or photoallergic reactions upon sun exposure. Examples include thiazide diuretics, antibacterial sulfonamides, sulfonylurea antidiabetic drugs, phenothiazines (especially chlorpromazine), griseofulvin, demethylchlortetracycline, and psoralens (methoxsalen). As soon as is practical, the drug should be discontinued. Otherwise, sun avoidance and clothing are necessary. Sunscreens should block the UV-A as well as UV-B.

Contact Photosensitivity Dermatitis. Table 2 lists contact photosensitizers. Patients photosensitized to halogenated salicylanilides may remain photosensitive for several years, even after the offending chemical is removed. Exposure to psoralens occurs in agriculture workers handling pink-rot celery or carrots. Treatment is to avoid exposure to both sun and the offending agent and treat as for any contact dermatitis.

TABLE 2. **Contact Photosensitizers**

Cosmetics
Perfumes, colognes, after-shave lotions (essential oils and psoralens)
Lipsticks (fluorescein derivatives)
Creams and hair preparations (coal tar derivatives)
Plants (phytophotodermatitis)
Persian limes
Pink rot-infected celery
Many plants of the Umbelliferae and Rutaceae families
(These problems are primarily due to psoralen compounds)
Therapeutic Agents
Phenothiazines and sulfonamides (usually used therapeutically)
Halogenated salicylanilides
Sunscreens
Blankophores (usually photoallergic)
Diuretics

LUPUS ERYTHEMATOSUS

method of
LOREN E. GOLITZ, M.D.
Denver, Colorado

Discoid lupus erythematosus and systemic lupus erythematosus represent variants of the same disease, with involvement limited to the skin in the former. Cutaneous lesions in discoid lupus erythematosus tend to produce scarring with hyperpigmentation, hypopigmentation, and cicatricial alopecia. Although it is uncommon for discoid lupus erythematosus to progress to the systemic form of the disease, patients with systemic lupus erythematosus may have "discoid skin lesions." Therapy in discoid lupus erythematosus should be conservative, with the goal being the prevention and treatment of disfiguring cutaneous lesions.

Discoid Lupus Erythematosus

General Measures. 1. A complete history and physical examination is indicated to exclude systemic lupus erythematosus.

2. Laboratory tests of significance include complete blood count, sedimentation rate, urinalysis, antinuclear antibody, and a lupus erythematosus cell preparation.

3. When photosensitivity is a factor, the avoidance of excessive sunlight is important. Sunbathing, skiing, and excessive outdoor activities between 9:00 A.M. and 3:00 P.M. may cause exacerbation of the rash. Long-sleeved shirts and hats with brims are helpful. A significant amount of ultraviolet radiation can be avoided by keeping the car windows closed.

4. A sunlight phobia should be avoided. Common sense will permit a moderate amount of outdoor activity.

5. Covermark Makeup by Lydia O'Leary is useful in hiding prominent scars. A wig covers areas of scarring alopecia and provides protection from ultraviolet radiation.

6. Bed rest is not necessary in discoid lupus erythematosus.

Local Therapy. 1. Sunscreens containing 5 per cent para-aminobenzoic acid in an alcohol base (PreSun, Pabanol) should be applied each morning and at mid-day in photosensitive persons.

2. Fluorinated corticosteroid creams or ointments (Lidex, Halog, Kenalog, Synalar, Aristocort, Cordran, Valisone) are highly effective agents for inflammatory lesions when applied four or more times daily. Topical hydrocortisone preparations (Hytone, Cort-Dome) are less potent.

3. Corticosteroid solutions (Synalar, Cordran) or gels (Flurobate Gel, Benisone Gel, Topsyn Gel) can be applied to hairy areas without producing matting of the hair.

4. Flurandrenolide impregnated tape (Cordran tape) enhances penetration of the steroid several-fold and is one of the most useful therapies for discoid lupus erythematosus. After washing the affected area to reduce bacteria, the tape may be left in place for 12 to 24 hours.

5. Fluorinated corticosteroid creams or ointments covered with Saran Wrap or plastic gloves are particularly useful at night for areas too large to be treated with Cordran tape.

6. Intralesional triamcinolone acetonide (Kenalog-10 Injection) may be injected into localized lesions. The preparation should be diluted with saline to 4 or 5 mg. per ml. and about 0.10 ml. injected per each square centimeter. Side effects include temporary atrophy and, in blacks, occasional hypopigmentation.

Systemic Therapy. 1. Antimalarial drugs are useful in severe scarring discoid lupus erythematosus that fails to respond to local therapy. Care is required in their administration because of the potential for ocular damage. (a) Hydroxychloroquine (Plaquenil) is the antimalarial drug of choice owing to a low incidence of ocular side effects. An initial dose of 200 mg. twice daily is usually adequate. If there is no response in 3 months, the dose may be increased to 600 to 800 mg. per day (this dose is larger than that mentioned in the manufacturer's official directive). (b) Chloroquine (Aralen), 500 mg. every other day, may be effective in individuals unresponsive to hydroxychloroquine; however, ocular side effects are more common (this use of Aralen is not listed in the manufacturer's official directive). (c) Quinacrine (Atabrine), 100 mg. per day, although helpful in some patients, produces yellow discoloration of the skin and rarely may cause exfoliative dermatitis or aplastic anemia (this use of Atabrine is not listed in the manufacturer's official directive).

Hydroxychloroquine and chloroquine may produce a reversible keratopathy and an irreversible retinopathy. Although the incidence of retinopathy is low, all persons receiving antimalarials should have baseline eye examinations and re-examination every 3 to 4 months while on the medication. The examination should include slit lamp, funduscopic, and visual field (red target) evaluations. Attempts to reduce or discontinue antimalarial drugs during the winter months may decrease the incidence of side effects.

2. Prednisone in low dosage may relieve some of the inflammation in discoid lupus erythematosus but is rarely indicated because of the side effects associated with long-term administration.

Systemic Lupus Erythematosus

Systemic lupus erythematosus is a disease characterized by variable combinations of joint symptoms, renal involvement, central nervous system manifestations, serositis, and a cutaneous eruption. The rash generally consists of erythematous, edematous patches on sun-exposed skin without significant scarring. About 20 per cent of patients, however, have scarring cutaneous lesions typical of discoid lupus erythematosus. Although arthralgia is the most common symptom in systemic lupus erythematosus, uremia and central nervous system involvement are the two most frequent causes of death.

General Measures. 1. A complete medical evaluation to determine the extent of systemic disease is indicated.

2. Drug-induced lupus erythematosus should be excluded by an adequate history. Procainamide, hydralazine, methyldopa, and chlorpromazine are drugs which may produce symptoms of systemic lupus erythematosus.

3. Rest plays an important role in the management of systemic lupus erythematosus. Hospitalized patients may require bed rest with bathroom privileges as tolerated. A 1 to 2 hour rest period daily is helpful in outpatients.

4. Excessive sunlight exposure may produce an erythematous rash or systemic symptoms. Generally, ultraviolet radiation is most intense from 9:00 A.M. to 3:00 P.M. A reasonable amount of outdoor activity is tolerated by most patients with the use of sunscreens and protective clothing.

5. Pregnancy should be avoided when the disease is active, as it may result in an exacerbation of symptoms. The incidence of abortions and

stillbirths is increased, and the transplacental passage of antibodies may cause transient features of lupus in the infant.

Local Therapy. 1. Sunscreens containing 5 per cent para-aminobenzoic acid in alcohol (Pre-Sun, Pabanol) should be applied each morning and again at midday in photosensitive individuals.

2. Topical and intralesional corticosteroids are usually not indicated in the erythematous, edematous rash of systemic lupus erythematosus. Scarring, discoid-type skin lesions can be treated as outlined for discoid lupus erythematosus.

Systemic Therapy. 1. Salicylates. Aspirin, 1 gram (15 grains) four times daily, is effective in controlling fever and joint symptoms in many patients. The dosage may be gradually increased to 2 grams (30 grains) four times daily or until symptoms of salicylism develop.

2. Indomethacin. The control of arthritis or arthralgia may be accomplished with indomethacin (Indocin), 25 mg. four times daily. A maximum dosage of 50 mg. four times daily is occasionally needed. (This use of indomethacin is not specifically listed in the manufacturer's official directive.)

3. Phenylbutazone. If salicylates and indomethacin fail to control joint symptoms, phenylbutazone (Butazolidin), 100 mg. three times daily, may be helpful; however, this drug is less desirable for long-term therapy because of the rare occurrence of blood dyscrasias. (This use is not listed in the manufacturer's official directive.)

4. Other nonsteroid analgesics: Although not listed in the manufacturer's official directives for use in lupus erythematosus, the following compounds appear to be effective in relieving arthritis in some patients: ibuprofen (Motrin), naproxen (Naprosyn), fenoprofen calcium (Nalfon), and tolmetin sodium (Tolectin).

5. Antimalarials. Antimalarial drugs are useful to reduce photosensitivity, to control symptoms not responsive to the nonsteroid analgesics, and to allow reduction of systemic steroids. Hydroxychloroquine (Plaquenil), 200 mg. twice daily, combines effectiveness with a low incidence of side effects. Other antimalarials as listed for discoid lupus erythematosus may also be helpful. Slit-lamp, funduscopic and visual field (red target) examinations should be performed initially and every 3 to 4 months while these patients are on antimalarial drugs. Although the incidence of irreversible retinopathy is low with 400 mg. of hydroxychloroquine daily, periodic attempts to withdraw the drug are indicated.

6. Corticosteroids. Acutely ill patients with systemic lupus erythematosus are best controlled with systemic corticosteroids. Prednisone, 40 to 80 mg. daily, is usually adequate, but higher dosages are occasionally necessary. Indications for systemic corticosteroids include progressive renal disease, central nervous system disease, hemolytic anemia, and thrombocytopenia. Patients who become psychotic while receiving systemic corticosteroids should initially be treated with a higher dosage of steroids to rule out lupus cerebritis. If the psychosis persists, the condition most likely represents steroid psychosis and the corticosteroid dosage should be reduced.

Disease activity while patients are taking systemic corticosteroids may be monitored by clinical symptoms, renal function tests, serum complement titers (total hemolytic complement, C_3) and anti-DNA antibody titers. The dosage of corticosteroids is gradually tapered as the clinical and laboratory findings improve. The addition of immunosuppressive agents or antimalarials may aid in the withdrawal of corticosteroids.

Patients with less acute symptoms may be controlled with 10 to 20 mg. of prednisone daily, with reduction to less than 5 mg. daily in some patients. The use of salicylates, nonsteroid analgesics, or antimalarials may allow the use of alternate day corticosteroids in relatively low dosages. Side effects of systemic corticosteroids include cushingoid features, peptic ulcer disease, cataracts, hypertension, aggravation of diabetes mellitus, and aseptic necrosis of the femoral head. Chronic herpes simplex infections are seen in patients taking systemic corticosteroids and immunosuppressives.

7. Immunosuppressive agents. Despite the widespread use of these drugs in systemic lupus erythematosus and the recent publication of several double-blind studies, their effectiveness remains controversial. The administration of immunosuppressive agents should be restricted to investigators familiar with their effects. Immunosuppressives generally are used in combination with systemic corticosteroids to control progressive renal disease, or to produce a steroid-sparing effect. The drugs most commonly used investigationally are cyclophosphamide and azathioprine.

The side effects of cyclophosphamide include leukopenia, thrombocytopenia, hair loss, gonadal suppression, and hemorrhagic cystitis. Because of the later effect, ample fluid intake should be encouraged in patients on cyclophosphamide. The main toxic effects of azathioprine are hematologic. An increased incidence of malignancy is reported in patients treated with immunosuppressive drugs. The development of opportunistic infections and the suppression of the febrile response in septic patients are other factors which should be considered during therapy with systemic corticosteroids and immunosuppressive agents.

DISORDERS OF THE MOUTH (BENIGN)

method of
ROY S. ROGERS III, M.D.,
and CHARLES M. REEVE, D.D.S.
Rochester, Minnesota

Disorders of the oral mucous membrane may be caused by conditions that are limited to the mouth or they may be oral manifestations of a systemic disease. Careful examination of the skin or a general medical evaluation may be necessary in some instances to correctly assess the scope of the problem. Treatment of oral disease without consideration of systemic factors may fail. Conversely, the administration of systemic treatment without control of local factors such as periodontitis, plaque or calculus accumulation, or the huge resident endogenous oral flora may predispose to a therapeutic failure. Thus close cooperation between the physician and the dentist can provide maximal care in many instances.

The possibility that a lesion may represent a premalignant or malignant condition is an excellent example of this cooperation. There is no substitute for adequate histopathologic sampling of questionable lesions. Indeed, multiple biopsy specimens obtained at the initial evaluation and at the follow-up examinations are a necessary part of the management of leukoplakia. In addition, histopathologic and immunopathologic examination of tissue is often a key to the diagnosis of inflammatory lesions of the oral mucosa. In these situations, the close cooperation of the physician and the dentist is very helpful.

As is the case with the skin, the oral mucosa is readily accessible for direct visual inspection and palpation by the clinician. The use of a dental mirror (or an ENT mirror) aids in visual examination of the tongue and oropharynx. The majority of oral cancers could be detected by careful examination before they become large or metastatic with the attendant poorer prognosis. Estimates of new oral cancer cases for 1977 are 23,900, with 17,000 in males and 6900 in females. Estimated deaths from oral cancer for 1977 are 8450, with 6000 for males and 2450 for females. Because most early oral cancers are mistaken for benign conditions and because they do not exhibit any particular morphology, complete clinical examination and histopathologic study take on even greater significance.

Good oral hygiene is an excellent starting point in the treatment of benign oral conditions. Regular tooth brushing with a soft-bristled toothbrush, using up and down strokes and a fluoride-containing toothpaste, adequate oral intake of fluoride in childhood, and the use of unwaxed dental floss to remove plaque and calculus are important to good oral hygiene. Proper alignment of occlusal forces prevents damage to the periodontium and oral soft tissues. Regular dental examination and correction of defects are a necessary part of good oral hygiene.

In general, inflammatory diseases of the oral mucosa should be treated with gentle measures such as avoidance of hot, acid, and irritant foods and fluids, frequent and gentle cleansing of the tissues with saline mouthwashes (1 teaspoon of table salt to 240 ml. [8 oz.] of lukewarm water), Cepacol mouthwash, or low pressure-pulsed water. Adequate hydration, topical or systemic analgesia, avoidance of tobacco, and rest all play a role in the recovery of inflamed oral tissues.

This article is organized by anatomic regions of the mouth—lips, tongue, other oral soft tissues, gingival and periodontal membrane, teeth, jaws and facial and masticatory musculature, and salivary glands and regional lymph nodes. Diseases that typically affect more than one region will be discussed under the region where they most commonly occur.

Lips

Anatomically, the lip is divided by the vermillion border into two regions: (1) a mucosal surface with a sparsely keratinized epithelium and a loose submucosa in which mucous glands are found, and (2) a cutaneous surface that is better keratinized with a denser dermis in which sebaceous glands are found. Ectopic sebaceous glands (Fordyce's spots) may be found on the mucosal surface. These grouped or clustered yellowish spots are benign and require no treatment.

Cleft Lip and Cleft Palate. This congenital anomaly occurs in approximately 1 in 1000 births. Paramedian pits or fistulas of the lower lip increase the hereditary risks for clefts. Management should be undertaken by specialized teams of physicians, dentists, and speech therapists. Surgical correction usually begins at 1 to 2 months of age; treatment must be individualized, and prompt referral is indicated.

Vascular Tumors. *Hemangiomas* may be limited to the lips or involve other oral tissues. They may represent isolated anomalies or a manifestation of various syndromes of cutaneous and visceral hemangiomas. A cautious approach with frequent examination and accurate measurements should be followed. If vital functions are compromised, a multidisciplinary approach of medical and surgical treatment should be pursued. *Lymphangiomas* are rarer tumors that may require surgical intervention. *Venous ectasias (lakes)* are common among the elderly. No treatment is required.

Mucoceles. These small cystic tumors occur most often on the lower lip. No treatment is indicated unless they do not involute spontaneously—which is apt to happen. Surgical excision presents the risk of damage to adjacent mucous glands resulting in a recurrence of the mucocele. Incision and drainage sometimes allows for resolution, as does intralesional injection of corticosteroids.

Trauma. *Lip lacerations* are a common result of facial trauma. Occlusal roentgenographs may be helpful in localizing foreign bodies in the wound. Debridement of devitalized tissue and apposition of the vermillion edges by marker sutures should be carried out before reconstruction of the laceration. The clinician should recommend face bars and mouthpieces for athletes to help alleviate traumatic injury to oral soft tissues and teeth during contact sports. *Physical trauma* from wind, sunlight, cold, lip-licking tics, and desiccation will cause desquamation. This may be prevented by zinc oxide paste, photoprotective lip balms, or petrolatum. Mouthguards may be utilized to offset nighttime lip-sucking in those afflicted with this tic. *Actinic cheilitis* is a premalignant condition from which a squamous cell carcinoma may develop. Aggressive photoprotection, appropriate biopsy specimens, and surgical procedures such as a lip shave to remove the affected area are therapeutic approaches to this condition.

Allergic Reactions. *Angioedema* may occur as part of an allergic reaction such as a bee sting or a drug reaction. Should the airway be compromised, injection of epinephrine (1:1000), 0.3 to 0.5 ml. subcutaneously or intramuscularly, is indicated. Cold compresses and systemic antihistamines may also be utilized. *Hereditary angioedema* is characterized by the deficiency of a complement enzyme, C1 esterase inhibitor. Angioedema of lips or other mucosal surfaces, including the gut, may be a life-threatening emergency (see pp. 582 to 584). *Contact cheilitis* is a contact dermatitis of the lips. Identification and elimination of the offending allergen are the cornerstones of therapy. Contactants such as dentifrices, mouthwashes, lipsticks, cosmetics, metals, and foods may be causative. Cool compresses, topical fluorinated corticosteroids, and protective salves are helpful in reducing the inflammation. *Erythema multiforme* often affects the lips and should be treated locally as for angioedema and contact cheilitis as well as systemically (see pp. 607 to 608). *Recurrent lip swelling* may be part of the Melkersson-Rosenthal syndrome or a recurrent angioedema.

Macrocheilia. Many conditions may cause macrocheilia. Acute causes include trauma, angioedema, and infectious processes. Chronic macrocheilia may be due to developmental defects, tumors, sarcoidosis, infectious processes, and lymphatic defects.

Angular Cheilitis. This condition is most often attributed to the loss of vertical dimension of the jaws after tooth loss or to a vitamin deficiency. Although some patients suffer from these problems or from Sjögren's syndrome, most patients have a low-grade intertrigo with or without candidiasis or infection with other microorganisms. Local treatment with nystatin, neomycin sulfate, gramicidin, and triamcinolone acetonide (Mycolog) ointment (the cream contains many contact sensitizers) and drying to prevent maceration is helpful. Correction of other local or systemic factors is necessary to forestall chronicity.

Infectious Diseases. *Candidal cheilitis* is rarely an isolated finding (see pp. 611 to 612). *Verruca vulgaris* may occur on the vermillion border or on the oral mucosa. Treatment with 25 per cent podophyllin in tincture of benzoin as for condyloma acuminatum or electrocautery or medical cautery may be utilized. *Primary syphilitic chancres* and *mucous patches of secondary syphilis* may affect the lips. The most common infectious disease of the lips is the *recurrent herpes simplex virus infection*, although *acute herpetic gingivostomatitis* may also affect the lips. There is no definitive treatment for recurrent herpes simplex virus infections. However, nihilism should not be allowed to pervade the therapist's thinking despite the absence of a definitive form of therapy.

Palliative treatment with topical medications from witch hazel to 70 per cent alcohol to ethyl ether has been helpful after unroofing of the vesicles. Topical 5-iodo-2′-deoxyuridine (idoxuridine [Stoxil]), which is marketed for ophthalmic usage, may be helpful in severe cases, but it is a topical sensitizer and may cause abnormalities in DNA. The same holds true for topical arabinoside A (vidarabine, Vira-A), which has recently been marketed for ophthalmic use. Topical heterotricyclic dyes and incandescent light have not been shown to be effective in double-blind trials and may have an oncogenic potential. Prevention of eliciting and provocative factors such as high fevers, sunburn, windburn, and other trauma by photoprotective lip balms and avoidance of exposure should be undertaken. A more extensive discussion of herpes simplex virus infections can be found on pages 613 to 616.

Tongue

The dorsum of the tongue is covered with filiform papillae that give the tongue a velvet-like appearance. Scattered irregularly over the dorsum and lateral borders of the tongue are the larger, vascular fungiform papillae. An increased number of fungiform papillae are sometimes seen in Behçet's syndrome. The circumvallate papillae are arranged in a V shape at the posterior portion of the tongue. The foliate papillae are really collections of lymphoid tissue along the posterolateral borders of the tongue. These can be quite prominent in inflammatory diseases of the oral cavity.

The undersurface of the tongue is smooth and has many prominent vessels. Varicosities of these vessels are common with aging and are of no diagnostic significance.

Furred Tongue. This condition is commonly seen with upper respiratory infections, fevers, and smoking. It is due to failure of normal desquamation or to hypertrophy of the filiform papillae, or both. Brushing the tongue with a soft-bristled toothbrush and a dentifrice is satisfactory in most instances.

Hairy Tongue. The cause for the hyperplasia and excessive length of the filiform papillae in this condition remains enigmatic. The pigmentation is attributed to pigment-producing oral flora that inhabit the tongue. Hairy tongue often occurs after a course of treatment with antibiotics. Simple tongue brushing as for the furred tongue may suffice. If not, application of 25 per cent podophyllin in tincture of benzoin once weekly for 2 to 3 weeks or brushing for 3 minutes after application of 40 per cent urea may be utilized.

Smooth Tongue. Atrophy or absence of filiform papillae is classically associated with nutritional deficiencies such as iron-deficiency anemia, sideropenic dysphagia (Plummer-Vinson syndrome), malabsorption states (sprue, celiac disease), pellagra, and pernicious anemia. Treatment is directed at correction of the underlying disease.

Scrotal Tongue. The fissured or scrotal tongue is a developmental defect. It is seen in mongolism, Sjögren's syndrome, and Melkersson-Rosenthal syndrome, but it occurs most often as an isolated defect that increases in prevalence with advancing age. No treatment is necessary.

Geographic Tongue. It is wise to record observation of geographic tongue, for the patient is often alarmed by its presence and can be readily reassured that it is benign. Unlike scrotal tongue, it is most commonly encountered among pediatric patients, in whom the prevalence may be as high as 15 per cent.

Median Rhomboid Glossitis. Traditionally said to represent a developmental defect of the tuberculum impar, this condition rarely appears until the third or fourth decade of life. The patient is often concerned about cancer. Median rhomboid glossitis is benign and may well represent a chronic hyperplastic candidiasis. If the lesion does not respond to anticandidal therapy, a biopsy may be indicated to exclude carcinoma.

Glossodynia. This is one of the most vexing problems of oral medicine, which afflicts middle-aged and elderly females almost exclusively. Unfortunately, in most patients no cause can be found for the burning paresthesias. Critical to the evaluation are the color, amount, and nature of the papillae and the state of oral hygiene. The "true" glossodynias have no morphologic aberrations, or they show only mild fortuitous changes (furred, geographic, scrotal). "Secondary" glossodynias have abnormal morphology or symptoms (diminution or perversion of the sense of taste). The differential diagnosis includes trigeminal neuralgia; referred pain from dental disease; pernicious anemia and various vitamin deficiencies; vascular disturbances such as thromboses of the central nervous system or the heart; and zinc deficiency, xerostomia, mercurialism, diabetes mellitus, hypothyroidism, recent antibiotic therapy, achlorhydria, gastric reflux, oral sepsis, periodontal disease, occult dental abscesses, and temporomandibular joint disease.

Macroglossia. A variety of conditions may lead to an enlarged tongue. It may be seen as a developmental defect and in mongolism. Tumors such as hemangiomas, lymphangiomas, neurofibromas, and neurolemmomas and thyroglossal duct cysts may cause an enlarged tongue. Infectious processes such as actinomycosis, tuberculosis, and syphilis and metabolic processes such as hypothyroidism, amyloidosis, multiple myeloma, and acromegaly are other causes of an enlarged tongue. Miscellaneous additional conditions are angioneurotic edema, the superior vena cava syndrome, and sarcoidosis.

Other Oral Soft Tissues

Tissues of the buccal mucosa, soft palate, uvula, tonsillar pillars, and sublingual mucosa are poorly keratinized and have a loose lamina propria. The hard palate is better keratinized with a more dense lamina propria.

Viral Infections. Small vesicles with an erythematous halo may be noted in *hand, foot, and mouth disease, herpangina,* and *infectious mononucleosis.* Local measures are appropriate for treatment, and attention is directed toward the primary process. *Recurrent herpes simplex virus infections* of the oral soft tissues occur more commonly than is generally appreciated. Lesions are usually limited to one quadrant of the mouth, are grouped, heal spontaneously in 7 to 10 days, and are recurrent like herpes labialis. Local palliative treatment is sufficient. *Acute herpetic gingivostomatitis* can affect the oral soft tissues, including the labial, buccal, gingival, palatal, and sublingual mucosa as well as the tongue. Fever, malaise, lymphadenopathy, oral pain, and anorexia are attendant symptoms. Treatment is supportive, and recovery is expected in 7 to 14 days (see pp. 613 to 616).

Candidiasis. Lesions caused by *Candida albicans* can present as thrush with curd-like plaques localized or diffusely involving the intraoral tissues. These plaques are removed readily by rubbing with a tongue blade or with a gauze pad which reveals an erythematous base with punctate bleeding points. Other lesions can present as a diffuse inflammation, as a hyperplastic indurated plaque, as atrophic inflamed plaques, or as a leukoplakic area. Candidiasis is an opportunistic infection, occurring in pregnant or debilitated patients, patients with diabetes mellitus or other endocrinopathies, and in immunosuppressed patients. Candidiasis is also associated with antibiotic, corticosteroid, anovulatory, or cytotoxic drug therapy.

The diagnosis is confirmed by direct visual examination of scrapings of the lesions or by culture. Treatment is directed at the underlying condition in conjunction with local therapy. The use of 4 to 6 ml. of nystatin suspension held in the mouth three times a day or sucking on 1 tablet of nystatin (500,000 units) three times a day will often suffice. Nystatin cream may be applied under the denture plate in resistant palatal infections. Failure to respond to therapy or rapid recurrence should stimulate evaluation of the patient for associated conditions or chronic mucocutaneous candidiasis (see pp. 611 to 612).

Denture Sore Mouth. Improperly fitting dentures are associated with two conditions of the oral mucosa—palatal papillary hyperplasia and denture stomatitis. *Palatal papillary hyperplasia* is a hyperplastic response of the palatal mucosa and palatal glands to suction pressure or irritation of ill-fitting dentures. Removal of the denture allows some regression of the lesions. The lesions may be removed surgically so that new dentures can be properly fitted. *Denture stomatitis* can occur with palatal papillary hyperplasia or by itself. This inflammatory condition is often associated with candidiasis. Removal of the denture relieves the condition. Anticandidal therapy applied to the oral mucosa and to the denture itself is often helpful. Frequently the stomatitis can be resolved by having the patient remove the dentures at night (as should be done anyway) and using anticandidal therapy. Occasionally, construction of a new denture is necessary.

Nicotine Stomatitis. Previously thought to have a premalignant potential, nicotine stomatitis is a benign condition that may affect as many as 1 per cent of the population of the United States. The squamous metaplasia of the palatine ducts and a sialadenitis of the palatine glands are directly related to smoking. Removal of the offending habit allows regression of the changes and provides an example to the patient of the need to stop smoking.

Leukoplakia. Although the term leukoplakia implies a premalignant lesion to some, the indiscriminate use of the word to apply to all white lesions of the mouth may be confusing. All keratotic white lesions of the mouth should be sampled histopathologically unless an infection (candidal) or other obvious cause is recognized. Classification of a lesion by the clinician as leukoplakia does not imply a diagnosis, only a morphologic observation. The histopathologist should classify the lesion as benign, dysplastic, or malignant, and the clinician should follow the patient appropriately.

Leukokeratoses are benign white plaques, usually caused by chronic trauma such as cheek-biting, pressure, sucking of the buccal occlusal linea alba, ill-fitting dentures, or malpositioned teeth. Benignity is recognized by the distribution of the lesions and not by their morphology and is best confirmed by biopsy if any question exists. Treatment by avoidance of tobacco, scrupulous oral hygiene, correction of dental abnormalities, and removal of irritating factors is followed by improvement. As with all "leukoplakic" lesions, induration, irregular thickening, ulceration, or erythroplasia should alert the clinician to the necessity for additional tissue samples to exclude malignancy.

Leukoplakia implies a premalignant condition, although only a small percentage of these lesions develop into a squamous cell carcinoma. Histopathologically, cellular atypia, disordered maturation, and thickened mucosa are often noted. Occasionally, it may be difficult to exclude in situ or invasive squamous cell carcinoma. Multiple sections and additional biopsy specimens may be necessary to assess the nature of the leukoplakia correctly. Frequent periodic examinations, additional tissue samples, removal of offending factors, and good oral hygiene are the cornerstones of a treatment program. Leukoplakic lesions of the tongue and floor of the mouth should be treated early surgically, for their potential for malignant transformation is greater than that for buccal, labial, or palatal lesions.

Lichen Planus. Oral mucosal lesions of lichen planus may be seen without skin lesions, although one third of patients who have skin lesions of lichen planus will also have oral lesions. Several types of oral lesions can occur. The most common are the reticulated, lacy hyperkeratotic plaques of the buccal mucosa. Atrophic, erosive, papular, bullous, linear, and ulcerative variants may also be seen. However, even with these variants, areas of reticulated, lacy hyperkeratosis may often be seen on the buccal mucosa. The lesions of the tongue are sometimes difficult to distinguish from leukoplakia. A biopsy is often helpful. Unilateral lichen planus does occur, but lesions are usually bilaterally symmetric.

The natural history of oral lichen planus provides the basis for therapy. Hyperkeratotic lesions are most likely to remit, whereas atrophic, ulcerative, erosive, and bullous lesions tend to persist. Remission in 1 to 2 years occurs in about one third of patients. Drug-induced lichenoid reactions (gold, thiazide diuretics, antimalarials, and rarely phenothiazine derivatives and methyldopa) must be excluded. Asymptomatic patients require no more than good oral hygiene. Symptomatic patients may be treated with topical fluorinated corticosteroid preparations applied five to six times a day to the affected areas. Local injections of 0.1 to 0.3 ml. of triamcinolone acetonide (5 mg. per ml.) may be helpful in localized or very painful areas. Griseofulvin, the antifungal antibiotic, has been recommended by some clinicians as being helpful in difficult cases of oral lichen planus. The reason for its benefit is unknown. Therapy should be instituted with 500 mg. of micronized griseofulvin or 125 mg. of ultramicronized griseofulvin twice a day. (This use of griseofulvin is not listed in the manufacturer's official directive.) Short-term treatment with systemic corticosteroids may be utilized when lesions are severe or especially painful and have not responded to local forms of treatment. Long-term treatment with systemic corticosteroids should not be undertaken except in extreme instances. Occasionally, hydrochloroquine (Plaquenil) in a dose of 200 mg. daily for 3 months may be attempted in severely disabling oral lichen planus. (This use of hydrochloroquine is not listed in the manufacturer's official directive.)

Longstanding oral lichen planus of the erosive, ulcerative, or bullous variety can be complicated by the development of a squamous cell carcinoma. This is a rare occurence, but patients with chronic disease should be periodically reexamined, and biopsy specimens should be obtained of any questionable lesions.

Lupus Erythematosus. Oral mucosal lesions of lupus erythematosus can occur with both the systemic and the discoid types. Approximately 15 per cent of patients with systemic lupus erythematosus may have oral lesions. These are usually inflammatory, erythematous, erosive, or ulcerative in nature and are associated with more severe systemic disease. Approximately 5 per cent of patients with discoid lupus erythematosus will have oral lesions. These lesions are similar to those of lichen planus or leukoplakia and are more chronic in nature. A biopsy specimen is often diagnostic; however, examination of the tissue by the direct immunofluorescent method for the deposition of immunoglobulins or complement components in a granular pattern at the basement membrane zone can be helpful in confirming the nature of the lesion. Local treatment as for lichen planus may be valuable for oral lesions of lupus erythematosus. Other forms of treatment should be instituted as for the basic disease.

Bullous Diseases. Oral lesions may be the presenting manifestation in up to half of patients who have *pemphigus vulgaris*. Persistent erosive, ulcerative, or bullous lesions should be sampled histopathologically and by direct immunofluorescent studies. Serum samples may show the antibodies to the intercellular substance which are so characteristic of pemphigus vulgaris. An early diagnosis of pemphigus vulgaris will facilitate early treatment, which may well prevent extensive lesions in this potentially fatal disease. Approximately one third of patients with *bullous pemphigoid* will have oral lesions. These bullae are less friable than those in pemphigus vulgaris, but as with all oral blisters they break easily to become erosions or ulcerations. Histopathologic and immunopathologic testing is helpful in establishing the proper diagnosis. Serum samples are also helpful in demonstrating the presence of the circulating anti–basement membrane zone antibodies that are associated with bullous pemphigoid.

Oral lesions are characteristically the first manifestations of *cicatricial (benign mucous membrane) pemphigoid.* Again, histopathologic and immunopathologic studies allow proper diagnosis. Treatment of these disorders is discussed on pages 644 to 646.

Recurrent Aphthous Stomatitis. Canker sores afflict at least 20 per cent of young adults; fortunately, relatively few are afflicted by severe, continuous ulcerations. Canker sores commonly affect the "movable," nonkeratinized oral mucosa, usually sparing the attached gingiva and hard palate. There are three types of canker sores, the classification of which is largely based on the size of the lesions. Minor aphthous ulcers are recurrent crops of one to five punched-out ulcers less than 1 cm. in diameter which usually affect the lips, buccal mucosa, mucobuccal and mucolabial sulci, and tongue. Major aphthous ulcers are recurrent, large—greater than 1 cm. in diameter—chronic, and usually solitary ulcers that begin as nodules, destroy deep tissue, and heal with scarring. Major aphthous ulcers also affect the movable oral mucosa and may also be found in the posterior mucosal surfaces. Herpetiform ulcers are recurrent, multiple, shallow, pinpoint lesions of 1 to 2 mm. that may affect any part of the oral mucosa. Minor aphthous ulcers are far more common than are major aphthous or herpetiform ulcers.

The cause of canker sores is not known. Canker sores may represent mucosal manifestations of diseases such as nutritional deficiencies of vitamin B_{12}, folate, and iron, Behçet's syndrome, chronic ulcerative colitis (see pp. 403 to 407), and Crohn's disease (see pp. 367 to 370). Patients who suffer from recurrent aphthous stomatitis but do not have any of the aforementioned associated diseases may well have a process that represents an autoimmune phenomenon.

Systemic diseases associated with recurrent aphthous stomatitis should be excluded. A complete blood count and determination of serum vitamin B_{12}, folate, and iron levels may define patients whose diseases will be responsive to replacement therapy. Trauma appears to play a permissive role in the development of canker sores. Reduction of trauma by avoidance of sharp-surfaced foods, the use of a soft-bristled toothbrush, avoidance of talking while chewing, and correction of any dental defects may be helpful.

Some female patients note a definite flare in the premenstrual phase of the menstrual cycle. Doses of estrogens or estrogen-dominated oral contraceptives may suppress these flares. Escharotics such as silver nitrate or negatol (Negatan) may be utilized for very early lesions that are few in number. These should not be used late in the course of the disease, as this will only increase the amount of tissue necrosis. Topical fluorinated corticosteroids may be applied during the first few days of the disease but should be avoided once the lesion has become fully established. Topical or systemic antibiotics may be used in the latter part of the disease or may be tried initially. Herpetiform-type ulcers often respond to topical or systemic administration of tetracycline. On occasion, systemic corticosteroid therapy or intralesional corticosteroid therapy may be helpful. Three ml. of 2 per cent viscous lidocaine (Xylocaine) held in the mouth for 1 minute before meals provides relief of pain for these patients.

Melanocytic Nevi. Occurrence of pigmented nevi in the oral mucosa is not uncommon, and they are rarely malignant. All types of nevi, including lentigines, dermal nevi, junctional nevi, compound nevi, blue nevi, and lentigo maligna, may be found. Removal of the pigmented lesion is the best treatment and is definitely indicated if the lesions are chronically irritated, enlarging, developing color changes, or ulcerative. Occasionally, an amalgam tattoo may be mistaken for a melanocytic nevus. At times, occlusal roentgenograms will demonstrate metallic fragments in the oral mucosa.

Gingival and Periodontal Membrane

Eruption Cyst. Eruption of the deciduous and permanent dentition may cause redness and swelling of the mucosa covering the erupting teeth. This reaction is an *eruption cyst,* and it may be treated merely by making an incision in the overlying tissue. The eruption of the deciduous dentition in young children may produce considerable discomfort, and topical anesthetic ointment may be necessary to relieve it. Aspirin may also be used for its analgesic effect.

Pericoronitis. This is an inflammatory reaction that develops around erupting third molar (wisdom) teeth. Occasionally, these inflamed areas will become infected and antibiotic treatment is necessary. Trismus and submandibular lymphadenopathy are clinical signs of severe pericoronitis. Removal of the offending tooth or teeth is necessary for relief.

Localized and Generalized Enlargement of the Gingival Tissue. Localized enlargement may be evidence of a periodontal abscess or a hyperplastic growth caused by local irritating factors (epulis). Plaque and calculus deposits are the most common form of irritation. However, faulty dental restorations may be responsible. Patients treated with phenytoin (Dilantin) may have generalized enlargement of the gingiva. If this tissue becomes a problem esthetically, interferes with mastication, or prevents adequate oral hygiene, the tissue must be removed surgically. After surgical treatment, the construction of a positive-pressure mouthguard may reduce the regrowth of the tissue. *Idiopathic gingival fibromatosis* may also cause a generalized enlargement of the gingiva. This enlargement is also treated surgically.

Leukemic infiltrates into the gingival tissue may be responsible for diffuse enlargement. Hemorrhage is a complicating factor, and surgery is contraindicated. Gentle cleaning of the teeth is helpful in reducing irritation from dental deposits. If hemorrhage occurs, topical hemostatic agents such as an absorbable gelatin preparation (Gelfoam) and a periodontal dressing are applied.

Acute Necrotizing Ulcerative Gingivitis (Trench Mouth, Vincent's Infection). This is an infectious process caused by *Fusobacterium fusiforme* and *Borrelia vincentii*. The lesions are usually localized to the interdental spaces between the teeth, but in severe instances lesions may involve the buccal mucosa and pharynx. Clinically, the lesions appear as craters or punched-out areas with a yellowish necrotic surface. There may be considerable discomfort, and analgesics (codeine) may be necessary to control the pain. In severe infections with fever and submandibular lymphadenopathy, antibiotic treatment (penicillin, erythromycin) is indicated. Pronounced improvement is usually noted 4 to 5 days after antibiotic treatment has been initiated. After the acute phase has passed, cleaning of the teeth and oral hygiene measures (brushing, flossing) must be started. Occasionally surgery (gingivectomy) is necessary to recontour the craters that have developed between the teeth. Mild infection may be treated by warm hydrogen peroxide mouth rinses and improvement in oral hygiene. Stress, fatigue, and heavy smoking are predisposing factors.

Gingivitis and Periodontitis. These diseases are the most common inflammatory reactions that involve the supporting structures of the teeth. *Gingivitis* is an inflammatory reaction involving the papillary, marginal, or attached gingiva and is caused by accumulation of plaque (bacteria plus mucinous deposits) and calculus (hard deposits) at the junction of the gingiva and the tooth surface. Treatment consists of thorough removal of all plaque and calculus deposits and meticulous oral hygiene by brushing and flossing.

When the inflammatory reaction spreads to the periodontal ligament and alveolar bone, *periodontitis* is present. Periodontitis, if untreated, may cause extensive bone resorption, separation of the gingiva from the teeth with eventual tooth loss, and infection (pyorrhea). In advanced periodontitis, there may be a separation of the gingiva from the tooth. This phenomenon is termed a "periodontal pocket" and if such pockets are more than 3 to 4 mm. deep, surgical correction will be necessary. The soft tissue is surgically separated from the teeth, and the tissue is elevated to expose the underlying bone and tooth roots. Granulation tissue and any deposits on the roots of the teeth are removed with curets. If bone destruction has occurred and bony craters and irregularities are present, the bone will need recontouring. The soft tissue is then repositioned and held in place with silk suture, and a zinc oxide periodontal dressing is placed over the wound to protect it during the healing phase. Healing is usually complete in 14 days.

Periodontosis. Destruction of the alveolar bone may also occur in periodontosis. This resorptive process usually involves the molar and incisor teeth, is more common in females, and usually starts at a young age (15 to 18 years).

Systemic Diseases. Systemic diseases such as diabetes mellitus, hyperparathyroidism, histiocytosis X, and scleroderma may be responsible for changes in the alveolar bone. Papillon-Lefèvre syndrome is characterized by early exfoliation of the deciduous teeth and rapid exfoliation of the erupting permanent teeth. The gingival changes include a fiery red attached gingiva. There is associated hyperkeratosis of the palms and soles. The teeth are lost at an early age, and dentures are necessary.

Diabetes mellitus has an adverse effect on the periodontal tissues. Longstanding diabetes causes a thickening of the capillary basement membrane, and this thickening has an adverse effect on local tissue metabolism. Usually diabetics are more prone to have periodontal disease and dental infection.

Chronic Desquamative Gingivitis. This diffuse inflammatory reaction is limited to the attached gingiva. The reaction is most often seen in postmenopausal women but is occasionally seen in males. The lesions are chronic in nature and may be confused with bullous pemphigoid, cicatricial pemphigoid, or pemphigus vulgaris. A biopsy should be performed in order to establish an accurate diagnosis. In patients with desquamative gingivitis, periodontitis and bone resorption do not develop even though the gingiva is severely inflamed. The inflammatory reaction can sometimes be suppressed by the application of a topical steroid such as fluocinonide (Topsyn Gel), 0.05 per cent.

Teeth, Jaws, and Musculature

Teeth. The *congenital absence of teeth* may present a problem with occlusion. The maxillary lateral incisors are missing most often. If detected at an early age by dental x-ray films, the space that would have been occupied by the tooth can be maintained by an orthodontic appliance until a permanent bridge can be constructed, or if necessary the space can be closed orthodontically. Multiple impacted and missing teeth may be present in *cleidocranial dysostosis*. *Ectodermal dysplasia*, such as epidermolysis bullosa, may cause extensive carious lesions to develop and lead to loss of the teeth.

Enamel hypoplasia may occur from excess fluoride in drinking water (fluorosis) or from disease states during childhood (chickenpox, measles). *Developmental anomalies* of the enamel (amelogenesis imperfecta) or dentin (dentinogenesis imperfecta) also make the teeth more susceptible to dental caries. These teeth may require extensive restorative procedures.

Pigmented teeth may be caused by a traumatic injury to the tooth which causes hemorrhage inside the tooth. If the pulp tissue becomes necrotic, it must be removed and replaced by a root-canal filling. Systemic administration of tetracycline during the formative stage of the teeth should be avoided, because staining of the tooth structure can occur.

Malposition and malocclusion of the teeth may present esthetic and functional problems. Discrepancies in occlusion require orthodontic treatment, and if severe problems of prognathism, retrognathism, or open bite exist, surgical correction is necessary to restore proper occlusion and esthetics.

Dental Caries. Dental caries affects all age groups. The disease is most prevalent in young persons (4 to 20 years). The administration of topical or systemic fluoride is an effective measure for reducing tooth decay. In areas where the municipal water is fluoridated (2 ppm), there may be a 50 per cent decrease in the incidence of tooth decay. If municipal fluoridation is not available, fluoride can be administered in tablet form or applied topically by a dentist. Toothpastes containing fluoride are also beneficial in reducing decay.

After a carious lesion has developed in a tooth, the lesion must be removed and a restoration placed in the tooth. If left untreated, a pulpitis or periapical abscess may develop. *Pulpitis* is treated by placing a medicated dressing (calcium hydroxide plus zinc oxide and eugenol) in the carious portion of the tooth after the carious lesion has been excavated. If the pulp becomes necrotic from the inflammatory reaction present, a *periapical abscess* may develop. This may be corrected by endodontic treatment (root-canal filling) or, if indicated, by removal of the tooth. Antibiotic therapy is often necessary to control the infectious process. If the infection is left untreated, facial cellulitis and fascial plane infections may develop. Large abscesses can develop which need to be incised and drained. Sometimes drainage can be established by drilling a hole in the occlusal surface of the tooth.

Ludwig's Angina. Ludwig's angina is an infection of the floor of the mouth and fascial planes of the neck. This infection, if left untreated, may be responsible for a compromised airway. If this develops, hospitalization of the patient is necessary with initiation of proper supportive therapy (tracheostomy, antibiotics, fluids).

Complications of Dental Extractions. Extraction of teeth is usually an uncomplicated procedure. However, excessive bleeding, osteitis (dry socket), perforated maxillary sinus, or even jaw fracture may occur. *Extensive bleeding from a socket* can usually be controlled by placing a hemostatic agent (Gelfoam, Oxycel) into the socket and suturing the socket closed. Initially the bleeding may be controlled by injecting a local anesthetic containing 1:100,000 or 1:50,000 epinephrine into the tissue surrounding the socket. *Localized osteitis or dry socket* is treated by placing iodoform gauze saturated with butacaine and nitromersol (Butyn Metaphen) ointment into the socket. The dressing may have to be changed daily until relief is obtained. Analgesics containing codeine may be necessary to control the pain. If *rupture of the lining of the maxillary sinus* occurs during the removal of a tooth, a surgical procedure may be necessary to close the defect. If the opening is small (1 to 2 mm.), it may close spontaneously. If a tooth root is left in the sinus, sinusitis may develop. *Jaw fracture* is relatively uncommon after the removal of teeth, but the removal of deeply impacted mandibular third molars (wisdom teeth) may result in fracture of the mandible. *Paresthesia* may also develop after removal of impacted mandibular third molars if the inferior alveolar nerve should be damaged during the procedure.

Osteomyelitis. Osteomyelitis can develop from chronically infected teeth or from organisms that may enter the oral cavity from an external source *(Actinomyces bovis)*. Patients receiving radiation therapy for tumors of the head and neck are also more prone to have osteomyelitis. Bacterial culture and sensitivity tests are needed to determine which antibiotic agent should be employed in the treatment of osteomyelitis.

Jaw Tumors. *Odontogenic cysts and tumors* develop from odontogenic epithelium that persists in the jaws after the teeth have developed. *Ameloblastomas* may develop into extremely large multilocular, cystic lesions, with destruction of large portions of the jaw. Large lesions may require extensive resection. Ameloblastomas are the most aggressive of the benign odontogenic tumors. *Odontogenic cysts* are slower growing but, if left untreated, can also be very destructive. In most instances, an odontogenic cyst can be treated by removing the cyst lining and the associated tooth if one is present. *Odontogenic keratocysts* are cysts that have a keratinized lining. Thorough removal of the lining is necessary, because these cysts have been known to undergo malignant transformation.

Periapical cementoma appears initially as a radiolucent area at the apex of the teeth, usually the lower incisors; it is more common in females. After the lesion has matured it may become radiopaque. Histologically, the lesion appears similar to *fibrous dysplasia,* except that the lesion is always associated with the tooth root. Fibrous dysplasia may be a generalized process and involve large portions of the jaws. The lesions of fibrous dysplasia may become disfiguring, and cosmetic surgery may be necessary.

Giant-cell reparative granuloma usually presents as a solitary radiolucent area, and if such a lesion is diagnosed histologically, blood calcium levels should be evaluated to rule out hyperparathyroidism.

Temporomandibular Joints. The temporomandibular joints may be involved in several systemic disorders. *Rheumatoid arthritis* may involve these joints, and if pain and limitation of motion are present, intracapsular injection of steroids may be necessary. Trauma may also be a factor in temporomandibular pathology. If the joints have been damaged severely, surgical removal may be necessary followed by a Silastic joint arthroplasty. Ankylosis may also occur from longstanding immobilization caused by trauma, but this can be corrected by surgical intervention.

Temporomandibular joint syndrome is a symptom complex consisting of pain, crepitation, and trismus. It may be due to faulty occlusion, improperly constructed dentures, or severe bruxism. Treatment consists of alleviating any contributing dental factors and initiating analgesic and muscle relaxant (diazepam [Valium]) therapy. Heat applied to the area is also beneficial. Occasionally, occlusal splints are necessary, and occlusal equilibration may be indicated in selected cases. Neurologic disease—e.g., trigeminal neuralgia or tic douloureux—must be ruled out in patients complaining of temporomandibular joint pain.

Salivary Glands and Regional Lymph Nodes

Sialolithiasis. Obstruction of a salivary gland duct by calcific stones within the duct is not uncommon. If the stone is small and close to the orifice, it can often be removed with a fine probe. If the stone is large and inaccessible, surgical removal of the entire gland is indicated. *Sialadenitis* is an inflammatory reaction involving the major salivary glands. The glands may become swollen and painful. The usual cause is obstruction of the major duct by a mucous or bacterial plug. Systemic antibiotics should be administered and fluid intake increased. Usually the gland will return to normal in 1 to 2 weeks. However, if the symptoms persist, surgical removal of the gland is necessary.

Xerostomia. This is a relatively common complaint of patients 50 years old or older. Drug therapy, often in the form of antidepressants, may be responsible for xerostomia. Patients with this complaint should always be questioned about any medications they are taking. In patients who have received radiation to the head and neck, xerostomia may develop because of atrophy of the salivary glands. Sjögren's syndrome and Mikulicz's disease must also be excluded. Xerostomia is a difficult disorder to treat, because there is no effective way to increase salivary fluid once a gland has atrophied. If the problem is drug induced, it may not be practical to withdraw the patient's medication. These patients are also more prone to have dental caries and candidal infections. Fluoride mouth rinses are helpful in reducing dental decay, and nystatin oral suspension is beneficial in oral candidiasis.

Lymph Node Enlargement. This should always be viewed with suspicion. If there is nodal involvement in the submental or submandibular area, dental infection should always be considered. A thorough oral examination should be performed to rule out any malignant lesions. Oral squamous cell carcinoma may present with metastasis to regional lymph nodes.

DISORDERS OF THE MOUTH (MALIGNANT)

method of
DONALD SERAFIN, M.D.
Durham, North Carolina

Malignant disorders of the mouth account for 7 to 8 per cent of all cancers in the United States. Approximately 20,000 new cases each year are reported. Squamous cell carcinoma accounts for over 90 per cent of these malignancies. In spite of ready availability and accessibility to examination, oral malignancies frequently are undiagnosed for extended periods of time. This is one factor which influences the relatively poor survival in this disease. Other factors which influence prognosis are location of the primary lesion, its size, and the presence of nodal metastases. The degree of tumor differentiation is of lesser importance in determining prognosis.

Any physician involved in the treatment of head and neck malignancies must be familiar with the tumor, nodes, and metastases (TNM) classification system for squamous carcinoma of the head and neck (Table 1). This system is provided

TABLE 1. **TNM Classification System for Squamous Carcinoma of Head and Neck**

T—Tumor
T_{is}—Carcinoma in situ
T_1—Tumor <2 cm.
T_2—Tumor >2 cm. but <4 cm.
T_3—Tumor >4 cm.

M—Metastases (distant)
M_0—None
M_1—Distant metastases

N—Regional lymph nodes
N_0—No palpable nodes
N_1—Ipsilateral lymph nodes (not fixed)
N_2—Contralateral lymph nodes (not fixed)
N_3—Fixed

Stage I—$T_1N_0M_0$
Stage II—$T_2N_0M_0$
Stage III—$T_3N_0M_0$
$T_1N_1M_0$
$T_2N_1M_0$
$T_3N_1M_0$
Stage IV—Remainder

by the American Joint Committee for Cancer Staging and End Results Reporting (1967). It is useful in determining both treatment and prognosis.

Common treatment modalities include cobalt-60 radiation, surgery, and adjunctive chemotherapy. The literature is replete with conflicting reports advocating one mode of therapy as opposed to another. Survival rates are cited supporting these conclusions. In general, however, favorable lesions (Stages I and II) have a good prognosis if treated with either mode of therapy, whereas unfavorable lesions (Stages III and IV) have a less favorable prognosis. It is in this latter group that a multidisciplinary approach is necessary to achieve the maximal result. Surgery and/or irradiation with adjunctive chemotherapy is frequently employed.

Malignant disorders of the oral cavity are further subdivided into different anatomic regions, each of which has a different malignant potential and patterns of extension. Treatment efforts therefore must take those differences into consideration. The oral cavity consists of (1) lips, (2) buccal mucosa, (3) gingiva and alveolar ridge, (4) tongue (anterior to circumvallate papilla), (5) floor of the mouth, and (6) hard palate. Any disease noted more posteriorly is best considered under oropharynx (e.g., soft palate uvula, base of tongue). Malignant potential in this region is greater than in the oral cavity and increases with more posterior tumor origin.

Lips

This is the most common site for a malignancy of the oral cavity, accounting for approximately 25 to 30 per cent of reported cases. There is a significantly high (95 per cent) male preponderance, the greatest incidence occurring in the fifth to seventh decade. The lower lip is involved 95 per cent of the time. Surprisingly, late diagnosis is the rule, an average of 2 years elapsing before medical attention is sought. Commonly, three histologic types occur: (1) exophytic, (2) ulcerative, or (3) verrucous. The ulcerative type tends to be the most aggressive, invading earlier, and is usually of a higher histologic grade of malignancy. The verrucous type is rare and carries a more favorable prognosis. The size and duration of the primary lesion influence prognosis the most. Regional lymph node metastases are uncommon (10 to 15 per cent), but when they occur it is usually to the submandibular region. The lesion can be treated with external irradiation or surgery. Survival statistics are about the same; there is approximately an 80 to 90 per cent 5 year survival rate with either mode of therapy. This is halved if regional nodal metastases are present.

Buccal Mucosa

Squamous cell carcinoma of the buccal mucosa is most frequently encountered at the commissures, occlusive plane of the teeth, and retromolar region. It has a similar sex and age distribution as outlined for carcinoma of the lip. In the southeastern United States, where local tobacco irritants are used by both sexes, the sex incidence is approximately equal.

Frank malignant changes are usually preceded by leukoplakia. The disease is frequently multifocal, as 31 per cent of the patients develop a second primary lesion. There are usually three histologic types: (1) exophytic, (2) ulcerative, and (3) verrucous. Verrucous carcinoma rarely metastasizes and carries the best prognosis (60 to 75 per cent 5 year survival), whereas 50 per cent of exophytic and ulcerative carcinomas have metastasized at the time the primary lesion is first diagnosed. The overall 5 year survival rate is 30 to 50 per cent. Early lesions can be treated with irradiation or surgery. The more anterior the lesion (e.g., commissure), the more favorable the prognosis. Certainly, the presence of positive nodes adversely influences survival (37 per cent). Verrucous lesions are best treated surgically, as irradiation tends to exacerbate regional spread.

Gingiva and Alveolar Ridge

Squamous carcinomas of the gingiva and alveolar ridge account for approximately 10 per cent of all oral malignant neoplasms. The lower edentulous jaw (premolar and molar region) is more frequently affected than the upper jaw.

As noted in other regions, there is a male preponderance in the later decades. Because of the proximity of the underlying bone, invasion occurs 50 per cent of the time.

Treatment with irradiation often results in bone devitalization. For this reason surgery is more frequently employed in therapy. The 5 year survival rate is approximately 50 per cent.

Tongue

Squamous cell carcinoma of the tongue accounts for 25 to 30 per cent of all oral malignancies and is second in frequency only to carcinoma of the lip. As in other oral malignancies, the disease is most common in men in their later decades of life. Seventy-five per cent of malignancies occur in the anterior two thirds of the tongue (i.e., anterior to the circumvallate papillae). The most common site of involvement is the middle third along the lateral border. Metastases to regional nodes occur more frequently than they do from tumors in other locations. On admission, 40 per cent of patients have positive ipsilateral lymph nodes and 20 per cent have bilateral involvement. Prognosis is influenced by (1) the location of the lesion (anterior lesions have the most favorable prognoses), (2) presence of positive nodes, and (3) size (lesions >2 cm. have poorer prognosis). The overall 5 year survival rate in lesions of the anterior two thirds of the tongue is 67 per cent. This is reduced by half if positive nodes are present. Posterior tongue lesions have the poorest prognoses, with a 5 year survival rate of 15 per cent. Treatment of the small early lesion without palpable nodes can be either irradiation or surgery. Since occult metastases exist (17 per cent) in the absence of clinically palpable nodes, the ipsilateral neck should probably be included in the ports of irradiation and a neck dissection done if surgery is undertaken. Larger lesions with clinically palpable nodes are best treated surgically with a composite resection consisting of a portion of the tongue, mandible, and a radical neck dissection. Unfavorable lesions with a poorer prognosis or with inadequate surgical margins should also have postoperative irradiation and possible adjunctive chemotherapy.

Floor of Mouth

Squamous carcinoma of the floor of the mouth accounts for 10 to 15 per cent of all oral malignancies and is the third most common location for development (lip and tongue are more common). Age and sex predilection are about the same as those of carcinoma in other sites. The most frequent location is anterior, adjacent to the frenulum. The tumor is frequently exophytic or papillary, and like malignancies of the buccal mucosa it is frequently multifocal. Unlike malignancies of the tongue, metastases occur later. Approximately 35 to 70 per cent of patients have palpable lymph nodes during the course of their disease, about half of which are positive.

Prognosis without nodal involvement is good (70 per cent 5 year survival), but this figure drops to 25 per cent if nodes are involved. Treatment can be with either irradiation or surgery, depending on the size of the lesion, presence or absence of nodes, and proximity to the mandible. Early lesions have the same prognoses with either mode of therapy.

Hard Palate

Squamous carcinoma of the hard palate, unlike other oral locations, occurs less frequently than other malignant neoplasms (e.g., salivary gland or mucous carcinomas). It is a disease of elderly men. Prognosis is influenced by the size of the tumor and the presence of positive nodes. The 5 year survival rate is 54 per cent in tumors <3 cm. and negative nodes. Lesions >3 cm. have a 5 year survival rate of 16 per cent. This is reduced in half (8 per cent) when nodes are positive. Squamous carcinoma of the hard palate can be treated successfully with either irradiation or surgery.

In the preceding paragraphs, an attempt has been made to coordinate existing modes of therapy to the behavior of squamous carcinoma in different anatomic regions of the oral cavity. In early stages, survival statistics are favorable; however, in more advanced stages the results with a single method of therapy are not good. If one considers the overall 5 year survival rate in all squamous cancers of the head and neck, it is quite low, approximately 20 per cent. In spite of considerable effort and variation in techniques, the survival rate has not improved in 15 years.

In an attempt to improve these deplorable statistics, a multidisciplinary approach has been designed to improve patient care, as well as the length and quality of survival.

In this institution a head and neck tumor clinic meets weekly with representatives from plastic surgery, otolaryngology, radiation therapy, and medical oncology, as well as representatives from nursing, dietetics, and social service. Patients with advanced malignancies of the head and neck (Stages III and IV) are carefully evaluated and combination therapy consisting of surgery and/or radiation and chemotherapy begun.

1. Surgical therapy varies, but the basic principle consists of an en bloc removal of the primary malignancy and associated node-bearing tissue. This frequently requires a composite resection, consisting of the malignant oral primary, a segment of mandible, and a radical neck dissection. Reconstruction, following such extensive extirpative surgery, is accomplished, when possible, during the same operative procedure in order to expedite the initiation of the other modes of the combined therapy protocol and to minimize the deformity. Thus the psychologic insult from the deformity is minimized and the quality of life improved.

2. Postoperative radiation is administered by a cobalt-60 unit in a fractional dose of 200 rads given in 5 treatments each week. Between 5500 and 6500 rads total tumor dose is administered. If no cervical lymph nodes are involved, 5000 rads is given to the neck. If cervical nodes are positive, 6000 rads is given.

3. Current chemotherapeutic drugs employed in this institution are bleomycin, methotrexate, vinblastine, and a nitrosourea compound (CCNU). Treatment with these drugs is initiated 3 weeks after surgery and/or radiation in six 28 day cycles.

Bleomycin is employed because of its demonstrated effectiveness in the treatment of patients with squamous carcinoma. It is administered subcutaneously in 10 unit aliquots on days 1 and 4 of the first course and repeated at a dosage of 2 units on the same days in successive cycles. Tissue toxicity is relatively low, as is bone marrow suppression.

Methotrexate, an antimetabolite, has also been demonstrated to be effective in the treatment of patients with squamous carcinoma. It is administered orally at 10 mg. per square meter of body surface on days 1 and 4 of each course. Bone marrow suppression must be carefully monitored.

Vinblastine, a mitotic inhibitor, is also beneficial in the treatment of squamous carcinoma. It is given intravenously at 8 mg. per square meter on the first day of each course. If neurotoxicity supervenes, dosages are correspondingly reduced by 50 per cent.

CCNU, an alkylating agent, has been demonstrated to have some effectiveness in the treatment of squamous carcinoma when employed in conjunction with other drugs. It is administered orally, 75 mg. per square meter only on day 1. Bone marrow suppression must be monitored carefully.

Initial results with this multidisciplinary approach are promising. Whether 5 year survival statistics will be altered can be answered only with time. Certainly, without question the quality of life of these unfortunate patients has improved.

DISEASES OF THE NAILS

method of
W. CHRISTOPHER DUNCAN, M.D.
Houston, Texas

Nail disorders, like disorders of the hair, are an important cosmetic defect, and therefore patients demand treatment for relatively minor deformities. Unfortunately, treatment is still unsatisfactory in many instances. However, the use of griseofulvin in fungal infections and local injection of triamcinolone for conditions affecting the matrix represent the treatment for almost 50 per cent of the nail deformities seen. Most changes in the nail plate reflect abnormalities in the nail matrix that occurred weeks to months before the nail changes are observed. All too frequently the causes of abnormalities of the nail matrix are unknown or are processes that do not respond well to therapeutic efforts. Nail diseases can be classified as those that primarily involve the nail matrix and nail plate, diseases of the nail bed, and diseases of the periungual tissues. Those conditions involving the nail bed and tissues around the nail are somewhat more responsive to therapy.

Diseases of the Nail Matrix and Nail Plate

Congenital Nail Dystrophies. Congenital abnormalities of the nails may range from the markedly thickened nails of pachyonychia congenita to the small friable atrophic nails of dyskeratosis congenita and congenital ectodermal defect. These conditions are examples of abnormalities in function of the nail matrix which cannot be altered by any known therapy. The mechanical problems caused by thickening of the nails can be remedied by avulsion of the nail and destruction of the nail matrix by curettage or application of phenol in order to prevent regrowth of the nail.

Koilonychia. In this condition, also known as spoon nail, the nail is concave instead of convex. Koilonychia is sometimes associated with hypochromic anemia, other nutritional deficiencies, or polycythemia, and may be reversible if these conditions are corrected. However, most cases are familial or idiopathic and do not respond to treatment.

Traumatic Nail Dystrophies. Injuries to the base of the nail and the nail matrix may result in longitudinal ridging or splitting of the nail plate. Removal of the nail plate, excision of the scar in the matrix and nail bed, and approximation of the normal tissues with nylon sutures will sometimes result in a less severely grooved nail. Onychogryphosis refers to the long, markedly thickened, clawlike toenails seen in patients who are old, obese, or otherwise unable to properly take care of their nails. The chronic minor trauma to the untrimmed toenails pressing against the shoes results in hypertrophy of the matrix, producing thickening of the nail plate. A superimposed fungal infection may occur. The best treatment is prevention by proper nail trimming. When the condition is severe and interferes with the wearing of shoes, removal of the nail and destruction of the matrix may be necessary.

The trauma of jamming the great and/or second toenail against the toe of sports shoes, e.g., as occurs in tennis, may cause lateral ridging and splitting. Treatment consists of better fitting shoes.

The chronic trauma of biting or picking at the nails can lead to abnormalities in the nail plate. The most frequent example of this habitual, self-inflicted trauma is the horizontal ridging of the thumb nail that results from continuous picking at the nail and the nail base with a finger of the same hand. Only sincere motivation on the part of the patient will enable him to cease habits of this type.

Tumors Involving the Nail Matrix. Benign tumors, particularly fibromas and myxoid cysts, may occur near the base of the nail and cause pressure on the nail matrix, resulting in longitudinal grooving of the nail plate. Myxoid cysts sometimes respond to aspiration of the mucoid material and injection of 0.1 to 0.2 ml. of triamcinolone acetonide (3 mg. per ml.) into the lesion. Multiple treatments may be necessary.

Inflammatory Dermatoses Affecting the Nail Plate. Dyshidrotic eczema, lichen planus, and psoriasis may involve the base of the nail and nail matrix, resulting in longitudinal and horizontal ridging of the nails and pitting of the nail surface. In dyshidrosis, the nail changes, usually a series of irregular ridges across the nail, are associated with small vesicles along the lateral aspects of the fingers which progress to scaling pruritic patches. In lichen planus nail changes occur in about 10 per cent of the patients and for the most part consist of longitudinal striations and notching of the distal nail. Psoriasis is probably the most common condition affecting the nails. Discrete small pits in the nail plate are the most distinct sign; however, involvement may resemble gross fungal infection with opaque, discolored, irregular, and thickened nail plates. Patients will frequently have typical psoriatic plaques of the elbows, knees, and scalp; however, there may be no other lesions of psoriasis. Patients with dyshidrotic eczema are more likely to respond to topical treatment than are those with lichen planus or psoriasis. Refractory inflammatory conditions can be treated by triamcinolone acetonide (3 mg. per ml.) injected just proximal to the posterior nail fold. A tuberculin syringe with a 30 gauge needle works well, or a jet injector (Derma-jet) may be used. Intralesional injections are reserved for severe nail deformities in psoriasis and lichen planus; they are rarely or never indicated in dyshidrosis.

Dermatophytosis. Clinically fungus infections of the nail are characterized by irregular thickening and softening of the nail plate with subungual keratotic debris. Separation of the nail plate from the nail bed (onycholysis) is common. Since the identical picture can occur in psoriasis and other nail dystrophies, potassium hydroxide preparations must be performed to confirm the diagnosis. Cultures of nail clippings are not as reliable. Dermatophyte infections of the fingernails respond well to oral griseofulvin (500 mg. of the micronized type twice daily). Griseofulvin should be given until the nails have grown out (3 to 6 months for fingernails). Toenail infections respond poorly; if asymptomatic, they are usually best left untreated. Otherwise, surgical management with debridement or avulsion may be (rarely!) indicated.

Striations. Longitudinal striations are common in perfectly healthy persons. They are usually of a minor degree in young persons, but become more prominent with increasing age. There is no effective treatment.

Twenty-Nail Dystrophy of Childhood. Twenty-nail dystrophy is an idiopathic nail dystrophy of all 20 nails that begins insidiously in early childhood. The nails are uniformly affected with excessive longitudinal striations with frequent distal splitting and notching. It is believed to be a self-limited abnormality that resolves slowly with age.

Leukonychia. White spots of the nail plate are due to imperfect keratinization of areas of the plate and can follow many acute and chronic systemic disease processes. Most commonly they are seen in otherwise normal persons, and the cause is unknown. There is no effective treatment, although in most cases the areas grow out as the nail grows and are spontaneously cured.

Nail Splitting. Nails may split either lengthwise or laterally in layers. It occurs most frequently in persons, such as housewives, who often have their hands in soap and water with subsequent excessive drying of the nail. The regular use of a good hand cream combats this. The patient should be advised to keep the nail trimmed (filed, not cut) as short as possible—i.e., it must not extend beyond the fingertip. Regular use of nail polish is protective and insofar as possible should be applied over old polish rather than frequently removing the polish with remover. Only oily removers should be used. Several layers of nail polish splint the nail in addition to protecting the nail from the effects of frequent soap and water exposure.

Diseases of the Nail Bed

Onycholysis. Onycholysis (separation of the nail plate from the underlying nail bed starting at the free margins and proceeding proximally) may occur in psoriasis, fungal infections, hyperthyroidism, impaired peripheral circulation, hyperhidrosis, and photo-drug reactions. It occurs most frequently without apparent cause, however. In the idiopathic variety there is simply a loosening of the plate from the nail bed without deformity of the nail plate or nail fold. Trauma, including picking with pointed instruments, contributes to the condition, and patients must be advised to trim the nail plate as far back as possible. This prevents further trauma and removes the roof from the space between the plate and nail bed, thereby reducing the possibility of secondary infection with Candida or Pseudomonas. Four per cent thymol in chloroform is useful to dry the space and to suppress growth of Candida and Pseudomonas. If the overlying nail plate becomes greenish-black, indicative of Pseudomonas infection, polymyxin ear drops may be effective. Injection of triamcinolone acetonide (3 mg. per ml.) into the posterior nail fold is frequently of benefit.

Subungual Hematoma. Acute trauma will frequently result in a painful hematoma between the nail plate and nail bed. Pain can be relieved by draining the collection of blood by carefully making a hole through the nail plate. This can be done most easily with the heated (red hot) end of a paper clip held in a needle holder, or with special drills.

Tumors of the Nail Bed. Bowen's disease, squamous cell carcinoma, basal cell carcinoma, and malignant melanoma all can rarely involve the nail bed, causing separation of the nail plate from the bed and subungual scaling. When these changes are seen involving a single nail with negative mycologic studies and absence of other skin lesions of psoriasis, the nail plate should be removed and the nail bed biopsied. Amputation of the digit is indicated if melanoma is present or if there is squamous cell carcinoma with invasion of the bone. The other conditions can be treated by local excision.

Diseases of the Periungual Tissues

Acute Paronychia. Acute paronychia, or inflammation of the folds surrounding the nail plate, is painful and usually associated with *Staphylococcus aureus*, but Pseudomonas and Streptococcus may rarely be responsible. If pus is present, the area should be incised and drained. This can be done by inserting a scalpel blade between the nail and the nail fold. Gram stain of the exudate and bacterial cultures and sensitivity studies provide guidance to appropriate antibiotic therapy. Cloxacillin or erythromycin, 250 mg. four times daily, should be continued until the pain, swelling, and redness subside completely. Pseudomonas paronychial infection may be treated with tetracycline, 500 mg. four times daily, or sulfisoxazole, 1.0 gram four times daily following an initial loading dose of 2.0 grams, provided the organism is sensitive to either of these. Severe infection, unresponsive to incision and drainage, may require parenteral carbenicillin.

Chronic Paronychia. Chronic paronychia is much more difficult to treat than the acute form. It usually starts with loss of cuticle (and, by the same token, is not "cured" until regrowth and adherence of the cuticle to the nail plate occur). This may be the result of constant contact with soap and water, but physical injury may be etiologic. The infection is a mixed one, but *Candida albicans* is present in most cases. The condition must be distinguished from a true fungal infection with which it is often confused, because griseofulvin has no role in the treatment of the usual paronychia.

Treatment, for the most part, is by frequent local applications to the nail fold. Four per cent thymol in chloroform is both antimonilial and antibacterial for a variety of organisms. Haloprogin (Halotex) or clotrimazole (Lotrimin) is also effective against both yeasts and bacteria, and the liquid formulations penetrate beneath the nail fold. Injection of triamcinolone (3 mg. per ml.) into the posterior nail fold is almost always followed by remarkable improvement. Occasionally, topically applied steroids in liquid formulations (betamethasone [Valisone lotion] or fluocinolone acetonide [Synalar solution]) will be effective. If there is evidence of Pseudomonas infection—e.g., green discoloration of the nail plate—polymyxin B, neomycin, and hydrocortisone (Cortisporin otic drops) or neomycin and hydrocortisone (Coly-Mycin S otic drops) are often effective.

Periungual and Subungual Warts. Warts of the nail fold frequently occur in those who chew their nails and can be spread by this habit, which should be discouraged. Warts involving nail folds or the distal nail bed can be treated by cryotherapy with liquid nitrogen, by curettage under local anesthesia, or by application of cantharidin in flexible collodion (Cantharone). All methods of treatment are fraught with failure. Prior to treatment the overlying nail plate should be trimmed so that the entire wart can be treated. The cantharidin in collodion is applied to the wart, allowed to dry, and then occluded with adhesive tape for 24 hours. This usually results in a marked inflammatory reaction involving the wart tissue with subsequent sloughing of the wart. Sometimes repeat treatment is necessary. It should be borne in mind that all destructive treatments may lead to scar tissue formation and permanent disfiguration, and the wart may recur in the scar. Sometimes warts involute spontaneously, and more conservative therapy such as 17 per cent salicylic acid and 17 per cent lactic acid in flexible collodion (Duofilm) or twice daily application of 10 per cent formalin may hasten this occurrence.

Ingrowing Toenails. Ingrowing toenails result when the lateral margin of the nail plate is trimmed in a curved fashion so that on regrowth the lateral free edge penetrates the lateral nail fold. This can be avoided by trimming the nail straight across. When the nail penetrates the soft tissue, local infection often occurs. This can often be treated with hot tap water or Burow's solution soaks for 30 minutes three to four times daily. A small wisp of cotton or dental floss is packed under the nail, gradually separating the nail from the injured tissue and preventing further penetration of the nail. More severe infections should be treated with systemic antibiotics. In recurring cases, excision of the lateral aspect of the nail under local anesthesia followed by curettage or chemical destruction of the nail matrix with liquefied phenol will prevent regrowth of the offending portion of the nail.

NEVI

(Common Moles)

method of
PEYTON E. WEARY, M.D.
Charlottesville, Virginia

There are few absolute rules that dictate whether a pigmented nevus merits removal. Often the physician is prompted to remove a lesion about which he is not apprehensive simply because it is a source of anxiety and the patient is unresponsive to reassurance, or because the lesion is cosmetically unacceptable. These are valid reasons for removal if the patient understands that the lesion will almost surely be benign.

A history of sudden change in size or appearance of a nevus is more important than the cosmetic appearance in deciding its malignant potential. All patients should therefore develop the habit of periodic self-examination every 3 to 4 months to detect any sudden subtle change. The word "sudden" should be stressed, however, because most nevi change gradually in size, shape, or color over the course of years, and such gradual changes need cause little concern. Rapid enlargement of a nevus, uniform or irregular darkening, particularly of a blue-black color, marked variation in coloration of a nevus from one area of the nevus to another area of the same lesion, the appearance of a smudged or indistinct margin or pseudopod-like projections of pigment at the margin, or the observation of macular pigmented satellite spots adjacent to the nevus should all prompt strong consideration of removal. When a nevus becomes malignant, in addition to changes in color, the surface of the lesion may gradually lose the normal skin lines which often overlie benign junctional nevi. Melanomas are often very vascular lesions and may be mistaken for pyogenic granulomas or angiomatous malformations on occasion. Bleeding, erosion, and ulceration are late signs of malignancy. Inflammation of a nevus does not necessarily indicate malignant transformation, as some nevi surmount inclusion cysts which may rupture and become inflamed.

Patients with red hair, green eyes, or very fair complexion who tan poorly have a somewhat greater incidence of melanoma than the average person. Also, there is an increased incidence of melanoma developing in certain families and in the skin of a patient who has had a previous melanoma removed. Such patients deserve particularly close scrutiny of their nevi.

Approximately 50 per cent of melanomas arise de novo instead of at the site of pre-existent nevi. When a melanoma arises in a nevus, it will ordinarily do so in one with microscopic evidence of junctional activity (the presence of nests of nevus cells at the dermal-epidermal junction). Nevi that are predominantly junctional in type are prevalent in childhood, and in adults are often located on the hands, feet, and genitalia. Most such lesions are flat or only slightly elevated. However, melanoma is rare prior to the age of puberty, and approximately 20 per cent of adults have pigmented nevi of the palms, soles, and genitalia. Indiscriminate removal of junctional nevi is not advisable, although the flat or slightly elevated nevus bears closer scrutiny than the brown or pale, dome-shaped, sessile, pedunculated, polypoid, or papillomatous nevus that is the most common adult type and generally intradermal (the nevus cells occupy the dermis exclusively). The compound nevus (the nevus cells are both junctional and intradermal) is a transitional type, often somewhat elevated, either smooth or verrucous, and frequently surrounded by a pale brown halo. Nevi are thought to regularly exhibit progression from junctional in childhood to compound and eventually intradermal in adult life.

The following pigmented nevi probably should be routinely removed because of greater than average malignant potential:

1. Nevi arising in the region of a nail matrix or nail bed which often produce a linear band of pigment in the nail plate.
2. Those situated on mucosal surfaces and transitional zones such as the lips, anus, labia, and glans penis.
3. Lesions at sites of unusually heavy and persistent trauma such as primary weight-bearing surfaces of the foot or hands of manual laborers.

Certain types of nevi deserve special consideration:

Juvenile melanoma: This misnomer refers to an uncommon, reddish-brown, dome-shaped, compound nevus, usually first appearing in childhood, which grows rapidly and may mimic malignant melanoma on cursory microscopic examination. Although they are clinically benign, excision of such lesions is usually advocated.

Giant "bathing-trunk" nevi: These extensive and bizarre pigmented nevi are present at birth, often associated with neural melanocytosis and spinal anomalies, and exhibit a very high incidence of malignant melanoma even in childhood. Although technically difficult, their early removal is advisable. Some experts recommend that all congenital pigmented nevi be excised.

Blue nevus: These deep dermal blue or blue-black nevi arise most often on the distal extremities and because of their dark color are occasionally mistaken for melanoma, although true melanoma arising in such a lesion is quite rare.

Halo nevus: Occasionally a pigmented nevus in the process of spontaneous involution will develop a surrounding halo of depigmentation. This is not a sign of malignancy. Some melanomas, however, do develop depigmented halos, as do occasional metastatic melanoma lesions. Removal should thus be based on the history and appearance of the pigmented lesion, not solely on the basis of whether or not there is a halo.

Removal of a pigmented nevus because of true concern for possible malignancy should be accomplished, when feasible, by simple excision with a margin, although biopsy of a portion of a very large lesion is acceptable and apparently does not increase the chance of metastasis. Lesions removed for cosmetic reasons or for reassurance can be shaved off flush with the surface under local anesthesia and the bleeding controlled with ferrous subsulfate (Monsel's solution). Such a procedure often yields a superior cosmetic result and provides a specimen adequate for histologic diagnosis. In some instances pigment will recur in the scar, but this alone should not cause undue concern.

OCCUPATIONAL DERMATOSES

method of
JAMES S. TAYLOR, M.D.
Cleveland, Ohio

Occupational skin disorders still account for almost half of all reported work illnesses, despite the fact that they are almost fully preventable. No industry, whatever its size, scope, or location, is immune to their occurrence. Occupational skin diseases are produced from old chemicals in processes both old and new, new chemicals in new processes, and a wide variety of biologic and physiologic agents. The major categories of work-related skin disorders are contact dermatitis (allergic, irritant, and photosensitivity), acne and follicular eruptions, and pigmentary abnormalities.

Contact Dermatitis

In this category are most occupational dermatoses. They may be caused by some of the hundreds of thousands of chemicals used in industry. About 80 per cent of contact dermatitis is produced by irritants, 20 per cent from allergic sensitization, and a small percentage, often overlooked, from photosensitivity. Most affected are the hands, but any part of the body may be involved.

Acute Contact Dermatitis. 1. Avoid contact with the offending agent. This may require several days away from work or temporary transfer to another job.

2. Avoid contact with potential aggravating factors such as excessive soap and water, alcohol, thimerosal, and sensitizers such as topically applied antihistamines, antibiotics (neomycin or nitrofurazone), and anesthetics ("caine" preparations). Other contributing factors to be avoided are heat, friction, and radiant energy.

3. Apply cool wet compresses to weeping and blistered areas 15 minutes two to three times daily. Isotonic saline solution may be used. With commercial preparations of Burow's solution (Bluboro powder or Domeboro powder or tablets), 1 packet or tablet per 500 ml. (pint) of water makes approximately a 1:40 dilution. Make certain the mixture is completely dissolved before application. A soft cloth such as Kerlix gauze, an old, clean thin white handkerchief, or a towel is immersed in the solution. The cloth is wrung slightly and applied to the affected area of the skin. When the cloth begins to dry, remove it completely and resoak in the solution before reapplying. Do not pour the solution directly on the dressing; a fresh solution should be prepared before each treatment.

As an alternative the patient may soak the affected part, such as a hand or a foot, directly in the solution for the same period of time.

For generalized involvement hospitalization may be necessary. Compresses may be applied to all affected areas of the body, and in some cases baths such as with Aveeno colloidal oatmeal may be preferable.

Treatment should be continued for no more than a few days (usually 3 to 4) to avoid excessive drying of the skin.

4. Immediately following the compresses, soaks, or baths, apply a topical corticosteroid spray (triamcinolone [Kenalog] spray or betamethasone [Valisone] aerosol). A 2 or 3 second spray to each affected area is sufficient. One of the many topical corticosteroid creams such as betamethasone valerate (Valisone), triamcinolone

(Kenalog), or fluocinolone acetonide (Synalar) may be used when the acute dermatitis is not extensively vesicular. Avoid ointments in the acute stages.

5. Oral antihistamines such as cyproheptadine (Periactin), hydroxyzine (Atarax), or diphenhydramine (Benadryl) help relieve itching. It is imperative that workers be warned not to drive or operate dangerous machinery while taking antihistamines.

6. Systemic use of corticosteroids is indicated in patients with severe, localized dermatitis, such as a vesiculobullous eruption of the hands or feet, or with severe, generalized dermatitis. An injection of triamcinolone acetonide suspension (Kenalog-40 injection) may be given, or oral corticosteroids such as prednisone (Deltasone), 30 mg. to 60 mg. daily in two or three divided doses, is begun initially and tapered over 10 to 30 days.

Subacute and Chronic Contact Dermatitis. 1. Avoidances as outlined in (1) above.

2. Do not compress or soak.

3. Use a topical corticosteroid cream or ointment two to three times daily and continue treatment for 2 to 3 weeks after the skin appears normal.

4. Oral antihistamines as in (5) above.

5. I wish to emphasize that frequently recurring cases of acute contact dermatitis should be considered "chronic," and frequent use (more than once every 3 months) of short courses of systemic corticosteroids should be avoided. In these patients a tireless search for precipitating and aggravating factors is necessary.

Secondarily Infected Contact Dermatitis. In my experience this is infrequent. A low grade bacterial infection such as from a coagulase-positive Staphylococcus may occur. In these patients compresses or soaks with povidone-iodine (Betadine Solution) are helpful, followed by application of oxytetracycline-hydrocortisone spray or ointment (Terra-Cortril). Bacterial cultures should be taken, and antibiotic therapy such as erythromycin stearate (Erythrocin), 250 mg. three to four times daily for 10 days, is initiated. Acute cellulitis with accompanying chills, fever, and lymphangitis may require more aggressive and closely supervised antibiotic therapy.

Ancillary Measures in Treatment of Occupational Contact Dermatitis

Resources to Identify Causative Agent(s). It is imperative that the causative agent(s) be identified in every patient. Unless this is done, treatment may be doomed to failure and the patient will experience recurrences of the dermatosis. A careful work history should be obtained to determine in detail all the patient's industrial contacts. Inquiry into exposures from second jobs, hobbies, and household contactants is essential. In this regard I have found it most helpful to consult the following sources:

1. Occupational Diseases of the Skin, by L. Schwartz, L. Tulipan, and D. J. Birmingham. 3rd ed. Philadelphia, Lea & Febiger, 1957.

2. Occupational Contact Dermatitis, by R. M. Adams, Philadelphia, J. B. Lippincott Co., 1969.

3. Contact Dermatitis, by A. A. Fisher. 2nd ed. Philadelphia, Lea & Febiger, 1973.

4. Occupational Dermatoses, by G. A. Gellin. Chicago, American Medical Association, Department of Environmental, Public and Occupational Health, 1972.

5. Chapters 14 and 15 on contact dermatitis by N. Hjorth and S. Fregert, *in* Rook, Wilson, and Ebling: Textbook of Dermatology. 2nd ed. Oxford, Blackwell, 1972.

6. Industrial Hygiene Toxicology, F. A. Patty (ed.). 2nd ed. New York, Interscience, 1958–63.

7. Division of Technical Services, National Institute for Occupational Safety and Health, United States Public Health Service, 4676 Columbia Parkway, Cincinnati, Ohio 45226.

8. The patient's employer (with the consent of the patient), such as the plant manager or industrial research department.

Together these resources may provide lists of chemicals contacted in various occupations, information on cutaneous and systemic toxicity of chemicals, suggested patch testing concentrations, and information on sources of products and processes which contain a particular chemical. The latter is extremely important, because a worker may be exposed to the same chemical at home and at work (e.g., rubber, metal, chromates, dyes, plastic resins) or in several sources at work.

Diagnostic Patch Testing. Patch testing, when properly performed and correctly interpreted, is unquestionably of great value in identifying the causative agent(s) of allergic contact dermatitis. Initial testing is usually done with the most frequent contact allergens (nickel, chromates, rubber, medicaments, preservatives, dyes, and resins). Other materials, found at home or work, may also have to be tested in appropriate concentrations in order to distinguish occupational and nonoccupational factors. Patch testing should be employed only by physicians highly experienced with this technique. Pre-employment patch testing should generally be avoided. The same recommendations and precautions apply to photopatch testing which is used to diagnose photoallergic contact dermatitis.

Preventive Measures. It is impossible to separate treatment from prevention. Personal measures such as wearing protective clothing may be required when they can be used safely. Barrier or protective creams should only be used as a last resort and should never be applied to inflamed skin. Environmental control such as good housekeeping, engineering controls, and removal of physical and chemical hazards is also important.

Fiberglass Dermatitis

This special form of papular, eczematous, and occasionally purpuric dermatitis is produced by mechanical irritation from glass fibers. Body folds and areas of tight-fitting clothing are common sites of involvement. Hardening usually occurs after several weeks of exposure.

Treatment. 1. Limitation of further exposure to fiberglass.

2. Wearing of loose-fitting clothing which is changed daily.

3. Frequent skin cleansing.

4. Topical corticosteroid creams (see Contact Dermatitis, above).

5. Workers with dermographism or urticaria should not work with fiberglass.

Oil Acne

Most cutting fluids used today are synthetic or semisynthetic and most frequently produce contact eczema. Treatment of these patients should follow measures described previously for contact dermatitis. However, exposure to insoluble, straight cutting fluids may produce folliculitis ("oil boils") in areas uncommon for acne vulgaris, usually the extremities.

Treatment. 1. Avoidance of contact with oils and grease.

2. Daily changes of work clothing.

3. Frequent cleansing of the skin with soap and water.

4. The worker should avoid cleansing his skin with his fabric waste, which is intended only for cleaning machines and tools.

5. Local acne medications (benzoyl peroxide 5 per cent lotion or gel or retinoic acid cream 0.05 to 0.1 per cent).

Chloracne

This extremely refractory form of industrial acne is produced by exposure to various chlorinated aromatic compounds, such as chloronaphthalenes, polychlorobiphenyls, polychlorodibenzofurans, and chlorophenol and aniline herbicide intermediates.

Treatment. 1. Absolute avoidance of chemical exposure through a totally enclosed manufacturing process.

2. Appraisal of possible systemic toxicity, including liver, kidney, and porphyrin analyses.

3. Work clothing should be laundered at work.

4. Double locker rooms (clean and dirty) with adequate shower facilities.

5. Protective creams should not be used.

Pigmentation Disorders

Staining. A number of chemicals stain the skin by direct external contact. The stain usually responds to attempts at cleansing, avoidance of chemical exposure, and the passage of time.

Hyperpigmentation. Exposure to tar, pitch, and chemicals such as psoralens in combination with ultraviolet light may produce increased pigmentation of the skin. Protective clothing and/or sunscreens may be helpful. Hydroquinone (Eldoquin), applied twice daily, may help reduce the pigmentation.

Hypopigmentation. Exposure to monobenzyl ether of hydroquinone (rubber industry), paratertiary butyl phenol or catechol, or paratertiary amyl phenol (germicidal disinfectants, oils, plastics, paints, or resins) may produce occupational leukoderma. Treatment involves avoiding chemical exposure and using stains for the skin (Vitadye, Dy-O-Derm). Photochemotherapy with oral psoralens (methoxsalen [Oxsoralen]) and black ultraviolet light is usually not effective in this form of leukoderma.

Other Dermatoses

Microbial infections, granulomatous reactions, ulcerations, and neoplasms may occasionally occur. The spectrum of these and other occupational dermatoses is wide, and therapy varies depending upon cause. The hallmarks for the successful treatment of occupational dermatoses are identifying the causative agent(s), early therapy, and prevention of further chemical exposure.

PEDICULOSIS

method of
ROBERT P. FRIEDMAN, M.D.
Tucson, Arizona

Throughout history, lice and man have coexisted. Indeed, these ectoparasitic, wingless, bloodsucking insects cannot survive for more than a few days away from the human host. Species infesting humans are (1) *Phthirus pubis* (crab louse) and (2) *Pediculus humanus,* with its two varieties, *P. humanus capitis* (head louse) and *P. humanus corporis* (body louse). All produce symptoms by injecting saliva during feeding. Local irritation and allergic sensitization lead to itching and the resultant excoriations, secondary infection, and dermatitis.

Phthirus Pubis (Crab Louse)

This species is chiefly transmitted by sexual contact. It localizes to the genital region, although other hairy areas such as the trunk, axillae, beard, and eyelashes can be affected. Here we find the occasional louse grasping the base of a hair shaft and the many eggs (nits) firmly cemented to the hairs.

Pediculus Corporis (Body Louse)

This variety is found chiefly in seams of undergarments, especially in pressure areas. The eggs are attached to clothing fibers (occasionally they are found on body hairs in severe infestations), where they remain viable for up to 1 month, hatching when the clothing is worn and they are exposed to body heat. Body lice are commonly associated with overcrowding and poor hygiene, dissemination occurring through contact with infested persons, clothing, or bedding. *Pediculus corporis* is the vector for rickettsial diseases such as epidemic typhus and relapsing fever.

Pediculus Capitis (Head Louse)

The head louse generally infests only the scalp, preferring the occipital and temporal areas. Infestation is more common in children, females, and individuals with long hair. Transmission is by contact with infested persons and fomites (e.g., combs, brushes, wigs, hats, towels).

Treatment

1. Gamma benzene hexachloride is the drug of choice for most louse infestations. Apply the lotion to hairy areas (excluding eyelids) and leave on for 24 hours. Although this is generally curative, re-treat heavy infestations in 4 to 7 days. Pediculosis capitis may also be treated with gamma benzene hexachloride shampoo.

Note: Recent concern over potential toxicity of gamma benzene hexachloride suggests that it should be avoided in pregnant women and infants.

2. Nits (eggs) remaining attached to hairs after treatment should be removed with a fine-toothed comb.

3. Pubic lice infesting the eyelashes can be treated with twice daily applications of petrolatum and careful removal of nits.

4. Lice and nits must be eliminated from clothing and bedding, particularly in body louse infestations. This is easily accomplished by laundering (hot water), dry cleaning, or careful pressing with a hot iron. Clothing may also be dusted with 10 per cent chlorophenothane (DDT) powder or gamma benzene hexachloride (lindane) powder. In infestation with *Pediculus capitis,* disinfect all fomites by overnight soaking in gamma benzene hexachloride shampoo or by boiling.

5. Secondary bacterial infection is best treated with appropriate systemic antibiotics.

6. For dermatitis remaining after treatment of the infestation, prescribe a topical corticosteroid.

7. If severe itching is present, oral antipruritics may be useful—e.g., cyproheptadine (Periactin), trimeprazine (Temaril), or hydroxyzine (Atarax).

8. Examine all family members and other close contacts for infestation and treat if necessary.

9. Evaluate patients with pubic lice for coexisting venereal disease.

10. Remind patients that pediculosis does not produce immunity and that therefore they can be reinfested at any time upon re-exposure to the organism.

PIGMENTARY DISTURBANCES

method of
JOHN A. KENNEY, Jr., M.D., F.A.C.P.
Washington, D.C.

Although research in pigmentation has made rapid strides in the past 2 decades and has provided new insight into the mechanism of pigmentation and many of its disorders, the therapy for such disorders is still far from satisfactory and empirical measures must be used. One dermatologic professor of my acquaintance would begin some of his lectures with a statement to the effect that disease affects man in three ways: it can cause disability, it can cause death, or it can cause disfigurement, and it is with the last of these that dermatology has most often to concern itself. Nowhere in the field of dermatology is this more true than in the case of disorders of pigmentation.

Hyperpigmentary Disorders

Postinflammatory Hyperpigmentation. Many inflammatory skin conditions—even banal ones such as acne or pityriasis rosea, as well as contact and atopic dermatitis and others—resolve only to leave residual and at times longstanding hyperpigmentation, often in cosmetically important areas of skin. If the condition is of recent origin, I ordinarily recommend that the patient wait a few weeks to months to see how much of the melanin pigment will be carried away through normal exfoliation and normal pigment excretory mechanisms. If therapy must be used, one might employ a low-potency steroid cream such as 1 per cent hydrocortisone. When more active therapy is desired, I recommend a trial first of a 2 per cent hydroquinone cream (often one of the inexpensive and commercially available over-the-counter preparations such as Artra is entirely satisfactory), directing the patient to rub this into the pigmented spots or plaques twice daily, but warning the patient that, since hydroquinone is a pigment inhibitor and acts slowly, he must allow 3 to 4 months for a therapeutic effect to be achieved.

If these measures do not result in the desired amount of depigmentation, then a higher percentage of hydroquinone must be employed and in a different formulation. I prescribe the following for my patients and have been relatively satisfied with the results: 2 per cent salicylic acid, 5 per cent hydroquinone, steroid cream q.s.ad. 100. If the lesions are on the face, because of the possibility of causing the persistent vasodilation and erythema reported to result from the long-term use of high-potency fluorinated steroid creams in such skin areas, one should employ hydrocortisone or a nonfluorinated steroid cream such as desonide (Tridesilon) as the ointment base. Because of the rare occurrence of sensitization to the hydroquinone, it is advisable to warn the patient of this possibility and to advise stopping use of the compound at the first signs of irritation.

The monobenzyl ether of hydroquinone (commonly available as Benoquin ointment) must be separately considered. Because of the inability to control the extent of depigmentation and the danger of producing an unsightly confetti-like depigmentation of skin areas adjacent to and even far distant from the site of desired depigmentation, I restrict the use of monobenzyl ether of hydroquinone to patients who have extensive vitiligo which has affected 50 per cent or more of the body skin and which has left islands of normal skin pigmentation on the face, the hands, the dorsa of the arms, or the anterior lower legs and other skin areas easily visible to others. Again, because of the danger of producing a primary irritant reaction or allergic sensitization with higher concentrations of the drug, I will often begin therapy with a 10 per cent preparation, made by diluting the commercially-available Benoquin ointment (which contains 20 per cent monobenzyl ether of hydroquinone) with an equal quantity of water-washable base (e.g., Unibase). Of course, just as with the use of the hydroquinone preparations previously described, the patient must be warned that months rather than weeks of therapy are required. The patient must also be advised to use appropriate sunscreens or to take other steps to prevent exposure of the treated skin to sunlight. If allergic sensitization does indeed occur, then of course further use of the drug is impossible.

Although there is some rationale for using time-honored ammoniated mercury preparations as a bleach or inhibitor of pigmentation (i.e., mercury supplants copper in tyrosinase, inactivating it and preventing the first chemical reaction in melanin formation, that of the conversion of tyrosine to dopa), considerations of toxicity and the possibility of sensitization to mercury make its use inadvisable. Trichloroacetic acid peeling and dermabrasion are considered questionable methods of therapy for hyperpigmentation for the average physician or even dermatologist, and should be reserved for special indications or for those uniquely skilled in their use.

Melasma. In many darker-skinned patients, especially in blacks, the condition termed melasma, in which there are deposits of melanin in variously shaped patches or plaques in the skin of the forehead and cheeks, constitutes a cosmetic problem of the first magnitude. One might attempt therapy with hydroquinone (*not* the monobenzyl ether of hydroquinone) as already described, but in many instances the melanin is located deep in the dermis, and it is questionable as to how much therapeutic effect can be obtained by locally applied ointments. Perhaps an attempt at such therapy is better than none.

Hypopigmentary Disorders

Vitiligo. Vitiligo constitutes the most important disorder of hypopigmentation from the therapeutic standpoint. Although many theories have been advanced as to its causation, evidence seems to be accumulating that it should be classed with the autoimmune diseases. Therapy, however, is still empirical and is based on the use of oral or topical psoralens plus long-wave ultraviolet light (UV-A).

One must be careful first of all to make certain of the diagnosis. I have seen patients suffering from progressive systemic sclerosis who have been misdiagnosed as having vitiligo, and others in whom tinea versicolor has been confused with vitiligo. The hypopigmentation produced by scleroderma is most often spotty and diffuse, leaving persistent areas of perifollicular pigmentation which is characteristic for this disease. In tinea versicolor a microscopic examination of skin scrapings which have been placed in a drop or two of potassium hydroxide will quickly reveal the true diagnosis. Examination of vitiligo patients with a Wood's light ("black light," a filtered ultraviolet light of 340 to 400 nm.) will readily reveal areas of skin which lack epidermal pigmentation.

Because we know that vitiligo can be associated with hyperthyroidism, diabetes, pernicious anemia, and Addison's disease, one must be on the alert for these in patients with vitiligo and their families.

If the vitiligo is localized to a small area or plaque, topical therapy is preferred. This is done by painting methoxsalen lotion on the skin (Oxsoralen lotion, 1 per cent), allowing it to dry and waiting 45 minutes to an hour (to permit penetration of the drug), and then exposing the area to long-wave ultraviolet light (UV-A), "black light." Keeping the distance from the light source to the skin constant (e.g., 20 cm.), one uses first 15 seconds, then 30 seconds, and then increasing increments of time for every-other-day or even once-weekly exposures until a visible erythema appears in the previously white areas of skin. When this exposure time level is reached, one then holds subsequent exposures to this same time, or slightly increases it to maintain the erythema and thus stimulate maximum pigment formation. With such therapy pigment will be seen to fill in from the normally pigmented skin borders and also from perifollicular melanocytes. I warn patients that occasional burns are to be expected and prescribe steroid lotions and creams and sedative antihistamines if burns occur. It should be emphasized that topical therapy must be closely supervised by the physician. I believe in following the directions on the package label and never give this potentially dangerous lotion to the patient to apply.

In southern latitudes where there is adequate sunlight, or in more northern regions in summertime and in patients whose vitiligo is more extensive, systemic therapy with oral psoralen is preferred. This may be done by utilizing the synthetic trioxsalen tablets (Trisoralen, 5 mg.) or the methoxsalen capsules (Oxsoralen, 10 mg.). For adults, I recommend the use of 4 trioxsalen tablets or 4 methoxsalen capsules taken 2 hours before sunlight exposure. The patient is directed to plan his treatment utilizing natural sunlight between the hours of 10 A.M. and 4 P.M. and to start with a 1 minute exposure, gradually increasing his every-other-day treatments until a visible erythema is obtained, just as with the local topical therapy just described. The psoralens give a delayed burn response, so that the every-other-day treatment schedule is preferred to avoid overexposure.

The trioxsalen is said to produce pigmentation without visible erythema, whereas the methoxsalen does produce marked erythema. Occasional patients will experience some nausea with methoxsalen. If this occurs, taking the drug after a glass of milk or a sandwich will usually allay this sensation.

In speaking of oral psoralen, a word should be said about two concerns, one old and one new. When the drug was first introduced in this country, about 1950, because laboratory animals given many times the equivalent human dose showed some liver function test abnormalities, the manufacturers of the drug were forced to include a warning regarding possible liver toxicity and advice to perform liver function studies on patients taking the psoralens for vitiligo. However, extensive use of the drug in this country and abroad has failed to reveal any liver toxicity caused by this drug. I have employed this drug in my practice since it was first introduced, even using it to treat vitiligo in young children (use in children is not listed in the manufacturer's official directive), and after years of finding entirely negative liver function tests in psoralen-treated patients, I no longer subject vitiligo patients to such testing.

The other, more recent concern is that of possible eye damage with high-dosage psoralen therapy plus the new intense long-wave length (UV-A) treatment of psoriasis (the so-called PUVA therapy). Because this therapy has been utilized only for the past 2 years and has yet to be approved by the Food and Drug Administration, and, although widely used by dermatologists, is still officially an experimental procedure, in the present medicolegal climate it is most likely advisable to have the patient about to undergo long-term therapy with oral psoralens to have a baseline ophthalmologic examination.

There is a recent report of using PUVA–psoriasis light treatment cabinets in the treatment of vitiligo as well as psoriasis; but although the method offers promise, final assessment cannot yet be made as to its efficacy.

It must also be pointed out that after the patient has used either topical or oral psoralen his skin is sensitive to ultraviolet light for at least 24 hours, and if further sunlight exposure is contemplated (e.g., a trip downtown) he must use cover-ups or sunscreens (e.g., Uval, PreSun, Blockout, Eclipse, RVP, Solbar) to prevent further ultraviolet light (UV-A) exposure.

Other Pigmentary Problems

Pigmented moles, pigmented basal cell carcinomas, seborrheic keratoses, and nevus depigmentosus are ordinarily treated by surgical or electro- or cryosurgical means or have no specific treatment, and they are not considered in this discussion.

PEMPHIGUS AND BULLOUS PEMPHIGOID

method of
S. JABLONSKA, M.D.,
and T. CHORZELSKI, M.D.
Warsaw, Poland

Pemphigus

Treatment of pemphigus consists mainly of the use of corticosteroids and immunosuppressive drugs. Treatment exclusively with high doses of steroids is still recommended by some doctors, but, in our opinion, this is much less effective and less safe than the combined use of corticosteroids and immunosuppressive drugs.

Combined Treatment with Steroids and Immunosuppressors. CORTICOSTEROIDS. Initially, doses of 100 to 120 mg. of prednisone (about 2 mg. per kg. of body weight) daily are given until all symptoms of active disease disappear—i.e., for about 3 to 4 weeks—and the dose is then gradually reduced.

IMMUNOSUPPRESSORS. Immunosuppressive drugs, preferably azathioprine, are either given from the beginning combined with corticosteroids or added after 2 to 4 weeks when the dosage of corticosteroids is gradually reduced. (This use of azathioprine is experimental in the United States of America.)

Dosage of azathioprine: At first, 2.5 mg. per kg. of body weight, i.e., 150 to 200 mg., is given daily for 6 to 8 weeks, together with steroids, until all disease symptoms have disappeared. When full remission sets in, the dose of azathioprine is gradually reduced to 100 and then 50 mg. daily; at the same time, the dose of steroids is reduced by 5 mg. every other day, leading to an alternate day regimen. On one day the patient receives the full dose of steroids with gradually decreasing doses of azathioprine, and on alternate days no drugs at all.

MAINTENANCE TREATMENT. After 2 to 3 months, the dose of steroids is reduced by 5 mg. every other day, until the maintenance dose of 15 to 20 mg. of prednisone, together with 50 mg. of azathioprine on alternate days, is reached. This treatment is continued for several months. Then the dose of steroids is reduced by 5 mg. every week, so that 5 mg. of prednisone and 25 mg. of azathioprine is given every other day for some months. Finally, 5 mg. of prednisone is given, at first twice and then once a week, together with 25 mg. of azathioprine.

There are no objective criteria as to when treatment can be stopped. In some patients remission lasting many years can be achieved (cure?), and in others recurrences are to be expected.

In patients refractory to treatment, azathioprine, which is the safest drug, can be replaced by methotrexate, 12.5 mg. twice weekly or 25 to 50 mg. once weekly intramuscularly or perorally, cyclophosphamide, 100 to 200 mg. daily perorally, or chlorambucil, 2 to 4 mg. daily. (This use of methotrexate, cyclophosphamide, and chlorambucil is experimental in the United States of America.)

Complications of Therapy. Side effects of azathioprine treatment are rare. After longer administration, however, bacterial or viral infections, leukopenia, and other hematologic disorders may occur. Methotrexate, cyclophosphamide, and chlorambucil, like all immunosuppressors, cause leukopenia, lowered resistance to bacteria and viruses, and liver damage, and may be teratogenic. Cyclophosphamide may cause marked, although reversible, loss of hair.

Immunofluorescence Studies in Evaluation of Treatment. At present, immunofluorescence studies are essential not only for diagnosis but also for evaluation of the treatment. Histopathology and immunopathology of the skin have only diagnostic significance, whereas fluctuation of the titers of pemphigus (IC [intercellular]) antibodies in serum reflects activity of the disease process. Periodic examinations of the serum can be helpful in determining dosage of drugs and duration of their administration.

Maintenance therapy should not be started until serologic tests have become negative.

Response. Response to treatment varies with each patient, but also depends on the form of pemphigus. *Pemphigus vulgaris* requires the most intensive treatment, mainly because the oral mucous membrane lesions are resistant to treatment. In *pemphigus erythematosus,* skin lesions recede rather quickly; abortive cases respond favorably to lower dosage of steroids in combination with immunosuppressive drugs.

In rare cases of *herpetiform pemphigus,* which is an atypical form of pemphigus with clinical symptoms resembling those of dermatitis herpetiformis, but with acantholysis and immunofluorescence findings typical of pemphigus (circulating and in vivo bound IC antibodies), sulfones are beneficial: dapsone, 100 to 200 mg. daily, or sulfapyridine, 1.5 grams daily; steroids in low doses, 10 to 30 mg. daily, may be additionally needed in some cases. (This use of dapsone and sulfapyridine is experimental in the United States of America.)

Topical Treatment. Topical treatment is only supplementary. Bullae should be incised and erosions treated with sprays or creams containing corticosteroids and antibiotics or antiseptics.

In *pemphigus vegetans* and *pemphigus seborrheicus,* betamethasone or other fluorinated steroids may be beneficial, but occlusive dressings are not recommended.

TABLE 1. **Combined Treatment of Pemphigus with Steroids and Azathioprine***

DRUG	TIME OF TREATMENT (MONTHS)				
	1 2	*3*	*4 5 6*	*7*	*8–12*
Prednisone	100–120 mg. daily	One day, full dose Every other day, reduced by 5 mg.	One day, 0 Another day, reduced dose up to 15–20 mg.	One day, 0 Another day, reduced by 5 mg. up to 5 mg.	5 mg. once a week
Azathioprine	200 mg. daily	100–50 mg. on alternate days	50 mg. on alternate days†	25 mg. on alternate days	25 mg. once a week

↑ Full remission ↑ IF titer 0

*The use of azathioprine in the treatment of pemphigus is experimental in the United States of America.
†On the same day as prednisone.

Mucous Membranes. The frequent secondary Candida infections should be treated with antifungal solutions; artificial dentures should be kept in antiseptic fluids. Pain may require the use of topical anesthetics, especially before eating.

Prognosis. Following our treatment schedule, it was possible to obtain full remission in some patients.

Provoked Pemphigus

It is now well recognized that pemphigus may be provoked by drugs such as phenylbutazone, D-penicillamine, rifampin (rifampicin), and others.

In some patients the lesions disappear when the drugs are withdrawn and corticosteroid or immunosuppressive therapy is not necessary, or low doses of steroids—10 to 15 mg. of prednisone daily—may be sufficient. However, in some patients the disease process becomes self-perpetuating, and the treatment is the same as for the idiopathic variety.

Bullous Pemphigoid

Bullous pemphigoid occurs most frequently in older age groups, but may be encountered in patients of all ages, including children.

In some instances in older patients, bullous pemphigoid may coexist with malignant tumors of the internal organs; according to some authors, this coexistence is entirely fortuitous or is due to a higher incidence of tumors in patients in these age groups. Nevertheless, we have observed disappearance of the cutaneous lesions after removal of tumor, and their reappearance with the recurrence of the tumor. Tumors were present in 15 per cent of our adult patients, and in two patients pemphigoid was associated with lymphoma, but no instances of coexisting tumor and pemphigoid were observed in children.

If tumor is found, surgery should be preceded by treatment with low doses of corticosteroids, 30 to 40 mg. of prednisone daily, until the cutaneous lesions are cleared.

Corticosteroids. The treatment of choice is corticosteroid therapy. Usually medium or low doses are sufficient, 30 to 60 mg. daily, administered until the skin lesions disappear, and, after that, maintained in gradually reduced low doses of 5 to 10 mg. daily. In some patients who have a severe course, high doses, 100 to 120 mg. daily, as in pemphigus are necessary, although usually the lesions regress sooner, often after several weeks.

Immunosuppressors. Corticosteroid therapy may be combined with immunosuppressive drugs, especially azathioprine, 2.5 mg. per kg. of body weight—i.e., 150 to 200 mg.—daily for several days or weeks until the lesions recede. (This use of immunosuppressive drugs is experimental in the United States of America.) Steroids may also be combined with methotrexate in injections of 12.5 mg. twice weekly or 25 to 50 mg. once weekly. However, in older patients these drugs may be dangerous because their use increases the incidence of bacterial and viral infections, may injure the liver, and, after longer use, may even provoke leukemia. Immunosuppressive drugs should not be used in patients with malignancy and are not indicated in children.

Sulfones. Some cases of pemphigoid, especially in children, respond to sulfones in doses of 100 to 200 mg. daily for adults and correspondingly lower doses in children, or sulfapyridine, 1.5 grams daily, although the response is not as dramatic as in dermatitis herpetiformis. (This use of sulfones and sulfapyridine is investigational in the United States of America.) Remission after use of sulfones is often incomplete, and the addition of steroids in low doses may be necessary, such as 5 to 20 mg. of prednisone daily; at the same time, the dosage of sulfones can be diminished to 25 to 50 mg. daily or every other day.

Immunofluorescence (IF) Studies in Evaluation of Therapeutic Results. The IF studies are fundamental for diagnostic purposes.

In a majority of patients (about 80 per cent) circulating antibodies against the basement membrane zone of the epidermis (anti-BMZ) are detectable, and in all patients in vivo bound IgG and complement in the basement membrane zone are detectable. On the other hand, monitoring therapy by repeated serum studies is here of less significance than in pemphigus, as titers are not distinctly parallel to disease activity. During remission, however, antibodies usually disappear from the circulation, and immunofluorescence findings in the skin become negative.

Topical Treatment. After the bullae are incised, corticosteroid sprays with antibiotics should be applied. In the localized form of the disease, topical treatment exclusively may be sufficient.

Cicatricial Pemphigoid. This variety of pemphigoid mainly involves the mucous membranes of the oral cavity and eyes, and less often the skin.

Topical treatment of ocular lesions consists in retrobulbar injections of corticosteroids. Steroid and antiseptic solutions may be applied to erosions in the mucous membranes. *Systemic treatment with steroids* is of little value. Some positive results have been reported using azathioprine (dosages as above). Apparently this form of pemphigoid is especially refractory to treatment.

The *Brunsting-Perry form* is an exceedingly rare variety of scarring pemphigoid. It appears mainly on the face, scalp, and neck, but does not involve mucous membranes. Treatment consists of systemic steroid therapy as in bullous pemphigoid and topical steroid ointments or sprays.

The immunofluorescence in cicatricial pemphigoid is analogous to that in bullous pemphigoid, but circulating antibodies are usually absent.

PITYRIASIS ROSEA

method of
RAYMOND L. CORNELISON, M.D.
Midwest City, Oklahoma

Pityriasis rosea is a common papulosquamous eruption. The disease is self-limited, is usually asymptomatic, and clears in most patients in 6 to 8 weeks. The cause is unknown.

Most cases begin with a single oval lesion (herald patch), 1 to 5 cm. in diameter, which is followed in a few days to weeks by a widespread eruption of similar but smaller lesions. The eruption is most commonly found on the trunk and proximal extremities.

If the patient is seen in the early single-lesion phase, KOH examination is advisable to rule out tinea corporis. Patients having systemic complaints of fever, malaise, and generalized lymphadenopathy may have secondary syphilis, and a VDRL is indicated. If the eruption persists over 8 weeks, dermatologic consultation is advised.

The cornerstone of therapy is frequent exposure to minimal erythema doses of ultraviolet light. This can be accomplished by artificial or natural sunlight. This therapy will clear many cases in 2 to 3 weeks. Those patients who have associated pruritus may be helped by diphenhydramine (Benadryl), 25 to 50 mg. orally every 4 to 6 hours. Other antihistamines, such as chlorpheniramine (Chlor-Trimeton), hydroxyzine (Atarax, Vistaril), or cyproheptadine (Periactin), are equally of value. Patients should be advised of antihistaminic side effects.

I frequently find that patients obtain symptomatic relief from 40 mg. of triamcinolone acetonide (Kenalog) added to 120 ml. (4 oz.) of a lipid-free skin cleanser (Cetaphil lotion) with 0.25 per cent menthol. This preparation spreads easily and is economical. I do not feel that it shortens the course of the disease.

POLYARTERITIS

method of
C. E. RUPE, M.D.
Detroit, Michigan

Accurate diagnosis as early as possible is essential if therapy is to be effective. The potential complications of therapy with corticosteroids or immunosuppressive agents preclude their use, unless the diagnosis is confirmed by biopsy. The first choice of a site for biopsy is an active superficial lesion with the underlying muscle. If there are no visible areas of involvement, a second choice would be an involved organ (kidney, liver, testicle, or lung). If neither choice is available, the best site for "blind biopsy" is the sural nerve, because involvement of the vasa nervorum is frequent. In the patient with clinical manifestations of polymyalgia rheumatica, the "asymptomatic" temporal artery is the biopsy site of choice. In view of the occurrence of skip lesions, a negative report calls for further sectioning of the block and/or biopsy of the opposite temporal artery if clinical suspicion is high.

The high mortality of polyarteritis nodosa and necrotizing angiitis justifies the risk of steroid therapy. Prednisone is begun at a dose of 1 to 2 mg. per kg. and adjusted upward if there is failure of control. Assessment of efficacy of therapy depends on having established some baseline data before starting therapy.

The selection of data depends on the individualization of the nature and extent of organ involvement, as well as on more general indicators, such as the sedimentation rate, white blood count, serum globulin, fever, or rash.

If there is evidence of control of the disease process over a period of several weeks or more, cautious stepwise reduction of steroid dosage may be undertaken. It seems to me that the increments in reduction should be a percentage of the dose, rather than a set amount. Stability of control with each dose over a period of 1 or 2 weeks sets a reasonable time scale during reduction of the dose. If a "breakthrough" occurs, it is my practice to increase the dose by several increments rather than just back to the last effective dosage.

If control is maintained during dosage reduction, one may then give consideration to alternate day therapy—e.g., giving the total dose for 48 hours at 8:00 A.M. every other day.

Better understanding of the "disimmune state" and further ability to manipulate the immune system should improve therapy. The use of the more toxic immunosuppressants is generally reserved for steroid failures and desperate cases. Reports of improvement with nephrectomy in a related condition—Goodpasture's syndrome—are interesting but apparently not applicable in polyarteritis.

Management of complications is largely that of support in organ failure or intervention in the event of organ infarction.

PRECANCEROUS LESIONS OF THE SKIN AND MUCOUS MEMBRANES

method of
ROBERT L. JETTON, M.D.
Greenville, South Carolina

Several epithelial neoplasms have the potential to undergo malignant transformation but do not invariably become cancerous. They are considered to be premalignant on the basis of microscopic cellular atypia. These lesions are (1) Actinic keratoses caused by chronic sunlight exposure; (2) arsenical keratoses caused by ingestion of inorganic pentavalent arsenicals (Fowler's solution, Asiatic pills) for medicinal purposes; (3) leukoplakia; (4) Bowen's disease; (5) erythroplasia of Queyrat, and (6) chronic radiation dermatitis. Bowen's disease and erythroplasia of Queyrat are actually intraepidermal squamous cell carcinomas.

Squamous cell carcinoma may develop in other cutaneous disorders such as lichen sclerosus et atrophicus of the female genitalia, giant condyloma acuminatum of Buschke-Loewenstein, oral florid papillomatosis, chronic ulcers, and chronic draining sinus tracts. Nevus sebaceus of Jadassohn, a lesion present at birth, may later develop into a basal cell epithelioma. The primary lesions in all these diseases do not show the microscopic cellular atypia of the premalignant epithelial diseases to be considered in this article. They must, however, be followed closely for signs of malignant degeneration, and prophylactic surgical excision is indicated for some of these diseases.

Actinic Keratoses

Approximately one fifth of these lesions develop into squamous cell carcinomas which are not usually locally aggressive and which do not readily metastasize.

Treatment. The method of treatment is determined by the number of lesions and the morphology of the individual lesions.

1. The patient with five to six lesions is easily and effectively treated by cryosurgery, using liquid nitrogen applied with a cotton-tipped applicator, or by means of a cryospray unit. The duration of freeze depends on the size and thickness of the lesion but usually requires 5 to 10 seconds with a spray and 10 to 20 seconds with a cotton-tipped applicator.

2. Individual and multiple lesions may also be treated by curettage with or without light electrodesiccation following local anesthesia. Curettage prior to electrodesiccation yields a specimen adequate for microscopic examination.

3. Larger, thicker, and inflamed lesions and cutaneous horns may be biopsied and definitive therapy determined by the pathology report. Otherwise, they are best removed by simple excision with microscopic evaluation of the excised specimen. These same lesions also respond well to curettage and electrodesiccation, but the curettage fragments from the entire lesion and base should be submitted to a pathologist.

4. Numerous actinic keratoses are usually best treated by topical application of a cream or solution containing 1, 2, or 5 per cent 5-fluorouracil (5-FU). Both clinical and preclinical lesions undergo a selective response characterized by various degrees of inflammation. 5-FU is usually applied twice a day for 2 to 3 weeks. The inflammatory reaction subsides rapidly during the next 1 to 2 weeks. If the reaction is especially

severe, a topical corticosteroid cream, preferably 1 per cent hydrocortisone cream, may be applied during and after the period of treatment. Sunlight exposure often accentuates the inflammatory reaction. Actinic keratoses on the hands and arms respond less well to topical 5-FU and require a longer period of therapy or adjunctive treatment with a keratolytic or desquamating agent such as tretinoin (Retin-A) cream, salicylic acid gel (Keralyt Gel), or a 5 to 10 per cent salicylic acid cream or ointment to enhance penetration.

Periodic examination is desirable following all methods of treatment. Lesions that persist or recur must be biopsied. Patients should be encouraged to avoid excessive and careless exposure to sunlight, and a good sunscreen should be prescribed to be applied to all exposed surfaces.

Arsenical Keratoses

Patients with arsenical keratoses are infrequently encountered, but most have numerous lesions which must be followed closely for malignant change.

Treatment. The numerous small palmar and plantar keratoses which may be present are usually left untreated except for the use of keratolytic agents to reduce scaling. Intermittent treatment with topical 5-FU, preferably with occlusion beneath a plastic film, would seem to provide a logical means to detect lesions requiring more serious attention.

Suspicious lesions should be biopsied. Therapy should be individualized, but surgical excision, cryosurgery, and curettage and electrodesiccation are all appropriate and effective.

Intraepidermal carcinomas not infrequently coexist and, because arsenic is a carcinogen, internal malignancy may occur. These associations further emphasize the need for periodic evaluation.

Leukoplakia

Lack of a uniform definition and inaccurate clinical and histologic correlation have created confusion about leukoplakia. Squamous cell carcinoma develops in about 25 per cent of patients with persistent leukoplakia, and these cancers have a poor prognosis.

Treatment. EARLY LESION. Elimination of external causative factors such as pipe and cigarette smoking or ill-fitting dentures and protection from sunlight with sunscreen may allow spontaneous resolution of early, mild, and noninfiltrated lesions. Superficial lesions may be treated by electrodesiccation and curettage, cryosurgery with liquid nitrogen, and topical chemocautery with 50 per cent trichloroacetic acid. Some physicians report satisfactory results on the lips with topical 5-FU.

ADVANCED LESIONS. Any persistent, infiltrated, hyperplastic, denuded, or ulcerated lesions should be biopsied at the most suspicious site. When the biopsy indicates a more advanced lesion, surgical excision is usually the best and most thorough treatment.

Bowen's Disease

Accurate diagnosis is often elusive, because the lesion frequently looks eczematous rather than neoplastic. A high index of suspicion is required. Biopsy is essential. Bowen's disease is a squamous cell carcinoma in situ (intraepidermal squamous cell carcinoma). These lesions are more aggressive and metastasize to regional lymph nodes more readily than the squamous cell carcinomas which develop from actinic keratoses. The disease occasionally involves mucocutaneous junctions and can involve mucous membranes such as the vulva, vagina, nasal mucous membranes, cornea, and larynx.

Treatment. Treatment is best accomplished by surgical excision. Curettage and electrodesiccation and cryosurgery are frequently used with good results. Topical 5-FU is also effective and in certain locations where surgery is difficult it may be the preferred treatment. The 5-FU should be applied twice a day for a minimum of 6 to 8 weeks, and the effectiveness will be improved by simultaneous use of agents to remove surface scale and crusts or by occlusion beneath a plastic film.

Some workers report a predisposition to other premalignant and malignant skin lesions as well as internal adenocarcinomas. This tendency has not been accepted by all who have studied Bowen's disease, but periodic general examinations are suggested.

Erythroplasia of Queyrat

This rare lesion occurs on the glans penis and prepuce and is more common on the uncircumcised phallus. It resembles Bowen's disease microscopically and is regarded by some as Bowen's disease of the mucous membrane of the penis. The rate of dermal invasion is greater than with Bowen's disease elsewhere, and the resulting cancers are more aggressive and metastasize more readily than Bowen's disease.

Treatment. Treatment, which should be preceded by a biopsy, is much the same as with Bowen's disease. Excision may be used for small lesions and is essential for invasive lesions which may require partial amputation. Topical 5-FU has produced excellent results on noninvasive lesions and does not sacrifice important tissue. The patient should be prepared for a vigorous inflammatory reaction. Cryosurgery and curettage and electrodesiccation are effective but probably less desirable.

Chronic Radiodermatitis

Progressive and irreversible changes occur once the skin tolerance for radiation has been exceeded.

Treatment. Small hyperkeratotic lesions may be removed surgically by excision. Excision and destructive methods such as curettage and electrodesiccation and cryosurgery should be used cautiously, because healing progresses slowly in areas of chronic radiodermatitis. At times, surgical excision followed by skin grafting is the best treatment for advanced lesions. Topical 5-FU is a logical and effective treatment for x-ray- and sunlight-induced keratoses which develop in areas of radiodermatitis. Further irradiation must be avoided, and the areas must be protected against sunlight by proper clothing and sunscreens.

MILIARIA
(Prickly Heat)

method of
ROGER H. STEWART, M.D.
Fort Lauderdale, Florida

Miliaria, first described in 1884, refers to the clinical situation related to closure of the sweat pore with resultant sweat retention in the skin. Its cause stems from the mechanical obstruction of the eccrine sweat duct, rupture of the duct proximal to the point of obstruction, and formation of a retention vesicle by the outpouring of sweat into the skin secreted by the intact, underlying sweat gland.

The clinical manifestations are determined by the level at which the retention vesicle occurs in the skin. In *miliaria crystallina,* clear, tense, nonpruritic vesicles occur from the trapping of sweat in the inert stratum corneum. In *miliaria rubra,* the retention of sweat within the well innervated cells of the living epidermis, followed by stimulation of itch receptors by enzymes released from these damaged cells, results in the aptly described syndrome of prickly heat. Bacterial overgrowth, usually staphylococcal, may result in the formation of *miliaria pustulosa.*

Deeper rupture of the duct, within the dermis, results in *miliaria profunda,* a nonpruritic papular eruption sometimes eventuating into tropical anhidrotic asthenia (heat distress syndrome).

Miliaria is seen clinically in situations of high environmental temperature and humidity in which large quantities of unevaporated sweat remain on the skin for long periods of time. It is initiated by poral occlusion, be it from apposition of warm, sweaty body surfaces in the delicate popliteal and antecubital fossae in the warmly dressed infant, the redundant folds of the obese patient hospitalized for a febrile illness, or under the elastic wristband of the summer athlete. It is frequently encountered in profusion in the victim of a diving accident subjected to the hyperbaric oxygen chamber.

Treatment

Physical. 1. Air conditioning is the best medicine.

2. A cool shower or bath followed by brisk toweling; the latter will often open the occluded sweat pore. Plain water is best, as harsh soaps, bath oils, detergents, and even salt may worsen the condition.

3. Rest.

4. Cool, loose-fitting clothing.

5. When the aforementioned methods are unavailable, a swim (preferably in fresh water), a shaded area, and the use of a fan are helpful.

Pharmacologic. 1. *Thin* application of a dusting powder (ZeaSORB powder) will suffice in mild cases.

2. Application of a shake lotion. Simple calamine will often suffice, or 0.25 per cent menthol and/or 0.25 per cent phenol may be added for further relief of pruritus.

3. Antibiotic-steroid lotion—e.g., 1 tablet (500 mg.) of neomycin per 30 ml. (1 oz.) of 0.025 per cent betamethasone benzoate (Flurobate) lotion, especially where pustules are present.

4. If pustules persist, carry out studies and start therapy for secondary infection. (a) Nystatin, miconazole, or clotrimazole lotion or cream for *Candida albicans.* (b) Cloxacillin, 250 mg. four times daily, or erythromycin, 250 mg. four times daily, for staphylococcal infection.

5. Discontinue cholinergic drugs.

6. Appropriate treatment of underlying febrile illness.

Environmental. Permanent change will be necessary if repeated attacks of miliaria rubra occur, or if miliaria profunda develops, to prevent heat distress syndrome.

PRURITUS

method of
STEPHEN B. WEBSTER, M.D.
La Crosse, Wisconsin

Pruritus is itching, and itching is certainly the most important symptom concerned with the skin. No physician can observe the torments of a patient with severe itching and not realize and appreciate the distress that this symptom can produce. Watching a patient with an intractable itch mutilate his skin with scratching and digging makes it obvious that pain is preferable to the itch. Indeed, few physicians have not themselves suffered from pruritus in one form or another. Hence, the understanding and therapy of this symptom is of importance to any physician.

The pathophysiology of pruritus is not totally worked out, and it is important that further research be carried out in this field, for it is critical to know the physiology of a symptom in order to treat it adequately. Briefly, we may state that itch and pain are related as they do travel over similar anatomic nerves, but they must be considered as separate sensations. Many chemical and physical stimuli may produce itch, probably acting through numerous different mediators. Enzymes such as the peptidases are important in the itch sensation, and histamine is certainly an important mediator of pruritus, but it is important to keep in mind that other vasoactive materials such as kinins, acetylcholine, and prostaglandins may also be important in the itch reaction. It appears that these various mediators stimulate nerve endings around the dermal-epidermal junction and impulses flow over the dermal nerve plexuses, primarily following the C fibers in a certain spatial and temporal pattern that is perceived by higher centers as itch. It is the pattern of impulses rather than specific nerve endings that produces itch. The pathway from the skin follows the sensory spinal nerve, ascends in the spinothalamic tract, enters the thalamus, and finally reaches the sensory cortex. These higher centers can affect the perception of itch, and anxiety, nervousness, and external distracting stimuli may all alter how the itch is perceived. Hence, pruritus is a complex sensation, not fully understood; but some appreciation of these points aids in the successful control.

Therapy of Pruritus

Obviously the successful therapy of pruritus depends on identification of the cause of pruritus and elimination of this cause if possible. A thorough history to attempt to identify what is causing the pruritus is essential, followed by a physical examination. This history and physical examination should establish if there is a systemic or cutaneous cause for the pruritus, and therapy can then be directed at the specific systemic or cutaneous disease. Although this is easy to say, it is frequently very hard to accomplish. Frequently, it is difficult to determine if there is an underlying cutaneous disease present or if the skin changes have been produced by the patient scratching the skin alone. However, this differential is important. If no definite cutaneous cause is found, then a systemic disease producing the pruritus must be considered, as is discussed at the end of this presentation. The symptom of pruritus must be treated with respect, and if an obvious cause is not found initially as the therapy of the pruritus is continuing, the patient should be carefully observed for any new symptoms that could indicate an underlying disease. Great care must be taken in calling the symptoms "psychosomatic."

The following discussion of pruritus will be quite general, and again it should be emphasized that if a specific skin disease is present, that specific skin disease must be primarily treated. Similarly, if a systemic disease is found, therapy should be directed at that disease.

General Aspects of Therapy. The most common response to itch is to scratch the area. Basically, scratching will change the aggravating itch to tolerable pain and will also fatigue or damage the receptor nerves. Scratching may also dilute the mediators of the pruritus. Obviously the patient may damage himself with scratching and may eventually aggravate the pruritus by altering the pattern of the nerve impulses. However, the patient may be unable to stop scratching with severe pruritus, and so simply telling the patient not to scratch the area is impossible advice to follow. Rather, the physician must work with the patient to abolish the sensation.

1. General rest and relaxation are important. At the cerebral cortex level, nervousness and fatigue will aggravate the itch.
2. A constant climate is important, as extremes of temperature and fluctuation may aggravate the itching. Particularly, a hot climate will aggravate the itching.
3. Avoid rough, irritating materials rubbing on the skin which tend to initiate the itch.
4. Avoid excessive drying of the skin such as by excessive washing of the skin with strong soaps. Dryness of the skin aggravating pruritus especially tends to be a problem in winter.
5. Avoid caffeine, alcohol, or spicy foods which may promote an initial vasodilation and aggravate the pruritus.

Specific Topical Measures. 1. Heat or cold applied to the area will convert the itch to a different sensation. Hot water will substitute a burning sensation for the itch, but as this causes vasodilation and increases local inflammation and lowers the threshold of the itch, the general effect is short lived. Cool compresses are preferable and should be applied early in the therapeutic course, using ordinary tap water or saline solution made by dissolving 1 teaspoon of salt in a pint of cool water. These should be applied as an open compress with a soft rag (not gauze), keeping the solution in the refrigerator until used. The cool temperature of the solution plus the evaporation produces the cooling effect which is very effective in the control of pruritus. If weeping is present, such as with an eczematous process, Burow's solution (Domeboro, Bluboro), 1 packet or tablet to a pint of water, can be used for its greater astringent effect. The combination of cool compresses with a topical steroid cream will be very effective if there is definite inflammation of the skin, again such as that seen in an eczematous process.

In generalized eruption, cool baths with Aveeno oatmeal, 1 cup to the tub, or cornstarch are very soothing.

2. If the skin is dry, it is very important to hydrate the skin adequately. An oil bath (preferably not containing lanolin) such as Lubath bath oil, 2 to 3 tablespoons per tub, is very effective. This oil bath should be followed by the application of a water and oil emulsion such as Eucerine, Lubriderm, or Cetaphil to the moist skin.

3. Antipruritic lotions are effective and allow the patient to apply something to the skin ad libitum for local relief.

Calamine lotion U.S.P. is effective but tends to be drying.

Crotamiton 10 per cent (Eurax) is an effective antipruritic cream and lotion and also is effective as an antiscabietic.

Schamberg's lotion is very satisfying to the patient for relief and is not drying.

Prescription:

Menthol	0.5
Phenol	1.0
Zinc oxide	20.0
Calcium hydroxide solution	40.0
Peanut oil to make	100.0

Phenol, menthol, and camphor in concentrations from 0.25 to 1 per cent may be incorporated into a wide variety of vehicles at the discretion of the physician.

4. Topical steroid (creams) are effective in the control of inflammation if it is present and is a cause of the pruritus. It should be emphasized that if inflammation is not present to a significant degree, the antipruritic effect of topical steroids is minimal. Therefore they should be used only if definite eczematous changes are present in the skin. Triamcinolone acetonide (Kenalog, Aristocort) 0.1 to 0.025 per cent or fluocinolone (Synalar) 0.01 per cent can be used. Many other steroid preparations are available. These tend to be expensive, and if large areas are involved or less severe inflammation is present, obviously the lower concentration of steroids should be used. If there is minimal inflammatory change, 1 per cent hydrocortisone (Dermacort) cream can also be used effectively.

Systemic Therapy. 1. Antihistamines are frequently used in the therapy of pruritus. These are specifically effective in pruritus caused by histamine-release, urticarial lesions, and it must be understood that they are of far less benefit when other mediators are involved. Indeed, the sedative effect of antihistamines may be the primary beneficial effect. Sleepiness as a possible side effect of the antihistamines must be stressed to the patient. (a) Diphenhydramine (Benadryl), 25 to 50 mg. four times daily. (b) Cyproheptadine (Periactin), 2 to 4 mg. four times daily. This medication is reported to have antihistaminic and antiserotonin effect.

2. Hydroxyzine hydrochloride (Atarax), 10 to 25 mg. four times daily, is very effective as a tranquilizer in patients with anxiety associated with the pruritus. A syrup is available and is effective in children (10 mg. per teaspoon). This medication also has had some antihistaminic effects demonstrated.

3. Tranquilizers are of benefit in patients who have considerable agitation associated with their pruritus. (a) Chlordiazepoxide hydrochloride (Librium), 5 to 10 mg. three to four times daily. (b) Diazepam (Valium), 2 to 5 mg. three to four times daily.

4. Systemic steroids should be reserved for conditions with an obvious inflammatory cause for the pruritus and the absence of any contraindications to the use of the steroids. Prednisone or its equivalent may be used in doses of 40 to 60 mg. initially and then in tapering doses over 7 to 10 days.

5. Aspirin has been advocated in the past, but as this tends to accentuate histamine-induced pruritus, it probably should be avoided in most patients with pruritus.

6. Sedatives have a place in the therapy of pruritus in allowing the patient to rest, but prolonged use should be avoided.

Systemic Pruritus

Persistent pruritus in the absence of the obvious cutaneous disease should suggest the possibility of systemic disease. Appropriate studies should be carried out to check for these conditions in addition to the control of the pruritus. Systemic causes of pruritus include hepatic and renal disease, lymphomas and other blood dyscrasias, internal cancer, pregnancy, hyper- and hypothyroid states, polycythemia vera, and psychiatric disease. Appropriate studies should be carried out to rule out any of these conditions if the pruritus is unrelenting or other causes are not found.

Control of the symptom of pruritus should be of primary concern to the physician, for it is a very disagreeable and disabling complaint for the patient. An understanding and sympathetic attitude by the physician toward the patient with pruritus should be added as a benefit to any therapeutic regimen.

PRURITUS ANI AND VULVAE

method of
REES B. REES, M.D.
San Francisco, California

Itching, chiefly at night, of the anogenital area is the presenting symptom. Up to 10 per cent of gynecologic patients may present with this complaint. There may be no skin reaction, or there may be inflammation of any degree, including leathery lichenification. Pruritus of the scrotum, the analogous condition in the male, is less common than pruritus ani in men; in women, pruritus ani by itself is rare and pruritus vulvae does not usually involve the anal area, although anal itching will generally spread to the vulva.

The pathways of the sensation of itching are not well understood.

Most cases have no obvious cause, or anogenital pruritus may be due to the same causes as intertrigo, lichen simplex chronicus, seborrheic dermatitis, psoriasis ("inverse psoriasis"), or contact dermatitis (from soap, colognes, douches, bubble baths, contraceptives, or the very medications being applied in the attempt to gain relief). The symptom may also be caused by irritating secretions, such as diarrhea, leukorrhea, trichomoniasis, or local disease (candidiasis, dermatophytosis). Diabetes mellitus is cited as the cause in some instances, but this must be rare. Uncleanliness or, conversely, compulsive overcleanliness may be the cause.

Assuming that all possible causes described above have been ruled out, one is left with the designation of idiopathic or essential pruritus, by no means a rare phenomenon.

In addition to ruling out or treating all possible systemic causes, one should follow general measures, such as the avoidance of spicy, highly seasoned foods and oral medications which might contribute. Soap should be avoided, and plain water used for cleansing. Moistened, unscented toilet tissue may be followed by dry tissue to pat the areas dry. Anal douching is the best cleansing method for all types of pruritus ani, and affected parts should be cleansed with plain water after urinating or defecating. All patients should be instructed regarding the harmful and pruritus-inducing effects of scratching.

Local measures include the use of a hydrocortisone preparation, but it is almost axiomatic that one must use an additional agent, such as mild tar or iodochlorhydroxyquin. An example of the former is 0.5 per cent hydrocortisone and coal tar (Zetone) cream and of the latter, 0.5 per cent hydrocortisone and diiodohydroxyquin (Vytone) cream or mild iodochlorhydroxyquin and hydrocortisone (Vioform-hydrocortisone) cream. Either is applied thinly morning and night, and then wiped clean. Both tar and iodochlorhydroxyquin may discolor underclothing, the latter more than the former. If these are not tolerated, one may use 1 per cent hydrocortisone ointment (Cortef). This contains no preservatives or other agents.

Potent fluorinated corticosteroid topical agents should be avoided, because of the likelihood of inducing atrophy and striations of the skin.

When candidiasis is demonstrated (with skin scrapings examined in 15 per cent sodium or potassium hydroxide under the high power of the microscope), one may use nystatin cream or amphotericin B lotion topically. The newer topical antifungals, including miconazole and clotrimazole, tend to be irritating in the anogenital area. For dermatophyte fungal infections ("jock itch," "ringworm of the groin"), also proved by microscopic examination of scales in hydroxide but under low power, 1 per cent salicylic acid and 3 per cent precipitated sulfur in an emulsion base may be gently rubbed in morning and night.

Topical anesthetics should not be used, because they are ineffective and because the "caines" are sensitizing.

A good office procedure is to paint the involved areas with Castellani's solution, and then to pat dry with cotton and dust over with talcum powder.

It may be necessary to prescribe an antihistamine, such as chlorpheniramine, 4 mg. given two to four times daily.

For intractable pruritus it may be necessary to give systemic corticosteroids, such as the intragluteal injection of triamcinolone acetonide suspension, 40 mg. per ml., using 30 to 40 mg. not oftener than every 3 to 4 weeks. This may disturb the menstrual cycle in premenopausal women, unless they are taking birth control medication. Prednisone may be used as an alternative, 10 mg. orally on awakening, 5 days each week, in 3 week courses.

One must always be alert to the possibility of an underlying malignancy or lymphoma. Extramammary Paget's disease, for example, may be inapparent clinically and yet may cause intractable pruritus.

PSORIASIS

method of
SIGFRID A. MULLER, M.D.
Rochester, Minnesota

Psoriasis is a relatively common chronic, scaling dermatosis that frequently involves the elbows, knees, lumbosacral area, genital region, or scalp. Atypical forms are occasionally seen, and the condition may be mistaken for seborrheic dermatitis, intertrigo, or other disorders. In a few patients, widespread lesions may progress to generalized involvement, or there may be an acute disabling illness characterized by sterile pustules and exfoliation. Remissions and exacerbations of psoriasis may occur unpredictably.

Arthritis may be significantly related to psoriasis in a few patients so that exacerbation of both diseases may occur together. Treatment of the psoriatic eruption can have important favorable effects on the arthritis.

General Measures

Although the cause of psoriasis is not known, possible aggravating factors should be looked for and corrected. These may include streptococcal infections, irritating external agents, drug sensitivity reactions, and severe anxiety and fatigue states. Patients who are overweight should reduce their weight, particularly for the treatment of intertriginous psoriasis.

Daily tub baths for 15 to 20 minutes with soap and a suitable bath oil, such as 15 to 30 ml. (½ to 1 oz.) of Robathol, Lubath, or Alpha-Keri, and a daily shampoo with green soap solution, Sebulex, or a tar shampoo help remove scales and topical medication. Lubrication of affected skin regions with a simple emollient, such as Eucerin cream or white petrolatum, may give significant benefit. Topical therapy as indicated below is the treatment of choice for the great majority of patients.

Usually psoriasis improves in the summer and worsens in the winter, so that worthwhile relief may be obtained by making effective use of exposure to the sun. Gradually increasing amounts of sunbathing are usually beneficial, especially when generalized tanning occurs. Severe sunburn must be avoided; in a few cases sunlight aggravates psoriasis, and therefore sunbathing might be contraindicated.

Topical Therapy

Fluorinated corticosteroids are the most helpful and commonly used agents in office practice, and they are available as liquids, creams, ointments, or gels. Creams are usually preferred by patients because ointments are too greasy and gels too drying, even though ointments and gels may be theoretically more effective. Such creams as 0.025 per cent fluocinolone (Synalar), 0.1 per cent triamcinolone (Kenalog), or 0.05 per cent betamethasone (Diprosone) are applied three or four times a day to the affected skin regions. Liquid preparations, such as 0.01 per cent fluocinolone (Synalar) solution or 0.1 per cent betamethasone (Valisone) lotion, are more suitable for use in the scalp. Care should be taken in the chronic use of these high-potency steroid preparations, especially on the face and intertriginous areas, because they may produce atrophy, persistent erythema, telangiectasia, striae, or acneiform eruptions. The effectiveness of the creams may be enhanced and the need for frequent applications reduced by the use of occlusive plastic dressings overnight. Plastic sweatsuits may be easier to use when there is widespread involvement. Adrenal suppression must be considered a possibility when large areas are treated for long periods.

A few localized lesions of psoriasis can be treated by intralesional injections of corticosteroids, which is a very effective treatment for more resistant lesions. Approximately 0.05 to 0.1 ml. of triamcinolone acetonide suspension (Kenalog) in a concentration of 5 mg. per ml. is injected into the middle or lower dermis with a 25 gauge needle at 1 cm. intervals in a psoriatic plaque. Atrophy of the skin may occur but is usually reversible after several months.

Keratolytics. The pronounced scaling of psoriatic lesions can be greatly reduced by the use of salicylic acid. This agent can be incorporated into a variety of corticosteroid creams and tar ointments in a concentration of 3 to 5 per cent. A salicylic acid gel (Keralyt Gel) is an effective commercial preparation that is particularly useful for psoriatic involvement of the palms and soles when used with occlusion for 3 or 4 hours, followed by its removal and the application of a corticosteroid cream and occlusion for 8 to 12 hours at night. Keralyt Gel can also be used on the scalp, which is covered with a plastic cap during sleep; the substance is then washed out in the morning with a shampoo.

Tar. Coal tar preparations are used mainly for inpatient treatment in combination with ultraviolet light. They are usually not used at home because they are messy and they stain clothing and furniture. New therapeutic tar gel preparations, such as Estar gel and PsoriGel, have recently become available and are much more acceptable cosmetically for outpatient use. They are frequently effective, though less so than coal tar ointments. They can be rubbed into the skin once or twice a day, but many patients complain of dryness, which can be relieved by lubrication. Five or 10 per cent liquor cabonis detergens in hydrophilic ointment or Nivea oil can also be used at night, followed the next morning by a soap tub bath and the application of a corticosteroid cream two or three times during the day. Ultraviolet light can be given daily in gradually increasing amounts five or six times a week for approximately 3 weeks, care being taken not to burn the skin excessively.

Anthralin Preparations. Anthralin derivatives are not popular in the United States because they discolor the skin and are quite messy. They may be compounded in a concentration of 0.1 to 0.5 per cent in a soft starch paste (salicylic acid, 20 grams; paraffin wax, 98.7 grams; white petrolatum, 1405 grams; zinc oxide, 234 grams; and starch, 234 grams) or purchased as Anthra-Derm in a concentration of 0.1, 0.25, 0.5, and 1 per cent. They are very effective in healing chronic, localized, stable psoriatic plaques of glabrous skin, but they frequently cause irritation of normal skin. Initially, 0.1 per cent anthralin compound is applied nightly to the psoriatic lesions, and this is followed the next morning by a cleansing tub bath and the application of a corticosteroid cream. The concentration of anthralin may be increased in stepwise progression for greater effect if there is not excessive irritation.

Inpatient Treatment. Patients with severe psoriasis unresponsive to outpatient treatment are candidates for the Goeckerman treatment given during a hospitalized period of approximately 3 weeks. An ointment consisting of 2 to 5 per cent crude coal tar in petrolatum with 1 per cent Tween 20 is applied to the skin three times daily. Minimal erythema doses of ultraviolet light are given daily. Individual large plaques that are most resistant can be treated by shielding normal skin regions and spotting additional ultraviolet light onto these severely affected areas. The Goeckerman treatment has been modified for daytime use in special psoriasis day care centers that are available in a few medical centers.

Systemic Therapy

Corticosteroids are rarely used systemically because of the significant side effects of these drugs after their prolonged use and because rebound flares of the disease often occur when use of the drug is discontinued.

Methotrexate. Complete clearing is not the goal of therapy with methotrexate, but rather the aim is to control the disease reasonably well while limiting the risk of possible toxicity. This drug has been used for more than 15 years and is approved by the Food and Drug Administration. However, it is a dangerous drug whose long-term side effects from prolonged use have not been determined. Methotrexate should be used only in cases of severe psoriasis when other methods have failed, and it is contraindicated in pregnant women or in women who are likely to become pregnant or when liver or renal impairment is present. Hematologic abnormalities are also a contraindication. Two dosage schedules are presently considered to be reasonably safe and effective: 2.5 to 5.0 mg. is given every 12 hours for three doses repeated once a week; alternatively, 15 to 25 mg. is taken as a single dose once weekly. A liver biopsy is suggested in all patients before treatment is started, and patients should abstain from alcoholic drinks. Blood and platelet counts should be obtained before each dose initially and then less often at 2 to 4 week intervals once the tolerance for the drug has been established, unless unusually large doses are being given. Liver function tests should be done also three or four times a year. There may be reason to repeat the liver biopsy at variable intervals in 1 or more years if hepatotoxicity is suspected or if the drug has been taken for several years. Photosensitivity reactions to methotrexate may also occur.

Photochemotherapy

The combined administration of a psoralen derivative, 8-methoxypsoralen or trimethylpsoralen, followed in 2 hours by irradiation with long-wave ultraviolet light (UV-A) has been shown to clear up or markedly improve psoriatic lesions. This form of treatment has not yet been approved by the Food and Drug Administration for the treatment of psoriasis, and is not listed in the manufacturer's official directions. Psoralen drugs may be administered orally or topically.

Oral. Photochemotherapy using 8-methoxypsoralen (8-MOP) has been evaluated during the past 2 years in a randomized cooperative clinical study at 16 medical centers in approximately 1300 patients with severe psoriasis and has proved to be safe and effective. No clinically significant abnormal laboratory findings have occurred as a result of the treatment. However, there is concern about the possibility of long-term side effects, principally the theoretical occurrence of increased numbers of cancers of the skin and cataracts. There is as yet no evidence of either of these side effects in humans. Because long-term maintenance therapy or frequent re-treatment sessions will be necessary in many patients, it is important to look carefully for any skin abnormalities or systemic effects that may develop. The administration of this form of treatment requires of the physician a basic understanding of photobiologic principles involved in the administration of photosensitizing drugs and ultraviolet light exposure.

In this treatment, 0.5 to 0.8 mg. per kg. of 8-MOP (available in 10 mg. capsules as Oxsoralen) is given orally 2 to 3 hours before total body exposure in a special UV-A therapy chamber. Treatments are given twice a week for those who sunburn easily and tan poorly and three times a week for those who tan well. The phototherapy chambers manufactured by GTE Sylvania and the National Biological Corporation have proved to be safe and effective and are maintained by the manufacturers in case of breakdown. The light source in these units provides relatively uniform high-intensity UV-A over the entire body surface, and it omits biologically significant amounts of short sunburn ultraviolet light or infrared irradiation. Built-in dosimeters, which permit the accurate measurement of the amount of UV-A given (in joules per square centimeter), are an indispensable part of any light therapy unit. Special goggles to protect the eyes should be worn during each treatment and for 8 hours after ingestion of the psoralen drug. Suitable goggles can be obtained from NOIR Recreational Innovations Company, Saline, Michigan.

The initial exposure dose of UV-A is less for those patients who sunburn easily and tan poorly. The usual starting dose is 1 to 3 joules per square centimeter, and a stepwise progressive increase of 0.5 to 1 joule per treatment is given once the patient's tolerance to the treatment has been established. At least 48 hours should elapse between treatments, because the psoralen-UV-A erythema reaction may not peak for 48 to 72 hours and consecutive daily treatments are likely to result in a severe phototoxic dermatitis. Most patients will show clearing of the skin in 10 to 20 treatments, reaching a maximum dose of UV-A of 8 to 15 joules per square centimeter. Severe sunburn-like reactions and blistering may develop from too much UV-A and may persist for 1 to 2 weeks or more, and this can result in severe exacerbation of the psoriasis. Excessive erythema or soreness of the skin (or both) should indicate to the physician the need to omit a treatment, to shield the affected area, or at least to reduce significantly the amount of UV-A administered. The development of severe phototoxic dermatitis requires cessation of therapy and is treated by soothing cool tap-water compresses, corticosteroid creams, and aspirin.

Maintenance treatments can be given with decreasing frequency, holding the UV-A dosage constant, once 95 per cent or more of the psoriatic lesions have cleared (excluding the scalp, which is protected from the light by the hair). Maintenance treatments can be given once a week for 4 weeks, then decreased to once every 2 weeks for four treatments, and then once every 3 weeks for two times before the treatments are stopped. Re-treatment may be required if there is a widespread recurrence of the psoriasis. The patient's suitability for this type of treatment will depend on his responsiveness and the length of time he remains free of psoriasis. Clinical assessment of chronic skin damage (possibly by skin biopsy) will be necessary until long-term side effects have been determined.

Sun exposure can provide sufficient UV-A for photochemotherapy, but the unpredictability of the UV-A intensity and the long treatment times make it more difficult to control and to clear up psoriatic lesions. It is important to remember that patients remain photosensitive for 8 hours after taking a psoralen compound and will need to protect themselves from extra, inadvertent UV-A exposure in sunlight also. Wearing wide-brimmed hats and long-sleeved shirts, avoiding exposure to the sun, and using sunscreen lotions such as UVAL or Solbar lotion applied to exposed skin areas are indicated.

Nausea is an occasional side effect and can be prevented or greatly reduced by having the patient take the psoralen drug with food or take half the prescribed amount at first and the remainder a half hour later. Pruritus is occasionally bothersome but can usually be controlled by appropriate lubrication of the skin between treatments and by the use of 50 to 100 mg. of diphenhydramine (Benadryl) at bedtime. Excessive tanning is a characteristic effect of the treatment; it may be quite intense in genetically predisposed persons. The hyperpigmentation fades with decreasing frequencies of treatment, and most patients do not object to it because it is generalized and even.

Topical. Topical photochemotherapy is also an effective treatment for psoriatic lesions. A 1 per cent solution of 8-methoxypsoralen (8-MOP) lotion is applied to psoriatic lesions and irradiated with small amounts of UV-A (0.2 joule per square centimeter) 2 hours later. This is done every 2 to 3 days for approximately 2 to 5 weeks. It is important to remember that there is a narrow margin of safety in the dosage of UV-A given, and painful blistering reactions may occur unless careful attention is paid to dosimetry. An intense, irregular hyperpigmentation develops at the treated sites and gradually fades after several weeks. Topical therapy of this type may be suitable for isolated, thick, resistant plaques of psoriasis.

INFLAMMATORY ERUPTIONS OF THE HANDS AND FEET

method of
WALTER G. LARSEN, M.D.
Portland, Oregon

Nonspecific General Treatment

Acute Vesicular Exudative and Crusted Phase. 1. Compress with Burow's solution (1 to 40), using Kerlix or bed sheeting. Compresses can be used continuously if the eruption is severe. Usually compressing for 30 minutes four times a day is sufficient.

2. After use of the wet packs, a drying lotion such as colloidal oatmeal (Aveeno) or calamine liniment can be used.

Subacute Phase. 1. Decrease or stop wet packs.

2. An emollient such as neutral aliphatic hydrocarbons (Nivea) or a corticosteroid cream may be used.

Chronic Phase. 1. Switch to a corticosteroid *ointment.*

2. Occlusion overnight with polyethylene gloves.

3. Avoid topical sensitizers such as neomycin, iodochlorhydroxyquin (Vioform), and benzocaine.

4. Flurandrenolide (Cordran) tape for fissures.

Specific Therapy

Dermatophytosis of the Feet with an Id Reaction on the Hands. 1. KOH and culture for fungus.

2. Griseofulvin, 0.5 gram, 1 tablet twice a day after meals for 5 days and then 1 tablet daily.

3. Antifungal agents twice daily to the feet: tolnaftate (Tinactin) solution, haloprogin (Halotex) solution.

4. Whitfield's ointment at bedtime if scaling is prominent.

Contact Allergic Dermatitis. 1. Patch test to a screening series plus specific materials with which the patient is in contact.

2. Avoid allergen.

3. Appropriate topical treatment (see above).

4. For severe eruptions, use oral prednisone, 40 to 60 mg. in one morning dose for 1 to 2 weeks.

Housewife's Dermatitis (Irritant Contact Dermatitis). 1. Avoid wetting and drying of hands.

2. Avoid irritants and sensitizers.

3. Lubricate frequently with urea (Carmol) cream or a eucerite base preparation (Aquaphor).

4. Hand protection with appropriate gloves.

Psoriasis. 1. Five per cent liquor carbonis detergens in a betamethasone (Valisone) or fluocinonide (Lidex) *ointment.* Apply three or four times a day and use occlusion with polyethylene gloves at night.

2. Grenz ray therapy.

3. Anthralin ointment 0.1 to 0.5 per cent.

4. Flurandrenolide (Cordran) tape.

Recurrent Pustulovesicular Eruptions ("Dyshidrosis," Pustulosis Plantaris et Palmaris, Pustular Psoriasis). 1. KOH and culture for fungus.

2. Gram stain, culture, and sensitivity for bacteria.

3. Fluorinated steroids topically.

4. Burow's compresses.

5. Treatment with systemic antibiotics such as penicillin, tetracycline, or erythromycin. Use 1 gram daily until improvement occurs and then decrease the dose. A low maintenance dose is sometimes needed.

6. For severe recalcitrant eruptions, use oral prednisone in a dose of 30 mg. given in a single morning dose for short periods of time.

Other Diseases. Other diseases with manifestations on the hands include secondary syphilis, scabies, porphyria cutanea tarda, photosensitivity reactions, collagen disease, erythema multiforme, and atopic dermatitis.

BACTERIAL INFECTIONS OF THE SKIN

method of
SIDNEY HURWITZ, M.D.
New Haven, Connecticut

Impetigo

Impetigo is a term used to describe superficial infections of the skin caused by streptococci, staphylococci, or both. The clinical distinction between impetigo caused by each of these two organisms has been stressed, but is not yet firmly established. Bullous impetigo is usually caused by a phage group II (usually type 71) Staphylococcus. Vesiculopustular impetigo with crusted lesions is caused by beta-hemolytic streptococci (alone or in combination with staphylococci). Staphylococci, when seen, are late colonists and accordingly play no role in the pathogenesis of streptococcal pyoderma.

Topical Therapy. 1. Gentle washing of lesions, removal of crusts, and drainage of blisters and pustules help prevent reaccumulation of crusts and spread of lesions. If crusts are firmly adherent, warm soaks or compresses are helpful.

2. Topical antibiotics are often effective in the early treatment of superficial staphylococcal pyoderma. Of these, bacitracin, polymyxin, gramicidin, and erythromycin are relatively free of contact allergy. Although a high incidence of allergenicity has been attributed to the topical use of neomycin, this probably has been exaggerated.

Systemic Therapy. 1. Patients with persistent or recurrent bullous impetigo caused by *Staphylococcus aureus* may be treated with erythromycin, 250 mg. orally four times a day (30 to 50 mg. per kg. per 24 hours in children) for 7 to 10 days. For those acutely ill or with severe forms of bullous impetigo, dicloxacillin may be administered, 250 mg. orally four times a day (12.5 to 25 mg. per kg. per day for children) for 7 to 10 days.

2. Systemic antibiotics are the treatment of choice for cutaneous streptococcal infection. They may be administered as oral penicillin G (400,000 units three to four times a day) or penicillin V (250 mg. four times a day) for 7 to 10 days, or as benzathine penicillin (600,000 to 1,200,000 units intramuscularly). Patients with penicillin sensitivity may be treated with erythromycin (250 mg. four times a day).

3. In areas where nephritogenic M-strains of streptococci are endemic, urinalysis should be performed and patients should be watched for signs of glomerulonephritis for at least 7 weeks after the cutaneous streptococcal infection.

Ecthyma

Ecthyma is a deep or ulcerative type of pyoderma commonly seen on the lower extremities and buttocks of children with thick overlying crusts, adenitis, and/or fever. Treatment, as in streptococcal impetigo, consists of warm compresses and appropriate systemic antibiotics.

Folliculitis

The term folliculitis refers to a superficial or deep infection of hair follicles. Coagulase-positive *Staphylococcus aureus* is the most common pathogen in this disorder. On occasion, streptococci, Proteus, Pseudomonas, or coliform bacilli may be responsible for the infection.

Treatment. 1. Superficial folliculitis usually responds to gentle cleansing and the application of topical antibiotics.

2. Persistent or recurrent folliculitis may require appropriate systemic antibiotics (penicillin, erythromycin, or tetracycline) for a period of 7 to 10 days or more.

Furuncles, Boils, and Carbuncles

A furuncle or boil is a painful circumscribed perifollicular staphylococcal abscess of the dermis and subcutaneous tissue which develops from a preceding superficial folliculitis. Carbuncles are deep staphylococcal abscesses created by an aggregation of confluent furuncles. Accompanied by intense inflammation in the surrounding connective and subcutaneous tissue, they eventually suppurate and drain through multiple openings in the cutaneous surface.

Treatment. 1. Mild furunculosis may be controlled by warm moist compresses which relieve discomfort, promote drainage, and aid in localization of infection.

2. Severe or persistent infections may require systemic antibiotics. Since penicillin-resistant staphylococci frequently are seen, cultures and sensitivity studies should be performed. Oral semisynthetic penicillinase-resistant penicillins (oxacillin, cloxacillin, dicloxacillin, nafcillin, or cephalexin) appear to be the antibiotics of choice. Erythromycin, lincomycin, or clindamycin may be given (dependent upon sensitivity studies) to patients allergic to penicillin and its derivatives.

3. When lesions are large, painful, localized, and fluctuant, incision and drainage is indicated and beneficial.

Pyogenic Paronychia

Acute pyogenic paronychia is an inflammatory reaction involving the folds of the skin surrounding the fingernail; it is usually due to hemolytic staphylococcal infection secondary to local injury. In the chronic form other organisms (Streptococcus, Pseudomonas, coliform bacilli, and Proteus) may be involved.

Treatment. 1. Therapy should begin with warm compresses to promote drainage and localization of infection.

2. Deep lesions are best treated by systemic antibiotics (as in the treatment of impetigo and furunculosis), with incision and drainage when lesions are painful, localized, and fluctuant.

Sycosis Barbae (Folliculitis Barbae, Barber's Itch)

Sycosis barbae is a term used to describe a

deep-seated folliculitis of the bearded area which involves the entire depth of the follicle and perifollicular region. Although other bacteria occasionally may be isolated, the infection usually is staphylococcal in origin.

Treatment. 1. Although relapses are common, warm soaks, compresses, and topical antibiotics often control minor forms of sycosis barbae.

2. Care in the technique of shaving should be taken by those persons susceptible to this disorder. Shaving should be light and infrequent, with use of a brushless shaving cream and a fresh blade with each shave. An electric razor, rather than a safety razor, is sometimes helpful in the prevention and management of this disorder.

3. When sycosis barbae is chronic, severe, or recurrent, systemic antibiotics may be required. Although erythromycin or tetracycline frequently is effective, persistent infections require culture and appropriate antibiotics dependent upon sensitivity studies.

Folliculitis Keloidalis Nuchae (Acne Keloid)

Folliculitis keloidalis nuchae represents a chronic perifollicular infection of the nape of the neck seen in men. The bacteriology varies from patient to patient and at different time intervals. Although pathogenic staphylococci often are found, they appear to be secondary invaders.

Treatment. 1. Treatment consists of long-term antibiotic therapy as in the treatment of severe acne vulgaris and chronic folliculitis, with intralesional triamcinolone (in an effort to minimize keloid formation) and incision and drainage of lesions.

2. In severe cases, excision and plastic surgical repair may be necessary.

Cellulitis and Erysipelas

Cellulitis is an acute suppurative inflammation of the subcutaneous tissue. Although group A beta-hemolytic streptococci and staphylococci are by far the most common causative agents, other bacteria occasionally are implicated. Erysipelas is a more superficial form of cellulitis, with a well demarcated border, caused by beta-hemolytic streptococci. A peculiar and severe cellulitis, caused by *Hemophilus influenzae* type B, occasionally may be seen in infants and young children. This disorder is characterized by a dusky red or reddish-purple tender and warm indurated area without elevated or sharply demarcated borders. Although detection of *H. influenzae* type B in nose and throat cultures is suggestive of the diagnosis, the only definitive method of diagnosis is by the use of blood cultures.

Treatment. 1. Cellulitis and erysipelas are treated with appropriate antibiotics, with penicillin as the usual drug of choice. Erythromycin, clindamycin, lincomycin, or cephalexin is indicated for those allergic to penicillin.

2. For patients with penicillin-resistant staphylococci associated with the Streptococcus, a semisynthetic penicillinase-resistant penicillin may produce a rapid clinical response.

3. Children with cellulitis caused by *H. influenzae* should be hospitalized and treated with intravenous ampicillin (150 to 200 mg. per kg. per day in divided doses at 4 to 6 hour intervals). Once the patient responds, therapy may be continued with oral ampicillin (50 to 100 mg. per kg. per day in four equal doses). Treatment should be continued until the patient has been afebrile for 7 to 10 days. For patients allergic to penicillin and its derivatives, chloramphenicol (50 to 100 mg. per kg. per day) may be used. Aplastic anemia, however, must be considered as a possible complication to use of this agent.

Erythrasma

Erythrasma is a superficial bacterial infection of the skin caused by *Corynebacterium minutissimum*. It is characterized by well demarcated, reddish-brown, slightly scaling patches in the groin or axillae, or by maceration and scaling in the interdigital spaces of the toes. Erythrasma shows a coral red fluorescence under Wood's light owing to the production of porphyrins by the bacteria in the stratum corneum.

Therapy. 1. The treatment of choice is oral erythromycin (250 mg. four times a day for 7 to 14 days).

2. Topical keratolytics (e.g., Whitfield's ointment twice a day) are suppressive rather than curative.

3. Antibacterial soaps may help prevent recurrences of this disorder.

Atypical Mycobacterial Infections (Swimming Pool Granuloma)

Abrasions sustained in swimming pools or fish tanks may become infected with atypical mycobacteria (*Mycobacterium marinum*—formerly known as *M. balnei*) and possibly other unclassified mycobacteria. Most lesions are seen as solitary (occasionally multiple) subcutaneous nodules, ulcers, or abscesses at points of trauma, usually on the elbows, knees, hands, feet, and nose.

Treatment. 1. Cultures on Löwenstein-Jensen medium can help clarify the proper diagnosis. The greatest yield of positive cultures is obtained by direct inoculation of freshly biopsied material.

2. Although minocycline has been used with varying degrees of success, there is no specific satisfactory treatment for swimming pool gran-

uloma. The response to therapy with antituberculous drugs is unpredictable and generally poor. Cryosurgery with liquid nitrogen may aid involution of small lesions. Surgical excision may be satisfactory for early or small lesions, but recurrences are not uncommon.

3. Most lesions eventually involute spontaneously, although the time period may vary from a few months to several years or more.

Toxic Epidermal Necrolysis Due to Staphylococci (Staphylococcal Scalded Skin Syndrome)

Toxic epidermal necrolysis due to staphylococci (staphylococcal scalded skin syndrome [SSSS]) is a distinctive dermatitis caused by an exfoliative toxin, "exfoliatin," elaborated by coagulase-positive Group II staphylococci (usually type 55 or 71). Although staphylococcal scalded skin syndrome is primarily a disorder seen in children under 10 years of age and toxic epidermal necrolysis, when seen in adults, is usually a drug-induced disorder, on occasion the staphylococcal form of this disease has been reported in adults.

Treatment. 1. Treatment of staphylococcal scalded skin syndrome requires prompt initiation of antistaphylococcal therapy to eradicate the focus of infection and eliminate further toxin production.

2. Since most of the organisms are resistant to penicillin and some are resistant to erythromycin, penicillinase-resistant antistaphylococcal agents are preferred. Dicloxacillin, 12.5 to 25 mg. per kg. per day in four equal doses, is given to children weighing less than 40 kg. (88 lbs.); for adults and children weighing 40 kg. or more, 250 mg. every 6 hours is usually an adequate dose.

3. Corticosteroids appear to be contraindicated, as they seem to enhance susceptibility of the host to infection.

4. Topical antibiotics are unnecessary and should be avoided.

5. In the late desquamatous phase the skin should be lubricated with bland ointments or lubricating lotions.

ROSACEA

method of
THOMAS J. RUSSELL, M.D.
Milwaukee, Wisconsin

Rosacea is a chronic recurrent acneiform eruption of the central face, involving to a variable degree the nose, forehead, cheeks, and chin. It is typically an eruption of the middle-aged fair-complected patient of Northern European or Anglo-Saxon descent and often persists into old age. Clinically it appears much like an inflammatory acne in a patient well past the usual adolescent and young adult age of acne vulgaris. Erythema, papules, and pustules of the face are present. Eventually telangiectasia and rhinophyma may develop, which, to an extreme degree, would have been exemplified by a W. C. Fields with pimples.

The pathologic mechanism for the disease is not clearly understood. It is not considered a simple extension of acne. Anything which produces a facial flush has an adverse effect on rosacea. Vasomotor lability of the menopausal female, the easily embarrassed person, and emotional stress may be significant contributing factors. Diet has been traditionally ascribed a major role in aggravating the eruption. This includes spices in highly seasoned foods, physically hot food, alcohol, and stimulants such as coffee and tea. An associated seborrheic dermatitis may be present, involving the scalp, brows, and nasolabial crease.

An iatrogenic role has become increasingly recognized as a major aggravating factor in the guise of potent fluorinated topical steroids, compared with the often beneficial effect of the relatively low potency hydrocortisone topical preparations. The fluorinated steroids comprise almost all of the well-known potent topical steroid preparations. Many patients see their physician about an irritation of the face, are given a prescription for these preparations, and become habitual users, resulting in steroid rosacea. The anti-inflammatory effect oscillates with the inflammatory effect on the sebaceous apparatus ascribed to the fluoride component. The more inflamed the skin appears, the more fluorinated steroids are used, and withdrawal inflammatory rebound becomes a problem. The use of fluorinated steroids is excellent on most areas of the body, but not on the face for a chronic problem such as rosacea.

Inflammatory eye lesions may be associated with rosacea, at times preceding skin signs. Blepharitis, conjunctivitis, and keratitis may occur, the last of these occasionally becoming severe with secondary staphylococcal corneal ulceration. Photophobia and persistent complaints of eye irritation may warrant a referral to an ophthalmologist for an evaluation.

Therapy

General Measures. All patients are advised on dietary management, which primarily is avoidance of aggravating stimulants, spices, and alcohol. Menopausal women with prominent vasomotor lability may need addition or alteration of replacement hormonal therapy. Tetracycline, 250 to 500 mg. per day, appears to be the most effective single therapeutic modality in most patients. It is given over several months on a regular basis, with gradual withdrawal to 250 mg. every second day before stopping. Repeated and prolonged courses of tetracycline may be necessary.

Topical Treatment. Topically, all patients are advised to avoid fluorinated steroids on the face. All patients are advised to adjust frequency and vigor of topical therapy to their individual tolerance, as most of them are susceptible to additional contact irritation and subsequent inflammation.

Fair-complected patients usually tolerate 1 per cent hydrocortisone cream with 1 per cent precipitated sulfur applied sparingly once or twice daily to the involved face with clean fingers. Individual judgment must be used, because areas of the face vary in ability to tolerate topical medication—e.g., the nasolabial crease is very sensitive compared to the relatively nonsensitive nose. In addition, a clear drying lotion containing a low concentration of hydrocortisone (Komed HC) applied principally to the nose once or twice daily decreases papules and pustules.

For the oily-complected patients, more vigorous applications of the same topical medications can be tolerated. One per cent hydrocortisone cream with 2 per cent sulfur may be necessary, as well as increased frequency of other drying lotions (Komed HC). Retinoic acid cream 0.05 per cent (Retin-A) applied to the nose at bedtime every 1 to 3 days has prolonged therapeutic effect and supplements the topical hydrocortisone-containing preparations by increasing turnover of epithelium in follicular orifices.

For patients who are not doing well with tetracycline or who have a relative contraindication to its prolonged use, e.g., diabetes, a trial of topical clindamycin (Cleocin) may be warranted. One 600 mg. ampule of intravenous clindamycin is added to a mixture containing 6 ml. of propylene glycol and equal parts of 91 per cent isopropyl alcohol and water sufficient to make 60 ml. This solution is applied twice daily with the fingers, relatively sparingly because of its expense. If the patient is judged to be excessively susceptible to minor irritation, the concentration of alcohol may be decreased. As a supplement to this regimen, the 1 per cent sulfur-hydrocortisone cream may be used at bedtime in more sensitive skin or the retinoic cream or gel can be used at bedtime in the more oily patient. Regardless of what topical therapy is used in rosacea, the skin always demands it be handled with care.

SCABIES

method of
ALEJANDRO MORALES, M.D.
Detroit, Michigan

Human scabies is a contagious disease caused by infestation and sensitization to *Sarcoptes scabiei* var. hominis. Sensitization occurs 20 to 30 days after infestation. Pruritus is due to sensitization to the mite and is usually intense at night. Therefore there is a period of 2 to 4 weeks during which infested individuals are asymptomatic carriers. Clinically, the disease presents various types of lesions. Burrows and vesicles are directly related to the presence of the mite and its eggs in the skin. Urticarial papules, nodules, and excoriations are due to sensitization, whereas pustules and crusts result from secondary infection.

The clinical diagnosis of scabies is best confirmed by finding the mite by microscopic examination of scrapings of the skin mounted in potassium hydroxide solution or with a drop of mineral oil on a No. 15 scalpel blade. Therapeutic trials may be unsuccessful and are not recommended, as the mite may be killed by the insecticide preparation but the pruritus may continue long after the eradication of the mite. Also, the preparations used as insecticides can act as irritants, and their prolonged use may lead to a secondary dermatitis.

It is essential to treat *all* the members of the household simultaneously, including those that are asymptomatic. It is absolutely mandatory that the insecticide be applied thoroughly to the skin from the neck to the toes, including the scalp in children under 1 year of age. (See precautions in manufacturer's official directive before using.) Routine washing of personal and bed clothes should be done at the same time. Fumigation and boiling of the clothing are not necessary.

The three most commonly used insecticides are as follows: (1) Sulfur ointment 6 to 10 per cent, applied on 3 successive nights after a shower or bath using a mild soap. In particular, this preparation in its lowest concentration is recommended for the treatment of children, as there is no danger if the children ingest it by sucking the fingers. (2) Benzoyl benzoate 12.5 to 25 per cent solution, also applied on 3 successive nights after a shower or bath using mild soap. (3) Gamma benzene hexachloride U.S.P. 1 per cent cream or lotion; one 24 hour application is usually sufficient. (See manufacturer's official directive before using.) Because of the potential for central nervous system toxicity of this preparation, I have limited its use to older children and adults.

In most patients, antihistamines and topical corticosteroid preparations may be needed for 1, 2, or more weeks after completing a course of the insecticide. It is not uncommon to observe pruritus and dermatitis after a successful treatment for scabies. In such patients, a short course of oral corticosteroids may be administered. Persistent postscabies nodules may require intralesional corticosteroid therapy injections.

If secondary infection of the lesions is suspected, bacterial cultures should be obtained and appropriate systemic antibiotic therapy should be instituted accordingly; my preference is either erythromycin or oxacillin.

Norwegian scabies is rare. It is usually nonpruritic. The recognition of this entity is important, as it has none of the clinical characteristics of common scabies and can simulate many other dermatoses.

Animal scabies is not a problem, because the host specificity of the mites leads to spontaneous cures, usually within 4 to 6 weeks. Symptomatic treatment with antihistamines or topical therapy with corticosteroids is effective. However, the animal source should be detected and treated or eliminated; otherwise, reinfestation will occur.

SCLERODERMA

method of
ALLEN R. MYERS, M.D.
Philadelphia, Pennsylvania

Therapeutic Strategy

Scleroderma or progressive systemic sclerosis is a member of the family of so-called collagen or connective tissue diseases, and like the other members of this group its cause is unknown. Although there are successful therapeutic modalities available for the treatment of many connective tissue diseases, no specific agents have been found to date which can halt the progression of scleroderma. This, however, should not deter the clinician from an expectant attitude toward treatment, because many approaches are available in the management of this disorder which can relieve specific symptoms and may prevent future complications.

In general, knowledge of the pathogenesis of a disease is helpful in designing a therapeutic approach. Unfortunately, this has not been the case in scleroderma. The present concept of the disease involves a primary microvascular abnormality, but just how this relates to increased collagen production is not clear. In any case, specific agents directed at the microvascular process are not available, and those aimed at increased collagen biosynthesis have met with variable responses. Therefore two major points must be kept in mind when approaching the therapeutic dilemma of scleroderma. The first is that the natural history of the disease may be quite variable. Although the disease is usually progressive, it may pursue such a course slowly, occasionally with spontaneous remissions. Second, the morbidity and mortality of the disease are related to its visceral involvement and not to its most obvious manifestation, the skin. Therapeutic decisions should be based upon the extent and type of involvement, which can be readily assessed by clinical and laboratory evaluations. The discussion to follow will be directed at an organ system approach and will assume that the physician has knowledge of the extent, severity, and rapidity of involvement of the specific system described.

Raynaud's Phenomenon

Prior to the institution of vasoactive drugs, it is imperative to instruct patients in the necessity for keeping generally warm, besides paying particular attention to the extremities. Patients are aware of what type and duration of cold exposure produce vasospasm, and this must be reviewed by the physician. Emphasis should be placed upon avoidance of specific vasospasm-inducing stimuli by keeping warm, using quality mittens and heavy socks, and keeping face, ears, and neck warm, which, if not protected, may lead to reflex vasospasm of extremities. Air-conditioned areas should be avoided.

If Raynaud's phenomenon occurs frequently after only brief exposure to cold temperatures, or is associated with digital ulcerations, a trial of medical therapy is indicated. It is our experience, however, that those patients with established obliterative vascular disease have little chance of responding to vasoactive agents, and therefore knowledge of peripheral blood flow may be helpful in predicting response.

Phenoxybenzamine (Dibenzyline) is a long-acting alpha-adrenergic blocking agent which produces a decrease in total peripheral resistance and hence increases blood flow to the skin. The usual daily dose is 20 to 60 mg., but treatment should be initiated with 10 mg. daily and increased by 10 mg. weekly with careful monitoring. Significant side effects include postural hypotension, tachycardia, inhibition of ejaculation, and nasal stuffiness, but these symptoms often disappear with continued use.

Tolazoline (Priscoline) is another adrenergic blocking agent which may produce increased blood flow to the skin, but is short acting. Dosage is 25 to 50 mg. four times daily. Side effects include nausea, vomiting, diarrhea, tachycardia, and flushing, which may clear with continued use.

*Reserpine** may act to increase blood flow through its depletion of body stores of catecholamines. Oral doses of 0.25 to 1 mg. daily have been used in Raynaud's phenomenon, but side effects are significant and frequently lead to cessation of use. These include nasal stuffiness, depression, nightmares, diarrhea, impotence, and activation of peptic ulcer. Intra-arterial reserpine has been used with variable success but usually without significant side effects. A dose of 1.0 mg.

*Unapproved use for an approved drug.

given directly into the brachial artery may result in immediate relief of digital ischemia, and increased blood flow may persist for 1 week or more. Repeated intra-arterial injections at regular intervals have not been as effective as initially suggested.

Guanethidine (Ismelin), alpha methyldopa (Aldomet), isoxsuprine (Vasodilan), and griseofulvin (Fulvicin) have been reported to increase blood flow and relieve Raynaud's phenomenon, but the general experience is that they are rarely effective clinically. Sympathectomy has likewise been discarded as a useful therapeutic modality owing to the transient nature of the relief produced.

It must be emphasized that extremities with reduced nutritional blood supply are more easily damaged following simple trauma, and care must be taken to assiduously avoid abrasions, lacerations, and puncture wounds of the fingers lest ulcerations develop.

Skin

Skin care is essential to prevent chronic ulceration, particularly of the fingers. Avoidance of Raynaud's phenomenon and trauma has already been emphasized. In addition, the use of lanolin creams to increase pliability and prevent fissuring is important and helpful. If digital ulcerations develop, they must be kept clean and lubricated. Careful attention to the ulcers generally results in healing.

The initial phase of the skin involvement is an edematous one, and a trial with salicylates as anti-inflammatory therapy is indicated. However, the use of corticosteroids is not advised because of the risk-to-benefit ratio—i.e., little benefit and more risks. Diuretics are unfortunately without value. Most often, the edematous phase is gradually replaced by skin thickening, which is then followed by a hidebound stage. Treatment of these primary manifestations of scleroderma is generally unrewarding, but recent trials have suggested a possible therapeutic approach with the use of D-penicillamine* (Cuprimine), an agent that inhibits collagen biosynthesis and collagen cross-linking and may have anti-inflammatory properties. Its use has been associated with softening of skin, decreased stiffness, and increased hair growth in some scleroderma patients. Unfortunately, large control studies are not available to document the therapeutic efficacy. The dose ranges from 250 mg. to 1.5 grams daily, and toxicity includes bone marrow suppression, skin rash, and membranous glomerulonephritis. Therapy is initiated with 250 mg. daily and increased by 250 mg. increments every 3 to 4 weeks. Careful monitoring for proteinuria, granulocytopenia, and thrombocytopenia is mandatory. Fortunately, the bone marrow and renal toxicities are reversible, and skin rash may not recur on reinstitution of therapy after a short hiatus.

Immunosuppressive agents, colchicine, potassium p-aminobenzoate, corticosteroids, dimethyl sulfoxide, and epsilon aminocaproic acid have not proved to have any therapeutic value in the basic disease process, and therapeutic trials are not recommended.

Extreme tightening of the skin may lead to flexion contractures, and physical therapeutic measures should be instituted for preventive purposes. Exercises directed at forced extension must be practiced, and the use of light sponge rubber or plastic putty balls to maintain hand mobility is recommended.

Calcinosis circumscripta, a common complication in the fingers, is not amenable to medical therapy, but rarely is it a significant clinical problem.

Musculoskeletal

Joint involvement is common and most frequently occurs early in the course of the disease. Treatment is best accomplished with aspirin (3.6 to 6.0 grams daily). Myositis is being recognized in progressive systemic sclerosis with increasing frequency and is the single indication for the use of corticosteroids in this disease. Doses in the range of 40 to 60 mg. daily may be indicated, depending upon the severity of the myopathy.

Gastrointestinal

Esophageal disease manifested by distal hypo- or aperistalsis and decreased lower esophageal sphincter pressure occurs in 80 per cent of patients with scleroderma, and may produce dysphagia, peptic esophagitis, or esophageal stricture. Severe involvement may lead to recurrent aspiration. Demonstration of asymptomatic or overt esophageal changes is a definite indication for peptic esophagitis–hiatal hernia–type therapy. Such therapy includes multiple small feedings, frequent antacids, and elevation of the head of the bed during sleeping. Recalcitrant problems may be considered for surgical intervention if the patient is otherwise reasonably healthy. If strictures develop, mechanical bougienage may be helpful.

Small intestinal involvement may lead to bacterial overgrowth and secondary malabsorption. Treatment with tetracycline, 250 mg. four times daily for 10 to 14 days, is effective in reducing the infection and clearing steatorrhea. Recurrences are frequent and require re-treatment. Pseudo-obstructive (adynamic ileus) episodes

---

*Unapproved use for an approved drug.

when the small bowel is involved are not uncommon, and conservative hospital treatment with suction and hydration will frequently suffice. If malabsorption secondary to bowel disease is severe and results in cachexia, intravenous hyperalimentation may be employed in order to maintain nutrition.

When colonic hypomotility and sacculations occasionally produce symptoms, a high roughage diet should be advised in order to increase intraluminal pressures.

Pulmonary

The pulmonary fibrotic lesions of progressive systemic sclerosis are reasonably slowly progressive, and no therapeutic agent has been demonstrated to be effective in controlling the process. Caution in the use of corticosteroids is warranted owing to toxicity and general ineffectiveness. Cor pulmonale and right heart failure should be treated in the appropriate manner. In instances of severe pulmonary hypertension, oxygen may help to slightly modify pulmonary artery pressure and may be advised for home use. Superimposed pulmonary infections are common and should be treated aggressively.

Renal

The development of hypertension, proteinuria, and/or microangiopathic hemolytic anemia is an ominous sign in progressive systemic sclerosis, because it heralds the presence of "scleroderma kidney." Rapidly progressive renal failure ensues and is uniformly lethal. Very aggressive antihypertensive therapy (propranolol and hydralazine) must be instituted immediately in an attempt to prevent renal insufficiency. However, this is usually impossible, and chronic dialysis should be considered early for selected patients without advanced involvement of other viscera. Notably, peritoneal dialysis may be impeded by sclerodermatous involvement, and isoproterenol has been helpful in such patients. Occasionally, bilateral nephrectomies may be necessary to control hypertension. Renal transplantation has been successfully carried out in a few patients and might be considered in specific situations.

Cardiac

No specific treatment is available for the occasional patient with myocardial involvement and left-sided failure other than a cardiotonic program. However, the most common cause of heart failure in scleroderma is cor pulmonale resulting from either pulmonary vascular or pulmonary parenchymal disease. Treatment with a standard regimen, including diuretics, digitalis, and salt restriction, is effective.

URTICARIA AND ANGIOEDEMA

method of
E. GEORGE THORNE, M.D.
Denver, Colorado

Urticaria, or "hives," is composed of transient, pruritic areas of local edema caused by histamine release from mast cells. Urticarial wheals are dynamic, ranging in size from a few millimeters to several centimeters and lasting only 24 to 48 hours. Wheals lasting longer than 48 hours may represent another form of allergic skin reaction (erythema multiforme or vasculitis). The most common factors triggering urticaria are listed in Table 1.

Angioedema is edema affecting primarily subcutaneous tissue, and is more frequently found about the face, occasionally with laryngeal symptoms. Occasionally angioedema may be difficult to distinguish from cellulitis, particularly angioedema following an insect bite. The treatment for angioedema is the same as for urticaria. If respiratory distress occurs, epinephrine is used as described for anaphylaxis (see pp. 000 to 000).

In most patients, acute urticaria resolves within a few days to a week. Occasionally the cause as listed in Table 1 can be found. History is usually more helpful than a battery of laboratory tests.

If no other cause is readily apparent, I screen patients for hepatitis B surface antigen. Although the HB_sAg is an uncommon cause of acute urticaria, it has important medical implications. HB_sAg screen is especially necessary for medical personnel, relatives of renal dialysis patients, and patients suspected of using illicit drugs. Adequate treatment with antihistamines usually controls the symptoms. Unfortunately, a few patients go on to develop chronic (lasting longer than 6 weeks), re-

TABLE 1. **Urticaria Trigger Factors**

1. Drugs—penicillin, opiates (all urticaria patients should avoid salicylates)
2. Foods—nuts, shellfish, strawberries, food additives
3. Infections—teeth, gallbladder, sinus, urinary tract, Hepatitis B infections, infectious mononucleosis (acute urticaria), yeast, and parasites
4. Physical agents—dermographism, cholinergic, cold, solar, pressure
5. Insect bites
6. Inhalant allergens (rare)
7. Contactants—animals, foods, plants
8. Emotional stress
9. Internal disease—vasculitis (watch for renal involvement), collagen vascular disease, endocrine disease (thyroid disease)

curring urticaria, which can be a torment to both patients and physicians. Chronic urticaria differs little from acute urticaria. It shares the clinical picture, pathogenesis, and treatment goals of acute urticaria. A treatment program may be outlined as follows:

1. Identification and elimination of the cause. Table 1 is a good starting point, but many causes have been described and almost anything from intrauterine devices (IUD's) to menthol cigarettes may be suspect. Even with a thorough history, diet diary, skin tests, and extensive laboratory work-ups, a cause may be found in only 10 to 20 per cent of patients. But the physician should be alert for clues which may lead to some obscure cause.

2. Patients need education about possible causes and should actively participate in the search for the cause of their urticaria. They should be reassured that urticaria rarely eventuates in a serious internal disease.

3. Antihistamines are the most useful agents to control urticaria. I usually start with chlorpheniramine maleate, either tablets (Chlor-Trimeton, 4 mg. three or four times daily) or slow-release forms (Chlor-Trimeton, Histaspan, or Teldrin, up to 36 mg. per day). This particular alkylamine antihistamine does not produce as much drowsiness as the ethanolamine antihistamine, diphenhydramine (Benadryl). However, this side effect could be useful in some patients, particularly at bedtime. The usual dose for diphenhydramine is 25 to 50 mg. three times daily and 50 to 100 mg. at bedtime. Another very useful antihistamine, particularly in treating physical urticarias (dermographism and cholinergic urticaria) is hydroxyzine (Atarax, Vistaril). Start with a low dose, 10 mg. three times daily, and gradually build up to 25 to 100 mg. three times daily and 50 to 100 mg. at bedtime. In some cases a single bedtime dose may suffice. With most cases of chronic urticaria, a constant course of antihistamines is better than treating when symptomatic. Occasionally, adding ephedrine, 25 mg. three times daily, may be helpful in some recalcitrant cases or when angioedema is associated with the urticaria. Although cyproheptadine (Periactin) is not a true antihistamine, it does seem to help some patients with urticaria—specifically, those with cold urticaria. The usual adult dose is 4 mg. three or four times daily.

4. Many patients, particularly those with dermographism, have dry skin which adds significantly to the symptoms. Dry skin should be treated with hydration, followed by an emollient (Lubriderm Lotion or Eucerin). Soothing baths of colloidal oatmeal (Aveeno oilated) may also help control pruritus.

5. A few patients who are incapacitated by their urticaria, in whom the cause has not been found, or who are not responding to adequate doses of antihistamine may need oral prednisone, 20 to 40 mg. a day, for acute flares and alternate day steroids for maintenance therapy. Follow the patient closely, looking for any side effects of steroids and always attempting to decrease the dose.

WARTS

method of

ROYAL M. MONTGOMERY, M.D.
Forest Hills, New York

Because all warts do not respond to the same type of therapy and because they may be confused with other skin lesions, their management often challenges one's diagnostic skill and patience. Warts occur on all parts of the body but in different guises, which makes it imperative to distinguish them from such lesions as a corn, keratosis, nevus, molluscum contagiosum, Kaposi's sarcoma, or even melanoma. All warts are caused by a virus of the papovavirus group. They can be transmitted by direct contact as well as by autoinoculation. Often they occur on many members of the same family. Trauma may also be a factor. All warts except flat warts contain capillaries rising perpendicularly to the skin's surface, which can be seen after the keratotic cover is pared away. All warts have sharp margins and may occur singly or in groups. Those on the palms and soles have a keratotic covering. Elsewhere, they have a hyperkeratotic, papillomatous texture, or they can be smooth and almost flat.

Many warts will disappear spontaneously on an immunologic basis, especially in children. Others will respond to psychotherapy, which probably stimulates the immunization process. Others will prove resistant to therapy. All warts will respond in time to the proper therapy for their particular type, so before I choose a method I determine the type. I avoid surgical excision because of the resultant scar and the high rate of recurrence.

Verruca Plana

These multiple flat warts occur most frequently on the face, arms, or hands of children, but adults are not exempt. They are slightly elevated, smooth papules that range from skin color to yellowish. These are difficult to cure, so if one type of therapy does not work within a few weeks, I try another. With children I choose methods that cause little pain.

Acids. Thoroughly wet a fine applicator with a saturated solution of trichloroacetic or bichloracetic acid. Then touch each wart lightly. Neutralize 1 minute later with alcohol.

Gels or Creams. Prescribe retinoic acid (tretinoin) 0.05 to 0.1 per cent to be applied to each wart twice daily. (This use of retinoic acid is not listed in the manufacturer's official directive.)

Psychotherapy. Children often can be cured by a convincing optimistic suggestion. I rub a bright new penny over each wart, wrap it carefully, and give it to the child with instructions to bury it while chanting some doggerel. If the ruse fails, I explain that the patient did not recite the chant properly. All practitioners have their own "magic modality."

Verruca Vulgaris

These common warts are hyperkeratotic papules and occur usually on the knees, elbows, dorsum of the hands, and fingers, especially about the periungual areas. To prevent scarring, choose acid therapy if the wart is large, near a cuticle, or under a nail.

Acids. Pare off the keratotic covering. Touch the wart with a fine applicator that has been dipped in a saturated solution of trichloroacetic or bichloracetic acid. Cover with 40 per cent salicylic acid plaster cut to the shape and size of the wart. Hold in place with adhesive tape. Advise the patient to keep the area dry. Repeat the treatment weekly. For a more caustic reaction, use acid nitrate of mercury (distilled water, 15 ml.; fuming nitric acid, 45 ml.; mix, then add red oxide of mercury, 40 grams). For home use prescribe a mixture of three acids in collodion (salicylic acid, 3 grams; acetic acid, 3 ml.; lactic acid, 3 ml.; flexible collodion q.s. ad. 30 ml.) twice daily. If the reaction to any of these therapies is severe, instruct the patient to remove the medication and soak the area in boric acid solution. If blisters are present, drain them and dress with antibiotic ointment.

Occlusive Bandage. Cover the warts on the fingers with three layers of adhesive tape down to the middle phalanx and keep in place for 6½ days. Remove for a half day. The patient rewraps the fingers for another 6½ days. See the patient in 2 weeks. Often the warts can be removed with macerated tissue. If the warts are still present, repeat until they are gone.

Blunt Dissection. Anesthetize the wart with an injection of lidocaine 2 per cent. Incise the skin about the wart with a No. 15 blade or iris scissor. A Williger curette is a good blunt instrument with which to loosen the wart from the surrounding tissue. It is imperative to remove all the wart tissue from the dermis to prevent a recurrence. Treat the base lightly with trichloroacetic acid 75 per cent or light electrodesiccation. Dress with antibiotic ointment. The wound heals well without scarring.

Electrosurgery. Used alone, without blunt dissection, this method is apt to destroy too much tissue and result in a disfiguring scar.

Cryotherapy. Solid carbon dioxide gives good results, and many warts can be treated with it at one time. However, the procedure is painful and should not be used with children. Cut the stick to the size of the wart. Apply with moderate pressure for 1 minute. Dress with antibiotic ointment. A blister will form, which should be drained. When the patient returns in a week, if any wart tissue remains, it is treated with acids. Many dermatologists use liquid nitrogen with success, but I prefer the convenience of solid carbon dioxide.

Verruca Plantaris

Verruca plantaris may be classified as single, mother-daughter (epidemic), or mosaic. Differentiation is important for therapy, for each is slightly different. All treatment starts with paring off the hyperkeratotic covering to see if the lesion is a wart, corn, or callus. Every wart will have capillary tips rising perpendicularly to the surface. The margin tends to be sharp and the papillary lines diverge around the wart. A corn has a translucent core devoid of blood vessels. A callus retains a normal papillary line pattern, although enlarged. A single wart varies in size from a small horny point to a large lesion 7 mm. in diameter. The mother-daughter type has one central wart surrounded by satellites which have a vesicular appearance. The mosaic type has patches of small individual coalescent cores so closely grouped that they resemble a mosaic pattern.

Acids. This is my preferred method, for it does not scar and is effective for all types. Pare the lesion to the bleeding point. Stop bleeding with an aqueous solution of 100 per cent silver nitrate (30 grams $AgNO_3$ in 30 ml. H_2O). Apply saturated solution of trichloroacetic or bichloracetic acid with a fine cotton-tipped applicator. Cover with 40 per cent salicylic acid plaster cut to the size and shape of the wart or warts. Cover the entire area with moleskin. Have the patient keep the foot dry. Repeat at weekly intervals until the normal papillary lines reappear in the warty area. Should a painful reaction occur, remove the dressing and soak the foot in boric acid solution. Drain any bullae that may appear and dress with an antibiotic ointment.

Electrosurgery. Use this method cautiously to avoid deep permanent scarring. Do not use it for large warts or mosaic warts, because the resultant scar will be painful and the warts tend to recur about the scar. Electrodesiccation alone will soften the wart and it can be easily curetted out. Then lightly desiccate the base. If the wart persists, change to acid therapy.

Blunt Dissection. This method is preferable to electrosurgery, as it avoids scarring. It should not be used for mosaic warts.

Cryotherapy. At times I use solid carbon dioxide to thin a large mosaic wart and then proceed at the next treatment with acid therapy. Small single and mother-daughter warts may also be treated with cryotherapy.

Verruca Filiformis

These small keratotic thread-like warts may occur anywhere but are usually found on the eyelids or about the mouth and chin. They are easily removed with electrosurgery.

Verruca Barbae

Small, usually 1 to 2 mm. in diameter, these warts may be single or grouped and are scattered about the beard. Each one is desiccated lightly, curetted, and desiccated again. Dress with antibiotic ointment. Caution the patient to sterilize his shaving equipment.

Verruca Acuminata (Condyloma Acuminatum)

These small papules, which may be single, multiple or clustered, occur on the penis, vulva, or anal area. At times they may be cauliflower-like masses. Because of the accumulation, they are macerated and malodorous. They are difficult to cure, and patients with extensive anal warts should be referred to a surgeon.

Podophyllin. Touch each wart with podophyllin 25 per cent in tincture of benzoin, using a cotton-tipped swab. Instruct the patient to rinse off with water within 5 hours. The patient is to keep the area clean and dry with powders. Repeat this procedure every 5 to 7 days. If ulceration occurs, apply an antibiotic ointment.

Acids. Touch warts with a fine applicator dipped in a saturated solution of trichloroacetic or bichloracetic acid. Dress daily with an antibiotic ointment. Repeat every week.

Electrosurgery. Use electrosurgery if there are a few small warts on the penis or in the anal area. Infiltrate with lidocaine. Desiccate lightly. Apply an antibiotic ointment.

XANTHOMAS

method of
JOHN C. LaROSA, M.D.
Washington, D.C.

Xanthomas are lesions in both skin and subcutaneous connective tissue resulting from the deposition of fat, particularly cholesterol and its esters. They may or may not be associated with elevated plasma lipid levels. They have been described in all forms of genetically determined hyperlipoproteinemia (primary HLP), as well as in HLP secondary to diabetes mellitus, pancreatitis, biliary cirrhosis, and hypothyroidism. They may be seen independent of HLP in the following forms:

1. *Xanthelasmas* are yellowish, flat xanthomas of the eyelids. In adults over 40 years of age they may be present without an elevation of plasma lipids in about 60 per cent of cases.
2. *Planar xanthomas* (see below) may occur in a generalized form in association with dysproteinemias, including multiple myeloma and various forms of lymphoma.
3. *Juvenile xanthogranulomas* represent granulomatous lesions of the skin, eyes, and lungs which regress spontaneously and require no therapy.
4. *Xanthoma disseminata* is a form of histiocytosis. These xanthomas occur in the skin of the neck and axilla as well as in the mucous membranes and in pulmonary, bone, and pituitary tissues.
5. *Hereditary tuberous and tendinous xanthomas,* occasionally associated with similar lesions in the lung or central nervous system, represent a genetic disorder for which there is no adequate therapy.

These forms of xanthomatosis, however, are rare. Xanthomas commonly seen in a general physician's office are almost always secondary to HLP. Medical therapy for the common xanthomatoses therefore is directed to reduction of elevated blood lipid levels. It is important to note that the surgical removal of xanthomas is generally unnecessary and ineffective, as they are likely to recur unless the underlying hyperlipidemia is corrected.

Medical Therapy of Xanthomatosis Secondary to Hyperlipoproteinemia (HLP)

General Comments. When a patient presents with xanthomas, the presence of HLP should be established in plasma taken after a 12 hour fast.

Causes of secondary HLP, including diabetes mellitus, hypothyroidism, and dysproteinemia, should be eliminated. If the presence of primary HLP is determined, a trial of diet, as outlined below, should be instituted first. If that is not successful in normalizing plasma lipids after about 2 months, an appropriate drug can be added. If a combination of diet and drug therapy does not effect a reduction of 15 per cent or more in plasma lipid levels after 4 to 6 months, drug therapy should be discontinued. These steps are summarized in Figure 1.

Xanthomas may be divided into five types, including tendon, tuberous, planar, eruptive, and tuboeruptive xanthomas. The occurrence of each of these in five major types of primary hyperlipoproteinuria is summarized in Table 1.

Tendon Xanthomas. These xanthomas occur in the extensor tendons. The most common is the achilles tendon. The tendon may be diffusely thickened and may exhibit firm, discrete nodules as well. The extensor tendons of the hands and feet as well as the knees and elbows may also be affected.

Tendon xanthomas are found almost exclusively in familial hyperbetalipoproteinemia (Type II HLP). They have also been identified occasionally in Type II HLP secondary to hypothyroidism.

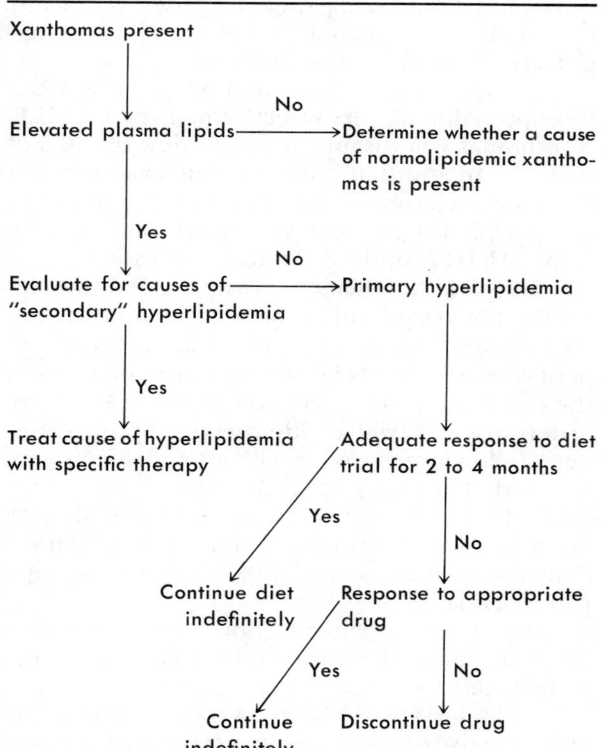

Figure 1. Sequential steps in the treatment of xanthomas.

TABLE 1. **Occurrence of Xanthomas in Primary HLP**

TYPE OF XANTHOMA	TYPE OF PRIMARY HYPERLIPOPROTEINEMIA I	II	III	IV	V
Tendon		+			
Tuberous		+			
Planar		+	+		
Tuboeruptive			+		
Eruptive	+			+	+

DIET. Treatment of Type II HLP should begin with a low cholesterol diet containing less than 300 mg. of cholesterol a day. The ratio of unsaturated to saturated fat in the diet should also be increased. In practice, this means the virtual elimination of some high cholesterol foods (egg yolks; whole milk and cream products; organ meats such as kidney, liver, or pancreas) and the limitation of animal fat in other forms. Additional polyunsaturated fat should be supplied in the form of corn, safflower, sesame, or cottonseed oils. Roughly 1 tablespoon (15 ml.) of oil should be taken for every 3 ounce portion of meat. A more detailed description of this and other diets designed for the treatment of hyperlipoproteinuria can be obtained from the National Heart and Lung Institute.* With strict adherence to such a diet, cholesterol lowering of about 10 per cent can be expected in patients with primary Type II.

DRUGS. Several drugs, including nicotinic acid (Nicalex), D-thyroxine (Choloxin), beta sitosterol (Cytellin), and neomycin, have been successfully used as hypocholesterolemic agents in Type II. In practice, however, only two drugs—cholestyramine (Questran) and clofibrate (Atromid S)—combine effective lipid lowering with a tolerably low level of side effects.

Clofibrate given in a dose of 1 gram twice a day may be effective in some patients with Type II who have associated mild increases in plasma triglycerides. Its mechanism of action is poorly understood. It appears to act by blocking sterol synthesis in the liver. Side effects are relatively mild and include gastrointestinal symptoms and the potentiation of oral anticoagulant and hypoglycemic drugs. In a few patients, a syndrome of

*Heart and Lung Information, NHLI, Building 31, Room 4A10, National Institutes of Health, Bethesda, Maryland 20014.

myositis associated with elevations of serum glutamic oxaloacetic transaminase (SGOT) and creatine phosphokinase (CPK) levels limit use of the drug. In Type II patients without associated hypertriglyceridemia, the drug is not useful.

Cholestyramine is effective in doses of up to 24 grams a day, usually given as 8 gram doses three times a day or 12 gram doses twice a day. It acts by interfering with bile acid reabsorption in the gut and indirectly enhancing the conversion of plasma cholesterol to bile salt in the liver. Internal side effects are uncommon. A few patients may develop transient elevations of liver function tests. In patients with pre-existing liver or intestinal disease, malabsorption of fats and fat-soluble vitamins (A, D, and K) may occur. Malabsorption of thyroxine, digoxin, and warfarin (Coumadin) may also occur if these drugs are taken simultaneously with cholestyramine. In a large number of patients (over 20 per cent), gastrointestinal symptoms may develop, including nausea, bloating, and constipation. These symptoms can be mitigated with the use of antacids and stool softeners. Proper education of the patient in taking the drug thoroughly mixed in a large volume of liquid is also helpful. Laxatives should be avoided. With careful instruction, a great majority of patients tolerate the drug well. A 20 per cent fall in cholesterol levels can be expected if the drug is taken regularly.

Diet and drug therapy may be very effective in lowering cholesterol levels in Type II, but regression of xanthomas is considerably less consistent. Although partial or complete remission of tendon xanthomas in properly treated patients has been reported, such results cannot be consistently expected.

Tuberous Xanthomas. Tuberous xanthomas are large cutaneous nodular xanthomas that occur on the skin overlying the extensor surfaces of the extremities and on the buttocks. Although they may occasionally occur in Type II secondary to myxedema, they are seen most commonly in familial Type II HLP. The treatment of tuberous xanthomas is the same as that for the tendinous variety. Again, although cholesterol lowering may be achieved, this will seldom result in complete resolution of the xanthomatous lesions.

Planar Xanthomas. Planar xanthomas are small, yellow, plaque-like lesions that may occur on the eyelids (xanthelasmas) and over the extensor tendons of the extremities. Xanthelasmas may occur in elderly patients independent of any lipoprotein abnormality (see above). They may also occur in primary Type II HLP. In that circumstance they are commonly associated with corneal arcus and tendon and tuberous xanthomas. Planar xanthomas occurring on the extensor surfaces of the extremities are commonly seen in the children with severe (homozygous) Type II HLP. The treatment for this disorder has been previously reviewed.

Planar xanthomas may also be seen in the palms, where they are sometimes associated with orange-yellow streaking of the palmar creases. These xanthomas are seen in primary Type III HLP (broad-beta disease, dysbetalipoproteinemia) as well as in the HLP which accompanies biliary cirrhosis. In the latter case, xanthomas can be expected to disappear when and if the biliary obstruction and resulting hyperlipidemia are adequately treated.

Diet. In Type III HLP, it is necessary to limit both cholesterol and carbohydrate in the diet, because both may elevate levels of the abnormal beta-lipoprotein which is characteristic of the disease. Cholesterol intake should be limited to 300 mg. or less a day and polyunsaturated fat increased as previously outlined. In addition, carbohydrates should be limited to less than 40 per cent of the total daily calories. In overweight patients, reduction to ideal body weight is an important therapeutic objective.

Drugs. Clofibrate, in doses of 1 gram twice daily, is the drug of choice in Type III HLP. Cholestyramine should *not* be used, because it is unlikely to benefit the hypocholesterolemia and may aggravate the hypertriglyceridemia.

A combination of diet and drug therapy can be expected to be very effective in Type III HLP. Xanthomas will disappear after a few months of therapy. In addition, there is some evidence that the atherosclerotic lesions commonly present in the peripheral vascular system of patients with Type III HLP undergo similar regression.

Eruptive Xanthomas. Eruptive xanthomas are discrete, small, yellow papular lesions that can appear anywhere on the skin but are most prominent over the buttocks and extensor surfaces of the extremities. They are commonly seen in disorders in which triglyceride-carrying lipoproteins, i.e., chylomicrons and prebeta-lipoproteins, are elevated. They may occur in Types I, IV, and V HLP. These forms of hyperlipoproteinemia may occur as primary disorders or may be secondary to diabetes mellitus, pancreatitis, nephrosis, or dysproteinemias.

Treatment regimens for these disorders must be tailored to the individual lipoprotein abnormality.

Type I Hyperlipoproteinemia. Diet is the only effective therapy. Because this disorder is one in which chylomicrons cannot be cleared from the plasma (presumably secondary to a deficiency of lipoprotein lipase), it is necessary to restrict all dietary fat to less than 25 grams per day. To some extent this diet can be made more palatable by the substitution of medium chain triglycerides for dietary fat. Medium chain triglycerides in the diet are not synthesized into chylomicrons in the intestine but rather are taken up directly by the portal vein. In practice, it is difficult to maintain triglycerides at normal levels in Type I HLP. Xanthomas, however, will disappear if triglycerides are normalized for several weeks and will not recur unless triglyceride levels rise again.

TYPE IV HYPERLIPOPROTEINEMIA. This disorder is characterized by the presence of elevated levels of prebeta-lipoprotein in the plasma. Prebeta-lipoprotein originates, for the most part, in the liver. Its synthesis is stimulated by excessive dietary carbohydrate. It is necessary to restrict the dietary carbohydrate to 40 per cent of total calories in order to control this disorder effectively. Limitation of alcohol intake is also important in the control of hyperprebetalipoproteinemia, as is reduction to ideal body weight. For most patients with Type IV HLP, a combination of weight reduction and careful attention to diet is sufficient therapy to normalize plasma triglycerides. In a few patients, clofibrate is an effective adjunct to dietary therapy. It can be expected that adequate therapy will result in disappearance of all eruptive xanthomas.

TYPE V HYPERLIPOPROTEINEMIA. This disorder is characterized by the presence of both fasting chylomicronemia and elevated levels of prebeta-lipoprotein. Total fat intake and carbohydrate intake must be restricted to 30 and 50 per cent of total calories, respectively. Weight reduction and alcohol restriction also play important roles in the dietary therapy of Type V HLP. As in Type IV, clofibrate may be a useful addition in patients whose response to diet is not optimal. Eruptive xanthomas will disappear completely after a few weeks of adequate therapy.

Tuboeruptive Xanthomas. As the name implies, these xanthomas have some of the characteristics of both tuberous and eruptive xanthomas. They are somewhat larger than eruptive xanthomas. Rather than being discrete lesions, they tend to occur in coalescent clusters. They are often surrounded by an inflammatory base and are the only xanthomas which are tender to palpation. They occur commonly over the elbows and less frequently on other extensor surfaces and on the buttocks. They are seen almost exclusively in primary Type III HLP. Adequate therapy of Type III HLP, as previously described, will result in their complete disappearance.

HERPES ZOSTER

method of
R. L. PITTS, M.D.
Kansas City, Kansas

Herpes zoster, or shingles, is an acute infection of the skin caused by chickenpox virus, herpesvirus varicellae, and it usually represents activation of latent infection of the posterior nerve root ganglia. It is most commonly seen in the older age group in otherwise healthy persons. Precipitating factors include lymphoma, leukemia, immunosuppression, intercurrent illness, and local trauma.

The first manifestation is unilateral, radicular pain followed by grouped vesicles on an erythematous base. These occur in a dermatomal distribution. The vesicles progress to pustules and at times become hemorrhagic and ulcerative.

The usual course is uncomplicated. Recovery takes 2 to 3 weeks. Rarely patients have more than one area of involvement, and a few have disseminated cutaneous involvement, with a minority of these having internal organ involvement. Disseminated disease occurs most frequently in immunosuppressed patients.

The most distressing and protracted source of morbidity in the herpes zoster patient is postherpetic neuralgia. This occurs predominantly in patients over 60 years of age. These patients experience persistent pain and occasionally paresthesia of the involved dermatomal area. Sequelae include scarring and transient paresis.

Treatment of uncomplicated herpes zoster is symptomatic.

Pain is usually controlled with analgesics such as aspirin or acetaminophen, and rarely requires a narcotic.

Topically, protection of the active lesions from minor trauma is usually all that is required. This can be accomplished by using nonadherent dressings such as Telfa or covering the area with zinc oxide paste with a soft cloth dressing.

Patients with severe involvement and patients over 60 years of age can be started on *systemic steroids* early, in the absence of contraindication. One controlled study suggests that this dose decreases the severity of the illness as well as the duration of postherpetic neuralgia. The usual dosage is prednisone, 40 to 60 mg. daily for 1 week, 30 mg. daily for 1 week, and then 15 mg. daily for 1 week.

Secondary infection is treated by culture and appropriate systemic antibiotics.

Lesions on the tip of the nose indicate involvement of the basociliary nerve and possible *ocular involvement.* Patients with herpes zoster ophthalmicus should be examined by an ophthalmologist early in the course of the disease.

The management of lower motor neuron lesions or paresis consists of supportive physiotherapy, including mobility and graded resistive exercise.

Disseminated zoster may be treated by the intravenous administration of cytosine arabinoside. (This use of cytosine arabinoside is not listed in the manufacturer's official directive.) The usual dose is 40 mg. per square meter of body surface for each 24 hour period for 5 days. The patient should be observed for hematopoietic suppression. More recently, adenine arabinoside has been used with efficacy. (This use of the adenine arabinoside is not listed in the manufacturer's official directive.) The usual dose is 10 mg. per kg. per day given in a 6 hour infusion. Culturable virus usually disappears after 5 days of treatment. Mild nausea and infrequent vomiting have been a problem, but these symptoms disappear after the fourth day of therapy. Meningoencephalitis tends to run a benign course and usually requires only supportive therapy. Varicella pneumonia can be managed by supportive therapy and maintenance of adequate arterial oxygenation.

Postherpetic neuralgia is usually a difficult clinical problem in management. Systemic steroids can be tried in the absence of contraindication—prednisone, 30 mg. daily for 2 to 3 weeks. Intralesional triamcinolone acetonide, 2 mg. per ml. of saline injected subcutaneously daily until the patient gains relief, has markedly benefited some patients. (This specific use of triamcinolone acetonide is not listed in the manufacturer's official directive.) Neurosurgical consultation for rhizotomy or cordotomy can be considered for intractable postherpetic neuralgia. These procedures should be preceded by local nerve blocks to determine potential effectiveness.

Prophylactic administration of zoster immune globulin appears to ameliorate this disease in immunocompromised persons who have been exposed to the virus. Three to 5 mg. of zoster immune globulin (ZIG) is administered within 72 hours of exposure. Zoster immune globulin is available only from the Center for Disease Control, Atlanta, Georgia.

HERPES GESTATIONIS

method of
ROBERT P. FOSNAUGH, M.D.
Southfield, Michigan

Herpes gestationis is characterized by an extremely pruritic polymorphous vesicular and papular eruption occurring most frequently during the fourth and fifth months of pregnancy. The eruption may occur as early as the first month and may last into the first few weeks post partum. Systemic manifestations are usually minimal. The maternal prognosis is good, but the incidence of fetal abnormalities and death is high (possibly 30 per cent). In my experience, the incidence of nausea of pregnancy is high in patients with herpes gestationis.

Treatment

When considering therapy for herpes gestationis, the physician must consider the possibility of drug-induced fetal damage, particularly in the first trimester. The many divergent treatments which have been proposed for herpes gestationis reflect the fact that little is known about the pathogenesis of the disease. Recent immunologic investigations, utilizing immunofluorescent techniques, may suggest a possible pathologic relationship between herpes gestationis and bullous pemphigoid rather than dermatitis herpetiformis, but the fact that herpes gestationis terminates after pregnancy, or shortly thereafter, differentiates them as separate entities. On the other hand, herpes gestationis and dermatitis herpetiformis have identical histopathologic findings.

The most reliable mode of treatment is corticosteroids; however, these drugs cannot be used safely in the first trimester. Prednisone, in dosage as high as 40 mg. daily, may be necessary for control of the eruption. Alternate day dosage technique is preferable to daily treatment. The dosage should be gradually reduced to a minimum during the final weeks of pregnancy to avoid adrenal suppression of the fetus. The patient should be monitored closely with regard to weight gain, blood pressure, and water retention.

Pyridoxine has been reported to be effective in some patients. Initially, it should be administered intravenously or intramuscularly in doses of

100 mg. twice daily. The intravenous route is by far the most effective method for establishing control of the disease. Simultaneous oral pyridoxine is administered in dosage varying from 100 to 400 mg. daily. The dosage can be reduced gradually by from 25 to 50 mg. daily. After control of the eruption, the dosage can be further reduced gradually to 25 mg. daily.

In my experience, the response to pyridoxine treatment is "all or nothing." If results of treatment are not seen within 10 days, continuing the treatment is pointless and it should be abandoned in favor of another modality. This "all or nothing" response to pyridoxine could indicate that more than one disease entity exists while exhibiting the clinical and histopathologic picture of herpes gestationis. The difference in immunologic findings by various investigators using immunofluorescent techniques could also suggest that herpes gestationis encompasses more than one clinical entity.

One advantage to pyridoxine therapy is that it can be administered safely when herpes gestationis occurs in the first trimester of pregnancy.

In some patients, 50 to 100 mg. of progesterone daily has been employed with some benefit. (This use of progesterone is not listed in the manufacturer's official directive.)

PAPULAR DERMATITIS OF PREGNANCY

method of
ROBERT P. FOSNAUGH, M.D.
Southfield, Michigan

The papular dermatitis of pregnancy may or may not be a distinct entity. The condition has several features in common with herpes gestationis but differs from it primarily in morphology and histopathology. Papular dermatitis is distinctly limited to pregnancy and is characterized by intensely pruritic, soft, red papules, 3 to 5 mm. in diameter, usually having a central papule. The lesions become crusted and eventuate into a pigmented macule. The condition terminates with pregnancy and tends to recur with subsequent pregnancies.

Treatment

In untreated cases the fetal mortality may be as high as 25 per cent. Very high doses of prednisone are required for control (up to 100 mg. daily); the steroid therapy results in a marked reduction in fetal mortality. In common with herpes gestationis, the condition presents a marked increase in chorionic gonadotropin levels; these gonadotropin levels fall to normal with prednisone therapy. Plasma cortisol levels may be lowered in papular dermatitis of pregnancy, which might account for the large doses of steroid necessary for control. Progesterone and sulfapyridine are ineffective. About 50 per cent of reported patients have been Rh factor negative. Patients with papular dermatitis have a positive skin test to placental extracts made from the placentas of other patients who have had the disease. I have seen two patients who appeared to have, both clinically and histopathologically, mild forms of papular dermatitis of pregnancy which responded to pyridoxine therapy as described for herpes gestationis.

A variant of papular dermatitis may very rarely occur in patients who are taking or who have recently discontinued contraceptive tablets. I have successfully managed two such patients with oral pyridoxine, 200 to 400 mg. daily; the therapy had to be continued for several months.

SECTION 12

The Nervous System

BRAIN ABSCESS

method of
RICHARD A. R. FRASER, M.D.
New York, New York

Despite current techniques which make their diagnosis relatively simple, 30 to 40 per cent of patients who develop a brain abscess will die. The introduction of antibiotics has not dramatically improved these survival statistics. Similarly, morbidity remains very high. Much of the problem lies in the nature of the site—the brain has inadequate antimicrobial abilities, no lymphatic system, and a very limited capacity for functional regeneration.

Various methods of surgical treatment—early excision, aspiration and later excision, and aspiration alone—have vigorous advocates. A comparison of reported clinical series, however, does not reveal a greater effectiveness of any one treatment method.

We advocate a therapeutic regimen based upon bacteriologic and pathophysiologic events common to brain abscesses, one which reduces morbidity and mortality to a minimum. Accurate and rapid diagnosis, recognition of septic foci, management of increased intracranial pressure, appropriate antibiotic therapy, and a properly designed surgical approach remain the basis of management.

Treatment

When a cerebral abscess is suspected after thorough physical examination and appropriate cultures, a CAT scan and skull x-rays are immediately performed. Subsequent management depends upon the findings of these studies and the patient's clinical status.

Pressure Reduction. Increased intracranial pressure is common, and rapid pressure reduction is necessary if the patient is severely obtunded or comatose. (1) *Osmotic diuretics* provide a safe and rapid means of reducing pressure. Mannitol in an initial dose of 100 grams intravenously in adults and 1 to 1.5 grams per kg. intravenously in children is recommended. Urea, a more toxic diuretic, is no longer used in this institution. (2) *Steroids* (dexamethasone, 24 to 32 mg. per 24 hours) may also help to reduce intracranial pressure by reducing edema and by potentiating and prolonging the effect of osmotic diuretics. Lower doses are used in children (4 to 6 mg. per 24 hours per 10 kg. of body weight).

Antibiotics. Most abscesses are caused by the gram-positive cocci, *Staphylococcus aureus* and streptococci (often microaerophilic). In chronic ear infections, these pathogens are often replaced by gram-negative bacteria, such as Proteus, Pseudomonas, and, more rarely, Klebsiella.

Until positive cultures are available and antibiotic sensitivities identified, broad-spectrum antibiotics are used. These must be started immediately while cultures are pending. Drugs recommended at this stage are as follows:

1. Chloramphenicol sodium succinate: In adults, 1 gram intravenously every 6 hours for the first 24 hours, and 500 mg. every 6 hours thereafter; in children, 100 mg. per kg. per 24 hours in divided doses. If concomitant meningitis occurs in adults, higher doses are necessary to achieve appropriate minimum inhibitory concentrations in cerebrospinal fluid (CSF). As soon as CSF and clinical examination indicate improvement, a reduction to 500 mg. every 6 hours is suggested. Prolonged administration of higher doses of chloramphenicol will lead to frequent episodes of toxicity which may be fatal.
2. Penicillin G: 20 million units per 24 hours in a continuous intravenous drip in adults, and 400,000 units per kg. of body weight per 24 hours in children.

Both these agents must be used for 4 weeks. Six weeks' administration may be necessary in some patients.

Special Circumstances

Contiguous Cranial Infections of a Chronic Nature. Because of the high incidence of Pseudomonas and Proteus infestations in these patients, the aforementioned antibiotic regimen is supplemented with intravenous gentamicin. Eight mg. per kg. of body weight per 24 hours is used as a loading dose. This is later reduced to 4 mg. per kg. per 24 hours and is given in divided doses every 6 hours in both children and adults. (These doses are higher than that listed in the manufacturer's official directive.)

Staphylococcal Endocarditis or Septicemia. The great majority of such patients will harbor penicillinase-producing penicillin-resistant *S. aureus.* If this situation is strongly suspected, nafcillin is substituted for penicillin G. Nafcillin is administered in divided doses intravenously, 8 grams per day. Twelve grams per day is used in adults if clinically significant meningitis is present. Nafcillin is preferred to methicillin because of its lower toxicity.

Obviously, the choice of these drugs may require revision when cultures become available. In the interim we have found that these agents provide maximum antibiotic effectiveness. An additional caveat must be described—approximately one fourth to one third of all intracranial abscesses never yield a positive culture. This is attributable to early use of antibiotics with subsequent cultures, as well as to inappropriate culture methods. In such patients one is forced to maintain these multiple agents unless the clinical picture suggests the need for a change.

Surgery. In 1893 McEwen reported only 1 death in 20 supratentorial abscesses treated surgically. This level of cure has not been experienced since.

Surgical treatment of intracranial abscesses takes two forms: (1) needle aspiration through a burr hole and (2) craniotomy and excision of abscess.

Needle aspiration is preferred as an initial form of treatment in all encapsulated abscesses. This is done under general anesthesia through a burr hole. The cortical surface of the brain is cauterized and incised. A 15 gauge blunt-tipped needle with a trocar is gently inserted toward the abscess. Firm resistance is felt when the abscess wall is reached. The needle is then pushed into the abscess cavity. Pus usually extrudes spontaneously, although gentle aspiration may be necessary. We prefer to perform gentle barbotage of the abscess contents with saline after an initial pus specimen is removed for culture. This allows for maximum removal of abscess contents. We then instill a saline suspension of barium-impregnated micropaque (1 to 2 ml.). This will be taken up in the abscess wall. The needle is then removed. Repeated percutaneous aspiration can thus be carried out under biplane x-ray control, with the patient awake. This is performed daily initially. Usually serial x-rays will reveal reduction in abscess size over the first week of such treatment.

Abscess excision: We prefer to excise all cerebral abscesses when this can be done without risking a substantial neurologic deficit. Abscesses in the sensory cortex, motor cortex, or speech areas are treated with serial aspiration only, as are those in or near the internal capsule or basal ganglia. All cerebellar lesions are excised. When excision is not carried out, the risk of recurrence is greater. Seizures are a common sequel of cerebral abscesses Some authors have claimed a reduction in seizure frequency when the abscess is excised, and use this as a further indication for excision. However, a review of our experience and reports of others reveal that seizure frequency is the same whether the abscess is excised or treated by serial aspiration.

A recent report describes quite satisfactory antibiotic levels in cerebral abscess aspiration specimens after administering systemic antibiotics. Assuming this is true, there seems to be no reason for maintaining the practice of instilling antibiotics into the abscess cavity.

In occasional patients one encounters the situation of focal cerebritis—acutely inflamed hypervascular cerebral tissue. This is simply a precursor to abscess formation. If the computerized axial tomography (CAT) scan suggests the presence of focal cerebritis, neither aspiration nor excision should be attempted. Aspiration will not produce a specimen and may be hazardous. Surgical excision at this stage will necessitate the removal of normal cerebral tissue and carries a substantial risk of producing additional neurologic deficit. Obviously this should be avoided. Management of focal cerebritis includes control of intracranial pressure and appropriate antibiotics. Maturation of the lesion and formation of a "ripe" abscess will be revealed by later CAT scans. At this time needle aspiration can be instituted. Excision, if warranted, is performed later.

If the abscess is caused by the tubercle bacillus, surgical methods remain as above. Appropriate antibiotics in such patients include so-called "triple therapy," utilizing streptomycin, 1 gram per 24 hours; ethambutol, 15 mg. per kg. per 24 hours; and isoniazid (INH), 300 mg. per 24 hours. Para-aminosalicylic acid is no longer used because of adverse gastrointestinal effects and hypersensitivity reactions. To minimize the risk of polyneuritis from INH-induced pyridoxine deficiency, pyridoxine in doses of 15 to 50 mg. daily is advocated.

Fungal infections must be treated with special agents. Amphotericin B may be required. Consultation with an infectious disease specialist is advised in such patients.

Follow-up of patients with brain abscesses is crucial. This is especially true in those patients in whom the lesion is treated only by repeated aspiration and antibiotics. If the abscess capsule remains, the risk of recurrence is higher. Late recurrence many years after the original diagnosis and treatment has been witnessed.

Anticonvulsants should be administered permanently to all patients with supratentorial abscesses. Epilepsy occurs in approximately 50 per cent of such patients.

Hydrocephalus may be encountered in a minority of abscess patients. This must be treated appropriately. A CSF shunt cannot be used until CSF and abscess contents are consistently sterile. Occasionally hydrocephalus follows rupture of the abscess (either spontaneously or subsequent to aspiration attempts) into the ventricular system. If rupture occurs into the fourth ventricle, death usually follows; if into a lateral ventricle, according to recent data, no increase in mortality occurs.

INTRACEREBRAL HEMORRHAGE *

method of
JULIAN T. HOFF, M.D.
San Francisco, California

Causes of Hemorrhage

Trauma is the main cause of brain parenchymal hematomas. Post-traumatic clots characteristically are found in the temporal and frontal lobes. Spontaneous hemorrhage in patients with hypertension or cerebrovascular disease is the next most common cause. Hypertensive hemorrhage typically occurs in the basal ganglia, subcortical white matter, pons, or cerebellum; more than half of the cases appear in the basal ganglia; the remainder appear equally often in the other three areas of the brain. Extravasation into brain tissue from a ruptured congenital or mycotic aneurysm or from an arteriovenous malformation ranks third in frequency. These vascular lesions usually bleed into the frontal lobes, basal ganglia, ventricles, or subarachnoid spaces. Less common sources of intracerebral hemorrhage include hematologic diseases, such as leukemia and thrombocytopenia; vasculitides, such as polyarteritis and lupus; and neoplasms, such as metastatic tumors and gliomas.

Early Treatment

Early treatment focuses on the mass caused by the hemorrhage. Mass effect is best assessed clinically. Improvement of neurologic function (consciousness, motor power, speech, brainstem reflexes), which is established by repeated examinations after the ictus, implies a favorable outcome and usually obviates emergency operation to remove the mass. If the patient fails to improve after the initial ictus, then clot removal may help. When the patient continues to deteriorate after the initial hemorrhage, operation becomes an obvious alternative treatment, depending upon the site, size, and source of the clot.

When is operation indicated? The question can be answered easily in certain circumstances. A hematoma in a cerebellar hemisphere or placed superficially in a nondominant cerebral hemisphere, particularly in the frontal or temporal region, should be removed if the patient fails to improve and if the clot is of sufficient size to deform the surrounding brain. Recovery in these patients may range from complete restoration of neurologic functions to severe disability, but with speech preserved. In contrast, a hematoma that is located superficially in the dominant hemisphere can be expected to render the patient hemiplegic and aphasic unless the clot is remote from the speech and motor areas of the cortex. Deep clots, their position determined by CT scan and/or angiography, usually cause profound neurologic impairment from which functional recovery is unlikely, regardless of their site and regardless of therapy.

Whether or not operation is done for an intracranial hematoma, treatment should include the following measures:

A Good Airway. Adequate oxygenation (PaO_2>80) and CO_2 control ($PAco_2$ 30 to 40) are fundamental to management. Hypoxia adds insult to injury. Hypercarbia ($Paco_2$ > 40) causes brain swelling, which aggravates the mass effect caused by the clot.

Blood Pressure Control. Patients with an intracerebral hematoma often develop arterial hypertension acutely, without pre-existing hypertensive disease. The elevated blood pressure probably results from the Cushing reflex (↑BP, ↓P, caused by increased intracranial pressure), which is the body's attempt to maintain adequate cerebral arterial perfusion. Therefore reduction

*Supported by grants from the National Institutes of Health, NS11051 and GM18470.

of blood pressure by medication must be done cautiously—e.g., methyldopate hydrochloride (Aldomet), 250 to 500 mg. intravenously every 6 to 8 hours—in order not to jeopardize cerebral perfusion pressure. Arterial blood pressure should not fall below 80 to 90 mm. Hg (mean) in patients who were normotensive, or below 100 to 120 mm. Hg in patients who were hypertensive, before the hemorrhage.

Temperature Control. Hyperthermia causes the brain to swell. While hypothermia reduces brain bulk and lowers intracranial pressure it can produce other management problems, such as shivering or hypostatic pneumonia. Normothermia (36 to 38° C.) (97 to 99° F.) is a reasonable compromise.

Diuretics. These drugs reduce brain bulk by dehydrating normal cerebral tissue. Furosemide (Lasix), 20 to 40 mg. intravenously, or mannitol, 1.5 mg. per kg. per 24 hours, is preferred. Close observation of serum osmolarity is necessary when these potent drugs are being used to prevent complications of hyperosmolarity (>330 mOsm. per liter). Diuretics are most effective during the first few days after hemorrhage, when brain swelling is intense.

Steroids. There is no conclusive proof that these drugs (dexamethasone, 20 to 40 mg. per day in divided doses, or methylprednisolone, 250 to 500 mg. per day) are of benefit to patients with intracerebral hemorrhage; however, most physicians use them when confronted with a patient who is deteriorating from an intracerebral hematoma. The decision to use steroids or not to use them should be made soon after hemorrhage if any possible beneficial effect is to be achieved.

Anticonvulsants. Many patients with intracerebral hemorrhage have seizures. Phenytoin (Dilantin), 300 to 400 mg. per day, is good prophylactic therapy, and a loading dose of 1000 mg. intravenously, administered slowly over 1 hour, can be given safely. Occasionally, seizures are continuous during the early posthemorrhage period. Diazepam (Valium), 10 to 50 mg. intravenously given in divided doses of 5 to 10 mg. will terminate most episodes of status epilepticus.

Antibiotics. Most physicians agree that antibiotics should be used for documented infections. Prophylactic antibiotics are not indicated.

Anticoagulants. These drugs are contraindicated in patients with an intracranial hemorrhage.

Supportive Measures. The required procedures are not unique for patients with an intracranial hematoma. Maintenance of good pulmonary, cardiovascular, and renal function is essential. Acid-base balance requires close attention. Inappropriate antidiuretic hormone (ADH) secretion, diabetes insipidus, and hyperosmolar states may develop quickly or insidiously unless serum electrolytes, osmolarity, urea nitrogen, and creatinine are measured periodically. Patients who have an intracranial lesion and receive steroids, anticonvulsants, diuretics, and/or hyperosmolar feedings are particularly susceptible to acid-base and osmolar disturbances. Good nursing care is fundamental throughout the illness. Decubitus ulcers, pneumonia, urinary tract infections, fecal impaction, contractures, and other complications of prolonged immobilization can be prevented by vigorous nursing and early mobilization of the patient. Weight loss is a common hazard that can be minimized by feeding the patient, either by mouth or by nasogastric tube, soon and regularly after hemorrhage.

Treatment of the Cause of Hemorrhage

Since intracerebral hemorrhage is a secondary phenomenon stemming from an underlying primary disorder, therapy must be directed at both the problems—the mass and its cause—at the same time. Traumatic intracerebral hemorrhage is usually accompanied by diffuse brain injury in addition to the localized clot. Often the head injury is only one of several injuries requiring intensive care. Patients with hypertensive hemorrhage must have their hematoma treated, and hypertension must be controlled promptly. Specific operative treatment of aneurysms and arteriovenous anomalies that are the source of hemorrhage usually is delayed until recovery from the hematoma appears likely. Excessive morbidity and mortality commonly accompany an emergency operation to remove a hematoma and obliterate the causative vascular malformation simultaneously. A mycotic aneurysm that bleeds into brain tissue must be treated immediately with antibiotics to control the infection that caused the aneurysm. Underlying systemic diseases, such as hematologic, vascular, or neoplastic disorders, that cause an intracerebral hemorrhage must be treated early in order to prevent additional hemorrhages.

Late Treatment

If the hematoma is favorably placed, and if early care has been optimal, then a combination of good nursing care, emotional support, physical therapy, occupational therapy, and speech therapy can restore a stroke patient to functional independence. Regardless of initial neurologic deficits, the patient's outcome cannot be predicted accurately until weeks, or even months, have passed. The potential for rehabilitation of patients who have intracerebral hemorrhages is influenced by their age and motivation for recovery, as well as by complicating illnesses, site of lesion, and adequacy of medical care. These patients may have good prospects for survival and functional recovery, provided that their posthemorrhage course is well directed.

ACUTE ISCHEMIC CEREBROVASCULAR DISEASE

method of
WILLIAM K. HASS, M.D.
New York, New York

The hallmark of acute ischemic cerebrovascular disease is the sudden onset of focal cerebral or brainstem dysfunction in a defined cerebrovascular territory usually reaching full development in minutes to hours. Computed tomographic brain scanning and/or cerebrospinal fluid examination performed acutely will assure the investigator that the problem is not a result of cerebral hemorrhage. In the elderly the incidence of ischemic events is 10 to 100 times greater than in patients under the age of 40. Further, in the elderly the range of diagnostic possibilities is more limited; most often ischemia is secondary to cholesterol, fibrinoplatelet, or mixed clot emboli arising from extracranial arteries, particularly from the origins of the carotid arteries in the neck.

The Transient Ischemic Attack

This most common form of acute ischemia may present as one or many transient episodes of dysfunction referable to the carotid or vertebrobasilar arterial territories, usually lasting several minutes or, rarely, several hours. These episodes are now called transient ischemic attacks (TIA's). TIA diagnosis is aided by the identification of an appropriate bruit in a carotid arterial territory in the neck, ophthalmoscopic evidence of cholesterol or fibrinoplatelet embolization, and lack of evidence of cardiac arrhythmia or valvular disease. *The basic aim of treatment in TIA patients is the prevention of a catastrophic stroke causing profound and persistent focal neurologic dysfunction.*

The usual therapeutic modalities employed have been anticoagulants, platelet inhibitory drugs, and carotid endarterectomy. None of these treatments as of this time has demonstrated a clear superiority in the prevention of stroke after TIA's; nevertheless, reasonable benefit-to-risk ratios can be achieved by the judicious application of one or more of these treatments in specific patient categories.

1. In the elderly patient with evidence of widespread arterial occlusive disease, a history of arteriosclerotic heart disease, and other risk factors, including diabetes and moderate hypertension, initial treatment with aspirin, 325 mg. four times daily, is preferred if TIA's are in the carotid arterial territory. If there is a history of peptic ulcer or aspirin intolerance, sulfinpyrazone, 200 mg. four times daily, is a suitable alternative. (This use of this agent is not listed in the manufacturer's official directive.)

2. When transient symptoms in the vertebrobasilar territory appear, most investigators favor immediate use of warfarin at dose levels sufficient to increase the prothrombin time to 1½ to 2½ times control prothrombin time for a period of at least 6 months if the patient is free of episodes. When anticoagulants are contraindicated, aspirin is a suggested alternative.

3. When transient ischemic attacks occur in patients in the age group of 45 to 65 who are otherwise healthy or who suffer from at most mild diabetes and/or systolic hypertension, primary treatment with aspirin is suggested, parallel with cerebral angiographic studies designed to demonstrate a surgically treatable arterial lesion if such is present. Stenosis of up to 99 per cent of the lumen of the carotid artery at its origin in the neck can now be successfully treated at recognized medical centers with a less than 3 per cent incidence of mortality and morbidity by the technique of thromboendarterectomy with or without vein patch. This procedure is suggested if an irregular or ulcerated arterial lesion is demonstrated in the *symptomatic vascular territory.* If no lesion is present in the symptomatic vascular territory, continuing therapy with aspirin only is indicated. If there is complete occlusion of the carotid artery in the symptomatic arterial territory and symptoms continue on platelet antiaggregant therapy, or if the occlusive disease is intracranial, consisting of either high grade stenosis or occlusion of the intracranial carotid or the primary stem of the middle cerebral artery, bypass microsurgery linking the superficial temporal artery to a branch of the middle cerebral artery can give excellent results with little risk. This procedure, however, is still considered innovative and should be performed only at major centers where appropriate microneurosurgical techniques are available.

4. In uncommon situations in patients in the age group of 50 to 70, TIA's may evolve into stepwise or progressive increases in focal deficit related to a specific vascular territory over a period of several days. When such an event occurs in the vertebrobasilar territory, the consensus is that an-

giography should *not* be performed and that therapy should be begun in a hospital with anticoagulants—e.g., intravenous heparin, 5000 units four times a day for several days, followed by oral warfarin at dose levels sufficient to increase the prothrombin time to twice the control value.

5. When a stepwise or progressive focal neurologic deficit appears in the carotid territory in younger patients who are considered to be good surgical risks, cerebral angiography is indicated. More often than not, high grade stenosis or frank occlusion of the appropriate carotid artery is disclosed. If progression has occurred during platelet inhibitory treatment with aspirin or sulfinpyrazone, treatment with intravenous heparin, 5000 units four times daily for a period of 2 weeks, is indicated, followed, if the patient has largely recovered, by an appropriate endarterectomy or bypass procedure.

6. As seizures are an extremely rare presenting symptom in this group of patients, it is usually necessary to employ only anticonvulsants, i.e., phenytoin, 100 mg. three or four times a day (sufficient to provide a phenytoin [Dilantin] blood level of 10 to 20 micrograms per ml.) for a period of at least 6 months after a superficial temporal artery–middle cerebral artery bypass procedure.

7. Concurrent hypertension should be initially treated with methyldopa (Aldomet), 250 mg. three times a day, and/or hydrochlorothiazide (HydroDiuril), 50 mg. daily.

8. TIA's are rare in patients who present with a cardiac arrhythmia. More commonly a cardiac arrhythmia is associated with episodes of global cerebral ischemia, characterized as Stokes-Adams attacks. Attention in these instances is most properly directed toward the treatment of the arrhythmia with appropriate drugs or with a pacemaker.

The Catastrophic Stroke

When a catastrophic stroke occurs with permanent and persistent deficit in the carotid–middle cerebral arterial territory in the absence of demonstrable cardiac disease, angiography and surgery are contraindicated in the acute period, especially if there is depression of the state of consciousness. Further, there is no compelling evidence that anticoagulant or platelet inhibitor therapy is of value in these patients. Some have suggested the use of corticosteroids in these patients, particularly when there is evidence of significant cytotoxic cerebral edema. The use of corticosteroids—e.g., methylprednisolone, 160 to 320 mg. intravenously daily for 10 days—has been suggested, but no clinical or experimental studies clearly support the use of steroids. The use of glycerol as a 10 per cent solution intravenously for this type of edema is currently under investigation.

During the period of acute catastrophic focal cerebral ischemia, feeding and administration of drugs by parenteral routes only is indicated. Frequent turning from side to side at 1 to 2 hour intervals and careful attention to skin care are mandatory. Tracheal suctioning with sterile tracheal tubes as necessary is indicated. Passive range of motion exercises of the paralyzed extremities should be begun as soon as possible. A sterile indwelling catheter connected to a sterile receptacle bag may be necessary for several days to weeks. Uncommonly after a period of several days unexpected significant recovery of function may appear. After 2 to 3 weeks in the hospital it may be determined that the patient is not able to care for himself and make his needs known adequately. At this time prevention of subsequent episodes should again be a major concern of the physician. Platelet antiaggregant therapy with aspirin should be begun, and cerebral angiography should be considered as described previously under item 5.

Cerebral Embolization from the Heart

Although TIA's often precede catastrophic strokes in patients with carotid or vertebrobasilar atherosclerotic disease, they are uncommon precursors of acute focal cerebral infarction secondary to embolism from the heart. When classic rheumatic heart disease with mitral stenosis and atrial fibrillation are present and acute massive cerebral hemispheric ischemia occurs, concern about recurrent embolization is matched by concern about the effect of breakup of a proximal large occluding embolus in the presence of anticoagulation within the first 48 hours, leading to lethal hemorrhagic changes in the established infarct. In these patients, therefore, initial attention should be restricted to parenteral feeding and appropriate antibiotic treatment if there is evidence of concurrent subacute bacterial endocarditis. Should significant recovery occur after the first 2 weeks, warfarin in doses sufficient to maintain the prothrombin time at twice the control value should be considered even if there is concurrent evidence of subacute bacterial endocarditis for which the patient is receiving antibiotic therapy. When there is evidence of only partial hemispheric involvement giving rise to a limited, noncatastrophic stroke and there is no evidence of endocarditis, warfarin therapy is indicated on the first day of hospitalization. In such a situation the therapeutic aim is prevention of further embolization.

Unlike persistent partial or severe focal ischemic episodes related to carotid arterial disease, those caused by emboli from the heart may evolve with apoplectic rapidity. There is often associated loss of consciousness. Not infrequently focal and/or generalized convulsive seizures occur. Seizures at onset require immediate treatment, because they further compromise brain tissue viability by increasing metabolic demand from a limited blood supply. Seizure treatment is always parenteral. If the seizures have persisted for 15 minutes or more at the time the patient is seen, phenobarbital, 200 mg., should be given intravenously, followed by the same dose at 20 minute intervals if seizures persist. When seizures cease, treatment may be maintained with phenobarbital, 45 mg. subcutaneously four times a day. When the patient is more alert, phenytoin may be added at a dose of 300 to 400 mg. a day by mouth to achieve a blood level of 10 to 20 micrograms per ml. Continuing lethargy may require the reduction of the phenobarbital dose or cessation of phenobarbital therapy when adequate phenytoin blood levels are established. Alternative initial treatment with intravenous phenytoin, 100 mg. per minute for 5 to 6 minutes, is of value.

When attacks of transient or persistent territorial ischemia are seen in patients with neoplasms, tumor embolus may be suspected. More commonly the cerebral embolus will consist of fibrinoplatelet material from cardiac valves demonstrating nonbacterial thrombotic endocarditis which often accompanies disseminated neoplastic disease. A concurrent chronic or acute disseminated intravascular coagulopathy may be present. It should be appropriately treated after a blood coagulation profile is obtained.

Perhaps the most common source for cerebral emboli from the heart now seen in large centers is the artificial prosthetic heart valve, particularly prosthetic mitral valves. Present evidence favors prophylactic therapy after surgical valve implantation, with warfarin, sufficient to maintain a prothrombin time at twice control values. There is evidence that addition of dipyridamole, 50 mg. four times daily, may provide an additional factor of safety. (This use of dipyridamole is not listed in the manufacturer's official directive.) When cerebral embolization occurs in patients with prosthetic heart valves, there is strong evidence that a bland infarction may quickly turn into a hemorrhagic infarction. If this occurs, anticoagulants should be stopped. If the area of hemorrhagic infarction is accessible, i.e., in the cerebellum, appropriate emergency neurosurgical decompression measures should be taken. Satisfactory recovery of a patient with either a bland or hemorrhagic infarction should raise the question of replacement of the artificial prosthetic heart valve with a glutaraldehyde-treated porcine heart valve. There is evidence that the incidence of cerebral embolization is reduced when these valves are used. Their limited supply prevents their universal employment as primary valve replacements. Up to one third of patients with emboli from artificial heart valves may exhibit a complicating endocarditis. As in the case of cerebral embolus in patients with subacute bacterial endocarditis with rheumatic heart disease and atrial fibrillation, there is still controversy about the concurrent administration of antibiotics and anticoagulants. At present, initial treatment with antibiotics only is suggested. After evidence of eradication of the infection in patients who show significant recovery, the physician should weigh a return to anticoagulant therapy against consideration of replacement of the artificial prosthetic valve with a porcine valve.

There is , in conclusion, little evidence to support the use of vasodilator drugs or carbon dioxide inhalation in the treatment of either transient ischemic attacks or completed strokes. In the rare patient in whom thrombocytosis is discovered alone or in association with polycythemia, the use of aspirin, 325 mg. four times daily, is recommended. Anemia when present should be treated but should not be considered causal in the vast majority of patients. When hypoglycemia is present at the onset of transient or persistent focal cerebral ischemia, it should be appropriately treated.

REHABILITATION OF THE PATIENT WITH HEMIPLEGIA

method of
ROBERT W. BRENNAN, M.D.
Hershey, Pennsylvania

Hemiparesis or hemiplegia is the most common neurologic disability seen in practice. With good medical care and intensive rehabilitation, all such patients can be helped to gain their full rehabilitation potential and many will regain a gratifying amount of self-sufficiency. Too often, feelings of helplessness or frustration dominate the attitudes of patients and their families, and occasionally those of physicians as well. What follows is a general plan for the care of the patient in both acute and chronic phases of hemiplegia, whether caused by ischemic vascular disease, trauma, or any other static brain injury. These guidelines focus on the supportive and rehabilitative aspects of total care for the patient with hemiparesis or hemiplegia. They presuppose an accurate diagnosis of cause and are complementary to any specific treatment measures that are appropriate.

Supportive Care

The goals of supportive care in patients with acute hemiparesis are (1) preserving life (although only a minority of patients with vascular hemiplegia will succumb as a direct consequence of it); (2) avoiding medical complications, particularly those that may extend or aggravate the original brain injury; and (3) recognizing and correcting secondary factors in the convalescent phase, which, if neglected, might limit the patient's ultimate rehabilitation potential. This last category of factors must be viewed as very broad, encompassing emotional, social, and economic issues as well as strictly medical ones.

Prevention of Life-Threatening Complications in the Acute Phase. Changes in respiratory rate or pattern are common in the acute phase, but airway obstruction is the particular danger, especially in patients with altered consciousness. Preventive measures include positioning on the unaffected side, insertion of an oral airway, and regular suctioning. Humidified oxygen may be delivered by a mask or nasal prongs if arterial hypoxia exists by clinical or laboratory evidence. A nasogastric tube may be useful to administer medication, but only clear liquids in small amounts should be permitted until the dangers of vomiting and aspiration are past. Intubation or tracheostomy should be reserved for that minority of patients with significant and persistent respiratory difficulties. When pulmonary infection or atelectasis is otherwise difficult to control, deep tracheal suctioning may be required regularly. The head should be turned from side to side to allow passage of a soft, sterile, fenestrated catheter into both mainstem bronchi. Cupping, turning into the semidecubitus position, and elevation of the hips will all contribute to pulmonary care in such patients.

Patients with acute vascular hemiplegia are frequently hypertensive, but rapid reduction of blood pressure is probably not required except in cerebral hemorrhage. In fact, it may be contraindicated, because a precipitous fall in blood pressure can increase cerebral ischemia in areas of low perfusion. This is a particular consideration if cerebral perfusion becomes abnormally pressure dependent, as it may in many forms of cerebral injury. Similarly, hypotension from any cause requires prompt evaluation. Treatment may require plasma volume expanders and pressor agents as well as management of impaired cardiac output from failure or arrhythmia. Because a few patients will develop symptoms of further ischemia when upright, strict bed rest in the supine position is the safest course.

Care of the Nonacute Patient. Bladder care must be instituted early, before the complications of retention, secondary bladder atony, and infection can begin. In males external drainage is preferable to chronic catheterization, but only if the postvoiding residual volume is not large. In many patients with acute hemiplegia, urinary retention is a self-limited problem and they can be tided over this period by serial sterile catheterization for decompression every 6 hours. Retention may respond to manual maneuvers, positioning, or the use of bethanechol chloride (Urecholine), 5 mg. subcutaneously. If an indwelling catheter is required for more than 4 days because of continuing incontinence, coverage with a bacteriostatic regimen such as methenamine mandelate (Mandelamine), 1 gram orally four times daily, ascorbic acid, 500 mg. twice daily, and adequate hydration become important. All such patients will manifest significant bacteriuria in time; the decision to treat with broad-spectrum parenteral antibiotics should be based on clinical criteria of infection.

Skin breakdown in an immobilized patient can best be avoided by regular repositioning, from side to side, and padding of protuberances, especially elbows, medial knees, malleoli, and heels. Frequent inspection for redness or abrasion is necessary. Use of a foam rubber pad or sheepskin will help control sacral skin breakdown. Dry, clean skin is less susceptible to pressure changes. Injections or intravenous catheters should not be applied on the plegic side. When an intravenous route is required, the risk of sepsis or local phlebitis can be minimized by changing the intravenous catheter every third day.

Bedbound patients with acute hemiplegia have a significant risk of systemic and pulmonary thromboemboli, This can be minimized by regular massage, exercising the extremities, and well-fitted elastic wraps or stockings to above the knee. Low dose heparin treatment on a regular basis can be administered through a well connected to a 20 gauge intravenous butterfly needle, or subcutaneously. Doses of 3000 units every 8 hours provide significant protection against the risk of thromboembolism, do not prolong bleeding times, and are usually well tolerated if no specific medical contraindication exists—e.g., active bleeding or a pre-existing coagulation disorder.

Constipation is common but temporary in hemiplegia; if regular bowel habits are not re-established by 5 to 7 days, an extenuating cause should be sought, e.g., ileus or fecal impaction. Persistent constipation will usually respond to increased hydration, increased roughage and fruit juice feeding, and the use of a stool softener such as dioctyl sodium sulfosuccinate (Colace). Increasing physical activity will often normalize bowel function. Milk of magnesia is useful also, but mineral oil should be avoided if there is any possibility of aspiration. If general nutrition and fluid intake by mouth are not adequate, they can be temporarily supplemented by regular small feedings introduced by nasogastric tube. In a few patients with severe and persistent dysphagia, a feeding pharyngostomy is a safe and effective way to maintain adequate intake with a low risk of aspiration.

Physical therapy can be instituted in this phase, with both passive and active range of motion of extremities, use of a padded bedboard to avoid plantar contracture, and padded splints to maintain a flaccid upper extremity in a physiologic position. The usual hospital program of progressive ambulation should be modified for the hemiplegic patient, to protect him from injury. Orthostatic hypotension and falling are common dangers in this setting; therefore close supervision is required.

Convalescent Care. The goal of care in this stage is to restore the patient to his previous life setting, with as much independence and self-sufficiency as possible given the kind and amount of his residual disability. Rehabilitation of the patient with hemiplegia is a continuous process, based on a structured plan of progressively increasing activity and self-reliance. To be most effective, the process must be instituted early in the patient's course. The understanding and assistance of the patient and his family are essential. Explain to all, in uncomplicated terms, the nature of the patient's disabilities, how these will affect ordinary activities, and what specific measures are planned to aid functional rehabilitation. The environment should be arranged to maximize the patient's ability and initiative to help himself in feeding, washing, and dressing. When in doubt about the patient's abilities to accomplish successive tasks, always give him a chance to try; even minor gains give patients the confidence and motivation they will need to achieve major ones. In a few hemiplegic patients, language disturbances or impairment of other higher integrative functions will limit the potential for rehabilitation. In others, the psychologic impact of a serious and disfiguring illness may provoke severe anxiety, depression, or agitation. Diazepam (Valium), in doses beginning at 5 mg. four times daily, is useful in anxious patients, but more seriously affected patients with agitation, delusional thinking, or self-injurious behavior will usually respond best to a phenothiazine agent. The apathy and depression of the patient with a cerebral lesion is most difficult to treat, but a few patients are improved by nonsedative antidepressive agents such as imipramine (Tofranil), 25 mg. three times daily or more as tolerated.

At this stage, all patients should be evaluated by a physiatrist or physical therapist, who will define a functional baseline in activities of daily living, assess the potential for benefit from physical therapy, and outline a treatment plan. Daily physiotherapy in an inpatient or outpatient facility will be required initially. In most instances of hemiplegia, leg function will be less impaired and will recover sooner than arm or face movement, permitting progressive weight bearing with assistance and increasing independence in transferring from bed to chair within a relatively short time. The appearance of spasticity in the lower extremity, which was previously flaccid, will often permit more secure standing and walking through an increase in reflex extensor tone. An ankle brace which provides dorsiflexion helps in avoiding toe scuffing or tripping. When patients can ambulate securely on parallel bars without assistance, training with a four-leg walker or tripod cane may be attempted. A sling should be used to support the arm until flexor tone returns. Grip strength and hand function may be improved by applying a splint to dorsiflex the wrist.

Common complications of spastic hemiplegia include spontaneous clonus of the extremities and muscle pain and spasm. Diazepam (Valium) is effective in suppressing such symptoms. Occasionally, patients may develop troublesome, spontaneous pain of central origin as a delayed complication of hemiplegia. A tricyclic antidepressant such as amitriptyline (Elavil), 25 mg. three or four times daily, can be of benefit in such patients.

Selected patients, typically those with significant residual disability but few underlying limitations to their rehabilitation potential, will benefit from prolonged intensive physiotherapy in a rehabilitation institution. When the patient with hemiplegia ultimately returns home, the services of a visiting nurse and the Vocational Rehabilitation Bureau in the community can be invaluable. Some modifications in the home environment may be necessary in the interest of the patient's safety and his physical independence. No list or formula of such aids would suffice, but simple and inexpensive devices such as handrails in bathrooms and along stairs, night lights, and specially designed eating utensils can do much to promote self-sufficiency.

EPILEPSY IN ADOLESCENTS AND ADULTS

method of
GAIL E. SOLOMON, M.D.
New York, New York

Epilepsy occurs in 1 to 2 per cent of the population. Ninety per cent of these patients with a convulsive disorder begin having seizures in childhood and adolescence. When the initial seizure is discovered, the physician must attempt to clarify the reason for the seizure.

Seizures may be the result of diverse causes, some of which are reversible without anticonvulsant therapy.

1. Metabolic imbalances secondary to hypoglycemia, hypocalcemia, hyponatremia, drug or alcohol withdrawal, or idiosyncratic reaction to medication are all reversible and do not require chronic anticonvulsant therapy.
2. Progressive structural lesions, such as brain tumor or abscess, which are often correctible by surgery may need anticonvulsant therapy at the onset and postsurgically.
3. Scars from brain lacerations, contusions, or subdural or epidural hematoma may lead to post-traumatic epilepsy.
4. Patients with infectious diseases, such as meningitis and encephalitis, can have seizures as a complication and need treatment for the acute manifestations and for the sequelae.
5. Occlusive vascular disease leading to stroke and vasculitis such as lupus erythematosus can produce seizures.
6. Genetic and idiopathic epilepsy require continued anticonvulsant therapy.

Each patient with epilepsy needs treatment, but by careful evaluation and neurologic follow-up with physical examinations and serial electroencephalograms, a structural lesion or a neurodegenerative disease may be revealed which was not apparent on initial evaluation.

Classification

The classification of epilepsy is central in the choice of therapy, because different medications are rather specific for certain types of seizures. There are many different classifications. The International Classification of Epileptic Seizures (Table 1) uses clinical and electroencephalographic (EEG) criteria to enable careful description of seizures, and to encourage the physician to use consistent terminology. Once the seizure is classified, appropriate therapy can be chosen.

For grand mal and partial cerebral seizures (focal, motor, sensory, and psychomotor), the general group of medications are the hydantoins (phenytoin, mephenytoin), barbiturates, and carbamazepine. For absences (petit mal), the drug of choice is ethosuximide (Zarontin). Second choice for absences (petit mal) would be trimethadione (Tridione). For bilateral massive epileptic myoclonus, atonic seizures, and akinetic seizures, the benzodiazepines, diazepam (Valium) and clonazepam (Clonopin), are useful. In some patients with such seizures, grand mal and petit mal drugs have limited usefulness.

TABLE 1. **International Classification of Epileptic Seizures***

I. Partial seizures (seizures beginning locally)
  A. Partial seizures with elementary symptomatology (generally without impairment of consciousness)
    1. With motor symptoms (includes jacksonian seizures)
    2. With special sensory or somatosensory symptoms
    3. With autonomic symptoms
    4. Compound forms
  B. Partial seizures with complex symptomatology (temporal lobe or psychomotor seizures) (generally with impairment of consciousness)
    1. With impairment of consciousness only
    2. With cognitive symptomatology
    3. With affective symptomatology
    4. With "psychosensory" symptomatology
    5. With "psychomotor" symptomatology (automatisms)
    6. Compound forms
  C. Partial seizures secondarily generalized
II. Generalized seizures (bilaterally symmetrical and without local onset)
    1. Absences (petit mal)
    2. Bilateral massive epileptic myoclonus
    3. Infantile spasms
    4. Clonic seizures
    5. Tonic seizures
    6. Tonic-clonic seizures (grand mal)
    7. Atonic seizures
    8. Akinetic seizures
III. Unilateral seizures (or predominantly)
IV. Unclassified epileptic seizures (due to incomplete data)

*Abstracted from Gastaut (1970).

In the adult, one deals mainly with partial seizures or grand mal seizures as the major manifestations of epilepsy. Seizures consisting of brief impairment of consciousness only, beginning in adulthood, are not absences (petit mal), but rather partial seizures with complex symptomatology (psychomotor, temporal lobe) emanating from limbic or temporal lobe. Petit mal seizures begin in children between the ages of 4 and 12 and are genetically inherited as an autosomal dominant with incomplete penetrance. In most patients with petit mal seizures, the seizures stop late in adolescence. Half of these patients do develop grand mal as a complication. A small percentage of patients with absences (petit mal) epilepsy have seizures persisting into adulthood and even have episodes of petit mal status. Eliciting an accurate history, asking the patient to hyperventilate for 3 minutes, and the presence of the classic 3 cycle per second spike and wave in the electroencephalogram (EEG) determine the diagnosis.

Most patients with epilepsy, in fact more than 70 per cent, can be well controlled on anticonvulsants. A few patients have intractable seizures and may require the use of newer medications currently being developed. In selected patients with uncontrolled epilepsy, surgery can be used to control seizures. Careful monitoring of drug blood levels is essential in the overall management of the patient with epilepsy. Knowledge of such levels and careful questioning of the patient enable the physician to determine if the patient is taking his medication or if the medication is being absorbed or metabolized too rapidly.

General Therapeutic Principles

General principles of therapy include the following:

1. Selection of appropriate medication for seizure type.
2. Use of a primary drug in increasing dosage until therapeutic effect occurs or toxicity develops.
3. Monitoring the drug level to assure compliance and the drug's absorption.
4. If there is inadequate control with the first drug or if toxicity is reached, the first medication should be lowered to nontoxic levels and an additional drug should be added to therapeutic levels. After the two drugs are in the therapeutic range, one should consider tapering the first and possibly discontinuing it.
5. Anticonvulsants should never be discontinued abruptly in patients with grand mal epilepsy, as this may precipitate grand mal status epilepticus, leading to irreversible brain damage.

The physician should be familiar with a few anticonvulsant drugs and know them well with their side effects. He should utilize the laboratory for drug levels, especially in the case of phenytoin (diphenylhydantoin, Dilantin, DPH) and phenobarbital, as the levels correlate so well with the clinical effectiveness. Other medications that can be readily tested for by gas-liquid chromatography (GLC) screening include primidone (Mysoline), carbamazepine (Tegretol), and ethosuximide (Zarontin). Although mephenytoin (Mesantoin), mephobarbital (Mebaral), methosuximide (Celontin), phensuximide (Milontin), diazepam (Valium), clonazepam (Clonopin), and trimethadione (Tridione) can also be determined by GLC, information relating to the correlation between the clinical control and the anticonvulsant level is not yet well established. Table 2 lists optimal therapeutic blood levels of commonly used anticonvulsants.

Several of the anticonvulsants are metabolized into products which themselves have anticonvulsant action. It is important to realize that these products contribute to good therapeutic control and are probably more relevant than parent drug levels. Examples of such medications include primidone (Mysoline), trimethadione (Tridione), and mephobarbital (Mebaral).

There is wide variation in the accuracy of determining anticonvulsant levels. Fortunately, the Epilepsy Foundation of America is attempting to standardize this procedure and to correct the variations in individual laboratories by sending specific samples to a laboratory to maintain standards of accurate determinations.

One must remember that prescribing a dosage alone is not entirely reliable, as compliance, absorption, and rate of metabolism influence the drug level. Therefore obtaining an anticonvulsant blood level is vital, particularly in the case of adolescents who are prone to experimentation by stopping and starting medication. Drug levels provide a helpful guide to compliance, especially when there is breakthrough. One should also remember that certain medications interact with the anticonvulsants and cause an increase or decrease in levels. (This will be discussed presently.)

Specific Therapy in Grand Mal and Focal Cerebral Seizures

Phenytoin (Diphenylhydantoin, Dilantin, DPH). Phenytoin (Dilantin) is the drug of choice for grand mal epilepsy and partial seizures (focal). If the patient has a well documented single grand

TABLE 2. **Optimal Therapeutic Blood Levels of Commonly Used Anticonvulsants**

SEIZURE TYPE	ANTICONVULSANT	USUAL DOSE RANGE	LEVEL (MICROGRAMS/ML.)	
Grand mal and partial (focal, psychomotor)	Phenytoin (Dilantin)	300–400 mg.		10–20
	Phenobarbital	100–150 mg.		20–40
	Primidone (Mysoline)	750 mg.–2 grams	Primidone	5–15
			Phenobarbital (derived from primidone)	15–40
	Carbamazepine (Tegretol)	1–1.2 grams		4–10
Absences (petit mal)	Ethosuximide (Zarontin)	750 mg.–2 grams		40–100

mal seizure, in general he is placed on phenytoin for 1 to 2 years in therapeutic dosage. With patients who have had repetitive convulsions, more prolonged anticonvulsant therapy is indicated, even when attacks are completely controlled by medication.

The usual adult dose of phenytoin is 300 mg. a day and can be given in a single dose or in divided doses. A therapeutic dose does not produce sedation and gives blood levels between 10 and 20 micrograms per ml. Phenytoin takes 7 to 10 days to reach therapeutic levels when given in standard daily dosage. If the daily maintenance dose is given three times (once every 8 hours) over the first 24 hour period and then followed by the first maintenance dose, therapeutic levels can be achieved within 1 day. This "Dilantinization" can also be achieved more rapidly, in fact, within 1 hour by the intravenous administration of phenytoin. It can be infused intravenously at a rate not exceeding 50 mg. per minute to a total dose in the adult of 1 gram. Severe cardiotoxic reactions from too rapid administration have been documented in elderly patients or in those with underlying cardiac disease. Intramuscular administration of phenytoin should be avoided, because the absorption is unpredictable and muscle necrosis can be caused by the injection.

Phenytoin is available in 100 mg. capsules, 50 mg. tablets, and the suspension containing 25 mg. per ml. of the active ingredient. The suspension is not recommended, because it is difficult to mix well and to avoid underdosing when medication is used from the top of the bottle and toxicity when used from the bottom of the bottle. Adult dosage can usually be achieved by giving the capsule. Excellent correlation between blood level and therapeutic response exists for phenytoin (effective when the blood value is more than 10 micrograms per ml., possibly toxic when it is more than 30 micrograms per ml.). The blood level should be obtained 2 weeks after starting the medication to make sure that the phenytoin level is within the therapeutic range. If the level is low and if there is definite evidence of good compliance, the dosage should be raised to therapeutic levels.

Adverse effects of phenytoin can be divided into three groups: (1) acute or chronic intoxication, (2) "allergic hypersensitivity reactions," and (3) rare metabolic side effects.

Intoxication with phenytoin closely correlates with elevated blood levels of the anticonvulsants. Most adults will show nystagmus at 20 micrograms per ml., ataxia at 30 micrograms per ml., and coordination difficulties and sedation from 40 micrograms per ml. Chronic phenytoin intoxication can be confused with dementia; choreoathetosis and tonic seizures have been reported in patients with toxic levels. A mild peripheral neuropathy which is usually clinically insignificant has also been reported in patients who have been on phenytoin for more than 10 to 15 years.

Allergic manifestations that are not correlated with dosage occur in 5 per cent of patients. A morbilliform rash may be seen between the tenth and fourteenth day. Stevens-Johnson exfoliative dermatitis is a rare side effect. If a rash is caused by phenytoin, the medication should be discontinued to avoid progression to exfoliative dermatitis.

Lymphadenopathy occurs in 2 to 5 per cent of patients, and a full-blown serum sickness picture has been reported. The lupus erythematosus syndrome may rarely occur; it is usually reversible when the phenytoin is discontinued.

Other side effects include a megaloblastic anemia related to folic acid deficiency which responds to folic acid.

Gingival hyperplasia occurs more often in children than in adults and in up to 40 per cent of patients who receive phenytoin. Good dental hygiene helps alleviate this problem. It is usually first seen within 2 to 3 months after starting the drug. It is exaggerated by orthodontic apparatus but is not seen in patients with dentures. Five per cent of patients have an increase in body hair (hypertrichosis), which is particularly unpleasant in adolescent girls and young women. Facial hair can also be seen as part of this side effect.

Hypocalcemia and osteomalacia have been occasionally reported in patients on multiple anticonvulsants, including phenytoin. These mainly occur in people with poor diets and who are not exposed to adequate sunlight.

Evidence suggests that phenytoin may have a teratogenic effect in that 2 to 3 times the incidence of congenital malformations is observed in infants born to mothers on phenytoin. The defects particularly noted are cleft palate, cleft lip, hypoplastic nails and digits, ptosis, coarse hair, hypertelorism, failure to thrive, psychomotor retardation, and congenital heart defects.

Clotting defects and clinical bleeding within the first few days of life have also been reported in infants born to mothers on anticonvulsants.

Rarely hyperglycemia has been seen in patients receiving phenytoin in large doses.

Interference with Metabolism of Phenytoin (Dilantin). Inherited and acquired disorders may impair tolerance to phenytoin. A genetic defect in parahydroxylation causes reduced phenytoin tolerance by reducing the patient's ability to metabolize it. Liver disease can also decrease the metabolism of phenytoin, leading to toxicity with the usual dosages. In about 10 per cent of patients who receive isoniazid (INH) and who are slow INH deactivators, phenytoin levels will rise to toxic levels despite normal dosage. Medications that have been rarely reported to interact and elevate phenytoin levels in patients receiving the anticonvulsant include coumadin, chloramphenicol, phenylbutazone, phenothiazines, propoxyphene hydrochloride, methylphenidate, and chlordiazepoxide.

Other Hydantoins. Another drug in the hydantoin group, mephenytoin (Mesantoin), is related to phenytoin chemically and is more toxic, particularly to the bone marrow. Aplastic anemia, pancytopenia, and leukopenia have been reported in as many as 5 per cent of patients receiving mephenytoin. Although the hematologic abnormalities are usually reversible, these can be fatal. Fever, rash, and lymphadenopathy can also occur. Monthly blood counts are desirable within the first 6 months and every 2 to 3 months thereafter in patients receiving this potentially toxic drug. Mephenytoin would be a drug to consider after phenytoin, phenobarbital, primidone, carbamazepine, and perhaps methsuximide have failed.

Phenobarbital. Phenobarbital is an excellent anticonvulsant for grand mal and partial seizures. However, the side effects of sedation often make it difficult to tolerate. It is readily administered by mouth, intramuscularly, or intravenously. In adolescents and adults, it can be administered as one dose daily at bedtime.

In adolescents who have absence (petit mal) seizures, even without clinical grand mal, phenobarbital should be started as the primary drug in therapeutic dosage and then ethosuximide (Zarontin) added. About half the patients with absence (petit mal) seizures develop grand mal epilepsy. The older the age of onset of petit mal, the more likely the patient is to have grand mal. Therefore all these patients should be initially started on phenobarbital before the petit mal drug is instituted to protect against grand mal. The phenobarbital therapeutic range is between 20 and 40 micrograms per ml. Clinical control correlates well with therapeutic blood level. Dose-related toxicity includes sedation, nystagmus, ataxia, and learning difficulties. A paradoxical reaction seen in some children and in brain-damaged persons is hyperkinesis. Allergic reactions, as with other medications, include drug rashes. Rarely folic acid–responsive megaloblastic anemia similar to that seen with phenytoin occurs with phenobarbital. Orally, phenobarbital takes 16 to 18 hours to reach peak concentration. Intravenously, brain peak concentration is achieved in 15 minutes. Intramuscular absorption is good, with an intermediate absorption time between that of the oral and intravenous times.

Within the barbiturate anticonvulsant group, mephobarbital (Mebaral) is similar to phenobarbital. The daily dose is about twice as much as that of phenobarbital to achieve therapeutic blood levels. The major active component in mephobarbital is the phenobarbital to which it is metabolized. Some physicians believe that mephobarbital has a less sedative action and causes less hyperkinesis, but there does not seem to be an important clinical difference. Since mephobarbital is metabolized in the liver to phenobarbital, it is the phenobarbital that acts as the major anticonvulsant.

Primidone (Mysoline). Primidone (Mysoline) is effective for treating grand mal and focal cerebral seizures, especially partial seizures with complex symptomatology (psychomotor seizures). Its major side effect is drowsiness. If one starts with small doses and builds up to therapeutic levels, often the drowsiness is averted and is easily overcome. An adult dose of 0.75 to 1.5 grams is given daily, with a maximum dose of about 2 grams. We start with the 250 mg. tablet given as a half or whole tablet a day, advancing every 4 days as tolerated to therapeutic levels. When one measures the blood level after 2 weeks, one should evaluate not only the primidone level but also the phenobarbital level. The primidone level (usually 5 to 15 micrograms per ml. in therapeutic doses) is related to when the medication was last taken, since it reaches a blood peak level in 3 hours and has a short half-life (6 to 9 hours). Although primidone itself probably has some direct anticonvulsant action, its major metabolites—phenylethylmalonic acid (PEMA) and especially phenobarbital—are the main anticonvulsants. The phenobarbital level is usually two to four times that of the parent drug and reflects the more constant level of the drug in the blood. About 20 per cent of primidone is metabolized to phenobarbital. With patients on both phenytoin and primidone, often more of primidone is converted to phenobarbital because of induction of enzymes.

Primidone can cause sedation, nystagmus, ataxia, and personality changes. Less often megaloblastic anemia, responsive to folic acid, or an allergic maculopapular rash or lupus erythematosus syndrome can occur.

Since primidone is available only as an oral preparation, if there is intercurrent illness or surgery which prevents the oral administration of the medication, parenteral phenobarbital should be substituted temporarily in therapeutic dosage to avoid withdrawal reactions and for anticonvulsant action.

Partial Seizures with Complex Symptomatology (Psychomotor Epilepsy)

Carbamazepine (Tegretol) is the drug of choice for psychomotor epilepsy in Europe, including England, France, Scandinavia, and Germany. Within the last 5 years, carbamazepine has been approved by the Food and Drug Administration in the United States of America for use as an anticonvulsant. It was used in the United States before that time for treatment of trigeminal neuralgia (tic doloureux). The recommended dose for seizures is to begin at 200 mg. a day, with usual therapeutic levels being achieved at 400 mg. three times daily. More than 1200 mg. a day generally does not provide any more effectiveness. Drug levels do correlate with clinical control, with therapeutic ranges from 4 to 10 micrograms per ml. The toxicity includes fatigue, nystagmus, dizziness, and slurred speech. The effects are additive with those of primidone, phenytoin, and phenobarbital. Agranulocytosis, depression of platelets and leukopenia, hepatic dysfunction, and allergic rashes have been reported in patients receiving this drug. Repeated blood tests and liver function tests are recommended every 3 months in the initial use of the drug.

At the clinic in The New York Hospital, phenytoin is the drug of choice for grand mal epilepsy. If this is unsuccessful, phenobarbital is added as a therapeutic combination. If the two are not effective, primidone is added to replace the phenobarbital, and phenytoin and primidone are continued. If there is still inadequate control, carbamazepine is introduced. If the patient does well on all three, occasionally the primidone will be slowly discontinued to allow the patient to remain on phenytoin and carbamazepine.

In the case of partial seizures with complex symptomatology (psychomotor epilepsy), at the current time either phenytoin or primidone is still used as the drug of choice in our clinic, and the same procedure holds as with grand mal. In a young woman or adolescent girl because of hirsutism and the potential teratogenicity of phenytoin, we use primidone as the initial drug of choice. Studies show marked success in reports from Europe with the use of carbamazepine as the drug of choice in partial seizures with complex symptomatology (psychomotor epilepsy). With more extensive use of this agent in the United States, it probably will become our drug of choice for partial seizures with complex symptomatology (psychomotor seizures), but at present it is not the first one used in our clinic because of the potential liver and bone marrow toxicity.

Drugs that are not first line but are used to help difficult patients include methsuximide (Celontin), an analogue of ethosuximide (Zarontin) which has a spectrum that includes partial seizures with complex symptomatology (psychomotor seizures). Adjunctive drugs, which are not in the primary armamentarium of therapy for grand mal and partial seizures, include the benzodiazepines, such as diazepam (Valium) and chlordiazepoxide (Librium), particularly in patients whose seizures are triggered by emotional disorders or patients with partial seizures with complex symptomatology.

Acetazolamide (Diamox) is occasionally used as an adjunct of therapy when there appears to be increased seizure activity during menses or in intractable absence seizures. When it is used around the time of the menses, it is usually used as a diuretic rather than a direct anticonvulsant.

Absences (Petit Mal Seizures)

Petit mal epilepsy begins in children between the ages of 4 and 12. If petit mal begins around the age of 12, then phenobarbital would be the first drug to administer and then ethosuximide (Zarontin) would be added.

The drug of choice in absence seizures (petit mal epilepsy) is ethosuximide, which is given orally in a dose of 250 mg. (capsules), starting with 3 capsules a day in the adolescent and advancing to as much as 2 grams if needed. Blood levels of ethosuximide over 40 micrograms per ml. are usually effective; those over 150 micrograms per ml. may be toxic. The drug is available in 250 mg. oil-filled capsule or syrup containing 50 mg. per ml. The dose-related toxicity includes nausea, vomiting, anorexia, and, less often, fatigue and headache. Skin rashes, leukopenia, and even aplastic anemia have rarely been reported, and blood counts should be monitored monthly for the first year and every 3 months thereafter. Rarely systemic lupus erythematosus and adverse behavior reactions have been reported.

If ethosuximide is unsuccessful in controlling the absence seizures, trimethadione (Tridione) is used. It was the first anticonvulsant used specifically for absences (petit mal epilepsy). However, its toxicity appears to be greater than that of ethosuximide. Trimethadione may affect the bone marrow or produce lupus erythematosus, and has also been reported to cause nephrosis. Precautious monitoring of blood and urine is necessary if this drug is taken. In some patients, trimethadione can activate grand mal seizures in a patient having both grand mal and absence (petit mal seizures).

Clonazepam (Clonopin), an analogue of diazepam (Valium), has been introduced as an anticonvulsant for absence (petit mal seizures) and minor motor seizures, including massive myoclonic epileptic discharges and akinetic and atonic seizures. Given orally, clonazepam should be started in very small doses because of the drowsiness it causes. Adults usually begin with 1.5 mg. per day, administered in three divided doses, with a 0.5 to 1 mg. per day increase every 3 days until therapeutic effect or toxicity is reached. Clonazepam is available in 0.5 and 1 mg. tablets. Drowsiness and ataxia can occur. Clonazepam can potentiate the drowsiness from barbiturates, so this should be taken into consideration when prescribing. Skin rashes are rare. No serious hematopoietic, hepatic, or renal toxicity has been noted. Tolerance to the drug has developed. As with diazepam, breakthrough may occur, with seizures occurring after several months in as many as one-third of the patients.

A new anticonvulsant recently being tested in our clinic and laboratory is called Depakene (dipropyl acetate, valproic acid), which has an excellent spectrum for absence (petit mal seizures). It also may be helpful in grand mal seizures. Its proposed mechanism of action is to decrease the breakdown of gamma-aminobutyric acid (GABA), a metabolite in the brain which helps raise the seizure threshold.

Minor Motor Seizures–Massive Myoclonic, Akinetic, and Atonic

Control of minor motor seizures or myoclonic jerks of the extremities caused by degenerative diseases, metabolic disorders, or anoxia is difficult. Most of these seizures do not respond to the conventional grand mal and petit mal drugs. Clonazepam has been helpful in this group, but, as mentioned before, there may be breakthrough in control.

Status Epilepticus

Repetitive seizures with incomplete recovery of the patient's baseline neurologic function between seizures is defined as status epilepticus. Generalized or partial (focal or ictal confusional states) status can occur. The point is that there is no let-up, placing the patient and his brain at potential risk for irreversible brain damage, especially in the case of grand mal status epilepticus in which anoxia may ensue. Cardiovascular arrhythmias and systemic acidosis in addition to the generalized brain anoxia can be fatal in uncontrolled grand mal status epilepticus. The most common precipitating cause of status epilepticus in an epileptic is abrupt withdrawal of anticonvulsant drugs in grand mal seizures. Meningitis, encephalitis, brain abscess, electrolyte disturbances, uremia, hypertensive encephalopathy, toxins, extremely high doses of penicillin in patients with renal failure, and head trauma have been among the causes.

The most important step in initiating treatment for grand mal status epilepticus is the establishment of an adequate airway and oxygenation. Placement of an oral airway, followed by insertion of an endotracheal tube, is needed if the subject is unconscious. Avoid aspiration. Use emergency anticonvulsant therapy to stop the seizures. Intravenous therapy is the method of choice. If there is a metabolic cause for the seizure, appropriate therapy should be instituted. With an unknown patient who presents with status epilepticus, blood should be drawn for metabolic toxic studies, an intravenous infusion started immediately, and 50 per cent glucose infused to make sure the patient is not hypoglycemic. If no response is achieved, give intravenous diazepam. Usually 10 mg. is needed in the adult to stop the seizure and is the treatment of choice. When one is treating status epilepticus, one must be ready to resuscitate for cardiac and respiratory arrest. Parenteral diazepam should not be diluted in large volumes of water or saline, because it will precipitate. One can administer the diazepam two or three times with 20 minute intervals between. Its action is short lived, and it cannot be used for maintenance therapy. Once the seizures have stopped, intravenous phenytoin can be given as a maintenance treatment. "Dilantinizing" the patient acutely, using intravenous phenytoin, can achieve therapeutic blood levels within 1 hour, as described for phenytoin.

An alternative mode of therapy for grand mal status epilepticus is to use intravenous phenobarbital administered slowly. Sometimes as much as 400 mg. intravenously may be required to control the seizures. The phenobarbital given as the drug to stop status epilepticus can also be continued as the maintenance drug. It is dangerous to use phenobarbital and diazepam together intravenously because they are synergistic and depress respiration.

If the grand mal status epilepticus is secondary to barbiturate withdrawal, barbiturates should be used to control the seizure, and then withdrawn gradually and stepwise over a 2 week period if abstinence is needed.

If the measures described to stop status epilepticus do not stop the convulsions, a short-acting barbiturate can be given intravenously, such as amobarbital sodium (Amytal), 500 mg. slowly intravenously. The short-acting barbiturate intravenously should be given without hesitation if needed, as sustained generalized status epilepticus carries a high risk of producing brain damage.

Absence (petit mal) status or "spike wave stupor" generally is self-limited, but is best arrested by giving diazepam intravenously. Maintenance therapy is then started as for absence seizures (petit mal epilepsy). It is important to make sure that the patient is supervised and will not sustain any accidental injuries from the confusional state. Petit mal status tends to stop spontaneously within a maximum period of 1 to 3 days.

Surgical Therapy

If the patient has intractable seizures, surgery is considered. This has been particularly important in patients with intractable partial seizures with complex symptomatology (psychomotor temporal lobe epilepsy) when the seizure can be localized to one specific area, and, in indicated cases, implanted electrodes (corticography) can determine whether this is the active focus. The patient should have already received an adequate trial of nontoxic medical therapy to guarantee that the seizures are really intractable and are functionally and seriously limiting or disabling the patient. Seizures should be present for at least 6 to 12 or more months before considering surgery. Surgery is performed to remove the anterior part of the medial temporal horn in these patients, and results are excellent in selected patients.

In some patients with intractable seizures associated with behavioral disorders and hemiplegia of childhood, removal of the damaged cerebral hemisphere (hemispherectomy) has been found to control intractable seizures and improve the behavior disorder without causing additional neurologic deficit. Unfortunately, in some of the patients, scarring, hydrocephalus, and hemosiderosis of the nervous system have occurred as late complications.

Other surgical procedures to relieve epilepsy have been attempted, including callosal commissurotomy, stereotactic ablation of selected diencephalic areas, and stimulation of the cerebellum. All these methods are in an experimental stage and require further study before their efficacy can be established.

Special Management of Pregnant Women

In a young woman with epilepsy who is contemplating pregnancy, the question of choice of anticonvulsants or change of therapy should be raised. Congenital malformations have been reported two to three times more often in infants born to mothers on phenytoin. Many of the patients, however, were on multiple medications. The question of change of anticonvulsants to phenobarbital should be contemplated in these patients. If the patient can be well controlled on phenobarbital without sedative effect, then this would be a reasonable drug of choice.

Trimethadione has also been reported to cause malformations, including congenital heart disease. It is important that the patient be removed from any anticonvulsants that are not necessary. In the case of trimethadione, usually petit mal seizures have ceased by late adolescence and early adulthood, so that very few patients would require this medication.

During pregnancy the patient should receive vitamins with supplementary folic acid. Some of the phenytoin-related malformations suggest a relationship to anti–folic acid medication, such as cleft palate, which can also be produced in animals on anti–folic acid drugs. However, in patients who are on phenytoin and who have delivered babies with malformations, folic acid levels have usually been normal. There may be some problem with folic acid metabolism, but the actual levels are not the answer. In any case an adequate folic acid level should be maintained in a pregnant woman.

If a woman is already on phenytoin for a seizure disorder, is well controlled, and discovers she is pregnant, we continue her on the phenytoin through the pregnancy. Switching drugs risks seizures during pregnancy and the possibility of anoxia to the fetus.

One study revealed that 50 per cent of women with idiopathic epilepsy have no change in the number of seizures during pregnancy; 45.2 per cent have an increase in frequency, and 4.8 per cent have fewer seizures. Hypotheses of hormonal changes, fluid retention, effects of folate supplementation or reduced effect of previously adequate anticonvulsant drug levels, or increased metabolism by the liver during pregnancy or by fetal tissues have been put forth. In a small study of pregnant women on phenytoin and/or phenobarbital or its congeners, one group found that anticonvulsant levels dropped during the latter part of pregnancy. The plasma protein binding of phenytoin does not alter significantly during pregnancy. The exact reason for the decrease in level in these patients is not known. The requirement in this small group fell during the puerperium. Levels should be monitored carefully to avoid increased seizures during the latter part of pregnancy and toxicity to the mother in the puerperium.

Infants born to mothers on anticonvulsants, especially phenytoin or combinations of anticonvulsants, can have bleeding in the neonatal period related to a decrease in vitamin K dependent clotting factors. The anticonvulsant-related complication occurs earlier than the usual hemorrhagic disease of the newborn, potentially even during the birth process. All pregnant women on anticonvulsants in our clinic are placed on a water-soluble vitamin K tablet, 5 mg. by mouth once a week for the final 4 weeks of pregnancy, and the baby is given vitamin K, 1 mg. at birth.

After delivery the question of breast feeding arises. The fraction of the anticonvulsant blood level that is not bound to albumin is excreted in the breast milk: 10 per cent of the blood level of phenytoin and 60 per cent of the blood level of phenobarbital. For example, if the blood level is 10 micrograms per ml. of phenytoin in the mother, concentration in breast milk would be 1 microgram per ml. The baby would be getting a total of less than 1 mg. of phenytoin in his total daily milk consumption. The amounts are very small and would not cause any problem in this dosage in the neonate if the mother's levels are in the accepted therapeutic range.

If the mother has one infant affected with a "phenytoin syndrome" of cleft palate, hypoplastic distal digits and nails, hypertelorism, coarse hair, cardiac anomaly, failure to thrive, and psychomotor retardation, there may be a higher incidence of its happening again in her future children as compared to a mother with epilepsy who has had normal babies while on phenytoin. Genetic studies are underway to evaluate this anecdotal observation.

Uremia

Phenytoin levels are unreliable in patients with uremia who have high blood urea nitrogen (BUN) and creatinine. The blood phenytoin levels are often low despite adequate clinical control. This observation may represent the fact that these patients are hypoproteinemic and have a relatively higher than normal unbound drug concentration. The unbound phenytoin is the fraction that protects against seizures.

Recent studies in children who have had renal transplants raise the possibility that those children on phenobarbital or phenytoin or combinations may have a greater tendency to reject the transplanted kidneys, possibly related to increased steroid metabolism or other factors. More information is needed, but if the medication is not essential and the seizures occurred only as a metabolic phenomenon in adults or children, chronic anticonvulsant therapy should be discontinued. If anticonvulsants are needed, the possibility of bromides as an anticonvulsant is raised. Bromides do not induce enzymes to increase steroid metabolism and do not have any specific effect on connective tissues.

Other Anticonvulsants

An additional and less often used anticonvulsant is acetazolamide (Diamox), which may be effective for only short periods of time. It has a limited effect in patients with petit mal epilepsy. As an adjunct to treatment with grand mal and partial seizures with complex symptomatology (psychomotor seizures), it can be used in women who have an increase in seizures before or during menses. Giving acetazolamide 1 week before and during the first few days of the menstrual period as an adjunct to the usual anticonvulsant regimen is helpful in some patients.

Bromide, the first anticonvulsant ever used, can be still helpful in patients allergic to other medications or in whom the other medications have been ineffective. Side effects are unpleasant and include acneiform rash, drowsiness, and mental blunting.

Paraldehyde as an adjunct to treatment of grand mal status epilepticus by direct intravenous injection can be hazardous. A safer means of administering it is as a 4 per cent intravenous drip, but the use of diazepam has supplanted paraldehyde in most institutions.

When to Stop Anticonvulsants

No one wants to take medication on a permanent basis. This is particularly true of adolescents who often rebel and stop the medications and do not comply. Even with good control, withdrawal of anticonvulsants in a fully controlled epileptic should be done with great caution, if at all, in some patients. Sudden withdrawal of anticonvulsant medication is the most common cause of status epilepticus. Another important observation, clinically, is that if seizures recur when anticonvulsants have been stopped, it often becomes more difficult to stop the recurrence with the same dose of anticonvulsants that was effective previously. Studies show that adults have poorer tolerance to withdrawal of anticonvulsants than children. The recurrence rate in adults in general is quoted as 80 per cent even if the remission has lasted for 2 years. We generally continue anticonvulsants indefinitely in most patients whose seizures began after the age of 9 and in whom clinical seizures were difficult to control for 1 to 2 years, or in whom there were focal components or multiple seizure types (excluding petit mal). Anticonvulsants are continued indefinitely if a structural lesion is demonstrated and also in those with partial seizures with complex symptomatology (psychomotor), beginning in adulthood in most cases. In patients with genetic grand mal and petit mal epilepsy starting in childhood, the recurrence rate is lowest, with 8 per cent in grand mal and 12 per cent in uncomplicated petit mal upon withdrawal after being seizure free for 4 years.

If the patient has been seizure free for 4 years and the EEG is normal or mildly abnormal, the question of tapering drugs can be discussed and, under supervision, can be attempted over a 3 month period.

After head injuries, the most common time for the occurrence of epilepsy is within the first 2 years after the head injury. If the patient has been seizure free for 2 years and the EEG is not epileptiform, tapering the medication over 3 months should be considered.

If the decision is made to withdraw anticonvulsants, it is advisable to obtain an anticonvulsant blood level to see if the patient has already started to withdraw himself from medication and has levels below the therapeutic range. If this is the case, then further withdrawal may not present a major problem.

Many patients in adolescence and adulthood want to drive cars, and this should be strongly considered. If the patient has a seizure, his license is revoked. The states vary in their laws, but in most states at least 1 seizure-free year is necessary before a license can again be obtained. The social implications of a seizure at a job may be too great to take the risk of stopping the anticonvulsants. These problems must be thoroughly discussed with the patient.

In the case of a single seizure and no recurrence for 2 years, the question of discontinuing the medication is raised, and this can be done under similar supervision over a 3 month period.

Social aspects and compliance, job restriction, and educational opportunities should be considered in the overall therapy of epilepsy.

The major reasons for failure of anticonvulsant therapy include the following:

1. Inadequate dosage of the anticonvulsant without monitoring blood levels.

2. Selecting the wrong drug for the particular seizure pattern—i.e., thinking partial seizures with complex symptomatology (psychomotor seizures) are absences (petit mal) and using ethosuximide (Zarontin) rather than phenytoin (Dilantin), primidone (Mysoline), or carbamazepine (Tegretol).

3. An overly complex regimen in which the patient has to take the medication multiple times during the day, leading to noncompliance.

4. Failure to consider the social problems and psychologic impact of the disease on the patient and his family, particularly in the case of adolescents.

EPILEPSY IN CHILDREN

method of
HENRY G. DUNN, M.B., F.R.C.P.
Vancouver, British Columbia, Canada

Epilepsy is not a specific disease but a term for conditions characterized by recurrent seizures. The present article is concerned chiefly with seizures caused by a primary abnormality in the structure or metabolism of the brain itself, with consequent paroxysmal electrical discharges. It is true that seizures may also occur symptomatically in metabolic disturbances originating outside the nervous system (e.g., uremia, tetany, overhydration, phenylketonuria), but the detailed management of such disturbances is beyond the scope of this article. Febrile convulsions will be considered, because they frequently result from a particular and often hereditary tendency of the brain to form discharges in the presence of fever, whatever its primary cause. With regard to secondary (or symptomatic) seizures it is not proposed to discuss the management of the underlying organic conditions such as brain tumors or meningoencephalitis. We are concerned only with the management of the seizure disorder per se.

Classification of Seizures

The classification of seizures has long been a controversial subject. The International Classification, proposed to the World Health Organization by Gastaut and published in 1970, forms a useful basis for rational management (Table 1).

TABLE 1. **International Classification of Epileptic Seizures**

I. Partial seizures (seizures beginning locally)
  A. Partial seizures with elementary symptomatology (generally without impairment of consciousness)
    1. With motor symptoms [includes jacksonian seizures]
    2. With special sensory or somatosensory symptoms
    3. With autonomic symptoms
    4. Compound forms
  B. Partial seizures with complex symptomatology (generally with impairment of consciousness) (temporal lobe or psychomotor seizures)
    1. With impairment of consciousness only
    2. With cognitive symptomatology
    3. With affective symptomatology
    4. With "psychosensory" symptomatology
    5. With "psychomotor" symptomatology (automatisms)
    6. Compound forms
  C. Partial seizures secondarily generalized
II. Generalized seizures (bilaterally symmetrical and without local onset)
    1. Absences (petit mal)
    2. Bilateral massive epileptic myoclonus
    3. Infantile spasms
    4. Clonic seizures
    5. Tonic seizures
    6. Tonic-clonic seizures (grand mal)
    7. Atonic seizures
    8. Akinetic seizures
III. Unilateral seizures (or predominantly)
IV. Unclassified epileptic seizures (due to incomplete data)

Management of Seizures

The most common seizure pattern in children is that of brief generalized convulsions, and these occur particularly at the onset of febrile infections at the age of 6 months to 4 years. The usual "benign" febrile seizure does not last more than 5 minutes, and the child will then rapidly regain consciousness. In such brief febrile attacks there is generally evidence of a causative infection, particularly in the upper respiratory tract, and only the following measures are required:

1. Loosen the child's clothing, particularly around the neck. Insert airway if necessary.
2. Turn him on his side or three quarters prone to avoid aspiration of secretions.
3. Protect him from injury—e.g., by blankets or padding.
4. Get suction equipment, oxygen, and bag if available.
5. Set up monitoring procedure for heart rate, blood pressure, respirations, and temperature (preferably rectal). Watch for cyanosis, respiratory depression, and changes in size of pupils.
6. Administer sodium phenobarbital intramuscularly in a loading dose of 10 mg. per kg. body weight (5 mg. per kg. if the child was already receiving the drug).
7. Keep temperature below 38°C. (101°F.) by sponging with tepid water; if necessary, use fan and wet sheets.

If the seizure continues for more than 5 minutes, a more determined effort must be made to bring it to a close. An intravenous injection of diazepam (Valium), given *slowly* over 2 to 5 minutes, is the treatment of choice. The dosage is 0.2 mg. per kg. of body weight, and this may be repeated after 20 minutes. The respirations should be observed carefully. When seizure activity stops during the injection, the complete dose need not be given. The solution of diazepam should not be diluted, and a Mantoux syringe should be used for amounts less than 2 mg. The safety of intravenous diazepam in the newborn is still controversial. In view of the short-lived effect of intravenous diazepam, it should always be accompanied by a more long-acting anticonvulsant such as intramuscular phenobarbital, which will protect the patient against a recurrence of seizures and may later be continued by the oral route. If diazepam is not available, phenytoin may be given intravenously in a dosage of 6 mg. per kg. of body weight in 5 to 10 per cent solution, also slowly. With such intravenous injections it is essential to have equipment for artificial ventilation available. If possible, an anesthetist should be at hand to insert an endotracheal tube and administer bag ventilation in case of need.

If an intravenous injection cannot be achieved—e.g., in an infant—a *deep* intramuscular injection of paraldehyde in a dosage of 0.3 ml. per kg. of body weight (up to a maximum of 5 ml. in any one site) will often be effective. In situations when no injections can be given, the injectable solution of diazepam or a 10 per cent suspension of paraldehyde in diluted peanut oil may be given rectally.

Status Epilepticus. When seizures merge into a continuous series representing status epilepticus, the patient's condition becomes serious and after 30 minutes there is an increasing risk of cerebral ischemia and edema. Status is particularly liable to occur after cerebral anoxia or when preventive anticonvulsant medication has suddenly been discontinued. If the initial injection of intravenous diazepam or diphenylhydantoin and of intramuscular phenobarbital or paraldehyde has been ineffective, the following further steps may now be required:

1. Blood should be taken for estimation of glucose, urea nitrogen, and electrolyte levels, including calcium and magnesium, and for acid-base studies. (The blood glucose level may be assessed roughly at the bedside by use of Dextrostix.)
2. The possibility of an acute organic disorder such as meningitis is investigated.
3. Fluid intake and output should be measured, and intake should be restricted to about 1200 ml. per square meter of body surface per day.
4. A further attempt is made to arrest the seizures by one or more of the following medications: (a) A third slow intravenous injection of diazepam, now 0.4 mg. per kg. if there was no untoward effect with 0.2 mg. per kg. previously. (b) A second slow intravenous infusion of phenytoin, 5 to 10 mg. per kg. (c) An intramuscular injection of paraldehyde, 0.3 ml. per kg., if not given previously.
5. When there are clinical indications of raised intracranial pressure, an intravenous infusion of mannitol (1.0 gram per kg. of body weight) is established so as to be completed in about 30 minutes. (See manufacturer's official directive concerning children under 12 years of age.) Dexamethasone may also be given intravenously in an initial dose of 2 to 6 mg., depending on the size of the child, followed by 1 to 2 mg. 6-hourly.
6. An anesthetist is called and may have to paralyze the patient and ventilate him. Alternatively he may prefer to administer thiopental (Pentothal) or another general anesthetic to stop the seizures. In an emergency situation, when no anesthetist is available, open ether by the drop method applied to a face mask is still one of the most effective and safest methods of arresting persistent seizures in children. It is particularly urgent to terminate prolonged seizures associated with cyanosis, marked tonic spasms, or high fever.

Prevention of Seizures

When the diagnosis of epilepsy has been established clinically, it will usually be confirmed by electroencephalographic (EEG) examination, and the main aim of therapy is the prevention of further seizures. In most patients this involves the use of suitable anticonvulsant drugs. The choice of the drug will depend on the type of seizure and on the EEG pattern (see Table 2), but some broad *principles concerning drug therapy* should be emphasized:

1. The parents should keep a record of the time, duration, and pattern of the child's seizures.

2. Treatment is started with one drug that is suitable for the type of seizure and least liable to cause side effects.

3. Tablets are generally preferable to suspensions or elixirs; if necessary, the tablets may be crushed between two spoons and given mixed with jam or other flavoring. In suspensions the drug is liable to be distributed unevenly, so that they need to be shaken before use. Also, small children may become nauseated by an alcoholic elixir, whereas they can take the tablet quite well. Capsules are also suitable, provided that they are not too big for young children to swallow.

4. In general, it is best to start with about half the maximal tolerated dose for the age (see Table 3) and to increase the dose gradually at intervals of about 1 week until the seizures are controlled and the therapeutic range of blood level is reached. If the blood level is adequate and the seizures are uncontrolled, another drug should be added gradually in a similar manner, but it is rarely advisable to use more than three different medications.

5. Anticonvulsants should never be discontinued or changed abruptly, but only gradually over a period of weeks. Different drugs vary in the number of days required to reach a steady state and thus a persistently high blood level, and those which accumulate slowly also tend to persist longer when their administration is discontinued. Drugs also interact in their metabolism, so that the blood level of one medication may be influenced by that of another.

6. The estimation of serum anticonvulsant levels should be repeated periodically. It shows not only whether the various medications are present in therapeutic amounts, but also whether the patient has taken his drugs as prescribed and which of them might be responsible for toxic effects. In the case of primidone (Mysoline) and mephobarbital (Mebaral), it must be remembered that both drugs are partly metabolized to phenobarbital and that this may be responsible for toxic effects rather than the level of the original compound.

7. Drugs that control petit mal may precipitate or aggravate major seizures, and vice versa. If both types of seizures are present in the same child, both kinds of drugs may have to be used together.

TABLE 2. **Anticonvulsant Therapy in Relation to Various Seizure Patterns**

TYPE OF SEIZURE	EEG PATTERN AND LOCALIZATION	MEDICAL TREATMENT (IN ORDER OF PREFERENCE)
Complex partial (psychomotor, temporal lobe, etc.)	Spikes, sharp or 4–7 per second slow waves over one or both temporal lobes	Phenytoin Carbamazepine Primidone
Other partial (focal)	Localized spikes, sharp waves, often phase reversals	Phenytoin Phenobarbital Carbamazepine
Generalized tonic-clonic (grand mal)	Symmetrical spikes, sharp waves, spike-wave or polyspike-wave complexes, or slow waves	Phenobarbital Phenytoin Carbamazepine Clonazepam
Absences (petit mal)	Symmetrical, frontally dominant 3 per second spike-wave	Ethosuximide Acetazolamide Clonazepam Trimethadione
Infantile spasms (generalized myoclonic)	Hypsarrhythmia—i.e., multifocal high-voltage asynchronous slow and poly-spike-wave discharges, or milder similar abnormalities	ACTH, prednisone Nitrazepam,* clonazepam Acetazolamide
Other generalized (atonic, akinetic)	Generalized, often multifocal 2.5 per second or slower irregular spike-wave or polyspike-wave discharges	Clonazepam Dipropylacetate* Acetazolamide ACTH, prednisone Ketogenic diet

*Investigational drug in the United States of America.

TABLE 3. **Commonly Used Anticonvulsant Drugs in Children**

DRUG	TRADE NAME	PREPARATIONS ADVISED	TOTAL DAILY DOSAGE (MG./KG.)	DOSES PER DAY	THERAPEUTIC BLOOD LEVEL (MG./LITER)	MAIN TOXIC EFFECTS	ALLERGIC REACTIONS*
Phenobarbital	Luminal	Tablets, 10, 15, 30, 50, and 100 mg.	4–5	1–2	15–30	Drowsiness, irritability, unsteadiness	Rashes
Primidone	Mysoline	Tablets, 125 and 250 mg.	10–20	3	5–12 (plus phenobarbital)	Drowsiness, nausea, unsteadiness	Rash, confusion
Phenytoin	Dilantin	Tablets, 50 mg. Capsules, 30 and 100 mg. Suspension, 30 mg./5 ml. (shake before use)	5–7	1–3	10–20	Gum hypertrophy, hirsutism, ataxia, nystagmus	Rashes, liver damage, hematopoietic effects
Acetazolamide	Diamox	Tablets, 250 mg.	10–30	2–3	—	Thirst, polyuria, hyperventilation	Confusion, hematopoietic effects (like other sulfonamides)
Ethosuximide	Zarontin	Capsules, 250 mg. Syrup, 250 mg./5 ml.	15–30	2–3	40–100	Nausea, abdominal discomfort, drowsiness	Rashes, hematopoietic effects
Carbamazepine†	Tegretol	Tablets, 200 mg.	10–20	2–3	2–8	Drowsiness, unsteadiness, nausea, diplopia	Rashes, hematopoietic effects, confusion
Trimethadione	Trimedone Tridione	Capsules, 300 mg. Dulcets, 150 mg.	15–20	2–3	10–30	Photophobia, nausea, drowsiness	Rashes, bone marrow depression, nephrosis
Clonazepam	Clonopin Rivotril	Tablets, 0.5 and 2 mg.	0.02 → 0.3‡ (in slow steps)	3	—	Drowsiness, ataxia, behavior problems, excess salivation	Liver damage, hematopoietic effects
Nitrazepam (investigational)	Mogadon	Tablets, 5 mg.	0.1 → 1.0	3	—	Drowsiness, excess salivation	Liver damage, hematopoietic effects

*The occurrence of allergic reactions makes it necessary to stop the causative medication immediately.
†The manufacturer's official directive does not list a dose for children.
‡This dose is higher than that listed in the manufacturer's official directive.

8. When satisfactory control of seizures has been established, effective medication should be continued for at least 3 years after the last attack. Thereafter medication may be discontinued gradually over at least 6 months, provided that the EEG no longer shows any paroxysmal features.

9. Most of the commonly used anticonvulsants have a sufficiently long action that they need to be given at most three times in one day; phenobarbital can be given once daily. Sometimes an extra amount of drug may usefully be administered prior to the usual time of the seizure—e.g., at bedtime in the case of nocturnal attacks.

10. The child should be observed closely for possible toxic effects, and the parents should be warned concerning their nature. The occurrence of even minor infections should be reported, particularly when drugs are used which may depress blood formation. Monthly blood counts are advised when the diones (trimethadione, paramethadione), carbamazepine, and clonazepam are used, and the drug should be discontinued if the granulocytes fall below 1600 or the platelets below 125,000 per cu. mm. Regular urinalyses are required for patients taking diones. The addition of a stimulant (e.g., dextroamphetamine, 5 mg. in the morning) may help children to tolerate sedative drugs, particularly barbiturates. In general, the combination of two anticonvulsants which may each cause drowsiness should be avoided—e.g., phenobarbital plus clonazepam. Drugs with a sedative effect are also disadvantageous if EEG studies show that the tendency to seizures is aggravated by drowsiness.

11. During the past few years it has been shown that long-term therapy with anticonvulsants may cause rickets in children (osteomalacia in adults) and also folate deficiency. Therefore the serum alkaline phosphatase, calcium (preferably ionized), phosphate, and folate levels may usefully be checked at least twice a year. If necessary, supplements of vitamin D (1000 to 2000 I.U. per day) or folate (5 mg. weekly to daily) may then be given.

12. When serum drug concentrations reach the top of the therapeutic range, any further increments in dosage should be made with caution, as they may cause a disproportionate rise to toxic levels.

Relationship to Age

Seizures below the age of 6 months are always cause for serious concern, as cerebral malformation, birth injury, and metabolic disorders are common underlying abnormalities. After that, febrile convulsions are the most frequent type until the age of 3 to 4 years, and breath-holding spells also occur particularly in this age group and have to be differentiated from seizures. After the age of 4 years cryptogenic epilepsy becomes the leading cause of seizures in childhood.

Neonatal Seizures

In the first month of life seizures may be difficult to diagnose. They are often of the fragmentary generalized type, and when they are partial (focal) they tend to shift from one side or pattern to another. They may also be myoclonic or tonic or may take the form of apneic spells. The causes of these seizures are listed in Table 4.

Neonatal seizures represent a clinical emergency and have a serious prognosis. On follow-up, about half the children have been found to be normal, about 30 per cent had a serious neurologic defect, and 20 per cent had died. The outlook is most serious if seizures occur in the first 48 hours. The possibility of an underlying treatable infection or metabolic disturbance should be investigated promptly. Blood, urine, and cerebrospinal fluid should be examined, and an emergency electroencephalogram should be obtained, because the latter may be of help in diagnosis and prognosis. Apneic spells and massive myoclonic spasms are particularly ominous. Pyridoxine, 50 mg., may be given intravenously during electroencephalography and will have a dramatic effect on seizures and EEG in cases of pyridoxine dependency or deficiency, thus helping prove the diagnosis. Dextrostix testing of blood will indicate quickly whether intravenous glucose is required. When neonatal tetany is suspected, intravenous calcium gluconate may be administered immediately after blood has been drawn for serum calcium and phosphorus determinations.

The neonatal seizures as such can usually be treated satisfactorily by intramuscular sodium phenobarbital in a loading dose of 10 mg. per kg., followed by 6 mg. per kg. daily with careful

TABLE 4. **Causes of Neonatal Seizures**

1. Congenital cerebral defects—e.g., porencephaly, vascular anomalies
2. Perinatal anoxia or intracranial hemorrhage
3. Metabolic disorders—e.g., hypoglycemia (particularly in "runt twins" and in "small-for-dates" infants), hypocalcemia, aminoacidopathies (e.g., maple syrup urine disease), pyridoxine dependency
4. Toxic and electrolyte disturbances—e.g., hyponatremia, narcotic withdrawal, bilirubin encephalopathy
5. Infections—e.g., bacterial meningitis, viral meningoencephalitis, congenital toxoplasmosis
6. Cryptogenic
7. Miscellaneous—e.g., cerebral edema with hepatic necrosis, anoxia with cyanotic types of congenital cardiac malformation

monitoring of blood level. Alternatively, paraldehyde, 0.3 ml. per kg. as a 10 per cent suspension in peanut oil, may be administered rectally or by nasogastric tube; this may be repeated at intervals of 4 to 6 hours. Intravenous diazepam, 0.2 mg. per kg. of body weight, is advised in the newborn only if the seizures are not controlled by phenobarbital and paraldehyde.

Infantile Spasms

These seizures represent brief generalized myoclonic spasms, also described as "salaam" (or jackknife) seizures or "cheerleader" attacks, depending on the predominance of flexion or extension movements. Such spasms, lasting only a few seconds, may recur in series and are associated with a gross abnormality of the EEG, often amounting to "hypsarrhythmia" (see Table 2). The attacks usually commence prior to the age of 6 months, and over 90 per cent of the infants are at least moderately retarded by the age of 1 year. Unfortunately drug control of these seizures is often hard to achieve, and if it is accomplished, it may not prevent the child from becoming mentally retarded. Other minor motor seizures, such as atonic collapse attacks, head drops, and localized myoclonic jerks in infancy, also have a serious prognosis. Here the EEG pattern may not amount to gross hypsarrhythmia, but there may be generalized irregular spike-and-wave or polyspike-and-wave discharges at a rate of about 2 per second.

In about half of these infants with minor motor seizures, a congenital cerebral defect, perinatal brain injury, or tuberous sclerosis is held responsible; in about 30 per cent the cause is unknown, and in the remaining 20 per cent a variety of metabolic disorders and prenatal infections have been found. Among the metabolic disorders which may be responsible are aminoacidopathies such as phenylketonuria which are amenable to dietary therapy, and therefore investigation for metabolic disorders must be pursued.

In the control of infantile spasms the administration of ACTH or of adrenocortical steroids, such as prednisone, is often markedly successful, at least as far as the seizures and the EEG are concerned. The trial of these medications should be considered a matter of urgency, because they may improve the long-term prognosis for brain function. ACTH is administered in a long-acting form by intramuscular injection, usually 40 to 60 I.U. daily for 2 weeks, and if there is a satisfactory response of the seizures and improvement in the EEG, we then tend to change over to oral prednisone, 3 mg. per kg. daily in two or three divided doses. The baby may then be discharged from the hospital on a maintenance dose of prednisone, and the dosage is gradually diminished and changed to an alternate-day regimen over the course of several months (somewhat as in the therapy of nephrosis). If ACTH or steroids are not effective, we add a benzodiazepine. Nitrazepam (investigational) has been found to be almost equally effective as ACTH, and clonazepam (Clonopin, Rivotril) is also useful. The latter should be started cautiously at doses of 0.02 mg. per kg. per day, and the dosage is then increased every 3 days to a final level of 0.3 mg. per kg. daily, usually in three to four divided doses. (This dose is higher than that stated in the manufacturer's official directive.) Acetazolamide and phenobarbital are also sometimes useful adjuvants, but standard anticonvulsants rarely control such seizures by themselves. Treatment with benzodiazepines should be maintained for a year or longer, depending on improvement or relapses in the clinical course and EEG.

Lennox-Gastaut Syndrome

This term has recently been introduced for a severe convulsive disorder of childhood which clinically consists of various forms of minor seizures, including myoclonic, akinetic (momentary arrest resembling absences), atonic (drop attacks), and tonic forms. They tend to occur at the age of 1 to 6 years, the mean age of onset being about 3 years, and they are usually associated with progressive mental retardation. The electroencephalogram is characterized by diffuse slow spike-waves with a frequency of 2.5 Hz or less; often there is also slowing of background rhythms, and the spike-waves tend to be accentuated by sleep. The causes are probably multiple, as with infantile spasms, and the seizures are similarly difficult to treat.

In the management ACTH and steroids are usually ineffective. The most useful drug is clonazepam (Clonopin, Rivotril), which is reported to control the seizures in one third to one half of the patients. It should be introduced slowly at a dosage level of 0.02 mg. per kg. of body weight daily, and increments of 0.25 mg. may then be added every 3 days to a maximum of 0.3 mg. per kg. per day, divided into at least three doses (see Table 3). (This dose is higher than that stated in the manufacturer's official directive.) Recently, a new drug, dipropyl acetate (sodium valproate), has been introduced in Europe and is reported to control such seizures in about one-quarter of the patients, but it is still investigational in North America. Combinations with phenobarbital, acetazolamide (Diamox), and ethosuximide (Zarontin) may also be useful. In this syndrome and in other minor motor seizures, a ketogenic diet still brings occasional successes when all medications have failed.

Febrile Convulsions

These represent the most common type of generalized seizure in children aged 6 months to 4 years. They generally occur when the child has a temperature of at least 38.5°C. (101°F.) and soon after the initial rise, rarely later than 6 to 10 hours after the onset of fever. When they are "benign," they last only 1 to 5 minutes and have a recognizable cause in an extracerebral infection such as acute tonsillitis or a urinary infection. They may recur, but rarely more than 12 hours after the initial seizure in any one attack of fever. The child's neurologic status should be normal. There is frequently a family history of similar febrile seizures in early childhood. An EEG may show some slowing during the fever, but no other abnormality. Lumbar puncture and other diagnostic procedures to rule out meningitis and brain infections should have negative results.

In the management of such convulsions every effort should be made to terminate the seizure as described above, because there is a risk of subsequent epilepsy—i.e., afebrile seizures and neurologic deficits resulting from cerebral anoxia, edema and gliosis, or even venous or arterial thromboses, particularly with prolonged seizure activity. Efforts should also be made to keep the temperature below 38.5°C. (101°F.) by the use of antipyretics, sponging with tepid water, or even aiming a fan at a wet sheet over the child.

One third to one half of children with "benign" febrile convulsions lasting less than 5 minutes have no further seizures, and it is doubtful whether anticonvulsants should be prescribed for those who have had only a single seizure of this kind. After two febrile convulsions, or if a nonfebrile convulsion supervenes, or if the EEG shows epileptiform discharges, regular anticonvulsant drug therapy should be given continuously with at least 4 mg. of phenobarbital per kg. of body weight daily, and blood levels of phenobarbital should be kept in the therapeutic range—i.e., above 15 mg. per liter. Phenytoin is not suitable for the prevention of febrile seizures. If the child exhibits irritability or other abnormal behavior on treatment with phenobarbital, primidone (Mysoline) may be substituted. To prevent recurrence of febrile convulsions, persistent septic foci (e.g., infection in tonsils or urinary tract) may also require suitable treatment.

Breath-Holding Spells

Genuine episodes of breath-holding are not truly epileptic in nature, but are generally precipitated by injury or frustration. They occur mostly at the age of 6 months to 3 years. The infant cries and holds his breath, becomes cyanosed, falls to the floor, stiffens, and may lose consciousness. He then either resumes respirations or may exhibit clonic movements, probably a convulsive response to anoxia. Unconsciousness rarely lasts for more than 2 or 3 minutes. The EEG is usually normal apart from slow waves during the actual attack. Affected children rarely go on to have spontaneous recurrent seizures, but they may develop behavior problems. Preventive treatment with anticonvulsant is usually ineffective, but tranquilizing medications such as thioridazine (Mellaril) or promethazine (Phenergan), both in a dosage of 5 to 10 mg. two or three times daily, may be helpful. The parents should be reassured that breath-holding spells are not serious and are likely to cease on their own as the child gets older. They should also be given guidance concerning infant management.

Generalized Tonic-Clonic Seizures (Grand Mal)

The full-blown grand mal seizure of adults with its tonic, clonic, and postconvulsive phases, frequently preceded by an aura and epileptic cry, is rarely seen in childhood. However, a generalized convulsion may result from a seizure discharge anywhere in the brain spreading to the motor cortex bilaterally, and such widespread epileptic activity is particularly liable to occur in small children. Depending on the site of origin, such generalized convulsions may be associated with a variety of EEG patterns. In older children, sudden generalized convulsions without aura or fever may originate in the frontal lobe, and interictal electroencephalograms may show focal spikes in that area. In younger children the electroencephalogram often shows irregular polyspike-wave discharges synchronously and symmetrically over both hemispheres, suggesting a subcortical origin. In generalized convulsions of cortical origin the most useful drugs are phenobarbital, phenytoin, and carbamazepine. In generalized convulsions of subcortical origin, with spike-wave discharges on the EEG or occasionally with normal interictal tracings, clonazepam may be more effective.

Phenobarbital is still one of the most useful drugs in the treatment of epilepsy, being both cheap and generally nontoxic. The dosage, blood levels, and toxic effects are shown in Table 3. Steady blood levels will not be reached for 2 to 3 weeks. Children who have cerebral dysfunction (formerly called brain damage) with overactivity and brief attention span are liable to exhibit more restlessness and disturbed behavior on treatment with phenobarbital; therefore the drug is best avoided in this type of child, or, if it is essential for the control of seizures, some tranquilizing medication may usefully be added.

Phenytoin (Dilantin) is often described as the most effective anticonvulsant in seizures of cortical origin. In young children the usual safe dosage is 7 mg. per kg. of body weight daily, divided into two or three doses, whereas in teenagers the blood level may be maintained adequately on single daily doses. Whenever possible, the actual blood levels should be checked when the drug has been in use for 7 to 10 days. Phenytoin is available in white capsules of 30 mg. (with pale pink cap) and 100 mg. (with orange cap). For young children I prefer chewable tablets of 50 mg. (Infatabs), which have a pleasant flavor and cannot be confused. Tablets are also preferable to suspensions, for the latter come in two strengths (30 and 125 mg. per 5 ml.) and require shaking before use, as the solid material tends to settle to the bottom. A common side effect is hypertrophy of the gums; this can be largely avoided by careful oral hygiene and nightly cleaning of gum pockets. Another side effect which does not necessitate discontinuation of the drug is the occurrence of hirsutism; this will subside when the drug is ultimately discontinued. Ataxia (accompanied by nystagmus) is usually due to overdosage. Megaloblastic and other types of anemia have also been described, as well as a syndrome resembling Hodgkin's disease, but these are rare.

Carbamazepine (Tegretol) has been introduced as an anticonvulsant in the past few years and appears to be effective in generalized tonic-clonic, partial (focal) motor, and complex partial (temporal lobe) forms of epilepsy. It is supplied in tablets of 200 mg., and the dosage for children is 10 to 20 mg. per kg. of body weight daily. (The manufacturer's official directive does not list a dose for children.) This should be divided into two or three doses, and it is best to start with small amounts in order to avoid initial drowsiness, unsteadiness, and diplopia. The therapeutic blood level of 2 to 8 mg. per liter should be reached within 3 to 4 days after the full dosage has been attained. Since hematopoietic effects have been reported, it still seems advisable to check the blood count every 4 to 6 weeks.

Clonazepam (Clonopin, Rivotril) is an important new anticonvulsant which has already been mentioned in connection with the treatment of infantile spasms and other minor motor seizures in young children. In our experience it may also be useful in generalized tonic-clonic seizures of subcortical origin. It suppresses spike-wave discharges, but as a benzodiazepine it also has sedative properties. Accordingly the dosage must be built up slowly, starting with 0.02 mg. per kg. per day and increasing this by 0.25 to 0.5 mg. every third day, until a total dosage of about 0.3 mg. per kg. per day is reached or the seizures are controlled. (This dose is higher than that stated in the manufacturer's official directive.) The maximum blood level after a single oral dose is reached within 1 to 2 hours, and it is best to give the daily amount divided into at least three doses. Apart from drowsiness and ataxia the patients may have excessive secretion of mucus, which may lead to aspiration pneumonia. Periodic liver function tests and blood counts should also be performed during long-term therapy with this medication.

Partial (Focal) Seizures

Focal motor seizures tend to start with movements in one particular part of the body, such as twitching of a thumb or one side of the face, and this is a useful indication of the point of origin in the contralateral motor cortex. The classic progression or "jacksonian march" to other parts represented in adjacent motor cortex is seen less frequently in children than in adults. Adversive seizures with turning of the head and eyes to one side frequently arise from a focus in the contralateral frontal lobe. Clonic twitching of one part of the body, such as the arm, may be followed by temporary Todd's paralysis in the affected limb. Recently it has been pointed out that partial seizures beginning with clonic twitching of one side of the face and head after the age of 4 years are a somewhat specific, benign form of epilepsy. It is usually associated with a spike or spike-wave focus (so-called rolandic spikes) in the opposite hemisphere above the sylvian fissure. Treatment with phenytoin (Dilantin) or phenobarbital usually controls these seizures promptly.

Somatosensory disturbances, such as numbness, tingling, or crawling sensations, may indicate a discharge in the postcentral sensory convolution of the opposite hemisphere. Visual, auditory, and vertiginous seizures similarly arise from other cortical foci, which may be further defined by localized discharges in the EEG. In general, such focal seizures require investigation to exclude a space-occupying lesion (tumor, vascular malformation, abscess) adjacent to their points of origin. However, in children the great majority of such focal seizures are due to atrophic lesions or congenital defects. When a space-occupying lesion has been excluded, the patients are usually treated by anticonvulsant drugs, the most useful being phenytoin, phenobarbital, and carbamazepine. With a distinct localized scar or other irritative lesion these seizures may be hard to control, and primidone may also be tried.

Primidone (Mysoline) is a barbiturate which appears to have a somewhat different action from phenobarbital, but is partly converted into it. It is prepared in tablets of 250 mg. and in more pleasant-tasting pediatric tablets of 125 mg. The dosage ranges from 10 to 20 mg. per kg. of body weight. The dosage should be built up slowly in order to avoid excessive initial drowsiness. Once the full dosage has been attained, the blood level may be checked within 4 to 7 days. The serum phenobarbital concentration should always be estimated simultaneously, as it may be abnormally high owing to the conversion from primidone, even when no phenobarbital as such is being given and when the blood level of primidone is within the therapeutic range. Lethargy, unsteadiness, and nausea are the most common toxic effects of primidone, whereas skin rashes, psychotic confusion, and acute vertigo are seen more rarely.

Complex Partial (Temporal Lobe) Seizures

This type of seizure ranges from brief periods of confusion to attacks manifested by peculiar thought disorders or emotions and to abnormal behavior or automatic stereotyped movements (psychomotor seizures). They may be associated with hallucinations, incoherent speech, chewing or smacking movements of the lips, temper outbursts, or sudden fear. The EEG may show spikes or 4 to 7 Hz slow waves from temporal electrodes, but such abnormalities may be hard to demonstrate; they are often best seen in sleep records, or with the use of special nasopharyngeal leads.

In the treatment, phenytoin, carbamazepine, and primidone are generally most effective (often in combination). However, these seizures may be difficult to control, and there is frequently disordered behavior between seizures which does not respond to anticonvulsant treatment.

Surgical treatment is occasionally indicated in the presence of persistent partial (focal) seizures, even in the absence of a space-occupying lesion. The following conditions are generally considered a prerequisite for surgical intervention:

1. The focus should be close to the surface and situated in a part of the hemisphere which is not vital for essential functions such as speech.
2. The focus should be clearly identified clinically and electrographically and should preferably be single.
3. The seizures should be resistant to drug therapy, even after a thorough trial of several medications.

The indication for surgical excision of such a focus is strengthened by concomitant intellectual or behavioral deterioration of the child.

Generalized Absence Seizures (Petit Mal)

True petit mal is the best-known variety of generalized seizure in children, arising deeply in "centrencephalic" structures in brainstem or diencephalon. It is usually "idiopathic" and frequently hereditary. Characteristically, petit mal occurs after the age of 4 years, most commonly at 7 to 12. It consists of brief loss of consciousness (lasting less than 30 seconds) without loss of posture and without involuntary movements except fluttering of the lids and slight twitching of the hand or jaw. The EEG will typically show bisynchronous 3 per second spike-wave discharges symmetrically, with somewhat greater amplitude over the anterior head regions. Hyperventilation may precipitate attacks clinically and spike-wave discharges on the EEG. Any twitching of the eyelids or hands also occurs at the rate of 3 per second. In some children there are associated automatisms, such as continued walking or buttoning up of clothes, or there may be associated myoclonic movements, and in practice such more complex seizures are usually harder to control than simple staring spells. Also, when the EEG pattern varies from that of characteristic absences, it may indicate so-called secondary hypersynchrony precipitated by focal discharges, and structural brain lesions may then have to be excluded by appropriate studies.

In the treatment, it is well known that true petit mal often responds very well to the diones (trimethadione and paramethadione), but in view of the serious toxic effects which may occur with these drugs it is considered preferable to use ethosuximide, acetazolamide, and clonazepam when possible.

Ethosuximide (Zarontin) is supplied in 250 mg. capsules and in a syrup containing 250 mg. per 5 ml. The dosage ranges from 15 to 30 mg. per kg. of body weight per day, and it is usually given two to three times per day. The blood level may be checked 7 to 10 days after the maximum dose has been reached (see Table 3). In general, this drug is quite well tolerated, but occasionally nausea and epigastric discomfort, headaches, dizziness, drowsiness, skin rashes, or even bone marrow depression have been encountered.

Acetazolamide (Diamox) acts by interfering with carbonic anhydrase and thus appears to reduce seizure activity both directly in the nervous system and indirectly by causing diuresis. It is supplied in tablets of 250 mg., and the dosage ranges from 10 to 30 mg. per kg. daily, divided into two or three doses. It appears to be particularly useful whenever seizures can be precipitated or aggravated by hyperventilation and may also be helpful in other types of generalized seizures. Usually there are few side effects, but anorexia, pallor, thirst, and polyuria may be encountered, and marked acidosis may be manifested by overbreathing.

Clonazepam (Clonopin, Rivotril) is useful in absence seizures which do not respond to suximides or acetazolamide. The slow gradual increase in dosage which is required with this medication has already been emphasized.

Trimethadione (Trimedone, Tridione) is available in capsules of 300 mg. and chewable tablets (Dulcets) of 150 mg. The dosage ranges from 15 to 20 mg. per kg. of body weight daily, divided into two or three doses, and blood levels should be checked. A common and relatively harmless side effect is photophobia, which may be remedied by the wearing of sunglasses. However, the insidious onset of nephrosis and the sudden occurrence of agranulocytosis represent more serious dangers. Hence the urine and blood count should be checked monthly, and any infections should be reported promptly, so that an underlying bone marrow depression may be detected and treated. Paramethadione (Paradione) has a similar dosage and is said to be less toxic but also less effective.

Social and Emotional Aspects

It must be strongly emphasized that the management of epilepsy involves much more than the control of seizures by drugs. It is well known that emotional disturbance and social maladjustment may prevent successful control of seizures, and many epileptic children are markedly conscious of their disability and tend to feel socially inferior. The parents must be told that these children should be treated like healthy youngsters and should not be spoiled or overprotected. Normal play and physical activity should be encouraged. Only a few restrictions are required; thus swimming should be permitted, but only under the watchful eye of an adult; epileptic children should be warned to keep away from open fires or machinery, not to climb to heights where a fall might be dangerous, not to ride a bicycle in busy streets, and, later, not to drive a vehicle until they have been free from seizures for at least 2 years. Apart from these restrictions they should be encouraged to take an active part in the social life, sports, and games enjoyed by other children of their age. The parents may suitably be given an explanatory pamphlet concerning epilepsy, and when the youngster reaches the age of about 10 years it is advisable to discuss the disease with him. The school teacher should be informed of the epilepsy, so that the child with petit mal is not blamed for inattention and complex partial seizures are not mistaken for peculiar behavior, and also in order to enable the teacher to manage any seizures satisfactorily in the classroom. Later, vocational training should take the handicap of epilepsy into consideration.

In general, the parents and the child can be reassured that the seizures are likely to diminish or to cease with increasing age, and a realistic appreciation of the disability should be combined with an optimistic attitude for the future. The physician should help to promote acceptance of the epileptic youngster at school and in the community. At the same time the physician should be frank with the family concerning possible genetic implications, and the child and his parents should be encouraged to express their feelings and apprehensions.

HEADACHE

method of
NEIL H. RASKIN, M.D.
San Francisco, California

The large majority of patients with recurring headaches do not have identifiable anatomic or metabolic abnormalities that are etiologically related to their problem. This article will focus on the management of these patients; it will be assumed that causes of headache such as pheochromocytoma, brain tumor, temporal arteritis, and the like have been considered and excluded.

General Principles

1. The physician's attitude toward his patients with headache will undoubtedly influence the results he achieves. Caring for and having an interest in these people are essential for any therapeutic program. Communicating enthusiasm, support, and a positive approach go a long way toward ameliorating cephalgia, whether the mechanism is primarily muscle contraction, vascular dilatation, or both.

2. A carefully elicited history will usually reveal evidence of vasomotor instability in the large majority of patients who appear to have cervical muscle contraction as their primary complaint. The neck muscles respond to pain by a mechanism similar to the one whereby the abdominal musculature responds to an inflamed appendix by becoming spastic or "rigid." Vasomotor instability (migraine) is far more responsive to specific therapy than is muscle contraction; do not overlook this treatable aspect of the patients' problems.

3. Vague, daily, constant headaches do not necessarily imply a psychogenic cause. Ask about the most severe headaches for clues as to the

mechanism involved. The paroxysmal episodes are more likely to be pounding, and associated with scintillating scotomas, vertigo, or vomiting.

4. Analgesics may be all that can be offered to some patients with headache. Become familiar with the dosage required to produce physical dependence (addiction); they are much higher than many physicians' estimates. Codeine is highly unlikely to produce dependence at doses under 1000 mg. per day; meperidine (Demerol) does not result in dependence when used orally in doses under 600 mg. per day.

5. Although emotional stress, anxiety, and life's tensions are certainly important aspects of the cephalgic patient's life, it is clear that none of us are free of anxiety and stress. Be circumspect about being simplistic in applying a universal attribute of human beings to the problem at hand. Establishing a meaningful relationship with a patient, based on caring, trust, and support, is certainly more important than focusing upon his vulnerabilities.

Migraine

Removal of Precipitants as Provocative Factors. These include dental problems, refractive errors, poor sleep patterns, hunger, high altitudes, bright lights, certain foodstuffs that contain tyramine (cheese, wine), nitrites (frankfurters, salami, ham), monosodium glutamate (Accent, wonton soup), and phenylethylamine (chocolate). Other foodstuffs may also precipitate headache by a mechanism that is still obscure and includes fried or fatty foods, coffee, tea, sucrose, and alcohol. Chocolate, alcohol-containing beverages, and cheese should be avoided for at least a 1 month trial.

Oral contraceptive preparations are known to precipitate vascular headaches; women should be exhorted to abstain from oral contraception for at least 6 months to assess this possibility. If this is not feasible, a low estrogen preparation such as norethindrone acetate and ethinyl estradiol (Loestrin) (1/20) may be used as an alternative. Supplementary estrogen preparations may precipitate migraine because of a dosage which is too low, too high, or of the wrong type. A chemically pure synthetic estrogen such as ethinyl estradiol, starting at 0.02 mg. per day and increasing gradually, if necessary, to 0.05 mg. per day over a period of months, will resolve many menopausal patients' headache disorders. Stop exogenous thyroid therapy, unless the patient is unequivocally hypothyroid.

Acute Attacks. The earlier these episodes are dealt with, the likelier the possibility that they can be aborted. If feasible, lying down in a dark room with a cold pack (Cryogel) and trying to sleep, whatever else is done, is a very useful adjunct for many patients. Inhalation of 100 per cent oxygen through a tight-fitting mask, at a high flow rate (8 liters per minute) is often helpful. For infrequent attacks, a potent analgesic, such as hydromorphone (Dilaudid) administered as a 3 mg. rectal suppository, may be all that is necessary.

Ergotamine tartrate rectal suppository is the most effective form of this drug short of parenteral preparations. Cafergot contains 2 mg. ergotamine tartrate and 100 mg. caffeine; Cafergot P-B suppository contains, in addition, 0.25 mg. belladonna alkaloids and 60 mg. pentobarbital and suppresses nausea in susceptible patients. Wigraine contains 1 mg. ergotamine tartrate, 100 mg. caffeine, 130 mg. phenacetin, and 0.1 mg. belladonna alkaloids. The dose range is from 0.5 to 2.0 mg. of ergotamine tartrate as soon as an attack begins. The initial dose may be repeated in 30 minutes if the attack is unaffected. The next time, instruct the patient to use the total dose at the onset of headache.

Ergotamine tartrate aerosol (Medihaler Ergotamine, 0.36 mg. per inhalation) is not in solution, so that *patients must shake the cannister vigorously* before each inhalation. This is a very rapidly absorbed preparation of ergotamine tartrate and is very effective for many patients for whom a rectal suppository is not feasible. The usual dosage is 1 or 2 puffs; this may be repeated in 5 minutes if there is no clear response. There are about 50 doses in each cartridge.

Ergotamine tartrate, sublingual (Ergomar, Ergostat) is probably more rapidly absorbed than the other oral preparations; it produces less nausea per mg. of drug. There is 2 mg. of pulverized drug per individually wrapped tablet. The usual dose is 1 or 2 tablets at the onset of headache.

Ergotamine tartrate tablets (Gynergen, Cafergot, Cafergot P-B, Wigraine): This is the least expensive and probably least effective mode of administration of ergotamine tartrate. It is most effective for patients with clear-cut premonitory symptoms several minutes before a headache appears. Wigraine tablets are individually wrapped and are possibly absorbed faster.

Isometheptene mucate, dichloralphenazone, acetaminophen (Midrin) capsules: The usual dosage is 1 to 3 capsules at the onset of headache; it is less nauseating than ergotamine tartrate and as effective as the other oral preparations.

Ergotamine tartrate, injectable (Gynergen): The usual dosage is 0.25 mg. to 0.5 mg. intramuscularly.

Dihydroergotamine mesylate (D.H.E.-45); 0.5 to 1.0 mg., is given intramuscularly or intravenously. It may produce retching; it may abruptly terminate a migraine attack.

Ergotism: Severe and persistent peripheral vasoconstriction, leading, at times, to gangrene, is a potential hazard when ergotamine tartrate is used on a long-term basis; its appearance is almost always heralded by acroparesthesia and claudication pain. Patients should be apprised of this; no more than 6 mg. of ergotamine tartrate in 24 hours and less than 12 mg. per week should be administered to lessen the risk of this problem. Patients are at heightened risk during severe systemic illness; ergotamine tartrate should be avoided altogether if a patient contracts pneumonia, for example.

Ergot dependence: Abuse of ergots may result in physical dependence, which is manifested by a worsening of the original headache problem. Hospitalization for withdrawal from ergotamine tartrate with analgesic support may be necessary.

Interval Treatment (Prophylaxis). For patients with frequent, severe headaches that occur more often than weekly, the risks of ergotism plus the effectiveness of a large variety of relatively effective agents dictate the use, in a sequential fashion, of one or more of the agents mentioned below. If a patient is nonresponsive to ergotamine tartrate, it does not follow that he will be nonresponsive to other agents; nor does it mean that he does not have migraine. Each of the following agents is effective in roughly 50 to 70 per cent of patients and may require 3 to 4 weeks before an effect becomes apparent. Therefore sequential trials of several agents over 3 to 4 months may be necessary before substantial amelioration occurs. During this interval, adequate analgesia and support are essential.

Ergonovine maleate (investigational for this use): The dosage is 0.2 mg. three times daily, gradually increasing to 2.0 mg. daily over a 2 to 4 week period. One to 3 weeks at the optimal dosage is often necessary before effects are apparent. Its minimal vasoconstrictor action renders this ergot drug acceptable for daily therapy.

Propranolol (investigational for this use): The dosage is 20 mg. three times daily for 1 week, and then 40 mg. three times daily. It is contraindicated in congestive heart failure and in patients with asthmatic attacks. It appears to be especially effective in combination with methysergide.

Amitriptyline (investigational for this use): 50 mg. at bedtime is a useful starting dose. Fifty mg. twice daily for the second week, if necessary, and 100 mg. twice daily thereafter for another 2 weeks constitutes an adequate trial. It is sometimes useful in conjunction with ergonovine. Amitriptyline is useful whether or not patients are depressed.

Cyproheptadine (investigational for this use): The dosage is 8 mg. twice daily for 1 week, and then 12 mg. twice daily thereafter. Sedation is common early, but tolerance to this occurs rapidly.

Clonidine (investigational for this use): The dosage is 0.1 mg. twice daily for 1 week, increasing to 0.3 mg. twice daily if necessary. Sedation is a common early side effect.

Phenytoin (investigational for this use): The dosage is 300 to 500 mg. daily. The effect is usually apparent within 7 days.

Phenelzine (investigational for this use): Forty-five to 60 mg. daily is the usual effective dose. This agent is a monoamine oxidase inhibitor, so tyramine-containing foods should be avoided; cheeses are by far the most common provocatives. Cottage and cream cheeses are permissible. Red wine, nuts, beans, chocolate, avocado, and alcohol should be avoided.

Methysergide (Sansert): The usual dosage is 6 mg. per day. Some patients do not respond unless the dosage reaches 12 mg. per day, which may increase the risk of cardiac, pleuropulmonary, or retroperitoneal fibrosis. This is the only prophylactic drug that carries Food and Drug Administration (FDA) approval and also has the most serious potential side effects. Patients should be instructed to taper off this drug slowly every 2 months to be sure that they still require it. The manufacturer recommends frequent 2 month drug holidays, but this may not be feasible for some patients (see manufacturer's official directive). Retroperitoneal fibrosis is generally reversible if detected early so that biannual intravenous pyelography, serum creatinine determinations, and chest x-rays are essential for all patients who use the drug for periods exceeding 6 months.

Muscle-Contraction, or Tension Headache

Treatment:

1. Local massage and heat.
2. Relaxation techniques—meditation, muscle tension biofeedback.
3. Antianxiety and muscle-relaxing agents—diazepam, 5 to 20 mg. daily.
4. Non-narcotic analgesics: combinations of acetaminophen, butalbital, and caffeine are especially useful (Esgic, Phrenilin).
5. Cervical traction.

Establishing a relationship with patients and supporting them through the source of their stress and/or anxiety are at least equally important as the measures outlined above.

Lumbar Puncture Headache

The incidence and severity of this disorder can be reduced if patients assume the prone position before the needle is removed. Simple analgesics and bed rest with 10 to 15 degree elevation of the legs is generally all that is required for this self-limited problem. However, for those few patients with severe and persistent headache, epidural blood patches have usually been dramatically successful.

EPISODIC VERTIGO

method of
THOMAS J. CARLOW, M.D.
Albuquerque, New Mexico

Vertigo can be defined as either a subjective or objective illusory sensation of movement. Whether the patient experiences subjective vertigo (internal rotation) or objective vertigo (external rotation) is not important clinically. Isolated vertigo has minimal localizing value, as it represents dysfunction anywhere in the vestibular system: semicircular canals, eighth nerve, brainstem, cerebellum, or cerebral cortex.

The nonspecific complaint of dizziness is frequently used interchangeably with vertigo, necessitating the establishment of the presence of a definite sensation of rotation or whirling. A thorough history and physical examination are mandatory to separate vertigo from dizziness. Dizziness has been found to represent impending faint, cerebellar ataxia, the dysequilibrium of a peripheral neuropathy, impaired vision, the hyperventilation syndrome, or a serious psychiatric disorder.

Once true vertigo is documented, it is helpful to determine if the lesion responsible has a central or peripheral locus. A detailed neurologic examination can assist in identifying central vertigo if brainstem, cranial nerve, or cerebral signs are evident. Unilateral hearing loss or tinnitus accompanying vertigo suggests eighth nerve or labyrinthine dysfunction. The absence of neurologic findings is not necessarily indicative of a peripheral localization. A thorough neuro-otologic examination should be performed, including audiometrics, electronystagmography, and, if available, an auditory evoked cortical response test.

Before considering the management of acute vertigo, a brief review of the common conditions causing vertigo will be discussed.

Peripheral Causes of Vertigo

Meniere's Disease. Severe vertigo, nausea, vomiting, tinnitus, and a sensorineural hearing loss form the constellation of symptoms seen in idiopathic labyrinthine hydrops. This disorder is discussed thoroughly on pages 703 to 705. It must be remembered that congenital syphilis, allergies, and endocrine disorders such as hypothyroidism can mimic Meniere's disease.

Labyrinthitis. Vestibular neuronitis, acute peripheral vestibulopathy, and labyrinthitis are synonymous terms used to describe a disorder characterized by explosive, spontaneous vertigo lasting for hours or days with nausea, vomiting, and preserved hearing.

Head Trauma. Mild to severe head trauma may result in injury to the labyrinth or its central connections. Vertigo may be present initially or may be delayed for hours to days and persist for several months.

Benign Positional Vertigo. Rapid change of head position, heralded by vertigo, nausea, vomiting, and nystagmus, is probably the most common cause of episodic vertigo. It is transient, fatigable, and easily elicited clinically by utilizing the Dix-Hallpike maneuvers. It commonly follows head trauma.

Cervical Vertigo. Cervical osteoarthritis or any disorder involving the cervical spinovestibular connections has been described as causing episodic vertigo. Cervical traction and a soft collar, along with the medical management as described below, have been helpful.

Drug-Induced Vertigo. Streptomycin, gentamicin, carbon dioxide, phenytoin (Dilantin), trimethadione (Tridione), indomethacin (Indocin), and alcohol are only a few examples of common drugs that can result in vertigo.

Impacted Ear Canal. Cerumen totally obstructing the external auditory canal has been associated with episodic vertigo.

Labyrinthine Ischemia. Isolated ischemia of the semicircular canals with secondary vertigo is not well documented. Vertebrobasilar insufficiency can cause ischemia to the labyrinth; however, other areas of the brainstem supplied by the vertebrobasilar system are typically involved.

Central Causes of Vertigo

Vertebrobasilar Insufficiency. Abrupt vertigo associated with transient diplopia, cranial nerve pareses, and other signs of brainstem ischemia in elderly patients is presumptive evidence of vertebrobasilar insufficiency. The medical management of cerebrovascular insufficiency is discussed elsewhere in this volume.

Acoustic Neuroma. Mild vertigo, hearing loss, tinnitus, and a unilateral canal paresis must be considered to be an acoustic neuroma until proved otherwise. Polytomography of the temporal bone, computerized axial tomography with and without contrast, and a posterior fossa iophendylate (Pantopaque) study may be warranted.

Multiple Sclerosis. Vertigo may be the first manifestation of the presence of multiple disseminated sclerotic plaques in the brainstem. It must be emphasized that the diagnosis of multiple sclerosis should not be made until multiple lesions both in time and space can be documented.

Epilepsy. Electroencephalography is indicated if a patient with vertigo has symptoms or signs suggestive of a focus in the temporal lobe. If vertigo precedes a generalized seizure, a sleep electroencephalogram should be requested.

Psychogenic Disorders. Anxiety neurosis, hysteria, and the hyperventilation syndrome are frequently associated with vertigo. Merely instructing the patient to hyperventilate before performing the Dix-Hallpike maneuvers may produce or exaggerate benign positional vertigo.

Infectious Disease. Meningitis and meningoencephalitis, both bacterial and viral, have been implicated with acute and chronic vertigo.

Management of Vertigo

Diuretics, vasodilators, vitamins, tranquilizers, streptomycin, and vestibular sedatives have all been advocated in the medical management of Meniere's disease (see pp. 703 to 705). Successful drug therapy for episodic vertigo usually follows a series of therapeutic failures and therefore requires the individualization of treatment. The careful search to uncover the causative factor for the *symptom* of vertigo should be instituted concurrently with a supportive drug program.

The management of vertigo can be divided into outpatient and inpatient protocols. Each of the following drugs or combinations listed should be prescribed for a minimum of 2 to 4 weeks before resorting to a new preparation. A trial of several different drugs or combinations is frequently necessary in order to obtain optimal symptomatic relief.

Acute Vertigo—Outpatient Management. 1. Bed rest with the head held in the position of least vertigo.

2. Reassurance that the symptoms are transitory.

3. Vestibular sedatives *(only one preparation or combination should be used at a time)*:

a. Anticholinergics: (1) Scopolamine, 0.6 mg. orally every 4 hours. (2) Atropine, 0.2 mg. orally every 4 to 6 hours.

b. Antihistamines: (1) Cyclizine, 50 mg. orally every 4 hours. (2) Meclizine, 25 mg. orally every 6 hours. (3) Dimenhydrinate, 50 to 100 mg. orally every 6 hours.

c. Phenothiazine (minor tranquilizer): (1) Promethazine, 25 to 50 mg. orally every 4 to 6 hours. (2) Diazepam, 5 mg. orally every 4 to 6 hours.

d. Sympathomimetics: (1) Amphetamine, 10 mg. orally every 4 to 6 hours. (2) Ephedrine, 25 to 50 mg. orally every 4 to 6 hours.

e. Drug combinations: (1) Scopolamine, 0.6 mg., with ephedrine, 25 to 50 mg., orally every 4 to 6 hours. (2) Scopolamine, 0.6 mg., with promethazine, 25 to 50 mg., orally every 4 to 6 hours. (3) Scopolamine, 0.6 mg., with amphetamine, 10 mg., orally every 4 to 6 hours. (4) Ephedrine, 25 to 50 mg., with promethazine, 25 to 50 mg., orally every 4 to 6 hours.

4. Antinauseants:

a. Trimethobenzamide, 250 mg. orally or 200 mg. rectally every 4 to 6 hours.

b. Prochlorperazine, 5 to 10 mg. orally every 4 to 6 hours.

Acute Vertigo—Inpatient Management. 1. Total bed rest.

2. The head should be maintained in the position of least vertigo, utilizing either a cervical collar or sandbags.

3. Prolonged vomiting may result in dehydration and the need for intravenous fluids.

4. Antinauseants. Oral medication may be attempted; however, intramuscular or rectal routes of administration are usually necessary.

a. Trimethobenzamide, 200 mg. intramuscularly or 200 mg. rectally every 4 to 6 hours.

b. Prochlorperazine, 10 mg. intramuscularly every 4 hours or 25 mg. rectally every 12 hours.

5. Vestibular sedatives:

a. Dosages are as outlined for outpatient management.

b. Dimenhydrinate, 100 mg. intramuscularly every 4 to 6 hours.

c. Fentanyl in combination with droperidol (Innovar), 1 to 2 ml. intramuscularly, has been advocated for violent vertigo even though it is not listed as one of the indications for the drug in the manufacturer's official directory.

d. Diazepam can be titrated in an intravenous drip.

MENIERE'S DISEASE

method of
CHARLES M. LUETJE, M.D.
Kansas City, Missouri

The salient features of Meniere's disease are as follows:

1. Fluctuating hearing loss with distortion of sound and speech discrimination, especially in the early stages.
2. Tinnitus, roaring or seashell type, in the affected ear.
3. Vertigo, whirling, and incapacitation, accompanied by nausea and vomiting.
4. Fullness and pressure in the ear.
5. Episodic attacks of these symptoms, usually lasting from 1 to a few hours.
6. Spontaneous recovery in a matter of hours to a day or so from the acute attack.

Initially, it is extremely important to obtain a history of these features, because without these symptoms the diagnosis of Meniere's disease is usually not tenable. Subvarieties of Meniere's disease occur which involve the vestibular system without cochlear symptoms and cochlear system without vestibular symptoms. Usually, in the early stages, the attacks of Meniere's disease are preceded by abrupt onset of fullness or pressure in the ear, tinnitus, and then the hearing loss and vertigo.

Management

The management of patients with Meniere's disease has changed dramatically over the past few years. The goal of any treatment should be the elimination of vertigo and improvement or stabilization of hearing. This can best be accomplished by a combination of medical and conservative surgical management early in the course of the disease. Aggressive therapy in Meniere's disease may eliminate the ultimate severe loss of hearing and balance function.

Treatment of the Acute Attack. An acute attack of Meniere's disease is an urgent matter, with violent vertigo, nausea, and vomiting. The patient does not want to open his eyes, he wants to lie as still as possible, and usually there is nystagmus. Examination of the ears will rule out any acute otitis media or obvious infection. A brief neurologic examination is indicated.

At this point, it is best to let the patient choose the position in which he is most comfortable.

Several medications may be used. Atropine sulfate, 0.4 to 0.6 mg., should be given subcutaneously immediately. An intravenous infusion of fluids should be started for the purpose of allowing access to a vein and for the administration of diazepam (Valium), titrated to a dosage that will bring the acute vertigo under control. This has considerable range and may vary from 2.5 to 20 mg. Diazepam should be given slowly intravenously, and the patient should be monitored carefully. A rectal suppository of dimenhydrinate (Dramamine), 100 mg., can be given and will potentiate the aforementioned medicines.

The patient should then be allowed to wait in the emergency room or office until alert, but should not attempt to drive an automobile.

Management Following an Acute Attack. The patient should be referred to an otologist or neuro-otologist for definitive diagnosis and evaluation to rule out any other diseases of the vestibular or central nervous system.

Having established the diagnosis of Meniere's disease, one should then institute complete medical management, including (1) niacin in flushing doses twice daily; (2) propantheline bromide (Pro-Banthine), 15 mg. four times daily, as an autonomic blocking agent; (3) sublingual histamine 1:10,000, 2 drops daily under the tongue; (4) a vasodilating agent such as papaverine (Pavabid) or ethaverine (Ethatab) three times daily; (5) symptomatic treatment with antivertiginous medication such as dimenhydrinate (Dramamine) or meclizine (Antivert); (6) proper dietary management, including dietotherapy for obesity, hypoglycemia, or hyperlipoproteinemia; and (7) cessation of nicotine use.

Long-Term Management. Many patients with Meniere's disease will respond to the medical treatment outlined above. However, if the hearing has diminished, has stopped fluctuating, and is progressively deteriorating, or if the vertiginous attacks are incapacitating and not responding to medical treatment, then one should entertain the idea of surgical intervention.

Early surgical procedures which preserve hearing include (1) endolymphatic subarachnoid shunt operation; (2) middle fossa vestibular nerve section; (3) endolymphatic sac decompression operation, with or without incision of the sac; and (4) the Cody tac operation. My preference is to direct surgery to the endolymphatic sac to reduce or eliminate vertigo and stabilize hearing. Middle fossa nerve section and the Cody tac operation have a higher incidence of further loss of hearing.

For decompensated cases of Meniere's disease in which the hearing has dropped to a nonuseful point and the patient is totally incapacitated by vertigo or dysequilibrium, a destructive surgical procedure is indicated. The most thorough destructive procedure which can be accomplished is the translabyrinthine vestibular nerve section. This allows observation of the contents of the internal auditory canal and, in selected cases, section of the cochlear nerve for tinnitus. Middle fossa vestibular nerve section may also be performed. Mastoid labyrinthectomy and transcanal labyrinthectomy can be performed, but these are not 100 per cent efficient operations.

Medical Long-Term Management. In some instances patients will respond quite readily to medical management, the symptoms of Meniere's disease disappear, and, with appropriate dietary treatment to correct any metabolic disorders, the patient may do quite well. In this situation, the same medications that are used for early medical management are continued and certain ones discontinued at the discretion of the physician. These patients should be monitored carefully with audiometric evaluations periodically to prevent progressive sensorineural hearing loss.

A certain number of patients will not respond to medical treatment initially or may, after a few months to years, begin to show progression. These are the patients who are candidates for surgical intervention. At times, however, acute flare-ups of Meniere's disease can be handled by administration of intravenous histamine phosphate injection, 2.75 mg. over a 90 minute period on 3 consecutive days, on either an outpatient or in-hospital basis. If the patient is hospitalized, the treatment should be given twice daily.

Summary

The cornerstone of treatment of Meniere's disease over the years has been medical treatment and dietary management. However, with new and improved surgical techniques which are nondestructive in nature, early combined medical and surgical treatment renders the best chance for elimination of disabling vertigo and stabilization of hearing. It is improper to tell the patient: "There is nothing we can do."

VIRAL MENINGOENCEPHALITIS

method of
JERRY S. WOLINSKY, M.D.
San Francisco, California

Acute viral diseases of the central nervous system (CNS) can be divided conveniently into three general types, each with its own implications for outcome and therapy. These include acute viral meningitis without clinical symptoms or signs of parenchymal involvement, viral encephalitis with direct replication of virus in brain tissue, and postinfectious encephalomyelitis presumably related to an immune mediated attack on the CNS and for which viral replication in neural tissue may or may not be an absolute prerequisite. Most cases of acute viral meningitis ("aseptic meningitis") in this country are due to mumps virus, picornaviruses (usually echo- or coxsackievirus), California encephalitis virus, or lymphocytic choriomeningitis virus. Although the course of aseptic meningitis is usually benign, all these agents have at times been implicated in causing severe encephalitis with significant neurologic sequelae or fatal outcome. Most cases of encephalitis occurring in this country are caused by togaviruses (St. Louis, eastern, and western equine encephalitis), herpes simplex type I virus, or a member of the picornavirus group. Severe neurologic sequelae or death is typical of viral encephalidites, although gratifying recovery occurs frequently enough to warrant aggressive medical care. The parainfectious syndromes are most commonly associated with exanthematous childhood diseases such as measles and chickenpox, although they also occur after other viral illnesses. Despite a stormy clinical course, the possibility of an excellent outcome warrants aggressive supportive medical care of these patients. Treatment of these acute viral syndromes will be considered in terms of both supportive and specific modalities.

Acute Viral Meningitis

Supportive Measures. 1. Bed rest is indicated during the acute phase of the illness. Isolation is preferred until the nature of the responsible agent can be reasonably well established. Stool precautions should be observed in patients suspected of harboring enterovirus infections. Fortunately, most agents causing meningitis or encephalitis in this country are common in our environment and present little risk to hospital personnel. Strict isolation of patients returning from other countries with aseptic meningitis or encephalitis is mandatory until the nature of the agent is clear.

2. Headache can usually be alleviated with aspirin or acetaminophen administered every 4 hours. Occasionally codeine may be necessary.

3. Fever usually can be controlled with aspirin as necessary; severe hyperpyrexia warrants alcohol sponging or the use of cooling blankets.

4. The occurrence of generalized seizures, at least in children, does not necessarily indicate parenchymal involvement. The seizures should be treated as noted below. In the absence of clinical evidence of encephalitis or significant neurologic sequelae, seizures during the acute phase of viral meningitis do not necessarily presage the development of an epileptic disorder.

5. Attempts should be made to identify the agent responsible for the viral infection. These should include the collection of acute and convalescent sera (3 to 6 weeks later) for serologic testing by the appropriate state health department and viral cultures of the posterior nasopharynx, blood, urine, stool, and spinal fluid. If the expected benign clinical course is not met, repeat lumbar punctures are mandatory. Appropriate smears and culture of the cerebrospinal fluid (CSF) to rule out tuberculosis, fungus, or other agents presenting as an "aseptic" meningitis must be carried out on the initial specimens of all cases.

Viral Encephalitis

Supportive Measures. 1. All the supportive measures noted for viral meningitis are necessary for the patient with encephalitis. Since lethargy, stupor, or coma almost invariably develops, additional measures must be taken.

2. Intensive nursing care of the lethargic or comatose patient effectively prevents many secondary complications of immobilization such as aspiration pneumonia, urinary tract infection, decubitus ulcers, and contractures. Viral signs must be closely monitored. The patient should be positioned semiprone with the bed kept in slight Trendelenburg position to allow for easier clearing of pulmonary secretions and to avoid aspiration of vomitus. Secretions should be cleared fre-

quently, using nasopharyngeal suction. If necessary, a nasotracheal tube should be inserted; if coma is prolonged, a tracheostomy should be considered. The patient should be frequently turned, and optimally a foam or alternating air mattress should be provided to prevent pressure necrosis of skin. Physical therapy must be started early to prevent contracture. Passive range of motion of all limbs can be handled by the nursing staff and supplemented by physical therapists. The use of high cut gym shoes or foam boots should prevent Achilles tendon contracture or decubitus ulcer formation over the heels.

3. An intravenous line for administration of drugs should be established. The comatose patient may be maintained on parenteral fluids alone for a few days. Adequate nutrition should be provided over longer intervals by frequent, small volume nasogastric tube feedings. If coma is prolonged, consideration should be given to parenteral hyperalimentation. Inappropriate antidiuretic hormone secretion may complicate encephalitis; therefore serum electrolytes must be monitored frequently. The use of condom catheters facilitates nursing care of male patients; repeated catheterizations with strict attention to aseptic technique is preferable to long-term use of indwelling catheters in female patients.

4. *Seizures* may be aborted with a slowly administered intravenous bolus of diazepam (10 mg.). The prophylactic use of anticonvulsants for encephalitis is suggested by some. Once seizures occur, anticonvulsant therapy should certainly be instituted. Rapid protection from further seizures can be obtained with either parenteral phenytoin or barbiturate. Loading doses consist of either 1 to 1.5 grams of phenytoin given intravenously by slow infusion, not to exceed 50 mg. per minute, or 200 to 600 mg. of phenobarbital, 100 to 200 mg. given intravenously at a rate not to exceed 25 mg. per minute and the remainder intramuscularly in divided dosages. Maintenance doses of 300 to 400 mg. of intravenous phenytoin or 200 to 300 mg. of intramuscular phenobarbital a day should prove adequate. Phenytoin should not be administered by the intramuscular route, and phenytoin suspension given by nasogastric tube may be erratically absorbed. Blood anticonvulsant levels should be monitored as a useful aid to effective therapy.

5. *Cerebral edema* constitutes a major threat. Incipient herniation syndromes can be temporarily managed with osmotic diuretics. For an adult, 500 ml. of a 20 per cent mannitol solution can be administered over ½ to 1 hour (7.5 to 10 ml. per kg.). The repeated use of osmotic diuretics is decreasingly effective, and rebound increases in intracranial pressure can occur. Therefore osmotic diuresis can be considered only a temporary measure and should be followed with more definitive therapy such as surgical decompression or corticosteroids. Dexamethasone, 10 mg. by vein initially, and then 4 mg. every 4 to 6 hours, provides more lasting effects on intracranial hypertension. The possible benefit derived from corticosteroids when cerebral edema is clinically significant appears to outweigh their potential for immunodepression.

6. Early surgical decompression may be useful both to alleviate increasing intracranial pressure and to provide a definitive diagnosis, especially when specific antiviral therapy is contemplated. In any case, if decompressive brain biopsy is considered, prior arrangements should be made for the careful virologic and morphologic evaluation of the surgical specimen.

Specific Therapy. Several experimental antiviral agents have been used, primarily in herpes simplex type I encephalitis. Initially promising reports for idoxuridine (IUDR) and cytosine arabinoside (Ara C) have not been confirmed, and the toxicity of these drugs has been substantial. The efficacy of vidarabine (Vira-A) has recently been assessed in a carefully controlled study of biopsy-proved herpes encephalitis type I encephalitis. Improved survival and negligible drug toxicity were noted with use of this agent. Reduction of significant neurologic sequelae, however, requires early institution of drug therapy. Currently, vidarabine (Vira-A) is licensed for use as a topical agent only for herpes infection of eye and mucosal membranes. Approval for its use as a parenteral agent is pending. It appears that vidarabine may soon become the drug of choice in biopsy-confirmed herpes simplex encephalitis. Its efficacy in other viral encephalitides is uncertain and would be unlikely to be of value in encephalitis caused by RNA viruses.

Parainfectious Encephalomyelitis

Supportive Measures. General measures include those listed for acute viral meningitis and encephalitis. In patients presenting with acute myelopathy, particular attention must be directed to bowel and bladder care and to the prevention of contractures in paralyzed limbs.

Specific Measures. The use of corticosteroids to suppress the postulated cellular immune pathogenesis of the syndrome is controversial. The infrequent occurrence of the condition and the difficulty of confirming the clinical diagnosis in nonfatal cases make it unlikely that a careful controlled trial of any form of treatment will be possible for this disorder. By analogy with the effect of immunosuppressive agents in preventing or reversing the severity of experimental allergic encephalomyelitis, the use of steroids in selected instances of postinfectious encephalitis (particularly the acute hemorrhagic form of Weston and Hurst) is advocated.

MULTIPLE SCLEROSIS

method of
ELLIOTT M. MARCUS, M.D.
Worcester, Massachusetts

Multiple sclerosis is the most common cause of progressive neurologic disability in young and middle-aged adults in the United States, Canada, Northern Europe, and Australia–New Zealand. From a pathologic standpoint, it is a disease characterized by multifocal areas of demyelination of variable age within the central nervous system.

The underlying etiology remains unclear, despite much recent research implicating possible viral or immunologic factors. (See Porterfield [ed.]: Multiple sclerosis, Brit. Med. Bull., *33*:1–83, Jan., 1977.) It is apparent that there are certain familial and racial differences in susceptibility to multiple sclerosis and other immunologic disorders which appear to relate to the human leukocyte antigen (HLA) haplotype distribution. It is apparent that there must also be significant environmental factors that are operative before the age of 15 years, because multiple sclerosis has a marked prevalence to particular geographic latitudes within North America, Western Europe, and Australia. The environmental factors may be a viral agent such as the measles virus (patients with multiple sclerosis have an elevated measles antibody titer in serum and cerebrospinal fluid) or the transmissible factor described by Carp et al. and Henle et al. but subsequently unconfirmed (Madden et al.: Neurology, *27*:371, 1977). The characteristic alteration in percentage of immunoglobulin G (IgG) and of oligoclonal bonds in cerebrospinal fluid (CSF) in patients with multiple sclerosis is consistent with an immunologic response to a viral infection.

The elucidation of what may be a complex immunologic response of the nervous system to an infectious process obviously provides hope for the future regarding possible prevention of the disease. In this context, one may cite the analogy of the relationship of streptococcal infection to rheumatic heart disease and glomerulonephritis.

Advice as to Prognosis

There is a stereotypic image of a progressive disabling disease which pervades the public mind whenever the diagnosis of multiple sclerosis is mentioned. It is important for the patient to have a clear understanding that there are, from a prognostic standpoint, several varieties of multiple sclerosis. Thus one encounters many patients who have one or two or even multiple attacks of what was very clearly multiple sclerosis who then are not seen or heard from for many intervening years. When contacted, such patients indicated that no additional attacks or exacerbations have occurred. Examination of such patients reveals minor neurologic signs without actual disability. The actual frequency of such cases is certainly underestimated in long-term follow-up series. Thus in the series of McAlpine (Brain, *84*:186, 1961), among 241 patients followed for a minimum of 10 years, approximately one third were dead after severe disability, one third were disabled to a lesser degree but able to carry on most activities of daily living, and one third had no physical restrictions or disabilities as to work and home life. As regards survival, statistics derived from autopsy-proved cases suggest an average duration of disease of 12 to 14 years. The follow-up of young men seen in Army hospitals during World War II with the diagnosis of multiple sclerosis (Kurtzke et al.: Arch. Neurol., *22*:215, 1970) indicates a more favorable prognosis, with 76 per cent survival 20 years after onset and 69 per cent survival 25 years after onset. Such statistics then provide a more optimistic picture as regards the overall life plans of the individual patient.

Management of the patient with multiple sclerosis may be divided into essentially three sectors: (1) management of the acute episode, (2) avoidance of or minimization of exacerbation and progression, and (3) management of chronic neurologic disabilities.

Management of the Acute Episode

Objective: To end the exacerbation as rapidly as possible with the maximal preservation of neurologic function.

There is no specific agent available for treatment. There are nonspecific measures which may be employed:

1. Often fatigue and stress have played a role in the exacerbation or onset of an initial episode. There is, then, an indication for a period of rest. This does not have to be strict bed rest; rather, partial bed rest, avoidance of fatigue and stress, and temporary removal from a stressful job or family situation certainly are of value.

2. A febrile illness often precipitates the first episode or triggers an exacerbation. There are several mechanisms: (a) excessive heat in the environment with a subsequent increase in body temperature will produce a temporary worsening of symptoms, the reappearance of old symptoms, or the onset of new symptoms. In general, such effects are temporary, with a return to previous level

of function when temperature subsides to normal. Conversely, cooling, local or general, with a reduction in body temperature will produce a temporary improvement (Symington et al.: Neurology, *27*:302–303, 1977; Watson: New Eng. J. Med., *261*:1253–1259, 1959). (b) Febrile illness, however, also may play a role in exacerbating or triggering various diseases characterized by significant immunologic features. (c) When dealing with compromised spinal cord function, it is clear, moreover, that the state of spinal shock may recur in relation to a febrile illness, such as a urinary tract infection.

Obviously then, the cause of infection must be determined and treated in a specific manner.

From the general standpoint, hot baths, steam rooms or "baking in the sun" on a hot beach must be avoided. Cool baths for 15 minutes or longer may produce a temporary improvement. An ice collar over the spine also may produce some temporary improvement.

3. Adrenocorticotropic hormone (ACTH) and adrenocortical steroids continue to be employed in the acute phase of multiple sclerosis, although well controlled studies have often reported equivocal results. The cooperative study (Rose et al.: Neurology *18*:1, 1968; *20*:1, 1970) suggests that ACTH hastened improvement in symptoms and signs, although the ultimate improvement was not significantly greater than in the placebo-treated patients. Acute lesions of multiple sclerosis often have a significant element of edema and perivenous cellular infiltration (Adams: Brit. Med. Bull., *33*:15–20, 1977). There should then be significant anti-inflammatory effects possible with ACTH or steroids in the acute lesion. There is no substantial evidence that ACTH will achieve any greater anti-inflammatory effect than steroids which are much more convenient. Prednisone may be administered by the oral route; ACTH must be administered by the parenteral route.

Short-term, high dosage treatment is employed as follows: The majority of patients are admitted to the hospital for initiation of treatment and remain during the period of highest dosage—usually 10 days. It is rare in these relatively young patients to find a disease that would contraindicate the use of ACTH or steroids, but tuberculosis, renal disease, diabetes, peptic ulcer, and hypertension may prevent the use of these agents. Routinely the patients are placed on a low salt, bland diet and antacids. Daily weight and blood pressure charts are kept. If possible, the patient remains ambulatory.

We use prednisone, 80 mg. daily for 7 to 10 days, reduce the dose to 60 mg. daily for 5 days, to 40 mg. daily for 5 days, to 30 mg. daily for 5 days, to 20 mg. daily for 5 days, and then to 10 mg. daily for 5 days to complete a 4 to 6 week course. If ACTH gel is preferred, we would follow the routine of the cooperative study—i.e., 40 units of ACTH gel intramuscularly twice daily for 7 days, 20 units twice daily for 4 days, and 20 units daily for 3 days. It must be admitted that the doses and courses selected are arbitrary and titrated according to the patient response.

Hypokalemia, increased susceptibility to infection, peptic ulcer, and psychiatric disturbance may be seen with short-term treatment.

We have been particularly impressed with the value of such short-course steroid therapy in relation to demyelinating lesions involving the optic nerve or chiasm. Do we routinely treat all acute episodes? No, but we do treat when there is significant disability or evidence of rapid progression. We are influenced by the experience of previous episodes in the particular patient.

4. During the acute episode, the patient who is restricted to bed must receive passive motion exercises so that contractures do not develop. Depending on the degree and type of disability associated with the acute episode, a more active program of physiotherapy and occupational therapy may be started once the neurologic condition has stabilized. Fatigue must be avoided in both situations.

5. Time alone in some patients often results in a significant improvement in an acute episode. At times, such improvement occurs in a matter of days or weeks. Such rapid remissions, of course, complicate the evaluation of various treatment programs.

Avoidance of Exacerbations and of Progression

Patients differ in their pattern of disease. Some will have discrete episodes with relatively total recovery between episodes. Others will pursue a relatively relentless progressive course from the first episode or after subsequent episodes. Still others will have a stepwise increase in disability with succeeding episodes. There is no specific therapy to prevent recurrences or progression.

Diet. During the past few years, there has been a rebirth of interest in specific diets that might influence the course of multiple sclerosis. Two diets especially advocated recently are a gluten-free diet with vitamin and mineral supplements and a diet with the use of linoleate supplementation.

Over the years, a multiplicity of diets have been advocated, usually based on individual experience rather than scientific investigation. This is the case with the gluten-free diet. The studies of Liversedge (Brit. Med. Bull. *33*:80, 1977) indicate no effect on relapse rate of the course of the disease.

A finding of low levels of linoleic acid in the serum of multiple sclerosis patients during exacerbations has led to a double blind study of linoleate supplementation to the diet. After 2 years it was determined that there was no clear statistical evidence that linoleate supplementation affected clinical deterioration, although exacerbations were said to be fewer and less severe and responded quicker (Millar et al.: Brit. Med. J., *1*:765, 1973).

The Swank diet* advocates a low animal fat diet based upon epidemiologic studies in Norway and Switzerland, in which it was noted that the incidence of multiple sclerosis was low in areas where animal fat consumption was low, and higher among a population that had a high animal fat diet. Swank theorizes that high fat intake causes adhesiveness and aggregation of red blood cells, slowing of the circulation, and tissue hypoxia. In addition, he proposes that breaks in the blood-brain barrier occur and allow toxic substances to cross that lead to demyelination.

Our attitude has been to counsel the patient against placing high hopes on a specific diet, to be permissive with those who wish to try a proposed diet provided it is not harmful, and to caution all that a well balanced diet consumed in amounts consistent with an ideal weight is probably best.

Long-Term Treatment with Corticosteroids or ACTH. Anecdotal case histories of patients who develop recurrent symptoms and signs when an attempt is made to discontinue steroids after short-term treatment cause some physicians to continue prednisone or equivalent steroids on a daily, low dose (5 to 20 mg.) basis or as an alternate day double dose (10 to 40 mg.). The alternate day treatment is believed to minimize suppression of the hypothalamic-pituitary-adrenal axis.

Although there is a place for individual judgment in the treatment of a patient who has multiple sclerosis, benefit from long-term treatment with ACTH or corticosteroids has not been confirmed by group studies.

The use of intrathecal therapy with steroid agents (methylprednisolone acetate) is to be avoided. No therapeutic value has been demonstrated. Moreover, significant adverse reactions—adhesive arachnoiditis, aseptic meningitis, and pachymeningitis—have been reported with this treatment (Bernat et al.: Neurology, *26*:351–352, 1976).

Immunosuppressive Agents. The use of immunosuppressive agents (azathioprine, cyclophosphamide, and cytosine arabinoside) alone or in a combination with steroids is under investigation. The use of antilymphocyte globulin as an experimental technique resulted in a significant but temporary decrease in relapse rate. Any improvement was balanced by significant adverse side effects (Liversedge: Brit. Med. Bull. *33*:78, 1977). From a practical point of view, these agents should not be used randomly until the nature of the immunopathologic process is better understood.

Exercise and Activity. During periods when the disease is quiescent, all ambulatory patients are advised that daily walking is essential, and time should be set aside each day to walk a distance just short of unpleasant fatigue. Other exercise should be tailored to the patient's capacity and skills. Pool swimming, gardening, and stationary bicycling are suggested if appropriate.

In general, patients with neurologic disease causing difficulties in mobility tend to avoid activity, and one must constantly struggle with them to maintain the highest level of activity within their physical means. As already discussed, the psychologic paralysis is often greater than the actual disability. Whenever possible, the patient should be encouraged to maintain useful employment and other outside interests as long as possible.

Avoidance of Fever and Infections. See page 707.

Management of Chronic Neurologic Problems

Bladder Dysfunction. In the past few years, much has been learned of the central nervous system control of bladder function, and as a result we have a much better understanding of bladder dysfunction in multiple sclerosis and other diseases of the nervous system (Urol. Clin. North Amer., February 1974). The management of bladder dysfunction in multiple sclerosis was discussed in a most comprehensive manner by Dr. John Sullivan in the 1977 edition of Current Therapy. The discussion which follows has been abstracted with modifications from his presentation.

Bladder dysfunction may create intolerable embarrassment and discomfort. Most importantly, it may lead to early debility and death of the patient from recurrent infection and by promoting the development of decubitus ulcers.

It is our custom to inquire about bladder function early in the course of the disease. Often, the patient is unaware of subtle changes that have occurred. Urgency and incontinence are noted, of course, by the patient, but decreased bladder sensation, diminished force of the stream, and a lengthening of the intervals between voiding may have gone unnoticed.

Formerly, we tended to oversimplify and to

---

*Swank, R. L.: A Biochemical Basis of Multiple Sclerosis. Springfield, Ill., Charles C Thomas, 1961.

think in terms of upper and lower motor neuron types of bladder disturbance. Thus urgency, frequency, and uninhibited incontinence implied a suprasegmental lesion, a spastic bladder. Conversely, a large bladder capacity, disturbance of bladder sensation, difficulty in initiating voiding, and finally frequency, dribbling urination, and overflow incontinence equaled a segmental lesion and an atonic insensitive bladder. Animal experimentation, study of spinal cord injury patients, cystometry, and electromyography have provided more detailed and accurate information. However, multiple sclerosis does not provide a complete, static, and permanent lesion as in spinal cord injury. All varieties of neurogenic bladder may be seen in patients with multiple sclerosis, and a patient may show evidence of incomplete lesions at more than one level in the nervous system. Cerebral, brainstem, cerebellar, cord, and conus medullaris lesions may influence bladder function in varying degrees in the same patient.

Uninhibited Neurogenic Bladder. Lesions that interrupt the pathways from the frontal cortex to the pontomesencephalic reticular formation may result in the uninhibited neurogenic bladder. Since this system receives input from the cerebellum, basal ganglia, thalamus, and hypothalamus, the potential for plaques to partially interrupt this system can be readily understood. Inhibition of the micturition reflex may be defective. The patient has a decreased bladder capacity, but no residual urine. Infection therefore is not a problem. The uninhibited contractions may be modified by anticholinergic medication such as oxyphencyclimine (Daricon). (This use of oxyphencyclimine is not listed in the manufacturer's official directive.) Therapy is begun at 5 mg. twice daily and the dose titrated as necessary. The patient is instructed concerning excessive effects resulting in urinary retention. Propanthelamine bromide (Pro-Banthine), 15 mg. two or three times a day, may be employed instead of Daricon. (This use of propantheline is not listed in the manufacturer's official directive.)

Reflex Neurogenic Bladder. Lesions of the spinal cord above the conus medullaris produce this type of disorder, i.e., a spastic bladder. In multiple sclerosis the total picture may be present or various fragments may be encountered, depending upon the degree of damage to the spinal cord. Voluntary initiation of urination may be lost. There are uninhibited contractions and a reduced bladder capacity, and there may be residual urine. The latter is due to outlet obstruction, often caused by increased tone of the periurethral musculature. Some degree of bladder sensation may be retained, particularly if the lesions are located above the midthoracic spinal cord.

Early recognition and treatment of fragmentary and minor degrees of reflex neurogenic bladder are essential, because infection and interstitial cystitis may lead to a small contracted bladder, ureteral reflux, and pyelonephritis. The patient is trained from the beginning to regulate fluid intake in evenly measured amounts throughout the day, and to void "by the clock," ideally at 2½ to 3 hour intervals. Uninhibited contractions may be alleviated by anticholinergic drugs, as in the uninhibited neurogenic bladder. In severe degrees of reflex neurogenic bladder in males, it may be necessary to reduce resistance to outflow by doing a sphincterotomy and collecting urine with a condom and leg bag. In females, there is no satisfactory external collection system, and we may be forced to use a balloon plastic catheter. The largest size should be used to reduce intravesical pressure and to minimize the danger of plugging of the catheter by accretions. A plugged catheter must be cleared immediately. The incidence of bacteriuria rises sharply with an inlying catheter; if clinical signs of infection occur, short-term treatment with antibiotics is indicated. The selection of the antibiotic should be based on the results of sensitivity studies. We have found the combination of trimethoprim and sulfamethoxazole (Bactrim) to have a wide-range effect and to be convenient in dosage and relatively free of side effects.

Autonomous Neurogenic Bladder. In multiple sclerosis, the autonomous neurogenic bladder represents involvement of the conus medullaris and interruption of the vesical reflex arc. As there are varying degrees of sensory and motor-paralytic bladder, clinically it may be confused with spastic urgency, because if sensation is partially retained, there may be a sense of urgency with frequency and overflow incontinence. Urologic evaluation reveals a loss of voluntary micturition, voiding by the Credé method and abdominal straining, a large residual, and impaired bladder sensation. There may be local signs, a change in sacral sensation, and a loss of the anal reflex. In patients with minor degrees of sensory and motor paralysis the use of bethanechol (Urecholine) four times daily will be beneficial. The patient must develop methods of initiating voiding by coughing, contracting abdominal muscles, and compressing the lower abdomen. More severe degrees of dysfunction may require removing any obstruction to outflow (bladder neck resection) and a condom and collection bag in the male. Females may be taught sterile catheter technique for intermittent self-catheterization four times daily. In multiple sclerosis patients, fine hand control may be lost and members of the family may have to assist the patient.

Bladder Shock. An acute exacerbation

causing damage to the spinal cord may cause bladder shock in multiple sclerosis patients. Infection or other trauma may also induce this in a patient who has previously had a reflex neurogenic spastic bladder. The shock bladder may persist for days or months and is characterized by inability to void, loss of bladder tone, and absence of bladder contractions. This will present a changing and often confusing picture, and repeated urologic monitoring will be necessary to recognize returning function. In the meantime, bladder drainage will be necessary, preferably by intermittent sterile catheter technique. If this is not available, a plastic tube suprapubic drainage or balloon catheter may be necessary.

Patients who are unable to completely empty the bladder and those who have an indwelling catheter will develop bacteriuria. If there are no clinical signs of infection, this is not terribly important, although patients may complain of the odor of the urine. Acidifying the urine by the use of ascorbic acid and methenamine mandelate (Mandelamine) should inhibit bacterial growth of both gram-positive and gram-negative organisms, but it is least effective for Proteus and Pseudomonas organisms. In general, it is not a good practice to use antibiotics prophylactically.

Bowel Management. The incidence of constipation and fecal impaction is high in multiple sclerosis patients. This is particularly true of the incapacitated patient and may be due to an inability to exert force to expel feces. When frequent small diarrheal movements are occurring, an underlying fecal impaction may be found. For the patient who is confined to bed and chair, it is usually necessary to establish a routine of enemas or contact suppositories twice weekly.

Fortunately, if there is no underlying cause for diarrhea, bowel urgency and incontinence are uncommon. The usual history is one of sudden urgency and incontinence in social situations when the patient is fearful that this very catastrophe will happen. Evacuation of the bowel by suppository an hour or two in advance of social gatherings should provide protection.

Spasticity and Flexor Spasms. There is no satisfactory agent. The reduction of spasticity in the extensors may make any underlying weakness more apparent and thus defeat the aim of increasing ambulation. Diazepam (Valium) in moderate dosage of 4 to 10 mg. per day will reduce flexor spasms. Larger doses of 10 to 20 mg. per day will have some effect on spasticity but often at the expense of sedation.

Dantrolene sodium (Dantrium) has some moderate effects on spasticity. Some have found the drug to have only limited usefulness (Tolosa et al.: JAMA *233*:1046, 1975). The significant hepatotoxic effects of this drug preclude its use for any significant period of time (e.g., greater than 45 days). For these reasons, the use of this agent has now been discontinued by a number of neurologists.

Baclofen (Lioresal) has significant effects on spasticity without the sedative effects of diazepam or the hepatotoxic effects of dantrolene. In double blind comparison studies baclofen was more effective than diazepam or dantrolene in reducing spasticity associated with multiple sclerosis (Levine and VanBrocklin: Neurology, *27*:391, 1977). This drug is related to gamma aminobutyric acid (GABA); it acts at a spinal cord level by inhibiting mono- and polysynaptic transmission. It is widely employed in Europe and England (Amer. J. Phys. Med., *54*:175, 1975; Drugs, *8*:1, 1974), and release of the drug for use in the United States is projected for late 1977.

In patients with severe spasticity and spasm, the intrathecal injection of phenol should be considered, with referral of the patient to an anesthetist, neurosurgeon, or physiatrist skilled in this method.

The Spastic and/or Ataxic Gait. Disorders of gait resulting from damage to pyramidal tract, sensory, or cerebellar pathways represent a major cause of partial disability in many patients with progressive types of multiple sclerosis. Whenever possible the patient should be encouraged to remain ambulatory. Prolonged sitting in wheel chairs when a sensory deficit is present over the buttocks area may lead to the development of decubiti. Simple canes are often too narrow to provide much support. The use of a broad-tip or a three or four point cane provides a broader area of contact when ataxia is a major problem. A forearm aluminum crutch (Lofstrand) also will provide more support than the simple cane. A walker is sometimes advised, but patients often are reluctant to make use of this aid.

General points of advice with regard to gait include the following:

1. Inactivity leads to increased stiffness; activity should be encouraged.

2. Spasticity will result in limited range of motion at joints. The patient should have full range of motion at all upper and lower extremity joints several times daily. A physical therapist should instruct the patient and family in these exercises, which should be carried out in the home situation.

3. In a patient with sensory or cerebellar ataxia, spreading the feet and widening the stance will provide greater stability. Vision may be used to substitute for a proprioceptive defect.

Problems in the Care of the Bedridden or Chair-Bed–Limited Patient. These relate to skin care (the prevention of decubitus ulcers) and to care of joints (the prevention of contractures).

The following measures are utilized to prevent *decubiti* at pressure points:

1. A water mattress or air mattress should be employed.

2. Pressure points should receive adequate padding.

3. Change the position of the patient every two hours.

4. At each change of position, inspect the skin. Maintain a clean, dry condition.

5. Avoid any abrasions, as from adhesive tape.

6. Once an ulcer forms, months of hospitalization may be required with surgical repairs eventually necessary.

Contractures are the result of spasticity and immobility at the joints; usually a position of flexion develops.

1. Full range of motion exercises should be carried out several times per day.

2. At times, if possible, straighten the legs at night and then maintain this position by a sheet across the extended legs or by posterior splints.

3. In many patients, this is not possible or results in additional complications of decubiti. In such situations, if recovery of motor function is deemed unlikely, the chemical rhizotomy with intrathecal phenol, as discussed above, should be considered.

The total care of the patient with such a severe degree of disability severely strains the emotional and financial resources of the patient's family. The community resources must be recruited, in terms of visiting nurses and social workers. Often such incapacitated patients can be more effectively maintained in their home environment than in nursing homes. The visit of a physical therapist or occupational therapist to evaluate the home situation in terms of problems of daily living—e.g., grabrails, handrails, bed trapeze, eating utensils—may be of help.

In many cases, however, the family and/or community are unable to cope with the magnitude of the problems presented in terms of decubiti, contractures, urinary difficulties, and—in most progressive cases involving the cerebral hemispheres—the development of dementia and of emotional lability. In such a situation, in which long-term skilled care is required, placement in a chronic care hospital must eventually be considered.

Other Neurologic Problems Occurring During the Course of or as an Initial Symptom of Multiple Sclerosis. Trigeminal Neuralgia. The patient may present with classic trigeminal neuralgia as the first sign of his disease. In other patients, the typical pains in the face develop during the course of the illness. The patient may have sensory symptoms or findings not usually noted during the course of idiopathic trigeminal neuralgia.

1. Evaluate the patient for actual dental pathology. Dental hygiene in patients with chronic neurologic disease is often not good.

2. Institute a trial of phenytoin, 300 to 400 mg. per day. Check the patient's blood level in 7 to 10 days (therapeutic range, 10 to 20 micrograms per ml.).

3. If phenytoin is not successful, a trial of carbamazepine (Tegretol) is undertaken. Begin with 100 mg. twice daily and titrate upward to 800 to 1200 mg. per day. Check the patient's blood level in 2 to 4 days (therapeutic range, 4 to 13 micrograms per ml.).

(Note that both phenytoin and carbamazepine have significant toxicity relevant to the cerebellar system and thus may not be well tolerated in the patient who already has a significant degree of cerebellar deficit.

4. If the trial of carbamazepine is not successful, consideration should be given to neurosurgical referral for a selective thermal rhizotomy (radiofrequency lesion of the trigeminal ganglion). Excellent results may be obtained with preservation of tactile sensation.

Paroxysmal Tonic Seizures. These may occur in multiple sclerosis. A tonic stiffening of the limb occurs, often associated with a painful burning or tingling in the limbs of the same side. At times, the sensory phenomena occur in a contralateral manner (suggesting a Brown-Séquard pattern). These symptoms appear to be more commonly reported in Japanese patients, perhaps because spinal cord syndromes appear to be the predominant syndrome of multiple sclerosis in Japan (Toyokura et al.: Neurology, *26*:[2]18–19, 1976; Shibasaki and Kuroiwa: Arch. Neurol., *30*:47, 1974). The explanation for such paroxysmal spinal cord phenomena is not certain, but the possibility of ephaptic transmission between adjacent demyelinated fibers or of the altered excitability effects of deafferentation have been proposed as an explanation. Paroxysmal ataxia and dysarthria may also occur (Osterman and Westerberg: Brain, *98*:189–202, 1975).

In such paroxysmal syndromes, hyperventilation often has a provocative effect. The use of phenytoin (Dilantin) or of carbamazepine (Tegretol) often proves very effective in relieving symptoms. The use of acetazolamide (Diamox) has also been reported (Voiculesau et al.: J. Neurol. Neurosurg. Psychiat., *38*:191–193, 1975).

Epilepsy and Multiple Sclerosis. Although abnormalities in the electroencephalograms are common in multiple sclerosis, actual seizures are not a common accompaniment. However, generalized or focal seizures occur in greater frequency in multiple sclerosis patients than in the general population (Elian and Dean, *in* Penry: Epilepsy, the Eighth International Symposium; New York, Raven Press, 1977, pp. 341–344). The explanation for such seizures probably relates to partial cortical isolation effect with alteration in excitability, which a demyelination lesion in cortex and subcortex would provide. The treatment of such partial (focal), complex partial (temporal lobe), or generalized convulsive seizures is as discussed on pages 682 to 690.

TREMORS. Several types of tremors may occur in multiple sclerosis. In general, such tremors reflect involvement of the cerebellar fiber systems. Most often the tremor is of intention type; at times, a sustained positive tremor is present. Limbs or head or trunk may be involved. In most patients in whom only a moderate tremor is present, no specific treatment is required. When tremor is severe, the use of several medications may be considered. Diazepam (Valium) or chlordiazepoxide (Librium) may reduce tremor by reducing the anxiety which exacerbates any tremor or movement disorder. Such medications, however, also have side effects relevant to the cerebellar system in the sense of increasing ataxia. The beta-adrenergic blocker propranolol (Inderal) has been employed in essential tremor and might be considered in some patients with postural tremor of other cause. (This use of propranolol is not listed in the manufacturer's official directive.) When the tremor is severe and primarily unilateral, consideration may be given to neurosurgical relief via a stereotaxic lesion in the ventral lateral nucleus of the thalamus.

CONCURRENT MYASTHENIA GRAVIS. There have now been several series of cases reported in which both of these presumed immunologic disorders were present (Aita et al.: Neurology, *24*:72–75, 1974). Such patients may manifest variation in strength, diplopia, and dysarthria as a function of fatigue. Such patients may improve in relationship to the use of anticholinesterase agents and thymectomy.

Pregnancy. Pregnancy, per se, has no definite harmful effect. Occasional patients may experience an exacerbation. An exacerbation, however, is most likely to occur in the first several months after delivery, perhaps related to fatigue and nonspecific stress factors which may occur at this time relevant to the care of a newborn infant. The presence of a newborn infant in a family situation in which several young children are already present would obviously additionally increase the stress and fatigue factor. In such a situation, consideration should be given to limiting the number of pregnancies. One may also wish to advise a delay of 2 to 3 years after the last exacerbation before pregnancy is considered.

Alterations in Affect. Although euphoria has been considered a classic symptom of multiple sclerosis, the physician more often encounters emotional lability or depression. The emotional lability reflects the bilateral corticobulbar involvement with release of bulbar centers concerned in emotional expression.

Patients with significant frontal white matter lesions may manifest considerable apathy.

Depression occurs in a number of patients, often unrelated to the actual severity of the disease. Depression is, of course, a common symptom in many chronic diseases.

A positive rehabilitation-physiotherapy program often has a considerable role to play in dealing with much of this depression which occurs as a reaction to the chronic disease state. In some patients, the use of amitriptyline (Elavil) may be considered. For more severe depressions, psychiatric consultation is indicated.

MYASTHENIA GRAVIS

method of
FRANK M. HOWARD, JR., M.D.
Rochester, Minnesota

Myasthenia gravis is a disease that can produce weakness in any skeletal muscle and it affects persons at any age and of either sex, although it has a predilection for young women and older men. The weakness is characteristically but not invariably made worse by exercise and is improved by rest. Patients with this illness learn that periods of rest play an important role in treatment. However, physicians who examine patients who complain of weakness should make certain to have them exercise if no weakness is demonstrated in the resting state.

The most common symptoms are ptosis and diplopia, and at times the disease remains confined to the extraocular muscles—ocular myasthenia gravis. Most often it also involves the bulbar, neck, and extremity muscles. It may present with symptoms in any of these areas, and the diagnosis is most often missed in two categories of patients: (1) young girls experiencing the onset of the disease in the leg muscles which causes them to fall and (2) older patients in whom the disease is manifested as dysarthria and dysphagia and who are erroneously thought to have had a stroke. A chronic fatigue state without weakness is not myasthenia gravis.

Approach to Treatment

Since the cause of the disease is unknown, there is no ideal method of treatment. Because there is no way of predicting which patients will undergo a remission after thymectomy, and because of the side effects of corticosteroids and immunosuppressive agents, I still start all newly diagnosed patients on anticholinesterase medication. They are re-evaluated in 3 to 6 months. If control of symptoms is not ideal and the patient has generalized myasthenia gravis and is less than 55 years old, thymectomy is recommended. Long-term steroid therapy is reserved for older patients or those who do not respond to thymectomy. Plasmapheresis and immunosuppressive agents are considered only when all else fails.

Anticholinesterase Drugs

This type of medication has been used for more than 40 years. Three preparations are available. Table 1 lists these drugs with equivalent doses for various routes of administration. All have the same action, and one offers little advantage over the others. There is no benefit in using combinations of these drugs, and it only confuses the patient. The number of receptor sites for acetylcholine on the postsynaptic muscle membrane of patients with myasthenia gravis is reduced. The enzyme acetylcholine esterase is concentrated in close proximity to this membrane and causes acetylcholine to hydrolyze and become ineffective. The anticholinesterase drugs temporarily block this action and allow the acetylcholine both to persist for a longer time and to diffuse more widely along the junctional area.

The aim of treatment is to restore strength to as nearly normal as possible and to allow full activities, including sports. Most patients, however, will have some degree of weakness despite optimal therapy. Because of variations in the severity of the disease and frequent fluctuations in strength throughout the day, the program of medication must have some flexibility. Patients are best managed when they are thoroughly instructed in the use of the medication and its potential side effects and then allowed to vary their dose as necessary. All myasthenic patients tend to be frightened, and they are very much dependent on their physicians; it takes a considerable number of visits before they learn to live in harmony with their illness.

My own preference is to begin therapy with one 60 mg. tablet of pyridostigmine (Mestinon) three times daily. For those who prefer neostigmine (Prostigmin), the drugs can be interchanged on a tablet-for-tablet basis, but ambenonium (Mytelase) should be avoided unless the physician is familiar with this drug, because the equivalent dose is less than the smallest available tablet. Patients who have difficulty in chewing and swallowing should take medication 1 hour before meals so that they are at maximum strength during the meal. Individual doses are gradually increased by one-half tablet until maximum benefit is obtained. It is rare that an increase in the individual dose to more than three tablets results in any significant increase in strength. Most patients are weakest in the late afternoon, and a fourth dose between 3 P.M. and 4 P.M. is usually necessary. The duration of drug action varies between 2 and 4 hours. The major mistake in treatment is to try to adhere to a rigid time schedule. Nothing except unnecessary disability results when the patient waits 4 hours between doses when weakness develops 3 to 3½ hours after the previous dose. The dosage schedule is, therefore, tailored to the individual patient's need. The edrophonium test can be of benefit at times in adjusting the dose. One hour after the last dose, 0.2 ml. (2 mg.) of edrophonium, and never more than this amount, is given intravenously. If there is definite improvement in strength, the dose of pyridostigmine is increased. If there is no change in strength or if weakness increases, the dose should not be changed. During this initial period of titration of the dose, the patient should be hospitalized, especially if there are significant bulbar symptoms.

Pyridostigmine bromide (Mestinon) Timespan, 180 mg., is a prolonged-release form that exerts its effect over 8 to 10 hours. It is given at bedtime if the patient experiences weakness during the night or has weakness of significant degree

TABLE 1. **Average Equivalent Doses of Anticholinesterase Drugs**

		ROUTE AND DOSE (MG.)			
DRUG	TABLET SIZE, MG.	*Oral*	*Intramuscular*	*Intravenous*	*Syrup*
Neostigmine bromide (Prostigmin)	15	15	—	—	—
Neostigmine methylsulfate (Prostigmin)	—	—	1.0–1.5	0.5	—
Pyridostigmine bromide (Mestinon)	60	60	2.0	1.5–2.0	60 mg./5 ml.
Mestinon Timespan	180	90–180	—	—	—
Ambenonium chloride (Mytelase)	10 and 25	5.0–7.5	—	—	—

on awakening in the morning. The use of this preparation during the day should be avoided because the rate of release is unpredictable, and regular tablets provide more flexibility in varying the dosage. Patients sometimes observe the Timespan tablet in their stool. However, this is just the carrier portion of the tablet and the active ingredient has been absorbed.

Pyridostigmine and neostigmine are available in other forms. Syrup of pyridostigmine (1 teaspoonful equals 60 mg.) is of limited use. It sometimes is given to small children or administered through a nasogastric tube. Injectable neostigmine is available in solutions of 0.25 mg. per ml., 0.5 mg. per ml., and 1.0 mg. per ml. The injectable form of pyridostigmine contains 2 mg. per ml. It is rarely necessary to give these drugs intravenously, but intramuscular injection is of benefit in patients who cannot swallow the tablets. For equivalent doses, see Table 1.

Side Effects of Anticholinesterase Drugs. Because acetylcholine is the neurotransmitter for the muscarinic receptors of the parasympathetic nervous system and sweat glands, a variety of side effects may occur (Table 2). The most common are gastrointestinal, including nausea, abdominal cramping, and diarrhea. In addition, many myasthenic patients have a lax anal sphincter and can experience rectal incontinence. These side effects can be minimized by administering the drug with milk or a cracker if the patient has no difficulty swallowing. Other patients may require an occasional tablet of atropine sulfate 0.4 mg. ($^1/_{150}$ grain), or diphenoxylate (Lomotil). Codeine sulfate, 16 mg. (¼ grain), is very useful for patients who have rectal incontinence, especially before social activities or trips during which bathroom facilities are not readily accessible.

TABLE 2. **Unwanted Effects of Anticholinesterase Medication (Cholinergic Reactions)**

Muscarinic	*Nicotinic*
On smooth muscle	On skeletal muscle
Epigastric discomfort	Fasciculations (twitching)
Abdominal cramps	Spasm
Anorexia	Weakness
Nausea	*Central nervous system*
Vomiting	Irritability
Diarrhea	Anxiety
Pupillary miosis	Insomnia
On glands	Unpleasant dreams
Increased salivation	Dysarthria
Cold, moist skin	Mental clouding
Increased lacrimation	Syncope
Increased bronchial secretion	Coma
	Convulsions

The most ominous reaction is an increase in muscle weakness 1 hour after the anticholinesterase medication has been taken. It suggests overdosage and may indicate impending cholinergic crisis. Patients should be thoroughly aware of this possibility, because the natural tendency is to take more medication.

The other side effects are seldom encountered; they were seen mainly with the use of prolonged-action anticholinesterase drugs, which are no longer available.

Other Medications

Several drugs have been used as adjuncts in treatment. An occasional patient seems to benefit from ephedrine sulfate, 25 mg. three times daily. Potassium chloride, calcium chloride, germine monoacetate, and guanidine have also been used; these agents are relatively ineffective, and guanidine has major toxic side effects, including aplastic anemia.

Drugs to Avoid

Various antibiotics have the potential of producing neuromuscular blockade, but standard doses of the commonly used antibiotics seldom produce any problem. Neomycin, polymyxin, kanamycin, and colistin should be avoided if at all possible; if these are used, the patient should be carefully observed.

Procainamide, quinidine, quinine, and chlorpromazine have been reported to cause exacerbation of weakness. Although tonic water contains quinine, it is present in small amounts and is safe unless large amounts are ingested.

Myasthenic patients are more sensitive than normal persons to morphine sulfate, and meperidine (Demerol) is preferred. These patients are also very sensitive to muscle-relaxing agents such as succinylcholine used at the time of surgery.

With the exception of smallpox vaccination, immunizations are well tolerated.

Nerve blocks utilizing local anesthetics, e.g., for dental extractions, can be safely used.

Management of Crisis

The term "crisis" implies a fairly rapid exacerbation of weakness, especially difficulty with respiration. It may be secondary to infection (for example, pneumonia), failure to take medication, or overdosage with anticholinesterase medication. Many times the cause is unknown. This condition is a true emergency. If the patient is unduly apprehensive, has labored breathing with the use of accessory muscles, or is unable to swallow saliva, either nasotracheal intubation or tracheostomy should immediately be considered. If equipment to measure inspiratory force, tidal volume, and vital capacity is available, this can be utilized to help make the decision. However, the decision is a clinical one, and undue delay in intubation can lead to death.

Although theoretically an edrophonium test might be of value, under these circumstances it is unsatisfactory. The patient is apprehensive and cooperates poorly, and the brief duration of action makes evaluation difficult. The clinical axiom—"if in doubt, intubate or do a tracheostomy"—can rarely be challenged. If possible, this should be performed by a physician who is experienced in these techniques, and it should not be done frantically at the last moment. A cuffed tracheostomy or nasotracheal tube is utilized and a respirator is attached. With adequate respiration established, the patient's examination can be completed with a search for possible infection or other medical problems. All anticholinesterase medication should be withheld for 24 to 48 hours while the patient remains in the respiratory care unit. This approach is effective whether the patient is suffering from an overdose (cholinergic crisis) or is refractory to anticholinesterase medication (myasthenic crisis). It also minimizes salivation and tracheobronchial secretions and obviates the use of atropine, which can lead to inspissated, tenacious secretions. The care of these patients is similar to that of any patient on a respirator: namely, precautions against infection, meticulous observation and nursing care, and the routine use of wide-spectrum antibiotics. Nasogastric feeding is used when necessary.

After 48 hours, a test dose of 1.0 mg. of neostigmine is given intramuscularly. If definite improvement is observed, a regular schedule of intramuscular neostigmine is established, with judgment being made whether the dose should be increased by 0.5 mg. increments. Conversion to oral medication is done as soon as the patient can swallow without danger. Patients who require respiratory assistance for more than 72 hours should be considered as candidates for steroid therapy. An optimistic, confident staff adds much-needed emotional support to these patients. The most desperately ill patient still has a good chance of improvement to the point of remission.

Thymectomy

The value of thymectomy in treatment has been established. The mechanism by which thymectomy induces a remission is unknown, although it is presumed that removal of the thymus acts in some beneficial way on the autoimmune mechanism. Controversy remains whether all patients should have this operation or whether there should be selection of patients. It is known that patients with congenital myasthenia gravis do not respond well, and elderly patients may not have any demonstrable thymic tissue. Except for patients with only ocular symptoms, we recommend thymectomy for patients less than 55 years old who are handicapped in some way despite the use of anticholinesterase medication. Males respond as well as females, and although results appear to be more favorable if the disease has been present less than 2 years, remissions can occur in patients who have had symptoms for many years. Most statistics indicate that thymectomy will result in prolonged complete remission in 40 per cent of patients and that an additional 40 per cent will be significantly improved.

Although some centers advocate a transcervical approach, the majority continue to utilize a substernal split procedure in order to remove all of the thymic tissue. The operation has a very low mortality, and the patient has the added benefit that he is free from the possibility that a thymoma will develop (15 per cent incidence) later in life. Patients who have myasthenia gravis and a thymoma have a poorer prognosis; only 10 per cent experience a remission, and before steroid therapy two thirds of these patients died of their disease within 5 years. Even with the use of steroids, they present very difficult problems in management.

Thymectomy is looked on as a relatively minor procedure for a skilled thoracic surgeon. However, it is imperative that postoperatively the patient be in a respiratory intensive care unit until respiratory function has been shown to be adequate. All anticholinesterase medication should be withheld until weakness clearly develops. This may not occur for 10 to 24 hours postoperatively, and an occasional patient never needs medication. Meperidine is the preferred drug for analgesia.

Some centers advocate corticosteroid therapy before thymectomy. This is rarely required except for patients who have severe bulbar myasthenia, but steroids should be used if convalescence from surgery is prolonged.

Corticosteroid Therapy. The use of ACTH intramuscularly has largely been replaced by the administration of prednisone orally. ACTH therapy was administered in a dosage of 100 units daily for 10 days; and in the latter half of the treatment period, increased weakness developed which often required use of a respirator. Within 2 days after ACTH was stopped, there was often a rebound in strength, but these remissions seldom lasted more than a few months. Prednisone, on the other hand, rarely causes a dramatic increase in weakness when therapy is initiated, and patients can remain on a relatively small maintenance dose, taken on alternate days, for prolonged periods.

Although a carefully controlled study of an adequate number of patients treated with alternate-day prednisone has not been carried out, there is now overwhelming evidence that this regimen has been very successful in restoring most handicapped myasthenic patients to a full life.

If thymectomy fails to produce a remission or if the patient is elderly and does not respond well to anticholinesterase medication, alternate-day prednisone therapy is advocated, and it has been beneficial even in patients who have only ocular involvement. The ocular symptoms typically respond poorly to anticholinesterase medication. A wide variety of dosage schedules are now employed, and all patients except those with only ocular symptoms should be hospitalized for the initiation of treatment, because there may be dramatic worsening with as little as 25 mg. of prednisone, although this is uncommon. Patients are best referred to a center that has had considerable experience for initiation of this treatment.

The general principle is either to start with a dosage of 25 mg. of prednisone on alternate days and gradually increase the dose or to begin with a large dose, 100 mg., on alternate days. At times, the patients are given small doses of prednisone on their "off" day to smooth out the course, because patients are usually weaker on the off day early in the course of the treatment. As muscle strength improves, the dose of anticholinesterase medication is gradually reduced. The patient is maintained on high-dosage, alternate-day prednisone for several months and then tapered to a maintenance dose of 25 mg. every other day for an indefinite period. If the dose is reduced below this level, myasthenic symptoms will usually recur and high doses will again be required to bring the symptoms under control.

The patients must follow the usual precautions for steroid therapy and have periodic follow-up examinations. The following program can be recommended for laboratory studies:

1. Every 3 months: hemogram, serum potassium, and fasting blood sugar. If the patient has a positive tuberculin test and is taking isoniazid, liver function studies are required.
2. Every 6 months: chest roentgenogram (posteroanterior and lateral).
3. Every year: stereoscopic view of the pelvis with a Singh index for osteoporosis. Ophthalmologic examination for cataracts.

The majority of patients who fail to respond to prednisone are either congenital myasthenics or patients who have had thymomas. In these situations, a small number of patients have been treated with immunosuppressive agents such as azathioprine, cyclophosphamide, and methotrexate, and, more recently, plasmapheresis. These are experimental forms of treatment and should be carried out only by clinical investigators because of the many potential hazards. The value of these types of treatments has not been established.

Other Diseases Encountered in Patients with Myasthenia Gravis

The most commonly associated disease is thyrotoxicosis. Approximately 5 per cent of myasthenic patients will experience this illness at some time. Both diseases are treated simultaneously. Other autoimmune diseases have been encountered at a higher incidence than in a normal population, and these include rheumatoid arthritis, systemic lupus erythematosus, pernicious anemia, Hashimoto's thyroiditis, and ulcerative colitis.

Surgery in Patients with Myasthenia Gravis

There is no contraindication to surgical procedures in myasthenic patients. If the patient's condition is well controlled on alternate-day prednisone therapy, the patient is given a steroid preparation and after surgery he is maintained on his alternate-day schedule. If the patient is receiving an anticholinesterase agent, this drug is withheld postoperatively (just as with a thymectomy) until there is clear weakness. For unknown reasons, the patient is stronger in the immediate postoperative period, and giving anticholinesterase too soon may lead to a cholinergic reaction. Transurethral resection of the prostate is apt to lead to urinary incontinence unless a smaller amount of tissue than usual is resected.

Menses, Pregnancy, and Birth Control Pills

Menses may lead to exacerbation of weakness; and during this time, the patient may require additional rest and increased amounts of pyridostigmine. Thymectomy and other operations should be planned in such a way as to avoid the time of menses.

Myasthenic patients generally tolerate pregnancy and delivery without major problems. There may be some improvement or worsening. Improvement, if it occurs, is usually seen in the later phase of pregnancy, and there may be exacerbation after delivery. Children born to myasthenic mothers may have transient neonatal myasthenia gravis, with a poor cry, impaired respiration, problems in sucking, and feeble movements. If this occurs, the baby is given 0.1 to 0.25 mg. of neostigmine intramuscularly 45 minutes before feedings or is fed by nasogastric tube. This self-limited condition lasts only a few days to a few weeks and is thought to be due to maternal antibodies passing through the placenta to the child. It is extremely rare for the child to experience myasthenia gravis at a later date. Every baby born to a myasthenic mother, even if she is in remission, should be observed for this possible complication.

Birth control pills are usually well tolerated. Occasionally, the patient may become weaker; if this occurs, other contraceptive methods should be employed.

Myasthenia Gravis in Children

This disorder may occur as a congenital syndrome—that is, the child is myasthenic at birth even though the mother does not have myasthenia gravis. Small doses of anticholinesterase medication are used, proportionate to the size of the child, either by injection or as syrup of pyridostigmine. Congenital myasthenia may be a different syndrome, for it does not respond well to thymectomy or to steroids. These children are usually restricted in their activities, but they seldom die of their disease.

Myasthenia gravis can also develop at any time after birth. The sex ratio of males to females is equal until puberty, when there is a dramatic increase in the number of females affected by myasthenia gravis. If the child does not respond well to anticholinesterase therapy, thymectomy is performed. Our youngest patient was 2½ years of age. Long-term follow-up of these children has failed to show any increased incidence of other diseases, and this approach is preferable to steroid therapy with its potential complications.

Prognosis

With the advent of respiratory intensive care units, the lowered mortality of thymectomy, and the effectiveness of steroid therapy, death from myasthenia gravis is uncommon. Most patients can lead full and active lives, and some have competed in college sports, including football and track. The goal of treatment is to allow the patient to lead a life free of restrictions if at all possible. This can be accomplished only if the patient thoroughly understands the disease and its management and is not treated as an invalid living in fear of an impending catastrophe.

TRIGEMINAL AND GLOSSOPHARYNGEAL NEURALGIA

method of
G. ROBERT NUGENT, M.D.
Morgantown, West Virginia

Trigeminal Neuralgia

Trigeminal neuralgia is a specific clinical entity which is usually easily diagnosed. It predominantly affects the elderly, with sudden attacks of severe but short-duration pain limited to one or more divisions of the fifth cranial nerve. It is rare for it to begin in or be limited to the region of the eye and forehead. Often there is a trigger area in the region of the pain where even light touch may set off a paroxysm of pain. The pain may also be initiated by eating, talking, brushing the teeth, or washing the face. Although the cause is obscure, there is evidence that in some cases vascular lesions affecting the fifth nerve in the posterior fossa may be an underlying cause of the condition. It may also be seen with neoplasms in the cerebellopontine angle and in younger patients who have multiple sclerosis.

Medical Therapy. In recent years carbamazepine (Tegretol) has replaced phenytoin as a mainstay in the treatment of trigeminal neuralgia. This is given in a starting dosage of ½ tablet (100 mg.) morning and evening first day, 200 mg. morning and evening second day, 300 mg. morning and evening third day, and 400 mg. (2 tablets) morning and evening fourth day. In some patients it can be increased to a total of 6 tablets a day. Although carbamazepine effectively relieves the pain within a few days in almost all patients, it is a drug that must be used with considerable caution. Side effects include rash, dizziness and ataxia, leukopenia, and aplastic anemia. It should not be used if there has been pre-existing heart, renal, or liver disease, and a complete blood count should be performed every 2 to 4 weeks during the course of therapy. Liver function studies should also be performed at the onset of therapy, as well as periodically thereafter. Now that patients have been on this drug for several years, it seems that many are experiencing incomplete relief of pain or are so bothered by the side effects that they seek other forms of therapy.

Phenytoin also offers relief for some in a dosage of 100 mg. three or four times a day. Periodic blood levels may have to be obtained to ensure that a level of 10 to 15 micrograms per ml. is obtained.

In our experience vitamin B_{12} has been of no value as a therapeutic agent.

Alcohol Injections. When the pain involves the region of the cheek with a trigger area in the upper lip or side of the nose, the pain can often be eliminated for several months by an alcohol block of the infraorbital nerve.

With a trigger area in the lower jaw or lip, the mandibular branch can similarly be blocked at the point where this nerve makes its exit from the foramen ovale at the base of the skull, or by making a radiofrequency lesion at the same place.

In skilled hands, alcohol can be injected in minute amounts into the gasserian ganglion itself for more permanent relief of pain. The danger here is that the alcohol may flow through the subarachnoid space and involve other cranial nerves—sometimes with disastrous results.

Intracranial Surgery. In the past few years two new methods of treating the disease have been introduced which may soon supplant the time-honored subtemporal operation of Frazier, in which pain relief is obtained by sectioning or traumatizing the nerve.

The operating microscope has permitted a much closer examination of the trigeminal nerve as it courses through the cerebellopontine angle. This has revealed, in a high incidence of cases, abnormal blood vessels which appear to be compressing the trigeminal nerve. With microdissection these vessels can be removed from the nerve and separated from it, relieving the pain with preservation of all sensation in the face. This would appear to be the ideal form of treatment. It requires, however, a microneurosurgeon who is skilled in these newer techniques and who is familiar with operations in the posterior fossa. Many elderly patients are not candidates for such major intracranial surgery.

The other new form of therapy involves radiofrequency ablation of the trigeminal nerve in the region of the ganglion. In this procedure, which we have performed over 500 times, an 18 gauge lumbar puncture needle is inserted, with radiographic guidance, through the cheek and ultimately through the foramen ovale at the base of the skull. This places it in the rootlets behind the ganglion. An electrode can then be inserted so that low voltage stimulation evokes a tingling sensation in the face, corresponding to the area of the nerve in which the electrode lies. In this way the awake patient helps the surgeon adjust the electrode so that the area of pain can be treated. A radiofrequency current, which generates heat, is used to partially destroy the nerve fibers behind the ganglion, thus preventing regeneration. With this method, controlled ablation of the nerve is possible, permitting the selective treatment of the area of pain with sparing of the unaffected areas. In most cases the pain can be permanently abolished with the preservation of touch sensation in the face. The corneal reflex can usually be spared even if pain to be treated involved the eye and forehead. In the past 320 procedures the corneal reflex has been lost only 4 times. There is no possibility of facial paralysis with this treatment, and the patient usually leaves the hospital the day after the treatment. This technique, which avoids an open operation, appears to be a most promising new approach to the cure of the disease.

Glossopharyngeal Neuralgia

This pain is similar in nature to trigeminal neuralgia, except that the pain is localized to the tonsillar fossa and ear and is precipitated by swallowing. The patient may be aided in eating by the topical application of 1 per cent tetracaine (Pontocaine) or 2 per cent viscous lidocaine (Xylocaine) to the tonsillar region. When surgery is necessary, as it often is, section of the glossopharyngeal nerve and upper branches of the vagus in the posterior fossa nicely relieves the pain.

OPTIC NEURITIS

method of
J. LAWTON SMITH, M.D.
Miami, Florida

Definition

Medical semantics often blows with the winds of popularity, and may depend more upon what is in vogue at the moment than on strict English etymology. One might think that "optic neuritis" should mean "inflammation of the optic nerve." That would be like saying that "tonsillitis" means "inflammation of the tonsil" or "appendicitis" means "inflammation of the appendix." However, today many clinicians use the term "optic neuritis" as having a broader scope. They use it to describe any acute or subacute involvement of the optic nerve due to any cause whatever. We must remember that the "itis" and "opathy" clubs are both active in the eye field just as elsewhere. Why does one man speak of "optic neuritis" and another prefer to say "optic neuropathy?" You might think that "optic neuropathy" would mean any pathologic process in the optic nerve that is *not* inflammatory—if one is going to use that term rather than "optic neuritis." Certainly "neuropathy" is a nonspecific term meaning simply that the nerve is sick or diseased—or even in "pathos!" You might recall "nephritis" versus "nephropathy," or "peripheral neuritis" versus "peripheral neuropathy," or, in the old days, "diabetic retinitis" versus "diabetic retinopathy." Before you give up and throw this article away, let me leave two suggestions with you. First, Dr. Frank B. Walsh has emphasized that the diagnosis of "*chronic* optic neuritis" is usually *wrong*. I agree with that so much that I say: "The commonest cause of *chronic* optic neuritis is a *meningioma!*" If you accept that, we now have something to hang our hats on; if it can't be *chronic,* we are left *only* with *acute* and *subacute!* Let us therefore arbitrarily restrict the term "optic neuritis" to something showing *clinical activity* in the optic nerve over a period of *less than 3 months.* Second, let's use the term "optic neuritis" when we believe the process is *inflammatory* or *demyelination,* and let's say "optic neuropathy" when we think something else is going on (ischemia, toxicity, degeneration, or neoplasia). These definitions may not be right, but at least they are definite—so let's move on!

Classification

There are several classifications of optic neuritis. The subject is so confused, and the terminology and literature so vast, that I am simply going to give you the following from my personal experience and try to keep this as simple as possible. There are two simple ways to look at optic neuritis, as seen in Tables 1 and 2.

"Neuroretinitis" means that both the optic nerve head (optic disc, or papilla) and the adjacent retina are involved. You can see all of this in the fundus. "Papillitis" means the process primarily involves that "papilla" or optic disc or optic nerve head. "Retrobulbar neuritis" means the process is behind the globe. You may recall the old adage taught to medical students for years: "If you see a choked disk and the patient can see, it's papilledema; if you see a choked disc and the patient can't see, it's papillitis; if you don't see anything and the patient can't see anything, it's retrobulbar neuritis!" There are a few exceptions to this (you certainly can see patients with optic neuritis who have good visual acuity!), but the general statement still contains a *lot of truth* and therefore is a helpful way to start looking at the subject! Chiasmal optic neuritis is really rare and simply means that the process in the optic nerve has extended on back to also involve the chiasm as well. It was put in Table 1 simply for completeness. The two *big* ones on that list are "papillitis" and "retrobulbar neuritis."

Another way to look at optic neuritis is to consider an etiologic or pathogenetic classification of the problem. There are many loopholes in this, and we even get into trouble with the nomenclature previously proposed, but Table 2 includes the *commonest* things encountered in the differential diagnosis of optic neuritis. Let's look at these briefly.

TABLE 1. **The Ophthalmoscopic Classification of Optic Neuritis**

1. Neuroretinitis
2. Papillitis
3. Retrobulbar neuritis
4. Chiasmal optic neuritis

TABLE 2. **Etiologic Classification of Optic Neuritis**

1. Inflammatory
2. Postinfectious
3. Demyelinizing
4. "Ischemic optic neuropathy"
5. "Toxic amblyopia"
6. Leber's optic nerve disease
7. Idiopathic
8. Others

Inflammatory Optic Neuritis

Although not really too common, this form of optic neuritis was put first on the list because no one has a problem appreciating the fact that purulent inflammation of the optic nerve and its sheaths can occur during the course of meningococcal meningitis or other forms of meningitis (such as staphylococcal, pneumococcal, fungal, and the like). Acute optic neuritis may also occur during the course of mumps, measles, and other viral infections. Optic neuritis may occur in syphilis, infectious mononucleosis, and other infectious illnesses. In these cases, the treatment for the optic neuritis obviously is to manage the primary illness. Inflammatory optic neuritis can complicate nasal sinus disease but this is rare, and for practical purposes does not occur unless suppurative sinus disease breaks outside the bony confines of the sinus itself; for example, purulent ethmoiditis may spread into the orbit, causing orbital cellulitis with concomitant involvement of the optic nerve and its vaginal sheath.

Postinfectious Optic Neuritis

This is a much more common form of optic neuritis as seen in office practice in ophthalmology. A young woman in her 20's presents with a rather sudden onset of blurred vision in the left eye. She may or may not have noted a bit of pain on motion of the globe on that side. Her vision is 20/20 right and 20/70-1 left—there is a 2 + Marcus Gunn pupil on the left—and the fundi are perfectly normal in both eyes. Careful history reveals that she had a "flu"-like illness about 2 to 3 weeks ago. She might even be on "the pill", too—for another complicating factor! This is a common picture of so-called "postinfectious" optic neuritis, which presumably is due directly to the viral infection that the patient had, or to some form of allergic reaction set up by the viral infection. The patient should be taken off "the pill" and advised to get more rest and to have a well balanced diet; the process probably will improve on its own within a few weeks. Six weeks to 3 months is about "par" for the course. I probably would give the patient 1 ml. (40 mg.) of aqueous triamcinolone (Kenalog) by sub-Tenon's injection to the left orbit in this case, hoping to expedite her rate of recovery. Since the outlook in such a patient is in general good, I'd not advise systemic or oral steroids in this patient on the first attack.

One needs to avoid excessive work-up in these patients. A good neurologic history is important. Hospitalization is not indicated on the first attack. One could simply wait 3 days on the sub-Tenon's Kenalog injection; if not definitely better by then, she should have a good general physical examination, routine hemogram, serologic tests for syphilis (VDRL and FTA-ABS), urine, and chest x-ray. The single injection of Kenalog often lasts 2 to 4 weeks and probably would not have to be repeated. One should not become concerned in retrobulbar optic neuritis if the vision drops even to no light perception, for it will still clear in about 90 per cent of the patients.

Demyelinizing Optic Neuritis

Multiple sclerosis always is a cause for concern when one sees a young patient (late teens to about 40 years) with optic neuritis. The incidence of developing multiple sclerosis after a bout of optic neuritis has varied in the literature between 10 and 50 per cent, and probably is about 20 to 25 per cent. A careful neurologic history can be of great help in these cases. One should always look for *Uhthoff's sign* and *Lhermitte's symptom. Uhthoff's sign* is a drop in visual acuity associated with heat or exercise. One should ask patients if they have noted any change in vision following a hot shower. The "real McCoy" patient may tell you: "Why, doctor, I took a steaming hot shower the other day, and when I got out of the tub, I couldn't even see to find my way back to the bedroom! I had to sit down on the side of the bed and rest for 10 to 15 minutes, and then my vision came back to where it was before!" Such a visual drop may occur after 5 to 10 minutes of playing tennis or other vigorous exercise (such as jogging) and has the same significance. This is definitely a vote *for* a demyelinizing disease. *Lhermitte's symptom* is the presence of "electricity" shooting down the patient's neck or back or extremities on flexing the neck. Now you must know how to ask for this symptom. *Don't* say: "Do you note electricity shoot down your back when you flex your neck?" You just suggest the answer if you do it that way! I ask patients to put their chin on their chest while I'm looking at them, and then ask them if this bothered them at all. They may then smile and volunteer the history that they have noted Lhermitte's symptom in the past. Again, this is not an absolute criterion, but it is very helpful for a diagnosis of demyelinizing disease. *Pain on motion* of the globe is helpful in the history of optic neuritis. It has been said to be present in about 20 per cent of cases (which is also to say that 80 per cent of cases of optic neuritis do *not* have pain on motion). It probably occurs more frequently than that, however, in patients with demyelinizing disease. I ask patients to "cut" their eyes all around the room while I'm looking at them and watch to see if this causes them any discomfort at all. Obviously, a history of previous paresthesias in a foot for 2 weeks, episodes of dizziness or vertigo in the past, or fleeting bouts of double vision a year or two ago are all very helpful when one is looking for demyelinizing disease as the cause of optic neuritis. A careful neurologic examination is obviously indicated in these patients.

The question always comes up about the *spinal fluid* examination. One may find mild changes in the cerebrospinal fluid in about one third of the patients with optic neuritis (a few cells, slight elevation in protein, or a slight gamma globulin peak on electrophoresis). However, the point I want to emphasize is that it is *very common* in multiple sclerosis to have an absolutely normal cerebrospinal fluid examination to all parameters. In other words, a spinal fluid electrophoretic pattern *may* be helpful if unequivocally positive, but is very often quite negative, and I am therefore quite conservative about asking for this. If one has a patient with a protracted course, or repeated bouts of optic neuritis and the like, that is a different question. I personally favor the use of *steroids* in these cases. Dr. Alan Bird did a control study on steroids in optic neuritis, and he concluded that steroids really don't improve the final visual acuity in these patients as compared with the natural course of the disease. He did find, however, that the time span of the course of the illness was shortened by steroids, and my clinical experience has been that steroids definitely help. One must individualize the route, dose, and duration of steroid therapy in such patients. It might be reasonable to give an adult patient 100 mg. per day of prednisone by mouth for 3 days, then 80 mg. per day by mouth for 4 days, and then either stop or taper quickly. If the patient does not respond within 5 to 7 days on large-dose oral steroids, I see no reason to continue this therapy. A sub-Tenon's steroid injection by an ophthalmologist has many advantages—the medicine gets to that optic nerve where it is needed, you know the patient has had the drug, and systemic side effects are virtually negated.

"Ischemic Optic Neuropathy"

A clear-cut clinical entity is the "ischemic optic neuropathy syndrome." A 45 to 55 year old patient suddenly notes the onset of painless blurring of vision in one eye. When seen, the corrected visual acuity is 20/25 to 20/40 in that eye and the optic disc has a characteristic appearance described as "vascular pseudopapillitis." The disc is swollen and has two or three small linear or flame-shaped hemorrhages on its edge, and the arteries appear rather narrow. A lower nasal or altitudinal optic nerve type visual field defect is found in that eye. The patient will have mild hypertension or chemical diabetes in about half the cases, or the family history will be positive for these in about half the cases, if looked into carefully. The course sputters along over several weeks to about 3 months, and the disc rapidly becomes pale. One never sees a recurrence of this picture in the same eye, in my experience, when the disease has finally run its course. However, the problem is that, months to years later, there is a definite tendency for the process to recur in the *other* eye. If one sees the patient at the time of involvement of the second eye, the pale disc in the first eye, combined with the swollen disc in the second eye with relatively intact vision early, may lead one to a false suspicion of Foster-Kennedy syndrome, and one must be alert to that possibility. A neuro-ophthalmologic consultation is indicated in such cases.

Other forms of optic nerve ischemia include embolism to the optic disc from carotid atheromatous disease or from a cardiac source (mural thrombi, bacterial endocarditis, and the like), hypertensive vascular disease, carotid-cavernous fistula, and the like. The most important thing to remember in the patient 55 years of age or above, and particularly above 60, is the possibility of *temporal arteritis.* A *sedimentation rate* should be obtained on all patients above 60 years of age with sudden visual loss, or headaches, or other suspicious symptoms (such as polymyalgia rheumatica, malaise, jaw claudication, or temporal artery tenderness). The majority of cases of temporal arteritis that I see are of the "occult" form with minimal constitutional symptoms, and although normal sedimentation rates can be seen in such cases, they are exceptional, and this is still the best screening test for the disease for the clinician. Temporal artery biopsy should be done when indicated, serial sections should be obtained, and the patient should be treated promptly with steroids. Oral steroids are used in temporal arteritis—*not* orbital injections. The dose used should eliminate symptoms and return the sedimentation rate to normal. Steroid therapy does *not* guarantee that the other eye will not become involved! I have heard of about five to seven cases in which one eye went blind due to temporal arteritis, the patient was placed on 80 to 100 mg. per day of prednisone, and the other eye then went blind within a few days or a week or so while the patient was still on the steroid therapy. Steroid therapy is definitely helpful in such patients, but one should tell them we are giving them this medicine to try to reduce the chance of involvement of the other eye and that it is the best therapy now available for the disease. Remember that patients on indomethacin, salicylates, and the like may have a spuriously low sedimentation rate, and one should inquire about any medications they are on at the time of obtaining this test.

Leber's Disease

This is rather rare but is a visual disaster when it occurs. It usually involves males in the early years of life—commonly teens to late 20's—with a sudden visual loss in one eye. One should ask particularly about the maternal uncle's being involved. There is a characteristic fundus picture in the acute case with (1) circumpapillary telangiectatic microangiopathy, (2) pseudoedema of the nerve fiber layer around the disc, and (3) lack of staining on fluorescein angiography. This can be confused with papilledema, and a neuro-ophthalmologic consultation should be obtained in these patients to try to avoid unnecessary neuroradiologic studies. There is no effective therapy for this disease, and the second eye will become involved in less than a year after the first.

Other Causes of Optic Neuritis

There are idiopathic cases and many forms of unusual types of optic neuritis. Carcinomatous optic neuropathy, optic neuritis due to *Toxocara canis,* toxic optic neuritis (such as from ethchlorvynol), and many other forms are known. A careful slit lamp examination by an ophthalmologist looking for cells in the vitreous is helpful in detection of these cases. It is hoped that these remarks will help you differentiate some of these cases. "Toxic amblyopia" is seen in patients who smoke and drink too much and has a characteristic visual field defect, the so-called "cecocentral scotoma," which is characteristically larger for red and green colored targets than for white targets. These patients should be advised to stop tobacco and alcohol for 3 months, and placed on a good diet with supplemental vitamins; I give them hydroxocobalamin (Neo-Betalin 12), 1000 micrograms per ml. by injection, 1 ml. weekly for 10 weeks to use up the 10 ml. vial. This process will improve within 3 months, if the patient adheres to proper therapy, in my experience. This is such a large subject that only a brief introduction can be given in this article, but I pray that this will help you and your patients!

IDIOPATHIC PERIPHERAL FACIAL PARALYSIS
(Bell's Palsy)

method of
L. P. HINTERBUCHNER, M.D.
Brooklyn, New York

Idiopathic peripheral facial paralysis, or Bell's palsy, is that condition in which isolated involvement of the facial nerve, usually on one side and without any apparent cause, produces weakness of all facial muscles, including the frontalis and the orbicularis oculi muscles. This may be accompanied by pain; inability to close the eye, subsequent tearing, and exposure of the cornea to potential injuries; inability to handle food and saliva; difficulty in speech; change of taste; and, in some cases, hyperacusis.

It would be a serious mistake to consider all cases of peripheral facial paralysis as instances of Bell's palsy. There are intracranial processes that involve the facial nucleus of the brainstem or the facial nerve as it leaves the brainstem. The treatment in these cases is determined by the respective cause, be it an intracranial tumor, a vascular disease of the brainstem, or any number of processes which can involve either the facial nucleus or the nerve.

Because the cause of Bell's palsy is unknown, the treatment is symptomatic and nonspecific. Prognosis is as important as the treatment in the management of this condition. The prognosis is of considerable concern, especially to a younger patient because of the disfigurement, impairment of speech, and inability to handle saliva and food.

Prognosis

Once the diagnosis of the peripheral facial palsy of the idiopathic variety has been established, the patient must be reassured accordingly. It will comfort him to know that about 60 per cent of all patients will recover fully and about 90 per cent sufficiently well to be satisfied with the results. But it is prudent to point out that there may be deficits, which may consist of facial contracture (which may improve the appearance of the face in repose), facial synkinesias (associated movements), and, rarely, the appearance of crocodile tears. The last two phenomena are the result of faulty reinnervation, common in recovery from Bell's palsy. Recovery usually takes place within 3 to 6 weeks, but it may take as long as 6 to 12 months.

A more definitive prognostic statement can be made after 5 days based on electrodiagnostic studies. Voluntary potentials are most important prognostically at this point. The nerve latency provides further information. It is the time it takes for a stimulus delivered to the facial nerve just in front of the ear to travel through the nerve and across the neuromuscular junction to the muscle, where it is recorded as an action potential. Normally it is less than 3.5 milliseconds. The latency may remain normal in the presence of facial paralysis, suggesting that a complete conduction block without structural damage has occurred proximal to the point of stimulation. In such cases, the prognosis for full recovery is excellent. If, on the other hand, the latency is prolonged or no response at all can be obtained, axonal degeneration has taken place and the recovery may take longer and may be incomplete. Serial determination may be needed, because in about 10 per cent of patients the latency may become impaired only during the second or third week.

If the nerve excitability is absent at any time, even if this should occur late, recovery may take months because the nerve regenerates at the speed of about 1 inch per month. Such patients will have residuals of the palsy, and some will recover very little. But even then the subsequent contracture of the muscles may make the appearance of the face more acceptable.

When axonal degeneration has occurred, electromyography will detect absence of voluntary potentials early and presence of fibrillation potentials later, usually 10 to 12 days after the onset. They are useful in the quantitative assessment of the damage.

Therapy

The essentials of the therapy can be listed as follows:

Reassurance. The discussion of the diagnosis and of the prognosis should reassure most patients, and it should brighten their outlook.

Control of Pain. If there is pain, which is usually retroauricular, it is necessary to make the patient comfortable. Salicylates usually suffice; however, in some patients stronger analgesics may be necessary. Application of heat to the involved side of the face will add to the patient's comfort. If there is considerable sagging of the muscles, particularly about the mouth and of the lower face, it may be useful to splint the face with Scotch Tape or with a simple wire loop from the corner of the mouth hooked over the ear lobe. In most patients, however, this is not necessary.

Protection of the Eye. Protection of the eye is extremely important, because the paralysis has abolished the necessary blinking of the eye and particles of dust are no longer removed from the cornea. The patient may be partially protected by so-called Bell's phenomenon, which consists of upward deviation of the eye when the patient is attempting to close the eye, causing the eye and the cornea to roll up under the upper eyelid. However, this may not be sufficient to protect the eye at all times. Therefore protective eyeglasses or an eye shield are recommended. An eye shield is particularly important at night when the possibility of injury by rubbing against the bedding is greatest. In very severe cases in which the recovery may be delayed and the lower eyelid may become everted, a temporary tarsorrhaphy may be needed.

Maintenance of the Muscle. It is important to maintain the muscles in good shape. Heat will contribute to this by stimulating a better blood perfusion through the muscles. Muscle exercise imitating the function of the muscles on the healthy side is useful. Movements to be imitated are wrinkling of the forehead, closing of the eyes, pursing of the lips, drawing of the mouth to one side, blowing the cheeks, and whistling.

Galvanic stimulation is a form of exercise that delays but does not prevent atrophy. It is used to maintain the muscles so that they would be in good condition at the time of neural recovery. Faradic stimulation at low frequencies of the facial nerve is also recommended. When, in the course of recovery, first synkinetic movements appear, all mechanical and electrical stimulation should be stopped. Stimulators can be purchased for home use. However, because of their expense and potential for injury, it is best to have the stimulation therapy supervised by a physiatrist.

Drug Therapy. Salicylates and other analgesics for pain have been mentioned. The value of thiamine chloride in doses of 25 to 50 mg. three times daily is questionable. There is considerable controversy as to the efficacy of steroids and ACTH. Prednisone was shown to be effective in some controlled studies and ineffective in others. Recommended dose is 60 mg. per day for 4 days, tapering to 5 mg. in 10 days. The sooner the treatment is started, the better the results to be expected. ACTH seems to be helpful but is more cumbersome because of parenteral administration. The customary precautions in its use must be observed. The recommended dose is 80 units of ACTH intramuscularly daily for 5 days, then tapered by daily steps of 20 units for a total of 9 to 10 days.

Surgical Therapy. This consists of decompression of the facial nerve in its canal. It seems to be a drastic measure for a condition with 60 to 90 per cent spontaneous recovery rate. Its value is controversial. It should be considered only in patients in whom the electrodiagnostic studies suggest extremely poor prognosis. Some recommend surgery if there are no voluntary potentials, if the electrical excitability of the nerve decreases progressively within the first 5 days, and when the cosmetic defect would represent a catastrophe, such as in actors. Availability of a capable surgeon familiar with microsurgical techniques is essential.

PARKINSON'S DISEASE

method of
HAROLD L. KLAWANS, M.D.,
Chicago, Illinois
and DONALD B. CALNE, M.D.
Bethesda, Maryland

Introduction

The first effective treatment to be introduced for parkinsonism was the use of belladonna alkaloids by Charcot. These drugs were known to cause dryness of the mouth, and Charcot initiated their administration to patients with parkinsonism in an attempt to alleviate the drooling of saliva commonly encountered in such patients. It was soon recognized that the belladonna alkaloids had an unexpected beneficial effect on the rigidity and tremor of parkinsonism. Unfortunately the least obvious but most disabling clinical feature of parkinsonism—the slowness and clumsiness of movement termed hypokinesia—did not improve to any significant extent.

The succeeding years were notable for the absence of any therapeutic advance. The sterility of the pharmacologic setting is illustrated by the redundant arguments on the relative efficacy of belladonna derived from different sources, the Bulgarian preparation somehow achieving a particular vogue.

Following the Second World War, synthetic congeners of the belladonna alkaloids were introduced and virtually replaced the traditional natural products. The major advantage of the new drugs was an apparent improvement in therapeutic index so that the same beneficial results were obtained with fewer adverse reactions.

Over the last decade, a spectacular change in neurologic therapeutics has occurred with the development of levodopa as a treatment of parkinsonism. Levodopa represents a totally rational approach to treatment. Its use in parkinsonism is based upon firm biochemical observations which lead to accurate predictions of clinical efficacy. Levodopa is of crucial practical significance, because shortly after its introduction it was recognized as by far the most potent therapeutic agent available for parkinsonism. Unfortunately the efficacy of levodopa is limited by rather prominent (albeit dose-related and reversible) adverse effects.

Amantadine, the next important drug to enter the therapeutic arena for parkinsonism, differed in every respect from levodopa. Its beneficial action was discovered by a chance observation; critical studies showed that its antiparkinson efficacy was much less than that of levodopa; nevertheless, it is extremely well tolerated.

Anticholinergic Drugs

All effective drugs used in the treatment of parkinsonism prior to the advent of levodopa had central anticholinergic properties. In 1967 Duvoisin conducted an elegant series of experiments which demonstrated that these anticholinergic agents ameliorate parkinsonism by blocking muscarinic receptors at cholinergic synapses within the central nervous system. He drew this conclusion from the following observations:

1. Physostigmine is an anticholinesterase agent which inhibits the destruction of acetylcholine in both the central nervous system and the periphery. Administration of physostigmine to patients with parkinsonism exacerbates the clinical features of the disease.

2. Edrophonium is another anticholinesterase drug, but unlike physostigmine it does not readily cross the blood-brain barrier, so its actions are limited to the periphery. Edrophonium does not exacerbate parkinsonism.

3. Scopolamine and benztropine are antimuscarinic agents which cross the blood-brain barrier. Both these drugs ameliorate parkinsonism and protect patients from the deleterious effects of physostigmine.

4. Methylscopolamine and propantheline are antimuscarinic agents which do not gain ready access to the central nervous system. Neither of these drugs is capable of inhibiting the exacerbation of parkinsonism induced by physostigmine.

Although muscarinic blockade is clearly a major factor contributing to the therapeutic action of anticholinergic agents, another mechanism which may play a role is inhibition of active reuptake of dopamine. Normally, the major process responsible for the inactivation of dopamine released into striatal synapses is reuptake by the presynaptic dopaminergic nerve terminal. This active reuptake mechanism is inhibited by many of the anticholinergic agents which are employed to treat parkinsonism. Blockade of this reuptake system allows the transmitter to remain in the synaptic cleft where it can continue to act upon postsynaptic receptors. These effects reverse the decreased dopaminergic transmission in the striatum, which is the chemical basis of parkinsonism.

Anticholinergic agents achieve a worthwhile therapeutic action on tremor and rigidity, but hypokinesia (the most disabling clinical feature of parkinsonism) and loss of postural reflexes do not usually respond well.

There is no satisfactory evidence that any one anticholinergic drug is specifically effective for any one particular parkinsonian deficit, although patients often report a preference among the various alternative agents which they are commonly given. Sometimes a combination of two anticholinergic agents seems better than one, but it is seldom advantageous to give more than two anticholinergics at the same time. The initial therapeutic response to anticholinergic drugs is sometimes poorly sustained, suggesting the development of tolerance.

Antihistaminic drugs are often prescribed for parkinsonism. All the antihistaminic agents that have been found to be of value in parkinsonism have central antimuscarinic properties. It is probably the ability of these drugs to antagonize the activity of acetylcholine within the brain that accounts for their therapeutic action. Dosages of each of these agents must be adjusted individually. It is usual to start patients on a low intake, which is gradually increased until a satisfactory response is obtained or unwanted effects are encountered. Minor side effects such as dryness of the mouth and slight blurring of vision are common and may have to be tolerated in order to have an antiparkinsonian effect. Older patients appear to be more sensitive to the central side effects of these agents, and great care must be exercised in increasing these agents in the elderly. Some patients are remarkably sensitive to the central side effects and experience hallucinations in very low doses.

The most common adverse reactions to anticholinergic drugs are produced by blockade of muscarinic synapses of the parasympathetic system. They include dryness of the mouth, defective ocular accommodation, mydriasis which can precipitate glaucoma, constipation, and retention of urine. This last problem can lead to acute retention in patients with prostatic hypertrophy. Unwanted effects can also be induced through effects upon the central nervous system and include a toxic confusional psychosis and hallucinations.

Amantadine

The therapeutic effect of amantadine in parkinsonism was discovered by serendipity, and its mechanism of action remains unknown. However, in studies employing much higher tissue concentrations than those encountered in routine therapy, a number of properties have been reported which may be relevant. These include (1) increasing the synthesis of dopamine, (2) augmenting the release of dopamine, and (3) inhibiting the active reuptake process responsible for inactivating dopamine.

Amantadine has one unusual pharmacokinetic property—it is scarcely metabolized. Some 86 per cent of an administered dose is excreted unchanged in the urine.

Amantadine is of similar therapeutic potency to anticholinergic drugs, but in contrast it also alleviates hypokinesia and loss of postural reflexes. Because of its efficacy against these manifestations of parkinsonism it is particularly useful in the management of patients who respond poorly to levodopa. About 50 per cent of patients derive worthwhile benefit from amantadine; there have been conflicting reports on whether the response is sustained.

Amantadine is generally given in an initial dose of 100 mg. daily, which is doubled after a week if, as is usual, there are no adverse reactions. Since one of the more common unwanted effects is restlessness, the second dose of amantadine should not be taken late in the day.

In addition to restlessness, amantadine can cause dizziness, confusion, hallucinations, mood changes, nausea, abdominal discomfort, headache, edema, pruritus, and rarely cardiac arrhythmias. All these unwanted effects are reversible by stopping treatment. Overdosage can precipitate convulsions, so amantadine is not usually given to patients with a history of seizures. There have been reports of livedo reticularis, a condition in which there is edema and shininess of the shins, with livedo above or below the knee or on the dorsum of the foot.

Levodopa

The therapeutic efficacy of levodopa in the treatment of parkinsonism was first demonstrated in the early 1960's. Using intravenous levodopa, Birkmayer and Hornykiewicz demonstrated a decrease in akinesia in 20 parkinsonian patients. At the same time, Barbeau independently reported improvement in parkinsonism following oral doses of levodopa. The overall impression of the usefulness of levodopa remained unclear until the efficacy of long-term oral therapy was demonstrated by Cotzias et al. These workers first used large oral doses of DL-dopa for long periods of time and were able to produce dramatic and sustained improvement. Because of the toxic nature of the racemic mixture, they substituted levodopa for DL-dopa. Using the single isomer, they produced marked beneficial effects in parkinsonian patients without the same serious toxicity. A number of investigators have substantiated these results in large series of patients, including some studies which were done as double blind trials.

Levodopa has been shown to be effective in ameliorating rigidity, hypokinesia, loss of postural reflexes, and tremor. Although it is often said that levodopa has less effect on tremor than it has on rigidity and akinesia, it has a significant antitremor effect and is clearly the most potent agent now available for the treatment of parkinsonian tremor.

Although levodopa is the most effective drug for the treatment of parkinsonism, its use is frequently associated with a variety of side effects which often limit its beneficial action. When properly managed, both the incidence and severity of these side effects can be reduced, resulting in greater therapeutic efficacy. Success of long-term use of levodopa depends to a large extent on the understanding and management of these side effects.

The major adverse reactions to levodopa can be divided into three classes. The first of these are the centrally mediated side effects which are thought to result from activity of amines formed from levodopa within the central nervous system. The second are the peripherally mediated side effects which are thought to result from the formation of active amines outside the central nervous system. The last are the mixed central and peripheral side effects. Both central and peripherally formed amines are considered to be of physiologic significance in the pathophysiology of these side effects.

The centrally mediated side effects include dyskinesias, myoclonus, and psychiatric effects.

The appearance of choreoathetoid involuntary movement, or dyskinesias, is one of the most frequent and troublesome side effects of levodopa therapy. The occurrence of the movements during chronic oral dopa therapy was first reported by Cotzias et al. in their initial study of the efficacy of long-term high dosage DL-dopa and levodopa in parkinsonism. The incidence reported during chronic therapy ranges from a low of 39 per cent to as high as 80 per cent.

The dyskinetic movements induced by levodopa are remarkably diverse. Lingual-facial-buccal movements, such as grimacing, gnawing, yawning, and choreoathetoid movements of the tongue, are the most commonly observed manifestations. Choreoathetoid movements of extremities, neck, and trunk are also common.

Barbeau et al. have made the most extensive study of these movements and have proposed an extensive classification of these dyskinesias, which includes some 47 different types of levodopa-induced abnormal movements. Their classification includes eye movements such as blepharospasms and lateral eye deviations, as well as numerous types of lingual-facial-buccal, cervical, truncal, and upper or lower extremity movements. Although the diversity of these movements is remarkable, their effect on the long-term efficacy of levodopa is much more significant.

The prevalence of these movements is definitely *related to the duration of high dosage levodopa therapy*. Very little else about these movements is clearly understood. Although there is a direct relationship between levodopa and dyskinesias, there is no absolute relationship between the onset of such movements and the daily dosage of levodopa. In many patients dyskinesias have occurred with daily doses of less than 2 grams per day of levodopa. Other patients can be on 6 or more grams per day for up to 5 years without manifesting such movements. Once the dyskinetic movements appear, their severity is related to the daily dose of levodopa. Decreasing the daily dosage of levodopa invariably reduces the dyskinesias, and increasing the daily dosage makes them worse. Unfortunately the beneficial effects of therapy may be diminished when the dose of levodopa is decreased.

Many observers have found that reducing the daily dose of levodopa by 0.5 or 1.0 gram frequently eliminates the dyskinesias or at least reduces them to an acceptable level. For many patients the most effective dose for controlling the parkinsonian symptoms is at or just below that dosage which produces the dyskinetic movements. Because of this many patients have to compromise between partial control of parkinsonian symptoms and disabling levodopa-induced choreoathetosis.

The exact mechanism by which these involuntary movements are produced is unknown. The observation that the average daily dosage of levodopa is the same in patients with and in patients without levodopa-induced dyskinesias suggests that some variable, possibly histopathologic or biochemical, may be related to the occurrence of these movements. There is evidence that levodopa produces dyskinetic movements by an effect within the central nervous system rather than peripherally. Peripheral inhibition of dopa decarboxylase decreases the various peripheral side effects of levodopa but does not reduce the incidence or severity of the movements.

It is thought that these dyskinesias are related to an abnormal response to dopamine and that the mechanism underlying such an alteration of neuronal response to dopamine is the development of denervation hypersensitivity of the dopamine receptors caused by degeneration of the dopaminergic nigrostriatal pathway. Because of this denervation these receptors may become hypersensitive to dopamine. Levodopa may elicit dyskinesias as a result of dopamine activation of these hypersensitive receptors.

If levodopa-induced abnormal movements are related to the action of dopamine at dopaminergic receptor sites, then it should be possible to alter the neuronal response to dopamine and the subsequent movements in several ways. The most direct way would be to decrease the amount of dopamine reaching the receptors, which should improve the movements. Decreasing the dosage of levodopa would effectively decrease the amount of dopamine reaching the dopamine receptors. As noted above, this does reduce the severity of levodopa-induced dyskinesias. Unfortunately, however, the beneficial effects of levodopa on parkinsonian symptoms of these same patients are usually diminished at the same time. As a result of this, levodopa-induced dyskinesias often limit both the dosage of levodopa a patient can tolerate and the therapeutic response.

Barbeau initially reported that neuroleptic phenothiazines were of value in ameliorating levodopa-induced dyskinesias. Later Postma claimed that haloperidol could relieve the dyskinesias without worsening parkinsonism. It is our firm belief that neuroleptics will improve dyskinesias only at the expense of increased parkinsonism. We therefore do not advocate the use of neuroleptic agents for the treatment of levodopa-induced dyskinesias.

Jameson has reported that pyridoxine (vitamin B_6) reduces levodopa-induced dyskinesias without causing a loss of the levodopa effect. In our experience pyridoxine reduces dyskinesias *only* at the cost of a very significant increase in parkinsonian deficit.

In many patients, anticholinergic agents appear to worsen levodopa-induced dyskinesias. We have found that decreasing the level of anticholinergic medication in parkinsonian patients with dyskinesias decreases levodopa-induced dyskinesias in about one third of patients. This improvement in dyskinesias is unassociated with any detectable increase in parkinsonian signs and symptoms in about half of these patients.

It has recently been suggested that deanol may be useful in ameliorating levodopa-induced dyskinesias. Miller used deanol in 11 patients with severe dyskinesias and reported remarkable improvement in these abnormal movements in 8 patients without any worsening of parkinsonism. This effect of deanol was attributed to the central cholinergic activity of this agent. It is hard to understand how a centrally acting cholinergic agent could decrease dyskinesia without any increase in parkinsonism, as physostigmine (see above) significantly increased parkinsonism. We have studied deanol in 20 patients with well established levodopa-induced dyskinesias and found it to be of little if any value.

In some patients these movements appear to be increased by amantadine. If they occur in patients already on amantadine, decreasing or withdrawing amantadine may reduce the severity of the dyskinesias.

The most reliable means of decreasing levodopa-induced dyskinesias is to decrease the level of antiparkinsonian medication, either anticholinergic or dopaminergic. Alteration in daily dosages should be done as soon as dyskinesias become prominent; since any alteration may be associated with an increase in parkinsonism, it is probably best to decrease dosages slowly and to decrease only one medication at a time.

Levodopa-induced myoclonus consists of brief, rapid, usually symmetrical muscle jerks which frequently occur during light sleep. Decreasing the daily dosage of levodopa invariably eliminates myoclonus, but in some instances this is associated with some increase in parkinsonism. Decreasing the last dose before bedtime has the greatest effect on these nocturnal movements. Anticholinergic agents appear to have no influence on levodopa-induced myoclonus.

Untreated idiopathic parkinsonism is now well recognized to be frequently associated with psychiatric symptoms. Dementia is seen in up to 40 per cent of patients with idiopathic parkinsonism, and diffuse cortical atrophy is a common finding in these patients. Patients with postencephalitic parkinsonism often show behavioral and psychologic abnormalities of many types which are felt to reflect the diffuse pathology of their primary disease. The incidence of significant depression in patients with parkinsonism of any cause is high, nearly 40 per cent in one series.

Modifying intracerebral levels of amines by the administration of oral levodopa has also been found to cause significant psychiatric side effects in parkinsonian patients. These have been reported to include agitation, confusion, depression, delirium, hypomania, delusions, paranoia, hallucinations, lethargy, vivid dreams, hypersexual behavior, and overt psychosis. These side effects may occur days to months following the initiation of levodopa therapy.

In our experience it has been useful to divide the psychiatric side effects of levodopa therapy into several types. Some patients develop a full-blown psychotic response to levodopa. These patients have hallucinations, usually of a frightening character. Reality becomes tenuous, and the patients often have paranoid delusions. Levodopa has to be decreased and often discontinued in these patients. Patients with a past history of schizophrenic reaction or paranoid psychosis appear to be particularly susceptible to such reactions. Because of this, past history of such psychiatric problems is a strong contraindication to the use of levodopa. A toxic psychosis can also occur and requires reduction or discontinuation of levodopa.

A third type of psychiatric side effect is less serious. The patients report nocturnal visual hallucinations which occur most frequently after sudden exposure to light following light deprivation, as when the patient gets up in the middle of the night to go to the bathroom. When a light is turned on, the patient may see bugs or small animals running about the room, but there are no threatening hallucinations and no clouding of the sensorium. The patient is aware that these are hallucinations and usually learns to "live with them" without difficulty. It is usually not necessary to stop levodopa therapy in such cases. Many patients reject reduction of levodopa which increases their parkinsonism, because they feel that this side effect is more tolerable than their parkinsonian motor disability.

The occurrence of all psychiatric side effects of levodopa therapy has been reported as ranging from 10 to 50 per cent, depending on the interest and acumen of the investigators and the patient population. The average incidence is about 20 per cent, making mental symptoms the third most common reaction to levodopa therapy (after gastrointestinal disturbances and dyskinesias).

The pathophysiology of levodopa-induced mental changes is unknown. As one would expect, they are a result of amine formation in the central nervous system, because the administration of a peripheral dopa decarboxylase inhibitor does not prevent them. The question has been raised of possible involvement of serotonin in the pathogenesis of these psychiatric side effects. Levodopa is known to cause a decrease in brain serotonin. Two investigators have claimed success in treating levodopa-induced psychosis with the serotonin precursor L-tryptophan.

Severe psychiatric side effects of levodopa are usually treated by reduction or discontinuation of levodopa. Neuroleptics themselves exacerbate the symptoms of parkinsonism, so that a reduction in levodopa is a more direct and physiologically reasonable choice of therapy. Patients with severe psychotic reactions may nevertheless require temporary neuroleptic therapy. Depression in parkinsonian patients on levodopa often responds to treatment with tricyclics. Conventional monamine oxidase inhibitors should not be used in patients receiving levodopa because of the possibility of hypertensive crises.

Another side effect thought to be mediated in the central nervous system is emesis. The symptom complex of anorexia, nausea, and vomiting is perhaps the most common reaction to levodopa administration. These are also among the first side effects to appear in initiating levodopa therapy and often limit both the starting dose and subsequent increments of levodopa therapy. Symptoms of nausea and revulsion from food usually occur within a half hour of taking levodopa. Nausea is usually most marked in the mornings, particularly if the levodopa is taken on an empty stomach. Nausea and subsequent vomiting are dose related in that a large initial dose or a sudden increase in dosage often initiates or exacerbates them. There is also, however, a tendency to develop tachyphylaxis to these side effects. It is our impression that there may be somewhat less tolerance to the feeling of anorexia or loss of appetite.

Treating levodopa-induced nausea by administering standard phenothiazine antiemetics is of no value. These neuroleptics reduce the patient's nausea and vomiting but also worsen his parkinsonism. As in the case of the levodopa-induced dyskinesias and psychosis, neuroleptics reduce side effects only at the cost of increased parkinsonism. Duvoisin reported successful treatment of levodopa-induced nausea and vomiting with diphenidol, a trihexyphenidyl analogue with no known antiparkinsonian effect. He used diphenidol because it had been shown to antagonize the effect of apomorphine (a dopamine agonist) on the emetic center. Duvoisin reported that diphenidol relieved symptoms of nausea and vomiting in 17 out of 25 patients who had been unable to tolerate levodopa because of these side effects. Diphenidol had no effect on parkinsonism.

The most reasonable approach to emesis is a preventive one. Levodopa should be started in very small doses, in combination with an extracerebral decarboxylase inhibitor (see below).

Cardiac arrhythmias and myocardial infarction have been reported in patients receiving levodopa. The significance of such reports is unclear, as these problems are relatively common in the parkinsonian age group. It is difficult to judge the exact contribution of levodopa therapy to the appearance of cardiac arrhythmias, and its contribution, if any, to the occurrence of myocardial infarction seems even more uncertain.

Levodopa-related arrhythmias are considered to be due to the effect of peripherally formed catecholamines on the beta adrenoceptors of the myocardium. Their incidence should be decreased by concurrent administration of a dopa decarboxylase inhibitor or by the use of a beta-adrenergic antagonist such as propranolol.

The only clinically significant side effect of levodopa in which amines formed in the periphery and in the brain are both felt to play a role is hypotension. Calne found that the resting systolic and diastolic pressures are decreased by about 10 mm. in supine parkinsonian patients taking levodopa. Since this same decrease occurred when patients were given a peripheral decarboxylase inhibitor, they proposed that this effect of levodopa on the set of the blood pressure was due to an effect on the central nervous system.

Peripheral baroreceptor reflexes are also modified by levodopa therapy. The ability of patients to sustain an adequate blood pressure on assumption of the upright posture is impaired by levodopa. This postural hypotension is mediated at least in part by peripheral mechanisms and is decreased by dopa decarboxylase inhibitors. Patients receiving levodopa often complain of lightheadedness, dizziness, or even syncope when rising from a bed or a chair. Hypotension has been seen in about a third of patients taking levodopa, and can be a serious problem in the patient with an already compromised cerebral or myocardial circulation. Fortunately, tachyphylaxis is common and most patients show no evidence of postural hypotension after 2 or 3 months on levodopa. If hypotension is a problem, it usually responds to decreasing the daily dosage of levodopa.

There are other side effects of levodopa therapy which are less common and usually of much less clinical significance. These include gout, distortions and hallucinations of taste, darkening of urine, polyuria, mydriasis, and glaucoma.

The most common problem encountered in patients who have been taking levodopa over several years is abrupt fluctuation between exacerbations of parkinsonism and dyskinesia. The cause of these "on-off" phenomena remains obscure, but many factors might contribute. At present there is no satisfactory way of alleviating "on-off" phenomena, although several manipulations of therapy have been advocated. These include (1) stopping levodopa temporarily and restarting at considerably lower dosage; (2) slight reduction of levodopa intake; (3) more frequent administration of levodopa without altering the total daily dose; (4) concomitant administration of extracerebral decarboxylase inhibitors (with reduced dosage of levodopa); and (5) administration of a dopaminergic agonist such as bromocriptine.

Extracerebral Decarboxylase Inhibitors

In 1967 Bartholini et al. suggested that the therapeutic action of levodopa might be improved by concomitant administration of an extracerebral inhibitor of L-aromatic amino acid decarboxylase, the enzyme required for converting levodopa to dopamine. Two such inhibitors have been introduced into routine therapy, carbidopa (in the United States and Europe) and benserazide (in Europe). These drugs block the conversion of levodopa to dopamine at the periphery and thus prevent certain toxic reactions such as cardiac arrhythmias. Since the inhibitors cannot cross the blood-brain barrier, levodopa can still be converted to dopamine in the striatum, where it is needed. It is probable that carbidopa and benserazide penetrate the area postrema (close to the "emetic center" in animals), because both drugs reduce the nausea induced by levodopa, which is thought to be of central origin.

Carbidopa and benserazide are both formulated in combination with levodopa, the former in a 1:10 ratio (Sinemet) and the latter in a 1:4 ratio (Madopar). A recent carefully controlled double blind cross-over study failed to reveal any significant difference in the therapeutic or adverse effects of Sinemet and Madopar.

From the previous discussion it is evident that the major advantage of using extracerebral decarboxylase inhibitors is reduction of nausea and decreased risk of cardiac toxicity. In addition, it is usually possible to build patients up to maximum tolerated dosage more rapidly when they are taking peripheral decarboxylase inhibitors. It is usual to start frail patients on Sinemet 100 or Madopar 125 thrice daily, increasing according to tolerance. In more robust patients Sinemet 250 or Madopar 250 may be used, with similar increments adjusted for each patient individually.

Which Drug for Which Patient?

Since an appreciable number of patients develop serious adverse reactions to levodopa after several years of therapy (in particular, "on-off" phenomena), most neurologists are growing more cautious with the use of this drug. It is probable that "on-off" reactions are related to the cumulative dose of levodopa. Therefore, instead of treating patients as soon as possible with as much as possible, there is a tendency to save levodopa therapy until the patient really needs it, and then to administer the minimal dose that will achieve adequate functional improvement. Each patient must be considered individually. For many mild new cases of parkinsonism, it is appropriate to monitor the patient's progress without giving any medication. Anticholinergics or amantadine should be tried in those whose deficits are more advanced, or whose income or psychologic well-being is threatened by their disease. When anticholinergics and amantadine prove inadequate, levodopa may be given in combination with a decarboxylase inhibitor; since the build-up of levodopa dosage is facilitated by blockade of L-aromatic amino acid decarboxylase, there is no longer any place for starting patients on levodopa alone.

Surgery

James Parkinson reported that tremor improved after a stroke, his account providing the basis for an attempt to help patients by producing selective lesions of the nervous system. Early surgical procedures involved deafferentation by posterior rhizotomy of the spinal segments concerned with the most florid involuntary movements. The results were inconclusive, and there followed an era in which it was fashionable to inflict lesions to the corticospinal pathways. Excision of the motor area of the cerebral cortex, ablation of the anterior limb of the internal capsule, section of the lateral segment of the cerebral peduncle, and division of the spinal pyramidal tract were all pursued with more enthusiasm among neurosurgeons than their patients. In the words of Mackay: "The surgical relief of extrapyramidal hyperkinesias seems to boil down to the artificial production of paralysis."

A more rewarding period resulted from surgical attacks on the basal ganglia. In 1954, Cooper noted that occlusion of the anterior choroidal artery led to improvement in parkinsonian tremor, and following an extensive evaluation of the relative merits of destructive lesions in various structures supplied by this vessel, the ventrolateral nucleus of the thalamus emerged the target area of choice.

Many thousands of parkinsonian patients had their tremor reduced by stereotactic procedures aimed at the ventrolateral thalamic nucleus, but the most disabling clinical feature, akinesia, was not alleviated. Attempts to correlate the postmortem findings after operation with the therapeutic outcome revealed extensive regions, including the globus pallidus, internal capsule, lateral ventricular mass of the thalamus, and the field of Forel, within which both large and small lesions can achieve satisfactory results, regardless of their precise localization.

The rationale behind surgical approaches to parkinsonism stemmed from the view that abnormal motor activity could be decreased by interfering with pathologic activity at one of the several links in the chain of events in the central nervous system which culminate in tremor and rigidity.

The risk of damaging essential pathways in the course of stereotactic procedures was recognized, but it was not until the long-term results were analyzed that the major limitations of all this surgical endeavor were recognized. In 1969, Hoehn and Yahr published figures which demanded a serious reappraisal of the indications for surgery, and this revelation coincided in time with the widespread availability of powerful new pharmacotherapy in the form of levodopa. In consequence, stereotactic operations for parkinsonism have declined. Neither of the present authors has referred a parkinsonian patient for surgery in the last 5 years.

New Approaches to Treatment

Developments in the management of parkinsonism are likely to arise from new approaches designed to increase the therapeutic index of treatment—the ratio of toxic to therapeutic dosage. Now that peripherally induced adverse reactions have been decreased by the introduction of extracerebral decarboxylase inhibitors, future efforts will be made to reduce unwanted effects generated in the central nervous system. In this context, the most common problems in current therapy are dyskinesia, psychiatric disturbances, and "on-off" phenomena. Although progress has been limited in attempting to ameliorate these difficulties, there have been important conceptual advances toward increasing the selectivity of response, and some practical progress has been made in managing "on-off" phenomena. Three new approaches are of sufficient interest to justify consideration here:

Dopaminergic Agonists. Agonists which act directly on the postsynaptic receptor may theoretically be predicted to have greater specificity than levodopa if there are different categories of dopamine receptor in the central nervous system. Accumulating evidence suggests that there are, indeed, several types of dopaminergic receptors in the brain, so there is likely to be a real possibility of developing agonists which selectively activate receptors at those striatal synapses that are abnormal in parkinsonism. It is also reasonable to anticipate that agonists will emerge which have fewer effects than levodopa on noradrenergic synapses, thus generating a further level of specificity. Another useful property which can probably be achieved is a longer biologic half-life than that of levodopa. Since the enzyme responsible for converting levodopa to dopamine (L-aromatic amino acid decarboxylase) is depleted in parkinsonism, it can also be predicted that agonists, which bypass this enzymic transformation, will have a more consistent therapeutic action.

Two types of agonists have yielded encouraging clinical results:

APOMORPHINES. Cotzias et al. have shown that apomorphine has a therapeutic effect in parkinsonism, but chronic high oral dosage leads to azotemia. A more satisfactory response has been achieved with N-propyl-noraporphine.

ERGOLINES. Two ergolines have yielded good results in the treatment of parkinsonism: bromocriptine (2 brom-α-ergocryptine) and lergotrile.

In our experience, bromocriptine is at least as effective as levodopa (with or without an extracerebral decarboxylase inhibitor). We have found that some patients derive more benefit from bromocriptine than any other therapy, particularly if previous treatment with levodopa has led to prominent "on-off" reactions. Optimal treatment has often been achieved with a combination of bromocriptine and levodopa.

Adverse reactions to bromocriptine are qualitatively similar to those of levodopa, but in addition we have encountered erythema, tenderness, and edema of the ankles, which are dose dependent and reversible. Occasionally bromocriptine may induce peripheral vasospasm when the extremities are cold.

Lergotrile has been studied less extensively than bromocriptine, but Lieberman's initial report was encouraging, and we have confirmed that this drug elicits a therapeutic response. More evidence is necessary before the efficacy and toxicity of lergotrile can be compared with those of other medications.

Selective Monamine Oxidase (MAO) Inhibitors. Collins et al. have shown that two forms of MAO exist in the rat, termed MAO_A and MAO_B. MAO_A oxidizes norepinephrine (NE), serotonin (5HT), and dopamine, whereas MAO_B destroys dopamine but not NE or 5HT. Hence a specific inhibitor of MAO_B can be expected to lead to elevation of brain dopamine, without concomitant effects on NE or 5HT. Deprenil, a selective inhibitor of MAO_B, has recently been investigated by Birkmayer et al. in parkinsonism. These workers have reported striking potentiation of the therapeutic response to levodopa (in combination with an extracerebral decarboxylase inhibitor) when deprenil is administered intravenously, intramuscularly, or orally. Further studies are needed to define optimal dose regimens and evaluate deprenil in a more prolonged therapeutic setting.

The Role of Peptide Transmitters. The concept of "peptidergic" transmission in the brain is now becoming accepted, and Barbeau has recently reported substantial potentiation of the therapeutic action of levodopa following intravenous injection of MIF (MSH release–inhibitory hormone). Confirmation and extension of these observations would be of considerable interest.

Acknowledgment

We wish to thank Miss Pat Gerdes and Miss Vernita Bergmeyer for typing the manuscript.

PERIPHERAL NEUROPATHY

method of
CHRISTIAN WERTENBAKER, M.D.,
and HERBERT SCHAUMBURG, M.D.
Bronx, New York

Recent advances in experimental neuropathology have yielded a more meaningful classification of peripheral nerve degeneration that greatly facilitates diagnosis and therapy. Neuropathies can be classified clinicopathologically into five large groups: (1) compressive neuropathies, (2) vascular neuropathies, (3) acute demyelinating neuropathies, (4) chronic familial neuropathies, and (5) axonal or "dying-back" neuropathies.

Compressive Neuropathies

Compression is the major cause of mononeuropathies. Nerves can be affected in many different locations. The most important factors in causing compression are (1) the course of the nerve through a canal, over a bony prominence, or close to the skin; (2) habitual or occupational trauma, such as leg crossing or squeezing the palm with tool handles; and (3) factors rendering the nerve more susceptible, such as subclinical polyneuropathy. The most common compressive neuropathies are as follows:

Carpal Tunnel Syndrome. This disorder is most often idiopathic, but may be associated with obesity, rheumatoid arthritis, hypothyroidism, pregnancy, acromegaly, and multiple myeloma, and sometimes is the presenting complaint in these disorders. Treatment should be directed first to the underlying disorder, if there is one; remission of the carpal tunnel syndrome may occur with successful therapy of these conditions. When associated with pregnancy, the syndrome generally disappears after delivery. If the wrist is subject by habit or occupation to repeated flexion and extension, this behavior should be stopped or modified. A splint to immobilize the wrist in the neutral position may be worn. Nocturnal pain and paresthesias are often relieved by such a splint. Local injections of hydrocortisone into the carpal tunnel may provide relief, although the relapse rate is high. If these measures fail to bring relief, definitive treatment, consisting of simple surgical decompression of the nerve by section of the transverse carpal ligament, should be undertaken.

Entrapment of the Ulnar Nerve at the Elbow. This may follow significant injury to the elbow, but more frequently there is no clear-cut history of trauma. Repeated leaning on the elbows may provoke this syndrome, and symptoms may be relieved by stopping this habit. Symptoms may increase either following repeated vigorous use of the arm, such as hammering or shoveling, or by sleeping with the elbow flexed at an acute angle. Changing these habits may relieve the symptoms. If these measures fail and the symptoms are sufficiently bothersome, or if significant weakness develops, surgery is indicated. The operative procedure is either transposition of the nerve antecubitally or, in some cases, simple decompression of the cubital tunnel.

Compression of the Lateral Femoral Cutaneous Nerve (Meralgia Paresthetica). This syndrome may occur in association with obesity, pregnancy, or diabetes, or following local trauma (rarely an inflamed cecum or abdominal tumor will compress the nerve). The symptoms may be aggravated by prolonged standing or walking and may be relieved by modifying these activities; sometimes a particular position of the affected leg during standing will cause aggravation of symptoms. There is a strong tendency for the condition to remit spontaneously. In the obese, weight loss and exercises to strengthen the abdominal muscles may be helpful. Other therapeutic measures are hydrocortisone or local anesthetic injections at the point where the nerve lies medial to the anterior superior iliac spine. Surgical section of the fascia lata or transposition of the nerve is indicated in severe cases. Usually these measures are not necessary, as many cases remit spontaneously or following conservative measures.

Compression of the Common Peroneal Nerve. This generally occurs at the fibular head, and is often secondary to habitual crossing of the legs while sitting or to pressure by casts, high boots, or obstetrical stirrups, or it may occur during sleep or anesthesia. Conservative measures usually result in recovery. A short leg brace should be used if there is significant foot drop to avoid contraction of the gastrocnemius and damage to the extensor tendons.

Vascular Neuropathies

These are generally due to disease of small blood vessels, which produce ischemic mononeuropathy or mononeuropathy multiplex. Atherosclerosis of large vessels, even when extreme, rarely affects peripheral nerves. The most common causes are the collagen diseases, especially periarteritis nodosa and rheumatoid arthritis, and diabetes mellitus. In periarteritis nodosa and rheumatoid arthritis, the development of acute, severe, or progressive neuropathy is an indication for the use of high doses of corticosteroids. Initially, 40 to 60 mg. of prednisone is given daily. The dose is then increased until progression of the neuropathy ceases and other signs of active vasculitis have subsided. Prednisone can then be slowly reduced to the lowest suppressive dose. Return of function in the already damaged nerves may occur but is often delayed. The usual precautionary regimen for a patient on high dose steroids should be observed. A bland diet and antacids should be used, and stool guaiac and hematocrit monitored. Electrolytes should be measured frequently, and a low salt diet with daily supplemental potassium will help prevent hypernatremia and hypokalemia. In the collagen diseases, there may also exist a subclinical electrically demonstrable polyneuropathy or a mild nonprogressive distal sensory polyneuropathy. Patients with these signs need not be treated beyond whatever therapy is being used for other manifestations of the illness. Diabetes mellitus is the most common cause of rapid onset, painful vascular mononeuropathy and mononeuropathy multiplex involving cranial nerves and peripheral nerves. There is no specific treatment beyond control of the blood sugar, and the neurologic deficits usually improve over a period of months.

Acute Demyelinating Neuropathies

The major disorder in this group is the Guillain-Barré syndrome (postinfectious polyneuropathy). The other is diphtheritic neuropathy.

Guillain-Barré Syndrome. The patient suspected of having the Guillain-Barré syndrome must be admitted to the hospital even if the symptoms are minimal, as the neuropathy often progresses rapidly and unpredictably. For this reason, the patient should be admitted directly to an intensive care or respiratory care unit until his condition has stabilized or is clearly improving. Autonomic involvement may produce abnormalities of heart rate, rhythm, and blood pressure. The vital capacity and ability to cough and swallow should be closely monitored, as they can change without warning. Other conditions producing acute symmetrical motor weakness, such as hypokalemia, tick paralysis, porphyria, botulism, and myasthenia gravis, should be rapidly ruled out.

If mechanical ventilation is necessary (as determined by the degree of respiratory effort, the vital capacity, and the blood gases), it should be instituted early rather than waiting until the last moment. Endotracheal intubation should be replaced by a tracheostomy after 5 to 6 days, and secretions must be removed compulsively. Postural drainage and chest percussion may be helpful in preventing atelectasis and pneumonia. Some patients will be unable to swallow or to gag. Feeding should be done through a small nasogastric tube. The patient should be sitting when a feeding is given, and kept sitting for 30 to 60 minutes afterward to minimize aspiration.

The patient may be unable to urinate because of abdominal muscle weakness or autonomic involvement. The Credé maneuver may be helpful, and catheterization is occasionally necessary. Fecal impaction should be avoided by the use of stool softeners, laxatives, and enemas as required. The paralyzed patient must be turned frequently to avoid decubiti. A sheepskin or water bed may be used. Passive range of motion exercises of the limbs must be given, and a footboard should be used to prevent Achilles tendon shortening. If the eyes do not close completely, corneal damage must be prevented with protective solutions and the eyes taped shut at night; an ophthalmologist should care for the eyes if possible. Elastic stockings and leg massage can be used to help prevent pulmonary emboli; miniheparinization is advocated by some.

The patient may be under severe psychologic stress because of his paralysis and the intensive care environment, and sedation may be necessary. He may be unable to communicate at all; if so, the hospital personnel must not forget that he can see, hear, and understand. If there is a question about the patient's state of consciousness because of complications which have occurred, an electroencephalogram may be helpful.

If the patient with the Guillain-Barré syndrome can be carried through the acute stage of progressive paralysis (usually 2 or 3 weeks) strength gradually returns, and 90 per cent of these patients make a complete or nearly complete recovery after months of weakness. Thus the importance of extremely fastidious supportive care in the acute stage cannot be overstressed.

Considerable controversy surrounds the use of steroids in this condition, as, in most cases, the natural course of the disease is recovery, and steroids may increase the risk of pulmonary infection in a tracheostomized, paralyzed patient requiring ventilatory assistance. Therefore in many centers steroids are no longer routinely used for Guillain-Barré syndrome. In severe, long-lasting, relentlessly progressing paralysis or in the rare patient with recurrent paralysis, a short course of prednisone, 60 to 100 mg. daily, should be given.

Diphtheritic Neuropathy. Treatment of the primary infection with antibiotics and administration of antitoxin as soon as possible after the onset of this rare disease are the only specific therapeutic modalities available. The neuropathy of diphtheria appears weeks to months after the primary infection; the earliest signs may be palatal weakness and paralysis of accommodation. Disturbances of cardiac function can appear much earlier. The general treatment is the same as that of the Guillain-Barré syndrome, with more emphasis on cardiac and circulatory function. Full recovery is the rule if the patient can be supported through the illness.

Chronic Familial Neuropathies

These disorders fall into several groups. In the hereditary sensory neuropathies therapy is aimed at prevention of painless ulcers of the feet and hands and consequent local infection, osteomyelitis, and septicemia. The cooperation and understanding of the patient are essential. Care of the feet and hands requires the avoidance of trauma and prolonged focal pressure (as with ill-fitting shoes) and meticulous cleansing. Heavy labor should be avoided. If plantar ulcers develop, weight bearing must be discontinued until they heal. Unnoticed fractures can occur and must be watched for. These principles apply also to other severe chronic sensory neuropathies. Some of the hereditary motor neuropathies are associated with foot deformities (pes cavus, hammer toes) which may require special shoes and/or corrective surgery. In general, only symptomatic therapies are available in the hereditary neuropathies. An exception is Refsum's disease, in which a special diet lacking in phytanic acid (see specific literature for details) has been shown to be useful. In the porphyrias, avoidance of contraindicated drugs is extremely important (see pp. 333 to 336). In all hereditary neuropathies, genetic counseling should be given. In Fabry's disease, prenatal diagnosis is possible.

Axonal Neuropathies

This category includes most of the toxic, nutritional deficiency, and metabolic neuropathies. Neuropathy caused by toxins is best treated by identification of the agent and removing the patient from the environment. If the toxin is an industrial compound such as acrylamide, n-hexane, methyl n-butyl ketone, or triorthocresylphosphate, there may be an epidemic of cases in the same factory, because many workers are often simultaneously exposed. In heavy metal intoxications (arsenic, lead, mercury, thallium) chelating agents can be used. The specific literature should be consulted for details. Thallium neuropathy may respond better to oral potassium, which displaces it from tissues, than to chelating agents. The neuropathy produced by isoniazid may be prevented by administration of 50 mg. of pyridoxine daily; this does not interfere with the drug's antituberculous activity. In the case of vincristine and vinblastine, mild neuropathy is an accepted side effect, because the drugs are used in cancer chemotherapy. The more severe neuropathic symptoms may remit when the dose is lowered. The neuropathy of alcoholism is nutritional and due to thiamine—and possibly other B vitamin—deficiency. Fifty mg. of thiamine and a B-complex vitamin tablet should be given daily. The neuropathy of pernicious anemia should be treated in the same way as in its other manifestations.

The prognosis for patients with the aforementioned axonal neuropathies caused by exogenous toxins, drugs, or nutritional factors is generally excellent if (1) the neuropathy is diagnosed at an early stage, and (2) the offending toxin, drugs, or nutritional deficiency can be identified. If both these conditions are met, the axonal degeneration will cease after treatment and effective regeneration will commence.

The distal sensorimotor neuropathy of diabetes mellitus may or may not respond to strict control of the blood sugar. Most authorities encourage strict control; however, there is no proof that strict control alters the variable course of diabetic distal neuropathy. Painful dysesthesias are very common in diabetic neuropathy and, if unresponsive to simple analgesics, may be treated with phenytoin (Dilantin), 300 to 400 mg. per day in single or divided doses. In occasional patients, Dilantin may increase the blood sugar level, so this should be monitored closely. If Dilantin is ineffective and the dysesthesias are severe, carbamazepine (Tegretol), 100 to 600 mg. twice daily, may be tried (starting at the lower dose and building up gradually), with periodic measurement of hematopoietic and hepatic function. This use of Dilantin and Tegretol is not listed in the manufacturer's official directives but, in our experience, has occasionally proved helpful.

The effect of dialysis on uremic neuropathy is variable. There may be slow improvement or stability, or the neuropathy may appear to worsen while the patient is on dialysis. Often increasing dialysis time leads to improvement. It has been suggested that the efficacy of dialysis in removing medium-sized molecules is important; this may vary with the particular system used. Successful renal transplantation, on the other hand, generally leads to gradual improvement of the neuropathy, and some patients recover completely.

ACUTE HEAD INJURIES

method of
WILLIAM E. HUNT, M.D.,
and JOSEPH H. GOODMAN, M.D.
Columbus, Ohio

Head injuries result in damage to the scalp, skull, brain and its meningeal coverings, and vasculature of the region, depending on the impact force and mechanical factors involved at the time of trauma. Scalp injuries and linear skull fractures are usually of no consequence unless there is underlying damage to the brain parenchyma or secondary hemorrhage. Basilar skull fractures are rarely seen on routine x-rays and are diagnosed clinically on the basis of cerebrospinal fluid (CSF) otorrhea or rhinorrhea. The "panda bear" sign of periorbital ecchymosis and Battle's sign are diagnostic of anterior fossa and petrous basilar skull fractures, respectively. Arteriovenous fistulas—particularly the carotid cavernous fistula which is sometimes seen following a head injury—should be considered when dealing with extensive fractures in the region of the base of the skull.

Cervical spine injuries are frequently found in association with head trauma and should be looked for with palpation of the anterior cervical spine and the spinous processes, as well as radiographs including the entire cervical spine. C7 *must* be visualized, however difficult this may be technically.

The mildest brain injury is concussion, which is defined as a loss of consciousness, period of amnesia, or any transient nervous dysfunction which rapidly and completely recovers. Contusions imply structural damage to the brain, and lacerations are associated with massive head injuries as well as penetrating head injuries.

Epidural hematomas are most often of arterial origin, the most common cause being a fracture through the middle meningeal groove. They are usually marked by a rapidly progressing neurologic deficit following a lucid interval, although occasionally a chronic epidural hematoma may be seen. Subdural hematomas are usually venous in origin, resulting from avulsion of the bridging veins from the cortical surface that communicate with the dura. These are considered acute if they occur within the first 24 to 48 hours following injury, subacute if they are discovered within the first 2 weeks, and chronic if they are found after that time. Traumatic arterial pseudoaneurysms form at the site of skull fractures and may require surgical correction.

Initial Evaluation

On first contact it is important to establish a good history of the incident and types of forces involved when the injury occurred. In the amnestic or comatose patient, this is best obtained from witnesses to the accident such as emergency squadmen, family members, or any witnesses who may be able to provide that information about the patient's initial condition and progression of symptoms. It is of particular importance, if a general anesthetic is planned, to know when the patient last ate and whether there has been recent alcohol intake.

Physical Examination

An adequate airway should be established and maintained as necessary. After a brief examination for adequacy of vital signs, including temperature, pulse, and respiration, as well as other obvious associated injuries such as bleeding points and extremity fractures, attention is directed at a comprehensive neurosurgical evaluation. The level of consciousness should be noted and described. The preferred terms are those that are easily understood, such as awake, alert, combative, or nonpurposeful. Decorticate and decerebrate posturing are well recognized clinical syndromes and should be used when appropriate. Terms such as obtunded, comatose, or stuporous are not recommended as part of an initial evaluation, in that subsequent examiners may have different interpretations of their meanings. The skull is then palpated for evidence of hematoma and lacerations. A gloved finger or sterile instrument inserted into a laceration may detect an underlying skull fracture, and occasionally one diagnoses brain lacerations in this manner. Palpation of the cervical spine for point tenderness as well as malalignment of the spinous processes is done as an initial search for a cervical spine fracture or dislocation. Cerebrospinal fluid, when present in the ear or nose, indicates a basilar skull fracture, and quantitative sugar determinations may be helpful in establishing whether or not the fluid in question is in actuality cerebrospinal fluid (CSF). Pupil abnormalities should be noted and funduscopic examination carried out. Frontal scalp abrasions and contusions may result in anisocoria with an enlarged poorly reactive pupil on the side of the injury, which should not be confused with a third nerve palsy seen in the herniation syndrome. Papilledema rarely develops acutely in head injuries, although it has been reported to occur within the first several hours following extensive brain injury with increased intracranial pressure. The remainder of the neurologic examination is to determine whether or not lateralizing motor, sensory, or reflex changes are present. Motor examination should be recorded as to the type of movement present in all extremities. A search for associated injuries should include the chest, with auscultation as well as observation for symmetry of chest wall excursions during respiration. Abdominal and genitourinary examinations as well as evaluation of the extremities for fractures should also be done.

Initial Management

1. Maintaining adequate ventilation is of prime importance. Adequacy of oxygenation is confirmed with blood gas determinations, and the patient is intubated if necessary to maintain adequate Po_2 levels and prevent hypercarbia. If a cervical spine fracture is suspected, nasal rather than oral intubation should be done. Tracheostomies are occasionally necessary when associated facial and laryngeal injuries are present.

2. An intravenous line is started and maintained for fluid administration and medications as considered necessary. Lactated Ringer's solution is considered the fluid of choice.

3. A nasogastric tube is useful in evacuating the stomach of recently ingested fluids and blood which the patient may have swallowed as a result of injuries to the nasopharyngeal region.

4. Blood samples should be sent to the laboratories immediately for a type and cross-match, complete blood count, prothrombin time (PT), partial thromboplastin time (PTT), platelets, electrolytes, and blood urea nitrogen. Serum glucose and alcohol levels should also be established.

5. Insert a Foley catheter for urinalysis and for bladder evacuation.

6. Radiologic examinations are then carried out if the patient's condition is stable and there is thought to be no immediate need for surgical intervention. A routine skull series consists of anteroposterior, right and left lateral, and Towne projections. Water's view is useful in detecting facial fractures and opacification of the sinuses. The cervical spine is x-rayed inclusively from C1 to C7. X-ray evaluation detects fractures as well as a shift of midline structures such as a pineal if it is calcified. The echoencephalogram is considered to be of no value in an emergency situation because of the inherent variability of presently available equipment. Computerized axial tomography (CT) is a recently developed noninvasive procedure which is considered extremely useful for detection of intracranial mass lesions. Angiography continues to be a valuable procedure, although to some extent it has been replaced by the CT scan as a diagnostic tool.

Initial Medical Management

1. Tetanus prophylaxis is given if indicated when lacerations and abrasions are present.

2. Intravenous fluid maintenance is carried out in the unconscious, combative, or uncooperative patient, using 5 per cent dextrose and 0.45 per cent saline solution at 1200 ml. per square meter per day. Fluid management is adjusted appropriately for diabetes insipidus or an inappropriate antidiuretic hormone (ADH) response should these occur.

3. Steroids are given on an empirical basis, assuming that they stabilize cellular membranes and prevent the formation of cerebral edema. Dexamethasone sodium phosphate (Decadron), with a loading dose of 20 mg. intravenously followed by 4 mg. every 6 hours, is used routinely when there is evidence of brain contusion or laceration. Antacids given in conjunction with high steroid dosages are felt to decrease the incidence of gastric hemorrhage from ulcers.

4. With brain contusions and lacerations it is also appropriate to start anticonvulsants. Acute seizures are treated with intravenous diazepam (Valium), 10 mg., with particular attention directed to any changes in blood pressure and respirations. Should this not control an acute seizure, an additional 30 to 60 mg. of intramuscular phenobarbital should be administered. It is occasionally necessary to use additional anticonvulsants if seizures persist. Phenytoin (Dilantin), 100 mg. injected intravenously, and paraldehyde are valuable for acute seizure control. Maintenance anticonvulsants consist of phenytoin (Dilantin), 100 mg. to be given orally or intravenously on an 8 hour basis. Intramuscular phenytoin (Dilantin) is absorbed inconsistently and is not the preferred route of administration. Phenobarbital, 30 mg. every 8 hours intramuscularly or orally, is used in addition. In severe head injuries the long-term administration of anticonvulsants is required for up to 1 to 2 years, with follow-up electroencephalograms and a gradual tapering before completely withdrawing anticonvulsant coverage.

5. Mannitol is indicated for cerebral decompression in two instances, the first being when massive cerebral edema is present with no surgically correctible mass lesion. The second instance is when a mass lesion has been diagnosed and medical decompression is indicated in order to allow time to prepare the patient for the operating room. It is not recommended that mannitol be given to all unconscious patients with evidence of head injury unless one is committed to pursue definitive diagnostic studies, because this will alter the natural course of the disease and may delay diagnosis. The initial dose of mannitol is 500 ml. of

a 20 per cent solution given as an intravenous bolus. For pediatric uses the dose should be calculated at 1.5 grams of mannitol per kg. of body weight. (The dosage for children under the age of 12 years is not listed in the manufacturer's official directive.)

Surgical Treatment of Acute Head Injury

Scalp lacerations can be debrided and sutured in the emergency room, using a standard two layer closure. The galea is approximated with interrupted 000 silk, the skin closure with interrupted 0000 silk. One often encounters copious bleeding during the course of debriding these wounds, and this is best controlled with direct pressure or hemostats and eversion of the scalp margins. Linear skull fractures require no treatment other than a period of observation to ensure that there is no associated expanding mass lesion. Basilar skull fractures with and without CSF leakage are treated with antibiotics. Penicillin, dosages of 1 million units every 6 hours intravenously or an equivalent oral dose, and sulfadiazine, 500 mg. every 6 hours, are given for meningitis prophylaxis. This treatment is maintained for from 1 week to 10 days or for as long as a CSF leak persists. Surgical repair of CSF leaks is rarely necessary, as most injuries of this type heal spontaneously within 2 weeks. Persistent leakage after this time requires operative intervention. Indwelling CSF drains in the lumbar cistern may be of value in decreasing the spinal fluid pressure in order to allow closure of a persistent leak. Skull fractures are elevated within the first 24 hours if the inner table is depressed more than 0.5 cm. They are also repaired if fragments are seen in proximity to the sagittal or transverse venous sinuses. Compound depressed fractures are debrided and repaired immediately, with the bone fragments being discarded because they are considered contaminated. Cranioplasty at a later date is performed to correct the skull defect. Any underlying dural laceration is closed in a watertight manner. Dural grafting may be necessary.

Epidural hematomas are diagnosed clinically by a rapidly progressive decrease in the level of consciousness and confirmed by neuroradiologic diagnostic studies. Sometimes surgical intervention is carried out purely on clinical grounds. A boggy temporalis muscle on the same side as a linear skull fracture, accompanied by rapidly developing signs of brain herniation, is enough justification to proceed immediately with surgery. This is caused by blood extruding through the skull fracture line from the middle meningeal artery. At the time of surgery the hematoma is drained through burr holes; or if a solid clot is encountered, a full craniotomy is then performed. The middle meningeal artery is controlled by a coagulation and clipping during the procedure.

Acute subdural hematomas should be treated according to the same principles outlined for the acute epidural hematomas. Coexistence of underlying brain injury from the impact and edema formation contributes to the clinical deterioration, and often there are more factors at play than simply a mass lesion causing brain displacement. The prognosis is poor in the acute subdural hematoma, with mortality in some series being reported as high as 90 per cent. We have attempted large bilateral decompressive craniotomies in hopes of alleviating the effects of brain edema but have not been encouraged by the results in a limited number of patients. Chronic subdural hematomas should be treated with burr hole drainage as soon as the diagnosis is established.

In-Hospital Management

During the first 24 to 48 hours following admission, attention is directed at establishing the patient's progress neurologically. Nursing care includes checks of neurologic function hourly. A decreasing level of consciousness or the development of lateralizing neurologic signs requires immediate initiation of diagnostic procedures and appropriate therapy. In severe head injuries ventilation is supported artificially until the patient is able to breathe unassisted. Hypothermia with reduction of body temperature to 90°F. (32.2°C.) is occasionally used, but the results of this mode of therapy are difficult to evaluate. High dose barbiturates, intermittent mannitol, and intracranial pressure and compliance recordings may be of value in acute management.

During the recovery period strict attention is directed at the patient's nutrition in order to fulfill metabolic requirements, and vitamin supplements are given routinely. Physical therapy prevents contractures, which might otherwise cause problems during rehabilitation.

Management of Post-Traumatic Complications

1. Headaches occur commonly after head trauma, and treatment is symptomatic with nonnarcotic analgesics being the drugs of choice.

2. A communicating post-traumatic hydrocephalus may occur and should be suspected if a patient begins to plateau during this course of recovery or begins to gradually deteriorate after initial improvement. Shunting will alleviate this problem.

3. Personality changes, when present, require understanding and support by family members. Psychiatric counseling may be of value.

4. Seizures, when they occur, require modification of the maintenance of anticonvulsants or addition of another agent such as primidone (Mysoline).

5. Discussion of the intensive rehabilitation necessary for the severely head-injured patient is beyond the scope of this article.

Summary

The head-injured patient requires a systematic approach designed to provide the following:

1. Life support during the early critical phase.
2. Rapid diagnosis on the basis of history, clinical findings, and neurodiagnostic procedures.
3. Appropriate medical and surgical therapy to prevent additional brain damage from increased intracranial pressure and inadequate cerebral perfusion and oxygenation.
4. In-hospital care designed for early detection of changes in neurologic status and modification of the treatment plan in accordance with these changes as they occur.

Prevention of head injuries is undoubtedly the most effective method of preserving life and function.

HEAD INJURIES IN CHILDREN

method of
ARTHUR B. EISENBREY, M.D.
Detroit, Michigan

The management of a head-injured child should be undertaken with a considerable degree of optimism. Recovery rate is high, and secondary complications are less frequent than in adults. In a child under 3 years of age, attention must be given to the possibility of child abuse, as other forms of serious head trauma are less common at this age. The open fontanelle in children under 1 year of age should be used to evaluate intracranial pressure by palpation, and subdural taps may be done to evacuate subdural blood accumulation.

Upon arrival in an emergency room (preferably in transit) the most important step is maintenance of an unobstructed airway. This may require tracheal intubation after thorough nasotracheal aspiration. The patient's future depends largely on prevention of anoxia to the cerebrum and other organs as well. Respiratory support should be used more often than it usually is to prevent increasing intracranial pressure secondary to respiratory obstruction and hypoventilation.

The control of bleeding is essential. Shock is not the result of cerebral trauma, but is a sign of profound bleeding elsewhere. Hemoglobin and circulating volume must be maintained.

Initiation of intravenous therapy, using 5 per cent glucose and 0.3 per cent saline solutions upon arrival at a hospital, reduces the potential difficulties of finding suitable veins if the blood pressure subsequently falls.

The entire body must be examined for lacerations, new and old injury, and fractures of the ribs, long bones, and pelvis. Massive blood loss may be hidden in soft tissues of the thighs and retroperitoneum, especially in children whose circulating reserve is limited.

After these problems are considered, more attention may be directed at the head injury itself. A history as complete as possible and a neurologic examination should be recorded. All treatment is based on the status of the patient over a period of time. Specific data are recorded serially, and a "flow sheet" can be of value. At 15 to 30 minute intervals essentials of the examination are recorded so that a change in the patient is identified. One must know if the patient is stable, improving, or deteriorating.

1. Response to verbal command: Does the patient talk?
2. Response to noxious stimulus, pin prick or pinching.
3. Movements of the face and extremities: Are they symmetrical? Reflexes: Tendon responses, plantar responses.
4. Eyes: equal pupils, large or small pupils, reaction to light, funduscopic examination.
5. Pulse, blood pressure, respirations, temperature.
6. Generalized muscle tone—flaccid or rigid: What posture does the patient assume?

Note that behavioral descriptions are understood better than eponymic or technical terms.

A deteriorating patient needs further diagnostic and therapeutic procedures by a neurosurgeon. Treatment with mannitol is rarely warranted unless to buy time when on the way to the operating room. Rebound of edema necessitates repeated administration of mannitol, which may produce secondary electrolyte imbalances. The value of steroids remains equivocal in acute trauma, but they are commonly used.

Bloody drainage from the ears is evidence of basilar skull fracture and cerebrospinal fluid (CSF) leak. This and other compound fractures require that antibiotics, usually ampicillin, be given.

A dilated unresponsive pupil suggests an expanding blood clot—epidural hematoma. Hemiparesis or paralysis is evidence of cerebral hemispheric damage.

Seizures are not uncommon in childhood head injuries and are not a cause for panic. They should be treated only if persistent, and then conservatively. The safest drugs are phenobarbital, intravenous phenytoin (Dilantin) (not intramuscular) and paraldehyde. Some unfortunate experiences with diazepam in head trauma would discourage its use in control of acute traumatic seizures.

Skull x-rays are rarely needed on an emergency basis, but can be obtained later to evaluate depressions of the bone and the position of linear fractures.

After complete evaluation for spine injury, fractures, bleeding, and pulmonary and visceral injury, ward observation and supportive nursing begin. Monitoring continues by physicians and nursing personnel, not by machine.

Nasotracheal suction is provided, turning the patient from side to side every 2 hours, as well as intravenous fluids at about 60 ml. per kg. per 24 hours in addition to replacement of loss from nasogastric suction. Excess fluids in the young are usually well handled, but dehydration should be avoided and this is common when there has been vomiting and blood loss. The use of a urinary catheter allows accurate measurement of urine output and the general state of hydration. Electrolyte values and blood counts are obtained daily.

As care progresses to the less acute stages and stability or improvement is established, maintenance of nutrition and hydration can be accomplished by tube feeding, using the same volumes that were given intravenously.

Lumbar puncture is almost never justified unless meningitis is suspected. An increasingly restless patient may have expanding hemorrhage. Loss of vestibulo-ocular responses (doll eye movement) is a prognostically poor sign. This means there is no drift of the eyes when the head is turned from side to side. Patients with skull fractures across the middle meningeal artery, major venous sinuses, and foramen magnum require close observation (2 to 4 days) regardless of their apparently bright mental state, as slow bleeding may become evident.

Signs of deterioration include (1) decreasing response to verbal or noxious stimuli; (2) dilated or fixed pupil; (3) increasing restlessness; (4) developing hemiparesis or developing asymmetry of reflexes or movement; (5) the appearance of extensor posturing of the arms or legs (decerebrate posture) and opisthotonus; (6) alteration of respiratory activity, persistent slowing or rapid hyperventilation activity, and finally jerking, irregular respirations; and (7) increasing blood pressure and slowing pulse.

In summary:

Provide an unobstructed airway and respiratory support.

Control bleeding; restore and maintain blood and electrolytes.

Treat fractures and lacerations.

Support the patient's metabolic needs.

Obtain neurosurgical treatment for the deteriorating patient.

BRAIN TUMORS

method of
WILLIAM A. KELLY, M.D.
Seattle, Washington

The frontispiece of the classic, *Intracranial Tumors,* by Percival Bailey has a quotation from Foster Kennedy: "He who cares for patients suffering from brain tumor must bring to his problem much thought and stout action. There is a need also of formidable optimism for the dice of the gods are loaded." The first concern is to dispel this cloud of pessimism that has been the heritage of the last half-century.

The historical perspective of the management of brain tumors is a fascinating subject. To review the classic texts of McEwen, Horsley, Cushing, Dandy, Bailey, and others can only reflect the dramatic steps taken in modern concepts of current therapy.

Tumor Types and Incidence

Brain tumors represent approximately 2 per cent of the mortality from neoplasms and approximately 4 per cent of hospital admissions.

The cause of tumors still remains a debatable and unclear issue. There is some value in categorizing these lesions by site of origin and the incidence of certain groups as they reflect the types of treatment and success of therapy.

Tumors of the skull include osteoma, fibroma, chondroma, and chordoma but are not common. Totally they represent less than 1 per cent.

A common tumor, meningioma, derives from meninges, and its frequency is about 20 per cent. Located over the vault, meningiomas are usually totally resectable. On the base of the brain, there is a greater technical challenge to achieve total removal. They can be multiple and on rare occasions are found in the ventricles.

Another group of benign tumors predominantly located at the base of the brain are neurinomas, pituitary adenomas, craniopharyngiomas, and cholesteatomas. Collectively they approach 20 per cent incidence. They are treated aggressively by surgery, but some of these lesions are problems by virtue of their anatomic locations and attachment to adjacent vital structures. Radiation is a common adjunct in craniopharyngiomas and pituitary lesions.

Ependymoma, pinealoma, and choroid papilloma are located centrally in ventricles or adjacent to them. In adults, the ventricular lesions are more benign, and with resection survival is fair to excellent. Pinealomas respond well to irradiation alone and only rarely require operative intervention.

Tumors of brain parenchyma are the most common, totaling nearly 50 per cent. The cells of origin are neurons and glial cells. The nerve cell tumors are very rare and will not be elaborated upon.

In the pediatric age group, 75 per cent of tumors are located in the posterior fossa. Cerebellar astrocytomas, medulloblastomas, and ependymomas are about equally represented. The astrocytoma is resectable with a very high cure rate.

Ependymomas and medulloblastomas are more malignant, requiring operative decompression and pathologic identification. In addition, they must have total axis, head and spine, irradiation for the best functional survival, as there is a tendency to seed in cerebrospinal fluid (CSF) pathways.

Brainstem gliomas and gliomas of optic nerves and adjacent structures are a special category. Usually diagnosis is made by x-ray procedures or operative exploration, but the primary therapy is irradiation, with some quite dramatic responses.

Adult gliomas, unlike the childhood lesions, are predominantly supratentorial in location. The most common posterior fossa tumor is the hemangioblastoma, responding well to total resection but with a definite recurrence rate. The gliomas have a complete spectrum of all cell derivatives, and vary from benign and totally resectable to very anaplastic malignancies with a poor prognosis.

In the benign tumors such as circumscribed astrocytomas and oligodendrogliomas, one attempts radical resection.

The general rule in malignant glioblastomas is decompression and radiation with or without chemotherapy. The objective is functional survival for the time left.

The central nervous system is not an uncommon site for metastatic disease. Thirty per cent may present primarily as brain tumor. It is worthwhile resecting solitary lesions and appropriate multiple nodules of colonic or renal cell cancers. Radiation can provide some palliation as well as primary treatment for most multiple deposits or in areas where operative intervention carries a high risk of function loss.

Operative Adjuncts

Sedation. Diagnostic procedures requiring intervention and increased risk are performed in the hospital. When faced with an uncooperative patient such as a demented or agitated adult or a small child, general anesthesia may be indicated, but most frequently these procedures are managed under local anesthesia with basal or supplemental sedation. The specific medication regimen will obviously vary with the amount of sedation or control required. The simplest adjunct is diazepam (Valium); in children, the dose is related to their size; in adults, usually 5 to 10 mg. is given, supplemented by intravenous amounts of 2 to 4 mg. as required. Infants and young children usually do well on a DPT cocktail (meperidine [Demerol], 25 mg.; promethazine [Phenergan], 6.25 mg.; chlorpromazine [Thorazine], 6.25 mg.) on a dosage schedule as varied by weight on the recommendation of the pharmacist. The ratio usually is 4:1:1. For more profound control (and usually managed by the anesthesiologist so that he can monitor vital signs and respirations and perhaps give assistance if necessary), methohexital (Brevital) is given rectally or droperidol and fentanyl (Innovar) intramuscularly. Usually added is atropine, 0.25 to 0.75 mg., again varying with the size of the patient.

Anticonvulsants. If the patient has seizures or the operative approach requires manipulation and/or retraction of cortical surfaces, particularly if the tumor removal requires resection of cortex, the use of anticonvulsants is indicated. Phenytoin (Dilantin) is usually the preferred anticonvulsant, and the usual calculated dose is 5 to 10 mg. per kg. of body weight; this is particularly helpful in children. The normal adult should be started on 300 mg. a day in divided doses, but one should obtain a blood level, as there is a significant variability in the metabolism of this medication; a therapeutic range is approximately 15 to 20 micrograms per ml.

Repetitive seizures or *status epilepticus* necessitates more rapid action, as phenytoin (Dilantin) orally requires a matter of hours to achieve satisfactory blood levels. If the patient has not been on anticonvulsants before, phenytoin (Dilantin) can be given intravenously to obtain a rapid blood level. A dose of 250 to 500 mg. is given slowly intravenously while one monitors the electrocardiogram (EKG) for the development of arrhythmias. In addition, more rapid-acting medication is necessary to arrest ongoing seizure activity. The most satisfactory medication for this is diazepam (Valium), also administered intravenously; 2 mg. is given in an initial dose and repeated as necessary, observing for arrest of the seizure activity; one must also observe respiratory rate, blood pressure, and pulse. Obviously, once the acute seizure manifestations are controlled, the patient should be hospitalized for observation, as recurrence of the seizure activity frequently occurs.

There are many other effective anticonvulsants, such as phenobarbital, carbamazepine (Tegretol), and primidone (Mysoline), which may be required for more specific seizure management. The appropriate dosage and blood level must be verified before instituting these agents.

This therapy is usually continued for a minimum of 6 months postoperatively and then the medication is discontinued, dependent on the lack of seizure activity and the resolution of abnormalities seen with electroencephalography.

Steroids. Almost routinely with any major intracranial surgery, steroid therapy is started 24 hours prior to craniotomy. Occasionally in the patient presenting with significant neurologic dysfunction and/or pressure symptomatology, the steroids have been started at that time. Frequently there is adequate improvement in the patient, allowing a complete diagnostic work-up and therefore avoiding the emergent and sometimes less than desirable approach that occurred frequently prior to the use of steroids.

Routinely 10 mg. of dexamethasone sodium phosphate (Decadron) is given orally as a loading dose, and the patient is maintained on 4 mg. every 6 hours thereafter. To avoid the complications of gastrointestinal bleeding, antacids are used prophylactically—magnesium and aluminum hydroxide (Maalox) or aluminum hydroxide (Amphojel)—four times a day, usually before meals and at bedtime. Postoperatively the medication usually can be discontinued abruptly in 5 days without having steroid withdrawal problems.

Occasionally patients with large, infiltrating tumors such as diffuse astrocytomas or large glioblastomas do not tolerate steroid withdrawal easily and require a very long tapering schedule. When one more nearly approaches the normal replacement levels, the patient is usually converted to prednisone as a more economical substitute. The usual daily maintenance of that medication is 5 to 10 mg. per day. The conversion equivalents are 0.75 mg. of dexamethasone (Decadron) = 5 mg. of prednisone.

Antibiotics. Antibiotics are infrequently used prophylactically in most craniotomies, but there are some occasions in which it is well considered: entry into the paranasal sinuses, as with some frontal craniotomies, into a mastoid with temporal approaches, and certainly with the transsphenoidal approach so commonly used with current pituitary surgery. Even under these circumstances, antibiotics are not used routinely, but in anticipation preoperative nose and throat cultures are usually obtained to sample the flora so that if gross contamination does occur, the appropriate antibiotics can be instituted.

Mannitol. There are occasional circumstances in which there is a rapid change in neurologic status with impending transtentorial herniation. Rapid decompression cannot be accomplished by steroids or ventricular or cyst decompression. To prevent progressive neurologic dysfunction, which may not be recoverable, hyperosmotic agents such as mannitol may produce a very rapid but transient decompressive effect. A single dose of 25 to 50 grams given intravenously over half an hour may produce enough diuretic effect to prevent further progression and allow better management of the brain tumor patient without precipitous emergent treatment.

Similar utilization of this medication is occasionally effective during operative procedures when brain retraction is difficult or acute cerebral swelling is encountered.

On rare occasions, in immediate postoperative periods this can be effective in control of postoperative swelling. It is obviously essential in this set of circumstances to verify that this is the exact cause of the problem and not that of postoperative hemorrhage, ventricular obstruction, or other acute postoperative complications which might well be covered up by the diuretic effect of hyperosmolar solutions.

It is important to recognize that with the use of these agents one must monitor the diuresis, and in the poorly responsive or anesthetized patient a bladder catheter must be inserted to volumetrically measure the diuresis and prevent distention. An obvious concomitant is the osmolar change in fluid and electrolyte balance. The postoperative course is usually managed by keeping patients on the "dry" side; but with the use of mannitol, solute loss as well as excessive water loss may produce a metabolic problem of dehydration and hyponatremia.

Ventricular Drainage. There are certain circumstances in which ventricular drainage can provide a significant decompressive effect of improvement of neurologic function. If it is maintained, elective completion of diagnostic work-up and significant enhancement of the ability to do a definitive operative procedure will occur, minimizing the problems of operation upon a tense, edematous, swollen brain in an acutely ill patient. A classic example is the patient with a posterior fossa neoplasm, with an acutely obstructed ventricular outlet, massive increased intracranial pressure, and associated cerebral edema. In this set of circumstances, one should place a ventriculostomy. This is done under sterile operative conditions, inserting a ventricular catheter in the frontal horn. This will maintain normal intracranial pressure, allowing overflow to be collected in the sterile reservoir. Usually this will accomplish acute decompression with a marked improvement in patient symptomatology; accompanied by steroid therapy, the patient's overall status will improve. This is usually maintained for at least 24 to 48 hours, and at the time of operation the exposure is done with relative ease as if dealing with normal brain tissue.

Ventriculostomy is a safe procedure if all sterile precautions are observed, the patient maintained on prophylactic antibiotics, and the ventriculostomy not utilized beyond a 5 day period. Complications arise from overmanipulation, such as frequent obstructions of the catheter system, and prolonged use in excess of 7 days.

This method of pressure monitoring and control has been found to have such value that it is frequently extended to those patients showing significant intracranial pressure problems preoperatively. It provides not only a monitor but also intraventricular pressure control during anesthesia as well as in the postoperative period.

There are occasional patients with obstructed ventricular systems who are not acutely ill or who have exceedingly high intracranial pressure. We have been able to perform an elective ventriculoatrial or ventriculoperitoneal shunt and delay the definitive operative approach to a future date.

Vascular Obliterations. This technique is most frequently utilized in highly vascular meningiomas. When angiography reveals a contribution from large external carotid to the vascular stain of intracranial tumors, our neuroradiologist has frequently been requested to occlude the external carotid supply by one of the various embolization techniques.

This can be performed with a retrograde femoral catheter using either pledgets of Gelfoam or Silastic beads. This can dramatically reduce the blood supply to the lesion, thus reducing blood loss on exposure and the total operative risk. Usually this is performed approximately 24 hours prior to the definitive operative approach.

This procedure has also been used preoperatively in certain arteriovenous malformations or on occasion as palliative treatment of these vascular anomalies which are inaccessible surgically.

Operative Magnification. The use of the operating microscope or loupes with fiberoptic light source has obviously added a totally new dimension to the operative approach of many tumors. It has become almost standard practice in transsphenoidal pituitaries, parasellar lesions, acoustic neurinomas, and intraventricular tumors, as well as other lesions.

In addition, in many other tumors it may be useful in certain parts of the operation to better define capsular margins, deep areas of vascular supply, and so forth. Added to this general category is the use of bipolar cautery, which also enhances vascular coagulation with reduced surrounding tissue damage.

To learn this technique one should start with cadaver dissection, and then use magnification on disc surgery. This will increase facility and speed with working under magnification and will probably provide the stimulus for more extensive utilization in other operative approaches.

Anesthesia

It is of utmost importance to work with an anesthesiologist who has some understanding of the problems of craniotomies in the face of intracranial pressure. A smooth induction, maintenance of proper CO_2 as measured by blood gases, and the knowledge of the use of such agents as mannitol, barbiturates, narcotics, and hypotensive agents such as nitroprusside are essential when encountering the varying risks and problems commonly associated with intracranial tumor surgery.

It is almost routine to have an intra-arterial line to monitor blood pressure, a central venous catheter to be aware not only of venous pressure but also of aspiration of air emboli encountered during operations in the sitting position, and an esophageal stethoscope. Respiratory rate and electrocardiogram (ECG) are carefully monitored and followed by an ink writer throughout the course of anesthesia so that early changes can be detected and managed acutely. When a ventriculostomy is available, intracranial pressure is added to the observations.

It is usually advisable to have a urinary catheter in place to monitor output, and this is required if one uses the hyperosmotic diuretics such as mannitol so that the bladder will not become overdistended.

Postoperative Care

All major craniotomies are best observed in an intensive care unit with sophisticated neurologic nursing. Most of the vital observations carried on during the anesthetic procedure are continued for at least 12 to 24 hours, depending on the responsiveness of the patient. Airway maintenance and assuring adequate ventilatory capacity are of prime importance to prevent the development of hypercarbia, and again a baseline blood gas analysis is of value after the patient has been extubated and away from ventilatory assistance of the anesthesiologist. Almost every neurosurgical unit now has some recognizable form of a neurologic monitoring or coma nursing sheet on which periodic observations are made of conscious level, pupillary size and response to light, and motor activity in response to stimuli, as well as the usual pulse, blood pressure, respiration, and temperature. It is wise to set limits on the observed abnormalities, so that when the respiratory rate drops below 14 to 15 per minute or anisocoria exists, or any other observations critical to neurologic status occur, you will be notified immediately.

Fluid replacement is usually managed intravenously during the first day and is restricted to 1500 to 2000 ml. With a baseline set of electrolytes and adequate hourly documenting of urinary output, one modifies this regimen to meet changes from normal levels. It becomes particularly acute when there has been large volume blood replacement, hyperventilation for protracted periods, or use of mannitol during the operative procedure. Compensatory replacement would obviously vary with the changes induced by these agents.

As stated previously, steroids are usually maintained through the first 4 to 5 days; if the patient is doing satisfactorily, these can be abruptly discontinued. Variations from this usually simple standard format would be significant in the severely ill comatose patient with marked irregularities in vital signs.

More anaplastic lesions usually receive postoperative irradiation. The standard therapy has been with cobalt and is usually instituted on the fifth to seventh postoperative day. There are certain tumors which one may well diagnose by varying techniques—CT scanning, angiogram, and/or pneumoencephalogram—which are not amenable to gross tumor resection or even needle biopsy without extreme risk. In particular, this includes brainstem gliomas and pinealomas, as well as deep thalamic gliomas. Often there is a segment of ventricular obstruction, and a VA shunt will be placed but irradiation therapy completed without a tissue diagnosis. It is usually advisable to verify the effect of radiation after 3 to 6 months by repeating the diagnostic studies, and certainly CT scanning may allow us to do this with a minimum of risk. If there has been little or no effect, then a more vigorous approach by an open exploration is usually performed to verify the lesion histologically. Medulloblastoma and ependymoma in children are usually benefited by surgical exploration and decompression but require total axis radiation to prevent and control the spread of subarachnoid seeding. Another tumor of variable response to radiation is the optic glioma, and it is best to obtain a tissue diagnosis by open craniotomy. Resections of these lesions have not been attempted, as they frequently respond quite dramatically to irradiation with long-term survival.

There are additional methods of treatment of the more malignant gliomas undergoing clinical investigation. Evaluations are currently being made on a series of patients with whole brain fast neutron beam irradiation, and some of the responses are promising.

In addition, BCNU, CCNU, and methotrexate are likewise under experimental investigation. Other forms of chemotherapy are being tested, but the variations in response for most of these newer techniques have not placed them in the realm of standard therapy.

Other Specific Tumors

This article has not been conceived as a treatise on specific surgical techniques but has followed the line of the general concepts of brain tumor management.

Pituitary adenomas are rapidly increasing in number, and their management is becoming relatively common at present. The reasons for this change of incidence are not readily available. A surprising number are microadenomas of a few millimeters in size which hypersecrete prolactin. In addition, endocrinologists are "finding" many other tumors producing acromegaly, Cushing's syndrome, and hypopituitarism. Many of these are still contained within the sella and are most frequently approached by transsphenoidal techniques. With increasing familiarity with this approach, neurosurgeons have become more aggressive in managing other pituitary tumors that have expanded outside the confines of the sella and are achieving very satisfactory results. The pre- and postoperative support of these patients does bear some additional mention. Usually the evaluation of suprasellar extension has been clarified by visual fields and CT scanning. If the presence or extent of a supradiaphragmatic pituitary lesion is uncertain, angiography and/or tomographic pneumoencephalography will define it.

Preoperative nose and throat cultures are obtained, and ampicillin, 500 mg. four times daily, is

TABLE 1. **Treatment and Prognosis—Summary**

Treatment / Tumor	Prognosis
Operation	
Neurinoma	Benign; possible cures
Meningioma	
Pituitary adenoma*	
Epidermoids	
Cerebellar astrocytoma	
Astrocytoma (focal)	Relatively benign; long term; some cures
Oligodendroglioma	
Craniopharyngioma	
Plexus papilloma	
Hemangioblastoma	
Ependymoma† (adults—ventricles)	
X-ray	
Pinealoma (rare condition)	Relatively benign
Optic glioma	
Brainstem glioma	
Metastatic‡—thalamic gliomas	Palliation
Surgery and X-ray	
Pituitary adenoma*	Relatively benign
Craniopharyngioma	
Ependymoma†	Prognosis guarded; rare survivors for 1 to 3 years
Medulloblastoma	
Metastatic‡	
Glioblastoma	

*,†,‡–double listings; variations in specific tumor.

given 24 hours preoperatively and maintained 5 days postoperatively because of the surgical approach through a contaminated space.

In addition, pituitary insufficiency is assumed and prednisone is started. Ten mg. is given the day before and the day of surgery, augmented by intravenous hydrocortisone as necessary. The prednisone is given for 1 to 2 days postoperatively, then gradually reducing to 5 mg. by the time of discharge.

These patients are subjected to a fairly thorough endocrine evaluation. If there are any indications of low thyroid levels, the patient should be given Synthroid, 0.1 to 0.2 mg. the day before surgery; this is continued until postoperative evaluation 4 to 6 weeks later. The close observation of the fluid intake and output and urine specific gravity of these patients is essential, as diabetes insipidus is a not uncommon complication, but in the great majority of patients it is transient. The intake and output balance can be maintained intravenously for the first 24 hours, but these patients respond quite readily and maintain excellent balance on oral liquids if they are allowed to satisfy their thirst. It is indeed the rare patient who requires vasopressin (Pitressin) controlled water balance, and this certainly at a delayed time, not in the immediate postoperative period.

SECTION 13

The Locomotor System

RHEUMATOID ARTHRITIS

method of
JOHN T. SHARP, M.D.
Danville, Illinois

Many therapeutic agents have been advocated for the treatment of rheumatoid arthritis, but all have serious limitations. Rheumatoid arthritis is a complex disease with many manifestations and a variable course. Successful treatment requires an understanding of the natural history of the disease and a careful analysis of the patient's problems.

It is especially important to determine whether the main symptoms are the consequence of active inflammation in the joints, are the result of systemic effects of the illness, or are due to destruction of articular cartilage and bone from prior long, continued inflammation. This requires the physician to appraise the status of the articular system by history and physical examination, usually without resorting to histologic study. The presence of synovial effusions and an excess of synovial tissue in the capsular and pericapsular areas is usually the consequence of persistent inflammation. In addition, the involved joints may be warm and slightly tender to pressure and may be uncomfortable with normal degrees of motion. On the other hand, the presence of instability and severe degrees of crepitation may represent destruction of the cartilage and the supporting capsular tissues which has reached an irreversible stage and does not reflect the presence of current inflammation. Additional information can be obtained by radiologic appraisal of the extent of cartilaginous destruction and bony erosion, although x-ray examination is less helpful in determining the extent of active inflammation. In general, early disease is associated with active inflammation, but it is important to appreciate that the "early" changes refer to the stage of illness and not to elapsed time from onset, as there is great variability in the rate of progression of disease in different patients. Patients with intermittently active arthritis—namely, patients who have periods with symptoms and signs followed by the complete disappearance of active inflammation—rarely have a progressive, destructive arthritis. In contrast, those patients in whom inflammation is continually present for many months or years usually develop serious sequelae.

The treatment of rheumatoid arthritis should be considered under several broad headings: the general program, physical therapy, analgesics and anti-inflammatory drugs, specific agents, and surgical therapy.

The general program utilized by most rheumatologists includes a regular, normal diet with some adjustment of calories according to whether the patient is normal in weight, requires some weight reduction, or is underweight. In addition, the patient should get a regular night's sleep. When the disease is particularly active and fatigue is an important symptom, added periods of rest during the day are helpful.

Physical therapy is regularly prescribed to maintain good muscle tone and a normal range of motion insofar as possible. Help of the occupational therapist is enlisted to give the patient hints on the protection of inflamed and weakened joint structures.

Drug therapy should be considered in terms of analgesics, anti-inflammatory agents, those drugs which appear to be relatively specific in reducing the inflammation of rheumatoid arthritis, and cytotoxic drugs.

Aspirin is the anti-inflammatory agent of choice in the majority of patients with rheumatoid arthritis. In some patients, gastrointestinal symptoms are prominent side effects and salicylates may not be tolerated. Those patients who have a history of gastrointestinal bleeding should be treated with aspirin only with great caution. Toxic hepatitis is a rare complication of salicylate treatment. Fortunately, most patients tolerate aspirin well when given together with an antacid. For those patients whose tolerance for aspirin is limited, a propionic acid derivative such as ibuprofen (Motrin), naproxen (Naprosyn), or fenoprofen (Nalfon) may be useful. Tolmetin and indomethacin are moderately potent anti-inflammatory agents that also may be used instead of aspirin or may be given with aspirin in patients whose relief is incomplete. Acetaminophen is of little benefit in the treatment of rheumatoid arthritis. In the past, phenylbutazone has been utilized by some for therapy of rheumatoid arthritis, but it is no longer recommended because of the high incidence and serious nature of toxic reactions.

Most of the anti-inflammatory agents are also analgesic. In some instances, an additional analgesic is helpful, but unfortunately most of the potent analgesics are addicting drugs. Even propoxyphene (Darvon) and pentazocine (Talwin) are habit forming and, if used to excess, can produce physiologic addiction. For this reason, only occasional use of propoxyphene is recommended, and the drug is never used on a regular schedule. Pentazocine has little or no advantage over narcotics and is rarely advised.

Gold therapy has been shown to have an effect on the rheumatoid inflammatory process in numerous controlled studies. These studies have shown that about two thirds of the patients treated with gold improve, and analysis of patients treated over a 2 year period has shown slowing or halting of progression of destructive lesions in bone and cartilage as assessed by radiologic examination. However, some placebo-treated patients also improve, so the net benefit—namely, the percentage of patients who are treated with gold who improve over and above those treated with placebo who improve—is somewhere between 40 and 50 per cent. In the past, gold has been recommended in doses of 50 mg. gold sodium thiomalate or gold sodium thioglucose weekly. In a recent study, it was demonstrated that 25 mg. of the gold salt weekly was as effective as 50 mg.

Chloroquine was introduced in the treatment of rheumatoid arthritis in the 1950s. Short-term controlled trials demonstrated a modest benefit from chloroquine when compared with placebo. Long-term trials have not been conducted to establish whether the progression of the disease is altered as measured by the development of deformities and radiologic changes.

In recent years, penicillamine has been given a thorough double-blind trial and has been shown to benefit rheumatoid arthritis. The effect on progression of destructive lesions has not been established.

Glucocorticoids, when given in sufficiently large doses, partly or completely relieve the inflammation of rheumatoid arthritis. Unfortunately, effective steroid doses usually induce manifestations of hypercortisonism. In many patients, these effects are worse than the original disease, and in some the side effects are disastrous. For this reason, systemic corticosteroid therapy is not recommended.

Cytotoxic drugs, including cyclophosphamide, azathioprine, 6-mercaptopurine, and chlorambucil, have been used by several investigators. Unfortunately, all these drugs are associated with an unacceptable incidence of tumors in the recipients, particularly lymphoproliferative disorders. Further, the types of tumors that have occurred in patients receiving these drugs have been resistant to drug therapy, so that the mortality from such treatment-induced tumors has been extremely high. These drugs are therefore unacceptable in the treatment of rheumatoid arthritis today.

The successful management of the patient with rheumatoid arthritis requires a thorough evaluation by the attending physician. An analysis of the role that each factor may play in the disease and the willingness of the patient and the doctor to accept the fact that long-term treatment is required to achieve any benefit are the important ingredients of effective treatment.

The patient who has early disease with prominent inflammation and progressive changes by x-ray examination over a period of 6 months or longer should be considered for gold therapy. Gold therapy is routinely given weekly for a period of 20 to 40 weeks, using a dose of 25 mg. gold sodium thiomalate or gold sodium thioglucose. If, during this time the disease goes into complete remission, the frequency of injections is reduced to every 2 weeks for a period of 4 to 6 months. If, at the end of that time, the patient remains in remission, the frequency of injections may be reduced further; but in case of recurrence of disease, weekly injections are resumed to further suppress the activity, and the optimal interval of injections is reassessed. If no benefit is derived during a period of 40 weeks of weekly injections, gold therapy is discontinued. During the period of time when the patient is receiving weekly gold injections, the patient is examined by the physician prior to each injection to exclude toxic reactions, including stomatitis, dermatitis, pruritus, and diarrhea. In addition, a weekly leukocyte count, differential count, platelet count, and urinalysis are obtained.

Although most patients have disease in many joints and gold therapy is the preferred mode of preventing progression of the disease, in some instances a synovectomy may be performed as a method of treating inflammation localized to a single joint. The number of joints that are easily accessible to thorough synovectomy, which is required to produce lasting benefit, is somewhat limited, and synovectomy is successful usually only in the knees, ankles, and elbows.

Patients who, when first seen, have moderately advanced disease that has already produced physical deformities and destruction of cartilage and bone, must be analyzed carefully to determine whether inflammation is a continuing process. At this stage, these patients usually have had disease for 6 months to several years. If, in addition to the permanent damage, there are physical signs of inflammation, these patients may also benefit from gold therapy. If surgical correction of deformities is recommended, it is often wise to delay surgery for several months to permit the suppression of active inflammation by the gold treatment.

In other patients with advanced disease, who have deformities and radiologic changes, the inflammation may have subsided. The permanent changes in the cartilage, bone, and supporting structures will not be affected by gold therapy, and surgical reconstructive procedures may be the only treatment to consider. Such procedures at present are generally extensive and often require total joint replacement with a prosthetic device. The most successful of these has been the total hip replacement. Somewhat less successful but remarkably good in properly selected patients has been the total knee prosthesis. Still under study are total joint replacement procedures for ankles, wrists, and elbows. Hand surgery often provides cosmetic benefit, but the functional improvement is usually limited.

Proper analysis of each patient's problems with application of the appropriate therapeutic regimen will provide some relief for most patients, will slow or halt the progression of the disease in many during the inflammatory phase of the disease, and can restore major degrees of functional ability to those with "burned-out" disease.

JUVENILE RHEUMATOID ARTHRITIS

method of
VIRGIL HANSON, M.D.
Los Angeles, California

The first task in the treatment of juvenile rheumatoid arthritis (JRA) is the establishment of the diagnosis, which has been materially aided by recognition of at least three distinct subtypes. The basic criteria for the diagnosis of JRA are (1) onset under 16 years of age; (2) persistence of arthritis in at least one joint for at least 6 weeks; and (3) exclusion of other chronic inflammatory joint disease—e.g., other collagen diseases and infection. Active arthritis is defined by swelling of one or more joints with or without other signs, or by the presence of two or more of the following signs: limitation of motion, tenderness (including pain on motion), and warmth. The three subtypes are defined by clinical findings noted during the first 6 months from onset, as follows: (1) pauciarticular onset with less than five involved joints during the first 6 months, (2) polyarticular onset with five or more involved joints observed during the first 6 months, and (3) systemic onset characterized by persistent daily intermittent fever elevations to greater than 39°C. (102.2°F.). Since objective joint disease may not appear for months in the systemic form of the disease, a diagnosis of probable JRA can be made in the presence of spiking fever associated with the characteristic evanescent rash, along with one or more findings such as marked adenopathy, hepatosplenomegaly, pericarditis, or leukocytosis.

Treatment

Since there is no specific cure for JRA, treatment is directed toward control of the known manifestations of the disease coupled with education and counseling. JRA is characterized by chronic or chronically recurrent inflammation of the joints and other tissues. Acute inflammation results in transient disability associated with marked swelling and pain, but deformity and long-lasting disability are the results of chronic inflammation resulting in erosion of cartilage and bone, the weakening of ligaments, and fixed contractures. Treatment is directed toward control of this inflammation and the prevention or reduction of the secondary deformity, contractures, and disability noted above. The major goal of therapy is the maintenance of joint position, function, and muscle strength in patients seen early in their disease and restoration of these factors in those seen later in the course. The physical methods of therapy are as important as the medicinal. The pharmacologic modes of treatment are directed toward reduction of the inflammation and thus enhance the administration of physical means of therapy and possibly reduce the damage of joint structures.

Education and Counseling of Family and Patient

The outlook for most children with JRA is excellent for recovery with minimal or no residuals with proper treatment, but most parents are alarmed by the diagnosis. Doubts should be allayed by further consultation at this point if needed, but most important is time to provide parents with answers to their questions and information concerning the disease and its treatment. Such educational efforts must be reinforced by additional opportunities for answering questions as time goes along in a relaxed, unhurried atmosphere and for reviewing knowledge of the disease.

Explaining what is known of the mechanisms of the disease removes the frightening aura of mystery of the unknown, and a well understood plan of therapy provides the assurance of activity directed toward control and improvement. Continued school attendance whenever possible is to be encouraged, and instruction and information should be provided for the school personnel. The reactions of other children to the increased attention given the arthritic child must be explored and the family prepared to meet the problems without loss of other satisfying activities. In children with marked or protracted disability, additional counseling by a social worker or other psychologically trained personnel can be helpful in resolving the problems secondary to marked disability.

Nonsteroidal Anti-Inflammatory Agents

Aspirin. Acetylsalicylic acid remains the drug of choice among the nonsteroidal anti-inflammatory agents for several reasons. First, it is effective in controlling inflammation and fever in the majority of children with JRA. Second, it is relatively safe and long experience has been accumulated in its use. Third, none of the new nonsteroidal anti-inflammatory agents have yet been shown to be definitely superior to aspirin in effectiveness or toxicity. Fourth, none of the new nonsteroidal anti-inflammatory agents have yet been approved for the treatment of children with JRA under 14 years of age. Fifth, it is the least costly of the medications. Once the diagnosis of JRA has been established, treatment is begun with aspirin in a dose of 80 mg. (1$^{1}/_{5}$ grains) per kg. of body weight per 24 hours divided into four or more doses. The aspirin dose may be increased to 100 or 120 mg. per kg. per 24 hours if needed to achieve suppression of signs of inflammation or serum salicylate levels of 20 to 25 mg. per 100 ml. It is often difficult to reach serum levels of this magnitude in children with systemic disease, but increasing the daily dose above 130 mg. per kg. frequently results in significant toxicity. Abdominal pain and vomiting may be controlled in some children by the administration of antacid preparations. Enteric-coated aspirin is sometimes beneficial to children whose intolerance is primarily gastrointestinal. Infrequently, either gastric or duodenal ulcers may occur on prolonged high dose aspirin therapy, even with little in the way of gastrointestinal symptoms. A marked drop in hemoglobin may be the first warning of this complication. Serum transaminase levels (serum glutamic-oxaloacetic transaminase [SGOT] and serum glutamic pyruvic transaminase [SGPT]) have been found to be elevated in as many as 50 per cent of children on therapeutic doses of aspirin and should be monitored at least weekly during the first 6 weeks of therapy and at monthly intervals thereafter. Abnormal levels below 100 I.U. are not an indication for discontinuing treatment, but at levels between 100 and 300 I.U. the dose should be decreased by about 20 per cent. If the SGOT or SGPT values increase or remain at high levels, aspirin therapy should be discontinued until they become normal, at which time treatment may be reinstituted at a slightly lower dose and gradually increased, usually without recurrence of the hepatotoxicity. Satisfactory control of inflammation will be achieved for most children with this regimen; but for those who cannot tolerate aspirin in doses of 75 to 120 mg. per kg. per day, or who do not show adequate response within a 3 to 5 month period, other drugs must be considered.

Other Nonsteroidal Anti-Inflammatory Agents. For children over 14 years of age, other nonsteroidal anti-inflammatory agents should be tried, such as tolmetin, 200 to 300 mg. four times daily; naproxen, 250 mg. twice daily; or ibuprofen, 300 to 400 mg. four times daily. Experience indicates that failure of one anti-inflammatory agent does not preclude the possibility of successful treatment with another, and these medications should be sequentially tried for periods of 2 to 4 weeks, as they are in general less toxic than those at the next level of therapy.

For children under 14 years of age the therapeutic choices are far more limited. In those with systemic disease the addition of acetaminophen in two or three doses of 325 to 650 mg. (5 to 10 grains) prior to and at the time of the usual temperature rise may be helpful in controlling both fever and pain. For most patients, however, more potent and therefore more toxic agents will be required. Gold therapy is generally considered the next step at this point. Gold sodium thiomalate is the most commonly used preparation. The basic dose is 1 mg. per kg. per week given intramuscularly, but the first dose should be 0.25 mg. per kg., with 0.25 mg. per kg. stepwise increases each week until the full dose of 1 mg. per kg. is reached. Treatment is then continued weekly for 20 weeks, and if satisfactory improvement or remission has been achieved, continuation at 2 to 3 week intervals for at least a full year after all signs of inflammation have subsided is indicated. A complete blood count and urinalysis should be obtained each week within 24 hours prior to the next injection and history or presence of rash noted. Decrease of the white blood cell count below 5000, decrease of the absolute neutrophil count by 50 per cent, proteinuria, hematuria, and rash are indications for at least temporary cessation of therapy. When these findings have returned to normal, therapy may be resumed at a lower dose with gradual increase to the full dosage level. Severe leukopenia, neutropenia, continued heavy proteinuria, and exfoliative rash are contraindications to continued therapy.

Corticosteroids

Systemic corticosteroid administration may be considered after an adequate trial of therapy, as outlined above, in patients with persisting severe systemic disease or severe active polyarticular disease with marked limitation of motion and wasting of tissues. Pericarditis, unless accompanied by evidence of marked impairment of cardiac function, is not of itself an indication for this form of treatment. For severe uncontrolled systemic disease with cachexia, wasting, and other severe symptomatology, prednisone (or equivalent amounts of other corticosteroid) may be started at a dose of 1 mg. per kg. per 24 hours in a single daily dose given in the morning and increased in 0.5 mg. steps until satisfactory control is achieved, with an upper limit approximately 2.0 mg. per kilogram. Rarely in some children a single daily dose may not be adequate, and divided doses may be required for a short period. Once satisfactory control is achieved, medication should be gradually returned to a single daily dose and shifted gradually to every-other-day therapy. The parents must be indoctrinated in the need to accept some symptoms in exchange for reduction of corticosteroid toxicity. Ansell (Still's Disease: Juvenile Chronic Polyarthritis, M. I. V. Jayson [ed.], Academic Press, 1976), prefers daily administration of ACTH gel (Armour Acthar gel) in doses of 20 to 40 units intramuscularly daily in the morning to orally administered prednisone, but there is no consensus on this point. Most children can tolerate continued aspirin therapy at doses below 80 mg. per kg. per day if not the larger doses, and this should be continued as an adjunct to minimize the steroid dose. For children with severe unresponsive polyarticular disease, prednisone may be given every other day in doses of 0.5 to 1 mg. per kg., with other therapy such as aspirin and/or gold continued. Additional analgesics such as acetaminophen (Tylenol) or propoxyphene (Darvon) may be required on the days off steroid therapy.

There is no indication for treatment of pauciarticular JRA with systemically administered corticosteroids. Persistent marked inflammation of one or two joints is best treated by injections of triamcinolone hexacetonide (Aristospan) in amounts of 10 to 30 mg. no more frequently than every 6 months. Care must be taken that this preparation is not deposited in the tissues outside the joint. For iridocyclitis the opinion is divided as to the value of systemic corticosteroid, but it is usually recommended for short periods, 4 to 7 days, if the eye disease is severe and unresponsive to locally administered steroid drops. The treatment is usually then continued on an every-other-day basis until the condition comes under control.

Antimalarials

Hydroxychloroquine and chloroquine are rarely prescribed in the United States for the treatment of JRA at present because of their known eye toxicity. Early studies in adults showed these agents to be effective in reducing joint inflammation when given in large doses, and Stillman has recently reported evidence of effectiveness in the treatment of JRA. Hydroxychloroquine is preferred, as it is thought to be less toxic, and its use can be considered for the treatment of children whose disease remains uncontrolled with the medication previously outlined. The dose is 5 mg. per kg. daily. (This use of hydroxychloroquine is not listed in the manufacturer's official directive.) The patient's eyes should be examined by an ophthalmologist for evidence of retinal toxicity prior to beginning therapy, at 6 month intervals during the first year, and every 3 months thereafter.

D-Penicillamine

D-Penicillamine has not been approved by the Food and Drug Administration for the treatment of children with JRA and should be administered on an approved protocol only. Current reports, however, suggest that it may be as effective as gold but no more toxic and therefore may be a potentially useful drug in the future. The maximum dose is thought to be 30 mg. per kg. per day up to a limit of 1 gram per day. The maximum dose is reached in six steps at 2 week intervals with close monitoring of complete blood counts, platelet counts, and urinalysis. D-Penicillamine may result in the formation of antinuclear antibodies and drug-induced lupus, and periodic serologic studies for antinuclear antibody are therefore indicated.

Immunosuppressive Agents

Immunosuppressive agents in the treatment of JRA must be considered strictly experimental and used only with carefully designed experimental protocols. The most commonly used agents have been azathioprine, cyclophosphamide, and chlorambucil. These agents are successful in suppressing rheumatoid disease, but exacerbations, often severe, within months after discontinuing therapy are almost universal. Leukopenia of a severe degree is a likely complication of all, and the potential for tumorigenesis is thought to be high. Treatment of JRA with cyclophosphamide has been followed by recurrent severe hemorrhagic cystitis as long as 5 years after therapy and may result in fibrosis and stenosis of the bladder. Sterility is associated with both cyclophosphamide and chlorambucil. The only indication for the use of immunosuppressives in JRA may be amyloidosis, a potentially fatal complication, which, although relatively frequent in Europe, is rare in North America.

Detection and Treatment of Iridocyclitis

Iridocyclitis in juvenile rheumatoid arthritis is almost entirely insidious in onset and is noted by the patient or family only when decreasing vision or lens opacities call it to their attention. This complication can be detected early by periodic slit lamp examination carried out by an ophthalmologist, and the diagnosis of JRA therefore requires ophthalmologic examination at its beginning, at 3 to 6 month intervals thereafter for at least 10 years after onset, and probably at least yearly thereafter. Iridocyclitis is most commonly associated with the pauciarticular class of disease and is progressively more likely with young onset, female sex, and antinuclear antibody; but it occurs in all three types of JRA and therefore must be looked for in all. The ophthalmologic examination should be carried out not less often than every 3 months for girls with pauciarticular onset and antinuclear antibody and at least every 6 months for others.

Treatment is prescribed by the ophthalmologist and usually consists of one of several forms of corticosteroid eye drops and a dilating agent for the pupil to prevent adhesions between pupil and lens. Acute glaucoma and retinal blindness may result, or vision may be lost through clouded cornea or lens if the condition is left unattended. Some of the latter problems can be corrected by appropriate ophthalmologic surgery when indicated.

Physical and Occupational Therapy

The physical management of JRA is of the utmost importance. Only the gentlest of therapy can be given in the presence of acutely swollen hot joints. Rest is helpful at this stage but can become deleterious if continued for more than a few days, and planning for a complete program of therapy should be started immediately. Extensor muscle atrophy of joints begins early with or without pain. It is mediated through reflex arcs which not only inhibit extensor function but also facilitate flexors. Generally the inflammation will be brought under partial control within 3 or 4 days with appropriate medical therapy, and physical management can be begun. Active extensor exercises with gradually increasing resistance or load are therefore important and need to be adapted to the level of the child's maturity. Swimming and bicycling or tricycle riding are excellent exercises which may require less motivation than repetitive drills. The tendency toward increasing contracture may be slowed by provision of night splints for wrists and knees particularly; and if the hips are involved, long sitting should be avoided. Fifteen to 30 minutes in the prone position on a firm surface three to four times daily is recommended to aid in prevention of hip flexion contractures. Children with longstanding disease often have extensive muscle atrophy and relatively fixed contractures. Active exercises are therefore important and may be begun in warm water in a walking tank or pool with water levels around the mid-chest at first. Gradual reduction of the water level provides a gradually increasing load on the muscles and therefore strengthening. For marked flexion contractures of the knees, wrists, or ankles, serial casting at 2 day intervals with active exercises on the day of removing the cast are more effective. The cast should be applied at the maximum extension achieved without pain, and no forced extension should be applied. Maintenance of the reduced contractures often requires the utilization of lightweight plastic splints for both night and daytime use. A variety of additional techniques can be used for restoration of function, and further consultation is recommended for the more difficult problems. It is important to notify the school of the child's physical problems and to make arrangements for adaptations to his needs. Stiffness after sitting is common, and a high table for working part of the time in a standing position can be helpful in alleviating this problem.

Surgery

There is no proof that synovectomy significantly affects the course of disease in any joint, and consultation with orthopedic surgeons who have worked with pediatric rheumatology teams is recommended before considering any orthopedic surgical procedure. Well planned reconstructive surgery can be of major benefit to children with marked disability resulting from deformity or ankylosis. Total joint replacement, particularly of the hips, may be considered when there is no further potential for bone growth near the affected joint.

ANKYLOSING SPONDYLITIS

method of
FRANKLIN KOZIN, M.D.
Milwaukee, Wisconsin

Ankylosing spondylitis (AS) is an inflammatory disease of unknown cause affecting primarily the axial skeleton (sacroiliac and apophyseal joints of the spine). Root (hips, shoulders) and other peripheral joints may be inflamed on occasion, usually in an asymmetrical distribution. Extra-articular manifestations are found in 10 to 25 per cent of the patients, involving eyes, urethra, intestines, or heart. Amyloidosis or cauda equina syndrome is a rare complication. The recent discovery of HLA antigen B27 in 90 per cent of Caucasian and 50 per cent of black American patients has been a helpful adjunct in diagnosis of AS and related spondyloarthritides.

Treatment

The three major goals of therapy in AS are (1) pain control, (2) reduction of inflammation, and (3) maintenance of maximal spinal and joint function. Since inflammation and pain frequently go hand in hand, control of inflammatory response will reduce pain and allow pursuit of an exercise program aimed at restoring normal posture and mobility.

Aspirin remains the drug of first choice in AS, although it often is not as effective as in rheumatoid arthritis (RA). A starting dose of 10 to 12 (5 grain) aspirin tablets daily usually is necessary to achieve anti-inflammatory serum salicylate levels of 18 to 25 mg. per dl. (100 ml.). The dose may be increased slowly until such serum levels are obtained or until toxicity supervenes (tinnitus, gastric intolerance). To minimize dyspepsia or risk of gastrointestinal bleeding, it is recommended that aspirin be taken with meals or bedtime snack and followed by a full glass of water or milk. Enteric-coated aspirin or other salicylate preparations may be used when plain aspirin is not tolerated. Improvement as diminished pain and morning stiffness and increased mobility should be apparent within 3 to 6 weeks.

If salicylates prove inadequate, one of the newer phenylalkanoic acids, such as ibuprofen (Motrin), naproxen (Naprosyn), or fenoprofen (Nalfon), or tolmetin (Tolectin), a pyrrole derivative, should be substituted. These drugs also are best given with food, as gastric intolerance is a major side effect. Again, response should be seen within 3 to 6 weeks.

Failure of the aforementioned drugs to control symptoms dictates a trial of indomethacin (25 to 50 mg. capsules) or phenylbutazone (100 mg. tablets). Initially 4 to 6 tablets (capsules) daily are given in divided doses for 1 to 2 weeks and then gradually reduced to maintenance doses of 2 to 4 tablets daily over the ensuing 2 to 6 weeks. Caution must be exercised in the use of these agents because of the frequency and potential severity of side effects. Indomethacin is known to produce gastric erosion or ulcer, a variety of central nervous system effects (vertigo, lightheadedness, headache), and mild salt and water retention; phenylbutazone is notable for its tendency to produce gastric ulcer, marked salt and water retention, and bone marrow suppression. Patients with hepatic or renal insufficiency or with underlying heart failure and hypertension must be watched carefully for adverse reactions; regular blood counts are essential to safe use. When control of symptoms is obtained with indomethacin or phenylbutazone, every effort should be made to find the lowest possible effective dose; addition of aspirin or the other agents discussed above may prove helpful in lowering the dose.

Non-narcotic analgesics (acetaminophen, propoxyphene) may be necessary for pain control but should not replace anti-inflammatory drugs, as the arthritis and its disabling sequelae may progress unabated. Spinal radiation, which was used to treat AS in the 1940s with variable success, has no role in current management, as its hazards far outweigh any potential benefit. Intra-articular steroids are effective in treating root or peripheral joint involvement. Choice of preparation, dose, and the precautions in its use are identical to those in the therapy of rheumatoid arthritis and are discussed on pages 745 to 747.

Certain patients require more intensive treatment because of extra-articular complications or severe articular inflammation. Use of ophthalmic (for iridocyclitis) or systemic steroids may be necessary in these patients. Occasionally other immunosuppressive agents such as azathioprine or cyclophosphamide are indicated in this group when corticosteroid doses exceeding 10 to 15 mg. of prednisone (or equivalent) are required. (This use of azathioprine and cyclophosphamide is not listed in the manufacturer's official directive.)

It is most important to initiate a therapeutic exercise program at the earliest possible time to improve posture and spinal or joint mobility. Regular exercises should become a daily ritual for patients with AS to maintain maximal spinal mobility, chest expansion, and full range of motion of all peripheral joints. Education of the patient is essential to successful therapy. He (usually) or she must understand the critical role of exercise in preventing ankylosis and permanent deformity, limited joint function, and restrictive pulmonary complications. They must understand the logical progression of anti-inflammatory drugs from those with lesser risk to those with greater risk.

Finally, regular visits to the physician are important to ensure compliance with the established regimen, to evaluate spine and joint mobility, and to detect extra-articular manifestations as early as possible. Objective measurements such as finger-to-floor or head-to-wall distances and chest expansion should be recorded and the exercise program adjusted when necessary.

BURSITIS AND CALCIFIC TENDINITIS

method of
THOMAS A. MEDSGER, JR., M.D.
Pittsburgh, Pennsylvania

Bursae are sac-like potential spaces limited by modified synovial lining cells; they are located at areas of frequent motion between various musculoskeletal structures and serve to reduce friction and protect these moving parts. The most commonly involved in clinical situations are the subdeltoid or subacromial bursa at the shoulder; olecranon bursa at the elbow; trochanteric bursa at the hip; and prepatellar and anserine bursae near the knee. Bursitis may be initiated by a number of pathophysiologic mechanisms, including nonspecific degeneration, inflammation caused by crystals (sodium urate crystals in gout and calcium hydroxyapatite crystals from adjacent tendinitis), inflammation caused by any systemic arthritis which affects synovial tissue (e.g., rheumatoid arthritis), and occasionally bacterial infection. Soft-tissue calcification has a predilection for tendons and may lead to a localized low-grade inflammatory reaction with pain and tenderness. The rotator cuff tendons of the shoulders, greater femoral trochanteric tendons, and Achilles tendons are favorite sites for this type of involvement, and often roentgenograms of these areas will reveal punctate calcific deposits.

There are four basic objectives in the treatment of nonseptic bursitis and tendinitis: relief of pain, decrease in inflammation, removal of an inciting stimulus (such as calcium deposits), and preservation of motion. Table 1 outlines methods used to achieve these goals in acute, subacute, and chronic inflammation of bursae and tendons.

Acute Bursitis or Tendinitis

1. (a) Immobilization: upper extremity (sling, splint or cast); lower extremity (cast, crutches or non-weight-bearing). (b) Analgesic equivalent to codeine, 60 mg. four times daily. (c) Moist cold or heat application.

2. Anti-inflammatory agents: choice of (a) prednisone, 20 mg. orally at once, 15 mg. on days 2 and 3, and 5 to 10 mg. on days 4 through 10; (b) indomethacin, 100 mg. orally at once; 150 mg. in divided doses on days 2 and 3, and 75 to 100 mg. on days 4 to 10 (all doses given with meals or snacks); or substitution of (c) other agents, such as phenylbutazone, aspirin, and the new nonsteroidal anti-inflammatory agents; each has its particular risks and limitations.

3. Procaine injection and "washing out" the bursa with two-needle irrigation (if calcareous deposits are evident on roentgenograms) or multiple punctures in the area.

4. No exercises are advised when inflammation is acute.

Subacute Bursitis or Tendinitis

1. Enforced rest of affected part, as above, or general rest; adequate analgesia; moist heat.

2. Choice of (a) injection of corticosteroid (equivalent of prednisone, 20 to 40 mg., depending on size of affected area), or (b) oral nonsteroidal anti-inflammatory agents, as described above.

3. Multiple punctures in the area during the corticosteroid injection.

4. Range of motion exercises once daily, as tolerated.

Chronic Bursitis or Tendinitis

1. Limited active motion of the affected part; non-narcotic analgesics; heat applications, including ultrasound or diathermy.

TABLE 1. **Treatment of Bursitis and Tendinitis**

OBJECTIVE	METHOD	ACUTE	SUBACUTE	CHRONIC
Relief of pain	1. Immobilization			
	Enforced	+	+	0
	General	0	+	+
	2. Analgesia			
	Narcotic	+	+	0
	Non-narcotic	0	+	+
	3. Topical application	+	+	+
Decrease in inflammation	1. Corticosteroids (oral)	+	0	0
	2. Corticosteroids (injection)	0	+	+
	3. Nonsteroidal anti-inflammatory agents	+	+	+
Removal of calcium deposit (if present)	1. Multiple puncture (surgical two-needle irrigation)	+	+	+
	2. Surgery	0	0	+
Preservation of motion	1. Range of motion	0	+	+
	2. Resistive exercises	0	0	+

2. Nonsteroidal anti-inflammatory agents—these may be used indefinitely.

3. (a) Multiple needling with procaine alone or procaine plus corticosteroid preparation or (b), in refractory cases, surgical removal of calcific deposits and/or reconstruction of damaged tissues.

4. Encouragement of active full range of motion and muscle strengthening with progressive resistive exercises.

OSTEOARTHRITIS

method of
ROBERT W. LIGHTFOOT, Jr., M.D.
Milwaukee, Wisconsin

Osteoarthritis, or degenerative joint disease, is a predominantly noninflammatory arthritis characterized initially by loss of stainable mucopolysaccharide from the cartilage matrix, followed by grossly and microscopically visible splitting and fraying of the cartilage. Subsequently, proliferative osteophytes appear at the margins of the involved joint, and ultimately sclerosis of the subchondral bone, occasionally with cyst formation, may occur. Symptoms may vary from none to severe pain and deformity. In population studies, a majority of persons in middle age or beyond may have roentgenographic changes of degenerative joint disease, most without any symptomatology. Current theories as to the cause of osteoarthritis suggest that the loss with age of the elasticity of bone, the major shock absorber of weight bearing in the young, results in a transfer of normal weight bearing stress onto the cartilaginous portion of the skeleton. This, coupled with an alteration in mucopolysaccharide content of cartilage with aging, may predispose to the cartilage degeneration mentioned above. There is also evidence to suggest that proteolytic enzymes present in cartilage cells may activate in stressed cartilage and secondarily accelerate the degenerative process. It is clear that repeated trauma to a given joint area predisposes to degenerative arthritis. Specific examples are the wrists in former jackhammer operators and osteoarthritis of the knee following a remote athletic injury. Certain forms of osteoarthritis, notably that which occurs in the hands, seem in some instances to result from a familial predisposition.

The treatment of osteoarthritis includes medical, surgical, and physical measures. Although some have reported roentgenographic detection of reconstitution of lost cartilage, it is generally felt that once cartilage damage occurs in this condition it persists to a greater or lesser degree. Thus "cure" of the osteoarthritic joint cannot be effected. Because the disease is not systemic and tends to localize to specific joints, the treatment modalities mentioned above are applied differently from their application in a more generalized condition. The use of the aforementioned modalities and their ultimate efficacy will depend to a considerable extent on the stage to which the disease has progressed at the time therapy is initiated. Accordingly, a careful appraisal of the anatomic and functional status of the involved joints is essential before attempting to initiate therapy.

General Treatment Measures

Patient Education. A major concern of most patients consulting a physician for this illness is that they have a progressive, destructive arthritis which will ultimately involve many joints. It is important, if the patient is to cooperate in the therapy program, that his fears be allayed and that he understand the arthritis as primarily a localized "wear and tear" arthritis. In addition, the patient must understand that there is no universally successful mode of management, and that it may be necessary to try empirically a variety of medicines and physical therapy measures before improvement occurs. This avoids undue disappointment should the initial program of treatment not result in dramatic relief.

Rest. Because microtrauma seems to play an important role in the development and progression of this disease, and because overuse of an involved joint generally results in a worsening of symptoms, avoidance of undue physical stress on such a joint is important. However, except for an occasional patient with degenerative arthritis in the spine, rest in bed is rarely needed. Recognition of the pathogenesis of osteoarthritis and the role of rest in minimizing progressive joint destruction is especially important for the patient who is eager to undertake a vigorous program of jogging, bicycling, or other stressful activity in a misguided attempt to help his joint disease. The patient with osteoarthritis should be advised to restrict any activity which subjects the involved joint to prolonged or sudden stress. In mild cases, minimal or no limitation in normal activities of daily living should be required. In more advanced cases, a physical therapy consultation should be obtained to acquaint the patient with techniques to minimize stress on joints while carrying out normal activities. Because the lower extremity joints are those most frequently involved, elimination of stress may include such measures as prescription for shoes designed to eliminate inequality of leg length or alignment, as well as the use of canes or other assistive devices. A cane is best used in the hand opposite the most symptomatic joint, as this permits a shifting of weight off the involved joint when it is in the weight bearing phase of the gait.

Drug Therapy. Although osteoarthritis is not typically an acute inflammatory condition, patients often respond dramatically to milder forms of anti-inflammatory medication. The response of an individual patient to any of these drugs is entirely unpredictable, and it may be necessary to try a variety of these before concluding that they are ineffective.

Aspirin. 1. Because aspirin is widely touted as a headache remedy and mild pain killer, most patients will take aspirin reluctantly, if at all, unless instructed as to the rationale of its use.

2. Patients must be told that aspirin, when taken consistently in order to establish a blood and tissue level, exerts an anti-inflammatory effect which can be of help in treating various forms of arthritis.

3. Patients must also be instructed not to anticipate an overnight effect from the use of aspirin. It is generally advisable to take regular doses of salicylate for at least 2 weeks before drawing conclusions about its efficacy.

4. A general principle of salicylate therapy should be to push aspirin to toxicity, subsequently backing off to a tolerable dose.

5. A small number of patients will develop side effects to aspirin, including gastrointestinal irritation and, especially in older patients, tinnitus.

6. If tinnitus occurs, the maintenance dose of aspirin should be lowered.

7. If gastrointestinal irritation occurs, the dose may be lowered or an alternative salicylate preparation tried. In order to minimize gastrointestinal side effects in symptomatic patients, they may try taking their salicylates on a full stomach. In addition, drinking several glasses of water immediately after aspirin ingestion may minimize irritative contact of the tablet with the gastric mucosa. If these measures are not successful, alternative salicylate preparations, e.g., aspirin mixed with an antacid or enteric-coated aspirin, may be used. For reasons not readily apparent, patients intolerant of regular aspirin often have no gastrointestinal symptoms when taking one of these other preparations.

8. The usual starting dose for aspirin is 975 mg. (15 grains) four times daily. If this is ineffective after 1 week, the daily dose may be increased by increments of 650 mg. (10 grains) until improvement or toxicity occurs.

Indomethacin. 1. This nonsteroidal anti-inflammatory drug can be of impressive benefit in selected cases of osteoarthritis. The nature of its action in this predominantly noninflammatory disease remains unknown.

2. The usual starting dose is 25 mg. three times daily.

3. The dose may be increased at weekly intervals by 50 mg. per day, the total dose not to exceed 150 mg. daily.

4. The most common side effects of this medication are gastrointestinal upset, headaches, dizziness, and mental aberrations. For this reason the drug should be given with meals or accompanied by milk or a snack.

Phenylbutazone and Oxyphenbutazone. Among the most effective nonsteroidal anti-inflammatory drugs, these pyrazalone drugs have restricted use in osteoarthritis. Doses of 100 mg. three to four times daily for periods not exceeding 1 week may be helpful in acute exacerbations. Because the side effects include agranulocytosis, marked fluid retention, and upper gastrointestinal ulceration, treatment for longer than 1 week should be avoided.

Phenylpropanoic Acids. 1. Of the several compounds in this category available, two, ibuprofen and fenoprofen, are currently approved for use in the treatment of osteoarthritis. There are no data currently available to suggest that one of these compounds is preferable to the other in treating this disease.

2. Ibuprofen, 400 mg. three to four times daily, may provide adequate control of symptoms.

3. The recommended dose of fenoprofen is two 300 mg. tablets four times daily, never later than a half hour before or earlier than 2 hours after meals.

4. Although these compounds may have a lower incidence of gastrointestinal irritation than salicylates, some studies have shown that when the dose of these drugs is increased sufficiently to produce comparable degrees of relief, the incidence of gastrointestinal side effects is similar to that seen with aspirin.

Corticosteroids. So severe are the side effects of these agents in a predominantly older population that their systemic use in osteoarthritis is rarely or never justified. Similarly, there is no evidence to support a role for gold compounds, antimalarials, D-penicillamine, immunosuppressive drugs, or immunostimulant agents in controlling osteoarthritis.

Intra-Articular Corticosteroids. 1. Intra-articular steroids appear to be of limited benefit in alleviating symptoms of osteoarthritis. An exception may be those patients in whom the arthritis is complicated by an inflammatory component.

2. The dose used varies with the surface area of the synovial cavity to be injected and can be determined by consulting the package insert accompanying these compounds.

3. Patients must be cautioned not to interpret relief of pain from such injections as "cure." There is evidence to suggest that corticosteroid injections, if given repeatedly, may predispose to a more accelerated cartilage destruction, and for

these reasons the patients are best instructed to avoid excessive use of an injected joint for several weeks irrespective of pain relief.

4. For the reasons outlined above, joint injection, if effective, should probably not be repeated more often than three to four times per year.

Analgesic Drugs. ASPIRIN. 1. Although aspirin is a most effective non-narcotic analgesic drug, if it is to be used at all, it should be tried at anti-inflammatory doses as outlined above.

2. If patients are intolerant of anti-inflammatory levels, analgesic doses of 325 to 650 mg. (5 to 10 grains) every 4 to 6 hours as needed for pain relief may be used.

ACETAMINOPHEN. 1. Doses of 325 to 650 mg. every 4 to 6 hours as needed may effectively relieve pain.

2. This drug may be especially helpful in those patients intolerant of even low doses of aspirin.

3. Although generally better tolerated than aspirin, this medication proably has little or no anti-inflammatory effect and therefore should be used only when aspirin has been tried unsuccessfully.

PROPOXYPHENE COMPOUNDS. 1. Propoxyphene hydrochloride, 65 mg. three to four times daily, or propoxyphene napsylate, 100 mg. in a similar regimen, may provide significant analgesia in patients with osteoarthritis.

2. These compounds should be used only as adjuncts to the more important anti-inflammatory medications mentioned above.

3. These compounds exert greater analgesic effect when administered in conjunction with aspirin or acetaminophen.

4. They can be addictive if taken chronically.

PENTAZOCINE HYDROCHLORIDE. Fifty mg. every 6 hours, with or without aspirin, may be of benefit.

NARCOTIC DRUGS AND ANALOGUES. 1. Because of their addictive properties, narcotic drugs should be assiduously avoided in the treatment of any chronic illness such as this.

2. These drugs should never be considered part of the definitive treatment of osteoarthritis.

3. The only role for these drugs in the management of this illness may be the alleviation of severe pain in a patient in whom definitive treatment, such as joint replacement, is planned in the immediate future.

4. The use of narcotics, even for short periods, in other than the aforementioned situation, may result in lifelong addiction.

Physical Measures. The use of physical therapy is important in both the inpatient and outpatient management of degenerative joint disease. Such measures will have greater chance of success if the patient is adequately educated as to the nature of osteoarthritis, especially as to the reasons for avoiding undue joint trauma. Physical therapy may be especially valuable in certain specific situations as outlined below.

HEAT. 1. The application of mild heat may significantly reduce myospasm, which can be a major contributing component to the pain in this illness.

2. Excessive temperature may increase spasm in addition to resulting in cutaneous burns.

3. The muscle relaxation afforded by heat may permit a more effective exercise program.

4. Subjectively, moist heat is more beneficial than dry heat, although proof of its superiority is lacking.

5. Local heat may be applied in a variety of ways, including electric heating pads, hydrocollator packs, and paraffin baths.

6. A more general application of heat to the lower extremities and low back may be effected by the use of whirlpool baths, Hubbard tank, or heated pool. By lowering the effective weight borne on the lower extremities, pool therapy may facilitate the performance of lower extremity exercises.

7. Modalities such as short wave diathermy or ultrasound may be of value in delivering heat to deeper structures in certain limited situations, e.g., osteoarthritis of the cervical spine.

8. The aforementioned deep heat modalities should be avoided in inflammatory conditions, as they may result in increased pain, and in areas near metallic prostheses. The latter may absorb significant heat and result in searing of adjacent tissues.

COLD. 1. Ice packs or other forms of cold to a local area may have a significant analgesic effect, probably from the inhibition of the reflex arcs that cause muscle spasm.

2. Whether a given patient will respond better to heat or cold can only be determined empirically.

3. Cold applications should be used for shorter periods of time than heat, not to exceed 5 to 10 minutes.

4. Application of cold to the terminal portions of the extremity should be done cautiously to avoid ischemic damage resulting from vasospasm.

5. Cold applications are less apt to prepare the patient for an exercise program.

EXERCISES. 1. Exercises which result in excessive motion between weight bearing surfaces of the involved joint should be discouraged for the reasons outlined above.

2. The primary role of exercise in the treat-

ment of osteoarthritis is to (a) maintain range of motion, (b) strengthen adjacent muscles on which the stability of the involved joint may depend, and (c) improve proper posture and positioning of the joint.

3. Muscle strengthening exercise should be isometric, in order to avoid the excessive motion mentioned above.

4. Range of motion exercises should require moving the involved joint through its range of motion only five to ten times several times a day.

5. Any exercise which results in increased symptoms should be reduced or eliminated.

Traction. In general traction has a limited but specific role in certain forms of osteoarthritis.

1. Intermittent cervical traction, especially following application of heat, may be of marked benefit in cervical osteoarthritis.

2. If cervical traction under the direct supervision of the physical therapist is effective, the patient should obtain and be instructed in the use of a traction apparatus for use at home.

3. Pelvic traction is of limited value in this condition. It probably does little more than immobilize the patient, thus enforcing bed rest.

Splints. 1. Splinting or bracing appropriate joints may be of use in discouraging unfavorable movement or positions. Such devices rarely provide true stability to abnormally unstable joints.

2. Cervical collars of either the soft foam or hard plastic variety may be of dramatic benefit in lessening the symptoms of cervical osteoarthritis, especially if worn during certain periods known to stress the cervical spine, e.g., sleep, working at a desk, or riding in a vehicle.

Weight Control. 1. A force many times the total body weight is transmitted to lower extremity joints during normal ambulation. Because of this and the known correlation of lower extremity osteoarthritis with excessive obesity, weight reduction, even of a few pounds, can lessen the rate of progression of joint damage in osteoarthritis.

2. Weight reduction will also minimize perioperative morbidity in those patients who are candidates for surgery.

Surgery. Those patients who do not respond to a comprehensive program of anti-inflammatory, analgesic, and physical measures should be considered candidates for orthopedic surgery. In situations in which malalignment results in an abnormal distribution of forces on the weight bearing surfaces, e.g., severe valgus deformity at the knee, osteotomy to distribute the weight onto a more normal medial compartment may be of dramatic benefit. Similar realignment has been used with less dramatic benefit in osteoarthritis of the hip.

In the severely damaged joint, the implantation of low friction prostheses in the hips, knees, and some smaller joints has resulted in dramatic and long-lasting alleviation of symptoms.

On occasion the degenerative process may result in the formation of cartilaginous and bony debris which not only interferes with joint motion but can also cause pain and acceleration of the degenerative process. Occasionally such materials can be removed through arthroscopy. In other instances an open procedure is necessary to permit adequate removal of this material.

Fusion of involved joints will eliminate pain, but results in immobility of the joint as well. Although this may afford relief in the involved joint, it may put undue stresses on more proximal or distal joints in the same or the contralateral extremity. These factors must be appreciated when considering arthrodesis of a given joint.

Summary

Because osteoarthritis is not a systemic disease, the principles guiding therapy vary with the anatomic areas which are most symptomatic. Simple drug therapy with nonsteroidal anti-inflammatory compounds along with physical measures will suffice in most instances. In more severely involved joints, surgical intervention may be dramatically effective. A major component in the success of any treatment regimen is the degree to which the patient has been educated about the nature of the degenerative process.

SECTION 14

Obstetrics and Gynecology

ANTEPARTUM CARE

method of
BEREL HELD, M.D.
Houston, Texas

Introduction and Objectives

The goal of the obstetrician today, as it has been always, is to deliver a healthy newborn of a healthy mother. Medical supervision of pregnancy ideally should begin prior to conception in order to make an intelligent appraisal of the woman's medical status.

The broad purposes of rendering prenatal care include (1) preparation and psychologic support for the patient and her family; (2) prevention of illness and disease during the antepartum course; and (3) recognition and treatment of disease present in the mother or fetus.

Initial Medical Visit

Patients should begin prenatal care within 2 or 3 weeks after the missed period. This initial visit represents the most important visit to the physician's office in the entire pregnancy; and because of findings during the past decade, there has developed the concept that many pregnancies requiring specialized care after delivery can be identified antenatally. Between one third and one half of patients who subsequently will develop problems during pregnancy can be recognized during the first prenatal evaluation.

Various scoring systems and indices of high risk have been established and described. The rationale is that by using such identification systems, one might be able to focus on a minority of antenatal patients who will have the majority of complications. Figure 1 indicates the system used at our institution for the identification and evaluation of high risk pregnancies and represents a modification of the high risk score reported by Aubrey and Nesbitt. The utilization of such a form to provide an objective method of assessing risk, with visual representation of the multiplicity of risk factors involved, forces the physician and health care team to evaluate each patient systematically. This assessment at the time of the first prenatal visit emphasizes certain important facts to be sought in obtaining a history and in the performance of a complete physical examination.

History. The history taking follows a conventional pattern that should include a complete past, social, and family history, a review of the systems, and a detailed gynecologic and obstetric history.

Menstrual History. Facts to be elicited include age at the menarche, interval between and duration of menses, and previous contraception; if contraception was used prior to pregnancy, a statement of the reasons for its discontinuance and the time prior to conception that it was discontinued should be noted.

Present Obstetric History. Any subjective or objective symptoms the patient may have should be noted, in addition to determination of the first day of the last menstrual period and first day of the previous menstrual period. If an estimated date of confinement had been given to the patient previously, this should be recorded, as well as the date of quickening, if quickening has occurred by the time of the first prenatal visit.

Previous Obstetric History. This ought to include documentation of all previous pregnancies and their outcomes, the weeks of gestation elapsed, duration of labor, condition of children at birth, birth weights, and present condition of all children. A detailed history of any complica-

HIGH RISK SCORE

Name ______________ LMP ________ EDC ________ Ab's ________

Hospital No. ______________ Gravida ________ Para ________

SCORE: Initial Visit	28 weeks	L & D

I. Age

Age	
Under 15	20
15–19	10
20–29	0
30–34	5
35–39	10
Over 40	20

Marital	
Single	10
Separated	5
Married	0

Parity	
0	10
1–3	0
4–7	5
7+	10

II. Social

Trimester of Registration	
1st	0
2nd	10
3rd a) 28–34 wks	20
b) 34+ wks	30

Broken Appointments	
0–1	0
2–4	10
5+	30

Desirability	
Planned	0
Unplanned	10
Unwanted	30

Pre-Conception Contraception	
Bcp's	0
IUD	0
in situ	30

III. Past Obstetric History:

Abortions	
1	5
2	15
3+	30

Prematures	
1	10
2+	30
IUGR	20

Fetal Death	
1	10
2+	30

Neonatal Death	
1	10
2+	30

Congenital Anomaly	
1	10
2+	30

Damaged Infants	
Physical	10
Neurological	20
HMD	20

Prior Delivery History:

Malpresentation	10	Oxytocin stimulation	10	Low Apgar (<6)	20
Cesarean section	30	Medical induction	10	Mid-pelvic forceps	20
Abruptio	20	Postpartum hemorrhage	20	Infection	10
Placenta previa	20				

IV. Medical Obstetric Disorders

Systemic Illnesses	
Acute, mild	5
Acute, serious	10
Chronic, mild	5
Chronic, debilitating (meds)	20

Endocrine	
Diabetes—Class A	20
Over Class A	30
Definitive thyroid disease	20
Irregular menses	10
Infertility <2 yrs	10
>2 yrs	20

Heart Disease	
Class I and II	10
Class III & IV	20

Hypertension, Chronic	
a) Mild	20
b) Severe (meds)	30

Nutrition

Pre-Pregnancy Weight
- Under 100 — 20
- 100–110 — 10
- 110–180 — 0
- 180+ — 10
- Acetonuria — 20

Specific Infections
- Urinary
  - Bacteriuria — 5
  - Pyelonephritis
    - Past history — 10
    - Current Preg. — 20
    - With anemia — 30

Anemia
- Hgb 10–11 — 5
- Hgb 9–10 — 10
- Under 9 — 20
- Sickle-trait — 20
- ss or sc — 30
- Above with bacteriuria — 20
- Parasites — 5

Rh
- Maternal sensitization — 30
- Prior affected neonate — 40

Weight Gain
- <10# at 20 wks — 20
- <20# at delivery — 10
- <10# at delivery — 20
- >30# at delivery — 10

- Gonorrhea — 10
- Syphilis — 10
- Vulvovaginitis — 5
- and H/O PROM — 10

Smoking
- <1 pack/day — 10
- >2 pack/day — 20
- Alcohol, drug abuse — 30

V. Generative Tract
- Prior pelvic surgery — 20
- Definite incompetent cx — 20
- Anomaly — 10
- Uterine disease (myoma, septum) — 20

Pelvis
- Borderline — 10
- Contracted — 30

Threatened Abortion
- 1st trimester — 10
- 2nd trimester — 20
- Decreased movement — 20

VI. Fetal
- Multiple Gestation — 20
- Date-Exam Disparity — 10
- Post-Datism (>42 wks) — 20
- I.U.G.R.
  - Suspected — 10
  - Definite — 30

VII. Intrapartum
- Premature labor — 30
- PROM <12 hrs — 5
  - >12 hrs — 10
  - >24 hrs — 30
- Malpresentation — 30
- Unengaged vertex — 30

- Fever — 30
- Bleeding — 30
- Hypertension
  - Mild — 10
  - Severe ($MgSO_4$) — 30

- Prolonged active phase — 20
- Active phase arrest — 30
- Medical induction — 20
- Uterine tetany — 10
- Meconium
  - Dark_____ — 20
  - Light_____ — 10
- Abnormal FHR pattern — 30

VIII. Delivery
- Date________________
- Weight________________
- Method ________________
- Apgar_______/_______
- Neonatal complications ________________
- Maternal complications ________________

Figure 1.

tions occurring during previous pregnancies should be sought, including such complications as bleeding, hypertension, abnormal edema, excess weight gain, eclampsia, hyperemesis, urinary tract infection, phlebitis, dystocia, and oxytocin induction or stimulation. Included in this section would be comments regarding infertility, or the difficulty with which pregnancy was accomplished.

Family History. A complete family history of illnesses is obtained, including specifically a history of diabetes mellitus, hypertensive disorders, congenital abnormalities, genetic diseases (e.g., inborn errors of metabolism, chromosomal abnormalities, and hemoglobinopathies such as sickle cell disease), and multiple pregnancy.

Review of Systems. A complete and detailed systems review at the time of the first prenatal visit is important, and special emphasis ought to be placed on such illnesses as previous urinary tract infections, hypertensive disorders, anemias or blood transfusions, history of infectious diseases such as rubella, neuropsychiatric problems, and past surgical procedures. It is important to record a history of drug allergies and any previous transfusions, and to list current medications.

Physical Examination. A complete physical examination is performed at the time of the first prenatal visit. The following items warrant particular attention:

1. Height.
2. Weight—present and prior to pregnancy.
3. Blood pressure and pulse.
4. Funduscopic examination for hemorrhages, arterial-venous ratios, hypertensive changes.
5. Thyroid enlargements, nodes, bruits.
6. Breasts—condition of nipples, masses, tenderness, discharge, axillary extension of breast tissue.
7. Abdomen—organomegaly, scars, masses, fundal height, location of fetal heart tones.
8. Extremities—varices, edema.

Pelvic Examination. The purpose of a complete pelvic examination at the time of the first antepartum visit is to establish the diagnosis of pregnancy and to determine the presence or absence of pelvic and adnexal abnormality or disease. This includes an estimation of the capacity of the bony pelvis and the obtaining of a Papanicolaou smear. Important signs to be noted during inspection and palpation of the genitalia include the following:

1. Vulva and perineum—Scars, anorectal lesions, Bartholin's and Skene's glands.
2. Vagina—bluish discoloration (Chadwick's sign), presence of discharge or inflammation, blood, leukorrhea, etc.
3. Cervix—lacerations, erosions, scarring, dilatation.

Bimanual Examination. 1. Uterus—size, consistency, position, and shape.

2. Adnexa—tenderness or masses.
3. Clinical pelvimetry—measurement of the diagonal conjugate (normally not reached), sacrosciatic notch (generally two to two and one half fingerbreadths), prominence of ischial spine, curvature of the sacrum, intertuberous diameter, and angle of the pubic arch.
4. Description of pelvic configuration (gynecoid, platypelloid, anthropoid, android).
5. Rectal examination—hemorrhoids, fistulas, or masses.

Laboratory Studies. The following studies are routinely obtained at the time of the first prenatal visit in our Unit:

1. Complete blood count.
2. Blood serology.
3. Rubella titer.
4. Blood type and Rh determination (indirect Coombs if Rh negative).
5. Papanicolaou smear.
6. Glucose-6-phosphate dehydrogenase and Sickledex screen for all black patients.
7. Endocervical gonococcal culture.
8. Urinalysis and screening culture for asymptomatic bacteriuria.

Urine specimens for examination are obtained by the clean voided midstream technique; radiologic evaluation of the chest is not performed routinely.

Postexamination Counseling. After the initial history and physical examination, the physician should counsel the patient and, if possible, the husband also, as to what to expect during the course of pregnancy, and he should detail those items needed to maintain a state of physical and psychologic well-being throughout gestation. The patient should have sufficient opportunity during this session, as well as during future prenatal visits, to express her concerns, have unjustified fears allayed, have "old wives' tales" dispelled, and receive a set of specific instructions in regard to physical activity, sexual activity, travel, and nutrition. The availability of community or hospital educational programs should be described (such as Lamaze classes or childbirth education classes, if appropriate). Postpartum family planning and contraceptive advice should also begin during prenatal care.

Physical Activity. In the uncomplicated prenatal patient, a reasonable amount of physical activity ought to be encouraged and the dictates of good common sense utilized. Sufficient rest is also necessary; as pregnancy progresses, a 1 hour rest period in mid-day is advisable.

Coital Activity. Sexual activity can be maintained throughout a normal pregnancy according to the patient's comfort and desires.

Nutrition. Adequate protein intake during pregnancy is essential for optimal fetal health. For a well nourished, uncomplicated gravida, recommended daily allowances during pregnancy include a diet containing at least 60 grams of protein and a total caloric intake of approximately 2500 calories. Under no circumstances should weight reduction programs be instituted during pregnancy, and the optimal weight gain in the average size woman during pregnancy ought to equal between 20 and 25 pounds. The asthenic, undernourished woman should be encouraged to gain more than this amount, however, for it has been shown that inadequate weight gain during pregnancy is as detrimental to neonatal outcome as excess weight gain. Optimal amino acid intake can be obtained by ingestion of meat, milk, eggs, fish, and cheese. The importance of adequate protein intake during pregnancy cannot be overstressed, particularly in light of accumulating evidence relating to deficiencies of both gray and white matter in the brain and of the heart, liver, kidney, and placenta in the face of protein deprivation. Significant nutritional deprivation during pregnancy may result in the delivery of small for gestational age neonates as well as infants with an absolute decrease in the number of brain cells.

Drugs. Unless essential, medications of all types should be avoided during pregnancy. The worth of vitamins during pregnancy is debatable, but it is our usual custom to prescribe prenatal vitamins with folic acid supplement routinely. In addition, all patients should receive iron supplementation in the form of ferrous sulfate, 300 mg. three times daily. For symptomatic nausea and vomiting in early pregnancy, we prescribe dicyclomine (Bendectin), 2 tablets at bedtime and 1 tablet in the morning.

Smoking during pregnancy ought to be avoided, both for maternal health reasons and because of evidence that infants of smoking mothers are smaller in weight than those of nonsmoking mothers. Alcohol also is best avoided during pregnancy.

Dental Care. Dental care should be encouraged during pregnancy, although elective procedures, particularly those involving inhalation anesthetics, ought to be postponed.

Routine Prenatal Care of Normal Patients

In those patients who are completely normal at the time of the initial history and physical examination and remain so during the course of pregnancy, routine prenatal visits are scheduled monthly during the first and second trimesters, bimonthly during the seventh and eighth months, and weekly in the last month of pregnancy.

During each of these prenatal visits, the following minimum information is obtained:

1. Weight and weight gain—if in excess of ½ pound per week, a detailed nutritional history is in order.
2. Blood pressure—a systolic blood pressure of 140 mm. Hg or diastolic blood pressure of 90 mm. Hg, a systolic rise of 30 mm., or a diastolic rise of 15 mm. Hg is regarded as abnormal. For these patients, and certainly those with edema or other signs and symptoms of toxemia, more frequent visits and further evaluation are appropriate.
3. Urine test for albumin and glucose.
4. Presence of edema—pedal, fingers, facial.
5. Location of fetal heart tones.
6. Height of uterine fundus in centimeters and in particular its correlation with gestational age by history.
7. Presentation and station of fetus during ninth month.

An hematocrit is obtained in the midtrimester of pregnancy and repeated at the thirty-sixth or thirty-seventh week because of the high incidence of iron deficiency anemia occurring during pregnancy. In Rh negative patients with negative indirect Coombs titers, a repeat titer is obtained at the twenty-eighth to thirtieth week and again at the thirty-sixth week of pregnancy if the husband is Rh positive.

In addition, the patient should be given every opportunity to have her questions answered. At an appropriate time during the course of pregnancy, discussions ought to take place regarding the proposed management of labor and delivery. The latter includes a description of what to do if, for example, the membranes rupture, bleeding occurs, or regular uterine contractions begin. Further, during the course of prenatal visits, the types of analgesia and anesthesia available during labor and delivery should be discussed.

Specialized Problems and High Risk Care

If a patient on either initial or a subsequent prenatal evaluation is considered to be high risk in nature, specialized and more intensive care is in order. This may involve specialized tests, more frequent prenatal visits, or referral to a special high risk clinic. In any event, extra time should be scheduled for each visit and additional resources should be available. Anesthetic considerations become important in the high risk patient, and the neonatology team should be aware of any potential problem looming in the future. In short, a team approach is to be encouraged in the management of the high risk gravida.

Diabetes Mellitus. The perinatal hazards associated with diabetes, including Class A (gestational diabetes mellitus), are well known. Hence careful questioning to determine if the patient has diabetes on the basis of her obstetric history, delivery of a previous infant over 9 pounds, previous stillbirth of unexplained origin, multiple spontaneous abortions, or repeated glycosuria is an important aspect of good prenatal care. Her age and family history should be recorded. Our criteria for the diagnosis of biochemical diabetes mellitus are as follows: Using a standardized 100 gram dose of glucose and processing the plasma in an autoanalyzer that measures true glucose, our limits are (1) fasting, 105 mg. per 100 ml.; (2) 1 hour, 190 mg. per 100 ml.; (3) 2 hours, 165 mg. per 100 ml.; and (4) 3 hours, 145 mg. per 100 ml.

Equaling or exceeding any two or more values, or any recording of 200 mg. per 100 ml. or greater, provides confirmation of disease.

All diabetics are followed at least bimonthly, and the most important aspect of their care is proper nutritional counseling. Uncontrolled diabetes requires hospitalization, and timing of delivery is dictated by a combination of clinical evaluation, assessment of the fetus in utero, and tests of fetal maturity, all of which will be described below.

Hypertensive Disorders of Pregnancy. Essential hypertension during pregnancy is treated with the same agents utilized prior to conception. If untreated essential hypertension is detected during pregnancy, antihypertensive therapy is not instituted unless diastolic pressures equal or exceed 110 mm. Hg and systolic pressures equal or exceed 160 mm. Hg in spite of bed rest. If antihypertensive therapy must be instituted, methyldopa (Aldomet), in dosages approximating 250 mg. four times per day, is utilized after obtaining appropriate baseline studies, including electrocardiogram, funduscopic evaluation, creatinine clearance values, and 24 hour urinary protein excretion. In those patients with essential hypertension but without superimposed toxemia, the decision for early delivery depends largely on fetal growth and development during pregnancy, placental function tests, and fetal maturity.

Toxemia of pregnancy other than the mildest form is best managed by hospitalization and judicious delivery after stabilization with magnesium sulfate.

Multiple Gestation. Once a suspicion of multiple gestation is confirmed by x-ray or ultrasonography, the following problems ought to be anticipated and, ideally, prevented: anemia, owing to the increased iron demands of both fetuses; prematurity, ideally prevented by increased bed rest as pregnancy progresses; and toxemia of pregnancy, prevented by increased bed rest and careful attention to proper nutrition.

Cardiac Disease. Ninety per cent of all cardiac disease in pregnancy is valvular, and most valvular disease is a result of acute rheumatic fever, a history of which should be sought during the initial prenatal visit. All patients with heart disease are categorized in the functional classification suggested by the American Heart Association, and are evaluated in conjunction with a cardiologist. Baseline studies include a posteroanterior (PA) and lateral chest film, electrocardiogram, phonocardiogram, and pulmonary function studies. All cardiac patients are seen weekly and their physical activities restricted. Diuretics are not utilized routinely; digitalis is instituted only for heart failure; and prophylactic antibiotics are not administered anew during pregnancy. Prevention of anemia, provision of adequate nutrition and ideal weight gain, and avoidance of infectious respiratory conditions are the basic tenets of management. There are no cardiac indications to induction of labor, and the indications for cesarean section in the cardiac patient are obstetric only.

Rh-Negative-Sensitized Patients. The current management of Rh-sensitized patients involves spectrophotometric determinations of bilirubin pigments in serially obtained amniotic fluid specimens begun at 24 weeks of gestation. Amniocentesis is performed on the basis of past obstetrical history and, in our laboratory, when the indirect Coombs antibody titer exceeds 1:8. Decisions to deliver at term, to deliver prematurely, or to perform intrauterine transfusion are based on the reported optical density of the amniotic fluid. The correlation of these tests with amniotic fluid determinations to assess fetal maturity is helpful in these complicated pregnancies. It must be remembered that the optical density of amniotic fluid can be spuriously lowered by exposure to light; therefore proper precautions must be observed in handling the specimens.

Prenatal Genetic Diagnosis. If prenatal genetic diagnosis is contemplated, abortion must be an acceptable alternative to the family. More than 50 fetal diseases can be diagnosed prenatally; they include chromosomal abnormalities, X-linked recessive diseases, and inborn errors of metabolism. The indications for amniocentesis in these latter two instances depend largely upon family history, whereas fetal chromosomal analysis between the fourteenth and seventeenth weeks of pregnancy is indicated on the basis of maternal age and/or family history. These specialized tests, which involve biochemical determinations or culturing of cells from amniotic fluid, require delicate handling of specimens. Obtaining specimens and counseling therefore should be performed in a center geared to such specialized studies.

Incompetent Cervical Os. Incompetent cervical os can be suspected on the basis of past obstetric performance, which may include previous trauma to the cervix (such as dilatation and curettage [D & C] or septic abortion), followed by a history of mid-trimester losses characterized by rupture of the membranes, followed by a short, painless labor. The diagnosis is confirmed during pregnancy by observing and palpating progressive cervical dilatation and effacement between the sixteenth and thirtieth weeks of pregnancy. In a patient with an incompetent os, cervical cerclage by either a Shirodkar or McDonald procedure results in an 85 per cent success rate. This procedure is performed under general anesthesia with avoidance of hypotension and hypoxia, and the patient is discharged 24 hours postoperatively if no complications ensue. Patients in our institution undergoing a cerclage procedure do not receive prophylactic antibiotics; nor are they placed on progestational therapy or alcohol infusion for precautionary reasons. The suture is removed at approximately 38 weeks of gestation and after fetal maturity is ascertained, and patients normally are allowed to deliver vaginally. An occasional patient who wishes additional children but who has a poor obstetric history but a successful cerclage procedure is delivered via cesarean section to retain the cerclage suture for a future pregnancy.

Hyperthyroid Disease in Pregnancy. Hyperthyroidism is 100 times more frequent than spontaneous myxedema in pregnancy. In most instances, hyperthyroidism antedates the pregnancy rather than being precipitated by it. Although there is little general agreement as to the effect of pregnancy on the course of hyperthyroidism in the mother, there is no doubt of the deleterious effects of maternal thyrotoxicosis on the fetus. Abortion, stillbirth, and neonatal death are common, particularly if hyperthyroidism is uncontrolled. Radioactive iodine therapy for hyperthyroidism is contraindicated during pregnancy, and our preference in the treatment of this disease is medical rather than surgical. Propylthiouracil, 100 mg. three times daily, is administered until the disease is controlled, and then the dose is halved for maintenance. Concomitantly, L-triiodothyronine (Cytomel) is begun at a dosage of 25 micrograms daily, to prevent fetal goiter and cretinism. In severe disease, with marked tachycardia and signs of impending high cardiac output failure, propranolol (Inderal), 10 mg. four times daily, is instituted for its beta-adrenergic receptor blocking activity. Hydrocortisone, 100 mg. per day, is administered only if there is danger of thyroid storm or if the patient comes to labor and delivery not totally controlled.

Premature Rupture of the Membranes

Premature rupture of the membranes should be determined by sterile speculum examination. Visualization of the os with leaking fluid is confirmatory; the fluid should be tested by nitrazine paper for its reaction. A fern test of the fluid examined under the microscope is often helpful in determining true rupture. The management of premature rupture of the membranes without chorioamnionitis is somewhat controversial and depends, to a large extent, on the neonatal and nursery resources of the hospital. In our institution, fetuses beyond 32 weeks of gestational age or larger than 1500 grams are delivered within 24 hours of rupture. When membranes rupture prior to this fetal weight and gestational age, patients are treated expectantly for 24 hours in the hospital and then discharged if labor has not ensued. Antibiotics are not administered prophylactically, repeated vaginal examinations are interdicted, and at this time we do not administer corticosteroids in hopes of accelerating fetal maturity. Pharmacologic agents to retard premature labor are not utilized in our institution in the presence of ruptured membranes.

Assessment of Fetus in Utero

Assessing the status of the fetus in utero continually tests the clinical obstetrician's judgment and acumen. In a variety of pregnancy complications with fetuses at high risk, the advantages obtained by early delivery must be weighed against the risks of prematurity. Outlined below are special tests to assist the physician in clinical management.

B-Mode Ultrasonography. When disparity exists between fetal size and growth as compared with gestational age by history, B-scanning can be of considerable assistance. This is a safe, nonradiating form of imaging. Disproportionate uterine growth, when compared to gestational age, caused by trophoblastic disease or multiple gestation can be definitively recognized utilizing this study technique. In addition, with suspected intrauterine growth retardation (as, for example, might occur with chronic hypertension, severe diabetes mellitus, chronic renal disease, or nutritional derangements), serial B-scans measuring fetal biparietal diameters can document fetal growth patterns in utero.

Ultrasonography is useful in localizing the placenta when placenta previa is suspected, is a helpful adjunct to the performance of amniocentesis in localizing the amniotic sac, and can be utilized for delineating adnexal masses and ovarian cysts.

Amniocentesis. Currently there are three indications for amniocentesis during pregnancy.

These are (1) prenatal genetic diagnosis, (2) management of Rh-sensitized pregnancies in which the maternal indirect Coombs test result is positive, and (3) determination of fetal maturity. The first two indications have already been discussed. The determination of fetal maturity is accomplished by measurement of the lecithin/sphingomyelin ratio as performed by starch gel electrophoresis. A ratio of two or greater has a 95 per cent correlation with fetal pulmonary maturity. The indications for the performance of this test are several: (1) prior to elective repeat cesarean section when duration of gestation is questionable; (2) in the management of Rh-sensitized pregnancies to assist in determining advisability of early delivery; (3) to avoid too early termination of pregnancies in a diabetic; and (4) to corroborate fetal maturity in the presence of intrauterine fetal growth retardation or placental insufficiency.

Urinary Estriols. Estriol is a metabolite of estrogen formed in large quantities by the fetal-placental unit, and the amount excreted in maternal urine rises progressively throughout normal pregnancy. The indications for performing serial urinary estriols include the suspicion of intrauterine growth retardation or placental insufficiency. These determinations are of greatest value when performed daily or on a thrice weekly basis. The usefulness of this determination with the logistic problems involved in accurate collection and measurement are problematic. Urinary estriols may be chronically low in anencephaly and falsely low during the ingestion of certain drugs.

Human Placental Lactogen. The indications for the performance of this test serially during pregnancy are identical to those outlined above for obtaining urinary estriols. The usefulness of this test as a prognostic indicator of the status of the fetus in utero has not been fully established; it is not utilized routinely in our unit.

Oxytocin Challenge Test. The purpose of the oxytocin challenge test is to assess fetal tolerance to a transient decrease in fetal oxygen supply. Uterine contractions, whether spontaneous or induced by a controlled infusion of oxytocin, result in a transient decrease in the uterine blood flow and thus a transient decrease in the oxygen pressure in the fetus. The oxygen pressure of a compromised fetus (that is, a fetus already faced with compromised maternal-fetal oxygen exchange) will fall below a critical level, resulting in postcontraction fetal bradycardia detectable with an external fetal monitor. A healthy fetus, on the other hand, will tolerate this transient decrease in oxygen supply without postcontraction fetal bradycardia.

To perform this test, an external ultrasound fetal monitor is placed on the abdomen to continuously monitor the fetal heart rate and an external tokodynamometer is placed on the abdomen also to monitor uterine activity. Once baseline uterine activity patterns are established, intravenous oxytocin is administered by infusion pump, starting at the rate of 0.5 milliunit per minute. (This use of oxytocin is not listed in the manufacturer's official directive.) This rate is doubled every 20 minutes until the patient is having three contractions per 10 minute period. If there are no late decelerations for 30 minutes, the test is considered negative. If repetitive late decelerations are detected, the test is read as positive. Although the significance of a positive oxytocin challenge test is unresolved, a well-performed test with the negative result may be validly interpreted as reassurance that the fetus will not die from placental insufficiency within the succeeding 7 days. A positive test, on its own, does not necessarily call for immediate intervention unless other parameters and clinical evaluation so indicate. At this time therefore the primary usefulness of the test is as reassurance when negative in the face of suspected placental insufficiency.

Miscellaneous Comments

The association of anemia with postpartum maternal morbidity, prematurity, and urinary tract infection warrants an aggressive program of detection and correction of anemia occurring during pregnancy. Most anemias during pregnancy are nutritional, of the iron deficiency type, and will respond readily to oral ferrous sulfate supplementation. A more rapid replenishment of iron stores may be obtained utilizing parenteral iron preparations, and this may be efficacious, particularly if the anemia is diagnosed late in pregnancy. All anemias, whether caused by iron deficiency or hemoglobinopathy, should be treated additionally with folic acid, 1 mg. per day. If the Sickledex tube test for hemoglobins is positive, of course, confirmation of hemoglobinopathy ought to be obtained by hemoglobin electrophoresis.

Asymptomatic bacteriuria occurs in 5 to 7 per cent of all obstetric patients. Symptomatic urinary tract infection will develop in up to one fourth of this group. Although screening for asymptomatic bacteriuria by routine urine cultures is optimal, laboratory availability and cost are deterrents. Our experience does indicate, however, that all anemic patients should be screened routinely for bacteriuria. Asymptomatic bacteriuria should be treated with a 10 day course of sulfisoxazole therapy (see warning of use in pregnancy in manufacturer's official directive), and recurrent urinary tract infection during pregnancy mandates suppressive therapy for the remainder of the pregnancy.

Rh-negative unsensitized patients who deliver an Rh-positive infant should receive Rh immune globulin within 72 hours of delivery if the mother's indirect Coombs test is negative post partum. All patients who deliver a fetus in which Rh determination cannot be performed should also receive immune globulin if they are unsensitized.

Patients with symptomatic vaginitis should be treated during pregnancy and efforts made to identify a specific causative agent. A Gram stain and culture for Neisseria are always appropriate in these patients, and in addition a hanging drop preparation of the vaginal secretions should be performed. If Candida is the offending organism, our treatment includes nystatin vaginal suppositories twice daily for 2 weeks. If *Trichomonas vaginalis* is identified, we treat with oral metronidazole (Flagyl), 250 mg. three times a day for 10 days (see warning of use in pregnancy in manufacturer's official directive). The husband is usually treated with this dosage twice daily for 10 days. *Hemophilus vaginalis* can be diagnosed by the presence of "clue cells" and responds well to a sulfa cream applied intravaginally twice daily for 10 days.

An abnormal cytologic smear during pregnancy represents a relatively uncommon but potentially serious complication. Attempts should be made to clear any infectious process medically; if the cytologic smear remains abnormal, histologic diagnosis is mandatory. Colposcopically directed biopsies in these instances have greatly reduced the necessity for conization of the cervix during pregnancy. The management of pregnancy in a patient with carcinoma in situ is no different than in the normal patient; however, in those patients with invasive malignancy, management is dictated primarily by duration of gestation.

Summary and Conclusions

Technologic and laboratory procedures described in this article are important aids in the management of certain pregnancies, but equally crucial are intelligent screening and communication which can improve the physician's ability to identify, prognosticate, and plan more rationally for patients requiring more consideration.

Also, one should note that pregnancies that do not occur cannot become high risk pregnancies. In an analysis of maternal deaths recorded during the Collaborative Project Study, only three of 28 mothers identified as being high risk had indicated antenatally that they desired the pregnancy. Twenty of those 28 identified had stated specifically that they did not want the pregnancy that ultimately resulted in their deaths. When one adds to this reports of reductions in prematurity and perinatal and maternal mortality rates from areas in which contraception and abortion have been made available, one must consider the preventability aspect of high risk obstetrics. In this regard, interconceptional care programs, stressing correction of dysfunctional nutrition and detection and treatment of correctable hypertensive disorders, must also include cognizance of the medical value of contraception and sterilization in promoting and ensuring the total health of the female in the reproductive age group.

In summary, diligence, thoughtfulness, and advance preparation are still the most important qualities of the dedicated physician who wishes to provide expert management for the pregnant woman and her fetus.

ABORTION

method of
JAMES A. BATTS, Jr., M.D.,
and SUNTHORN BUNYAVIROCH, M.D.
New York, New York

General Principles

Expulsion of a fetus that has not attained a weight of 500 grams or has not completed 20 weeks of gestation may be a spontaneous complication of pregnancy or an induced event. In either case infection is always a possibility; therefore close observation and a well planned treatment regimen are essential.

Spontaneous Abortion

Threatened Abortion. Uterine bleeding is usually mild; cramps are mild or absent. The cervix is usually closed.

1. Exclude other causes of vaginal bleeding.
2. No coitus or douching.
3. If patient is apprehensive, prescribe bed rest and mild sedation, e.g., phenobarbital, 30 mg. three times daily.
4. If gestation is over 12 weeks, progestin therapy may be helpful, especially if pregnanediol test shows low pregnanediol excretion.
5. If bed rest had been advised, allow the patient to be up and about the house after 2 days of no bleeding and/or pain.
6. No douching or coitus until the patient has been free of all symptoms for 2 weeks.
7. Observe for evidence of continuing progression of the pregnancy.

Inevitable Abortion. Loss of the pregnancy usually is certain when there is (1) cervical dilatation, (2) a portion of products of conception passed or presenting at the os, or (3) moderate to heavy or persistent bleeding.

1. Complete the abortion as soon as possible to prevent further blood loss and infection.
2. Hospitalize. Type and cross-match 2 units of blood.
3. Remove any products of conception present in the vagina or cervical canal.
4. Start an oxytocin infusion, 20 units in 1000 ml. 5 per cent dextrose in water.
5. Suction and/or dilatation and curettage is done as an emergency if bleeding is heavy—otherwise, at the next operating room session.

Complete Abortion. When all the products of conception of an intrauterine pregnancy have passed or have been evacuated, there is no further bleeding.

Incomplete Abortion. Bleeding and/or uterine cramps continue when portions of the products of conception are retained.

1. Hospitalize; cross-match blood as indicated.
2. Transfuse if the hematocrit falls below 25 ml. per 100 ml.
3. Provide oxytocin infusion to make the uterus smaller and firmer and to encourage expulsion of loose products of conception.
4. Suction and/or curettage is performed as an emergency if bleeding is heavy—otherwise, as soon as can be electively scheduled in the operating room.
5. Give methylergonovine maleate (Methergine).
6. The patient may be discharged when her condition is satisfactory (usually 4 to 6 hours after the operation).

Septic Abortion. Infection is always a possible complication of abortion whether it was spontaneous or induced. It should be suspected when (1) oral temperature is 100.4°F. (38°C.) or over or (2) there is a foul vaginal discharge.

When the infection extends beyond the endometrium, it has direct access to the maternal vascular compartment; in the presence of peritonitis secondary to uterine perforation, the stage is set for sustained septicemia.

1. Nothing by mouth. Give intravenous fluids through an 18 gauge needle or intracatheter.
2. Check vital signs every 4 hours or more frequently if condition requires.
3. Record fluid intake and output.
4. Complete blood count; urinalysis; SMA 6 and 12; fibrinogen and split proteins; clot observation test; arterial blood gases; cross-match 2 units of blood. Gram stain and culture of specimen from cervix.
5. Antibiotic therapy. The initial choice is penicillin plus kanamycin. Give ampicillin intravenously, 6 to 12 grams daily, or, if no sensitivity, aqueous penicillin G, 30 to 50 million units per day. Add kanamycin, 15 mg. per kg. per day in two divided doses—usually 500 mg. intramuscularly every 12 hours. The total dose is not to exceed 15 grams.
6. If Gram-stained smears show numerous organisms but there is no culture growth, if culture identifies *Bacteroides fragilis*, or if there is no response to initial antibiotics in 48 hours, use clindamycin to replace kanamycin, 600 mg. by intravenous Soluset every 6 hours.
7. Remove any tissue from the cervical canal; look for vaginal or cervical trauma.
8. Take flat and upright films of the abdomen and chest x-ray. Look for a foreign body or signs of pneumoperitoneum.
9. If the uterus is over 12 weeks' size, attempt evacuation by intravenous administration of oxytocin.
10. After 3 to 12 hours of antimicrobial therapy, carry out curettage. Suction is unsafe if the uterus has been previously perforated. In the case of excessive bleeding or evidence of septic shock, the uterus must be emptied without delay.
11. Emergency laparotomy is required in the presence of (1) an intraperitoneal foreign body, (2) evidence of uterine perforation, (3) generalized peritonitis, (4) bowel injury, or (5) clostridium infection. Hysterectomy and repair of injured bowel are mandatory.
12. Antimicrobial therapy is reviewed as culture and sensitivity results become available.
13. If persistent spiking temperature continues and especially if accompanied by disproportionate tachycardia, suspect pelvic thrombophlebitis and give a therapeutic trial of heparin.

Management of Septic Shock. Shock that is not due to blood loss or that does not respond to adequate blood replacement is probably due to endotoxin. The diagnosis becomes more certain if cervical and/or blood cultures show *Bacteroides fragilis* or *Escherichia coli*.

1. Perform immediate dilatation and curettage (D&C) if uterine size is 12 weeks or less to remove any retained necrotic placental tissue.
2. Attempt oxytocin evacuation if the uterus is over 12 weeks' gestation size.
3. Hysterectomy is indicated in the following circumstances: (a) uterine size over 12 weeks and failure of oxytocin to evacuate the uterus in 4 hours; (b) insignificant retained products of con-

ception obtained at D&C; (c) failure to improve after evacuation by either curettage or oxytocin infusion; (d) foreign body in the peritoneal cavity; (e) presence of pus or blood on culdocentesis; (f) diagnosis of clostridial infection; or (g) generalized peritonitis.

4. Central venous pressure (CVP) monitoring.

5. Adequate circulating blood volume maintenance.

6. Correction of lactic acidosis by intravenous bicarbonate.

7. Intravenous glucocorticoids, 30 mg. per kg. per day of methylprednisolone over a 15 minute period, may be employed.

8. Use vasoactive drugs according to circulatory status. Dopamine hydrochloride (Intropin), 200 mg. diluted in 250 to 500 ml. of isotonic saline, 5 per cent dextrose, or lactate, and infused at rates of 2 to 20 micrograms per kg. per minute, usually produces satisfactory blood pressure and urine flow responses. When it does not, the addition of another agent may improve the response (e.g., isoproterenol (Isuprel), 2.0 mg. in 500 ml. of 5 per cent dextrose in water). Blood volume requirements may be markedly increased when vasodilating drugs are used. Carefully monitor central venous pressure (CVP) to avoid overplacement.

9. Oxygen for dyspnea and/or cyanosis.

10. Digitalization may be used as indicated.

Missed Abortion. In missed abortion the abortus has been dead for at least 8 weeks and retained in the uterus.

1. Do not intervene if the diagnosis is not certain.

2. Beginning with the third week after apparent fetal death, check the fibrinogen level weekly. Advise the patient to report any bleeding or bruising.

3. If a coagulation defect develops, correct and evacuate the uterus.

4. When the diagnosis is definite, evacuate the uterus.

5. Since the uterus shrinks and loses its soft consistency, curettage or suction may be safely carried out if the uterus is 12 weeks' size or smaller. When the uterus is over 12 weeks' size, use an oxytocin infusion. Increasing dosage is administered, preferably by constant infusion pump; observe fluid intake and output closely to avoid water intoxication.

6. Other effective approaches include an intra-amniotic prostaglandin.

Therapeutic and Voluntary Abortion

The United States Supreme Court's decisions of January 22, 1973, made elective abortion during the first and second trimesters legal nationwide, thus making it a decision to be made by the patient with the guidance and care of her physician. Elective abortions have increased rapidly since then, so that in 1976 about 1,115,000 were performed in the United States.

The following factors will determine choice of method as well as outcome: (1) accurate diagnosis of uterine pregnancy; (2) the detection of extrauterine pregnancy; (3) assessment of uterine size; (4) adnexal masses; (5) multiple pregnancy; (6) uterine anomalies, especially duplication; and (7) position of the uterus, especially anteflexion and retroflexion. Ultrasonography is helpful in clarifying some of the diagnostic difficulties.

The available options are as follows: (1) Menstrual extraction—first 4 weeks of pregnancy (up to end of seventh week past last normal period). (2) Suction—fifth to twelfth weeks of pregnancy; easier, quicker, and less traumatic than sharp curettage. (3) Intra-amniotic instillation—sixteenth to twentieth week. (4) Hysterotomy—because of risks, rarely done, unless a viable infant is anticipated. (5) Hysterectomy—occasionally justified when there is sufficient uterine pathology. (6) Laminaria and oxytocin or prostaglandin.

Menstrual Extraction (Induction or Aspiration) (Outpatient Procedure). 1. Wait until the second week after missed period. Perform pregnancy test and/or ultrasound study if available.

2. Local anesthesia—paracervical block.

3. Use a flexible plastic cannula; this usually eliminates the need for cervical dilatation. Use the largest size cannula that will slip into the cervical canal without forcing. Attach a syringe or suction pump. Move the apparatus in and out of the uterus with a rotary motion of the hand while aspirating all areas of the cavity until no more tissue can be obtained. Check the retrieved tissue with a hand lens to identify the frond-like villi of the placenta. If the tissue is uncertain, send to laboratory for microscopic study.

4. Examine the patient in 2 or 4 weeks to make certain that she is not having a continuing pregnancy.

Induced Abortion of Pregnancies of 12 Weeks' or Less Duration. 1. General anesthesia or paracervical block may be used.

2. Eight weeks or less—no cervical dilatation is required with Karman cannula; paracervical block alone is adequate for most patients.

3. Suction curettage with equipment developing required 25 inches of mercury vacuum.

4. Curette exploration to see if the cavity is completely evacuated.

5. Inspect contents in suction apparatus tissue receptacle.

6. Submit the tissue to pathology.

7. Patient may be discharged when fully recovered from anesthesia (3 to 6 hours).

8. Detailed instructions on possible complications (hemorrhage, infection) and how to reach medical help are given to the patient.

9. Routine postoperative examination at 2 weeks.

Induced Abortion Beyond 12 Weeks. From the twelfth to the sixteenth week the pregnancy is too large for safe suctioning but not big enough to be found transabdominally. At present, although there is a high incidence of emesis, diarrhea, and drug fever, dinoprost tromethamine (PGF_2) given as a vaginal suppository seems to offer a reliable and safe way to evacuate the uterus during this lag period. Recently, a few have claimed that dilatation, curettage, and evacuation can be safely done up to 20 weeks of gestation by a properly trained physician.

Induced Abortion at 16 to 20 Weeks. 1. When there is no cardiac or renal contraindication, the intra-amniotic instillation of 200 ml. (100 to 250 ml.) of 20 per cent sodium chloride solution augmented by intravenous oxytocin usually works well. *Do not* (1) inject intravascularly; (2) inject in the presence of a "bloody tap"; (3) overdistend the amniotic cavity by injecting a volume of solution in excess of the amniotic fluid volume removed; or (4) fail to discontinue immediately if the patient complains of pain, especially a burning sensation, thirst, "heat," or other unusual symptoms suggestive of intravascular hypertonic saline administration.

2. Prostaglandin (Prostin F2 alpha), in a single dose of 40 mg. placed in the amniotic cavity, is also a very satisfactory method. Although this method avoids the risk of hypernatremia and disseminated intravascular coagulation (DIC), the patient has to contend with the unpleasant side effects (vomiting and diarrhea) of prostaglandin. It is contraindicated in patients with asthma and those who have unusual reactions to a test dose of prostaglandin. A second dose of 40 mg. is required in some patients.

3. If the placenta is retained for more than 3 hours or if bleeding is excessive, it is removed operatively.

General. 1. Rh immune globulin is administered within 24 hours to all patients who are Rh negative and who do not have evidence of isoimmunization.

2. Contraceptive education and services should be an integral part of the management of abortion.

RESUSCITATION OF THE NEWBORN

method of
ELIZABETH J. JAMES, M.D.
Columbia, Missouri

Rapid and effective resuscitation of the asphyxiated newborn infant is essential for intact survival. In the past, the delivery of such an infant was often an unexpected and catastrophic event. Today with modern obstetric techniques, intrauterine distress can be detected and prompt treatment can avert an unfortunate outcome.

Identification of the Infant at Risk

It is absolutely essential that high risk infants of all types be identified before delivery so that maternal transport can be carried out whenever optimal neonatal care is not available at the referring hospital. Likewise, it is advantageous for the infant at risk of perinatal asphyxia to be identified before delivery so that obstetric intervention and/or prompt neonatal resuscitation can be performed. Both obstetric and pediatric teams must be involved in the decision to deliver and must attend these deliveries to assure optimal neonatal outcome.

A maternal history (Table 1) is essential for identification of the infant at risk. Previous

TABLE 1. **Identification of the Infant at Risk for Perinatal Asphyxia**

- Previous pregnancy history
  - Neonatal deaths
  - Isoimmunization
  - Dystocia
- Medical history
  - Hypertension
  - Diabetes
- Current pregnancy complications
  - Age
    - Under 16
    - Over 40
    - Primipara over 35
  - Pregnancy-induced hypertension
  - Hypotension
  - Bleeding
  - Multiple pregnancy
  - Intrauterine growth retardation
  - Polyhydramnios
  - Greater than 42 weeks from last menstrual period
  - Breech
  - Meconium-stained amniotic fluid
  - Greater than 24 hours ruptured membranes
  - Preterm gestation
  - Infertility history

neonatal deaths, isoimmunization, difficult vaginal deliveries, hypertension, or diabetes should always alert the physician to potential problems in the infant. Complications of the pregnancy which should warn the physician of impending problems include multiple fetuses, polyhydramnios, maternal age extremes, breech presentation, prolonged rupture of membranes, and prematurity. It should be remembered that as many as one third of infants with hyaline membrane disease are the result of inappropriate preterm delivery, as in elective repeat cesarean sections performed without maturity studies. Problems which frequently result in or indicate uteroplacental insufficiency include pregnancy-induced hypertension (toxemia of pregnancy), hypotension, abnormal vaginal bleeding, intrauterine growth retardation, and meconium-stained amniotic fluid.

It is imperative that fetal heart rate monitoring be done whenever any of these risk factors is present; the routine use of fetal heart rate monitoring will reveal unexpected cases of fetal distress, a fact which argues strongly for the practice of monitoring all labors. Risk infants are also detected by fetal heart rate abnormalities before labor, as in the case of a positive oxytocin challenge test or positive nonstress testing.

Intrapartum Resuscitation

Fetal Heart Rate Abnormalities. With the use of fetal heart rate monitoring the obstetrician has become involved in active resuscitation of the infant in utero. Variable deceleration patterns may be responsive to maternal position changes, removing pressure from the umbilical cord. Late deceleration (uteroplacental insufficiency) may be alleviated by decreasing uterine activity, correction of maternal hypotension, maternal oxygen inhalation, or maternal position change removing inferior vena cava compression and improving cardiac output.

Meconium Staining of the Amniotic Fluid. Prevention of meconium aspiration by means of intrapartum suctioning of the meconium-stained infant is now possible. Mortality in the meconium aspiration syndrome approaches 25 to 30 per cent in most centers, or about 0.5 per cent of all infants with meconium staining. Visualization of the larynx with tracheal suctioning after delivery has been shown to decrease the problem but does not eliminate it, as the first breaths will pull oral and pharyngeal meconium into the lungs. It is therefore recommended that the physician delivering the infant perform nasopharyngeal and oropharyngeal suctioning with a sterile disposable DeLee trap as soon as the head is delivered and before the delivery of the chest. When this is done, we have seen virtual elimination of meconium aspiration pneumonia as a cause of neonatal mortality. If meconium is obtained during intrapartum suctioning, the larynx should be visualized after delivery, and any intratracheal meconium should be suctioned under direct vision by applying negative pressure directly to the endotracheal tube as it is withdrawn.

Acute Fetal Blood Loss. It is frequently assumed that blood flowing from a maternal orifice is maternal blood. In the case of vaginal bleeding, this may not be true. Fetal blood loss in the amount of 120 ml. will represent half of the term infant's blood volume, and must be treated vigorously if the infant is to survive. Fetal-to-maternal hemorrhage, twin-to-twin transfusion, and enclosed hemorrhage may show no visible blood loss and challenge the diagnostic abilities of the physician called upon to resuscitate the infant. The exsanguinated infant may present with a weak, rapid heart rate and gasping respirations if the blood loss has been acute, but rapidly progresses to apnea and bradycardia. Cyanosis may be absent in the face of extreme asphyxia, and should suggest the diagnosis. Volume expansion in such instances is lifesaving, and the ideal volume expander is placental blood in the amount of 10 to 20 ml. per kg. of body weight, or the amount necessary to restore blood pressure. It is therefore recommended that, in the presence of risk factors such as maternal bleeding, placenta previa, placental abruption, twin gestation, extreme low birth weight (less than 1200 grams), or intrauterine asphyxia, the obstetrician obtain at least 20 ml. of placental blood via sterile puncture of an umbilical vessel (prior to placental separation to avoid high concentrations of tissue thromboplastin in the placental blood) for administration to the infant if signs of hypovolemia appear in the first hour of life. The blood should be drawn in a 20 ml. syringe containing 0.1 ml. of heparin (concentration 1000 units per ml.), so that it contains 5 units of heparin per ml. of blood. If 25 per cent albumin is used, 4 ml. should be diluted with 16 ml. of 5 per cent dextrose, or with 3 ml. (3 mEq.) of sodium bicarbonate and 13 ml. of sterile water for injection.

Neonatal Resuscitation

Equipment for Resuscitation. Table 2 details the equipment necessary for effective resuscitation. It is essential that the presence of each item be confirmed at the beginning of each nursing shift.

Priorities of Treatment. It is helpful to use the alphabet for management of the asphyxiated infant:

Delivery room
- A—Airway
- B—Breathing
- C—Circulation
- D—Drugs

Nursery
- E—Evaluation for cause
- F—Follow-up for:
- G—Glucose
- H—Hypocalcemia
- I—Irritability and other central nervous system (CNS) symptoms

Stepwise, the procedure (outlined in Fig. 1) is as follows:

1. Timing is begun at delivery.

2. Place the infant in a head-down position on a warm surface under a radiant heat source, towel-dry, and gently suction the nose and mouth with a bulb syringe. For most infants, this is all that will be required. If the infant is meconium stained and meconium has been recovered on intrapartum suctioning, the pharynx and vocal cords must be visualized and tracheal suctioning must be performed before any positive pressure ventilation is begun.

3. If the infant is apneic, expansion of the lungs is next accomplished after clearing the airway, using bag and mask ventilation. The mask must fit securely, and the bag should be capable of delivering peak inspiratory pressures of 30 cm. of water (as measured by an attached manometer under optimal conditions). The bag should also have the capability of delivering continuous positive airway pressure. A maximum respiratory rate of 40 per minute should be employed in order to allow the poorly compliant newborn lung to empty, to avoid overexpansion, and to prevent hypocapnia with rapid changes in cerebral blood flow. Simultaneously, the infant's heart rate should be made audible, either by means of a cardiac monitor or by an assistant tapping out the rate while listening to the chest with a stethoscope.

4. If the heart rate response is not immediate (four to six inflations) or if the infant is extremely small (less than 1200 grams), an oral endotracheal tube should be placed and bag-to-tube ventilation should be instituted with immediate assessment of the bilateral adequacy of breath sounds by chest auscultation. Heart rate and color should respond immediately with adequate ventilation. In the case of the very low birth weight infant, 4 to 6 cm. of water continuous positive airway pressure (CPAP) should be used.

5. If the heart rate remains less than 60 beats per minute after four to six inflations via the endotracheal tube, external cardiac massage is given, using two fingers over the mid-sternum while palpating for a femoral pulse to assess adequacy of massage. Massage and ventilation should be alternated, with a ratio of three or four cardiac compressions to one ventilation, thereby avoiding simultaneous chest compression and lung expansion, and allowing time for exhalation between breaths.

6. With continued need for ventilatory and circulatory support, an umbilical vessel is catheterized. It is desirable to use the umbilical artery, as volume expanders and bicarbonate solutions may be infused through it, central aortic pressure may be measured, and arterial blood gas monitoring can be accomplished. If a catheter cannot be placed in the umbilical artery after one attempt, the umbilical vein may be used, but it should be remembered that a catheter placed in the vein may enter the liver or the portal system, and all hyperosmolar solutions such as sodium bicarbonate infused through such a catheter must be greatly diluted and given slowly.

7. Sodium bicarbonate, up to 3 mEq. per kg., may then be given slowly (10 to 15 minutes), diluted at least 1:2 with sterile distilled water. A preferable dilution is 3 mEq. (3 ml.) $NaHCO_3$ diluted to 20 ml. with sterile water for injection. Arterial blood gases will indicate whether a respiratory acidosis is present, requiring improved ventilation, or a metabolic acidosis is persisting, indicating the need for improved oxygenation and/or perfusion. With signs of hypovolemia

TABLE 2. **Equipment for Resuscitation**

Overhead radiant warmer with adequate light*
Under-baby heat source†
Oxygen: wall and/or portable
Suction: wall or portable (50 to 80 cm. water negative pressure), DeLee trap, and bulb syringe; suction catheters
Ventilatory bag: anesthesia or self-inflating, with CPAP capability‡
Masks: term and preterm sizes
Endotracheal tubes: Foregger and Portex, 2.0, 2.5, 3.0, and 3.5 mm., with stylets and adaptors to fit bag
Laryngoscope: infant, with straight and curved blades, sizes 0 and 1, spare batteries, and bulbs
Stethoscope
Tape, benzoin, iodophor solution, 2 × 2 gauze pads
Umbilical catheterization tray with catheters and stopcocks
Nasogastric tubes, 15 inch, sizes 5 and 8 Fr.
Blood pressure apparatus
Drugs: albumin 25% salt-poor; heparin, 1000 units per ml.; sodium bicarbonate, 1 mEq. per ml.; sterile water; epinephrine 1:10,000; Narcan Neonatal, 0.02 mg. per ml.; dextrose 10%

*E.g., Ohio Neonatal Intensive Care Center or Isolette Infant Care System.

†E.g., Circulating warm water mattress, Gorman-Rupp Industries, Inc., Bellville, Ohio, or Porta-warm mattress, Kay Laboratories, P.O. Box 676, Moberly, Mo.

‡E.g., Jackson-Reese Modification, Ayers T-Piece No. 330-15HFSC, Medical and Industrial Equipment, 655 73rd St., Niagara Falls, N.Y.

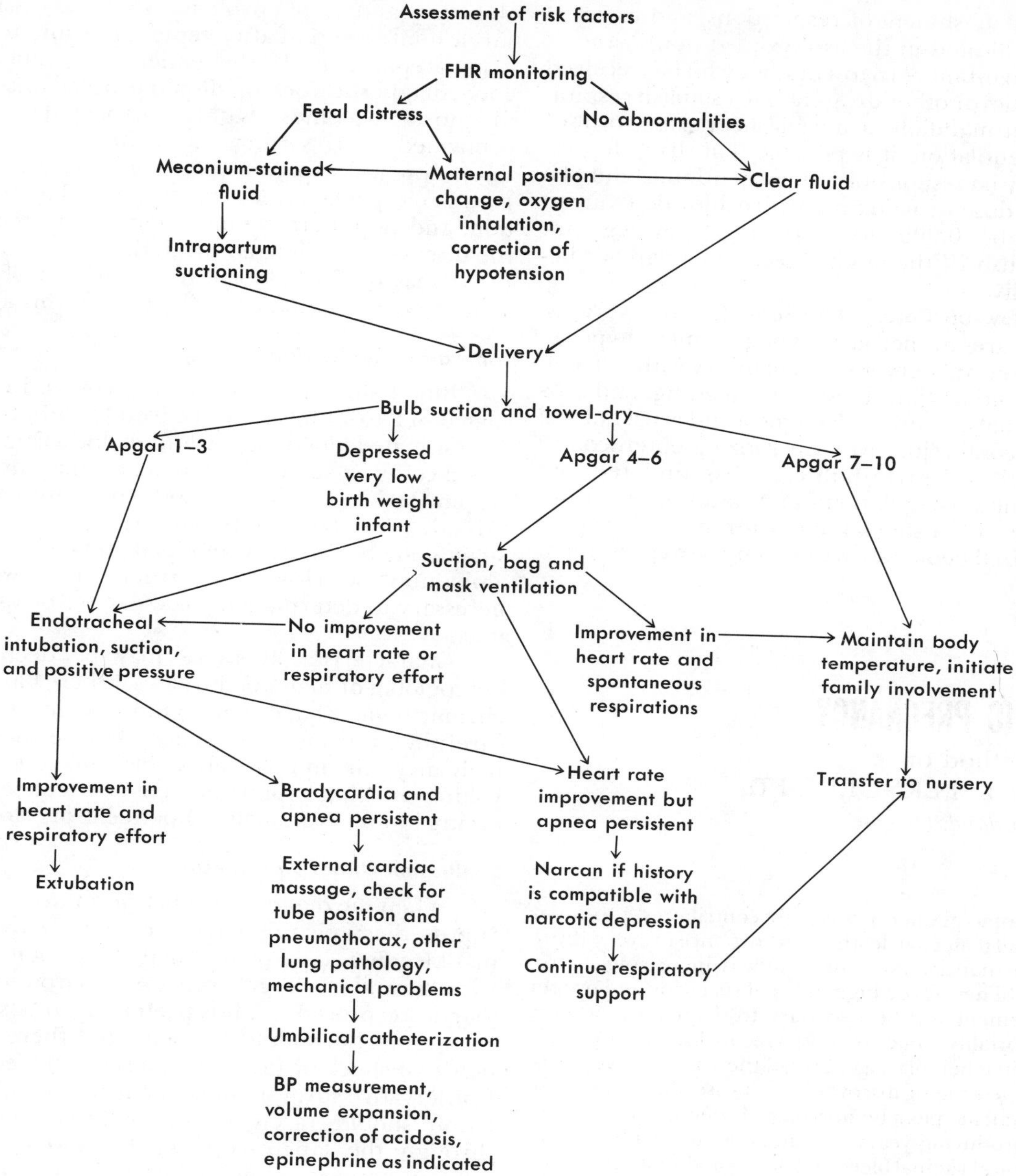

Figure 1. Perinatal resuscitation.

(hypotension below 30 mm. Hg systolic and poor peripheral perfusion), fresh heparinized placental blood (10 to 20 ml. per kg.) or albumin should be given.

8. With lack of cardiac response, epinephrine, 0.5 ml. of 1:10,000 solution, is given by intracardiac puncture or via the umbilical venous catheter if the tip has entered the inferior vena cava (as indicated by a fall in pressure as the diaphragm is crossed). It is important to remember, however, that the most common cause for persistent bradycardia is ineffective ventilation; whenever heart rate fails to improve, malposition of the endotracheal tube or pneumothorax should be looked for.

9. Stress depletes liver glycogen stores, and it is therefore desirable to infuse a 10 per cent dextrose solution (55 to 65 ml. per kg. per day) after resuscitation has been accomplished to prevent hypoglycemic sequelae.

It should be emphasized that the injection of so-called respiratory stimulant drugs is not helpful in the establishment of respirations, and in fact is contraindicated in the asphyxiated newborn.

If an infant born to a mother who has received anesthetics or other drugs fails to establish respirations but maintains a normal heart rate with assisted ventilation, it is possible that drug depression may be responsible. Such an infant should be given a dose of naloxone hydrochloride (Narcan Neonatal), 0.005 to 0.01 mg. per kg. intravenously, if the mother received a narcotic before delivery.

Follow-up Care. The sequelae of severe asphyxia are numerous: hypoglycemia; hypocalcemia; central nervous system injury with irritability, hypotonia, jitteriness, poor feeding, and seizures; renal necrosis with oliguria and renal failure; gut mucosal injury with necrotizing enterocolitis; congestive heart failure; disseminated intravascular coagulation; and pulmonary insufficiency with a shock lung syndrome. All require specialized neonatal care by competent personnel.

ECTOPIC PREGNANCY

method of
M. L. PERNOLL, M.D.
Portland, Oregon

Ectopic gestation currently contributes 3 to 5 per cent of all maternal deaths. It occurs once in every 120 to 200 pregnancies and apparently is increasing in frequency. Therefore a high index of suspicion and proper management will be necessary to decrease morbidity and mortality. The greatest risk to life from ectopic gestation is hemorrhage. Even if there is no active bleeding at the time of discovery, each case should be managed as an incipient hemorrhage. Indeed, any woman in the reproducing years with amenorrhea (with or without atypical vaginal bleeding), lower abdominal or pelvic pain, and an adnexal mass should be suspected of ectopic pregnancy. The average age of patients with ectopic pregnancy is 30 years, and 40 per cent occur between 20 and 26 years of age. More tubal gestations are found on the right than on the left.

The definitive management for ectopic pregnancy is surgery, which should follow diagnosis as soon as possible. Delay in diagnosis or procrastination in surgical treatment poses a grave risk to the patient. Most patients with ectopic pregnancy either obviously require immediate care or present a problem in differential diagnosis; therefore immediate management is determined by the patient's status. Symptoms and signs of acute surgical abdomen and/or hypovolemic shock necessitate surgical intervention after rapid, appropriate patient preparation. If the patient's condition is good, diagnostic work-up should proceed until the diagnosis becomes highly suspected or is confirmed. Recognizing these differences, this discussion will separate the diagnostic management, emergency management, surgical intervention, and postoperative management. Moreover, the discussion is directed primarily to the ectopic pregnancy of the fallopian tube, for over 98 per cent of ectopic gestations will occur in this area.

Laboratory Evaluation

Blood should be drawn for type and crossmatch of 2 to 4 units of whole blood in addition to the estimated blood loss. Additionally, a complete blood count, β-subunit human chorionic gonadotropin (HCG), blood type, and Rh should be obtained. Amylase determination has been suggested, because the fallopian tube is rich in alpha amylase. However, further studies will be necessary to determine its true diagnostic usefulness.

Characteristically there may be decreased hemoglobin or hematocrit values if there has been chronic hemorrhage. Values must be interpreted carefully in acute hemorrhage because they initially may remain relatively stable while the blood volume is being rapidly depleted. A leukocytosis occurs in approximately 50 per cent of patients.

Evaluation Under Anesthesia

When the diagnosis is unclear, in cases of unruptured ectopic pregnancies or those with minimal bleeding, laparoscopy may be absolutely invaluable and has largely replaced laparotomy as a diagnostic procedure. It is preferable to posterior colpotomy, but should not be used if there is evidence of shock or gross intraperitoneal bleeding. Conservative surgical therapy for the ectopic gestation should rarely or never be undertaken through the laparoscope or by posterior colpotomy, because neither method offers as good an opportunity for reproductive conservation as does laparotomy.

Pelvic examination under anesthesia should be conducted extremely gently because of the possibility of rupture of the ectopic gestation. Dilatation and curettage has been used in the past, but is of less value at present. Characteristically, the endometrium with ectopic gestation will demonstrate the Arias-Stella phenomenon.

Emergency Management

Thirty-three per cent of all patients with ectopic gestation will present in shock. In such cases it is necessary to have a plan of immediate management.

Admission to Hospital and Preparation for Surgery; Large Bore Indwelling Intravenous Catheters. One or more 16 gauge intravenous catheters should be placed in the patient presenting in shock. Additionally, it may be necessary to initiate central venous pressure monitoring.

Blood. Type and cross-match 2 to 4 units of whole blood or packed red cells in addition to the estimated blood loss and obtain blood for complete blood count. Clotting studies may also be useful.

Volume Expander. If the shock is mild to moderate, administer 5 per cent dextrose and Ringer's lactate (D5RL) and await fully cross-matched blood. In more severe shock, blood volume expanders (such as albumin) coupled with rapid infusion of D5RL will allow sufficient time for a rapid (20 minute) cross-match. In the rare patient without obtainable blood pressure, the wait necessary for type-specific blood should not be undertaken, and type O Rh negative blood may be necessary to sustain life. It is important, however, to recognize that surgery before blood transfusion in the patient in shock appreciably increases mortality. Therefore blood should nearly always be available and be administered before the time of surgery.

Foley Catheter. An indwelling Foley catheter should be placed to record the intake and output.

Counseling. Even in the critical case the patient and/or family should be queried to learn their desires regarding future reproduction.

Surgical Intervention

As rapidly as possible after diagnosis, the patient should be moved to the operating suite and an exploratory laparotomy performed.

Anesthesia. Anesthetic management is critical in the patient with shock. It is important to use inhalation (not conduction) anesthesia, and the anesthesiologist should utilize a high percentage of oxygen in the inspired air. Additionally the anesthetic should be maintained at minimal levels, because cardiac arrhythmias are a risk during or after induction of anesthesia and are a common cause of death in patients not adequately prepared by preoperative treatment of shock.

Incision and Exploration. In patients in whom there is very chronic bleeding or none at all, a low transverse incision may be utilized. It is important that the pelvis be explored immediately and that blood loss be controlled. If blood is encountered and the cause is not found in the pelvis, the upper abdomen must be explored immediately. In patients in shock the vertical midline incision is preferred.

Assessment of the Problem and Evaluation for Fertility. As soon as blood loss is arrested, both ipsilateral and contralateral tubes and ovaries should be carefully inspected and any abnormalities noted before the definitive surgery is performed. Conservative surgical therapy should be possible more than 50 per cent of the time and may increase as diagnostic and operative skills increase.

The majority of tubal pregnancies occur in the ampullary region (47 per cent). The other areas of the tube involved are as follows: isthmic (21.6 per cent), fimbrial (5.8 per cent), interstitial (3.7 per cent), and infundibular (2.5 per cent). Conservative surgery may be especially important if the involved tube is the patient's only one remaining or if the contralateral tube is irreparably damaged.

Conservative Surgery. SALPINGOSTOMY. Conservative therapy is most successful with early unruptured ectopic gestations when linear salpingostomy may be performed. All bleeding points should be carefully ligated, using fine chromic catgut suture (5–0). Further attempt at tubal repair is discouraged at this point so that later, under more optimal conditions, reconstructive surgery may be performed. Thorough but gentle evacuation of the blood and blood clots should be performed.

EXPRESSION. Occasionally, when the pregnancy is in the distal half of the tube, the products of conception may be expressed through the ostium. Care must be taken to guarantee hemostasis, and evaluation for tubal patency or defects is mandatory before another pregnancy is undertaken.

UTERINE SUSPENSION. Uterine suspension may be very useful in conservative therapy. It is designed to keep the fallopian tubes from falling back onto raw or denuded surfaces and thus forming adhesions.

Extirpative Surgery. SALPINGECTOMY. Salpingectomy may be necessary if there is extensive tubal damage and hemostasis cannot be obtained. This will most frequently be true in those patients with shock. In such patients desiring sterilization, the ipsilateral salpingectomy should be combined with a contralateral tubal ligation.

CORNUAL RESECTION. If salpingectomy is necessary, a small wedge-shaped resection of the myometrium assists in the prevention of interstitial ectopic gestation. The small (approximately half the myometrium) resection is favored, for it will prevent the most distal implantation and yet not run as great a risk of uterine rupture with subsequent pregnancy as is the case if the entire myometrial portion of tube is removed.

UNILATERAL OOPHORECTOMY. This procedure has been advocated in the past on grounds that it would eliminate migrations, a possible mechanism in future ectopic pregnancies. However, there are documented cases in which pregnancy was achieved by this method. Moreover, a subsequent problem may destroy the other ovary, and therefore conservation of ovarian tissue is favored.

HYSTERECTOMY. Hysterectomy may be justifiable in some patients with ectopic gestation. For example, it may be useful when both tubes are irreparably damaged, an interstitial pregnancy has created extensive uterine damage or difficulty with hemostasis, the patient is near the menopause, her family is complete, she desires sterilization, sterilization has been attempted, or there are uterine leiomyomas or ovarian tumors. It is of course important that the patient has had a full discussion prior to the surgery and has also had a negative Papanicolaou smear within 6 months, good cardiovascular status, satisfactory anesthesia, satisfactory exposure, and no technical problems.

Incidental Appendectomy. Except in a rare patient in whom there is coincident evidence of appendiceal adhesions, fecalith, mucocele, or inflammation, removal of the appendix is discouraged.

Culture. Anaerobic and aerobic cultures of the intraperitoneal surface should be obtained at the time of surgery in the event that subsequent infections develop.

Postoperative Management

Antibiotics. Currently antibiotics are used only in the presence of infection. However, with controlled investigation, it may be proved that antibiotics are warranted.

Rh Immune Globulin. In those patients who are Rh negative, Rh immune globulin should be administered within 72 hours.

Intraperitoneal Therapy. Several reports have indicated that intraperitoneal steroids may be useful. However, more controlled studies are necessary before a definition of their usefulness can be made.

Hydrotubation. Twenty ml. of sterile isotonic saline solution containing 100 mg. of hydrocortisone acetate may be administered through the cervix on the third and fifth postoperative days. This should not be done when there is uterine bleeding. In theory it has the advantage of flushing out blood clots and keeping the fimbria nonadherent.

Hysterosalpingography. Hysterosalpingography may be useful if the patient's course has been entirely within normal limits and she has not had evidence of infection. It may be obtained as early as the fifth postoperative day and should be repeated at 6 to 8 weeks following surgery.

Counseling. Currently the woman who has a tubal pregnancy has a 50 to 60 per cent chance of never becoming pregnant again. Her chances of having another ectopic pregnancy are at least 10 per cent and possibly more. Only one third of women who have a tubal pregnancy will subsequently have a healthy child. It is hoped that with better diagnostic tools, earlier diagnosis, and more conservative therapy, the chance of this unfortunate prognosis may be lessened.

Other Ectopic Pregnancies

Cervical implantations may be treated most effectively with suction curettage (8 mm.). If hemostasis is not possible, hysterectomy may be necessary. Ovarian pregnancies usually require oophorectomy but occasionally may be treated by a wedge resection. Abdominal pregnancies constitute a dire threat of hemorrhage. Therefore prompt surgical intervention is recommended upon diagnosis. The placenta is commonly left in situ unless partial separation and hemorrhage necessitate attempted removal.

HEMORRHAGE IN LATE PREGNANCY

method of
GERALD A. GLOWACKI, M.D.
Baltimore, Maryland

Hemorrhage in late pregnancy is more aptly stated in terms of "third trimester bleeding." In the past few years, we have seen great advances in the perinatal care of the premature newborn, and it is now feasible in intensive care neonatal centers to save more than 50 per cent of infants delivered after the twenty-sixth week of gestation. This, together with the knowledge and ability to accelerate fetal lung maturation with glucocorticoids, has allowed us to revise our thinking on management of the third trimester bleeding patient and, more specifically, the expectant management thereof.

Causes of Third Trimester Bleeding (in Order of Frequency)

1. Rupture of cervical vessel(s) (2 degrees to eversion of cervix).
2. Placenta previa.
3. Abruptio placentae.

*If the patient is admitted with active contractions, a careful speculum and digital examination may be warranted to determine if bleeding is not secondary to cervical dilatation.

4. Vaginal vessel rupture (spontaneous from varices or traumatic secondary to coitus).
5. Cervical neoplasm.
6. Vasa previa.

Outline of Ideal Management of the Patient with Third Trimester Bleeding

1. Prompt admission to hospital with appropriate vital signs and bed rest.*
2. Start intravenous infusion with volume-expanding solution—i.e., Ringer's lactate (not D5W).
3. Type and cross-match (preferably packed cells).
4. Hematocrit (HCT).
5. Placental localization via ultrasound or radionucleotide scanning. Soft tissue techniques are too inaccurate. If placenta previa is adequately ruled out, do speculum and digital evaluation of cervix and vagina.
6. External fetal monitoring should be initiated before and after placental localization studies have been performed.
7. If vasa previa is suspected, a sample of the blood should be obtained on speculum examination and submitted for fetal red cell determination by the Kleihauer-Betke technique. If positive, prompt cesarean section should be performed.
8. Colposcopic evaluation of cervical lesion is done if one is suspicious of malignancy on visualization. Indiscriminant biopsies may lead to further profound bleeding.
9. Packing with application of microfibrillar collagen hemostat (Avitene) on visualized cervical or vaginal bleeding sites. By use of these hemostatic materials, packing can be removed after a brief time (1 to 2 hours), thus eliminating need for hospitalization, bed rest, and an indwelling catheter.

Management of Placenta Previa

Total Placenta Previa (Pregnancy Between 27 and 34 Weeks).* If the magnitude of bleeding is sufficiently severe (> 100 ml. per hour), cesarean section is performed.

If bleeding has stopped or is <100 ml. per hour:

1. Initiate glucocorticoid therapy with dexamethasone, 6 mg. intramuscularly every 12 hours for four doses.
2. If HCT initially is or falls below 32 per cent or Hgb <10.5 grams per 100 ml., transfuse with 2 units of packed cells.
3. Give O_2 by mask or intranasally at 5 liters per minute to prevent any hypoxic episodes.
4. Constant fetal monitoring (external).
5. Keep the patient on her left or right side—not flat on her back.
6. Perform cesarean section 72 hours from initiation of glucocorticoid therapy.

Partial Placenta Previa. If more than 34 weeks' gestation, do a prompt cesarean section. If amniotic fluid can be obtained with ultrasonic guidance to avoid the placenta, this is desirable. In the event of an immature L/S ratio of less than 1:1.8, the glucocorticoid therapy protocol as previously outlined should be followed with subsequent cesarean section after 72 hours.

If less than 34 weeks' gestation, initiation of glucocorticoid therapy, with reinforcement every 7 days from completion of the previous course, is necessary. If partial placenta previa persists owing to lack of placental migration after 34 weeks, do a cesarean section.

Marginal Placenta Previa. 1. Initiation of glucocorticoids in all gestations of less than 34 weeks. Reinforce therapy as stated above.

2. Uteroplacental sonography is done every 2 weeks to relocate the placenta. The earlier the gestation, the greater the probability that the placenta will migrate high in the lower uterine segment because of continued uterine enlargement.

Abruptio Placentae

Diagnosis of abruptio placentae can be established conclusively by uteroplacental sonography with determination of uteroplacental clot. The presence of fibrin split products produces a secondary indication of clot formation and some dissolution with suspected abruption.

The status of the patient (uterine rigidity) and fetus (by monitoring) will enter into the following decisions:

1. Active bleeding and rigid uterus: (a) Cervix favorable—i.e., >2 cm. dilated and at least 50 per cent effaced—rupture membranes and augment with oxytocin as needed. (b) Cervix unfavorable—cesarean section.
2. Bleeding remitted, definite diagnosis established: (a) More than 34 weeks—cesarean section. (b) Less than 34 weeks—glucocorticoid therapy and then cesarean section.

All patients should have fetal monitoring with a consideration of transabdominal pressure catheter placement under sonography control. In almost all circumstances, a direct fetal scalp electrode should be placed. All breeches and other malpositions of the fetus should be handled appropriately. The complications of abruptio placentae, including disseminated intravascular coagulation (DIC) and renal failure, are discussed

*Gestational age should be reconfirmed by ultrasonic fetal head biparietal diameter measurement. If gestational age is 34 weeks or more, prompt cesearean section is performed.

elsewhere. The Couvelaire uterus may not contract properly post partum and may need higher than normal amounts of oxytocic agents. Occasionally, either uterine or internal iliac ligation or hysterectomy may be necessary when medical therapy fails.

Most of these remarks are predicated on the availability of specific instruments and laboratory studies. In emergency situation, prompt therapy must be accomplished at facilities where these are not available. In situations in which it seems feasible to transport the patient to a facility where such equipment is available, it is advisable to do so to benefit both mother and fetus.

TOXEMIA OF PREGNANCY

method of
FREDERICK J. HOFMEISTER, M.D.,
Milwaukee, Wisconsin
and NOBLE DOSS, Jr., M.D.
Austin, Texas

An awareness of the fundamental fact that hypertension is not specifically a condition related to a certain age group, the older patient, is important. It is also important to recognize that hypertension may be related to any one of several coincidentally existing conditions, such as pregnancy.

It is essential that a concerted effort be made by all physicians to detect and diagnose the existence of hypertension during all routine physical examinations regardless of age, physical status, or the reason the patient has sought medical advice. The blood pressure must be taken and should be recorded on all the patient's records. This minimal effort may reveal the fact that a hypertensive state exists in a very young, apparently healthy woman. The cause of this condition may be cardiovascular. It may be neurogenic. It may be nephropathic. Finding this chronic hypertensive state may influence the physician's counsel to the patient regarding the advisability of her becoming pregnant. It may relate to advice concerning methods of contraception. It may influence the patient's conduct of her life.

Thus we also lay the ground rules for an approach to the management of the normotensive, primigravida patient who, by testing with the Gant "roll over technique," may be determined to be a hypertensive risk when her pregnancy advances. This evaluation and management are based upon one fundamental that must be the basis of all medical evaluations: an exacting, complete history and physical examination of every patient; in this case, every woman, and specifically, every obstetrical patient. Only by this approach is one able to establish the basis upon which abnormal conditions, such as toxemia, related to and associated with hypertension can be detected and adequately combated. In fact, prevention of toxemia of pregnancy may begin when a complete premarital examination is done on the nonpregnant woman, when the physician enlightens the bride-to-be concerning her physical status—the existence of good health or the existence of a chronic hypertensive state.

Hypertension, edema, proteinuria (albuminuria), and epigastric pain before the thirtieth week of gestation must direct the clinician's attention toward therapy planned to combat essential hypertension, kidney disorders, or the existence of placental hydatidiform degeneration or mole. The last of these can be associated with hypertension and toxic symptoms.

Hypertension of pregnancy, or toxemia, is now fairly conclusively shown to be a chronic disease starting as early as the mid-second trimester. With special angiotensin infusion studies, one can demonstrate as early as 28 to 32 weeks, and before onset of the triad of elevated blood pressure, weight gain, and proteinuria, a loss of angiotensin resistance in the pregnancy destined to be complicated by toxemia. This has been semiquantified by the "roll over" screening test of Gant et al. Chronic toxemia may lend itself to antepartum discovery and hospitalization prior to the acute episode and need for immediate delivery. Unless astute awareness continues through pregnancy, toxemia may seemingly appear to occur suddenly as postpartum eclampsia. This can be fatal in as many as 20 to 25 per cent of patients because of its surprise appearance and, therefore, the unpreparedness of the nursing staff and physicians.

Thus in all forms of toxemia, awareness of its potential existence and prevention by careful, exacting antepartum and immediate postpartum care are the keys to complete patient control. The "roll over" screening test will help alert the obstetrician to impending problems. In this test, which is done between the twenty-eighth and thirty-second weeks of gestation, the patient is placed in the left lateral recumbent position for about 15 minutes, during which time her blood pressure presumably stabilizes. She is then rolled over into a supine position. An increase of 20 mm. Hg or more in diastolic pressure at that point is considered indicative of pregnancy-induced hypertension. This test has as its chief value the fact that it enables clinicians to treat the condition before hypertension threatens both mother and fetus, thus avoiding the necessity to resort to premature induction of labor. The suggested treatment for test-positive women is simply bed rest. This approach has been seconded by a fellow professor of obstetrics, Dr. Peggy Whalley. It has been indicated that since multigravidas produce a high percentage of false positive-results, the Gant test is best reserved for primigravidas. The test is time consuming and requires that someone supervise the patient during the 20 to 30 minute procedure.

Preeclampsia

The presence of any one of the following triad is a warning. The existence of any two of the three requires intensive treatment. Exacting observation during antepartum visits, spaced as indicated at from 1 to 4 weeks as determined by the patient's condition and the existence of early symptoms, is essential.

Excessive Weight Gain. The ideal weight gain should be limited to approximately 240 grams (8 ounces) per week, or about 9 kg. (20 pounds) during the gestational period. Weight gain in excess of 0.45 kg. (1 pound) per week points to the necessity for caution. Weight gain is often the earliest sign of preeclampsia. It usually precedes significant edema, an increase of blood pressure, and proteinuria (a late and grave sign). A low calorie, salt-poor diet is not indicated in view of the fact that in preeclampsia blood volume is relatively contracted—i.e., in the preeclamptic, the usual physiologic hypervolemia of pregnancy does not occur. Presently, salt restriction and especially the addition of diuretic agents do nothing but further reduce an already contracted blood volume. As shown by Shoemaker and Gant, the effect of thiazide diuretics on placental function is detrimental to fetal well-being by lowering placental perfusion.

Blood Pressure. By accepted standards, a blood pressure of 140/90 requires careful observation and a recheck within the week. Probably a more exacting approach would be to emphasize the importance of a rise of 30 mm. Hg in systolic pressure and 15 to 20 mm. in diastolic pressure. Sudden changes indicate the necessity for caution. The antihypertensive drug, methyldopate hydrochloride (Aldomet), can be used cautiously only when severe, chronic hypertension is present. It must be noted that, while on medication, signs and symptoms of hypertension can be controlled; however, the fundamental pathology smolders and the process can become more progressive. Regular periods of rest can greatly aid in the reduction of blood pressure. When blood pressure rises with a diastolic greater than 110 mm. Hg, the patient is advised to rest in bed and can be given hydralazine hydrochloride (Apresoline) in small intravenous doses, 5 to 10 mg. This is mandatory so that the patient may be accurately observed and prepared, as necessary, for termination of the pregnancy.

Proteinuria. The presence of proteinuria, determined by urine examination during an office visit, requires that instructions be given in the mechanism of obtaining a clean catch of urine or the examination of a catheterized specimen. Verification of proteinuria requires more exacting investigation. Bacteriuria and pyelonephritis must be eliminated as causes. The presence of 0.5 gram demands caution. The presence of 1 to 3 grams daily is serious. When an amount over 3 grams daily is detected, serious involvement is present.

Associated Warning Symptoms

The presence of cerebral signs, visual disturbances, gastrointestinal upset, and/or epigastric pain can be attributed to multiple causes and often erroneously treated. When these exist and pregnancy is present, the potential of sudden, severe preeclampsia or increasing preeclampsia must be the prime consideration.

Treatment When Preeclampsia Progresses

A recent publication by Dr. Peggy J. Whalley indicates that hospitalization with bed rest is the suggested primary approach. Dr. Whalley states: "Termination of pregnancy is the only effective therapeutic modality known for treatment of the woman with pregnancy-induced hypertension. Fortunately, the majority of these women develop hypertension late in pregnancy at a time when the fetus is mature and delivery can be safely effected. There are, however, an appreciable number of women who first manifest hypertension earlier when the fetus is too immature to survive or would require a prolonged stay in the premature infant nursery if delivered. It is in these women that postponement of delivery would be justified, provided that delay is without signifiant risk to the mother or without detriment to her fetus." In her presentation, Dr. Whalley discusses the management offered 346 nulliparous women with pregnancy-induced hypertension. This management included ambulation as desired. With this management, it was concluded that the nulliparous patient with pregnancy-induced hypertension prior to term can be safely managed by hospitalization and close observation as a viable alternative to prompt delivery.

An outline of suggested management of the preeclamptic condition is shown in Table 1.

TABLE 1. **Management of the Preeclamptic Condition**

CLINICAL CONDITION	THERAPY
Preeclampsia with mature infant	Prevention of convulsions; delivery
Preeclampsia with immature infant with any of the signs of severe preeclampsia, severe fetal growth retardation, or impending fetal death	Prevention of convulsions; delivery
Incipient or mild preeclampsia with immature infant	Expectant therapy—(1) ambulatory; (2) hospitalization

Orders. Upon admission to the hospital for observation as a high risk patient, the following orders are suggested:

1. Admit to high risk unit for observation.
2. Routine vital signs (blood pressure, pulse, and temperature every 4 hours while awake) and fetal heart tones.
3. General diet (do not restrict).
4. Ward privileges (ambulation—relative bed rest).
5. Complete blood count, blood urea nitrogen, creatinine.
6. Sonography (repeat every 2 weeks).
7. Urine protein (every other day).
8. Daily weight.
9. Twenty-four hour urine collection for protein creatinine (repeat weekly).
10. Iron, 1 tablet orally twice daily.
11. Dalmane (flurazepam hydrochloride), as necessary for sleep.

Blood Pressure. Antihypertensive drugs should be used with great caution, because they have been known to lower the perfusion of the placenta and thus compromise the fetus. Magnesium sulfate has been given with great advantage to prevent and to control convulsions. The suggested method of administration is as follows:

1. Loading dose of $MgSO_4$ is 10 ml. of 50 per cent $MgSO_4$ deep intramuscularly in each buttock.
2. Maintenance dose of $MgSO_4$ is 10 ml. of 50 per cent $MgSO_4$ deep intramuscularly every 4 hours if patellar reflexes are present and if urine output is above 100 ml. per 4 hours.
3. Vital signs with blood pressure every 4 hours.
4. Urine output every 4 hours.

Eclampsia:

1. Intravenous $MgSO_4$ dose—4 grams of 20 per cent $MgSO_4$ slowly; may repeat once if necessary.
2. Intramuscular loading dose, same as for preeclampsia.
3. Maintenance.
4. Vital signs every hour.
5. Urine output every hour.

Edema. Diuretics are not routinely employed but are indicated only when evidence of congestive heart failure is present. Urinary output should be 2000 ml. daily. It is mandatory that intake and output records be kept. Fluids should be restricted only when cardiac complications occur.

Management of Pregnancy. First, control the toxemia. Second, evaluate the status of the product of conception. Third, choose a method of delivery. Indications for delivery of a high risk patient near term are (1) term gestation, (2) favorable cervix near term, or (3) clinical worsening of hypertension.

The method of delivery depends on the status of mother and infant. These are as follows: (1) Induction by amniotomy and/or oxytocin induction, unless obstetrically contraindicated. (2) Cesarean section under balanced anesthesia, using a combination of sodium thiopental (Pentothal), nitrous oxide, and succinylcholine chloride (Anectine). The indications for cesarean section include failed induction, cephalopelvic disproportion, fetal distress, and fetal malpresentation.

Caution—Prolonged medical management, i.e., over several weeks, can compound the management problem and, indeed, can result fatally for both infant and mother. If the systolic blood pressure exceeds 170 mm. Hg, the diastolic approaches 100 mm. Hg, and the pulse exceeds 120 per minute in spite of treatment, eclampsia is imminent.

Preeclampsia and Eclampsia. Consultation is always helpful; in fact, it is mandatory when the patient has had a convulsion. The rule is to (1) control the convulsion, (2) maintain oxygenation, (3) maintain urinary output, and (4) terminate the pregnancy as indicated by the condition of the patient and her obstetrical status. All management is based on exact and expert nursing and the availability of knowledgeable physicians.

GENERAL PROCEDURES. 1. Establish an immediate intravenous route by insertion of a No. 18 needle or an Angiocath.

2. Insert an indwelling Foley catheter to ensure accuracy in measuring output.

3. An eclampsia tray should be available, containing a mouth gag, magnesium sulfate, calcium gluconate, and amobarbital (Amytal).

4. Check vital signs by constant monitoring and nursing care.

5. Oxygen for cyanosis. Airway must be maintained.

6. Tracheostomy may be necessary and lifesaving. Consultation must be readily available.

7. Use of magnesium sulfate as outlined for control of hypertension and convulsions.

CONTROL OF RENAL AND CEREBRAL SYMPTOMS. Expert monitoring of electrolyte evaluation is essential. Injudicious use of fluids can result in acute congestive heart failure. It is advisable that no hypertonic solution or diuretics be used despite oliguria. Oliguria is expected because of vasospasm. It may be severe even up to 24 hours after delivery. Attempts to force fluid into the vasospastic vascular tree can easily lead to pulmonary edema. Five per cent dextrose in water given 60 to 100 ml. per hour, alternating with 5 per cent dextrose in lactated Ringer's solution, can assist in keeping the patient in balance. Electrolyte evaluation is helpful and may assist in preventing water intoxication (hyponatremia) secondary to oxytocin (Pitocin) induction plus free water in the intravenous solution.

CONTROL OF HYPERTENSION. It should be noted that any antihypertensive agent which lowers maternal blood pressure will also lower perfusion of the placenta. It is important to note that because of the risk of a cerebrovascular accident it is probably wise to lower maternal blood pressure to more acceptable levels if the diastolic blood pressure is above 110 mm. Hg. Attempts should never be made to lower the blood pressure to the normal range. At times, hydralazine (Apresoline) can be used in small push doses. The antihypertensive action of this drug is probably less severe than that of other agents. It may be given in small, intravenous doses of 5, 10, or 15 mg. as needed to maintain the diastolic pressure below 110 mm. Hg.

CARDIAC FAILURE AND PULMONARY EDEMA. Medical consultation is advisable to assist in medical management and digitalization after oxygen has been started and an airway established. Furosemide (Lasix), a powerful diuretic, may be given 20 to 40 mg. intravenously as a single dose slowly. This may be repeated in 20 mg. doses intravenously every 2 hours until the desired effect is obtained (see package insert). Sodium ethacrynate (Edecrin), 50 mg. intravenously, is even more rapid acting. Only fluids are given, and these only by the intravenous route, until the patient is conscious.

MANAGEMENT OF PREGNANCY. Medical management should be provided to control convulsions as soon as possible and then, as indicated, induction or cesarean section. Although severe eclampsia has a 35 to 40 per cent mortality rate in the antepartum and postpartum periods, the management as outlined and based upon the methods employed at Parkland Hospital, Dallas, Texas, by Dr. Pritchard has been successful. There was no mortality in 154 cases managed. The most valuable treatment in the prevention of this condition in the postpartum period is accurate observation and nursing care. A sudden rise of blood pressure along with evidence of minor irritability and/or albuminuria is the signal that magnesium sulfate, as previously outlined, should be initiated.

OBSTETRIC ANALGESIA AND ANESTHESIA

method of
MIGUEL COLÓN-MORALES, M.D.
San Juan, Puerto Rico

Morton's demonstration of ether anesthesia, in 1846, initiated what soon made possible the separation of pain and surgery. Unfortunately, and in spite of all efforts, similar complete separation of pain and childbirth has not yet been achieved.

There are fundamental considerations responsible for the difficulties encountered with the relief of pain during labor and delivery. They must be well understood prior to any attempt to provide analgesia or anesthesia for the obstetric patient, lest more harm than good result.

The change in emphasis from mother to fetus during recent years and the concern for the long-term effects of depressant drugs on the newborn, together with the manpower shortage in well trained obstetric anesthesia personnel, have complicated the present situation even more.

Recently there have been favorable changes in the practice of obstetric anesthesia and analgesia. The introduction of new drugs and techniques, the increased knowledge concerning the alterations in physiology of the pregnant woman, the more accurate assessment of the fetus through monitoring and the increasing availability of well trained and experienced personnel to provide analgesia and/or anesthesia to the obstetric patient have modified to a certain extent our attitudes toward the problem of pain relief during childbirth and its potential hazards. There is at present no ideal anesthetic agent or technique for childbirth. All known analgesics or anesthetic drugs pass through the placental barrier to the fetus with its immature organs and in its state of hypoxia and acidosis.

There is, however, enough evidence to suggest that *properly* administered analgesia and/or anesthesia reduces mortality and morbidity of the newborn. This represents a challenge to all physicians concerned, especially to obstetricians, anesthesiologists, and pediatricians.

Basic fundamental knowledge and special skills are essential for the proper management of pain during labor and delivery and should be part of the armamentarium of every physician who assumes the responsibility for participating in the care of the obstetric patient during childbirth.

Fundamental Considerations

Pregnancy causes physiologic alterations of great importance in the respiratory and cardiovascular systems. Such alterations must be kept in mind in order to provide safe obstetric anesthesia or analgesia.

Respiratory System Alterations. During the later part of pregnancy, respiratory rate and depth are increased to cope with the rise in O_2 requirements. The dyspneic-like effect is the result of the pressure of the enlarging uterus on the diaphragm. When the fetal head engages in the pelvis—"the lightening"—around the thirty-sixth week of gestation, the condition improves. Because of the increased O_2 requirement, any respiratory depression resulting from increased dosages of sedatives, analgesics, or anesthetics may lead to maternal hypoxia and its hazards to the already hypoxic fetus.

Cardiovascular System Alterations. Increase in blood volume occurs early in pregnancy. There is a greater rise in the plasma than in red blood cells. The result is the anemia of pregnancy, which must be corrected by means of iron. The increase in volume will serve to compensate for the loss of blood during delivery. This must be kept in mind in patients with heart disease because of the greater burden imposed on the heart. There is also a gradual rise in cardiac output and pulse rate.

During the last trimester of pregnancy, pregnant women lying in the supine position may suffer from hypotension caused by a decrease in venous return resulting from the pressure of the gravid uterus on the inferior vena cava and pelvic veins. This is called the inferior vena cava syndrome. Although compression of the inferior vena cava occurs in 85 per cent of pregnant women, during the last trimester, when in the supine position, severe symptoms are manifested in only 8 to 10 per cent; this is due to compensation by an increase in heart rate and by diversion of the blood through the paravertebral veins and into the azygous vein. A rise in vasomotor tone and peripheral resistance compensates and often prevents a fall in maternal blood pressure but does not necessarily correct an impairment with uteroplacental perfusion. Regional anesthesia with resultant peripheral vasodilation may prevent adequate compensation to maintain maternal blood pressure. Compression of the aorta (Poseiro effect) may maintain maternal blood pressure in the upper extremities but may result in a drop in blood pressure of the uterine arteries.

The Placenta

The placenta serves as the lungs, liver, and kidney of the fetus during pregnancy and parturition. Anything interfering with normal placental circulation will affect the growth and development of the fetus and its adaptation to the external independent environment after birth. All drugs used for obstetric analgesia and anesthesia will cross the placental barrier—with the one exception of the muscle relaxants, when used in small doses.

Obstetric Maternal Deaths

Causes: (1) Hemorrhage, (2) infection, (3) toxemia, (4) heart disease, and (5) anesthesia.

Obstetric Anesthesia Deaths

Causes: (1) Aspiration of vomitus (most common), (2) hypotension, and (3) respiratory failure.

Aspiration of Vomitus

1. "Prepare for the worst and it will seldom happen."

2. All parturients must be considered to have full stomachs. The onset of labor slows emptying of the stomach, and continued gastric secretions accumulate in the stomach during labor.

3. Fifty per cent of the obstetric deaths caused by anesthesia are attributable to the aspiration of vomitus.

4. Prevention—"an ounce of prevention is worth a pound of cure." During her prenatal visits, both the obstetrician and the anesthesiologist should warn the patient against taking solids or liquids by mouth once labor has started. During labor, the use of antacids is recommended to serve the specific purpose of neutralizing acidity of the gastric secretions. A pH above 2.5 is a must to reduce mortality and morbidity in the event of aspiration. Recommended dosage is 15 to 30 ml. (one half to 1 ounce) of antacid a half hour before delivery time. Emptying the stomach artificially by stimulation of the gag reflex or with apomorphine is rarely used and is not considered effective or practical.

When anesthesia is needed, for the sake of safety a regional or inhalational *analgesia* technique should be used, preserving tracheolaryngeal reflexes to protect against aspiration if vomiting occurs.

If anesthesia is needed, rapid endotracheal intubation is essential. A "crash intubation" is performed, using, if necessary, the Sellich maneuver (pressure on the cricoid cartilage to close the esophagus) while the trachea is intubated and sealed by inflating the cuff.

The endotracheal tube is left in place until the patient is completely awake and able to protect her airway in the event that vomiting occurs.

Predelivery Anesthesia Visit

Relief of pain during labor and delivery does not start in the labor room.

If we are determined to improve obstetric analgesia and anesthesia, the predelivery visit to the anesthesiologist must be encouraged. It should be done well before the scheduled delivery date (EDC) or date scheduled for elective cesarean section.

1. A preanesthetic evaluation adapted to the obstetric patient should be done at that visit, preferably by the anesthesiologist.
2. The different types of analgesia and anesthesia available for delivery, as well as the psychologic methods, should be discussed and a tentative choice or plan of action described to the patient. A slide-type presentation may be satisfactory.
3. The final decision about what method of pain relief will be used is not determined until the patient is actually in labor because of the many factors that must be considered in making this decision. Such an interview should help remove all fears and misconceptions that the expectant mother might have. A well informed patient should be a well behaved patient through more confidence in those responsible for her pain relief during labor and delivery.

Causes of Pain During Labor

1. Myometrial anoxia—contraction of muscle during a period of relative anoxia causes pain.
2. Stretching of the cervix—a painful sensation is felt, mainly in the back.
3. Traction on tubes, ovaries, or peritoneum.
4. Stretching of supporting ligaments.
5. Pressure in the urethra, bladder, and rectum.
6. Distention of the muscles of the pelvic floor and perineum.

Mechanism of Pain

Nerve fibers carrying painful sensations during the *first stage* of labor enter the spinal cord at the T10, T11, and T12 levels. The painful sensations during the *second stage* of labor enter the spinal cord at the S2, S3, and S4 levels.

Pain relief during labor and delivery may be accomplished through (1) psychologic methods, (2) pharmacologic methods, or (3) a combination of both.

Psychologic Methods of Pain Relief

These include (1) natural childbirth (childbirth without fear, Dick Read method), (2) psychoprophylactic method (Lamaze, Vellay), and (3) hypnosis.

Unfortunately psychologic methods for pain relief during labor and delivery are not suitable for everyone. The decision to use natural childbirth should be made several months before the estimated date of confinement. It takes time to learn the special exercises and to condition the mind in order for this method to be most effective. The ultimate objective should be to minimize the use of pharmacologic analgesia and/or anesthesia.

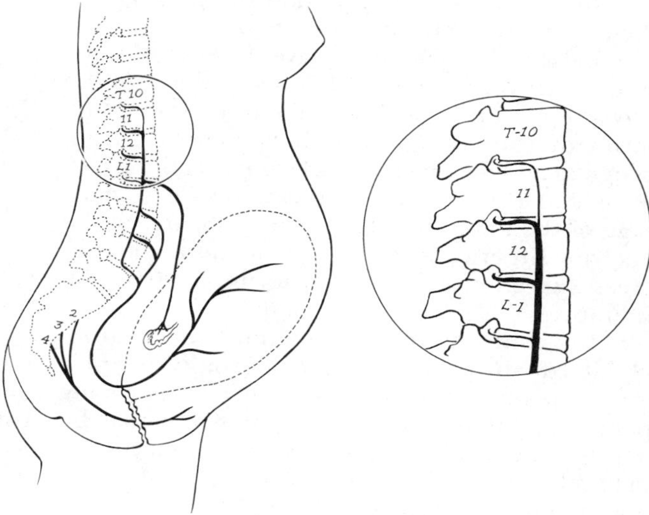

Figure 1. Parturition pain pathways. The uterus, including the cervix, is supplied by sensory (pain) fibers which pass from the uterus to the spinal cord by accompanying sympathetic nerves in the following sequence: uterine, cervical, and pelvic plexuses, the hypogastric nerve, the superior hypogastric plexus, the lumbar and lower thoracic sympathetic chain, and thence through white rami communicantes and posterior roots. The primary pathways (shown as thick lines in the inset) enter the eleventh and twelfth spinal segments, whereas the secondary auxiliary pathways enter at T10 and L1. The pathways from the perineum pass to the sacral spinal cord via the pudendal nerves. (Modified from Bonica, J. J.: Principles and Practice of Obstetric Analgesia and Anesthesia. Philadelphia, F. A. Davis Company, 1967).

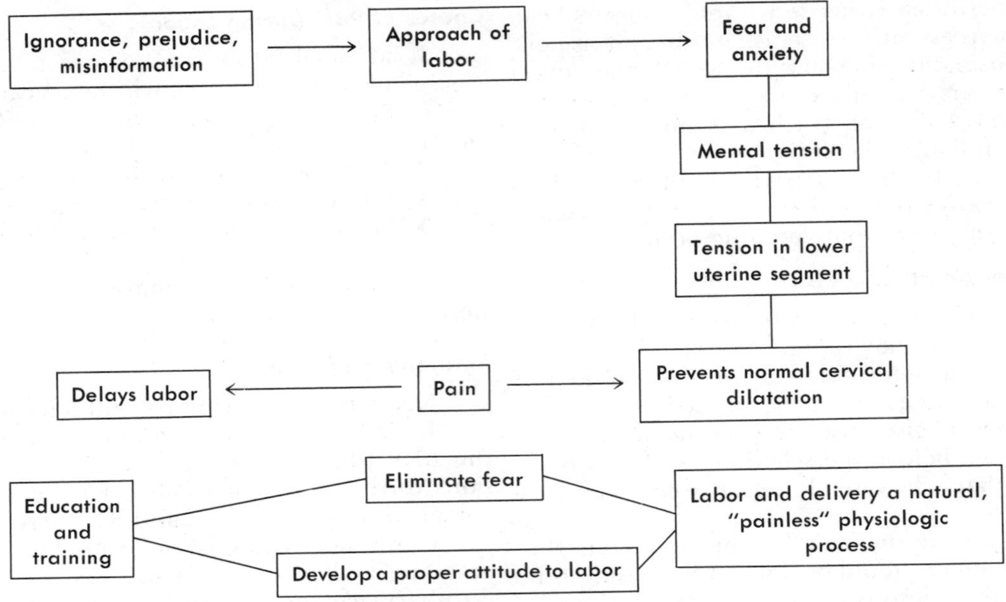

Figure 2. Natural childbirth (Dick Read method).

Preparation for Natural Childbirth. 1. Eight lectures in the basic anatomy and physiology of pregnancy.

2. A program of exercises and relaxation to be practiced throughout pregnancy.

Unfortunately great emphasis is placed on *conscious* and *spontaneous* delivery, and this can lead to severe psychologic trauma to patients who require operative delivery.

Psychoprophylaxis. Psychoprophylaxis was started in Russia, but was later developed in France by Lamaze and Vellay. It is based on the pavlovian concept of conditioned reflex training. Since women associate childbirth with pain, psychoprophylaxis aims to decondition the patient and then create new positive reflexes.

Method: The patient receives a series of illustrated lectures on the conditioned reflex and the physiology of normal labor. Then she is taught a series of exercises, which she practices during pregnancy. These include different breathing patterns and pain-reducing procedures—e.g., massage of the lower abdomen; and pressure on the anterior superior iliac crest when contraction increases in intensity. This is a form of distraction therapy.

In contrast to the method of natural childbirth, the patient in a psychoprophylaxis program is made aware that labor may be abnormally painful and that other forms of analgesia may be necessary. In the event she asks for pharmacologic pain relief or requires operative delivery, she does not feel that she has failed.

Hypnosis. Hypnosis is defined as a state of altered consciousness characterized by heightened suggestibility. Its exact mode of action is not known. Fifteen to 20 per cent of patients cannot be hypnotized. Only about 30 per cent of those who have been trained in the method achieve a relatively pain-free labor. The technique is very time consuming. Some patients may learn self-hypnosis. The majority require the presence of the hypnotist at the onset of labor and during the second stage.

Hypnosis should not be used in psychiatrically disturbed patients.

To summarize: Each one of these psychologic methods has its enthusiastic followers. At present, perhaps an individualized application of these techniques, alone or as an adjunct to the judicious use of the pharmacologic methods might come closest to the ideal goals we are searching for in the management of pain relief during childbirth.

Systemic Analgesia

A combination of narcotics and tranquilizers serves very well in obtaining pain relief during the first stage of labor.

Meperidine (Demerol), 25 to 50 mg., combined with promethazine (Phenergan), 25 mg., given slowly intravenously or by the intramuscular route, is used most often. It may be repeated every 3 to 4 hours. Avoid giving narcotics within 2 hours of the estimated time of delivery to avoid neonatal depression.

Alphaprodine (Nisentil), 20 mg. by intramuscular injection, is a potent respiratory depressant. Short lasting, its action is about 1 hour.

Scopolamine, 0.2 to 0.3 mg., may be used if amnesia is desired. It may cause restlessness and disorientation.

Diazepam (Valium), 5 to 10 mg. intravenously, may be very effective in allaying apprehension.

Promethazine (Phenergan), 25 mg. intravenously, an antihistaminic tranquilizer and antinauseant, will potentiate the effects of meperidine (Demerol).

Inhalational Analgesia

A low concentration of anesthetic agents may be administered for short periods to provide pain relief during labor and even delivery. The mother remains conscious and maintains her airway, and her protective reflexes are active. The progress of labor is not affected. There is no effect on the fetus because of low concentration. The effect of these agents may be reinforced during the second stage of labor by using a pudendal block or by local infiltration of the perineum.

The agents used are N_2O and O_2 in a 50-50 mixture. Methoxyflurane (Penthrane), 0.3 to 0.5 per cent, may be added for more profound analgesia. These agents may be self-administered under close supervision by a nurse or physician.

Types of Anesthesia

1. Local infiltration of the episiotomy site.
2. Pudendal block.
3. Paracervical block.
4. Low spinal or saddle block.
5. Epidural block—lumbar epidural or caudal.
6. General anesthesia—inhalational or intravenous.

General anesthesia is generally used only when there is a contraindication to regional anesthesia such as central nervous system disease or hypovolemia, or when delivery is imminent.

The least potent agent should be used to avoid a depressant effect on the fetus and newborn. There should be at least 25 per cent O_2 in the anesthetic mixture. Recommended mixtures are (1) N_2O and O_2 in a proportion of 3:1, or (2) an N_2O-O_2 mixture in 1:1 proportion with methoxyflurane 0.3 to 0.5 per cent.

To avoid the consequences of vomiting and aspiration in the obstetric patient, endotracheal intubation is highly recommended once a patient is given general anesthesia. This should be undertaken only by those highly skilled in crash intubation and with the necessary assistance. It must be kept in mind that the lighter and shorter the anesthesia, the less depressant drugs will reach the infant before birth.

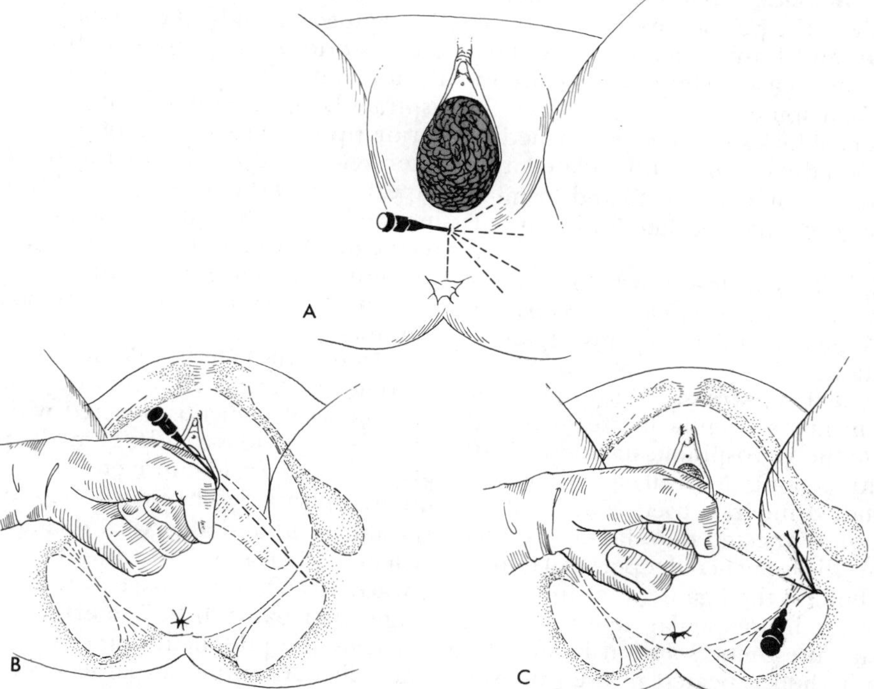

Figure 3. *A,* Local anesthesia: direct infiltration. *B,* Pudendal nerve block: transvaginal route. *C,* Pudendal nerve block: percutaneous transperitoneal approach. (Redrawn from Oxorn, H., and Foote, W. R.: Human Labor and Birth. 2nd ed. © 1968 by Meredith Corporation, Appleton-Century-Crofts, New York.)

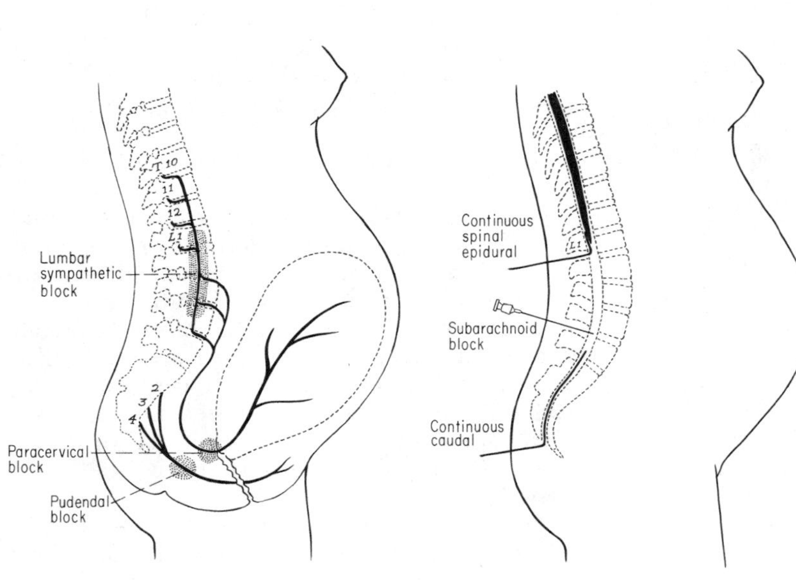

Figure 4. The most common regional anesthetic techniques used for obstetric analgesia-anesthesia. On the left are shown the site of injection and the diffusion of the local anesthetic (depicted by the stippled area) for "minor" blocks. Both paracervical block and pudendal block can be achieved by inserting a needle transvaginally, whereas lumbar sympathetic block is achieved by the paravertebral technique which entails insertion of a 3 to 4 inch needle 4 cm. lateral to the tip of the spinous process of the second lumbar vertebra and advancing it so that its point comes to lie on the anterolateral surface of the vertebra anterior to the attachment of fascia or iliopsoas muscle. Injection of a maximum of 10 ml. of solution on each side will interrupt labor pain pathways and produce relief of pain associated with uterine contractions. Bilateral paracervical block achieves the same effect, whereas bilateral pudendal block will relieve perineal pain caused by distention of the perineum by the presenting part. (Modified from Bonica, J. J.: Atlas of mechanisms of pathways of pain and labor. What's New, 1960, pp. 216–217.)

Pudendal Nerve Block. The pudendal nerve is the main supply of the perineum. It arises from the second, third, and fourth sacral nerves. The nerve is blocked most easily where it lies close to the tip of the ischial spine.

Pudendal nerve block should be performed in primigravidas when the cervix is fully dilated and the presenting part is at station +2, and in multiparas when the cervix has reached 7 to 8 cm. of dilatation.

Pudendal block provides satisfactory anesthesia for spontaneous delivery, low forceps extraction, breech delivery, and episiotomy repair or repair of laceration.

Transvaginal Technique. With the tip of the index finger inside the vagina, locate the ischial spine and palpate the sacrospinous ligament. A 10 ml. syringe, with a long No. 20 spinal needle guided by the index finger, is used. Three ml. of anesthetic solution is injected into the sacrospinal ligament. The needle is pushed deeper; as it enters the loose tissue behind the ligament, aspiration is attempted to avoid intravascular injection, and then 7 ml. of the anesthetic solution is injected. The procedure is then repeated in the opposite side.

Transperineal Technique. A skin wheal is raised with local anesthetic midway between the anus and the ischial spine. With the index finger in the vagina as a guide, the needle is directed toward the posterior surface of the ischial spine's inferior tip and into the pudendal canal. If no blood is aspirated, inject 3 ml. of solution beneath the inferior tip of the spine; another 3 ml. is injected after relocating the tip of the needle under the superior tip of the ischial spine. The needle is then inserted a little beyond the spine into the greater sciatic notch and 4 ml. of solution is injected. The procedure is then repeated in the opposite side.

Satisfactory anesthesia should take place in 15 minutes.

Paracervical Block. Paracervical block is used to relieve uterine and cervical pain. The local anesthetic of choice is injected within the lateral fornices at 4 and 8 o'clock 1 cm. deep. Precautions are taken to avoid intravenous injection by frequent aspiration. The injection is done once labor is established and a cervical dilatation of 4 cm. is reached. Duration of anesthesia is 1 hour. Paracervical block is used for the relief of first stage labor pains. It has no effect on areas innervated by the pudendal nerve (vagina, perineum, and vulva). Continuous paracervical block may be used by placing plastic catheters in the paracervical areas. At present no helpful instruments are available to facilitate this technique.

Fetal bradycardia sometimes follows paracervical block (incidence, 10 to 85 per cent). It may be followed by neonatal depression and even death.

TOXICITY OF LOCAL ANESTHETICS. Local anesthetics are rapidly transferred across the placenta into the fetus. Once in the fetus there is rapid uptake by the heart, the brain, and the liver. Susceptibility of the fetal heart to local anesthetics administered to the mother may be explained by the relatively high concentrations of the local anesthetic in the fetal heart, similar to that in the mother.

Myocardial toxicity of local anesthetics is enhanced by *hypoxia* and *acidosis*. Therefore drug levels well tolerated by the mother may be responsible for severe myocardial depression observed in the partially asphyxiated fetus. Similarly, local anesthetics may accumulate in the fetal brain and later result in respiratory depression at birth.

Factors of importance in toxicity include the dose and the rate of drug absorption from the site of injection.

In paracervical block the drug is injected in a highly vascular area and may result in transiently elevated drug levels in fetal blood associated with fetal *bradycardia* and *acidosis*.

To reduce the hazards of toxicity to the fetus and newborn:

1. Use less toxic drugs.
2. Reduce maternal and fetal blood levels of anesthetic by (a) using the smallest dose that will provide adequate analgesia, (b) using rapidly metabolized drugs (e.g., chloroprocaine), and (c) using long-acting drugs (e.g., bupivacaine), which will require less frequent reinjection.

TOXIC REACTIONS TO LOCAL ANESTHETIC DRUGS. True hypersensitivity to the local anesthetic drug, causing sudden death after injection of a small dose, is extremely rare. Allergy occasionally develops in dentists or pharmacists after repeated contact.

Toxic reactions usually result from (1) overdose from too large volume or too high concentration, (2) inadvertent intravascular injection, or (3) very rapid absorption. They may also occur when the rate of absorption of the drug exceeds the rate at which it is neutralized.

Signs and symptoms: Central nervous system (CNS) stimulation, as manifested by restlessness, dizziness, fine muscular twitching (e.g., facial muscle), or generalized convulsions; leading to hypoxia, loss of consciousness, obstruction of airway, vomiting, aspiration, further obstruction, further hypoxia, depression of vital centers in medulla, and at last respiratory and circulatory failure.

It must be remembered that most local anesthetics are rapidly detoxified by the liver and that blood concentration soon falls below toxic levels.

Treatment consists of the following measures:

1. Maintain an airway.
2. For apnea, give artificial respiration, either mouth-to-mouth or by bag and mask.
3. For pulselessness: artificial circulation, external cardiac compression, epinephrine (Adrenalin), sodium bicarbonate, calcium gluconate or chloride.
4. Hypoxia must be treated promptly by giving O_2 by mask.
5. Convulsions may be controlled by diazepam (Valium), 5 to 10 mg. intravenously, or by thiopental (Pentothal), 50 to 100 mg. intravenously. If immediate intubation is available, a short-acting muscle relaxant may be used to stop convulsions and allow ventilation and adequate oxygenation promptly.
6. Consider the possibility of a reaction or sensitivity to epinephrine (Adrenalin) in the anesthetic solution. This should be short lasting if treated promptly with oxygen, reassurance, and adequate ventilation.

Low Spinal Anesthesia (Saddle Block Anesthesia). After adequate preparation of the back, with the patient in the sitting position, the subarachnoid space is entered with a No. 26 or 25 spinal needle.

A hyperbaric mixture of equal volumes of tetracaine (Pontocaine) 1 per cent solution and dextrose 10 per cent solution is injected: tetracaine (Pontocaine), 4 mg. (0.4 ml.); dextrose, 40 mg. (0.4 ml.). The patient remains in the sitting position for at least 5 minutes after injection.

The injection should not be made during a contraction to avoid a higher level of the anesthetic.

This anesthetic technique is used when the cervix is fully dilated and when low forceps can be used easily to extract the head.

Lumbar Epidural Analgesia and Anesthesia. The pain of the first stage of labor may be very effectively relieved by blocking the afferent impulses from the uterus to the eleventh and twelfth thoracic segments via sympathetic pathways. Blocking the sacral roots at this stage is unnecessary and also undesirable. Relaxation of the pelvic floor muscles will affect proper flexion and rotation of the baby's head as it passes through the birth canal.

Lumbar epidural anesthesia may be given by single injection or by continuous technique. The latter is used more frequently, as it provides analgesia for the greater part of the labor. The optimal time to use it is when labor is well established and the cervix is dilated 4 to 6 cm. in primigravidas and 3 to 4 cm. in multiparas.

The *technique* for this procedure is as follows:

1. The patient lies on her side or sits up.
2. Her back is prepared with povidone-iodine (Betadine) or pHisoHex.
3. A No. 17 Tuohy needle is inserted in the second or third lumbar interspace with the bevel pointing cephalad.
4. Epidural puncture is made by the loss of resistance technique.
5. A test dose of 5 ml. of the solution of the local anesthetic of choice is injected into the epidural space.
6. After a 2 minute interval, if there is no evidence of intrathecal injection, a vinyl plastic tube is inserted through the needle for a distance of about 3.75 cm. (1½ inches). The needle is removed over the catheter. The catheter should never be pulled back lest it be severed by the sharp tip of the needle.
7. Antibiotic ointment is applied around the tubing and skin and properly covered, using gauze and tape so as to avoid kinking of the vinyl plastic tubing.
8. A needle and syringe filled with the local anesthetic of choice is connected to the distal end of the plastic tubing.
9. The patient lies on her back, and a second dose of anesthetic, 10 to 15 ml., is injected to avoid unilateral analgesia.
10. During labor the patient should lie on her side to avoid inferior vena cava compression.
11. When labor pain returns, more of the local anesthetic agent is injected through the catheter.
12. When the patient starts feeling pelvic pain and is fully dilated, the perineal dose, 10 to 15 ml., is given while she is in the sitting position. The patient remains sitting for about 5 minutes to allow the anesthetic solution to descend by gravity toward the sacral roots.

Anesthesia for Cesarean Section. There is no "ideal" anesthetic for cesarean section. There is a risk to the mother and fetus inherent in all known techniques. The final decision will depend on the needs of the patient and the skill of the anesthesiologist or obstetrician.

ELECTIVE CESAREAN SECTION. Regional anesthesia is strongly recommended—local, lumbar or sacral epidural, or spinal anesthesia. Our preference is *spinal anesthesia.*

Technique: Intravenous infusion is started with a 16 gauge indwelling catheter. Initial blood pressure and pulse are taken and recorded. Five hundred to 1000 ml. Ringer's lactate solution is given rapidly. Spinal anesthesia is administered with the patient sitting or on her side. The drug used is tetracaine 1 per cent solution diluted in 10 per cent dextrose, 50 : 50 mixture. The dosage is 6 to 10 mg., depending on the position used (sitting up, lateral decubitus) and the height of the patient. The patient is then placed in a supine, 10 degree Trendelenburg position for approximately 30 seconds. The Colón-Morales (C-M) uterine displacer is applied, displacing the uterus to the left. Blood pressure and pulse are taken repeatedly. The displacer is readjusted if necessary. If there is a drop in blood pressure below 100 mm. Hg systolic, the uterine displacer is readjusted. If the blood pressure drops below 90 mm. Hg systolic in spite of the intravenous fluids and uterine displacement, 12.5 to 25 mg. of ephedrine is given intravenously.

EMERGENCY CESAREAN SECTION. Spinal or general anesthesia is used, depending on the cause for the emergency situation.

In hypotensive states or in fetal distress, regional anesthesia may not be applicable. In such an urgent situation, general anesthesia may be favored.

The *technique* for emergency cesarean section is as follows:

1. The patient is placed in the supine position.
2. The uterine displacer is applied, displacing the uterus to the left.
3. Blood pressure and pulse are taken.
4. The patient is draped.
5. When the obstetrician is ready to start surgery, a sleeping dose of thiopental (Pentothal) is given intravenously (150 to 250 mg.); an N_2O–O_2 analgesic mixture (50:50) is started, and 40 to 60 mg. of succinylcholine is given intravenously, followed by endotracheal intubation. After delivery of the infant, 0.3 to 0.5 per cent methoxyflurane (Penthrane) is added to the analgesic mixture, or meperidine (Demerol) in small repeated doses is given intravenously to provide analgesia.

Postspinal Headache. Postspinal headache is due to leakage of cerebrospinal fluid through the puncture hole; it usually starts on the second or third day after administration of spinal anesthesia. The patient feels relief from the headache when recumbent, but the headache gets worse when she is sitting up or standing. It may be short- or long-lasting, mild or severe. The incidence is markedly reduced if 24 to 26 gauge spinal needles are used for the puncture.

Treatment encompasses the following measures:

1. The patient should be kept flat in bed for 12 to 24 hours.
2. The foot of the bed may be raised slightly to reduce cerebrospinal fluid (CSF) hydrostatic pressure at the site of the puncture hole.
3. One thousand ml. of intravenous fluid

(isotonic saline or Ringer's lactated) is given, and the patient is asked to drink plenty of fluids.

4. Vasopressin (Pitressin) may be given in a dosage of 0.5 to 1.0 ml. intramuscularly to speed up rehydration.

5. Analgesics and tranquilizers should be given—codeine, 30 mg. (½ grain), or diazepam (Valium), 5 to 10 mg. intravenously, intramuscularly, or orally.

6. If headache persists in spite of the aforementioned treatment, an injection of isotonic saline solution into the caudal or epidural space should be tried.

7. A blood patch in the epidural space has also been advocated and has been claimed to be very effective.

Caudal Anesthesia. Blocking the sacral nerves provides complete analgesia of the lower uterine segment as well as the vulva and perineum.

Technique: The patient is placed in the knee-chest position or in the lateral position with her bottom leg straight and top leg flexed.

Landmarks include the sacral cornua, tip of coccyx, and sacral hiatus.

The area is prepared, leaving a plug with antiseptic over the anus. With the middle finger and thumb, identify the sacral cornua. Then identify the tip of the coccyx with the index finger. Slide the finger cephalad, identifying the sacral hiatus. Inject a local anesthetic into the skin over this area.

For a single caudal injection, insert a No. 20 or No. 18 gauge needle into the sacrococcygeal membrane at an angle of 45 degrees, recognizing the sacral canal by the loss of resistance. Depress the tip of the needle toward the intergluteal cleft until it lies almost parallel to the dorsum of the sacrum and advance the needle 2 cm. along the sacral canal. Aspirate to check for blood or cerebrospinal fluid; if negative, inject air or saline, with fingertips over the sacral area feeling for swelling or crepitus. If present, reinsert the needle until no crepitus is felt or no blood is aspirated. If spinal fluid is aspirated, abandon the procedure. When the needle is in the correct position, inject the local anesthetic solution slowly after a preliminary test dose of 3 ml. has been used to make sure the dura has not been entered. Wait 5 minutes after the test dose injection and check for weakness of the legs. If the test dose is negative, inject the local anesthetic—e.g., lidocaine (Xylocaine) 1.5 per cent, 20 to 25 ml. with repeated aspiration, or bupivacaine 0.5 per cent, 20 to 25 ml.

For the continuous technique, use a Tuohy No. 18 needle and thread a vinyl catheter into the caudal canal.

Intravenous Anesthesia. Ketamine has been used for pain relief in vaginal delivery. Dosage is 12.5 to 25 mg. administered intravenously at crowning. This dosage may be repeated if indicated to a maximum dosage of 100 mg. If necessary, local anesthesia may be used for the removal of the placenta or repair of episiotomy. With the aforementioned dosage schedule, Akamatsu reports that "No untoward effect was encountered in mother or infant."

The Colón-Morales (C-M) Uterine Displacer—"the Third Hand"

The administration of spinal and/or epidural anesthesia prior to cesarean section relaxes abdominal muscles, causing the pregnant uterus to fall to the right, resulting in compression of the inferior vena cava. Cardiac output is decreased owing to inadequate venous return, and the uteroplacental perfusion may be impaired.

The C-M uterine displacer (left uterine displacement device) was specifically designed for the physiologic management of the supine hypotension syndrome reducing the need for use of intravenous fluids or vasopressors. Properly adjusted, the C-M uterine displacer will reposition the uterus, relieving pressure on the inferior vena cava, thus increasing venous return, central venous pressure, cardiac output, mean arterial pressure, and systemic vascular resistance. Maternal normotension and uteroplacental perfusion are restored.

Initial Care of the Newborn After Vaginal or Abdominal Delivery

In every cesarean section a physician highly skilled in newborn resuscitation should be present with the necessary equipment to provide the best possible care during those important first few minutes of life.

An accurate Apgar scoring of every newborn at 1 and 5 minutes of life should be done by the physician in charge of the initial care of the newborn. In the words of Dr. Virginia Apgar: "Nine months' observation of the mother surely warrants one minute's observation of the baby!"

Analgesia and Anesthesia in Special Obstetric Situations

Multiple Delivery. Be very careful with the administration of sedatives, analgesics, or tranquilizers because of the effect on the fetuses and the progress of labor.

Avoid the supine position at all times to prevent the hazards of aortocaval compression.

The possibility of prematurity must be kept in mind.

Regional anesthesia—saddle block or pudendal block—is given after the cervix is fully dilated and the presenting part is at least at the +2 station.

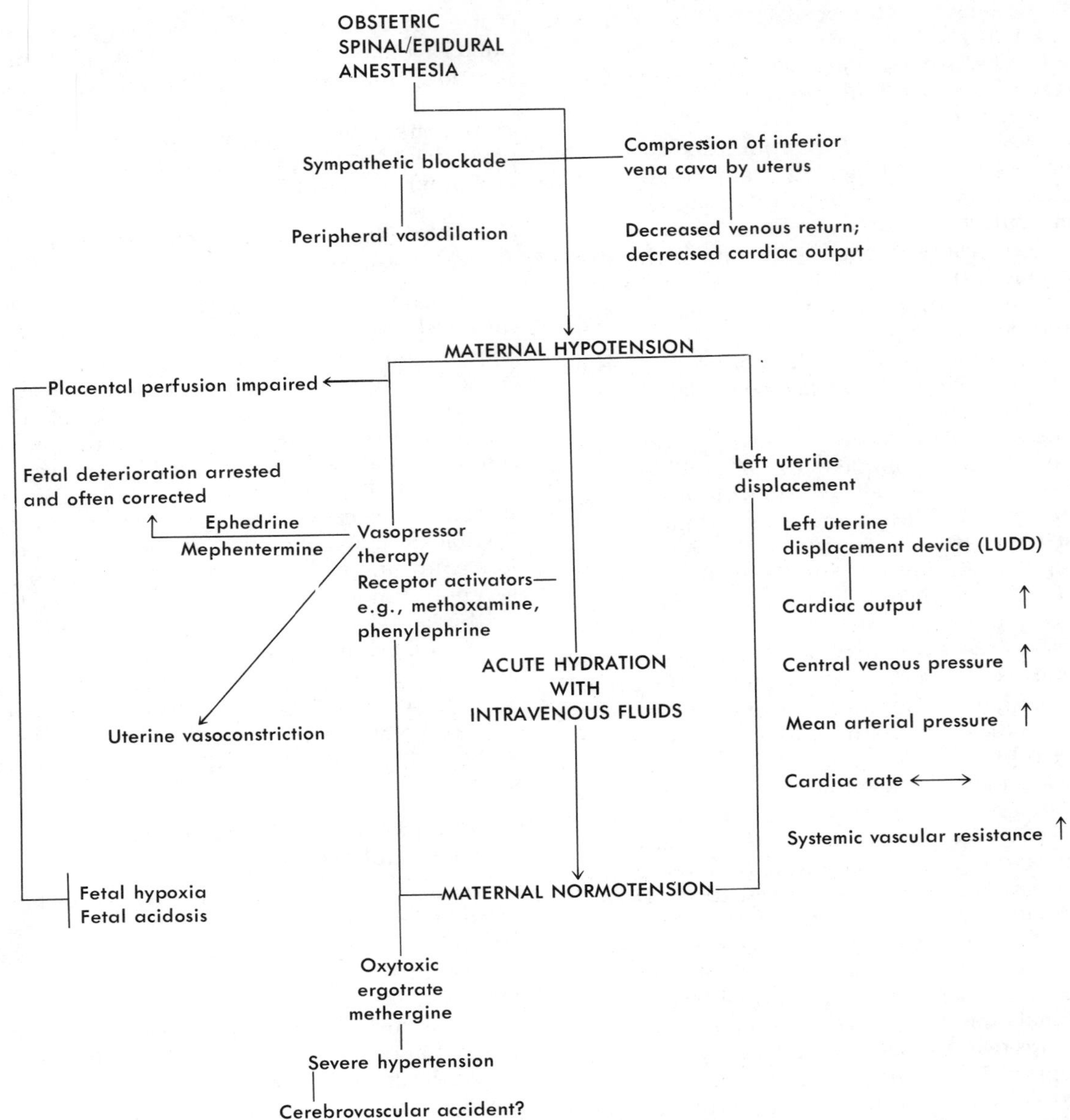

Figure 5. (From scientific exhibit of supine hypotensive syndrome, physiologic versus pharmacologic management. Presented by Miguel Colón-Morales, M.D., during annual meetings of American Medical Association and American Society of Anesthesiologists.)

If intrauterine manipulation is necessary, halothane or ether anesthesia may be necessary to relax the uterus.

Breech Delivery. Avoid overdosage with systemic analgesic drugs during the first stage of labor.

Regional anesthesia—saddle block or pudendal block—is given when the cervix is fully dilated and the presenting part is at the +2 station.

If the aftercoming head becomes trapped, be ready to relax the uterus with deep halothane anesthesia.

Prematurity. Avoid analgesics. Regional anesthesia—lumbar epidural or spinal—is safe, but avoid maternal hypotension by uterine displacement or hydration or with ephedrine, 12.5 mg. intravenously, if needed. General anesthesia should be avoided. Paracervical block is too risky. Pudendal block is used for delivery.

Preeclampsia. The presence of uteroplacental insufficiency should caution one against any techniques causing hypotension.

Care must be taken with vasopressor drugs. There is increased sensitivity in these patients.

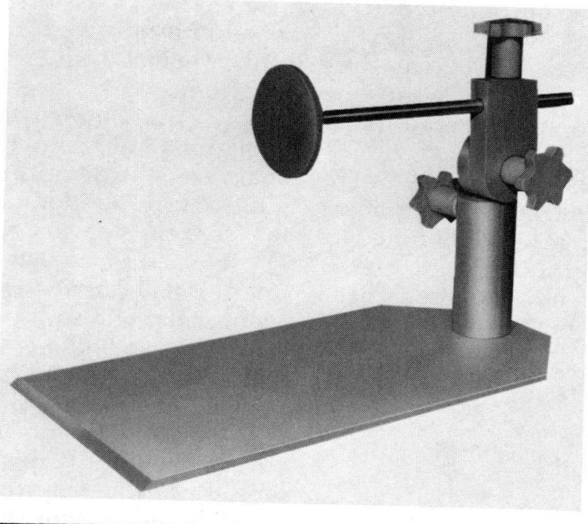

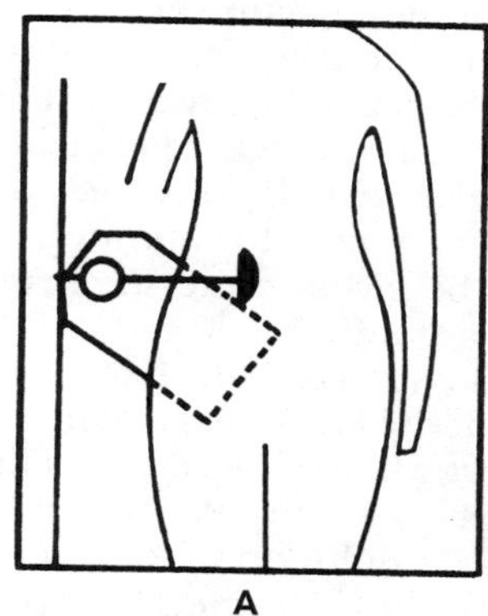

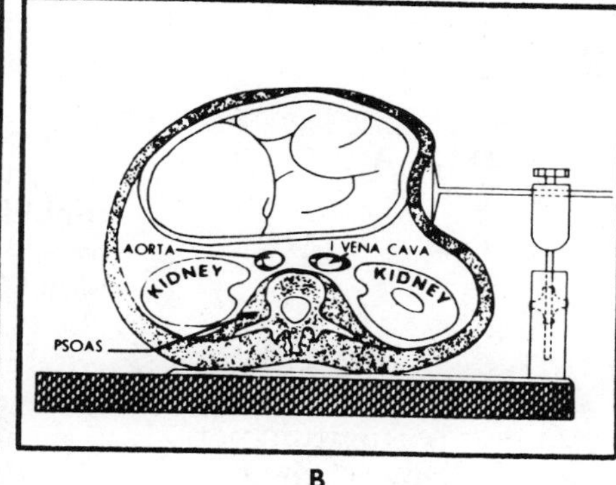

A B

Figure 6. The C-M uterine displacer. Instructions for use: After regional anesthesia is administered, place patient in supine position. Raise patient's right side enough to allow for placement of plate under right lumbosacral region (or mattress), positioning the vertical post cephalad to minimize interference with the surgeon *(A)*. Displace the uterus manually to the left and adjust pressure pad so as to gently maintain the uterus in the desired position *(B)*. As soon as the peritoneal cavity is opened, the horizontal rod may be released so as not to interfere with intra-abdominal manipulation by the surgeon. (Developed by Miguel Colón-Morales, M.D.)

Diabetes. In all forms of diabetes the fetus should be considered at risk. Regional anesthesia is preferred for cesarean section. Paracervical block should be avoided.

Rheumatic Heart Disease. Avoid any increase in oxygen consumption—e.g., tachycardia or myocardial depression. Provide some analgesia. In the first stage, segmental epidural block or paracervical block may be used. In the second stage, pudendal block, saddle block, or caudal block is used for terminal delivery.

Mandatory Safety Measures in Obstetric Analgesia and Anesthesia

1. Well secured indwelling intravenous cannula.

2. Ready availability of blood. (a) Type and cross-match every obstetric patient when admitted in labor. (b) Have 500 ml. of type O Rh-negative blood available in the delivery room at all times.

3. Suction equipment in good working condition.

4. A rapid-tilting delivery table.

5. Strict observance, through patient education, of nothing by mouth (solid or liquid) with onset of labor contractions, with the one exception of recommended alkali oral therapy.

6. Administration of antacids throughout labor and about 1 hour prior to scheduled cesarean section, to neutralize acidity of stomach contents.

7. Presence of an anesthesiologist or anesthetist capable of performing a rapid endotracheal intubation under difficult conditions and of treating the complications of local anesthetics and regional techniques.

Conclusion

The fact that, in spite of all efforts, childbirth and pain have not yet been divorced is good evidence of the serious difficulties encountered so far in solving this problem.

Great progress has been made, especially during the last 2 decades, but such progress must be considered partial solutions to a very difficult problem.

Let us all hope and work for a breakthrough in the not too distant future. In the meantime let us make the best possible use of all the knowledge, the skills, and the manpower available, to do the best we can with what we have to protect the mother, the fetus, and the newborn. We will be protecting future generations and perhaps even mankind.

POSTPARTUM CARE

method of
TAKEY CRIST, M.D., F.A.C.O.G., F.A.C.S.
Jacksonville, North Carolina

Introduction

The term puerperium or postpartum period includes the period elapsing between the end of the third stage of labor and the return of the genital tract to its normal nonpregnant state.

Management of the patient during this time span can be divided into three phases: (1) hospital care, including the delivery room, recovery room, and postpartum unit; (2) home care; and (3) the postpartum office visit.

Hospital

Delivery Room. The puerperium begins with the delivery of the placenta. This period requires careful management and attention to ensure an uneventful and uncomplicated recovery period. Immediately after expulsion of the placenta, care should be taken to ensure that the uterus is well contracted. The placenta should be carefully inspected to determine that membranes and placenta are intact. Manual examination of the uterus is carried out to rule out retained fragments as well as uterine abnormalities.

The fundus is gently but firmly massaged to help express clots and to ascertain that it remains firmly contracted.

If intravenous infusion is used, oxytocin may be administered by this route in the amount of 20 units per 1000 ml. of 5 per cent dextrose in water.

The cervix is inspected for lacerations and repaired if indicated. Further inspection is made of the vaginal vault for lacerations or hematoma formation.

The episiotomy is repaired with 2–0 chromic interrupted and running sutures. An estimate of blood loss is made, and, along with blood pressure, pulse and respirations are recorded before transfer from the delivery room.

Testosterone enanthate and estradiol valerate (Deladumone OB) is administered intramuscularly to suppress lactation in the mother who wishes to bottle-feed. It may be administered with the delivery of the infant's head or immediately before transfer from the delivery room.

Recovery Room. Ideally, postpartum recovery should take place in a separate recovery area. Regardless of areas of recovery, the procedure should remain the same. For patients who have no complications, this intensive care period should be carried on for at least 2 to 4 hours. Care should include a sterile perineal pad with T-binder. The pulse, blood pressure, and respirations are recorded every 15 minutes. Careful attention should be given to uterine firmness. The fundus must be gently massaged every 15 minutes and blood loss recorded. Excessive bleeding or inability of the uterus to remain firm should result in administration of intravenous fluids, along with 20 units of oxytocin (Pitocin) per 1000 ml. of intravenous solution and/or ergonovine maleate (Ergotrate) or methylergonovine maleate, (Methergine) intramuscularly.

The bladder region should be palpated frequently to detect distention. Bladder distention must be prevented, by catheterization if necessary, to avoid prolonging the time required for recovery of normal bladder tone and function.

Following spinal or epidural anesthesia, the patient must be able to move her legs before she is transferred to the postpartum unit.

Visitors in the recovery area should be limited to the child's father.

If the patient desires to breast-feed immediately following delivery, this may be allowed so long as the baby's normal body temperature is maintained.

Postpartum Nursing Unit. It is felt that for both the physical and psychologic well-being of the patient, the hospital stay should be at least 72 hours. In most cases, 3 to 5 days is the normal hospital stay, depending on the condition of both infant and mother and the establishment of a satisfactory feeding routine. The routine orders that must be included are as follows:

1. Routine vital signs, including temperature, pulse, respirations, and blood pressure, are recorded at least four times a day.

2. A regular diet is given unless contraindicated.

3. Early ambulation is encouraged.

4. The patient may shower on the second postpartum day.

5. Catheterization is advised every 6 to 8 hours if the patient is unable to void.

6. Instruction should be given as to proper perineal care.

7. A heat lamp is provided three times daily for 15 minutes beginning the first postpartum day. If the patient desires, sitz baths twice daily may be used.

8. Complete blood count (CBC) is taken the morning after delivery.

9. Urine culture is also taken the morning after delivery.

10. Empirin compound with codeine, 30 mg. (Empirin No. 3) can be given every 3 to 4 hours as desired for pain. If the patient is allergic to codeine, propoxyphene (Darvon), 65 mg. every 3 to 4 hours as necessary, may be substituted.

11. Dioctyl calcium sulfosuccinate and danthron (Doxidan), 2 capsules, can be given at bedtime beginning the day of delivery as a laxative.

12. Secobarbital sodium (Seconal), 100 mg., may be given at bedtime for sleep.

13. Unless contraindicated, methylergonovine maleate (Methergine), 0.2 mg. three times daily, can be given.

14. Breast-feeding mothers are instructed to wear good supportive brassieres, preferably a nursing brassiere. Emollient cream (Massé Cream) may be applied to the nipples and areolae three times daily.

15. Bottle-feeding mothers are instructed to wear snug-fitting supportive brassieres. If engorgement becomes uncomfortable, ice packs may be applied.

16. If indicated in Rh-negative mothers, a RhoGAM work-up is done and immune globulin (human) RhoGAM is given intramuscularly after satisfactory laboratory cross-match.

It is important that the patient be observed for any postpartum complications. The most important of these are hemorrhage, puerperal infection, thrombophlebitis, mastitis, and cystitis and pyelitis. Careful attention to the temperature is important at this time. A temperature of 100.4°F. (38°C.) on two consecutive occasions should result in further thorough investigation as to the cause, followed by the appropriate treatment.

Excessive bleeding should be immediately investigated and appropriate action taken, which usually includes administration of intravenous therapy and, if necessary, whole blood replacement.

Home Care

The 4 to 6 week period after discharge is a continuation of the patient's transition to her normal nonpregnant state. It is important that she be given specific instructions before discharge as to how to care for herself. Before being sent home, an examination should be done, including inspection of the breasts and nipples and examination of the perineum for healing, the uterus for involution, and the abdominal wall for relaxation.

Discharge instructions should be discussed and written instruction sheets given to the patient. Activity may be gradually increased, beginning with light activity and 1 to 2 hour rest periods per day for the first 10 to 14 days, and gradually increasing to full normal duties at 6 weeks. Light exercises may begin in 2 weeks and these, also, gradually increased. Continuation of prenatal vitamins and iron for approximately 6 weeks is advised for bottle-feeding mothers and as long as nursing continues in breast-feeding mothers.

Sexual intercourse may be resumed at the discretion of the couple, making sure that the patient and her partner have been instructed in the use of birth control. No restrictions as to shower or tub baths are given. The patient is advised to maintain a well balanced diet. Contraception is discussed with the patient. If the nonbreast feeder desires oral contraceptives, she is instructed to begin pills. If she is not breast feeding and engorgement occurs, she is instructed to wear a good light supportive brassiere day and night. Any stimulation to the breast is to be avoided. Ice packs and acetaminophen (Tylenol) are given for discomfort. She is told to report at once any increase of pain in her episiotomy, localized pain or reddened areas in the breasts, excessive bleeding, abnormal pain, or fever. An appointment for a return visit to the office in 6 weeks is mandatory.

Postpartum Office Visit

The postpartum visit is necessary to determine the rate of return to a normal nonpregnant state, and to be sure there has been a healthy adjustment between mother, baby, and the family unit. Family planning measures are discussed.

During this visit, weight, blood pressure, temperature, pulse, respiration, urine sugar, and protein are recorded. An evaluation of breast, abdomen, and lower extremities is made.

A pelvic examination is done, giving special attention to healing of the perineum, vagina, and cervix. A careful bimanual examination is done to determine uterine involution and absence of any adnexal disease. A Papanicolaou smear is also done at this time.

Resumption of menstruation should be discussed and the breast-feeding mother instructed that menstruation may not occur while she is lactating, but may occur at irregular intervals. It should be emphasized to her that breast feeding is not a form of birth control.

The bottle-feeding mother should be reassured that normally periods will not resume for 8 to 10 weeks.

Contraception is discussed at this visit. If oral contraception has already begun, instructions are reinforced. If the patient is breast feeding, oral contraception is not used until the baby is weaned. If a diaphragm is chosen, proper fitting and instruction for proper use are carried out. If the patient chooses an intrauterine device (IUD), it can be inserted at this time. If nonprescription contraception is desired, she is encouraged to use foam and condoms.

A pelvic examination is usually repeated after 6 months and 1 year. Adequate postpartum care over a year may prevent or even cure conditions that would otherwise cause trouble in later years.

CARE OF THE LOW BIRTH WEIGHT INFANT

method of
ROBERT S. MENDELSOHN, M.D.
Chicago, Illinois

Despite all the highly publicized "advances" of the past decade, the medical management of premature infants remains, at best, unsatisfactory. Treatment of the major pathologic conditions occurring in prematures is still uncertain and controversial. Therefore maximum effort must be invested in prevention of premature births.

Prevention

1. The major cause of prematurity is maternal malnutrition. The incidence—particularly of the most troublesome smaller prematures—is estimated by authorities to be 10 to 20 times higher among those in low socioeconomic circumstances than among the well-to-do. Therefore the prevention of the overwhelming proportion of premature births depends on the elimination of hunger, malnutrition, slum housing, unemployment, poor sanitation, inadequate medical care, and other concomitants of poverty. However, as Tom Brewer, M.D., and others have emphasized, even in the middle and upper social classes, low-birth-weight infants may result from the common, though unwise, obstetric practice of undue limitation of weight gain during pregnancy.

2. Other causes of prematurity (maternal infection, placenta previa, and so forth) are statistically of less significance and may be managed according to established practice.

Evaluation of Technologic Advances

The modern management of prematurity differs from that of several decades ago primarily in the extensive utilization of technology. A concomitant of this has been a change in nomenclature. Thus the old titles of premature nurseries or premature stations have been replaced by new designations such as "newborn intensive care units" or "high risk nurseries." Watchful waiting of previous years has given way to active intervention, necessitating an impressive array of devices for artificial ventilation and other measures, as well as extensive machinery for monitoring. A physician who has not been in a premature unit for the past 20 years would indeed be startled at the jungle of apparatus.

Yet the value of these "advances" in preventing mortality and morbidity is far from clear. There are various reports attempting to demonstrate the improvement in outlook resulting from modern therapy. However, the great majority of these investigations are subject to the usual shortcomings of statistical studies, and there is an almost total absence of carefully designed and executed double blind studies. Furthermore, characteristically, every report arguing for the superiority of modern management has been conducted and published by those in the field of neonatology, obviously a group highly vulnerable to the charge of harboring, consciously or otherwise, a vested interest in the outcome of their work. Thus the possible bias introduced by a more than potential conflict of interest throws a cloud of suspicion over even the most well-intentioned investigation.

Few reports exist describing the dangers of high risk nurseries, although exceptions include the risk of deafness from noise levels in incubators as well as observations of later behavioral disorders associated with lack of mothering. Understandably, no studies have been completed at this time seeking the long-term effects of early treatment, 10, 20, or more years later.

It is therefore reasonable to conclude that, at this point, monitoring, artificial ventilation, drug management, and other modalities of present-day premature care remain in the category of the experimental. The possible benefits—or disadvantages—of new, stylish (i.e., modern) therapy over old-fashioned management remain to be established.

This being the case, some of the time-tested basic principles will now be underscored.

Delivery

1. Do not give analgesia or anesthesia if there is any hint that the child may be premature. The infant will be exposed to narcotization, which may result in immediate or subsequent damage. The physician may be exposed to a malpractice suit.

2. Do not depend on interns or inexperienced residents. The premature newborn deserves a pediatrician or other experienced physician on the spot at the time of delivery.

3. Keep the baby warm but do not be surprised at subnormal temperatures in very small infants.

4. Avoid unnecessary handling.

5. It is not necessary or advisable to immediately remove the vernix.

6. Do not let the incubator become overheated; this is a common cause of hyperthermia in the infant.

Nursing Care

1. Ask nurses experienced in premature care for advice on the following items: type of incubator; temperature of incubator; level of humidity; type of soap or other cleansing agent preferred (being sure to avoid hexachlorophene); handling, bathing, clothing, and turning of infant; placement of infant on abdomen or back; frequency and amount of feedings; and type of bottles and nipples.

2. Medical judgment on the aforementioned matters is available, but in general is not so practical or soundly based as that of a good nurse. A valuable textbook for general reference is that by Evelyn C. Lundeen, R.N., and Ralph H. Kunstadter, M.D.: Care of the Premature Infant, published by the J. B. Lippincott Company. Although published almost two decades ago, it describes many practices and attitudes far superior to those in vogue today.

3. Keep nursing simple; caps are not necessary; changes of gowns are not necessary; the usual careful handwashing is sufficient.

Feeding of Prematures

1. Breast milk is best for the premature infant; artificial milk is at best an inadequate substitute, and its disadvantages are well documented.

2. Encourage mothers to breast feed; discourage them from bottle feeding.

3. Feed the baby as soon as possible after delivery; there is no magic number in 24, 48, or 72 hours and no need to keep the baby hungry; early feeding diminishes the occurrences and severity of hyperbilirubinemia and hypoglycemia.

4. Milk from one mother will often supply several infants; it may be necessary to promote the establishment of a breast-milk bank.

5. If human milk is not available, a variety of artificial products may be used. No commercially available formula offers a scientifically proved significant advantage over its competitors.

6. Intermittent tube feeding may be necessary for short periods of time. Indwelling tubes or prolonged use of gavage is discouraged; it usually indicates inadequate staffing of the nursery or inexperienced personnel.

7. Vitamin supplements are not necessary in the breast-fed infant.

Parent Participation

Many developmental problems afflict the premature in later years. These include learning disability, perceptual handicaps, pseudomental retardation, and emotional disorders. Of major significance in the production of these serious conditions is the prolonged period of separation of the premature infant from his mother. The following measures are helpful in overcoming the effects of this separation.

1. Encourage the mother to visit inside the nursery as soon as she is ambulatory. Allow her to hold the baby (in the case of large prematures) or stroke his skin (in the case of small prematures).

2. Have the nurses instruct her in feeding techniques and also in the technique of pumping her breasts. Have her feed the baby whenever possible.

3. Encourage the father to participate in feeding, bathing, and general care of the infant.

4. Remember that the best nursing staff is never the equal of the child's mother.

Discharge

1. There is no magic discharge weight—5 lbs., 5½ lbs., 6 lbs., and so forth.

2. Many infants weighing about 4 lbs. have been discharged with no untoward results.

3. Remember that the danger of epidemic disease lurks in every hospital nursery; therefore the premature station cannot always be considered safer than the home.

4. The decision to discharge should be made individually for each child. Important factors include the child's clinical condition (exclusive of his weight), the capability of his parents, and the availability of community services (public health nursing, homemaker service, and so forth).

Diseases

1. The sick premature infant does not show signs of disease typical of full-term, heavier babies. Lethargy or failure to suck properly may often be the first and only sign of sepsis, pneumonia, or meningitis. Therefore early diagnosis depends crucially on the observations of an experienced nursing staff and on good communication between physician and nurse.

2. Treatment for some of the major diseases of prematurity is not firmly established. Many different regimens, for example, have been used in hyaline membrane disease. These include steroid hormones, intravenous fluids, aerosol administration, hyperbaric pressure, enzyme therapy, and a host of others. All have their hazards and side effects, and there is general agreement that none has demonstrated clear-cut superiority.

3. Oxygen should be given with caution in view of the possibility of causing retrolental fibroplasia if it is given in high concentrations. In addition, low concentrations (below 40 per cent) have not clearly been shown to be effective in either saving lives or preventing future disability.

4. The management of erythroblastosis follows the same principles in prematures as in the full-term infant. With the widespread use of ultraviolet light, there is an increased appreciation of its hazards as well as its benefits; this type of therapy therefore should still be considered as experimental and approached with caution.

5. Conditions requiring surgical intervention are common and, in general, carry a high mortality.

6. The dosage of most drugs in prematures is highly uncertain, and individualization is the rule. In some cases (e.g., chloramphenicol) lower dosage schedules than in adults are recommended for the premature; in others (e.g., digitalis) relatively greater amounts are required.

7. Recommendations for management of premature infants keep changing; it is important to keep current with the opinions and advice of the experts. It is also important to remember that yesterday's fact may be today's falsehood; therefore one's own judgment and feeling must always guide one's practice.

Prognosis

1. Present the pertinent statistics to the parents, indicating that the mortality among premature infants is in the order of 90 per cent in those weighing below 1000 grams, approaches 50 per cent in those weighing in the 1000 to 1500 gram range, and is lower at higher weights. These statistics have changed very little over the past few decades.

2. Be aware of the difficulties the surviving premature faces in later life. These include growth retardation, mental retardation, learning disorders, perceptual handicaps, and so forth. It is neither wise nor necessary to acquaint parents of newborns with these conditions.

3. Be cautious and indefinite in prognosticating the future of any individual child. The premature is full of surprises.

4. A certain amount of optimism is justified even when the outlook is bleak, because it is important for the family to maintain hope even in the face of overwhelming odds, and medical tradition suggests that the outcome of therapy may often depend on the attitude and enthusiasm of the physician.

NORMAL INFANT FEEDING

method of
MABELLE DORA D'AMODIO, M.D.
New York, New York

Infant feeding is by far the most common problem that mother, infant, and pediatrician have to face within the infant's first few months of life and first year. One should always keep in mind that feeding times must be pleasant experiences for both mother and child and that the purpose of feedings encompasses much more than merely meeting caloric requirements and ensuring somatic growth. The human infant is born relatively premature in comparison with other animals. Unable to satisfy his own needs in this respect, he depends on the placenta during his intrauterine life and on the breast or its substitute during exterior gestation to meet his caloric requirements.

The human infant will be able feed himself only at 1 or 1½ years of age when his neural maturation allows it.

Fluid Requirements

The need of a determined amount of water per 24 hour period stems from the expenditure of this element through (1) insensible water loss, which reflects the pulmonary and skin evaporative losses—30 ml. per kg. per 24 hours; (2) urinary losses—50 ml. per kg. per 24 hours; and (3) fecal losses—10 to 20 ml. per kg. per 24 hours. Exceptions should be made for the small premature infant and the normal newborn, who need smaller amounts of water in the first few days of life because of a significant decrease in the extracellular compartment and therefore a large endogenous water load.

Caloric Requirements

With reference to caloric requirements, the aim is to give about 120 to 130 cal. per kg. per 24 hours. The balanced distribution of calories should be as follows: proteins, 7 to 16 per cent; fats, 30 to 55 per cent; and carbohydrates, 35 to 65 per cent. In very special circumstances infants will require caloric intakes of about 150 to 200 cal. per kg. per day, such as infants of drug-addicted mothers or infants with hyperactivity, to establish a satisfactory growth curve.

In small premature infants one should not exceed the gastric capacity in an attempt to force feedings and promote growth. The consequence of these eager procedures will lead to problems of regurgitation, aspiration, and pneumonitis.

Proteins, carbohydrates, and lipids are the major sources of energy. As the child grows, the original requirement of 120 cal. per kg. per 24 hours decreases to about 108 cal. per kg. per 24 hours at age 6 months.

The aforementioned caloric requirement features stem from the following expenditure sources:

Resting caloric expenditure	50 cal. per kg. per 24 hours
Intermittent activity	15 cal. per kg. per 24 hours
Cold stress	10 cal. per kg. per 24 hours
Specific dynamic action	8 cal. per kg. per 24 hours
Fecal losses	12 cal. per kg. per 24 hours
Growth allowance	25 cal. per kg. per 24 hours
Total	120 cal. per kg. per 24 hours

Proteins

Proteins are a good source of energy and they provide amino acids for growth and tissue repair. They play a role in osmotic equilibrium and acid-base balance. They are present in hemoglobin, enzymes, hormones, and nucleoproteins. The essential amino acids are leucine, isoleucine, tryptophan, valine, histidine, methionine, threonine, and phenylalanine.

Proteins should be provided in a total of 2.4 grams per kg. per 24 hours at birth or soon after and 1.5 grams per kg. per 24 hours at 6 months of age. The concentration of protein in cow's milk is about 3.5 grams per 100 ml., as opposed to maternal milk, which contains 1.5 grams per 100 ml. The casein fraction in cow's milk is extremely rich in phosphorus. The young infant is unable to handle so much phosphorus through the kidneys effectively. As a result of this, there is an increase in solute load, and phosphorus retention and calcium decrease occur with or without clinical manifestations.

One need not worry about the loss of nitrogen through the gastrointestinal tract in the first few days of life. Infants do not go into negative nitrogen balance, for practical purposes, until after the first week of life.

Carbohydrates

The greatest bulk and almost 50 per cent of the caloric intake are provided by carbohydrates. They are oxidized to glucose, stored as glycogen, and metabolized to lactic acid.

The main carbohydrate in the infant's diet is lactose. This carbohydrate provides glucose, which is readily available for tissue metabolism, and galactose, which is used in the synthesis of galactolipids, important elements in the development of central nervous system tissue, particularly in the first year of life.

Newborn infants are usually born with adequate glycogen stores and are able to maintain carbohydrate homeostasis. Exception should be made for intrauterine fetally malnourished infants (IUM), infants of diabetic mothers (IDM), and infants with enzyme deficiencies. Lactose has the ability to enhance calcium absorption through the intestinal tract, thus contributing to a more stable Ca-P equation. The curd of human milk also has a lower surface tension, making it more digestible.

Lipids

Lipids are: (1) a very concentrated source of energy; (2) carriers of liposoluble vitamins A, D, E, K; and (3) carriers of linoleic acid. This last characteristic relates to dermic integrity. Deficiency in linoleic acid produces skin desquamation, intertrigo, and failure to thrive in pediatric patients. Although linoleic acid is not synthesized by the human body, human milk is richer in this acid than cow's milk.

Lipids produce a feeling of satiety and delay the emptying time of the stomach. The emptying time is less in infants that are breast fed, probably because of the different fat composition of human and cow's milk. Maternal milk is much richer in polyunsaturated fatty acids, and these are more readily absorbed. Breast milk contains 60 per cent polyunsaturated fatty acids and 40 per cent saturated fatty acids; cow's milk contains 40 per cent polyunsaturated fatty acids and 60 per cent saturated fatty acids. Human milk has the most variable range with regard to lipids, but the unsaturated fraction usually reaches 60 per cent of the total. In general, breast-fed infants have a higher concentration of plasma fatty acids, cholesterol, tocopherol, and vitamin A.

Vitamins

Liposoluble. VITAMIN A. A deficiency of vitamin A is associated with the development of xerophthalmia, blindness, and impairment of rhodopsin conversion. The daily requirements are 400 retinol equivalents or 2000 I.U. Human milk contains 1700 I.U. of vitamin A per liter; cow's milk contains 1000 I.U. per liter.

VITAMIN D. Vitamin D is formed in the skin by action of the sun on 7-dehydrocholesterol. Daily recommended doses of 400 I.U. suffice to avoid clinical manifestations of its deficiency. Breast milk contains 22 I.U. of vitamin D per liter; cow's milk contains 400 I.U. per liter (fortified milk).

VITAMIN E. Vitamin E deficiency in the premature infant is associated with edema, hemolytic anemia, and thrombocytosis. The recommended daily allowance is 4 I.U. until the child is 6 months of age and 5 I.U. up to 1 year of age. There is an increased serum value of vitamin E in the first weeks of life of breast-fed infants. Breast milk contains 2.5 I.U. of vitamin E per liter; cow's milk contains only unsatisfactory amounts of this vitamin.

VITAMIN K. Vitamin K increases synthesis of prothrombin and other clotting elements. It is synthesized in the gastrointestinal tract by bacterial activity and should be administered immediately at birth in doses of 0.5 to 1 mg. intramuscularly to avoid hemorrhagic disease of the newborn.

Water-Soluble Vitamins. THIAMINE. Recommended daily allowance is 0.03 mg. per kg. per 24 hours. Its deficiency is associated with beriberi, cardiac failure, and neurologic deficit.

RIBOFLAVIN. Recommended daily allowance is 0.4 mg. per day. Its deficiency is associated with dementia, diarrhea, and dermatitis.

Both thiamine and riboflavin are within normal required ranges in both human and cow's milk.

VITAMIN C (ASCORBIC ACID). The daily requirement is about 50 mg. Human milk contains 43 mg. of ascorbic acid per liter, and cow's milk contains 50 mg. per liter.

Minerals

The ash content of the fetus is very low. At birth it is 3 per cent and increases to 4.4 per cent. Thereafter, the solute load we impose on an infant should always be kept in mind when we introduce cow's milk in his feedings. To have an accurate idea of this matter, one should consider the following figures: Breast milk produces about 12 mOsm. per 100 cal. metabolized. Glucose produces 10 mOsm. per 100 cal. metabolized. Cow's milk produces 35 to 40 mOsm. per 100 cal. metabolized.

Requirements. SODIUM. The average sodium intake is 35 mg. a day. Human milk contains 7 mEq./L. Cow's milk contains 21 mEq./L.

POTASSIUM. The average potassium intake is 20 mg. per day.

CALCIUM. The daily requirement of calcium is 350 mg. About 40 mg. of calcium is provided when an infant is breast fed in the course of 1 day. About 70 mg. is provided if the infant is fed cow's milk. The calcium content of human milk is 300 mg. per liter, and that of cow's milk is 600 mg. per liter. Infants retain only 20 to 30 per cent of these amounts.

MAGNESIUM. The daily requirement of magnesium is 60 mg. The magnesium content of human milk is 4 mg. per 100 ml., and that of cow's milk is 12 mg. per 100 ml. Magnesium deficiency leads to irritability, tremors, and convulsions.

IRON. The daily allowance of iron should be within the range of 10 to 15 mg. Only 10 per cent of the administered iron is absorbed as ferrous sulfate, depending on intestinal wall integrity, acidity, and enzymatic participation.

Iron deficiency anemias appear mostly when there is low intake of this element or significant loss. Infants are bound to develop iron deficiency anemias at about 5 to 7 months of age or when they grow rapidly if the diet is not supplemented. Interestingly, breast-fed infants have less tendency to develop nutritional anemias.

COPPER. The decreased concentration of serum copper will lead to anemias, neutropenias, and osteoporosis. This is seen in caloric malnutrition, absorptive problems, nephrotic syndrome, and hypochromic anemias, and it will lead to hypotonias and learning disability. The daily requirement is 80 mg. Human milk contains 0.05 to 0.15 mg. of copper per liter, and cow's milk contains 0.015 to 0.18 mg. per liter.

ZINC. A deficiency of zinc will lead to loss of appetite and failure to thrive. A very serious clinical entity known as acrodermatitis enteropathica is associated with zinc deficiency. It is characterized by a pustulovesicular rash around the oral and anal orifices. Hypoalbuminemia can also occur. Serum values of zinc range from 70 to 90 mg. per 100 ml.

If one reads carefully all the aforementioned material, one will come to a conclusion about the advantages of breast feeding. The psychologic and immunologic elements should also be kept in mind as advantageous. However, in today's society, one cannot deny the practicality of artificial feedings, particularly considering the daily schedules of the young working or studying mother.

Artificial Feeding

Most of the proprietary milks will provide 20 cal. per 30 ml. (1 ounce) after being reconstituted. Easy computations will answer the questions of inexperienced mothers as to how much milk to give in each feeding.

The frequency of feedings will be decided by keeping in mind the emptying time of the stomach; every 3 to 4 hours seems to be suitable for most infants.

If one is dealing with relaxed parents, one can encourage them to feed the infant on demand. With anxious parents the pediatrician will do better to encourage feedings on schedule. In these cases it is not advisable to weigh the infant more than once a week. Somatic growth and development are left for the pediatrician to assess.

Solid Foods

There is a tremendous pressure on the pediatrician to start solid foods in the infant's diet as early as possible. It is my opinion that instead of complying easily with this, one should spend more time with the young mother and explain that (1) there is an extrusion reflex of the tongue in the first 2 months of life, and this would make solid feedings difficult for both infant and mother; (2) vegetables, most fruits, and cereals have no caloric advantage over milk feedings comparing mass to mass; and (3) the addition of cereals, fruits, starch foods, and sugars will create an imbalance in the calorie distribution, with increases in carbohydrate, osmolal concentration, and chronic hyperelectrolytemia which are not beneficial or desirable.

If it is decided that an infant is ready for solid foods at 3 months of age (not earlier), we usually add cereals and fruits. Vegetables are added at 4 months and meats at 5 months. Egg yolk is introduced into the diet at 5 to 6 months.

It is at this time that iron deficiency anemias of nutritional origin appear (or body weight is doubled), and a hemogram is called for.

In the presence of allergic predispositions, it is advisable to take a careful history and observe the relationship of symptoms such as emesis, diarrhea, and abdominal distention and the appearance of these when milk is given. If this is observed, one can resort to hypoallergenic milks such as ProSobee, Soyalac, Nutramigen, or goat's milk.

Far too much freedom exists in changing the patient from one proprietary milk to another, even in hospital settings, without investigating stools for pH in series and eosinophilic counts in the peripheral smear or taking a complete nutritional history.

DISEASES OF THE BREAST

method of
WILLIAM R. JEWELL, M.D.
Kansas City, Kansas

Introduction

Because of extensive publicity and public discussions in an effort to diagnose breast cancer at an early stage, women are developing a near-neurotic fear of breast disease. This fear must be constantly kept in mind by the physician. A recent controversy concerning a possible carcinogenic effect of mammography has contributed to the fear that most women have. Treatment of breast disease, therefore, starts with the patient. It is always necessary, regardless of the diagnosis, to thoroughly discuss the disease with the patient in terms of treatment and prognosis.

Anomalies

Asymmetrical Breast Size. Most women will vary up to 10 per cent in breast size from one side to the other. Usually simple reassurance is all that is required. Biopsy in the prepubertal child is contraindicated.

Precocious Development. Breast enlargement before the age of 8 or 9 is abnormal. Abnormalities in ovarian, adrenal, or central nervous system function should be sought.

Supernumerary Breast. Excision for cosmetic reasons.

Hypertrophy. Marked hypertrophy in females may require reduction mammoplasty. This should be done only after all anticipated pregnancies have been completed. Hypertrophic breasts in male patients, gynecomastia, should be removed both for cosmetic benefit to the patient and for excluding the possibility of carcinoma. In selected cases of obvious cause—e.g., cirrhosis, estrogen therapy, hypertrophy-producing drug therapy—conservative management may be selected.

Inflammation

Infections. Acute mastitis occurring in the postpartum female should be treated with warm soaks and broad-spectrum antibiotics. Fluctuants should be treated with incision and drainage. Breast feeding is discontinued.

Chronic Mastitis. The most common type is residual infection following acute mastitis. This disease is usually limited to one or two ductal systems, which should be defined and excised in total, using a formal quadrant resection if conservative management fails. Rare causes such as tuberculosis and other fungal disease should be excluded by culture.

Skin

All skin lesions that are suspicious for any reason or that are of concern to a patient—e.g., because of rubbing on a garment—should be excised.

Melanoma. Clark's level I or II and/or lesions less than 0.75 mm. depth of penetration should be treated by wide excision and skin graft only. Clark's level III, IV, and V lesions or lesions greater than 0.76 mm. depth of penetration should be treated by wide excision and skin graft plus axillary node dissection. Formal radical mastectomy is rarely indicated. Interquadrant high risk melanomas should be treated with internal mammary node dissection as well as axillary node dissection.

Nipple and Areola

Nipple Discharge. Premenopausal milky discharges are associated with breast function and require no therapy. A greenish discharge is usually associated with fibrocystic disease with intraductal hyperplasia. Any bloody discharge must be explained. Most bleeding lesions are within 2 cm. of the nipple and can be found by palpation with expression of blood through the nipple. The appropriate duct should be totally excised by a formal quadrant excision. Most bleeding is caused by intraductal papillomas, 85 per cent of which are benign.

Postmenopausal. Any discharge in a postmenopausal female is of significance and must be explained. If mammography and physical examination are negative, quadrant excision of the appropriate duct should be performed.

Nipple Erosion. Always be suspicious of Paget's disease. Biopsy of the skin is definitive. This is always associated with a deep malignancy, and therefore all patients with Paget's disease should be treated for breast cancer. When nipple erosion develops in a nursing patient, breast feeding should be discontinued and the skin lesion treated with topical antibiotic–steroid ointment.

Nipple Retraction. Inversion is always normal. A history of recent development, however, arouses suspicion of new disease and indicates the necessity of retroareolar biopsy.

Skin Retraction. This is caused by retraction of Cooper's ligament and is produced by carcinoma, fat necrosis, plasma cell mastitis, or old bacterial infection.

Painful Breast

Most often caused by fibrocystic disease, painful breast is usually related to menstrual periods. Mammography should be performed and the pain treated with reassurance. The patient is advised to wear a tightly fitting brassiere at all times until the pain disappears. Patients on birth control pills or other estrogen substances should discontinue the medication. Severe unrelenting pain may require quadrant excision or even simple mastectomy with or without Silastic implants. Heat is sometimes beneficial.

Any mass should be treated as below. If infection is expected, heat and antibiotics can be curative. Incision and drainage of fluctuants is indicated.

Mass

Any definable breast mass must be explained.

Cysts. Mammograph should be obtained; if no suspicious areas exist, aspiration of the cyst with a 20 gauge needle is indicated. Complete disappearance of the mass must occur. Fluid should be sent for cytology.

Solid Mass. Biopsy is always indicated and usually should be done under general anesthesia. If the patient is 30 years of age or younger, or in older patients who prefer it, biopsy only should be planned. A circumareolar incision is used.

Suspicious Area on Mammography. If the physical examination is negative, localize the lesion by mammographic measurements and excise. If calcification is present, obtain a mammogram of the specimen to confirm that the lesion was removed. If the lesion is not calcified, this step is omitted.

Carcinoma. PREOPERATIVE EVALUATION. A chest x-ray and routine admission laboratory work-up are the only tests ordered. Isotope scans are indicated only when clinical symptoms are present. Careful examination of the supraclavicular fossa should be performed. Biopsy-proved nodes in this location contraindicate surgery for cure.

PRIMARY CARCINOMA: OPERABLE FOR CURE. If there is minimal breast cancer (lesions less than 0.5 cm.), a modified radical mastectomy, including complete axillary dissection with removal of the deltopectoral fascia overlying the pectoralis major and minor muscles, is indicated. Lesions greater than 0.5 cm. should be treated with radical mastectomy. Inner quadrant or subareolar lesions should be treated with an Urban type internal mammary node dissection with complete repair of the chest wall, using anterior rectus abdominis fascia. Inflammatory carcinoma of the breast (defined as greater than one third of the breast involved with peau d'orange and proved subdermal lymphatic involvement with carcinoma) is treated with radiation therapy; adrenalectomy should be considered in the event of recurrence.

ADJUVANT THERAPY. There is no proved adjuvant therapy in patients with routine primary operable breast carcinoma regardless of normal status. If the operating surgeon is sure that tumor is left behind in patients with massive nodule involvement, the patients are benefited by radiation therapy. Adjuvant chemotherapy is indicated for patients in cooperative group studies only. Prophylactic oophorectomy should be condemned.

Recurrent Carcinoma

Triage: Premenopausal. 1. With chest wall recurrence, wide excision and a skin graft should be done if it has been more than 3 years since the primary tumor was excised and no spread has occurred. Radiation therapy of the chest wall and oophorectomy should be done if less than 3 years have elapsed since the primary tumor was excised or if spread beyond the chest wall is present.

2. In disseminated disease, oophorectomy is carried out and is followed in responders with adrenalectomy when relapse occurs, and then, finally, with chemotherapy consisting of cyclophosphamide (Cytoxan), 50 mg. daily by mouth, methotrexate, 25 mg. intravenously each week, and fluorouracil (5-FU), 500 mg. intravenously each week, continued for 8 weeks with a 4 week rest period. This cycle may be repeated if indicated.

Postmenopausal. 1. Chest wall recurrence is treated the same as in the premenopausal group.

2. In disseminated disease, if the patient is less than 5 years postmenopausal, start with fluoxymesterone (Halotestin), 10 mg. three times daily, and observe for response for 2 or 3 months. If no response occurs, stop the Halotestin, observe for 4 to 6 weeks and start an estrogen (diethylstilbestrol), 15 mg. a day in divided doses. If the patient is more than 5 years postmenopausal, start estrogen as above and treat for at least 2 to 3 months to observe for response. If no response to estrogen withdrawal occurs, start Halotestin as above. Responders to hormone manipulative techniques should be considered for adrenalectomy. Adrenalectomy should be performed anteriorly if the ovaries are still in place, and a bilateral oophorectomy should be performed. A posterior approach, removing the twelfth rib, is preferred if previous oophorectomy was performed. Replacement therapy with 50 mg. of cortisone acetate daily, 37.5 mg. in the morning and 12.5 mg. in the afternoon, is favored. Chemotherapy should be employed after all hormone manipulative therapy has been used.

Special Problems

Lymphangitic Pulmonary Spread with Shortness of Breath. Prednisone, 60 mg. by mouth daily.

Hypercalcemia. Prednisone, 60 mg. daily infusion, or mithramycin.

Pleural Effusion. If little disease exists elsewhere, open thoracotomy and pleurectomy is preferred. Instillation of nitrogen mustard through a chest tube, using systemic therapy dose levels, can be utilized to lessen effusion. Intrathoracic quinacrine hydrochloride (Atabrine), 200 mg. a day for 5 days, can also be tried. Great caution should be exercised in treating patients with intracavity nitrogen mustard who are also on systemic chemotherapy.

Isolated Bone Lesions. Radiation therapy.

Cerebral Metastasis. Neurosurgical excision or radiation therapy if multiple lesions are present.

Cortical Destruction of Weight-Bearing Bone. Orthopedic intervention with internal fixation if possible.

ENDOMETRIOSIS

method of
LAMAN A. GRAY, SR., M.D.
Louisville, Kentucky

Occurrence

Endometriosis occurs in the private practice of gynecology in at least 10 per cent of the patients and probably in 15 per cent. The uncommon finding of endometriosis in charity clinics and ward services has never been clearly explained.

Therapy

No treatment is required if the symptoms are insignificant or mild, except in the case of the adherent ovarian cyst, when operation may be indicated. For moderate symptoms, only analgesics are indicated.

For the past 20 years or more, the use of hormone therapy to cure or cause regression of endometrial implants has been under investigation. This has resulted in considerable controversy and difference of opinion. At first it was thought that large doses of stilbestrol would destroy endometrial implants, and, later, that large doses of progestins (in extraordinary amounts, such as norethynodrel with mestranol [Enovid] up to 120 mg. daily over periods of 9 months or a year) could replace surgical treatment. It is true that the progestins especially cause softening of the endometrial nodules, but these always reappear in the same degree when the progestins have been removed; at least, this has been my experience. Recently a new drug, danazol, has been recommended for treatment. Apparently this synthetic compound is not only antigonadotropic but also a weak androgen, and presumably it neutralizes the presence of estrogen. Its evaluation will require more time, but I am doubtful of its efficacy.

In summary, hormone therapy offers no cure for endometriosis and, in fact, may be dangerous because of the risk of emboli when the progestins and estrogens are given in large doses. In my opinion, the only hormonal treatment that should be used is that of the ordinary birth control pill in low dose for the prevention of ovulation. Strangely enough, the prevention of ovulation reduces or removes the pain of endometriosis in a surprising number of patients, but it is not curative.

Surgical Treatment. When patients have severe symptoms, especially that of dyspareunia, caused by the nodules of endometriosis in the cul-de-sac and uterosacral ligaments, and when ovarian masses of not completely clear origin are present, surgical operation is indicated. In addition, conservative surgical operations may be indicated for infertility when other causes of sterility have been excluded. Less than half the patients with endometriosis are infertile. In conservative operations in young women, the diseased tissue is resected from the ovaries (and it is important that one may be able to shell out a chocolate cyst and leave a reasonable portion of normal ovary), and various implants throughout the pelvis are excised if possible, especially from the uterosacral ligaments and the wall of the bowel. Combined with suspension of the uterus, which is always performed because adhesions tend later to pull the uterus into retroversion both from the irritating effects of the endometriosis and the operative procedure, the patient may experience remarkable improvement in symptoms, with a reasonable chance of pregnancy. There is always the possibility that the endometriosis may recur and a second complete operation may be necessary. By no means should radical operations be avoided when necessary, even in relatively young women. To leave behind an extensive endometriosis with functioning ovarian tissue generally leads to an unsatisfactory postoperative result.

Malignancy. A gradually increasing number of case reports of cancer occurring in patients with endometriosis and endometrial cysts are appearing. These have been difficult to document, because when the ovarian cancers are discovered, they are so widespread and have destroyed the ovaries so completely that no vestige of normal ovarian tissue, to say nothing of a vestige of endometriosis, can be found. Yet a considerable number of ovarian tumors are of the endometrioid type and even represent adenoacanthomas. How many of those may have arisen in endometriosis remains conjectural. I suspect that if endometrial carcinoma occurs in the intact uterus in 3 per cent of women, then one might expect that 3 per cent of the 10 or 15 per cent of women who have endometriosis may develop carcinoma. This makes the risk quite small, but nevertheless it is there. I continue to subscribe to the conservative approach; avoid operation when possible; encourage pregnancies (which does not cure endometriosis but, more importantly, does provide a progeny); prescribe birth control pills of the low dose type when indicated for the relief of pain and when pregnancy is not desired; and, finally, do not avoid operation when the pathology is obvious and the symptoms are marked.

DYSFUNCTIONAL UTERINE BLEEDING

method of
CHARLES B. HAMMOND, M.D.,
and MICHAEL R. SOULES, M.D.
Durham, North Carolina

Dysfunctional uterine bleeding (DUB) is abnormal menstrual bleeding secondary to endocrine (hormonal) dysfunction. It presents as vaginal bleeding that is abnormal in amount, duration, or periodicity in a female of reproductive age (menarche to menopause). Prepubertal and postmenopausal vaginal bleeding are separate problems that usually warrant a different approach. DUB can be present in ovulatory as well as anovulatory women, although the latter is much more common.

Dysfunctional uterine bleeding must always be defined against the background of normal menstrual physiology and terminology. When irregular vaginal bleeding is secondary to neoplasm, infection, trauma, anatomic derangements, pregnancy, medications (hormones, anticoagulants), intrinsic uterine diseases (leiomyomas, polyps, adenomyosis), or systemic abnormalities (clotting disorders), then the diagnosis of dysfunctional uterine bleeding is eliminated. It is incumbent upon the physician to adequately exclude these other, nondysfunctional, causes of abnormal bleeding before initiating a therapy plan.

Evaluation

All patients who present for persistent symptomatic irregular vaginal bleeding should have the following evaluation: (1) history, (2) physical and pelvic examination, (3) Papanicolaou smear and cervical mucus fern test, (4) endometrial biopsy, and (5) hematocrit. If these items are used to yield the maximum amount of information, the cause of the abnormal vaginal bleeding can be achieved most of the time. Even if this technique distinguishes only whether the problem is "functional" (i.e., leiomyoma uteri) or "dysfunctional" (endocrine related), a great stride will have been made and appropriate therapy or further diagnostic tests can be initiated.

This five-point approach should aid in the differentiation between the ovulatory and anovulatory types of DUB. Ovulatory patients will have secretory endometrium and lack of a fern pattern; anovulatory patients will have proliferative endometrium. The appearance of the tissue at the time of endometrial biopsy gives other important therapeutic clues which are immediately available. A "lush," thick sample of tissue easily obtained indicates an endometrium under the continued influence of estrogen; a small biopsy specimen that is obtained with more difficulty implies either that proliferative endometrium has nearly sloughed or that progesterone has been present.

Initially we stated that all patients with irregular vaginal bleeding should be evaluated by this five-point scheme. It may seem controversial to include an endometrial biopsy for the adolescent patient and to withhold an initial dilatation and curettage for the patient approaching menopause. The information obtained regarding the hormonal stimulation of the uterus more than justifies the small amount of discomfort in the adolescent. In the female at the opposite end of her reproductive life, a Papanicolaou smear, an endometrial biopsy, and an automatic dilatation and curettage with failed hormonal treatment will not let any neoplasms progress or remain undiagnosed.

The serious endocrine problems causing anovulation, such as thyroid disease, hormone-producing neoplasms, or pituitary adenoma, should be apparent after a careful history and examination. Obviously these disease entities require specific therapy beyond that for simple anovulation.

Treatment

Ovulatory Type. Luteal Phase Deficiency. If fertility is desired, treat with progesterone vaginal suppositories (25 mg. twice daily). Regulation of vaginal bleeding can be achieved with artificial cycles of standard dosage oral contraceptives (50 to 80 micrograms of estrogen).

Persistent Corpus Luteum. This is an unusual problem without the tendency for recurrence in any given patient. The treatment is expectant observation rather than hormonal. Ovulatory suppression with oral contraceptives may be used for patients with recurring problems.

Irregular Shedding. If symptoms warrant, treat with standard dosage oral contraceptives (usual regimen) or estrogen (conjugated estrogens, 1.25 mg., or ethinyl estradiol, 0.025 mg.), plus progesterone (Provera, 10 mg., or Norlutate, 5 mg.) in cyclic fashion—estrogen is given once daily for 25 consecutive days, with progesterone given once daily on days 21 through 25; rest 7 days; and begin again.

Midcycle Spotting. Midcycle spotting is best treated by estrogen and progesterone in cyclic fashion or by proliferative phase estrogen supplementation (0.3 mg. conjugated estrogen or 0.01 mg. ethinyl estradiol daily during days 5 to 15 of the cycle). Oral contraceptives can be utilized.

Anovulatory Type. The category we have labeled anovulatory DUB encompasses the majority of these patients. The approach to anovulatory DUB varies whether it is *acute* (heavy vaginal bleeding with orthostatic changes in vital signs and hematocrit <30 per cent) or *chronic* (moderate vaginal bleeding with no orthostatic changes and hematocrit >30 per cent).

Acute. 1. Admit to hospital—nothing orally until bleeding has been controlled.

2. Complete blood count (CBC) with red cell indices and estimation of platelets.

3. Intravenous fluids (5 per cent dextrose in lactated Ringer's solution or 5 per cent dextrose in isotonic saline).

4. Estrogen—7 day course. Conjugated estrogen (Premarin), 25 mg. intravenous "push" every 4 hours for three doses. Then begin oral estrogen (conjugated estrogens, 2.5 mg. twice daily, or ethinyl estradiol, 0.05 mg. twice daily) for 6½ days.

5. Progesterone—5 day course. Oral progesterone (Provera, 10 mg. twice daily, or Norlutate, 5 mg. twice daily) is given on days 3 to 7.

6. Vaginal bleeding should become insignificant after 24 hours on this regimen; the patient can be discharged the next day.

7. Iron replacement therapy: ferrous sulfate, 300 mg. twice daily or its equivalent for 6 to 12 months to replace iron stores.

TABLE 1. **Treatment of Acute Anovulatory Bleeding**

Days	1	2	3	4	5	6	7	Wait 7 days	Cyclic estrogen and progesterone for 6 months	Progesterone alone for 6 months
Estrogen	I.V./P.O.	P.O.	P.O.	P.O.	P.O.	P.O.	P.O.			
Progesterone			P.O.	P.O.	P.O.	P.O.	P.O.			

8. Estrogen and progesterone given for 6 months in a lower dosage 25 day cyclic fashion (as described under ovulatory type) after a 1 week withdrawal from the acute hormonal therapy.

9. Progesterone (Provera, 10 mg., or Norlutate, 5 mg. per day) for 5 days each month during the second 6 months. Then re-evaluate the need for further hormonal therapy.

10. Dilatation and curettage (D&C) is performed if further abnormal bleeding occurs after the acute therapy protocol is completed.

If this acute regimen fails to control the bleeding within 24 hours, then an immediate D&C should be performed (the final diagnosis will likely not be simple anovulatory DUB). The red cell indices with a complete blood count (CBC) give a good indication of chronic iron deficiency and the state of the patient's iron stores. A platelet estimation on the routine CBC is a good screening test for clotting disorders. Although we prefer intravenous estrogen to initiate the therapy of acute DUB, multiple dose oral contraceptives (4 combination tablets per day for 7 days) can be substituted. Also, combination oral contraceptives could be substituted in standard doses for the cyclic monthly therapy if contraception is desired. In addition to the benefit of the close observation of the therapy, the brief hospital admission enables the physician to obtain a more thorough history and physical examination, which are often not available in the setting of acute bleeding. The first several menstrual periods during the cyclic therapy will still be heavy but self-limited as the endometrial lining progessively sheds down to normal thickness.

CHRONIC. The therapy here depends on the desires of the patient for (1) *pregnancy*—clomiphene citrate (50 mg. per day), days 6 to 10 of menstrual cycle; (2) *contraception*—oral combination birth control pills in standard fashion; or (3) *regularity*—progesterone (Provera, 10 mg., or Norlutate, 5 mg. per day) 7 days per month. When clomiphene citrate is used, it is active only in the cycle under treatment and is indicated only for the infertile patient. A basal body temperature record should be used during each treatment cycle, with a pelvic examination to evaluate ovarian size before each cycle. Iron therapy should be liberally employed to combat chronic anemia in any patient with dysfunctional uterine bleeding. Progesterone alone is sufficient, as these patients by definition have sufficient levels of unopposed endogenous estrogen.

In either the acute or chronic therapy of anovulatory or ovulatory dysfunctional bleeding when the hormonal regimen employed is clearly unsatisfactory, the following steps are necessary:

1. Re-evaluate the diagnosis in the light of a failed response to the therapy for dysfunctional uterine bleeding. Further history and examination are probably warranted.

2. More extensive laboratory testing is reasonable, but the physician should avoid a "shotgun" approach. Some available tests are clotting studies, liver and renal function tests, thyroid index, maturation index, serum gonadotropins, laparoscopy, and hysterosalpingogram.

3. After the re-evaluation of the diagnosis and further testing, dilatation and curettage must be scheduled. The examination under anesthesia and the tissue obtained will certainly aid in the proper diagnosis.

4. Finally, a rare patient will have apparently true dysfunctional uterine bleeding which is refractory to all therapy. A hysterectomy may be indicated and curative in these patients, but should only be considered after other efforts are exhausted.

In summary, dysfunctional uterine bleeding is a common disease for which treatment has remained problematic. The treatment method outlined above has been quite successful if one realizes that it is based on proper diagnosis. The physician who takes the time and effort to make the correct diagnosis in the patient with irregular vaginal bleeding will be the successful therapist.

AMENORRHEA

method of
I. G. ANCES, M.D.
Baltimore, Maryland

Amenorrhea, the absence of menstruation, is a symptom relating to a variety of entities, the nature of which may be either pathologic or physiologic. The primary approach must be one of the diagnosis of the underlying causative process before any consideration of therapy can be entertained. Pregnancy, lactation, and menopause have been classified as "physiologic" in origin. Severely symptomatic persons with menopausal syndrome may be treated with any form of estrogen replacement. The controversy surrounding this modality of therapy has, in previous years, arisen secondary to a possible statistical correlation between endometrial carcinoma and continued use of estrogenic compounds. The patient should be advised of this association in the discussion of risks versus benefits of this therapy. Mild to moderate symptoms of vasomotor instability may be treated with such entities as phenobarbital, ergotamine tartrate, and alkaloid of belladonna (Bellergal) or diazepam, a chlordiazepoxide, in individual doses. Estrogen replacement in this age group should be continued for only a short period of time, usually a year or two, with a cyclic regimen and then gradually stopped. The addition of a progestational agent in the latter part of the monthly therapy cycle has recently been advocated to help prevent any hyperplastic changes within the endometrium. Patients are to be followed at regular intervals, with medication given only for the period of time between scheduled visits.

In the diagnosis as well as management of the remaining causes of amenorrhea, it is of importance to approach the problem in a systematic manner. Many plans have been advocated; one which has gained popularity in recent years is that by compartments as suggested by Speroff, Glass, and Kase (Table 1).

TABLE 1. **Classification of Amenorrheas**

I. Systemic
  A. Chronic debilitating condition
  B. Extragonadal endocrine diseases
    1. Adrenal: hyperplasia, Cushing's syndrome, tumor
    2. Thyroid: hypothyroidism
    3. Diabetes mellitus
  C. Iatrogenic
II. Reproductive system abnormalities
  A. Compartment I—outflow tract and end-organ failure
    1. Imperforate hymen
    2. Congenital absence
      a. Uterus and vagina
        i. Müllerian agenesis
        ii. Androgen insensitivity
      b. Cervix
    3. Unresponsive endometrium
      a. Synechiae
      b. Agenesis
  B. Compartment II—gonadal incompetence
    1. Agenesis
    2. Dysgenesis
      a. Turner's syndrome
      b. Variants
      c. Mosaics
    3. Tumor functioning
    4. Polycystic ovaries
    5. Failure
      a. Prepubertal
      b. Postpubertal (premature)
      c. Menopause
  C. Compartments III and IV—hypothalamic-pituitary axis
    1. Delayed pubescence
    2. Psychogenic
    3. Neoplasms
    4. Panhypopituitarism
    5. Hypogonadotropism
    6. Inappropriate lactation

Systemic Conditions

Chronic Illness. The treatment of the underlying illness will accomplish the goal of correcting the symptom of amenorrhea. The return of menses must await the gradual correction of the underlying illness. Evaluation of cervical mucus as to estrogenic effect may give one insight as to gradual correction of the illness.

Extragonadal Endocrinopathies. ADRENOGENITAL SYNDROME. Treatment is by replacement of corticosteroid sufficient to effect normal urinary ketosteroid excretion—i.e., dexamethasone, 0.5 mg., or prednisone, 5 to 10 mg. per day. Ovulatory cycles will occur. The dose need not change during pregnancy, but, as with all surgical procedures, supplemental parenteral medication should be administered for the stress of labor and delivery.

ADRENAL TUMOR. Surgical excision.

CUSHING'S SYNDROME. Surgical therapy is usually required, followed by appropriate replacement therapy with gluco- and/or mineralocorticoids as needed for life.

HYPOTHYROIDISM. Although an unusual cause of amenorrhea, it should be screened for. It is treated with desiccated thyroid or the synthetic derivatives in an individualized regimen.

DIABETES MELLITUS. Individualized care with diet and insulin will correct the amenorrhea as the disease is adequately controlled.

Iatrogenic

The discontinuation of hormonal contraceptives may not be followed by menstrual function. The majority of these patients will resume regular ovulatory cycles within 6 months, with 95 per cent returning to normal within 12 months. If conception is desired, the patient is best treated with clomiphene citrate if endogenous adequate estrogen stimulation is present or with human menotropins and chorionic gonadotropins if total gonadotropin suppression has occurred (Table 2). Following explanation of the mechanics concerned with her symptoms, she may be placed on substitutional progestin or estrogen-progestin if conception is not desired.

Reproductive System Abnormalities

The patient's desire for reproduction (Table 2) must guide the therapy of reproductive endocrinopathies. Cyclic hormonal therapy is quite sufficient if reproduction is not desired. The presence of adequate estrogen stimulation will necessitate only the use of progesterone or derivatives to

TABLE 2. **Therapy of Endocrinopathies**

MODALITY	DRUG	DAILY DOSE (MG.)	REMARKS
Estrogen	Conjugated	0.3–0.6 1.25–2.5	Patients with uterus; lower doses for menopause; cyclic days 1–25 of month; patients with gonadal dysgenesis may require higher doses
	Diethylstilbestrol	0.2–0.5 0.5–2.0	As above
	Ethinyl estradiol	0.02–0.05 0.05–0.15	As above
Progestin	Medroxyprogesterone	10	Days 21–25 when used with Estrogen days 25–30 of every 2–3 months for withdrawal
Estrogen plus progestin	Combined oral contraceptives	Variable	21 days of 28
	Combination of 1 and 2	—	As above
Induction of ovulation	Clomiphene citrate	50 mg. increments	Days 5–10 of cycle
	Human menopausal gonadotropins	0.50 I.U. by increments	When estrogen excretion is 100–150 mg./24 hours
	Chorionic gonadotropin	5000–10,000 I.U.	If greater than 200 mg./24 hours, withhold

accomplish the goal of cyclic menses. Sequential therapy or combined products may be used if estrogen production is deficient. Hypogonadotropic persons, specifically those with inappropriate lactation, must remain under periodic surveillance for a possible central nervous system neoplasm even though the initial evaluation is negative. If conception is desired, those women with low endogenous estrogen production will respond best to menopausal gonadotropins—follicle-stimulating hormone and luteinizing hormone (FSH-LH), followed by human chorionic gonadotropin (HCG). Prior to therapy with the latter agent, the patient is closely supervised, including a laboratory report of estrogen production every day correlated with cervical mucus production, because of the danger of hyperstimulation of the ovary with subsequent ovarian cystic enlargement and multiple ovulation.

Compartment I: End-Organ–Outflow Tract. Management of these conditions is surgical in most instances. A history of postabortal or puerperal curettage is helpful. Uterine synechiae are treated by cervical dilatation, disruption of the synechiae, and insertion of an intrauterine device (IUD). This is followed by high doses of estrogen. If the basalis layer of the endometrium remains, proliferation will occur. Conjugated equine estrogens, 2.5 mg., diethylstilbestrol, 1.0 mg., or comparable medication is given for periods of 30 days, with discontinuation for 5 to 7 days to allow for withdrawal bleeding. Such bleeding would demonstrate the success of this regimen.

Patients with androgen insensitivity (testicular feminization) will not have a uterus, and thus would fall into this category. These patients should have the gonads removed (after the onset of puberty) to allow the development of secondary sexual characteristics. Estrogen replacement therapy must be instituted following surgery (Table 2). These patients are psychologically, socially, and phenotypically female and should not be informed of their genetic sex.

Compartment II: Gonadal Causes. Patients with incompetence of the gonads are managed mainly by substitution therapy (Table 2). A regimen of estrogen with progesterone added at the end of the cycle has been most recently preferred secondary to the potential for endometrial carcinoma with prolonged unopposed estrogen therapy. Recent statistical studies have also implicated sequential preparations in the production of endometrial carcinoma, albeit not as commonly as with estrogen alone. The physician may prefer to give combination pills to obtain cyclic bleeding and institute appropriate diagnostic procedures if abnormal bleeding occurs. Replacement therapy should continue only until such time as the natural menopause is expected to occur, and then the patient should be gradually weaned from the medication.

Ovarian tumors are treated surgically, with appropriate replacement therapy if castration ensues.

Polycystic ovarian disease responds well to clomiphene citrate therapy if adequate estrogen production is present. If reproduction is not desired, the patient should be given combination therapy (norethindrone, 2.0 mg.; estrogen) to suppress androgen production.

Compartments III and IV: Hypothalamic-Pituitary. DELAYED PUBESCENCE. The woman who demonstrates good secondary sexual development and primarily has anovulation is best treated with progesterone (intramuscular or oral) every other or every third month to effect withdrawal bleeding. This schedule will allow spontaneous menstruation to appear in the interval if she begins to ovulate. Oral contraceptives are quite controversial in the treatment of these patients, for they may perpetuate the problem.

PSYCHOGENIC. Women under stress (e.g., fear of pregnancy, illness or death in the family, final examinations) will at times have amenorrhea of hypothalamic origin. This form of amenorrhea will usually respond to office reassurance and counseling. Occasionally, in more resistant cases, progesterone, clomiphene citrate, or menotropin gonadotropin is required for management. Anorexia nervosa requires hospitalization, intensive psychotherapy, and dietary management. Return of gonadal function can be followed by the return of cervical mucus, which will precede any return of menstrual events.

NEOPLASMS. Neoplasms are treated by surgery or radiation as appropriate. In many instances enough pituitary function will remain or subsequently reappear that substitution therapy is not required.

Panhypopituitarism

Panhypopituitarism may result from therapy of tumors as above or from postpartum necrosis. Substitutional therapy as indicated by loss includes (1) thyroid extract or synthetic derivatives, (2) adrenal steroid replacement, or (3) substitutional therapy with estrogenic compounds. If pregnancy is desired, menotropin gonadotropins are used as indicated.

Hypogonadotropic Hypogonadism

Hypogonadotropic hypogonadism does not respond well to clomiphene, owing to an estrogen lack, and therefore management is with sequential therapy or menotropin gonadotropins if pregnancy is desired. Repeated courses may be necessary to accomplish the desired effect. Precautions as described above to prevent hyperstimulation and multiple ovulations must be followed.

Inappropriate Lactation

Inappropriate lactation may be seen post partum, unrelated to pregnancy or secondary to a central nervous system tumor. X-ray studies of the sella turcica and visual field determinations should be done yearly if they are originally negative, as a significant number of patients will eventually show evidence of tumor. Clomiphene citrate has not been consistently successful in the management of these patients. Levodopa, 0.5 gram four times daily, is under investigation and appears to be effective in preliminary reports, although not approved for use in the United States of America. Bromo-ergocryptine is used in European countries with great success in the management of these patients, but the drug is not commercially available in the United States. The use of gonadotropin-releasing hormone remains only investigational as to use and availability.

PRIMARY DYSMENORRHEA

method of
ALVIN F. GOLDFARB, M.D.
Philadelphia, Pennsylvania

Painful menstrual function or pain in association with the menstrual period is defined as dysmenorrhea. There are two types of dysmenorrhea, primary and secondary. This presentation will not deal with secondary or acquired dysmenorrhea, but will comment only on primary dysmenorrhea. Women with secondary, or acquired, dysmenorrhea have it in association with pelvic pathology. The treatment of this problem requires the treatment and the removal of the pathologic cause which might lead to pain as a symptom in association with pelvic pathology.

Definition and Incidence

Primary dysmenorrhea occurs in young adult women, most notably during their teenage years. Approximately 50 per cent of all females in this age group will complain of some type of menstrual discomfort which may or may not require treatment. Many of the women with dysmenorrhea do not even confide or complain of this symptom to their physician. The incidence of dysmenorrhea tends to diminish as the female approaches her 20s and 30s. Many persons feel that this is a result of the maturation of the uterus and that dysmenorrhea per se is a part of this growth process.

Etiology

Primary dysmenorrhea is usually a symptom that is associated with ovulatory function. Many teenagers describe some menstrual periods as being painful and others as not. This type of scatter pattern with reference to dysmenorrhea would tend to support the observation that some menstrual cycles are ovulatory and others are not. From the behavioral standpoint, the symptom of dysmenorrhea can be described to the patient in a positive fashion. In doing this, we usually indicate to the patient that this is a symptom of a normal ovulatory cycle, stressing the fact of its normality. In describing this normality, we indicate that the patient ovulates and when she is interested in achieving a pregnancy later in life there should be no difficulties. It would appear that if this symptom is associated with ovulation, then an underlying endocrinopathy cannot account for this problem. There has been some discussion that severe painful uterine contractions might well be implicated in the etiology of dysmenorrhea. Some persons indicate that the maturation of the cervix and the fundal portions of the uterus has not been completed, and this also might cause the presenting symptom of pain.

Evaluation

In order to evaluate dysmenorrhea, the patient should be studied for ovulatory function. A simple technique for this is to request that the patient keep a basal body temperature chart to note whether or not she ovulates. This inexpensive technique for evaluating ovulatory function can be done by most women. In order to further evaluate the patient, after studying whether or not she ovulates, one should inhibit ovulation to see whether or not there is relief of pain.

Should there be no relief of pain when ovulation is inhibited, then the differential diagnosis should now include the possibility of endometriosis or psychogenic factors. Occasionally it becomes necessary in the adolescent to perform a laparoscopy to evaluate the anatomy of the pelvis. This step is not carried out unless the patient fails to get relief of her dysmenorrhea on ovulation inhibition.

Treatment

In the treatment of dysmenorrhea, many patients respond to the use of simple analgesics such as acetylsalicylic acid (ASA) by itself or in combination with phenobarbital or caffeine. Occasionally one progresses to combinations of ASA in conjunction with narcotic agents such as codeine sulfate or meperidine. In the past, ASA was combined with amphetamines to give the patient relief of the symptoms.

In discussing the cause of this problem it was suggested that painful uterine contractions might account for dysmenorrhea. These painful myometrial contractions might well be the result of the effect of the prostaglandins on smooth muscle. Recently, prostaglandin-blocking agents have been indicated as being of value in the management of dysmenorrhea. Indomethacin has been tried and found to be effective. It is a potent inhibitor of prostaglandin synthesis. The ideal dose appears to be indomethacin, 25 mg. given three to four times daily, starting the regimen 4 to 5 days prior to the onset of the flow, and continuing during the first 2 days of the flow. (This use of indomethacin is not listed in the manufacturer's official directive.) The usual side effects of this program should be discussed with the patient before she begins the treatment. Among the problems that may develop are persistent headaches, blurred vision, or unusual gastrointestinal symptoms. In the sexually active teenager with dysmenorrhea, ovulation inhibition using an oral contraceptive should give relief of the symptoms and at the same time serve as a contraceptive method.

Rarely is it necessary to use surgical intervention in the management of primary dysmenorrhea. Cervical dilatation has been advised and does give relief for a few cycles. However, there is return of the symptoms after this period of time. As a rule, we do not use this approach for the treatment of dysmenorrhea; nor do we sanction the use of presacral neurectomy as a method for managing the problem.

Most patients respond to the treatment of dysmenorrhea in the hands of a physician who has an understanding and an empathy for the problem. As a part of the management of any primary dysmenorrhea complaint, the patient should be thoroughly evaluated with both a complete physical examination, including a pelvic and rectal examination, and a study of ovulatory function should the dysmenorrhea be severe. In explaining a treatment program to the patient, the expectations of the physician and the patient should be reviewed and the modality of therapy discussed before the patient is placed on a treatment program.

THE MENOPAUSE

method of
RICHARD H. OI, M.D.
Sacramento, California

General

The menopause, by definition, is the cessation of menstruation. It occurs during the period of declining gonadal function, designated as the climacteric. It is the gradual decline of ovulatory activity and estrogen production to the level that the endometrium is unable to respond in cyclic fashion, resulting in irregularities of menstruation and finally amenorrhea. Estrogen production continues as a product of peripheral conversion of androgenic compounds produced by the ovarian stromal tissues and the adrenal glands, but is apparently insufficient in quantity or quality to induce endometrial proliferation.

Other specific changes associated with estrogen deficiency are vasomotor symptoms and genital atrophy. About two thirds of postmenopausal women have vasomotor symptoms represented by hot flashes, flushes, and sweats. These occasionally occur before the menopause, but other causes for these symptoms should be ruled out in these women. The vasomotor phenomena are usually self-limited, dissipating after 1 or 2 years and rarely continuing beyond this period of time. The atrophic genital changes in the vulva and vagina produce distressing symptoms of pruritus, dyspareunia, vaginal discharge, or bleeding, and the estrogen deficiency may also contribute to pelvic relaxation and subsequent urinary incontinence. Urethral caruncle formation is also estrogen related.

Osteoporosis is another condition of the postmenopausal woman. Generalized reduction in bone mass begins even before cessation of menses, and the relationship of osteoporosis to estrogen deficiency is not as substantial as its relationship to proper diet, mineral intake, and physical activity.

Recent epidemiologic studies have demonstrated that estrogen appears to be associated with an increased risk of endometrial carcinoma and that this risk is related to the duration of use and to the amount of estrogen used. There are no data to indicate that estrogen therapy incites the development of human breast or endometrial carcinoma, but the previously suspected association or predisposition has now been reinforced.

Contraindications

Estrogens should not be used, or should be used only after careful evaluation, in patients with (1) a history of estrogen-dependent neoplasia (breast and endometrial neoplasia), (2) thrombophlebitis or thromboembolic phenomena, (3) active liver or gallbladder disease, or (4) hypertension.

Risk-Benefit Assessment

1. Specific symptoms that are estrogen related are vasomotor instability and atrophic vaginitis.

2. There is no conclusive evidence that estrogen therapy prevents atherosclerosis.

3. Estrogens may have a potential value in preventing osteoporosis and are of value in providing relief of bone pain and perhaps prevention of the progression of osteoporosis.

4. There is little evidence to support the view that emotional disturbance at the time of menopause is related to decreased estrogen level.

5. There appears to be an association with or predisposition for endometrial carcinoma in patients on estrogen therapy.

It appears, then, that with the exception of specific contraindications, estrogen therapy may be used, particularly for the relief of vasomotor symptoms and genital atrophy. It should be used cyclically, in the lowest effective dose for the shortest possible time, with the patient being carefully observed for hypertension, venous thrombosis, and breast and endometrial neoplasia.

Treatment

Oral. The most convenient and simplest method of administration is the oral route; 0.625 to 1.25 mg. of conjugated estrogen per day is given cyclically on a regimen of 3 weeks of therapy and 1 week off therapy, or taken every day except for the first 5 days of the month. Occasionally, patients will become symptomatic during the 5 to 7 nontreatment days. An alternate schedule of 5 days on therapy with 2 days off may then be utilized. Equivalent dosages are estrone sulfate, 0.625 to 1.25 mg., ethinyl estradiol, 0.02 to 0.05 mg., and stilbestrol, 0.1 to 0.25 mg. After 6 months of therapy, the dosage may be reduced and the patient observed at this lesser dosage for another 6 month interval. Therapy should be gradually discontinued and therapy entirely stopped every 2 years if possible.

If bleeding occurs during a period of no medication, estrogen withdrawal may be suspected, but persistence of bleeding or any irregular or prolonged bleeding requires a thorough evaluation for uterine neoplasia.

Injectable Estrogen. Injectable estrogen may be used for those patients who experience nausea or gastrointestinal discomfort with the oral preparation. Estradiol valerate, 10 to 20 mg. intramuscularly, is given at intervals of 3 weeks or more. The usual precautions with deep intramuscular injections should be taken.

Topical Estrogens. Topical estrogens may be used for atrophic vaginal changes and dyspareunia. Dienestrol cream, one applicator full intravaginally, is used at bedtime for 2 weeks, followed by maintenance use of 1 applicator full once or twice a week. The cream should also be used externally on the introital tissues.

Estrogen-Androgen Combinations. There appears to be no advantage to using estrogen-androgen combinations. Androgens may increase the sense of well-being, but may have some virilizing effects, specifically hirsutism and acne formation.

VULVOVAGINITIS

method of
JAMES L. BREEN, M.D.,
and THEODORE COHEN, M.D.
Livingston, New Jersey

Introduction

The comparative importance of vulvovaginitis may appear minimal among the vast number of diseases that afflict women; however, the symptoms and signs which appear can produce severe distress in the person afflicted. Appropriate therapy is facilitated by the expediency of direct examination of the vulvar infection or inflammation. The relative ease of diagnosis is enhanced by the accessibility of sample material for testing.

Vulvovaginal Candidiasis

Introduction. Susceptibility to infection is related more specifically to host factors than to the mere contamination of the vagina by a species of Candida. The disease occurs primarily in women of childbearing age and is seldom observed before the menarche or after the menopause. The candidal organisms are indigenous to humans and are usually commensal, becoming pathogenic when favorable conditions develop in the host. The most prevalent offender is *Candida albicans,* although *C. tropicalis, C. pseudotropicalis, C. krusei, C. parakrusei, C. stellatoidea,* and *C. guilliermondi* have been implicated in the development of clinical disease.

Host factors that affect vaginal secretions and alter the vaginal environment appear to play a significant role in the causation of vulvovaginitis. Inclusive among the predisposing factors are the following: (1) Pregnancy. The high hormone levels in pregnancy lead to a pronounced increase in the glycogen content of the vagina, which constitutes a favorable environment for the growth of candidal organisms. Glycosuria, lowered glucose tolerance, and elevated blood sugar contribute to the increase in susceptibility to disease. Clinical disease usually dissipates at the conclusion of pregnancy. (2) Contraceptive pills. The incidence of infection is observed to be higher in patients taking cyclic hormones for contraception than in similar patients not adhering to this type of contraception. (3) Menstrual cycle. The intensity of the clinical manifestations of infection is usually more severe prior to menstruation because of available vaginal glycogen, with some relief experienced during and after the menstrual flow. (4) Antibiotics. A probable explanation for the increased incidence of candidiasis is that antibiotics act to reduce bacterial competition, thus allowing candidal organisms to multiply. (5) Intestinal tract. A frequent source of Candida organisms may under certain conditions perpetuate infection and reinfection of the vulvovaginal area. (6) Corticosteroids. These can reduce resistance to bacterial infection by diminishing inflammatory response. However, a full understanding of a causal relationship of systemic corticosteroids with vaginal candidiasis has not yet been completely clarified. (7) Diabetes mellitus. (8) Glycosuria (nondiabetic). Recurrent vaginal candidiasis may exist in patients with sugar in their urine caused by a low renal threshold. (9) Male factor. Reservoirs of organisms, especially beneath the foreskin and on the genitocrural tissues of males, act as transmitters of infection through sexual contact.

Treatment. Various regimens can be adhered to: (1) Nystatin (Mycostatin) vaginal suppositories, 1 daily for 2 weeks is most effective. (2) Miconazole nitrate (Monistat) vaginal cream, one applicator full daily at bedtime for 2 weeks. (3) Candicidin (Candeptin), 1 tablet inserted high in the vagina daily for 2 weeks, or one applicator of the cream inserted daily for 2 weeks. (4) Chlordantoin (Sporostacin) cream, one vaginal application twice daily for 2 weeks. (5) Proprionic acid gel (Proprion gel), one vaginal application daily for 3 weeks. (6) Gentian violet, 2 per cent aqueous solution applied topically to the vulva, vagina, and cervix twice weekly for 3 weeks. Patients may object to the color stain on their clothing.

For these treatment modalities to be effective, certain principles of treatment should be adhered to: (1) The presence of candidal organisms in the absence of clinical disease does not warrant therapy and should be construed in its proper context. (2) Therapy should be continued uninterrupted for the full interval of treatment, including during menstrual flow. (3) Male partners and other cohorts should receive appropriate treatment if indicated. (4) Achieve better control of those factors which perpetuate or predispose to recurrent vulvovaginitis, such as prolonged antibiotic therapy or uncontrolled diabetes.

Trichomoniasis

Introduction. Although categorized as a venereal disease because it is transmitted by sexual contact, trichomoniasis is an infection involving the vulvovaginal tissues of the female, including Skene's ducts, urethra, and occasionally bladder. The acute form of infection is characterized by distinct gross tissue changes in the vulva and vagina. The vulva exhibits redness and edema in response to irritative symptoms. The vagina is described by abnormal vaginal secretion, erythema of the mucosa, petechiae, and, rarely, a thin pseudomembrane. The vaginal flora is essentially devoid of lactobacilli, and the vaginal pH is elevated. Other, less severe forms of infection exist in the chronic and asymptomatic states. The causative agent is *Trichomonas vaginalis*, a unicellular protozoan flagellate, fusiform in shape and larger than a leukocyte.

Factors implicated as predisposing to infection are (1) hyperestrinism—for example, in pregnancy; (2) hypoacidity of the vagina, which enhances infection; (3) bacterial flora—certain gram-positive cocci and gram-negative bacilli function symbiotically with trichomonads to intensify the infection, whereas a predominance of lactobacilli discourages development of clinical infection; (4) menstrual flow, which exacerbates infection by altering vaginal pH; and (5) emotional and nervous disorders.

Treatment. 1. Metronidazole (Flagyl). Proper administration can achieve a cure rate approaching 100 per cent. The dosage schedule utilized is 250 mg. by mouth three times daily for 10 days, or 500 mg. twice daily for 5 days. (See also manufacturer's official directive for dosage recommendations.) Withhold treatment during the first trimester of pregnancy.

2. Treatment of the male partner is imperative, as he acts as a continuous source of infection. The dosage schedule employed is 250 mg. twice daily for 10 days.

3. Topical medicaments seldom effect complete eradication of vaginal trichomonads. They may be utilized in selective cases in which there is drug sensitivity or during the first trimester of pregnancy—e.g., furazolidone-nifuroxime (Tricofuron) suppositories. Recommended use is for 30 days or longer, including the period of menstrual flow.

4. Prophylaxis. (a) Contraceptive measures, condoms and creams, as a safeguard against infection. (b) Postcoital douching with vinegar in water solution or other acid preparations in instances when trichomoniasis is highly suspect. (3) Proper attention devoted to autogenous sources of reinfection; e.g., Skene's ducts, urethra, and paraurethral glands are harborers of organisms and can serve as continual sources of reinfection.

Hemophilus Vaginalis Vaginitis

Introduction. *Hemophilus vaginalis* vaginitis is primarily a disease of women in their reproductive years and is of less severity than the inflammations produced by candidal and trichomonad agents. The organism, *Hemophilus vaginalis*, operates by parasitizing surface vaginal epithelium and thereby altering the normal vaginal environment. The inflammatory tissue response is of a lesser degree, accounting for a paucity of pus cells and exudate in the vaginal discharge. *H. vaginalis* is a small, rod-shaped gram-negative bacillus which assumes heavy growth patterns in clinical infection. Microscopically, the organisms arrange themselves in dense aggregates about vaginal epithelial cells, which are, consequently, referred to as "clue cells." The infection is predominantly transmitted by sexual intercourse. Natural or exogenous estrogens predispose a favorable environment of enriched vaginal epithelial cells to support growth of *H. vaginalis* organisms. Gross tissue changes of vulvovaginitis do not manifest, because the infecting agents are surface parasites and do not invade tissues or evoke an inflammatory response. A vaginal discharge may present which is gray colored and malodorous and ranges in pH between 5 and 5.5.

Treatment. TOPICAL AGENTS. 1. Oxytetracycline and polymyxin B (Terramycin) vaginal suppositories, 1 suppository inserted daily at bedtime for 10 days. Unfavorable after effects include development of candidal or bacterial infections.

2. Sulfonamide preparations—sulfanilamide (AVC), a sulfathiazole, sulfacetamide, and sulfbenzamide (Sultrin) cream or tablets inserted twice daily for 10 days.

SYSTEMIC AGENTS 1. Ampicillin, 500 mg. every 6 hours for 5 days.

2. Oral tetracyclines are partially effective.

MALE PARTNERS. Male partners should receive simultaneous treatment, consisting of ampicillin, 500 mg. every 6 hours for 5 days.

Herpes Genitalis

Introduction. Herpes genitalis, an affliction of the genitalia, is caused by the herpes simplex virus type II. The disease is primarily venereal and may infect the cervix and vagina either independently or in association with the vulvar disease. Primary lesions of herpes genitalis consist of vesicular eruptions, which can be easily traumatized and secondarily infected by bacteria or fungi. These become transformed into painful shallow ulcers covered with exudate. A painful regional lymphadenopathy may result. Presumably, the person exposed to infection responds by making antibodies. However, the immune response is generally incomplete. The virus, seldom eradicated, may exist in a dormant state in the tissues of the lower genitalia and provoke recurrent disease under favorable circumstances. Constitutional symptoms of fever, malaise, headache, and anorexia can be experienced.

Treatment. Therapy is essentially palliative, as no single regimen exists to completely eradicate disease and block viral replication.

1. Application of neutral red dye followed by exposure to ultraviolet light may achieve symptom relief and healing. However, recent studies demonstrate oncogenic transformation by photodynamic dyes in hamster embryonic cells.

2. Sitz baths, boric acid solution, Burow's solution, or wet compresses may provide symptom relief.

3. Corticosteroids are not recommended because of their potential for inhibition of the immune response.

4. Theoretical assumptions: (a) Bacille Calmette-Guérin (BCG) vaccination is presumed to stimulate the immune response. (b) Repeated inoculations with smallpox vaccine may be beneficial because of an immunologic resemblance between smallpox and herpes viruses. (c) Ultimately, a vaccine may be produced from inactivated herpes simplex virus.

5. With regard to pregnancy, cesarean section is the preferred method of delivery to ensure against fetal contamination. If serologic studies determine no cross-reacting antibodies to herpes virus type I and amniocentesis confirms fetal infection, then delivery by the abdominal route may be unnecessary.

Atrophic Vulvovaginitis

Introduction. Estrogen deprivation brought about by the natural menopause, surgical castration, or functional ovarian failure causes atrophic changes in the vaginal epithelium, which then becomes vulnerable to infection. The extent of menopausal atrophy varies according to the ability of the ovaries and adrenal glands to serve as limited sources of estrogen supply. The onset of infection is usually unrelated to Candida, Trichomonas, or *Hemophilus vaginalis,* as the vaginal milieu is devoid of glycogen-laden mucosa. Instead, contaminant bacterial organisms establish a new vaginal flora which allows itself to proliferate and incite infection. The earliest demonstrable change of diminishing estrogen is evidenced in the vaginal cytologic smear. A shift in the maturation index is detected as the number of intermediate and parabasal cells increases. In advanced atrophy, large numbers of red cells, leukocytes, and mixed bacteria comprise the vaginal smear. Symptoms of atrophic vaginitis may first manifest as vaginal spotting.

Treatment. A course of adequate therapy can result in dramatic relief of subjective symptoms. Desired cornification of the vaginal mucosa returns, and pH and flora revert to normal.

Conjugated estrogens (Premarin) or dienestrol creams, inserted intravaginally nightly for 1 week and then maintained once or twice weekly, are very effective. If systemic administration is desired, Premarin tablets (0.625 mg., 1.25 mg., 2.5 mg.) and ethinyl estradiol (Estinyl) tablets (0.02 mg., 0.05 mg., 0.5 mg.) are available.

Trichomonads and Candida organisms, if present, may be potentiated by estrogens to proliferate.

Estrogens are contraindicated when there is a history of breast, endometrial, or ovarian tumors.

Pediatric Vulvovaginitis

Introduction. Pediatric vulvovaginitis applies to all cases of leukorrhea and vulvovaginal infections encountered in premenarchal patients. The vulvovaginitides commonly observed in older age groups (e.g., trichomoniasis, candidiasis, *Hemophilus vaginalis* vaginitis) seldom affect children. The gonococcus must be excluded as a causative agent. Most cases of pediatric vulvovaginitis cannot be attributed to a specific microbial agent and are thus classified as nonspecific. At birth the vaginal canal is well cornified and high in glycogen content as a result of maternal estrogen stimulation. Shortly thereafter, the vaginal epithelium progressively atrophies, cellular glycogen is lost, vaginal acidity decreases, and the cytologic smear is primarily parabasal. At the time of prepubescence a gradual process toward vaginal maturity is attained. It is important to understand physiologic leukorrhea in the right perspective; otherwise it may be misconstrued as products of infection and mistakenly treated. Neonatal leukorrhea is a transient discharge which dissipates as the influence of maternal estrogens declines. Premenarchal leukorrhea results from an increase in vaginal secretions in response to endogenous estrogen production.

Vulvovaginal Inflammations. NONSPECIFIC VULVOVAGINITIS. Nonspecific vulvovaginitis includes those cases in which abnormal vulvovaginal changes and irritative signs occur without specific demonstrable cause. Predisposing factors include hypoestrogenism, fecal contamination of the vulva, and tight-fitting underclothing. Treatment measures entail (1) hygienic habits and utilization of loose-fitting cotton undergarments; (2) application of estrogenic creams—conjugated estrogens (Premarin), 0.625 mg., or dienestrol 0.01 per cent, 1 gram applied nightly for 2 weeks and thereafter every 3 nights for an additional 6 weeks; and (3) oral estrogens according to the following regimen: Premarin, 0.3 mg. daily for 2 weeks and then twice weekly. In general, the response of nonspecific vulvovaginitis to antibiotics and sulfonamides is poor. Effective response implies a specific bacterial agent.

GONORRHEAL VULVOVAGINITIS. The diagnosis is usually confirmed by cultures on Thayer-Martin media or by immunofluorescent methods. Sex play is an important factor in dissemination of infection. The thin vaginal mucosa in childhood predisposes to infection by the gonococcus. Symptoms of itching, burning vulvar dysuria, and chafing may develop. The discharge is characterized by a creamy yellowish green secretion.

TRICHOMONIASIS, CANDIDIASIS, AND HEMOPHILUS VAGINALIS VAGINITIS. The immature vagina is generally not suitable for development of these infections. Candidiasis may arouse the suspicion of diabetes or suggest the recent administration of antibiotics or estrogens.

WORM INFESTATIONS. Pinworms *(Oxyuris vermicularis)* and roundworms *(Ascaris lumbricoides)* have been retrieved from the vaginal canal in certain cases of vulvovaginitis. Irritative symptoms and pruritus may be distressing. Treatment consists of administration of pyrvinium pamoate (Povan) in a single dose equivalent to 5 mg. per kg. of body weight. Piperazine hexahydrate (Antepar) may be given once daily for 7 days as an adjusted oral dose according to body weight.

FOREIGN BODY. The combination of persistent slight bleeding, vaginal discharge, and bad odor should arouse suspicion of a foreign body–induced vulvovaginitis. Treatment consists simply of removal of the foreign object. General anesthesia may be required in certain circumstances.

Miscellaneous Bacterial Vulvovaginitides

Various types of bacteria are recoverable from the vaginal canal and are just as heterogeneous in the normal state as in the abnormal state. Vaginitis is sometimes caused by one or more organisms, including streptococci, staphylococci, *Escherichia coli,* Hemophilus species, Pseudomonas, Proteus, Bacteroides, and Mycoplasma. Not infrequently one observes bacterial vaginitis manifest from antibiotic use, debilitating diseases, leukemia, and carcinomatosis. After excluding the common pathogens—Trichomonas, *H. vaginalis,* and Candida species—as causative agents, a thorough investigation consisting of wet mount preparations, stained smears, and bacteriologic cultures should be performed. In addition, a thorough understanding that the vaginal milieu of reproductive years contains a predominance of lactobacilli and mature epithelial cells, and that hypoestrogenism causes a thin vagina low in glycogen content with a mixed flora and immature cells, may provide a clue that an abnormal process is ensuing.

Streptococcal Vaginitis. Common inhabitants of the normal vaginal flora rarely act as independent pathogens. The clinical disease, beta-type streptococcal vaginitis, responds to treatment with estrogens and antibiotics in the pre-and postmenopausal states. Systemic antibiotics can be administered in the reproductive years.

Staphylococcal Vaginitis. Opportunistic situations arise from long-term use of antibiotics and from spread of skin conditions—e.g., vulvar folliculitis. Treatment consists of administration of appropriate antibiotics.

Escherichia Coli. Most abnormal discharges in which *E. coli* predominate usually do not require treatment. However, if a remedy is considered necessary, local application of sulfonamides is effective.

Pseudomonas and Proteus Infections. These organisms can be recovered from the vagina in opportunistic situations. Correction of the situation usually restores the natural flora.

Infection with Mycoplasma. This organism is rarely ascribed to urinary tract infections and septic abortion. Little evidence exists to implicate these organisms as a cause of vulvovaginal infections.

Corynebacterium in Vulvovaginitis. Corynebacteria (diphtheroids) are a normal component of vaginal flora. The only species of pathogenic potential, *Corynebacterium diphtheriae,* can give rise to diphtheritic vaginitis.

Tuberculosis of the Vulva and Vagina. Tuberculosis of the vulva and vagina should be suspected when lesions of the vulva, such as chronic ulcerations, draining sinuses, and adenopathy, are present. Primary infection in women, although rare, has been reported following intercourse with men afflicted with tuberculous epididymitis. The affected tissue reveals central caseation, epithelial cells, and giant cells. *Mycobacterium tuberculosis* may be recovered from scrapings obtained from the lesions. Treatment principles should adhere to therapy of tuberculosis in general.

PELVIC INFLAMMATORY DISEASE

method of
EDUARD G. FRIEDRICH, Jr., M.D.
Milwaukee, Wisconsin

Inflammation of the female pelvic viscera may follow obstetric delivery or abortion, intrauterine device (IUD) insertion, and gynecologic surgery; most cases, however, are related to sexually transmitted infection by *Neisseria gonorrhoeae.* Increased promiscuity and decreased use of condom contraceptives have significantly contributed to the current epidemic of gonorrhea in the United States.

Only a minority of women infected with gonorrhea will develop upper tract involvement of the tubes, ovaries, and pelvic peritoneum. Further reduction of this number can be achieved by early diagnosis and adequate treatment of the asymptomatic patient.

Asymptomatic Patients

1. Routine Thayer-Martin cultures of the endocervix should be performed on all sexually active women regardless of socioeconomic status.

2. Patients with positive cultures should be treated with a single intramuscular dose of 4.8 million units of procaine penicillin G, preceded by 1 gram of probenecid orally. Nonpregnant, penicillin-allergic patients should be given 2.0 grams of spectinomycin intramuscularly in a single dose. Pregnant penicillin-allergic patients should be treated with erythromycin, 1.5 grams orally immediately, followed by 0.5 gram four times daily for 4 days.

Resistance to penicillin has developed in some beta-lactamase-producing strains of *N. gonorrhoeae,* mutation resulting in spectinomycin resistance has been reported, and the efficacy of erythromycin is not yet firmly established.

3. Follow-up culture, 1 or 2 weeks after therapy, is therefore mandatory.

4. If retreatment is necessary, the oral administration of ampicillin, 3.5 grams in a single oral dose, preceded by 1 gram of probenecid; or tetracycline, 1.5 grams initially, followed by 500 mg. four times daily for 4 days, must be used.

As these oral regimens have higher reported failure rates, their use on a first-line basis is not justified. Few treatment failures result from antibiotic resistance; most represent true reinfections. Therefore:

5. Cultures of sexual partners should be made and, if positive, the partner should be treated.

6. Finally, a careful search for other sexually transmitted disease is warranted in all patients because approximately 15 per cent are found to harbor more than one disease. This search should include a serologic test for syphilis. If therapy other than penicillin is chosen, serology, if negative, should be repeated in 6 weeks.

Gonococci gain access to the endometrial and tubal mucosae at the time of menses and possibly by physical attachment to migrating spermatozoa. As a result, approximately 10 per cent of infected women suffer invasion of the upper tract and become symptomatic. Once present in the endosalpinx, the gonococcus invades the entire thickness of the fallopian tubes, causing cellular damage to the mucosa and scarring of the underlying fibromuscular layers. Partial or complete blockage of the tubal lumen may occur, along with clubbing and closure of the fimbriated portion of the tube. The stage is then set for subsequent infection of these damaged areas by other organisms from the cervix and vagina, notably streptococci, *Escherichia coli,* and Bacteroides. Pus, formed by these bacteria, may spread to involve all the pelvic viscera and adjacent structures. This sequence of events results in symptomatic disease represented by four distinct clinical entities: acute primary infection, acute recurrent infection, abscess formation, and chronic infection.

Acute Primary Infection

The initial episode of tubal infection caused by the gonococcus is marked by the onset of lower abdominal pain, pelvic tenderness, fever, and an elevation of the erythrocyte sedimentation rate (ESR). Cultures of the endocervix are frequently positive for *N. gonorrhoeae,* although Gram stain of cervical exudates is of little help. Such patients are managed on an ambulatory basis as follows:

1. Initial treatment is the same as for the asymptomatic patient, with the addition of oral analgesics and instructions for bed rest and sexual abstinence.

2. Ten days of oral doxycycline, 100 mg. per day, or ampicillin, 2.0 grams per day, in divided doses is added to the initial antibiotic treatment, and the patient is scheduled for follow-up examination within 1 week.

However, any of the following constitutes indication for hospital admission: (a) initial temperature of 101°F. (38.3°C.) or greater; (b) diffuse peritonitis, nausea, or vomiting; (c) presence of a pelvic mass; (d) uncertain diagnosis; (e) failure to respond to outpatient management; or (f) pregnancy. Such hospitalized patients require the following measures:

1. Bed rest in semi-Fowler's position to prevent upward spread of infection along the colic gutter, which may result in perihepatitis (Fitz-Hugh syndrome).

2. The degree of peritoneal involvement and ileus dictate the need for restriction of oral intake and use of nasogastric suction.

3. Serial determination of vital signs, erythrocyte sedimentation rate (ESR), leukocyte count, and urine output provides the best gauge of therapeutic response.

4. Intravenous fluids are given, along with the following antibiotics: Aqueous penicillin, 5 million units by Volutrol intravenously every 4 to 6 hours for a total of 20 to 30 million units per day. Nonpregnant penicillin-allergic patients receive doxycycline, 100 mg. intravenously every 12 hours. Acute salpingitis in pregnancy is unusual, but such patients, if allergic to penicillin, may be treated with intravenous sodium cephalothin, 2 grams every 6 hours, provided the danger of cross-allergenicity is recognized.

If the infection is truly an acute primary gonococcal salpingitis, such therapy should result in rapid resolution of the disease process manifested by overall clinical improvement within 48 to 72 hours, a concomitant decline in fever, and a slower decline in ESR. Once the patient has been afebrile for 72 hours, a repeat pelvic examination is performed and tenderness should be minimal or absent. Provided that there is no recurrence of fever during the 24 hours following repeat pelvic examination, the patient is discharged and continued on oral antibiotics for 10 days, as for the ambulatory patient. The prognosis for future fertility in such patients is good. If the repeat pelvic examination reveals the development of a pelvic mass or increase in size of a pre-existing mass, or if there is no improvement after 48 to 72 hours of therapy, then the diagnosis should be suspect and the patient managed as below.

Acute Recurrent Infection

Patients with a previous history of salpingitis and those whose initial episode does not respond promptly to intravenous penicillin alone frequently have a mixed bacterial infection which has spread beyond the tubes. Culdocentesis can be extremely helpful and should be performed whenever possible unless a suspected tubo-ovarian abscess is adherent in the cul-de-sac. A Gram stain of the peritoneal fluid obtained in this manner may show a mixed flora indicative of anaerobic infection, and the material should be cultured appropriately. Appendicitis, ruptured ovarian cyst, degenerating uterine myomas, diverticulitis, uterine perforation, and septic abortion may all result in similar clinical pictures. Laparoscopy has proved to be a safe and effective method of confirmation, and should be considered if the diagnosis is in doubt. Adequate material for anaerobic and aerobic culture can also be obtained in this manner. The inpatient management of such patients is basically similar to that described for acute primary infection, but additional gram-negative coverage is necessary.

1. An aminoglycoside is added to the antibiotic regimens outlined above after culture material has been obtained. We prefer tobramycin, 1 mg. per kg. intramuscularly every 8 hours.

2. If there has been no significant clinical improvement after 48 to 72 hours on the combined antibiotic therapy, a change of antibiotics or the addition of anaerobic coverage should be instituted, guided by the sensitivity reports from the culture material.

3. Pelvic thrombophlebitis may develop and result in septic embolization. For such patients, the addition of heparin, 5000 to 10,000 units intravenously every 4 to 6 hours, to the treatment program should result in a rapid improvement. Failure of response within 72 hours should lead to the suspicion of pelvic abscess formation.

Pelvic Abscess

The development of a pelvic abscess recognized at the time of initial presentation or arising during the subsequent management of a patient with pelvic inflammatory disease is an infrequent but ominous sign. Ultrasound determinations may be of great help in the diagnosis and localization of such a mass, and abscess formation should always be suspected in the patient who fails to respond to intravenous antibiotics. Septic shock may develop, and the danger of intraperitoneal rupture is ever present. Rupture will occur in approximately 15 per cent of such patients and carries with it a significant mortality. The close monitoring of all clinical and laboratory parameters is essential. *E. coli,* peptococci, peptostreptococci, and Bacteroides species are frequently involved.

1. Blood cultures, aerobic and anaerobic, should be taken during fever spikes and are helpful if positive.

2. Clindamycin, 600 mg. intravenously every 6 hours, or chloramphenicol, 2 grams intravenously every 6 hours, must be added to the antibiotic regimen. The potential side effects of these drugs must be monitored but are outweighed by the necessity for anaerobic coverage.

3. Most patients with pelvic abscess will respond to medical therapy, and the use of pelvic diathermy may accelerate resolution of the abscess. A decline in ESR and decrease in cavity size on serial ultrasound studies are good prognostic indicators.

4. If the abscess is located in the cul-de-sac, it may dissect the rectovaginal septum and point into the posterior vaginal fornix. Such abscesses, if fluctuant and in the midline, may be drained through a colpotomy incision. Two thirds of patients so treated quickly recover and remain asymptomatic.

5. Patients whose abscess lies higher in the pelvis and who show no signs of improvement on medical therapy after 72 hours become candidates for laparotomy.

Aggressive surgical management is indicated as an emergency procedure whenever intra-abdominal rupture of a pelvic abscess is suspected. Total abdominal hysterectomy and bilateral salpingo-oophorectomy are performed whenever possible. The increased risk of ureteral and bowel injury should be recognized. The desire to preserve childbearing function may be respected in some patients with removal of unilaterally involved adnexae, but the recurrence rate of additional inflammatory episodes is high, the fertility rate is low, and the incidence of subsequent ectopic pregnancy is increased.

Chronic Infection

Pelvic inflammatory disease that resolves after medical therapy may result in residual scarring, adhesion formation, and the development of hydrosalpinx. Chronic pelvic pain, dysmenorrhea, dyspareunia, and infertility may all be present. Oral analgesics, anti-inflammatory agents, and pelvic diathermy may temporarily control symptoms. A course of oral broad-spectrum antibiotics is added when mild pelvic tenderness is present, and continued until the ESR has returned to normal levels. Occasionally, surgical reconstruction of distally involved tubes may improve fertility. However, patients with chronic infection may develop acute exacerbation of their disease at any time, particularly after uterine instrumentation. Acute recurrent episodes may even develop after menopause. When the patient and her physician agree that the symptomatology and risks of exacerbation warrant definitive therapy, surgery is indicated.

Total abdominal hysterectomy and bilateral salpingo-oophorectomy (pelvic cleanout) should be performed during a quiescent period of the disease when the ESR is below 40 mm. per hour. The desire to preserve ovarian tissue must be balanced against risks of recrudescence of infection.

Although such surgery may seem extreme in younger patients, it represents the only long-term form of "cure."

UTERINE MYOMAS

method of
R. RICHARD MURRAY, M.D.
Albuquerque, New Mexico

Rationale for Management of Uterine Myomas

Uterine myomas are very common, being present in 20 to 30 per cent of women approaching the perimenopausal years.

Uterine myomas have a very low chance for malignant transformation, and their removal is not indicated for diagnosis or prevention of malignancy. Leiomyosarcoma is the rare malignancy associated with myomas. The presence of uterine myomas does not exclude the possibility of coexisting endometrial carcinoma (which must be ruled out, if suspected). Likewise, uterine myomas do not increase the chance for coexisting neoplasms.

Uterine myomas do not require active management unless they cause symptoms. Asymptomatic myomas should be followed by pelvic examination every 6 months, looking for increase in size. Rapid growth is suggestive of sarcoma.

Uterine myomas are estrogen dependent. They often become symptomatic in the perimenopausal years because of anovulation and high continuous estrogen levels. They usually decrease in size and become asymptomatic when the patient becomes postmenopausal. Oral contraceptives should be used advisedly because of the possible growth of myomas. Estrogen therapy for postmenopausal symptoms carries the added risk of growth in existing myomas.

Coexisting Factors Influencing Management of Uterine Myomas

Uterine Myomas Versus Adnexal Disease. Because of the much higher possibility of malignancy in ovarian masses, it is absolutely imperative that uterine myomas be differentiated from adnexal disease. Both ovaries must be identified separately from the myomas by pelvic examination. When some doubt exists, ultrasonography may establish a definite diagnosis. If not, examination under anesthesia, laparoscopy, and/or laparotomy is indicated.

Uterine Myomas Associated with Pregnancy. Myomas usually enlarge during pregnancy but may cause no symptoms or problems. Occasionally a myoma develops carneous or "red" degeneration in pregnancy or the immediate postpartum period, owing to alteration in blood supply. Such a myoma produces pain and may stimulate uterine contractions and premature labor. Management should be conservative and surgery avoided if possible. The pain is treated with medications, including codeine or meperidine (Demerol), if necessary. Premature labor can usually be stopped with appropriate therapy, but frequently will recur. The goal of management is to allow the fetus to obtain lung maturity before delivery.

Uterine myomas may cause soft tissue dystocia in labor by preventing the descent and delivery of the presenting fetal part. This situation should be anticipated before labor, or diagnosed early in labor, and the baby delivered by cesarean section.

If a cesarean section is performed on a patient with uterine myomas, myomectomy is to be discouraged unless the myomas exist in the line of the primary uterine incision. Additional uterine serosal incisions are contraindicated.

A cesarean hysterectomy may be performed if the patient has symptomatic or large myomas in the nonpregnant state, (1) if she must have a cesarean section for obstetrical indications and (2) if she desires no further children. The surgical risks are much less if hysterectomy is delayed 6 months, during which time the myomas will decrease in size and thus the uterus is more easily removed. Cesarean hysterectomy is associated with a significantly higher blood loss than cesarean section alone, and risk of urinary tract injury is higher. In favor of the cesarean hysterectomy is the increased risk to the patient associated with a second anesthesia in 6 months. This decision will depend on the surgeon's training, experience, and ability, plus consultation with the patient and her husband about the relative risks.

Management of Symptomatic Myomas

Abnormal uterine bleeding typically occurs in the form of heavy prolonged menses.

Examination under anesthesia and dilatation and curettage (D&C) are indicated for a single heavy bleeding episode or recurrent, moderate to heavy menses. Endometrial carcinoma must be ruled out. Submucous myomas, if present, should be diagnosed. Definitive surgery is indicated for submucous myomas. This surgery may be performed at the time of the D&C if the patient is in good condition and psychologically prepared, or the surgery may be delayed, even to the time of the next abnormal bleeding episode.

Definitive surgery is indicated if abnormal bleeding reoccurs after the second D&C.

Heavy bleeding caused by myomas may result in acute or chronic anemia. Supplemental iron therapy is indicated if anemia is due to chronic excessive blood loss. Blood transfusion may be necessary to replace blood loss in preparation for surgery. Bleeding may be stopped temporarily by intravenous conjugated estrogens (20 mg.), thus giving time to prepare for definitive surgery.

Pelvic pain may be primary, resulting from ischemia of the myoma, or secondary to the pressure of the myomas on other structures. Other causes of pelvic pain must be ruled out. This may require a laparoscopy. Persistent and significant pain requires definitive surgery. A large myomatous uterus may cause hydronephrosis or hydroureter because of pressure on the ureter, usually as it passes over the pelvic brim. The only symptom may be low or mid-back pain.

A uterus with myomas that are enlarging, especially in a postmenopausal woman, demands definitive surgery.

If the combined size of uterus and myomas is comparable to a 12 to 14 week gestation, hysterectomy is indicated. Although these patients may have no specific complaints, they usually have vague complaints of fatigue and abdominal and/or pelvic fullness, and feel much better after the hysterectomy.

Infertility may result when myomas distort the fallopian tubes or the uterine cavity. Recurrent spontaneous abortion may result because of distortion of the uterine cavity. In these circumstances, a myomectomy, or multiple myomectomy, should be considered. Myomectomy has a higher risk of postoperative adhesions and bowel obstruction than hysterectomy, and there is a significant chance of recurrence of myomas in the future. These risks must be understood by the patient. The patient must also understand that the myomectomy may not result in a pregnancy carried to term, and that if a pregnancy is carried to term, the method of delivery will be cesarean section. If the delivering physician was also the operating physician and/or there is good documentation that the myomectomy involved only the superficial myometrium, the patient may be allowed to labor and deliver vaginally under close observation.

A pedunculated submucous myoma passed through the cervical canal must be differentiated from a spontaneous abortion. A myomectomy may be performed using a wire snare, followed by a vigorous curettage of the base of the myoma. Blood should be available for transfusion and preparations ready for hysterectomy. Since there is almost always infection following incision of a pedunculated submucous myoma, antibiotics may be indicated.

Definitive Therapy of Uterine Myomas

Total hysterectomy is the definitive treatment of choice when the situation makes surgery desirable. As stated above, myomectomy is reserved for women who desire further childbearing and who understand the potential risks involved.

Hysterectomy for myomas is usually technically easier by the abdominal route. Depending upon the surgeon's training and ability, and if other advantages of the vaginal approach (i.e., need for repair of pelvic relaxation) exist, a uterus with myomas up to 12 weeks of gestational size may be safely removed vaginally, utilizing a morcellation technique.

Summary

Uterine myomas are very common and therefore are the most common pathologic finding at the time of hysterectomy. However, the presence of a myomatous uterus is not an indication for surgery unless it produces symptoms. Because of the high frequency of uterine myomas, physicians must be cognizant of the myomas that need treatment and those that only need to be followed by pelvic examination. Unnecessary surgery must be eliminated, but the quality of life of the patient, hampered by symptomatic myomas, must also be protected. This requires both the art and science of medicine.

CANCER OF THE UTERUS*

method of
HUGH R. K. BARBER, M.D.,
IRVING BUTERMAN, M.D.,
and RAJYALAKSHMI KAKARLA, M.D
New York, New York

Cancer of the Cervix

Cancer of the cervix is a disease of the inner city. On the basis of the incidence rates of cancer recorded in the Third National Cancer Survey, it

*Sponsored by the New York City Division of the American Cancer Society. Supported by the John C. Kilroe, M.D., Memorial Fund.

is calculated that 1.6 per cent of newborn girls, about 1 out of 63, will develop invasive cancer of the cervix uteri at some time during their lives. The probability of developing invasive cancer of the cervix uteri increases with age until menopause, and then, after a slight dip, levels off in older ages.

Diagnosis. There are no symptoms characteristic of cancer of the cervix. A high index of suspicion is necessary. Bleeding is probably the most common symptom associated with cancer of the cervix, and is usually bright red and "lawless."

An accurate histologic diagnosis is essential before definitive treatment is instituted. A differential diagnosis should rule out chancres, tuberculosis, granuloma inguinale, lymphogranuloma venereum, and condyloma acuminatum. A point to emphasize is that each of these lesions can be present concurrently with cancer, and this argues strongly for biopsy proof of disease.

The Papanicolaou smear is merely a screening method and has its greatest application in the asymptomatic female. Any visible lesion present on the cervix *should be biopsied,* as an obvious lesion may result in a negative Papanicolaou smear despite the invasive nature of the lesion.

The patient should be staged according to the international classification established by the International Federation of Obstetricians and Gynecologists (FIGO). It is shown in Table 1.

TABLE 1. **Clinical Staging for Cancer of the Cervix**

Stage 0:	Carcinoma in situ, intraepithelial carcinoma.
Stage I:	Carcinoma confined to the cervix (extension to the corpus should be disregarded).
Stage Ia:	Microinvasive carcinoma (early stromal invasion).
Stage Ib:	All other cases of Stage I. Occult cancer should be marked "occ."
Stage II:	The carcinoma extends beyond the cervix but has not extended to the pelvic wall. The carcinoma involves the vagina, but not the lower third.
Stage IIa:	No obvious parametrial involvement.
Stage IIb:	Obvious parametrial involvement.
Stage III:	The carcinoma has extended to the pelvic wall. On rectal examination there is no cancer-free space between the tumor and the pelvic wall. The tumor involves the lower third of the vagina. All cases with hydronephrosis or nonfunctioning kidney.
Stage IIIa:	No extension to the pelvic wall.
Stage IIIb:	Extension to the pelvic wall and/or hydronephrosis or nonfunctioning kidney.
Stage IV:	The carcinoma has extended beyond the true pelvis or has clinically involved the mucosa of the bladder or rectum. A bullous edema does not classify as Stage IV.
Stage IVa:	Spread of the growth to adjacent organs.
Stage IVb:	Spread to distant organs.

It is important to have an accurate histologic diagnosis once positive or suspicious cells are reported on Papanicolaou smear examination. Our plan for work-up is as follows:

1. Repeat smears, if no visible lesion is present, are taken, including the endocervix and the external os.

2. Colposcopic study is indicated in the presence of abnormal cytology. (a) If findings are normal and cytology remains suspicious, a diagnostic cone biopsy is indicated. (b) If abnormal findings are present, directed biopsies are indicated. (c) If unsatisfactory findings are present and suspect cytology is again reported, cone biopsy and diagnostic curettage should be carried out.

3. An alternative plan, if colposcopy is not available, is to carry out punch biopsies of the Schiller's or toluidine blue treated cervix and vagina. Endocervical curettage with a small curette is performed. Hospital admission for fractional curettage, further biopsies, or conization of the cervix should be done if it is deemed necessary.

4. Biopsy revealing invasive cancer avoids the need for conization.

Pretreatment Evaluation. It is important to know the exact extent of the disease before treatment is started. The patient should have a detailed history and complete physical examination. The laboratory studies should include the standard work-up with a metastatic series. The patient should be staged carefully, under anesthesia, by two examiners. Once the cancer of the cervix is assigned a stage, it cannot be changed after treatment has started.

Treatment. A method of treatment is outlined below. The question is not whether radiation or surgery is better but, rather, which is better for a given patient, surgery or irradiation. Instead of treating a stage of cancer, it is more enlightened to treat a volume of cancer in a given patient. Recently, the philosophy of treatment has swung from standardization to individualized therapy.

DYSPLASIA. Marked dysplasia is usually adequately treated by conization or multiple biopsies plus endocervical curettage. It is then followed postoperatively by Papanicolaou smears.

CARCINOMA IN SITU. The proper treatment is based on the clinical and histologic findings. It is important to re-emphasize that carcinoma in situ may occur in multiple sites and may be found in the cervix, vagina, vulva, perineum, and urethra. Therefore careful clinical evaluation (adequate exposure, use of Schiller's test, and histologic evaluation) must be carried out in each patient and treatment individualized. At this point, careful, planned, and systematized follow-up over a long period is necessary. It is obvious that all suspicious smears and even positive smears should be carefully repeated, because laboratory errors happen occasionally. Repeat positive smears require additional evaluation.

In young women desirous of having children, a well-planned cone (following outline by Schiller's stain) is carried out, anticipating that it will be a therapeutic cone. This form of therapy is acceptable only if the patient is cooperative and will accept careful long-term follow-up. There is universal agreement that therapy should be surgical and not by irradiation. Following the cone it is permissible to follow the patient if the smears remain negative. However, with positive smears indicating residual disease, the patient is a candidate for either another cone or hysterectomy. In those patients treated by hysterectomy, it is important to include approximately 2 cm. of vagina in the resection, which we believe is best done by the vaginal route. Attempts to obtain additional cuff by the abdominal route have an increased urinary fistula rate unless the ureters are exposed and carefully dissected. The ovaries should be preserved in young patients. In patients over 40 years of age with a positive smear, either multiple biopsies with careful curettage of the endocervix or a cone biopsy is indicated. If invasive cancer is ruled out, a total hysterectomy with vaginal cuff and bilateral oophorectomy is indicated. The presence of an invasive lesion requires more aggressive surgery.

Stage Ia: (1) Early stromal invasion: In general, this lesion is to be treated as invasive cancer. In cases in which the invasion is indefinite or only 1 to 2 mm. in depth and does not cover a wide area, and in which there is no vascular or lymphatic involvement, the treatment is then the same as that suggested for carcinoma in situ. (2) Occult cancer (carcinoma hidden in the cervix): In general, the treatment is radical hysterectomy and bilateral pelvic node dissection *or* primary radiation therapy. (3) Postsurgical: The management is best individualized and will consist of a combination of radical surgery, including bilateral pelvic lymphadenectomy, and a radiation therapy *or* primary radiation therapy.

Stage Ib: Radical hysterectomy and bilateral pelvic lymphadenectomy. Radiation therapy in those patients in whom surgical therapy is not to be performed because of age or general health.

Stage IIa: The same treatment as for Stage Ib.

Stages IIb, IIIa, and IIIb: Primary radiation therapy.

Stage IV: (1) Primary radiation therapy. This therapy may require preradiation diversion of the fecal and/or urinary stream. (2) Primary pelvic exenteration may be selected for those patients with central disease which extends into the bladder and in whom it is possible that the disease can be totally removed.

There are some problems and controversies related to this management outline. Microinvasion in Stage Ia is defined in different ways, leading to some differences in opinion regarding the optimal type of operative procedure indicated for this group of patients. Microinvasion has a predominant histologic picture of carcinoma in situ but has, in addition, a focus of invasion which is confined to the most superficial stroma. Microinvasion is found in about 6 to 10 per cent of those patients presenting as carcinoma in situ. A review of the literature reports only a handful of such patients in whom there was involvement of submucosal lymphatics or lymph nodes. The survival rates in patients with microinvasion treated by total hysterectomy and a cuff of vagina have been excellent. The infinitesimal risk of node metastases is adequately balanced by the small mortality associated with radical hysterectomy. If, on serial or step biopsies, there is lymphatic involvement, or the invasion is more than 5 mm. in depth, the patient should be treated as having Stage I cancer of the cervix. Our own preference for treating microinvasion is a classic Wertheim hysterectomy with a cuff of the paravaginal and paracervical area and the upper one fourth of the vagina. The ovaries are managed according to the age of the patient.

An apparently normal-appearing cervix that proves to have invasive carcinoma is not necessarily a "microcarcinoma." A sizable lesion may be hidden within the endocervical canal, and these should be termed "occult" carcinomas. Cases of occult cancer may be found in a cone or in the specimen from a large wedge biopsy performed in patients with carcinoma in situ or dysplasia. Obviously, they are invasive and should be treated with the appropriate radical operation or planned cancericidal radiation therapy.

Radiation therapy: Most plans of treatment are modified forms of one of the three leading schools—i.e., Paris, Stockholm, or Manchester. Todd and Meredith (Manchester) reported that the dosage should be related to two theoretical points: i.e., *A*—defined as 2 cm. lateral to the axis of the uterine canal and 2 cm. above the vaginal fornix, and *B*—3 cm. lateral to *A*. The rationale for this approach was that the dosage at point *A* would represent a convenient method of expressing the dosage received by the primary carcinoma located in the cervix, and that the dosage at point *B* would represent the dosage received in the lymph-bearing area. Although it provides a convenient plan to follow, it has not been universally accepted.

In order to achieve successful irradiation of

cancer of the cervix, it is necessary to deliver a high dose of radiation to the tumor and the tumor-bearing areas. The cervix and the vagina can tolerate very high doses, whereas the bladder and the rectum have a lower radiation tolerance. Careful calculation of the dosage to be administered as well as well planned and executed technique is essential if radiation damage to normal tissue is to be avoided. A systematic and careful pelvic and rectal examination should be carried out under anesthesia. Fractional curettage and biopsies must precede the insertion of radium. A rigid application—i.e., Campbell, Ernst, or Henschke—should be employed in order to minimize the variation in dose. It permits better distribution of the radium and permits delivery of 12,000 rads to the cervical canal, 6000 rads to point *A*, and 2000 rads to point *B* without an inordinately high morbidity. Scintillation probes and ionization chambers should be used immediately to check the dosage being delivered to the bladder and the rectum. A flat plate of the abdomen should be done to check the position of the radium. Afterloading techniques have been introduced which eliminate radiation exposure to the personnel in the operating room. By means of a computer, it is now possible to acquire information on dose distribution around an applicator within the pelvis far beyond the limited information available by using points *A* and *B* as the only references.

Recently, there has been a swing from the use of radium to be followed by pelvic external radiation to radiation of the whole pelvis by megavoltage technique (delivering 4000 rads in Stages I and II) and then following with radium insertion 5000 to 6000 mg. hours). The technique is changed for Stage III, cutting down the mg. hours of radium and supplementing an additional 1000 or 1500 rads to the involved side, whereas Stage IV is treated with 7000 rads, reducing the size of the field after 5000 mg. hours to the cervix. However, in most clinics, radium is inserted in divided doses (Stockholm or Manchester techniques) and is left in place for 36 to 50 hours at 2 to 3 week intervals, attempting to deliver a total dose of 6000 mg. hours at point *A*. Two or 3 weeks after the final radium application, external therapy is started.

Recurrent or persistent cancer of the cervix is best managed by a surgical approach. Radiation or re-radiation has little to offer in terms of cure and is accompanied by a high complication rate and augmentation of symptoms. A point to be emphasized in the surgical treatment of recurrence is that not all patients require pelvic exenteration to encompass disease. Approximately 20 per cent can be managed by less than a pelvic exenteration. For those requiring a pelvic exenteration, the 5 year survival rate is 20 per cent, and it jumps to 40 per cent among those treated by less than a pelvic exenteration.

Carcinoma of the Endometrium

Approximately 2.2 per cent of newborn girls, about 1 out of 45, will develop cancer of the corpus uteri at some time during their lives. It is a disease of suburbia. The greatest number of cases is found in age group 55 to 59 years, with a mean age of 61.1 years.

The first symptom is abnormal vaginal bleeding. Although cancer of the endometrium is predominantly a disease of the peri- and postmenopausal age groups, abnormal bleeding in any group should be accorded special attention. In the postmenopausal patient with abnormal uterine bleeding, a fractional curettage should be carried out. The patient must have a metastatic work-up prior to the curettage (fractional) and is staged under anesthesia.

The preoperative work-up includes routine history and physical examination, complete blood count, urinalysis, SMA-12 (urea nitrogen, glucose, calcium, phosphorus, and so forth), chest x-ray, intravenous pyelogram, and metastatic x-ray studies. *Optional* measures include proctoscopy, barium enema, cystoscopy, bone scan, and lymphangiogram.

After January 1971, a new classification was adopted (FIGO, International Federation of Gynecologists and Obstetricians), and this article follows the new classification. In the new classification, a case should be classified as carcinoma of the corpus uteri when the primary site of the growth is the corpus. Cases of mixed mesenchymal tumors and so-called carcinosarcoma should be excluded. The staging is shown in Table 2.

Treatment. The patients will be discussed according to the FIGO classification listed in Table 2.

Stage 0: Carcinoma in situ: The management should be guided by the definition established by the pathology department of a given hospital, and should be tailored to fit the needs of the patient, her age, and her desire for future childbearing. In selected young patients with minimal disease, an alternative to hysterectomy may be repeat curettage in 3 or 4 months, or a course of progestational agents followed by repeat curettage. The danger in this approach is that the carcinoma starts in the basal layer, and with the progestational agents only the compact and spongy zones are shed.

Stage Ia G1: Total hysterectomy and bilateral salpingo-oophorectomy, followed by postoperative vaginal radiation, is given.

Stage Ia G2 or G3: External pelvic radiation should be given preoperatively, followed by total

Table 2. **Clinical Staging for Cancer of the Endometrium**

Stage 0:	Carcinoma in situ. Histologic findings suggestive of malignancy. Stage 0 should not be included in the therapeutic statistics.
Stage I:	The carcinoma is confined to the corpus.
	Stage Ia: The cancer is present in a uterus measuring up to 8 cm. in length from the external os to the upper limits of the uterine cavity.
	Stage Ib: The carcinoma is present in a uterus measuring more than 8 cm. in length from the external os to the upper limits of the uterine cavity.
G1:	Highly differentiated adenomatous carcinomas.
G2:	Differentiated adenomatous carcinomas with partly solid areas.
G3:	Predominantly solid or entirely undifferentiated carcinomas.
Stage II:	The carcinoma has involved the corpus and the cervix (simultaneous presence of normal cervical glands and cancer in the same field will give the final diagnosis).
Stage III:	The carcinoma has spread outside the uterus but not outside the pelvis.
Stage IV:	The carcinoma has extended outside the true pelvis or has seriously involved the mucosa of the rectum and/or bladder. A bullous edema as such does not permit allotment of a case to Stage IV.

hysterectomy, bilateral salpingo-oophorectomy, and vaginal radiation postoperatively.

If preoperative external radiation has not been given and the surgical specimen reveals moderate or extensive myometrial invasion (one third or more of myometrial penetration), postoperative external radiation should be given. In those patients in whom the histologic grade is G2 or G3, instead of G1, external therapy should be given postoperatively.

Stage Ib: Preoperative external pelvic radiation is given, followed by total hysterectomy and bilateral salpingo-oophorectomy 6 weeks later. Postoperative vaginal radiation is indicated. The alternative to total hysterectomy may be a randomized selection of a type of radical hysterectomy.

Stage II: Preoperative external pelvic radiation is followed in 6 weeks by a modified radical hysterectomy and pelvic node dissection or a total hysterectomy. Postoperative vaginal radiation should be given. Since there is an increased incidence of pelvic nodes (up to 37 per cent) among this group, careful biopsies should be taken of the para-aortic nodes.

Stage III: If the lesion involves only the adnexal structures, preoperative x-ray therapy followed by total hysterectomy and bilateral salpingo-oophorectomy should be the treatment. Postoperatively, vaginal radiation is given. An alternative plan to total hysterectomy is to substitute a modified radical hysterectomy.

Stage IV: If the spread is limited to the pelvis with bladder and/or rectal involvement, the patient should be treated with external x-ray treatment as well as intravaginal and intrauterine radium insertion. In 4 to 6 weeks the patient should be evaluated for radical surgery. Initially, some patients may qualify for radical surgery, and if the disease is limited to the midline, pelvic exenteration should be considered as a modality of treatment.

Progestational therapy may be used in highly selected patients with advanced disease or recurrent disease. High dose progestational agents have been of benefit, especially in patients with well differentiated lesions and/or whose disease has recurred 2 or more years after initial treatment, or among those with pulmonary metastases.

In the presence of widespread disease and no response to progestational agents alone, the addition of cyclophosphamide, doxorubicin (Adriamycin), and 5-fluorouracil has given palliation. Localized symptomatic treatment that does not respond to the chemotherapy may derive benefit from x-ray therapy.

Although there are fewer indications for pelvic exenteration among patients with cancer of the endometrium than in those with cervical cancer, there is a place for pelvic exenterations among the methods of treatment used as definitive therapy for cancer of the endometrium.

CARCINOMA OF THE VULVA

method of
PAUL B. UNDERWOOD, Jr., M.D.
Charleston, South Carolina

Carcinoma of the vulva is primarily a disease of the geriatric patient and represents less than 5 per cent of the gynecologic malignancies. The majority are epidermoid carcinomas arising from the skin or mucous membranes of the vulva, although they may originate from skin appendages, Bartholin's glands, clitoris, or underlying stroma. As was not the case in the past, increasing numbers of women are seeking early medical attention for vulvar irritations and lesions. The physician should be familiar with certain premalignant conditions, even in the young female, because prevention and/or early diagnosis is the present-day answer to survival.

Premalignant Lesions

Premalignant lesions of the vulva may be classified into four categories: (1) granulomatous lesions, (2) white lesions, (3) premalignant lesions, and (4) nevi. Any vulvar irritation that does not heal with appropriate therapy must be biopsied. The accuracy of biopsy will be increased by staining the vulva with toluidine blue, which will delineate areas of epithelial hyperactivity. This technique involves the following measures: (1) wash the vulva with 1 per cent acetic acid to remove all mucus and excretions, (2) dry, (3) paint with 1 per cent toluidine blue, (4) dry, and (5) wash with 1 per cent acidic acid. Toluidine blue is a nuclear stain; hence, areas that remain blue have nuclear hyperactivity and represent areas to be sampled. Vulvar biopsy is an office procedure performed under a local anesthetic. If small, bleeding can be controlled by pressure; however, occasionally a suture of absorbable material is required for hemostasis.

The profound chronic infectious state of granuloma inguinale and longstanding condylomata acuminata with the resultant tissue reaction and scarring should be recognized as a carcinogen. Emphasis should be placed on chronicity, because in my experience, if treated early, these granulomatous lesions rarely result in carcinoma. The edematous, scarred, leather-like vulva of healed granuloma inguinale should be examined every 4 months for any ulceration. Condylomata acuminata are considered benign papillomatous lesions; however, when present for long periods of time, especially if chronically inflamed and/or ulcerated, they should be biopsied prior to the usual therapy.

The white lesion precipitates marked confusion between the terms kraurosis, lichen sclerosus et atrophicus, and atrophic and hypertrophic leukoplakia. Most authorities have recently agreed to classify these lesions as epithelial dystrophies prefixed with the words atrophic or hypertrophic. The atrophic dystrophies seldom develop malignant changes, whereas approximately 5 per cent of the hypertrophic vulvitides undergo carcinomatous changes. The management of dystrophies should be directed toward the relief of symptoms, specifically itching and dyspareunia: (1) keep the area clean and dry; (2) apply estrogen cream with 1 per cent hydrocortisone twice daily; (3) if dyspareunia is present, provide surgical relief of the introital stenosis by a midline episiotomy closed transversely; (4) with hypertrophic lesions, observe every 4 months for ulcerations or tumorfaction. Simple vulvectomies and "skinectomy" procedures should be used only when all conservative attempts fail, because in most cases a recurrence of the lesion will develop at the skin margins.

The preinvasive lesions are Bowen's disease, intraepithelial carcinoma, and Paget's disease. The eponym Bowen's disease denotes a specialized form of intraepithelial carcinoma that appears to grow more slowly; however, from the clinical standpoint, the two should be considered the same disease. These neoplastic changes usually develop in multiple areas upon the vulva, although an isolated lesion may be seen. The treatment of the solitary neoplasm should await histologic evaluation of multiple biopsies of the normal-appearing vulva. If they confirm a single abnormality, wide local excision is the treatment of choice. The typical patient with multifocal vulvar involvement can be managed either by a "skinectomy" procedure with skin graft or by a simple vulvectomy. The "skinectomy" produces excellent cosmetic results without introital stenosis. In the young female, the donor site should be from the buttocks in order to avoid embarrassing questions.

Topical 2 and 5 per cent 5-fluorouracil applied twice daily for 4 to 8 weeks has been effective in some patients. The neoplastic vulvar tissues will become ulcerated and miserable. Therefore, in my opinion, since the results are poor and the side effects high, this means of therapy should be utilized only for those patients who are believed to be medically inoperable.

Paget's disease of the vulva should not be managed by the "skinectomy" procedure, as it represents an intraepithelial spread of invasive adenocarcinoma and has a tendency to follow hair shafts. Also, truly invasive carcinoma below the epithelium can be found in approximately 10 per cent. A simple vulvectomy is therefore the treatment of choice. If invasive carcinoma is discovered after removal, a bilateral groin dissection should be performed at a later stage. The neoplastic cells involve the epithelium far beyond the gross lesion; therefore very wide margins should be obtained. If available, frozen sections of the margins for confirmation of adequacy should be obtained at the operating room table.

Five per cent of all melanomas are found on the perineum, which represents only 1 per cent of the body's skin surface. Since the majority occur after the age of 35, all vulvar nevi should be removed at the time of delivery as a worthwhile means of preventive medicine.

Invasive Carcinoma

The prognosis of a patient with invasive carcinoma is directly associated with the degree of differentiation, the size of the lesion, and its location. Most vulvar carcinomas are well differentiated; however, those arising from the clitoris are notoriously poorly differentiated. Malignancies of the clitoris or Bartholin's glands have a worse prognosis. Those occurring on the perineal body and posterior vestibule require wide labial excision, because the lymphatic drainage of the vulva swings farther lateral the more posterior the lesion. Carcinomas involving the distal urethra and lower vagina require a more radical approach. The size of the lesion is directly related to the incidence of lymph node metastasis.

The lymph drainage of the vulva is to the inguinal and femoral nodes. These nodes drain through Cloquet's nodes (a lymph node lying medial to the femoral vein and beneath the inguinal ligament) to the deep pelvic nodes. Vulvar carcinomas always involve the groin nodes before they involve the pelvic nodes, except for lesions of the clitoris in which the groin may be bypassed and the carcinoma metastasize directly to the deep pelvic nodes. Lymphatic drainage may extend to the contralateral groin, especially from the anterior vulva. The incidence of nodal metastasis varies from approximately 5 per cent for lesions less than 2 cm. in diameter to over 50 per cent for those greater than 7 cm.

With these facts in mind, therapy can be planned accordingly. The basic procedure is an en bloc radical vulvectomy and bilateral groin dissection. Cloquet's nodes should be resected separately and sent for frozen section. If positive, a deep pelvic lymphadenectomy is performed at the same sitting. If negative, the additional surgery and its complications do not warrant the pelvic lymphadenectomy. For reasons previously described, clitoral lesions are exceptions. Because of skin lymphatics, a 1 to 2 inch segment overlying the inguinal ligament and continuous with the vulva should be removed.

The technique for the groin dissection that I prefer is to undermine the abdominal skin for about 3 inches above the inguinal ligament and the skin of the thigh to the apex of the femoral triangle. All fatty and lymphatic tissue over the external oblique fascia is cleaned to the inguinal ligament. The fascia lata is incised along the sartorius muscle from the inguinal ligament to the apex of the femoral triangle, followed by its incision over the abductus longus muscle to the same apex. The saphenous vein is identified and double ligated as it exits this tissue mass. The fascia lata is incised from the inguinal ligament, beginning laterally and extending medially. By this technique, the femoral nerve, artery, and vein are cleaned of their lymphatic tissue without disturbing the more superficial lymph canals. This mass of fatty tissue is resected en bloc with the vulva. The more anterior the lesion, the more mons pubis one removes. The farther posterior, the farther lateral the labia majora are incised. If the urethra is involved, its distal one third can be excised without incontinence ensuing. All vulvar tissues external to the urogenital diaphragm are removed. The usual specimen is terminated distal to the hymen; however, the lower one third of the vagina can be excised by this approach. A finger in the rectum will permit a deeper dissection over the bowel without fear of entering it.

The technique for closure of this enormous defect is vital to prevent morbidity and complications. The sartorius muscle is excised from its origin and sutured to the inguinal ligament overlying the femoral vessels for their protection. The perineal skin and the vaginal mucosa are undermined for 2 to 3 cm. This permits closure without tension and places the suture line outside the vaginal orifice, thereby decreasing introital stenosis. A Z-plasty closure is also beneficial. Caution should be taken not to pull the urethra over the symphysis, as this may produce stress incontinence.

Suction catheters should be placed beneath the groin flaps. The groin incision should be closed with subcuticular absorbable suture to prevent folding of the skin at the suture line which may produce slough. Pressure dressings are contraindicated.

The secret to primary wound healing is immaculate wound cleanliness for 10 to 14 days. I emphasize cleaning all suture lines every 8 hours (not three times a day) with hydrogen peroxide. The patient is maintained at bed rest with feet elevated 15 degrees (to prevent thrombophlebitis) for 7 days. Suction drainage to the groins and bladder catheter is continued for a similar time. Prophylactic antibiotics are utilized. An over-the-bed cradle with a light bulb aids in maintaining dry suture lines.

If necrosis develops in the skin flaps, keep the area dry and observe as long as tensile strength of the devitalized tissue exists. This permits time for the skin flap to stick. Debridement is performed only after separation has occurred. At this point, wet soaks with one quarter strength Dakin's solution aids in wound granulation. Only rarely is skin grafting necessary.

Chronic lymphedema of the leg is another complication. For prophylaxis, elastic stockings are to be worn during awake hours for at least 3 months. Lymphangitis will contribute to permanent leg edema; therefore since most infections are streptococcal, prophylactic penicillin or erythromycin should be maintained for 1 year.

Radiation plays only a minor role in therapy of vulvar malignancies owing to its poor tolerance. Enormous lesions can be shrunk with 3000 rads delivered through a perineal port prior to radical surgery. Prophylactic irradiation to the groin and pelvis may be utilized with incomplete resection of tumor but usually produces permanent lymphedema of the leg.

Primary exenterative procedures are indicated for enormous lesions involving over one third of the urethra and vagina, or any part of the rectum. In special instances, an ileal conduit or colostomy can be utilized to permanently divert the excretory stream, permitting radical excision without the morbidity of the exenteration.

Other rare malignancies of the vulva are worthy of mention. Basal cell carcinomas do occur in the vulvar area, but usually in women over 60 years of age. Treatment is local wide resection. A low grade fibrosarcoma is occasionally seen in the subepithelial tissues. It generally metastasizes only in late stages; therefore radical local excision is adequate therapy. To the contrary, a rare, highly malignant rhabdomyosarcoma may develop in the inferior labia majora of teenagers. One should consider this diagnosis when an apparent Bartholin gland cellulitis does not heal by the usual means of therapy. A radical vulvectomy with bilateral groin and deep pelvic node dissection followed by postoperative chemotherapy with doxorubicin (Adriamycin) or VAC (vincristine, actinomycin D, and cyclophosphamide) for at least 1 year is the treatment of choice. Unfortunately, this tumor is usually beyond resection at the time of diagnosis. In such instances, local radiation plus the aforementioned chemotherapy becomes the treatment of choice. The prognosis for survival approaches zero. Another uncommon malignancy of the vulva is a melanoma. Therapy should be ultraradical excision extending to the depth of the urogenital diaphragm along with radical groin and deep pelvic node dissection.

PREOPERATIVE AND POSTOPERATIVE CARE FOR ELECTIVE GYNECOLOGY SURGERY

method of
MICHAEL K. KOWALSKI, M.D., MAJ, MC,
and ROBERT C. PARK, M.D., COL, MC
Washington, D.C.

Introduction

Many of the problems and diagnostic tests in gynecology are accomplished as outpatient or office procedures involving minor surgical or nonsurgical methods.

Once a decision to perform major surgery is made, it is assumed that all alternatives to conservative methods have been exhausted or at least discussed. Because the majority of gynecologic surgery is elective, frequently both patient and physician lose sight of the seriousness of a surgical procedure. Thus our first principle of elective surgery is set forth—that principle is adequate and thorough preoperative counseling.

Counseling

In the present medical-legal atmosphere, the concept of informed consent cannot be overemphasized. Some of the key elements of adequate counseling include the following:

Diagnosis or Differential Diagnosis. A gynecologic diagnosis can be difficult to explain to a patient in nonmedical terminology. We try to place the diagnosis in layman's terms, reflecting the pathophysiology, eventual outcome, and prognosis of the disease process in surgical and nonsurgical approaches.

Hazards of Surgery. Potential risks of the proposed surgical procedure are discussed in detail, with emphasis on the more common complications. This part of the counseling process is extremely variable and depends much on patient rapport, patient understanding, and intellectual level.

A patient can never be overcounseled, but inappropriate details can be overemphasized. Therefore care must be used not to generate undue anxiety.

Extent of Surgery. The patient should enter surgery with a reasonable expectation of how much surgery is to be accomplished. This is especially true of gynecology, because a large percentage of our procedures are extirpative. Too often a patient becomes a "psychologic cripple" because of unexpected extensions of the basic operation. Only in an extreme emergency should extirpative procedures be considered without adequate counseling and consent.

Expected Results. As gynecologists we realize that the result of reconstructive and extirpative surgery is not always predictable. We must, however, give attention to detail, especially in areas of sexual activity, convalescence, physical limitations, and desired objective of the surgical procedure.

Anesthesia. Although discussion of anesthesia properly rests with the anesthesiologist, some comment should be included by the surgeon regarding risks and choice of anesthesia. The surgeon has more extensive understanding of the patient's fears and anxieties and will help bridge any gap between the anesthesiologist and patient.

A husband, family member, or consort is encouraged to be present at the counseling session.

This proves to be very valuable, especially if the unexpected arises during surgery.

Patient Evaluation

The second basic principle of elective gynecologic surgery is adequate patient evaluation. Because we perform mainly elective surgery on a relatively young, healthy population, minor but very significant concurrent problems can be overlooked. It is not unusual to have a female patient attend only her gynecologist, and therefore the responsibility for detection and surveillance of routine medical problems rests with him.

A complete history, physical examination, and review of all organ systems is an absolute necessity prior to any surgical procedure. A thorough review of past medical history and previous records, if available, is valuable. Only in this manner can consultations be chosen for areas out of the gynecologic specialty.

Laboratory Evaluation. Laboratory evaluation consists of complete blood count, urine analysis, colony count, VDRL, and chest x-ray. In addition, an electrocardiogram is frequently indicated. Other laboratory tests are ordered on an individual basis. The value of screening with routine preoperative prothrombin and partial thromboplastin on all patients is questionable and can never substitute for an adequate bleeding history.

A recent Papanicolaou smear of the cervix is a requirement. In patients who have abnormal uterine bleeding, diagnostic endometrial sampling by aspiration or dilatation and curettage (D&C) is accomplished prior to hysterectomy.

When abnormal, a systematic evaluation with colposcopy and directed biopsy, prior to admission for surgery, is indicated.

Situations Which Deserve Special Evaluation. PELVIC MASS. An intravenous pyelogram or retrograde cystogram and barium enema should be performed. If there is any indication of possible bowel involvement, a general surgeon is consulted and a bowel preparation is initiated.

URINARY STRESS INCONTINENCE. Additional work-up prior to the decision of surgery includes intravenous pyelogram (IVP), cystoscopy, stress test, and urethroscopy. A chain cystourethrogram is rarely performed, as we depend mainly upon urethroscopy and bladder cystometrics.

Surgery Scheduling. Every attempt is made to schedule surgery in the proliferative phase of the menstrual cycle. Pregnancy tests are ordered when adequate contraceptive history is missing, menstrual history is irregular, or uterine enlargement is present.

In situations in which diagnostic or therapeutic minor surgery is performed prior to hysterectomy, as in the case of D&C or cone biopsy, major surgery is accomplished within 48 hours or after 6 weeks to avoid the effects of inflammation or healing.

No attempt is made to discontinue birth control pills prior to a surgical procedure; however, surgery is avoided during the menstrual period.

Routine Orders

Orders are needed to communicate desired objectives. They should be clear, concise, and well conceived. This is especially true of elective surgery.

Preoperative Orders. 1. Admission for elective procedure.

2. Diagnosis.

3. Diet: based on condition of the patient and on the problem.

4. Nothing by mouth: required for a period at least 8 hours preoperatively to allow the stomach to empty and reduce the risk of vomiting and aspiration.

5. Activity: maximum consistent with diagnosis.

6. Vital signs—pulse, blood pressure, respiratory rate—once per day. If temperature is desired more than once daily, this should be so stated.

7. Antibacterial douche (povidone-iodine).

8. Antibacterial shower and shampoo the evening prior to surgery (povidone-iodine or hexachlorophene).

9. Cleansing enema: Fleet's or saline.

10. Sleep medication.

11. Abdominal-perineal preparation in major surgery and diagnostic laparoscopy when abdominal procedure may follow.

12. Signing of permit: ensure that the name of the operating surgeon and indication that the patient was counseled is present, as well as the procedure proposed.

13. Foley catheter to be inserted, if indicated, or void on call to operating room (OR).

14. Prophylactic antibiotic. We feel these have been proved of value for at least vaginal surgery, and use a broad-spectrum antibiotic prior to surgery and 24 hours postoperatively—e.g., vibramycin, 100 mg. orally on the evening prior to surgery and 100 mg. intravenously on call to the operating room, followed by 100 mg. intravenously twice daily for 24 hours.

15. Preoperative medications as ordered by anesthesia.

16. Special orders, such as bowel preparation, catheter care, and central venous pressure are individualized.

Postoperative Orders. The orders written postoperatively void all prior orders.

1. A statement of the operative procedure and condition of patient, indicating the surgical procedure and complications, informs the staff of the general nature of care that is going to be required postoperatively.

2. Vital signs should be recorded frequently until stable and then less often as they stabilize—e.g., every 15 minutes until stable, then every 30 minutes for 2 hours, then every 4 hours.

3. Diet: depends upon type of surgery and anesthesia. Patients are usually kept on no oral intake (NPO) until bowel activity is present. Intravenous fluids are ordered to maintain adequate fluid and electrolyte balance.

4. Intake and output record.

5. Activity: depends upon type of surgery and anesthesia; early ambulation is encouraged.

6. Medications: pain medication augmented with sedation is individualized to provide pain relief and allow maximal activity.

7. Special instructions: (a) Usually the Foley catheter can be removed when the patient is ambulatory except in urethropexy or an extensive extirpative procedure. When cystotomy is performed, double drainage of the bladder is desired for 8 to 10 days. (b) Every effort is made to employ suprapubic catheterization when long-term drainage of the bladder is required. The care of the suprapubic catheter depends upon the physician and should be delegated to others only when responsibility and ability have been established. (c) Incentive respirometry and pulmonary toilet are used routinely on all major procedures.

8. Laboratory tests: individualized.

9. Special circumstances—tubes, drains, and packs: instructions should be included to make the staff aware of required care.

10. If infection is present, a note should be included in the orders to provide care appropriate with infection control.

Discharge Instructions

Discharge counseling is considered an integral part of postoperative care. Time is taken to explain in detail postoperative instructions, medi-

TABLE 1. **Example of Discharge Instructions**

GYNECOLOGY
WALTER REED ARMY MEDICAL CENTER

NAME__________________ DATE____________

DISCHARGE INSTRUCTIONS
FOLLOW-UP APPOINTMENT IN THE OUTPATIENT GYNECOLOGY CLINIC

Please obtain an appointment for a follow-up examination in the Gynecology Clinic in ________ weeks. Make this appointment through the Ward Secretary before leaving (if discharged during the week) or by calling ________ on the first working day after discharge (if discharged on a weekend). Please have your Outpatient Card available so you can give your number to the secretary making the appointment.

It is important that the following instructions be carried out after discharge from the hospital:

1. Take your temperature orally *twice* daily for *10* days and report any elevation over 100°F. (37.8°C.).
2. Report any *unusual* or disturbing symptoms at once. Should any complication arise prior to your appointment, call ________.
3. Refrain from sexual intercourse and douching for ________ weeks.
4. You may start taking tub baths after ________ weeks. Until then take a shower or sponge bath daily. You may wash your hair, preferably in the shower if you have an abdominal incision.
5. Any prolonged tiring exertion should be avoided. Do not permit yourself to become exhausted for the first few days.
6. Riding short distances in a vehicle is permissible now. However, riding long distances and driving should be avoided for ________ weeks.
7. Major surgery patients should usually limit stair climbing to one or two times a day when first arriving home and progressively increase this activity as their strength improves.
8. Activity should increase gradually and progressively within your limits of tolerance. Common sense should be used liberally.
9. You should be able to resume all your former activities gradually, starting in ________ weeks.
10. If your doctor gives you vaginal cream, apply one-half applicator at night as instructed.
11. Medications: ____________ Directions: ____________
12. Other:

____________ M.D.

cations, and reinforcement of the appropriate items of preoperative counseling.

Because this is a period of anxiety and stress in the patient, written instructions are provided for referral at home. This greatly reduces postoperative misunderstanding.

As with any large clinical service, we provide the patient with phone numbers for follow-up and ensure that the patient has an appropriate postoperative visit schedule.

An example of discharge instructions is listed in Table 1.

Postoperative Care

The postoperative visit completes the patient's operative care. At this time documentation of the diagnosis, pathologic findings, and operative procedures is included in the patient's record for further reference. Interim history and examination for operative healing and result should be accomplished. The patient should be counseled regarding activity and return appointment.

THROMBOPHLEBITIS

method of
ALAN L. KAPLAN, M.D.,
and SAM T. SCALING, M.D.
Houston, Texas

Venous thrombosis is generally classified as superficial or deep. If a thrombus affects a superficial vein, the symptoms and findings differ greatly from those found when a major deep vein of an extremity is involved. Moreover the implications, the risks, and the therapeutic measures for each vary tremendously. Superficial vein thrombosis usually runs a short course of gradual improvement. It rarely is of major significance or results in any significant complications. The treatment is conservative and symptomatic.

Deep vein thrombosis is a serious problem, and the discussion to follow concerns itself with this entity in obstetrics and gynecology.

Septic or suppurative pelvic thrombophlebitis is an uncommon but potentially grave complication of pyogenic, usually gestational, pelvic infection. This entity will be considered separately.

Gynecology

For the gynecologist, deep thrombophlebitis is essentially a postoperative problem, although since the advent of the birth control pill, he now not infrequently encounters it in a setting unassociated with surgery. The treatment method is directed toward the postoperative patient.

Prophylaxis. 1. Discontinue oral contraception. Retrospective studies report an increased risk of postsurgery thromboembolic complications in oral contraceptive users. It is recommended that therapy be discontinued at least 1 month prior to elective gynecologic surgery.

2. Early ambulation.

3. Compression bandages or stockings. This should be done routinely in the patient with varicosities but is not always necessary in the ordinary patient.

4. Mini-dose heparin. This should be considered in the patient who may be at risk for a thromboembolic complication. Five thousand units of heparin is given subcutaneously 2 hours before surgery and then every 8 hours for 7 days postoperatively. With this regimen, a slight increase in intra- or postoperative bleeding may be noted.

Active Treatment. CONSERVATIVE MEASURES. Ambulant interrupted activity, compression stockings, and proper elevation of the legs while at rest.

ANTICOAGULANTS. Anticoagulant drugs have proved of great value in reducing the progression of thrombosis, in shortening its course, and in preventing pulmonary embolism.

1. Heparin. This can be given by continuous intravenous administration; by single bolus intravenous injections at repeated intervals, usually every 4 to 6 hours; or by a third route, intramuscularly, and then usually in a slow absorption medium (Depo-Heparin). The continuous intravenous administration is preferred. This is given at a rate to maintain the Lee-White coagulation time within the desired range of 15 to 25 minutes or two and one-half to three times control. This usually necessitates 5000 to 10,000 units every 8 hours.

2. Warfarin sodium (Coumadin sodium). If a prothrombinemic drug is used, warfarin is the preferable one at present, as it is a much easier drug to manage than dicumarol. Its effectiveness can be induced much more rapidly, and it is much more controllable. If the patient shows signs of a bleeding tendency, cessation of the drug and administration of vitamin K_1 (phytonadione) orally or intravenously promptly bring about a shift toward normal in the prothrombin time, and the bleeding tendency is obviated within 2 hours, a control which, with dicumarol, would require at least 24 hours. The dose of warfarin is 35 to 50 mg. a day as an initial dose and as little as 5 mg. a day for a maintenance dose, depending on the prothrombin time.

SURGERY. Surgery can be lifesaving in many patients and in these instances is clearly indicated. The single objective of surgery is to prevent recurrent pulmonary embolism. Proximal major vein ligation is considered in that patient who has shown evidence of one episode of pulmonary embolization.

Obstetrics

When seen prenatally, deep vein thrombophlebitis should be treated aggressively, followed by consideration of prophylaxis or continued active therapy throughout the remainder of pregnancy. Determinant factors in this decision are (1) the severity and duration of the signs and symptoms, (2) the presence of complications such as pulmonary embolism, and (3) a recurrent episode.

Prophylaxis. 1. Compression stockings.

2. Adequate exercise and activity.

3. Mini-dose heparin.

Active Therapy. CONSERVATIVE MEASURES. Identical to those utilized for the postoperative patient; ambulant interrupted activity, elevation, and compression stockings.

ANTICOAGULATION. As previously described, the two drugs commonly used are heparin and warfarin (Coumadin). Heparin is preferred prenatally for several reasons: (1) it does not cross the placental barrier as does warfarin, and it does not appear in breast milk; thus the potential risk of perinatal or neonatal hemorrhage is alleviated by using heparin; (2) anticoagulation with heparin is more rapidly reversed than with warfarin; and (3) the question has been raised regarding the possible teratogenicity of warfarin when used in the first trimester.

1. In administering heparin, continuous intravenous administration is preferred.

2. In patients in whom warfarin is used prenatally, the goal is to keep the prothrombin time at two and one-half to three times control.

3. Intrapartum anticoagulation. It is desirable to stop active anticoagulation prior to or at the onset of labor, especially if warfarin is being used. This process can be facilitated if elective induction or operative delivery is planned.

4. Postpartum anticoagulation. This should be continued for 10 to 14 days. Warfarin is preferable unless the patient is breast feeding.

Septic Pelvic Thrombophlebitis

Heparin. This is administered by continuous intravenous infusion identically to its use with deep vein thrombosis.

Antibiotics. Broad-spectrum coverage should be administered. The bacteriology of this problem has not yet been precisely defined; however, the anaerobic Streptococcus is known to be a common offender, and the importance of other anaerobes, particularly Bacteroides species, has been appreciated in recent years. Our preference is a combination of penicillin, clindamycin, and an aminoglycoside.

Surgery. If there is no significant response to medical therapy within 48 to 72 hours, exploratory laparotomy is indicated. Total abdominal hysterectomy with bilateral salpingo-oophorectomy and ligation of the inferior vena cava and ovarian veins is the procedure of choice.

CONTRACEPTION

method of
AQUILES J. SOBRERO, M.D.,
and JOHN J. SCIARRA, M.D.
Chicago, Illinois

Presently available methods of fertility control can be considered as a spectrum ranging from relatively ineffectual techniques such as the vaginal douche to highly effective methods such as surgical sterilization and voluntary interruption of pregnancy which afford virtually absolute protection.

Patients seeking contraception are interested in regulating or controlling their fertility, usually temporarily and in a reversible manner; physicians and patients alike are concerned about use effectiveness, systemic effects and risks, convenience, reversibility, and cost.

The ideal contraceptive is highly effective, safe, aesthetically acceptable, reversible, and inexpensive. It has no deleterious side effects and is easy to store and simple to use. Further, it does not require special skills or professional intervention—i.e., it is easily self-administered. Its physical properties make it easily stocked and distributed. It has a long shelf life and is light, inconspicuous, and not bulky. Finally, its application is independent of the sexual act. As yet, for a large segment of the population, the imminence of coitus and the fear of its possible consequences are the only stimuli that arouse interest in contraception.

As with all ideals, the contraceptive that will satisfy the various needs of all women and all men does not now and perhaps never will exist, because personal situations and requirements change from time to time and are subject to many social, cultural, and economic influences.

Effectiveness

Users of contraceptive methods can be classified either as *spacers* (those who are temporary or occasional users, postponing pregnancy to a later time) or as *limiters* (who consider that they have completed their family or do not want a pregnancy, or who medically or economically cannot afford one). Patients in this category are quite determined to make a method work or, if an accidental pregnancy occurs, to obtain a pregnancy termination. Because of the motivational factor, there is a difference between these two groups in use effectiveness, with the best results occurring among the limiters and occasionally even matching theoretical effectiveness.

The term use effectiveness means "protection from unwanted pregnancy achieved by users under real life conditions, including the effects of carelessness, ambivalence, and other manifestations of human frailty"; theoretical effectiveness, on the other hand, refers to "the antifertility action of a method under laboratory conditions. Outside the laboratory, theoretical effectiveness implies perfect usage, without omissions or errors of any kind" (Tietze, 1971).

There are great variations in the reported rates of effectiveness of presently available contraceptives. The best rates are shown in clinical studies utilizing careful patient selection by the investigative team, with a considerable input of resources to diminish losses to follow-up and thus to increase the reliability of the data; this investigative approach serves also to reinforce instructions for correct use and to counter weakening motivation. Thus the results of most clinical studies tend to be better than the actual performance of any given method in general use, wherein a method is more subject to human failure.

The effectiveness of contraceptive methods is most often expressed according to the Pearl formula, in pregnancies (accidental or unwanted) per 100 woman years of use (or 1200 months). The Pearl formula is stated as follows:

$$\text{Failure rate} = \frac{\text{Number of pregnancies} \times 1200}{\text{Total months of use}}$$

A more modern expression of contraceptive effectiveness is calculated by the life table method, as recommended by Tietze.

According to the data of the 1970 National Fertility Study, analyzed by the life table procedure, younger women in the U.S.A. had accidental unwanted pregnancies more often than older women, and 26 per cent of couples failed in the first year to delay a pregnancy they would have preferred later, whereas 14 per cent failed to prevent a pregnancy that was never intended. Only 66 per cent of those couples who did not intend to have additional children were successful in avoiding pregnancy after 5 years of contraceptive use, Catholics and the young having the largest percentage of failures.

These national figures indicate a need for continuing follow-up of users, reiteration of instructions, change of method as necessary, and information for limiters about the availability of male and female sterilization and, for women with an unwanted pregnancy, about the availability of elective pregnancy interruption as a backup method, at a medically opportune time.

Contraception properly prescribed and intelligently used contributes to a lowering of the number of children who are unwanted, to a reduction in maternal and infant mortality, and to better control of genetically transmitted disorders.

Choice of Method

Table 1 lists the presently available contraceptive methods. Not included are methods still under study or not available in the United States.

In general, in the absence of contraindications, the patient's choice should be followed, because continuation of successful use of a contraceptive method is basically dependent on personal motivation and on the individual acceptability of the method. Discontinuance is often due to psychologic factors, such as fear of side effects, doubt of efficacy, ambivalence about pregnancy, shame or guilt (pregnancy as self-punishment), need to prove sexual identity through pregnancy, coital "gamesmanship" or hostility ("getting even" with the sexual partner, parents, or family), and equating love with risk-taking. The availability and acceptability of abortion may also be an important factor in both selection of method and the degree of dedication toward its continued use. The patient should always be informed that effective alternative methods are available and that the physician is willing to provide them in case of dissatisfaction with the one chosen. Benefits, undesirable side effects, and potential risks should be explained in terms comprehensible to the patient, without exciting unnecessary fears which might be conducive to the abandonment of contraception. An important consideration that both physician and patient should bear in mind is that maternal mortality risks are 5 to 15 times higher than all the risks attributed to contraceptive use.

It is estimated that, in the United States, between 28 and 34 per cent of women of reproductive age who are coitally active use oral contracep-

TABLE 1. **Relative Effectiveness of Various Contraceptive Methods, Expressed as Number of Unwanted Pregnancies per 100 Woman Years* (Estimates Based on Clinical Studies)**

METHOD	THEORETICAL EFFECTIVENESS	USE EFFECTIVENESS
Oral contraceptives		
Combination pills	0.1	0.2
Progestogen alone	1	3
Intrauterine devices	2	5
Barrier methods		
Condom and spermicide	1	5
Diaphragm and jelly	3	13
Condom alone	3	15
Foam or jelly alone	5	20
Coitus interruptus	3	15–23
Rhythm or periodic abstinence	14	35–40
Douche		35–40
No method	80	80
Surgical methods		
Vasectomy	0	<0.15
Tubal ligation—surgical	0	0.04
Tubal sterilization—electrocoagulation	0	0.01
Hysterectomy	0	0.0001
Abortion	0	0

*Modified from Meeker, C. I., and Gray, M. J.: Birth control, abortion, and sterilization. *In* Romney, S. L., et al. (eds.): Gynecology and Obstetrics: The Health Care of Women. New York, McGraw-Hill Book Company, 1975.

tive (OC) agents; in about 16 per cent of couples one spouse has been sterilized; 14 per cent use the condom, 7 per cent use the intrauterine device (IUD), and 6 per cent use the diaphragm.

In prescribing a contraceptive, the physician should take into consideration the patient's life style and ethical values, and should be nonjudgmental and unbiased in discussing the various methods available.

The Sexually Active Young Adult Woman

The provision of reliable reversible contraception to sexually active teenagers or single young adults is a controversial and difficult matter for the physician. Since many such patients have not yet established regular menstrual cycles or demonstrated their fertility, there are medical reasons for reluctance to prescribe oral contraceptives. All OC preparations exert a powerful pharmacologic effect on the hypothalamus, and the degree of functional maturity and ability to resume normal function on discontinuance of the OC is unknown for many of these young patients. Even if a regular menstrual pattern exists, casual and inconsistent use of an OC by teenagers and young women is very common, with the subsequent consequence of an unwanted pregnancy.

Theoretically, the IUD would seem to be a better choice for such patients, as only initial motivation is required and discontinuation demands a positive action. But insertion of an IUD in a nulligravid uterus is not always easy; it may require cervical dilatation, with inordinate pain and even vagotonic syncope. Also, the high incidence of coitally transmissible diseases among sexually active unmarried young adults makes these patients more susceptible to pelvic inflammatory disease with its complications, which in turn may affect future fertility.

Although this group of patients presents the physician with some particularly difficult problems, clinical investigators have had good results using either OCs or IUDs in teenagers and young adult women. It cannot be too strongly emphasized, however, that such results cannot be obtained without sensitive medical personnel providing a friendly and nonjudgmental atmosphere and careful and frequent follow-up so as to reinforce motivation and ensure repeated instruction for correct use.

In general, it is preferable to prescribe OCs for coitally active teenagers or young adult women who have demonstrated a regular menstrual pattern, provided that there is some basis for believing that regularity in OC intake can be expected. But if the physician is concerned that ovulatory dysfunction may be present or if an unwanted pregnancy has already occurred with OC use, the IUD may be preferable.

In some contraceptive programs for young adults, especially those involving "emancipated" teenagers, those with one or more pregnancies already, or patients with limited intelligence and education, an injectable progestogen (medroxyprogesterone acetate) has been recommended; however, this pharmacologic agent is not marketed for this purpose in the United States.

Hormonal Contraceptives

Clinical studies of oral contraceptives began in 1956, and in 1962 OCs were made available to the physician for prescription. Initially, they were approved for use for not longer than 2 years, but rapidly this limitation was extended to 4 years, and in 1967 all limitations were lifted. OCs have fulfilled and even surpassed many of the hopes regarding their effectiveness; however, as their use has involved larger segments of the population, a long list of undesirable side effects has been attributed to or associated with them. According to some estimates, OCs have been used at one time or another by 100 million women since they became available, and approximately 50 million women worldwide are using them currently. When a powerful drug has been so widely used, it is no surprise to find that a certain number of women will experience untoward side effects and be forced to seek other forms of contraception. Economic factors, inaccessibility of medical care, or the necessity for periodic medical examinations and other personal considerations may also lead to discontinuation.

The number and composition of OCs have changed over the years, and some preparations are no longer available. Combination type OCs (those in which every tablet contains fixed amounts of a synthetic estrogen and a synthetic progestogen) and "minipills," containing progestogen alone, are available in the United States; the sequential type of OC has been withdrawn from the market. The "once-a-month" OC never advanced beyond limited field studies. The two synthetic estrogens used in pill formulations in the United States are ethinyl estradiol (EE) and mestranol. The five progestogens used in the United States in contraceptive formulations are all derivatives of 19-nortestosterone.

Combination type OCs have a theoretical effectiveness of 100 per cent; their accepted failure rates in use (use effectiveness) are given in Table 1. Since all the formulations provide excellent contraceptive effectiveness, the current clinical trend is to prescribe the lowest dosage that will provide cycle control and regularity of withdrawal bleeding without breakthrough bleeding. Minimizing undesirable side effects is also an important consideration. It remains to be demonstrated, however, that lowering the dose will substantially reduce serious side effects or, equally important, provide better continuation rates.

When an OC has been used correctly for several months, and especially toward the end of a medication cycle, the missing of a few tablets (1 to 4) will probably result not in unwanted pregnancy but only in unscheduled uterine, or breakthrough, bleeding. This, however, may not be the situation with the low dose preparations, because the control of the hypothalamus may be borderline and ovulatory "escapes" and pregnancy might occur, especially when a few tablets are missed early in the medication cycle. For this reason, whenever 2 or more tablets have been missed, it is advisable to resume the medication, meanwhile adding a barrier method for the remainder of the medication cycle.

The combined type of pill is most often administered as 1 tablet daily, in cycles of 21 tablets, with 7 days free of medication—i.e., 3 weeks on medication and 1 week off. With the first OC cycle, medication should be initiated on the fifth day from the beginning of menstruation following a nonmedicated cycle. Thereafter, the first pill is taken after 7 days without medication. Some physicians advise adding a second method of contraception, such as foam, during the first OC cycle, especially when a very low dose OC is prescribed. Other physicians modify the first OC cycle by adding or subtracting a few tablets so that the first medication cycle ends on a Sunday, and thus all therapeutic cycles will continue to begin on a weekly basis, with the initial tablet always taken on a Sunday.

The same combined OC preparations may be found in packages containing 28 tablets, of which 21 contain the estrogen and progestogen and 7 are devoid of medication; these 7 tablets occasionally contain iron or multivitamins.

The "minipill," containing progestogen alone, is dispensed in a continuous regimen, 1 tablet daily without any time off the medication.

In general, it is advisable for the patient to take the OC at the same time each day, preferably after a meal or before retiring, to minimize gastrointestinal effects. Many women, however, prefer taking the pill on a daily basis every morning. This is a matter of individual preference which does not influence the efficacy of the medication.

A follow-up visit should be scheduled 1 month from the initiation of OC therapy. This visit provides an opportunity to find early intolerance of the OCs, to dispel unfounded fears, to answer questions that may have arisen since the OC was prescribed, to reiterate instructions, or to recommend an alternative form of contraception that may be better tolerated or accepted by the patient. Subsequent follow-up visits may be scheduled every 6 months, at which time blood pressure and weight should be recorded, breasts, abdomen, and legs should be examined, and a pelvic examination performed. Some physicians prefer yearly follow-up visits once the patient is comfortable with the chosen medication. An annual cervical smear for cytology should be performed. Some physicians also include an office urinalysis and SMA-12 and a gonorrhea culture or smear on a semiannual or annual basis, depending on age and social situation of the patient.

The benefits to be expected from the use of OCs are a high degree of effectiveness, coital independence and freedom from genital manipulation, regulation of menstruation, decrease of dysmenorrhea and premenstrual tension, decrease of menstrual flow, possible palliative effect on endometriosis, and possible improvement of acne and of hirsutism.

Accepted contraindications for OCs—those indicated by the FDA and those listed by most clinical investigators—are shown in Table 2. Despite the long list of contraindications, after a careful history and physical examination, approximately 85 per cent of women wishing to use OCs can safely use them, and of this group, 70 to 90 per cent tolerate them well.

TABLE 2. **Contraindications for Oral Contraceptives**

Absolute
- History of thrombophlebitis or thromboembolic disorders; deep vein, pulmonary, or myocardial thrombosis or cerebrovascular accidents; or predisposing conditions to any of these conditions
- Active liver disease; history of idiopathic jaundice or pruritus of pregnancy
- Known or suspected carcinoma of the breasts or estrogen-dependent neoplasia
- Progressive malignant hypertension
- Severe cardiorenal disease
- Congenital hyperlipidemia
- History of diabetes of pregnancy
- Sickle cell disease
- Vaginal adenosis

Relative
- History of migraine headaches
- Hypertension
- Obesity
- Diabetes mellitus or strong family history of diabetes
- History of cholecystitis, cholelithiasis or gallbladder disease, or cholecystectomy
- Active cardiac or renal disease
- Sickle cell trait
- Chloasma
- Submucous leiomyomas
- Epilepsy
- History of depression
- Forgetfulness, casualness, unreliability, mental retardation
- Irregular menstrual cycles: oligomenorrhea, amenorrhea
- Period of growth not completed
- Age of 40 years or over

Temporary
- Known or suspected pregnancy
- Immediate puerperium (4 weeks)
- Nursing
- Elective surgery planned within 4 to 6 weeks
- Postsurgical convalescence
- Undiagnosed abnormal vaginal bleeding

Mechanism of Action of OCs. All commercially available OCs (Table 3) utilize one of two estrogens, either ethinyl estradiol (EE) or its 3-methylether, mestranol. Controversy continues as to whether EE is pharmacologically superior or is equal to mestranol in potency and toxicity. There is a tendency, however, to attribute more activity and possibly less liver toxicity to EE, but this is not conclusive. Note that several preparations are similar chemically, but are marketed with different names by different pharmaceutical companies.

In assessing the various preparations, the physician should recognize that, in the body, additive effects may occur between the different progestogens and the two estrogens. The effects of the different combinations vary from patient to patient, according to numerous factors independent of the drugs. Thus potency ratings, which are in general based on pharmacologic action in different species, have only partial relevance to human use and should be considered subject to these limitations.

The contraceptive action of OCs of the combined type occurs primarily through a suppression of gonadotropin release. This occurs mainly through a negative feedback of the estrogen and the progestogen on the hypothalamus, with the exogenous hormones decreasing gonadotropin release and suppressing the preovulatory estrogen peak. The net effect on the patient therefore is to inhibit ovulation. Other effects attributed to OCs are alteration of tubal transport, assumed to occur especially with more estrogenic progestogens (norethynodrel) and pills high in estrogen content; changes in the endometrium, characterized by a regression of the proliferative phase, with incomplete gland development and overt progestational changes resulting in an exhausted or mixed type endometrium; and rapid progestational changes in the cervical mucus, which becomes scant, thickened, tacky, opaque, and hostile to sperm penetration and migration. With norethynodrel, however, one may find mucus which is not hostile to sperm penetration or survival.

Common Side Effects. The most frequent side effects experienced with OC use are gastrointestinal symptoms; most commonly, nausea, sometimes accompanied by headaches, and occasionally vomiting occur as pill use is started. On rare occasions, diarrhea may occur. The problems usually disappear after two to four medication cycles. An antiemetic preparation may bring relief. For some patients, change to a lower dose estrogen preparation is helpful.

Another mild but annoying side effect that

TABLE 3. **Commonly Prescribed Oral Contraceptives Available in the U.S.A., 1977**

TRADE NAME	PROGESTOGEN CONTENT	(MG.)	ESTROGEN	(μG.)
Enovid (Searle)	Norethynodrel	5	Mestranol	75
Ortho-Novum, 2 mg. (Ortho)	Norethindrone	2	Mestranol	100
Norinyl 2 mg. (Syntex)	Norethindrone	2	Mestranol	100
Enovid-E (Searle)	Norethynodrel	2.5	Mestranol	100
Ovulen (Searle)	Ethynodiol diacetate	1	Mestranol	100
Ortho-Novum 1/80 (Ortho)	Norethindrone	1	Mestranol	80
Norinyl 1/80 (Syntex)	Norethindrone	1	Mestranol	80
Ovral (Wyeth)	Norgestrel	0.5	EE	50
Norlestrin 2.5 (Parke-Davis)	Norethindrone acetate	2.5	EE	50
Norlestrin-1 (Parke-Davis)	Norethindrone acetate	1	EE	50
Zorane 1/50 (Lederle)	Norethindrone acetate	1	EE	50
Demulen (Searle)	Ethynodiol diacetate	1	EE	50
Ortho-Novum 1/50 (Ortho)	Norethindrone	1	Mestranol	50
Norinyl 1/50 (Syntex)	Norethindrone	1	Mestranol	50
Modicon (Ortho)	Norethindrone	0.5	EE	35
Brevicon (Syntex)	Norethindrone	0.5	EE	35
Lo-Ovral (Wyeth)	Norgestrel	0.3	EE	30
Zorane 1.5/30 (Lederle)	Norethindrone acetate	1.5	EE	30
Loestrin 1/20 (Parke-Davis)	Norethindrone acetate	1.5	EE	30
Zorane 1/20 (Lederle)	Norethindrone acetate	1	EE	20
Loestrin 1/20 (Parke-Davis)	Norethindrone acetate	1	EE	20
Micronor (Ortho)	Norethindrone	0.35	—	—
Nor-QD (Syntex)	Norethindrone	0.35	—	—
Ovrette (Wyeth)	Norgestrel	0.075	—	—

frequently occurs is intermenstrual spotting or bleeding, usually called breakthrough bleeding (BTB) when it occurs during the tablet days. If BTB occurs, most experts advise simply continuing with the OCs until the therapeutic cycle is completed, then waiting 7 days and beginning again, if this is acceptable to the patient. If BTB persists in subsequent cycles, a more estrogenic preparation may be considered. Traditionally, the recommended approach has been to double the dose for 2 or 3 days after the bleeding or spotting is controlled. Then the patient either reverts to the 1 tablet per day schedule until the end of the cycle or continues with the 2 tablets daily until the medication cycle is completed and then reverts to the 1 tablet daily schedule for the next cycle. Another approach of value is to add supplemental estrogen in the form of EE when BTB occurs.

Amenorrhea occurs in some women taking OCs. When the OC has been taken without omission, the amenorrhea, especially after the second cycle of medication, is virtually never due to an accidental pregnancy. One cannot, however, be sure of actual total compliance with the instructions for tablet intake; therefore after two consecutive OC cycles with persistent amenorrhea, the possibility of pregnancy should be considered and ruled out by a pregnancy test and pelvic examination. If the amenorrhea is of concern to the patient, withdrawal bleeding may be induced and a more estrogenic type of OC can be substituted or another contraceptive method prescribed.

Systemic Effects. Physiologic alterations resulting from OC use resemble, for the most part, the physiologic changes of pregnancy. The ovaries look quiescent, with follicular growth arrested; no developing follicles, no corpora lutea, and no luteinized follicles have been described in ovarian biopsies of OC users.

There are clinically measurable alterations in protein, lipid, and carbohydrate metabolism. The patient's glucose tolerance is diminished. Serum triglycerides, serum alpha 2 and beta globulins, plasma insulin, and serum carrier proteins are elevated. Thyroid binding globulin is increased, resulting in an increase in PBI and T_4 and a decrease in T_3 resin uptake; free thyroxine is normal, however, indicating that thyroid function is unchanged. Plasma cortisol is elevated owing to a similar increase in transcortin. Plasma renin substrate, angiotensin I, and angiotensinase, as well as some coagulation factors, are also increased. These tests revert to normal in 2 to 4 months after OCs have been discontinued.

Effects of OCs on the liver vary according to the estrogen and progestogen components, but it is difficult to separate them in pill users. Estrogens increase BSP retention, SGOT, and alkaline phosphatase; there is also an increase in plasma triglycerides and plasma phospholipid levels. These changes are dose related and reversible when the drug is stopped. Cholestasis and cholestatic jaundice have been reported as the result of metabolic changes in the proportion of liver pigments, leading to gallbladder disease and a doubling in the incidence of gallstones (Boston Collaborative Drug Surveillance Program). Hepatoma or hepatic cell adenomas, characterized by great vascularity and friability, with serious danger of hemorrhage and hemoperitoneum, have recently been reported. A registry of this infrequent serious entity has been established, and approximately 150 cases are currently registered; only one of these was a malignant hepatoma.

OCs may intensify pre-existing diabetes or cause recurrence of symptoms in women who developed gestational diabetes. It is possible that OCs may induce diabetes in women who have a pre-existing tendency to the disease. Increased risk of diabetes is found in obese women, those who give birth to an infant heavier than 4000 grams, those who report unexplained stillbirth, and those who have a family history of diabetes or previous abnormal blood glucose levels. The diabetogenic effects are usually reversible; occasionally, however, they are not.

Women taking OCs may present a deficit of pyridoxine (vitamin B_6). Pyridoxine prevents excessive xanthurenic acid excretion. Xanthurenic acid binds to free insulin, interfering with its metabolic action and affecting carbohydrate metabolism in certain women taking OCs. Fasting insulin values and the increase brought about by glucose loads are elevated in a substantial number of OC users. Growth hormone is also elevated in OC users and may result in amplifying the peripheral resistance to insulin and, in some women, in increased insulin release in response to glucose. This seems to be due to the 19-nortestosterone derivatives, whose effect on the liver is apparently potentiated by the concomitant use of the synthetic estrogen. Plasma levels of folic acid, ascorbic acid, niacin, riboflavin, and vitamin B_{12} have been found to be lower in OC users, resulting in an increased need for them and for zinc. The need for calcium, copper, iron, and vitamin K, however, may be reduced.

Thrombophlebitis, Cardiovascular, and Related Effects. The risk of deep vein thrombosis and embolism has received much attention. This risk seems to be dose related to the estrogen in the OCs at the 50 microgram level and above.

Increases in blood coagulation factors VII, VIII, IX, and X and in platelets, including altered platelet function and associated occlusive thrombi with clinically silent circulating microthrombi, are four times as common in OC users as in control women (Irey et al., 1970). The risk of death resulting from thromboembolic disease in pill users is given as 1.5 to 3.9 per 100,000 women, or 7 to 8 times as great as that for nonusers. This risk is increased for women with predisposing factors (smoking, history of toxemia, obesity, hypertension, diabetes) and for women over 40 and those with blood types A, B, or AB. Table 4 details death rates from various causes for women in their reproductive years in the United Kingdom, and Table 5 indicates the risk of death in the United States from various causes. Note that the mortality risks for complications of abortion and/or pregnancy, auto accidents, and cancer are significantly higher than the mortality risks associated with the use of oral contraceptives.

The risk of cerebrovascular accident or stroke seems to be about 4 times as great in OC users;

TABLE 4. **Estimated Annual Death Rates from Various Causes for Women 20 to 44 Years of Age in the United Kingdom***

	RATE PER 100,000 WOMEN	
	Age 20–34	*Age 35–44*
Cause of death:		
Pulmonary and cerebral thromboembolism in healthy married nonpregnant women		
Nonusers of oral contraceptives	0.2	0.5
Users of oral contraceptives	1.5	3.9
Motor vehicle accidents	4.9	3.9
Cancer	13.7	70.1
All causes	60.1	170.5
	RATE PER 100,000 LIVE BIRTHS	
	Age 20–34	*Age 35–44*
Cause of death:		
Puerperal phlebitis, thrombosis, embolism	1.3	2.3
Abortion	5.6	10.4
Complications of pregnancy	7.5	13.8
Complications of delivery	7.1	26.5
All risks: pregnancy, delivery, puerperium	22.8	57.6

*Modified from Meeker, C. I., Gray, M. J.: Birth control, abortion, and sterilization. *In* Romney, S. L., et al. (eds.): Gynecology and Obstetrics: The Health Care of Women. New York, McGraw-Hill Book Company, 1975.

TABLE 5. **Risk of Death, U.S.A.—Various Causes, Various Years**

Cardiovascular/renal disease	1970	493.9/100,000 population
Cancer	1970	166.6/100,000 population
Motor vehicle accidents		27.5/100,000 population
Diabetes	1970	18.8/100,000 population
Pregnancy	1973	16.0/100,000 live births
Murder/manslaughter	1972	8.9/100,000 population
Oral contraceptive users, aged 15–45		0.3–3/100,000 women
IUD users		0.3–1.5/100,000 women
Syphilis	1970	0.2/100,000 population

again, this seems to be dose related to the estrogen component.

An increased risk of myocardial infarction has been reported for OC users, stated as 2.8 per 100,000 for the 30 to 39 year age group, and 4.7 per 100,000 for those women over 40 (Mann et al., 1975).

Hypertension may appear in about 5 to 6 per cent of OC users. This hypertension is related to length of OC use and is reversible. There is no way to identify women susceptible to this undesirable side effect. Some women with prior hypertension may use the pill without any change in the previously controlled hypertension, and some women who were hypertensive during pregnancy are more susceptible to this complication, but not all.

The frequency and intensity of migraine episodes may increase; also, increased frequencies of epilepsy, asthma, and sickle cell crisis have been reported, but these data are not statistically well supported.

Other Effects. OC use increases breast size and sensitivity in about 10 per cent of users, but this effect is not permanent. Milk production is reduced, its composition is altered, and the presence of the synthetic contraceptive steroids has been reported in breast milk. Consequently, it is advisable for OCs not to be used if the woman desires to nurse her infant.

Weight gain of up to 2 kg. is relatively common, and gains of up to 5 to 10 kg. have been reported in 4 to 50 per cent of women taking OCs. Apparently, weight gain is greater with the high dose preparations. Mild sodium and water retention is related to estrogenic action and possibly also to a long-term progestational effect; however, in many instances, weight gain seems to be related more to a positive nitrogen balance than to fluid retention.

Uterine leiomyomas may become apparent and enlarge under the influence of the estrogen in the OCs. Skin pigmentation (melasma, chloasma) may also occur. This pigmentation may partly disappear upon discontinuance of OCs; however, it may remain.

Acne and dysmenorrhea usually improve with pill use, especially if one of the more estrogenic types of progestogen, such as norethynodrel, is prescribed. Menstrual flow is diminished in amount, with consequent conservation of iron.

Changes in libido in both directions have been reported and, like depression, seem to be directly related to the personality type of the user as well as to her social and sexual adjustment.

OCs should be discontinued 4 to 6 weeks preceding elective surgery in order to minimize the chance of thromboembolic complications. Contraception with OCs can be reinstated 4 to 6 weeks following surgery. Meanwhile, interval contraception with a barrier method should be prescribed.

A question frequently asked is whether OCs should be stopped periodically for two or three cycles to give the user a respite and let her body system return to "pre-pill" homeostasis before resuming pill use. There is no evidence that such a policy is effective in decreasing the incidence of complications. During the two or three months off OCs the woman may have to use a less reliable contraceptive method that is unfamiliar to her, with consequent risk of unwanted pregnancy, which is always higher in the first few cycles of any contraceptive experience. Furthermore, she will have to adjust once again to the OCs, with the possible recurrence of early symptoms.

Malignant Disease. Prospective and retrospective studies thus far reported have indicated no link or sustained trend in the incidence of neoplasia of the cervix, uterine corpus, or breast. There is no evidence of an increase in the incidence of precancerous lesions or in the aggravation of existing ones.

Return of Fertility. No study has demonstrated that return to regular menstrual cyclicity and subsequent fertility is affected by the duration of OC use, when age is controlled. At least 90 per cent of women who were previously ovulatory will resume ovulation within 3 months. Amenorrhea after discontinuation of the pill does occur in a few women (approximately 1 per cent, according to Shearman; some, 11 of 69 in Shearman's series, have galactorrhea); however, usually these women had a history of irregular menstrual cycles before OC use.

In most women with postpill amenorrhea, menstruation, although frequently irregular, returns spontaneously in about 6 months. In women presenting with amenorrhea, but without galactorrhea, who do not resume spontaneous menstruation in 6 months, it is advisable to perform assays of serum gonadotropins (LH and FSH, usually low) and prolactin (occasionally high) and radiologic study of the sella turcica for a possible chromophobe microadenoma (benign) of the pituitary gland. When galactorrhea is present, these exploratory studies should be initiated immediately.

When postpill amenorrhea occurs, if conception is not desired, a barrier contraceptive should be prescribed, and progesterone, 100 mg. intramuscularly, or medroxyprogesterone acetate (Provera), 10 mg. per day orally for 5 days, may be given every 6 weeks to induce menstruation. If pregnancy is desired, induction of ovulation with clomiphene citrate is indicated. When appropriate doses have been tried unsuccessfully for at least 6 months, treatment with menotropins and HCG is indicated. Recently, it has been reported that an ergonovine derivative, bromergocryptine, is effective in controlling the increase in prolactin and restoring ovulation. This drug, however, is not currently available in the United States.

Nova and Nova (1975) reported a slight increase in fetal malformation when the mother conceived immediately after discontinuing OC use, and Carr (1970) reported an increase in triploidy in women who became pregnant within 6 months after stopping OCs. However, in an extensive follow-up study of accidental and planned pregnancies after OC use, the incidence of congenital anomalies was 4.8 per cent (Rice-Wray et al.).

Progestogens Alone. These preparations, called "minipills," differ from combined OCs by using a very low dose of a progestogen alone in an uninterrupted daily intake schedule. Three such products are available, two containing 350 micrograms of norethindrone and one with 75 micrograms of norgestrel (Table 3). Their contraceptive efficacy results from suppression and/or alteration of LH secretion, physical changes in cervical mucus, and progestational changes in the endometrium; they do not consistently inhibit ovulation. The attributed failure rate is approximately 3 to 8 per 100 woman years. The major problem with this modality is irregular and unpredictable uterine bleeding. Amenorrhea is also a frequent concern.

Postcoital Contraception or "Interception." Large doses of estrogen administered within 72 hours of unprotected coitus during the presumed fertile period seem to protect from unwanted pregnancy. The preparations used are diethylstilbestrol, 25 to 50 mg. twice daily for 5 days, ethinyl estradiol, 1 to 5 mg. per day for 5 days, or conjugated estrogens, 20 to 25 mg. per day for 5 days. Acceleration of egg transport and/or changes in the endometrium are assumed to be the mechanisms of action. The failure rate has been reported as 0.3 per 100 woman years, 10 per cent of the unintended pregnancies being ectopic. If interception fails and a pregnancy occurs, it should be terminated because of the potential teratogenicity of the estrogens at the dose and time given.

A similar use of a copper-clad IUD has been reported with excellent results and no failures (Lippes, 1976). These clinical studies are being extended.

Regardless of the evident success reported in studies of postcoital contraception, this method should be used only in emergencies.

Injectable Contraceptives. No injectable hormone preparation has been approved for contraceptive use in the United States. Extensive clinical studies with medroxyprogesterone acetate have been conducted, and this product is in use in Canada, England, the Scandinavian countries, and elsewhere. The most common dose is 150 mg. intramuscularly every 90 days.

Vaginal rings, subdermal Silastic implants, and biodegradable implants using various progestogens are presently being evaluated.

Intrauterine Contraceptive Devices (IUDs)

Although a bewildering number of IUD types have been developed, few are widely available commercially in the United States. The FDA was recently authorized to regulate these devices, and as a result all "closed" IUDs were recalled. Hence, those that either by themselves (Gräfenberg, Hall-Stone ring) or together with their transcervical appendage (Majzlin spring) form a ring, and also the Dalkon Shield, are no longer commercially available in the United States, owing to potential problems with uterine perforations and intestinal occlusion. In addition, there is concern regarding the possibility of obstetrical sepsis and septic shock during the second and third trimesters of accidental pregnancy with this type of device in place.

In the United States and throughout the world, the Lippes loop remains the most widely used IUD. Extensive clinical studies of this device have been made, and its performance is frequently used as a standard to which newer devices are compared.

Several models of loop devices are available; the smallest, Loop A, is distinguished by a transcervical appendage (tail) of blue threads. Loop B is of a medium size and has a tail of black threads.

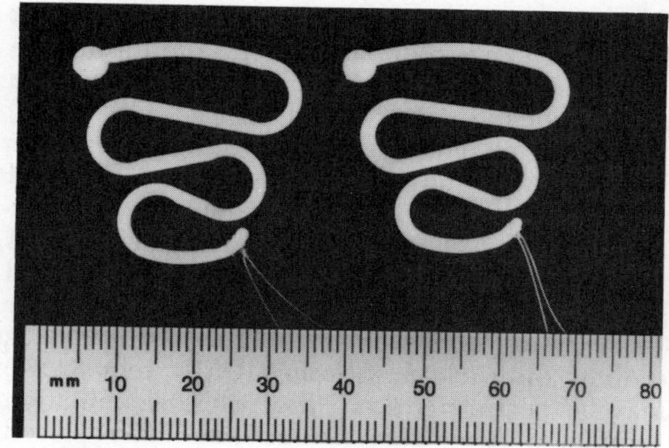

Figure 1. Lippes Loop C (left) and Loop D (right). Both are 30 mm. wide. The thicker, stiffer Loop D has a tail of white threads. It is generally the first loop fitted and is recommended for women with one or more children. Loop C has a tail of yellow threads, and is selected when Loop D must be removed for bleeding and pain.

Loop C is the largest size; Loop D is the same size, but is thicker and stiffer. These latter two are virtually the only ones used in the United States (Fig. 1). Less frequently found are the Saf-T-Coil, the Cu-7, and the Progestasert. Recently, the Copper T has also been approved by the FDA for commercial distribution. Both copper-bearing IUDs have been approved for a period of use of up to 3 years (Figs. 2 and 3).

The IUDs made exclusively of biologically "inert" plastics depend for their contraceptive effect mostly on the local foreign body reaction which they generate in the contiguous endometrium. As for the copper-bearing IUDs (Cu-7 and Copper T), their contraceptive action depends mostly on localized chemical changes in the uterine environment and in the cervical mucus;

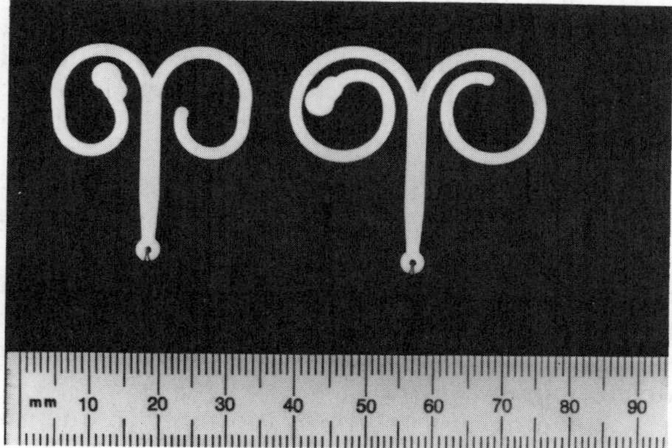

Figure 2. The Saf-T-Coil devices have tails of blue-green threads. The standard 33-S coil is at right; the intermediate-sized 32-S (left) is recommended for the patient who cannot accommodate the standard size, and for the nulliparous woman.

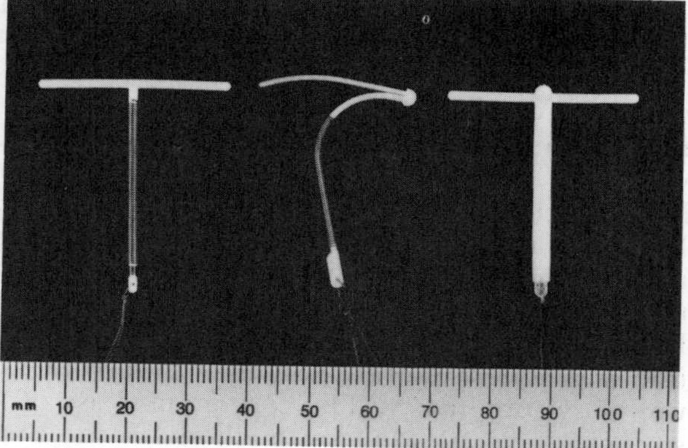

Figure 3. The Copper T model (left); the Cu-7 (center); and the Progestasert (right).

the endometrial secretions associated with these devices are thought to be somewhat spermicidal and also may have a blastolytic effect on any fertilized egg, thus preventing pregnancy.

In the Progestasert, the contraceptive effect may be provided by the combined local effect of the endometrial foreign body reaction created by the hormonal effect of the progesterone, which is continually diffused from a chamber in the shank of the device into the uterine lumen at the rate of 65 micrograms a day. This makes the endocervical mucus hostile to sperm migration and modifies the endometrium to a secretory type. Uterine motility may also be decreased. If accidental fertilization occurs, the chance of successful nidation is minimized because of the local endometrial changes. Since the progesterone bypasses the portal circulation, it can be effective at a much lower dose than if it were administered by mouth. In some studies, no alteration of the secretion pattern of LH and FSH was demonstrated. Thus the drug apparently does not interfere with ovulation.

One advantage of the Progestasert is its small size, which makes it more acceptable to the nulligravid and nulliparous patient. Other reported advantages are a lessening of menstrual flow and a decrease in dysmenorrhea. The main problems with this intriguing new device are its cost and the need for periodic replacement, because the load of progesterone becomes exhausted in time. Currently, the FDA has approved the Progestasert for a 1 year period of use, after which the device should be removed and, if the patient chooses, replaced. Progestogen- and progesterone-loaded IUDs are being tested that may provide contraceptive protection for as long as 2 or 3 years; similar devices with a drug load that may last for 10 years or more are planned.

The indications and contraindications for

selection of the IUD for contraception are listed in Table 6.

Insertion of the IUD. Insertion of an IUD is done preferably during menstruation. This affords the advantage of a more open cervical canal, while the ongoing bleeding camouflages any bleeding that may be caused by the procedure. Insertion at this time or immediately following menstruation also provides some assurance that the patient is not pregnant. The physician should be aware that some patients request IUD insertion into a pregnant uterus, hoping to interrupt an unwanted pregnancy. The concomitant use of a spermicide as an adjuvant method for the first cycle or during the fertile period is sometimes advisable.

Although immediate postpartum and postabortion insertions are recommended by some investigators and in certain social and medical circumstances may be advisable, in general, IUD insertion is not done until 4 to 6 weeks post partum and 1 to 2 weeks postabortion; this diminishes the chance of spontaneous expulsions and of uterine perforations.

TABLE 6. **Indications and Contraindications for IUD Use**

Indications
- Need for a coitus-independent and highly effective method
- Contraindication or unacceptability of hormonal contraceptives for medical, psychologic, personal, or social reasons

Contraindications
- Absolute
  - Cancer of cervix or uterine corpus
  - Recent or recurrent pelvic infections
  - Small uterine cavity (less than 5 cm.)
  - History of rheumatic cardiopathy
  - History of endocarditis
  - History of ectopic pregnancy
  - Anticoagulant therapy
  - Immunosuppressive therapy
- Relative
  - Nulligravidity
  - Nulliparity
  - Dyspareunia
  - Severe dysmenorrhea
  - Immediate puerperium
  - Psychologic or physical incapacity to check for transcervical appendage
  - History of PID
  - Submucous or intramural leiomyomas that are symptomatic or that deform uterine lumen
  - Prolonged uterine bleeding disrupting personal and/or sexual life
  - Anemia
  - Blood dyscrasias
- Temporary
  - Pregnancy or suspected pregnancy
  - Acute purulent cervicitis, even under treatment
  - Cervical polyp or other benign cervical pathology
  - Active or suspected PID, even under treatment
  - Venereal disease
  - Dysfunctional uterine bleeding
  - Herpes genitalis

Note: Genital anomalies are not a contraindication, provided that coitus, pregnancy, and insertion of an IUD are all possible.

In highly nervous or very young patients, or in nulligravid or nulliparous women, a mild analgesic (aspirin, Tylenol) 30 minutes prior to insertion may be helpful in allaying discomfort and associated anxiety. At this time, the cervical smear for cytology, GC culture (Thayer-Martin or Transgrow), and wet smear for Trichomonas (saline) and *Candida albicans* (10 per cent KOH) may be performed, and the pelvic examination completed. After the speculum has been replaced and antisepsis of the vagina and cervix performed, a tenaculum is delicately but firmly placed on the anterior lip of the cervix. Sounding of the uterus before insertion is standard procedure in the United States. Although in most women a competent pelvic examination would indicate the position and approximate size of the organ, it is best to follow a prescribed routine.

Loading of the device into the inserter should be done immediately preceding insertion, because plastic IUDs have poor elastic capacity and may be deformed by a prolonged stay in the inserter tube.

Most IUDs are inserted by the withdrawal technique, whereby the device is placed so that its broadest part is in the frontal plane of the uterine cavity. As soon as the loaded inserter touches the fundus, the inserter is withdrawn, while simultaneously the plunger within the inserter (which is kept in contact with the proximal end of the IUD) is held firmly. Thus the inserter slides out over the stationary plunger, gradually releasing the IUD at the fundus.

Presently available IUDs are equipped with a "tail" made of a monofilament thread which forms a transcervical appendage. After insertion of the IUD, these threads should be cut to a suitable length, leaving not less than 5 cm. protruding from the external cervical os; otherwise, the tail may be pulled into the canal or even into the uterine cavity by the movement of the IUD in utero.

Side Effects. The side effects most often associated with IUD use are bleeding, pain, expulsion, infection, excessive vaginal discharge, accidental pregnancy, translocation of the IUD or perforation of the endometrium, and anxiety in the patient because of fear of cancer or other deleterious side effects.

Bleeding and pain are the most frequently seen problems. In general, they are reported together, because in the majority of instances they occur simultaneously. Intermenstrual spotting or bleeding in the form of a sero- or mucosanguineous discharge may follow insertion and persist for several weeks. Menstruation, especially the first few periods after insertion, may be more copious and prolonged. Menstrual flow has been measured at more than twice that before insertion. Occasionally the change of menstrual pattern may be permanent. This is an important consideration in women who have iron deficiency anemia or who are susceptible to this condition. If spotting or bleeding disrupts sexual activity, or if the discharge is particularly distressing to the patient, a different form of contraception should be advised.

Lower abdominal discomfort, uterine cramps, and/or low backache can occur after insertion, but these are not as common as the changes in menstruation noted above, and if these latter symptoms are tolerated by the patient, they usually disappear in a few weeks. A mild analgesic taken by the patient during this period may bring relief and may help avoid early request for removal. Severe uterine cramps and even syncope may occasionally occur, mostly among nulligravid and nulliparous patients or women who have not had a delivery in many years. The significance of pelvic discomfort or pain depends on the pain threshold of the patient and her psychologic adjustment to contraception, the size of the device in relation to the uterine space, and the position of the device in the uterus. This complaint may be minimized if clear explanations precede insertion, the procedure itself is gently performed, and the device is carefully placed in the plane of the uterine cavity.

Pain or uterine cramps occurring after several asymptomatic months are significant, because they may indicate expulsion of the device or perforation of the adjacent surfaces or pelvic organs.

IUD expulsion occurs in approximately 20 per cent of insertions for some types of IUDs. Expulsions are frequent during the first month after insertion, and approximately 50 per cent occur within the first 3 months; they are more frequent in young women of lower parity. Most occur during a menstrual period. The chance of expulsion is inversely related to the size of the device, and IUDs that have been reinserted after expulsion have a higher expulsion rate.

Because there are no reliable statistics regarding the incidence of pelvic inflammatory disease (PID) in the sexually active population, it is difficult to determine whether or not the frequency of pelvic inflammation is increased in IUD users. Approximately 1.5 to 2 per cent of IUD users may develop a local infection, but in only 25 per cent of these patients is the infection severe. There is no agreement as to whether a device should be removed in the presence of PID before or during treatment of the infection. In the United States, however, the tendency is to remove the IUD at the time the PID treatment is initiated.

The current IUD failure rate of approximately 2 per 100 woman years (reports range from 1.8 to 3.6 per 100 woman years) appears virtually impossible to improve, although failures tend to decrease as duration of use increases. Accidental pregnancies are more frequent with smaller devices; however, this holds true only for the "inert" plastic models; IUDs with copper (Cu-7 and Copper T) and the progesterone carrier device (Progestasert), which are the smallest in current use in the United States, have shown as good or better effectiveness against unwanted pregnancy than the standard C or D loop. The manufacturer of Progestasert quotes a pregnancy rate of 1.9 per 100 woman years for parous women and 2.5 for nulliparous women, and expulsion rates of 3.1 and 7.5, respectively.

Most pregnancies occur early in the IUD experience, during the first year after insertion, and especially in the first cycle or first trimester. Two thirds of the pregnancies occur with the device in situ, the remainder after unnoticed spontaneous expulsion.

Pregnancy with the device in situ is complicated by spontaneous abortion in a 2 to 3 times higher proportion than when pregnancy follows expulsion. The relative incidence of ectopic pregnancy is increased, and this condition should be ruled out whenever pain is associated with an adnexal mass, even in the presence of a device in situ and a "normal" menstrual history. Removals of tailed devices from a pregnant uterus when the tail is still visible are not followed by a higher rate of spontaneous abortion than when the device is left in situ.

Currently, the standard policy is to remove an IUD as soon as an accidental pregnancy with the device in situ is diagnosed, as septic shock and death may occur in women with a device in the uterus during the second or third trimester of pregnancy. From 1972 through the first half of 1975, after a nationwide study, the Communicable Disease Center (CDC) reported 42 such deaths, 17 (43 per cent) among women who were wearing an IUD. Of these, 13 (76 per cent) were Dalkon Shield users (Cates et al., 1977) (Table 7).

No increase in fetal malformation has been reported in pregnancies going to term with a device in situ. The device remains outside the amniotic sac, and is frequently delivered with the placenta or membranes.

Perforation of the uterus and placement of the device in the peritoneal cavity, or parauterine spaces or organs, occurs mostly at insertion, but may also happen later as a result of pressure, necrosis, and uterine activity, generally called translocation. Perforation and translocation are most frequent with larger and more rigid devices, when immediate postpartum or postabortion insertions

TABLE 7. **Maternal Deaths Associated with Septic Spontaneous Abortion, Whether or Not IUD Was in Uterus, by Type of Device, United States, 1972–75***

TYPE OF IUD	1972	1973	JAN.–JUNE 1974	JULY–DEC. 1974	1975	TOTAL
Lippes Loop	2	0	1	0	0	3
Dalkon Shield	7	3	3	0	0	13
Saf-T-Coil	0	1	—	0	0	1
Non-IUD related	14	5	6	8	12	45
Total	23	9	10	8	12	62

*From data by Cates, J. W., Grimes, D. A., Ory, H. W., Tyler Jr., C. W.: Family Planning Perspectives 9:138–140, 1977.

are performed, and when the position of the uterus is not properly diagnosed; however, the majority of perforations result from improper and hasty insertions performed while using other than the recommended technique.

No relationship has been reported between the use of IUDs and the frequency of cervicitis or vaginitis, or in the frequency of abnormal cervical cytology. The incidence of premalignant or malignant lesions of the cervix and endometrium is not increased in IUD users. In discussing the side effects, the physician should stress this point, because the thought that the IUD may cause cancer occurs to most women at one time or another. A careful history, examination, and cervical smear for cytology, along with patient education at every follow-up visit (twice a year) should provide sufficient safeguards as to early diagnosis and treatment of any deviation from the norm. Some physicians allow annual follow-up visits in patients using IUDs without difficulties.

Removal of IUDs. Removal of some IUDs may prove a taxing experience for both the physician and the patient, especially if the device is embedded in the myometrium or if the tail is missing or breaks during the procedure. Dilatation of the cervix and local anesthesia may then be necessary. Occasionally removal may require surgical intervention. A careful evaluation of the situation should be made, taking into consideration the FDA recommendations regarding removal, the desire of the asymptomatic patient for future fertility, and the risk involved in removal of an inert device. These should be discussed frankly with the patient.

Because all IUDs available in the United States are radiopaque, x-ray search is facilitated and may be appropriate in some cases. In searching for an IUD with a missing or broken tail, it is useful to obtain frontal and lateral views of the pelvis. If translocation is suspected, another IUD or a uterine sound or dilator in the uterine cavity may provide a reference point against which the position of the device may be studied. Rarely, a hysterosalpingogram is needed to determine the presence of a "missing" IUD in the uterus, outside the organ, or lost through unnoticed expulsion.

Removal of a "lost" IUD from the cul-de-sac has been accomplished through posterior colpotomy or culdoscopy; removal from the abdominal cavity has been accomplished by laparoscopy, although occasionally laparotomy is necessary. Copper-bearing IUDs discovered in the abdomen require prompt removal by laparotomy, which may demand considerable surgical skill, because adhesion or agglutination of intestinal loops and omentum around the device may be extensive. IUDs "lost" in utero because the transcervical appendage broke or was cut too short may be brought to the vagina with the assistance of an endometrial curette (Novak, Randall, Garcia-Rock); when this method fails, such devices may be removed by hysteroscopy (Sciarra, Valle).

Almost always, when "lost" IUDs lie in the uterus, the removal can be performed in the office or outpatient facility, although the procedure requires rapport between the patient and operator, patience on both their parts, a competent, unhurried approach, and proper equipment (paracervical block equipment, cervical dilators, tenaculum, uterine sound, endometrial biopsy curette, IUD hook, uterine packing forceps, polyp forceps). Aseptic technique must be carefully followed.

After difficult removals or those requiring invasion of the uterine cavity, it is best not to insert another IUD immediately, because of possible infection (endometritis, PID) or bleeding. The patient's desire for immediate replacement, or her social need, do not justify the risk of these potential complications.

Continuing IUD Use. Discontinuation of IUD use is often associated with spontaneous expulsion of the device, uterine discomfort, or unacceptable bleeding. The latter two problems tend to decrease with continued use. Therefore continuation rates improve somewhat after the first 3 months of use, and even more after the first year.

Plastic IUDs can be left in utero indefinitely. There are well documented reports of successful continuous use for 20 or more years, although occasionally the plastic may become encrusted with salts and other precipitates that increase the rigidity of the device and subsequently cause pain and bleeding. When this occurs, removal of the symptomatic device and replacement by a new one are advisable. There is no need for an interval between removal and reinsertion, but in such cases the physician may wish to perform an endometrial biopsy in addition to the customary cervical smear for cytology and GC culture.

Copper IUDs should not remain in utero longer than the 3 years currently approved by the FDA, although approval for an extension of this time period is expected, and clinical studies of some experimental copper-bearing IUDs indicate that they may afford protection for as long as 20 years or more.

The superior continuation rates generally found in IUD studies, in comparison with other contraceptive modalities, may result not so much from a better adjustment of the user to the method, or from fewer or milder side effects, as from the fact that removal of the device requires the user to return to the physician.

The contraceptive protection offered by the IUD in the general population is second only to that afforded by the correct use of OCs and by sterilization. However, *careful regular users* of the diaphragm or condom can expect similar contraceptive protection from these traditional methods (Lane et al., 1975).

Barrier Methods

Although oral contraceptives remain the most popular method of contraception, in recent years a definite increase has been noted in the popularity of the diaphragm and the condom. This renewed interest in classic contraceptive methods may result from the concern with which many patients view the side effects and metabolic changes accompanying the use of OCs, or from the reluctance of some physicians to prescribe OCs or IUDs for women who consider their families complete but who have perhaps 20 years of fertility remaining. Further, a more liberal attitude toward pregnancy termination provides the necessary backup for methods with which the risk of pregnancy may be somewhat increased.

Diaphragm. The diaphragm was the first reliable contraceptive method available to women. It was introduced in America in the early part of the twentieth century and was popularized by the noted feminist, Margaret Sanger, in an attempt to liberate women from the burden of unwanted pregnancy. The diaphragm was originally utilized primarily by upper middle class women who had not only the sophistication to recognize their sexual rights but also the means and privacy to take advantage of them. With the development and availability of other contraceptive methods, the diaphragm lost some of its popularity for a number of years. Recently, however, an increasing number of women, concerned about reports of serious side effects associated with OC and IUD use, are again turning to the diaphragm for contraception.

TABLE 8. **Indications and Contraindications for Diaphragm Use**

Indications
- Desire for female control
- Hormonal or IUD contraception contraindicated or unacceptable
- Coitus during menstruation practiced or desired

Contraindications
- Absolute
  - Psychologic or physical incapacity to master correct use
  - Poor pelvic support, marked uterine prolapse
  - Aversion to handling genitals
  - Marked obesity
  - Fingers too short
  - Vagina too deep or too short
  - Vaginoplasty or rigid vaginal walls
  - Chronic local allergies, genital contact dermatitis, eczema genitalis, genital psoriasis, other genital dermatoses
  - Allergy to latex, rubber, or spermicidal preparations in either partner
  - Vaginismus
- Relative
  - Need for a contraceptive method of higher effectiveness
  - Lack of privacy
  - Moderate cystocele and/or rectocele
  - Dyspareunia
  - Fixed retrodisplacement of uterus
- Temporary
  - Acute or subacute vulvovaginitis of any cause
  - Pruritus genitalis
  - Herpes genitalis
  - Active or suspected venereal disease
  - Urethritis, cystitis, dysuria, pyuria, or hematuria—until cause is established
  - Condyloma acuminatum

Indications and contraindications for diaphragm use are listed in Table 8, and effectiveness is shown in Table 1.

Several types of diaphragms are available. The classic types are the coil spring, the flat spring or Mensinga, and the arcing diaphragm. These last two are particularly useful in women with a slight relaxation of the vaginal wall or a minor cystorectocele. A newer type of arcing spring diaphragm, the all flex, has a rim which can be easily bent in any direction; it has an external rim diameter of from 55 to 105 mm., and is available in sizes increasing by increments of 5 mm. Difficult to find but useful is the Matrisalus type with a rather rigid rim, which resembles a moldable Hodge pessary to which a rubber dome has been attached, and the Dumas rubber cap; these come in three sizes and are most useful in the rare but serious cases of poor pelvic support.

The physician fitting a diaphragm should select the largest one that will fit snugly into the space between the posterior fornix of the vagina and the retropubic groove without being felt by the patient. When the correct size is used, only the tip of the physician's index finger will fit between the vaginal wall in the retropubic groove and the rim of the diaphragm. Careful patient instruction about insertion is paramount, as is the assurance that the patient comprehends the need to use the device prior to each coital act and before sexual foreplay. A spermicidal preparation may be used with the diaphragm; the jelly type will give more lubrication, and a cream or foam can be used when less lubrication is desired. The patient should be taught to feel the cervix through the rubber of the diaphragm dome and to place the anterior part of the device snugly behind the pubic bone in the mucosal groove found in most women. We do not favor the use of a diaphragm inserter, because it tends to discourage the important post-insertion digital check. This step is essential to be certain that the diaphragm is properly positioned in the vagina. It also greatly decreases the chance of method failure.

Insertion of the diaphragm may become part of the daily routine of the sexually active woman. The device should be inserted several hours before coitus, and should not be removed for 4 to 5 hours following intercourse; when subsequent intercourse occurs, a fresh application of the spermicide may be inserted with a special syringe or a finger, without removing the diaphragm. Douching is not necessary, but the patient may do so if she wishes. The diaphragm may be left in place overnight, and for as long as 1 or 2 days at a time.

Condom. After OCs and sterilization, the condom is the most popular method of fertility control in the United States. It has the added advantage of preventing the transmission of venereal infection. A great variety of condoms are available in various textures and colors; thinner condoms permit greater sensitivity to tactile stimulation and temperature, and lubricated condoms also permit increased sensitivity.

Understanding how to use the condom effectively is important, and the female partner as well as the male should be familiar with its proper use. Two and a half to 4 cm. (1 to 1.5 inches) should be left free at the tip of the condom, collapsed and empty of air, to provide room for penile coital movements and the ejaculate. The condom should be placed on the erect penis before it is rubbed on the vulva or inserted into the vagina. A spermicide may be used to provide lubrication and add effectiveness.

Indications and contraindications for condom use are listed in Table 9. Theoretical and use effectiveness are shown in Table 1.

TABLE 9. **Indications and Contraindications for Condom Use**

Indications
- Male: genital or penile skin disease
- Female: vaginitis, even under treatment
- Couple: male control preferred
- Casual sexual encounter or infrequent intercourse
- Active or suspected venereal disease
- Herpes genitalis
- Condyloma acuminatum
- Urethritis of all causes, even under treatment
- Cystitis, dysuria, or pyuria—until cause is established
- Interim method before use of OC or IUD

Contraindications
- Absolute
  - Sexual irresponsibility
  - Disruption or interruption of sexual foreplay precluding sexual interest and/or expression
- Relative
  - Interruption of sexual foreplay interfering with sexual expression

Vaginal Spermicides

Although the list of available vaginal topical contraceptives was long a few years ago, currently it has been reduced to a few jellies, creams, foams, and one suppository. The indications and contraindications for this contraceptive modality are given in Table 10, and the acknowledged failure

TABLE 10. **Indications and Contraindications for Topical Contraception/Spermicides**

Indications
- Adjuvant to mechanical method (diaphragm, condom)
- Adjuvant to calendar rhythm method
- Adjuvant to IUD during fertile period
- Adjuvant to hormonal contraceptives at start of the first medication cycle or when 2 or more tablets have been missed
- Temporary or transient method prescribed before sexual relations are initiated, before a systemic method can be started or IUD inserted
- Low fertility or presumed infertility of woman unable or unwilling to use a mechanical method
- Casual sexual encounter or infrequent intercourse

Contraindications
- Absolute
  - Necessity for a method of high effectiveness for health, personal, or social reasons
  - Disruption or interruption of sexual foreplay precluding sexual interest and/or expression
  - Aesthetic unacceptability to either partner
  - Allergy to spermicidal preparations
  - Chronic local allergy, genital contact dermatitis, eczema genitalis, genital psoriasis, and other genital dermatoses
- Relative
  - Interruption of sexual foreplay interfering with sexual expression
  - High fertility
  - Dyspareunia
  - Vaginismus
- Temporary
  - Acute or subacute vulvovaginitis of any cause, treated or untreated
  - Pruritus
  - Herpes genitalis

rates are shown in Table 1. Vaginal spermicides are used primarily as an interim or occasional contraceptive method or while awaiting menstruation prior to the insertion of an IUD or initiation of OC use. The patient is instructed to insert the spermicidal preparation into the vagina prior to penile insertion, is advised that coitus should take place within an hour, or preferably 30 minutes, from the insertion of the spermicide, and is told that the dose (about 5 ml.) should be repeated before each coital event. Douching is not necessary, but if it is desired, the woman should wait for 3 or 4 hours after coitus to do so.

Most of these products have excellent shelf life when properly stored; they should not be refrigerated and never frozen, but kept tightly closed at ordinary room temperature. Their contribution to the control of coitally transmitted diseases is currently being studied, and laboratory studies indicate that vaginal spermicides have been effective against *Neisseria gonorrhoeae, Treponema pallidum, Trichomonas vaginalis, Candida albicans,* and herpes simplex II virus (Cutler, 1976). Should clinical studies support these findings in even 50 per cent of the patients, an important step will have been taken toward controlling the spread of these sexually transmissible diseases.

Rhythm or Periodic Abstinence

Recently, with a new awakening of interest in the rhythm method, some lay religious groups have offered careful instruction in its use, and provide the considerable psychologic support the successful practice of this method demands.

There are two basic ways of practicing periodic abstinence: the calendar method and the temperature method. Standard instructions for the calendar method are (1) to keep a record of the length of menstrual cycles for 12 cycles and (2) to subtract 18 from the shortest cycle and 11 from the longest cycle. The resulting figures indicate the period during which coitus without contraception may be practiced, the cycle day when abstinence should start, and the day when coitus may safely be resumed.

The more rigid and effective temperature method demands total abstinence until the basal body temperature has shown a sustained rise for at least 3 consecutive days in the absence of illness or other intervening factors.

Recently it has been reported that a higher incidence of anencephalia, Down's syndrome, and other defects of the neural system occur among Roman Catholics in England and the Netherlands and may possibly be due to failures of the rhythm method (Jöngbloet, 1977). The indications and contraindications for this method are listed in Table 11, and the failure rate in Table 1.

TABLE 11. **Indications and Contraindications for the Rhythm or Periodic Abstinence Method of Contraception***

Indications
- Personal or religious

Contraindications
- Calendar method
  - Lack of privacy
  - Sexually irresponsible partner
  - Partner cooperation not assured
  - Need for higher effectiveness
  - Irregular menstrual periods
  - Inability to perform necessary calculations with confidence
- Temperature method
  - Lack of privacy
  - Sexually irresponsible partner
  - Partner cooperation not assured

**Note:* The use of the *calendar method* to calculate the start of the period of sexual abstinence and resumption of sexual relations when indicated by the *temperature method* may assist in shortening the period of abstinence by allowing coitus during certain days of the follicular phase.

When a method of high effectiveness is indicated or requested and voluntary interruption of pregnancy is unacceptable or not legally available, only the rhythm method by *basal body temperature* should be advised and taught.

Surgical Contraception (Sterilization)

In the United States, couples generally have completed their family (two or three children) by the maternal age of 25 to 30, if not earlier. Under these circumstances, there remain another 20 to 25 years of reproductive potential requiring control. Although OCs afford virtually full contraceptive protection for such women, many physicians consider it socially unjustifiable and medically unsound to prescribe these compounds, with their powerful metabolic effects and the probability, increasing with age, of serious thromboembolic and other vascular complications. However, the alternative approach, using a less powerful or less effective method of contraception, carries the risk of accidental pregnancy, with additional potential risks to mother and child increasing with parity and maternal age.

For young couples who have a stable relationship and consider their family complete, when their youngest child is already 2 or 3 years old, voluntary sterilization may be considered as a possible method of fertility control that precludes these problems. There are no laws in the United States forbidding voluntary sterilization of consenting adults, and sterilization may be performed even in single persons, with or without children. The physician must, however, carefully inform the prospective candidate of the permanence of the operation, and must explore patient reaction to the possible loss of children or death of the spouse. Also to be considered are the patient's religious, family, and social background, and the potential reproductive desires of a possible future sexual partner. The performance of voluntary sterilization in one spouse cannot be legally impeded by the other, but whenever possible, both partners should participate in the decision.

Sterilization can be performed in the male—*vasectomy*—or in the female—*tubal sterilization* or *tubal ligation.*

Vasectomy. The bilateral division and ligation of the vasa deferentia is a simple surgical operation. It is performed under local anesthesia and can be done in any outpatient facility as an office procedure. There are several techniques for severing the continuity of the vasa to prevent the passage of sperm from the testes and epididymides to the penis.

After local anesthesia of the skin and spermatic cord and a small incision on each side of the scrotal skin, isolation of the vas from the spermatic cord is performed (a rather simple surgical procedure), cutting and tying the vas with unabsorbable suture. Some operators remove a piece of the vas; others bury the cut end under the fascia or reverse and tie the end of the severed vas; others cauterize the vas lumen. The purpose of these procedures is to prevent the formation of sperm granulomas and the potential recanalization of the vas and subsequent presence of sperm in the ejaculate.

The patient should be told that vasectomy does not immediately cause sterility; a lapse of several weeks and a number of ejaculations may be necessary to render the man azoospermic. At least one semen analysis totally devoid of sperm, even immotile sperm, is necessary before sexual relations can be resumed without additional contraceptive protection.

Assurance should be given that this procedure has no known effect on the gonads but leaves them intact; also that male hormone production, libido, and potency are not affected. Since the contribution of the testes and epididymides to the ejaculate is minimal (the bulk being provided by the accessory sexual glands, the prostate and seminal vesicles), the volume of ejaculate remains virtually the same.

A subtle but careful scrutiny of the psychosexual personality of the candidate should be made; once an informed decision is reached, a positive attitude should permeate all discussions.

Female Sterilization. There are numerous techniques to sever the continuity of the fallopian tubes and thus interfere with egg and sperm transport and fertilization. In the traditional abdominal operation, the tubes may be severed immediately post partum either at the time of a cesarean section or through a small infraumbilical or paraumbilical incision (minilaparotomy). In the absence of a recent pregnancy, a suprapubic minilaparotomy may be performed. Tubal ligation can also be performed vaginally by posterior colpotomy.

Probably the most popular current approach is by laparoscopy. Tubal sterilization through the laparoscope requires the performance of a pneumoperitoneum with CO_2, most commonly, or with N_2O. The abdomen is penetrated in the umbilical area, sometimes with a single puncture instrument that permits introduction of the accessory instruments (e.g., probe, forceps, scissors, cauterization attachments) through the same laparoscope, although more frequently the procedure involves a two puncture technique; a second puncture, in the suprapubic area, is used to introduce the accessory instruments. The two puncture technique permits additional manipulation of equipment and tissues. The sterilization may be accomplished by electrocoagulation, with or without cutting, or special clips or a Silastic ring may be applied to a loop in the isthmic or ampullary portion of the tube. In general, this procedure takes only a short time and may be performed under local anesthesia with good sedation, or, more commonly in the United States, under general anesthesia. Frequently laparoscopic sterilization can be performed on an ambulatory basis without hospitalization.

It is obvious that vasectomy can be performed more simply and inexpensively, but it does not have the same popularity as tubal sterilization. Reasons for this are lack of available referral services and lack of understanding by the public about the vasectomy procedure; many men are insecure about their sexual capacity and are afraid of losing potency and masculinity as a result of vasectomy.

TABLE 12. **Indications and Contraindications for Voluntary Sterilization**

Indications
- Desire for permanent contraception
- Family completed with many remaining years of potential fertility
- Medical or emotional illness making pregnancy and childbearing hazardous or undesirable
- Serious genetically transmissible disease

Contraindications
- Absolute
  - Strong religious or moral upbringing
  - Sexual identity associated with ability to reproduce
  - Desire for possibility of reversal
- Relative
  - Objection by spouse
  - Age below 25 years
  - No children; 1 or 2 very young children, the last less than 1 year old

Table 12 outlines the indications and contraindications for selection of voluntary sterilization.

Reversibility of Sterilization. With regard to reversibility, encouraging results have recently been reported with vasovasostomy, affording not only restoration of the capability for passage of sperm in from 30 to 90 per cent of the patients but also, more significantly, with subsequent impregnation of the spouse in 11 to 29 per cent of cases.

Female sterilization techniques offer difficulties when restoration of fertility is desired. Following tubal reconstructive surgery, only a 15 to 25 per cent pregnancy rate is achieved. Following salpingoplasty, 75 per cent of the pregnancies end in live births and 10 per cent are ectopic (Siegler).

Newer surgical techniques may improve these statistics, but they are not as yet well established or generally available.

Conclusion

The existence of so many methods and procedures to achieve a single and clear objective—the control, temporarily or permanently, of fertility—is an indication that as yet there is no ideal contraceptive or sterilization technique that is applicable for all men or all women in every clinical or cultural setting. The variety of methods and techniques presently available, however, should allow the physician effectively to assist his patients in finding an appropriate means of controlling their fertility.

SECTION 15

Psychiatry

ALCOHOLISM

method of
KENNETH H. WILLIAMS, M.D.
Pittsburgh, Pennsylvania

The principal role of the physician in the management of alcoholism is to diagnose this illness when it presents in his patients in one of its many disguised forms and to recruit his patient into treatment. The primary care physician is in an excellent position to accomplish these tasks, whether or not he decides to undertake part or all of the long-term treatment himself or to refer his patient to other sources of help. The goals of treatment are to achieve a state of productive and contented existence without the use of alcohol or other mind-altering (especially sedative) drugs.

Definition

Alcoholism can be defined as a chronic, progressive illness which involves the use of alcoholic beverages to such an extent that it interferes recurringly in the functional life of the individual, as manifested by health, family, job, legal, or emotional problems. If untreated, a mortality rate of 5 per cent per year can be anticipated. Alcoholics have a life expectancy approximately 14 years shorter than the average American. Most alcoholics in this country at present never have their disease diagnosed by a physician, and directly or indirectly die of their disease (from medical complications such as cirrhosis, automobile or home accidents, or suicide). In addition alcoholism contributes to the morbidity and mortality of other common diseases (such as diabetes and heart disease) and complicates their treatment. It may be this country's greatest (and most neglected) health problem.

Although there is no universally accepted definition of alcoholism, most definitions involve all three of the following criteria: (1) large or excessive quantity of alcohol consumed over a period of years, (2) abnormal, chronic loss of control over the ability to regulate consumption of alcohol, and (3) chronic damage to physical health or social standing. Thus to diagnose alcoholism we must examine not how much the person drinks but the consequences of the drinking—i.e., the functional problems associated with using alcohol. Perhaps the single most important characteristic of alcoholics in this country is their inability to consistently regulate their intake of alcohol once they begin an episode of drinking.

Treatment

If the diagnosis of alcoholism has been made or even if it is suspected, it is essential that this information be shared with the patient. Getting the alcoholic patient to accept his illness is probably the most important aspect of treatment. It also may be the most difficult. The goal of treatment is the establishment of a contented state of sobriety.

Confrontation. Directing the patient's attention to his "drinking problem" or "confronting" him with his diagnosis is the key to further treatment. How can a patient cooperate with treatment for a disease he does not know he has? In this discussion all the physician's skill and ability to practice the art of medicine may be tested.

However, having just diagnosed (or highly suspected) a chronic, progressive, often fatal illness, it is the physician's obligation to inform the patient. (If a physician had diagnosed diabetes, he would be under a similar obligation.) Learning to live with this condition will certainly greatly affect the quality and duration of the remainder of the patient's life. It will also greatly affect the lives of his family and friends.

In proceeding with the confrontation it is suggested that the physician attempt to get the patient to make his own diagnosis by asking him a question such as: "Have you ever wondered if you might have a 'drinking problem'?" It is surprising how often alcoholic patients will respond affirmatively. Many will be relieved to have this difficult subject discussed openly. Most alcoholics have, at some level, suspected their problem, but most also believe it to be hidden from others.

It is most helpful if the physician can progress objectively in this discussion with his patient, presenting the evidence for his diagnosis in objective, scientific, and easy-to-accept terms. He should present the evidence by showing the patient his concerns as revealed in the history, physical examination, laboratory findings, or x-rays. If the physician has utilized the Michigan Alcoholism Screening Test, simply informing his patient of how he has scored in relation to other alcoholics and normal persons will sometimes be very helpful. It is suggested that the physician be supportive yet persistent in this confrontation and to initially anticipate denial on the part of some patients.

The physician may elect to make a simple statement such as: "In my medical opinion you have a drinking problem, the disease of alcoholism." He should be persuasive, yet supportive, patient yet persistent, conveying his concerns and backing them up with facts.

It is suggested that an excellent time for this confrontation is at the time of a crisis or at the time of hospitalization. It is probably in times of crisis, when he has active problems with his drinking, that the alcoholic is most amenable to acceptance of his disease and most willing to do something about it.

If the doctor feels uncomfortable or for some other reason feels he cannot take the step of presenting to the patient the evidence for the diagnosis, he should at least find someone else who will. Although it is probably most effective and most easily done by the patient's primary care physician, a knowledgeable consultant can effectively take this step (and the next) with the patient. However, the physician is still obliged to bring in this consultant and present to the patient the reasons for doing so.

Education. Because of the stigma still associated with alcoholism, it is important for the patient and his family to become educated about the nature of this disease. This can usually be accomplished by suggesting the following methods:

1. Readings. I usually suggest Mann, M.: New Primer on Alcoholism, New York, Holt, Rinehart and Winston, 1958 for the patient; and/or Johnson, V.: I'll Quit Tomorrow, New York, Harper and Row, 1973 for the patient and his family; and/or Maxwell, R.: The Booze Battle, a Frank E. Taylor Book, New York, Praeger Publishers, 1976 for the family.

2. Attendance at an open Alcoholics Anonymous (AA) meeting (for the patient and his family) or an Al-Anon meeting (for the family of the patient). I know of no better way to educate a person about alcoholism than to suggest that he attend an AA meeting. To see many active members of AA, representing all walks of life and all social classes, happily involved in a meeting is also one of the best ways of destigmatizing the disease for the patient (and introduces the patient to a most important treatment modality). (For further suggestions on getting a patient to an AA meeting, see p. 850.)

Overdose. Acute alcohol overdose, whether done as a suicide attempt or by a young person as the result of a dare by others, is a relatively uncommon phenomenon. It may occur in alcoholics or in persons who cannot be diagnosed as alcoholic. If the person lives long enough, treatment, as with any other sedative overdose, is usually attempted in an emergency room setting. The primary risk of death is through respiratory depression.

1. Establish an adequate airway.
2. Ventilate the patient mechanically or by mouth-to-mouth artificial respiration if spontaneous respiratory efforts are insufficient.
3. Start intravenous fluids.
4. Obtain blood samples to check electrolytes, kidney and hepatic function, and glucose.
5. Lavage gastric contents when the patient is conscious if less than 2 hours have elapsed since ingestion. Examine gastric contents.
6. Suspect multiple sedative overdose and obtain historical and laboratory evidence (such as serum barbiturate level) to confirm diagnosis.
7. Consider hypoglycemia in a malnourished or hypothermic patient and administer 50 ml. of 50 per cent glucose intravenously.
8. Consider hemodialysis if the patient has not adequately responded to the aforementioned measures, if there is evidence for concomitant methanol intoxication or intoxication with another dialyzable sedative, or if severe acidosis (pH less than 7) is present.
9. Consider administration of 1 liter of 10 per cent fructose in isotonic saline solution intravenously over 1 hour. Fructose increases ethanol metabolism and may be helpful in certain situations. It is important to evaluate the patient every 30 minutes and to check for circulatory overload. It will be helpful to monitor blood lactate and uric acid levels. The primary danger is lactic acidosis; patients particularly susceptible to this complication will be those with liver disease, uncontrolled diabetes, hypoxia, and/or shock.
10. Consider other coexisting, contributing causes if coma is deep or prolonged.

Alcohol Withdrawal Syndrome. As with any addictive drug, regular heavy use of the sedative alcohol is accompanied by physiologic changes in the central nervous system which result in the phenomenon known as the withdrawal syndrome when ingestion of the drug is abruptly stopped or greatly diminished. The clinically significant alcohol withdrawal syndrome does not occur in the absence of alcoholism; its occurrence establishes the diagnosis. The ultimate goal of therapy is to enter the patient into long-term treatment for alcoholism.

The alcohol withdrawal syndrome may be conceptualized as an expression of the release phenomena from the depressant effect of alcohol on the brain. As in the withdrawal syndrome from other addictive drugs, the manifestations of the alcohol withdrawal syndrome can be seen to be, in many ways, opposite from the immediate direct effects of the drug on the brain. Thus in acute intoxication we typically find diminished psychomotor activity, with relaxation, hypothermia, depressed respirations, decreased rapid eye movement sleep, increased delta (stage 3 or 4) sleep, and an increased seizure threshold; in alcohol withdrawal we find increased psychomotor activity, with agitation, nervousness, hyperthermia, stimulation of the respiratory center producing hyperventilation and respiratory alkalosis, increased (or constant) rapid eye movement sleep, decreased delta sleep, seizures, hallucinations, and delirium.

The withdrawal syndrome is seen in all gradations of severity, from the very mild tremor requiring no treatment to the severe delirium tremens, a life-threatening emergency requiring hospitalization.

The severity of the alcohol withdrawal syndrome depends upon at least six factors: (1) the amount of alcohol consumed, (2) the duration of the drinking episode, (3) the individual's previous experience with alcohol withdrawal (those who have previously suffered convulsions or delirium tremens are much more at risk of experiencing them again), (4) coexisting disease problems (other things being equal, a patient with pneumonia is more likely to suffer a severe alcohol withdrawal syndrome), (5) nutritional factors (coexisting deficiency states tend to aggravate the condition), and (6) age (older persons will have a more severe withdrawal syndrome).

Generally speaking, the duration of the alcohol withdrawal syndrome will be proportional to its severity. The incidence of the most severe alcohol withdrawal syndrome, delirium tremens, has been decreasing in recent years.

The physician is often faced with the consideration of whether or not to admit an alcoholic patient to a hospital for management of the withdrawal syndrome. The more severe the syndrome, the more likely it is to require hospital management. The Physician's Task Force of the State of Pennsylvania's Governor's Council on Drug and Alcohol Abuse has devised guidelines for determining admission of an alcoholic patient who presents primarily because of alcohol withdrawal symptomatology to a general hospital. These guidelines state in part that "a patient with alcoholism should be admitted if he or she has been drinking recently and (a) demonstrates an acute alcohol withdrawal syndrome with hallucinations (visual, auditory, or tactile) or serious confusion, (b) has a history of recent convulsions or exhibits a poorly controlled convulsive disorder, or (c) manifests signs of impending or active delirium tremens—the autonomic syndrome of fever, tachycardia, hypertension, dilated pupils, sweating, with extreme agitation, disorientation, and hallucinations, especially if worsening 2 to 4 days after cessation of alcohol consumption." A decision regarding admission should also be based on other coexisting disease problems in the patient and on the availability of a residential-setting detoxification program in the community.

The following treatment considerations are recommended in management of the alcohol withdrawal syndrome:

1. Provide a nonthreatening, supportive, quiet environment in which the patient can relax and feel comfortable. A calm, supportive, and reassuring attitude provided by those caring for the patient may be the most important factor in avoiding the more serious manifestations of the withdrawal syndrome. Restraints are to be avoided whenever possible.

2. Reality-orient the patient, maintaining as much as possible his links with reality. Sensory deprivation predisposes toward illusions and hallucinations; therefore it is recommended that the patient be kept in a lighted environment with provision of company (friend, relative, or staff), a radio or television set, and a clock. As much as possible it is helpful to engage the patient in simple, purposeful tasks, encouraging ambulation and participation in daily activities.

3. Administer sedatives if the aforementioned measures fail to halt the progression of symptoms to a more severe withdrawal state. Evidence from several recent studies would suggest that the drugs best suited for sedation in the hospitalized alcoholic undergoing withdrawal are the benzodiazepines, diazepam and chlordiazepoxide. (However, other sedatives such as the barbiturates, chloral hydrate, and others are used with success in some centers.) The goal is to administer enough of the chosen drug early enough to prevent progression of symptoms (this may require, in unusual cases, as much as 1400 mg. of chlordiazepoxide in the first 24 hours) yet not so much that the patient's link with reality is completely severed. (This dose is higher than that listed in the manufacturer's official directive.) The

benzodiazepines should preferably be given orally or intravenously, as intramuscular doses produce slower, more unpredictable, and lower blood levels. The patient's response to these drugs is not completely predictable; it will vary with the degree of tolerance to sedative drugs in general, age, smoking history, and liver function. It is generally recommended that treatment begin with as small a dose as seems reasonable to effect the desired clinical response, with the patient and his vital signs being monitored closely (especially in the first 48 hours) and a re-evaluation being made hourly as to the necessity for additional doses of sedative medication. As soon as the patient is assessed to be improving, the sedative medication should be administered in diminishing doses. It is important to withdraw these drugs as rapidly as is deemed safe and to discontinue them as soon as possible, certainly prior to discharge. The benzodiazepines produce a sedative withdrawal syndrome of their own, and it is not conducive to continued sobriety to have the patient experiencing withdrawal symptoms from these drugs as an outpatient. I prefer to discontinue all sedative medication at least 48 hours prior to anticipated discharge, and do not discharge until the patient is able to sleep at least one night in relative comfort without any sedatives.

4. Administer vitamins. Thiamine (vitamin B_1), 50 to 100 mg. parenterally, is advised. If macrocytosis is present, or if the nutritional history would indicate a high risk of multiple vitamin deficiencies, it is suggested that a folic acid and vitamin B_{12} level be drawn, and that additional folic acid and B complex vitamins be administered orally.

5. Administer magnesium if desired. Definitive studies demonstrating the value of magnesium therapy in alcohol withdrawal have not yet been done; however, it may assist in reducing seizures, tremor, and cardiac arrhythmias. If desired, 2 ml. of magnesium sulfate 50 per cent solution may be injected intramuscularly every 8 hours for the first 3 days.

6. Administer phenytoin (diphenylhydantoin) if desired. If the alcoholic patient has experienced withdrawal seizures previously and is evaluated to be at high risk of experiencing them again, consideration should be given to administration of phenytoin, 100 mg. orally three times daily for 5 days. This appears to provide adequate blood levels and assists in prevention of seizures (Sampliner and Iber: JAMA, *230*:1430–1432, 1974).

7. Correction of electrolyte imbalance. Because of the frequent occurrence of acid-base and electrolyte abnormalities, every alcoholic entering a hospital should have a determination of serum electrolytes, which may include a serum magnesium level. The most frequent findings will be an excess of total body water (a typical alcoholic diureses a few pounds during detoxification) and a low serum potassium. If the clinical situation warrants (such as the existence of cardiac arrhythmias), potassium replacement may be given, preferably orally if vomiting is not a problem. Because of the likely existence of an excess of total body water (and the likely discomfort to the patient), it is suggested that intravenous fluids be avoided whenever possible. Intravenous glucose can precipitate a thiamine deficiency and increase the problems with hypokalemia. Oral fluids containing potassium, such as fruit juices, are to be encouraged.

8. Take a careful history regarding recent use of all sedative drugs. Recent studies have shown that it should be assumed that all alcoholic patients have been taking at least one other sedative drug in addition to alcohol. If a history of regular use of any "sleeping pills" or "tranquilizers" is obtained, the withdrawal syndrome from these drugs must be anticipated and treated appropriately. (For example, the withdrawal syndrome from diazepam does not generally begin until 3 to 5 days after cessation of use.)

If the patient is not considered sick enough to require hospitalization, or if hospitalization is refused and a "residential-setting" detoxification program is not available, an attempt may be made at ambulatory detoxification. This procedure may be successful if the patient is highly motivated and there is another supportive caretaker (spouse or friend) in almost constant attendance. In this situation drugs are best avoided; however, if used, consideration should be given to use of hydroxyzine, phenobarbital, or the benzodiazepines. The patient must be seen daily and only enough medication provided to last the subsequent 24 hour period.

Long-Term Treatment. The primary care physician is an excellent candidate to assist the alcoholic patient in long-term recovery from this chronic disease. An established, good doctor-patient relationship is a sound basis for assistive management of the patient to recovery. If the patient respects his doctor, feels confidence in him, and can confide in him, therapy can proceed naturally and easily.

However, after examining his own attitudes toward the alcoholic and assessing his own skills in a type of therapy which involves close, open, and honest contact with his patient in the doctor-patient relationship, it may be that the physician would elect not to treat the alcoholic person but to refer him elsewhere for assistance. This decision, arrived at after careful self-scrutiny, is to be commended. It is much better to do this than to become involved with alcoholic patients in a negative and antitherapeutic manner.

Such a physician cannot responsibly do nothing, however. His tasks with the alcoholic would be simplified. For this physician responsibilities would be limited to recognizing the disease of alcoholism, referral to other sources of help, and avoiding placing problems in the path of his recovering patient (for instance, by prescribing addictive, sedative medication or by advising him to resume drinking).

For the physician who is able to assist in providing long-term treatment for his alcoholic patients, a satisfying reward of assisting his patient to recovery may be realized. Most physicians who have participated in the long-term treatment of one of their alcoholic patients consider it to be a highly rewarding experience.

Those things a physician can do to assist his patients in long-term treatment of alcoholism would include the following:

PRESCRIBE PSYCHOTROPIC DRUGS WITH GREAT CARE, IF AT ALL. The detoxification of the alcoholic may appropriately utilize sedative medication. However, the long-term outpatient management of alcoholism (a type of sedative drug abuse) does not ideally involve prescribing another sedative drug. Some authorities in treatment of the alcoholic consider this the greatest disservice a physician can perform for his alcoholic patient and feel that it would be better if the doctor did nothing at all. Most physicians involved with large, outpatient alcoholism treatment programs agree that prescription sedative drugs are an almost total obstacle to recovery for the alcoholic.

This is not to say that the alcoholic will not want sedative drugs prescribed for him. Many will specifically request them and be very skillful in manipulating the doctor into prescribing them.

The dangers in prescribing sedative drugs on an outpatient basis for alcoholics are at least four: (1) The patient can become addicted to the sedative medication ("cross-addiction"). When a physician prescribes sedative drugs, he is simply substituting one sedative-hypnotic chemical in solid form for another (i.e., alcohol) in liquid form. Since alcoholic patients are already prone to become dependent upon their favorite sedative-hypnotic drug, alcohol, they are quite susceptible to dependence upon sedative-hypnotics. Just as with alcohol, they can quickly build up a tolerance to larger and larger doses of any of these other sedative-hypnotics. (2) The patient can accidentally kill himself or seriously overdose with a combination of alcohol and the sedative drug. (3) It isolates the patient from a very important source of help, Alcoholics Anonymous. (4) It tends to reinforce the notion in the patient's mind that if there is a problem—i.e., if he is nervous or upset—the answer lies in putting something in his mouth to make him feel better.

Experience has shown that the alcoholic outpatient tends to do very poorly on diazepam (Valium). Many alcoholics will seek out the "heady" high and abuse diazepam more readily than they would other, related sedatives.

The value of prescribing other, nonaddictive psychoactive drugs such as the phenothiazines or tricyclic antidepressants for the alcoholic would be negligible unless the alcoholic has another specific indication for use of this drug—i.e., a cognitive disorder or an identified depression. The value of lithium in the treatment of alcoholism is being tested.

PRESCRIBE DISULFIRAM. Consideration should be given for every alcoholic patient to take disulfiram (Antabuse). Experience with this drug now covers over 20 years and includes thousands of patients. In spite of the fact that doctors with the most extensive experience in prescribing this drug consider it to be extraordinarily safe, many practitioners are fearful of prescribing disulfiram. The dangers have probably been overemphasized. Very few deaths attributed to it have been recorded in the medical literature.

Disulfiram should be prescribed only with the patient's (and the family's) full knowledge and consent. To assist the physician in this educational process, Ayerst Laboratories, the company that manufactures Antabuse, has published a helpful patient education booklet. The contraindications to disulfiram administration are few: (1) If a person has brain damage or mental deficiency to such a degree that he cannot comprehend the significance of the instructions, he should not take the drug. (2) If a person is strongly suicidal, prescribing disulfiram would provide another potential means of committing suicide. (3) If a person manifests an allergic reaction to the drug, it should not be prescribed for him. (4) It should not be given to anyone who has alcohol in his blood. (5) Severe coronary artery disease should be at least a strong relative contraindication, as most of the deaths in those who have drunk alcohol while taking disulfiram have occurred in those with coronary artery disease. (6) There are five medications that a person should not take while on disulfiram. These include isoniazid (INH), sodium warfarin, hydantoin, paraldehyde, and metronidazole.

The indication for disulfiram is alcoholism. It can provide considerable benefit to an alcoholic who elects to take it. The physician should not hesitate to encourage patients to take it. One of the advantages to using Antabuse is that the drug stays in the body at least several days after the last dose.

Alcohol-Antabuse reactions have been experienced as long as 2 weeks after the last pill has been taken. As a result, the patient is forced to plan the drinking in advance. It can help eliminate the sudden impulse to drink, as many alcoholics drink on sudden impulse.

UTILIZE ALCOHOLICS ANONYMOUS. Involvement with Alcoholics Anonymous (AA) may be the best treatment available for the alcoholic. It is responsible for the recovery of more alcoholics than any other treatment modality. The doctor should make every effort to utilize this key resource for every one of his alcoholic patients. It may be the only treatment that the patient needs.

It is suggested that the doctor make it as easy as possible for identified alcoholic patients to get to their first meeting. The following specific suggestions may help in accomplishing this:

1. Arrange for telephone or personal contact with an individual AA member. If the doctor has among his patients a member of AA with some degree of knowledge and experience about the AA program, the physician can (with the AA member's permission) give the newly identified alcoholic this phone number; or the doctor can suggest that an AA member will phone him. If the doctor does not have such an AA member among his patients, the doctor can encourage the newly identified alcoholic to phone AA. In almost every city phone directory will be found a number for Alcoholics Anonymous. Many cities have a 24 hour answering service and can provide an experienced and knowledgeable member to speak to a newcomer on short notice.

2. Suggest that the newly identified alcoholic go to an AA meeting in his local area. This is usually a more difficult step for a person to take. Since specific AA groups vary considerably in the ethnic and socioeconomic composition of their members, it is helpful if the physician can direct his patient to a specific group which the newcomer will find easy to relate to and identify with. The newly identified alcoholic will be more likely to attend his first meeting if his physician agrees to go with him.

3. Provide the newly identified alcoholic with AA literature. Alcoholics Anonymous has many excellent pamphlets designed to introduce the newcomer to the program. Two excellent ones are "Is AA for You?" and "This is AA." These pamphlets are available at a cost of approximately 15 cents by writing AA World Services, Inc., P.O. Box 459, Grand Central Station, New York, N.Y. 10017; or by phoning (212) 686-1100. They are often provided to physicians free of charge by local AA groups. The doctor should consider phoning his local AA answering service to obtain literature.

4. The doctor himself can go to an AA meeting. If the doctor has been to one or more AA meetings and can speak knowledgeably about his first-hand knowledge of AA groups in the local area, his chances of getting his patients to AA meetings are greatly improved. It may be the single most important factor in the doctor's being able to convince his patients to go to an AA meeting. Unless a person has been to an AA meeting, it is very difficult for him to understand what AA is all about. Understanding AA begins with going to an AA meeting. There are other benefits to be had by the doctor going to an AA meeting: (a) It is an excellent way to learn about alcoholism, an educational experience. (b) It can demonstrate to the doctor that there is hope of recovery. (I had been a physician for 8 years, had treated medical complications in hundreds of alcoholic patients, and yet had not seen a single alcoholic who had recovered until I visited my first AA meeting.) (c) It will probably be an enjoyable experience. The speakers at AA meetings are generally very good and may be funny, sad, inspirational, or a combination of all three, but meetings are seldom unenjoyable. The friendliness and spirit among the members is infectious, and has to be experienced to be appreciated. (d) It might provide the doctor with a place he can receive some therapy for his own problem.

A physician wishing to attend a local AA meeting should identify his desires to the local answering service, listed in his phone directory. Attendance at an AA meeting should be suggested for the alcoholic patient who says that he has tried AA before. There is a tendency for alcoholics still in the active phase of their illness to downgrade every treatment program they have previously had contact with, including AA. A second or third try at affiliation may have a much different effect, especially if suggested by a physician.

AA can provide the alcoholic patient (1) a nondrinking peer group in an otherwise drinking society; (2) friendship and warm, personal support; (3) a simplified prescription for living a sober and happier life; (4) group therapy and resocialization; (5) education about the disease of alcoholism; and (6) hope of recovery by the example of many who have successfully arrested their disease, and probably much more.

INVOLVE THE FAMILY. Alcoholism has been called the family disease because of its characteristic manner of involving all family members. It is beneficial to involve families as early and as extensively as possible into the patient's treatment plan. In addition to improving the patient's chances of recovery, involvement of the family is specifically suggested for the following reasons: (1) To confirm or negate the history obtained from the patient. (2) To evaluate the spouse for alcoholism. It is true that alcoholics are much more likely than others to find a spouse who is alcoholic. One of the few reliable methods to identify this double problem is to interview the spouse. (3) To evaluate the spouse for other disease. Many times it will be discovered that the spouse is "sicker" and more in need of help than the identified patient. (4) To assess "game playing," "enabling," or other pathologically reciprocal relationships between the alcoholic and the spouse. The family is going to be with the patient 7 days a week. The doctor will probably have the patient for only a few minutes a week. If the family is not playing a therapeutic role, it is going to be very difficult for the alcoholic to proceed in treatment; the family can undo what the physician is trying to accomplish.

Al-Anon is a fellowship, patterned after the AA program, designed for the families of the alcoholic. Referral to Al-Anon should be considered for the spouse. As with referral to AA, referral to Al-Anon should be made with an expression of positive regard for this self-help organization. All the suggestions previously made about getting a patient to an AA meeting would apply to getting the spouse to an Al-Anon meeting. Make it as easy as possible for them to do this. If the doctor knows someone in Al-Anon, he can arrange for telephone or personal communication prior to attendance at the first meeting. The doctor may also provide the spouse with Al-Anon literature to read.

Refer to Alcoholism Treatment Facilities. Several authorities in the field of alcoholism have argued that the ideal treatment for alcoholism, a multifaceted problem of multiple causes, involves an interdisciplinary team. In considering other sources of help, the doctor will be assisted by a knowledge of other alcoholism treatment facilities in his area.

Most sections of the country are fortunate to have specialized alcoholism treatment facilities available locally. The facilities and services vary considerably, ranging from outpatient services to long term (2 years or more) residential facilities. A practitioner desiring to know what services are available locally to him should consult the Alcoholism Treatment Facilities Directory, published by Alcohol and Drug Problems Association of North America, 1130 Seventeenth Street N.W., Washington, D.C. 20036. This directory provides descriptive information (including name of facility, address, phone number, name of director, description of type of program and services available, and admission requirements) for over 2500 alcoholism treatment facilities, listed by state and city. The doctor may also find out what treatment facilities exist locally by contacting his local office of the National Council on Alcoholism, listed in the telephone directory.

NARCOTIC POISONING

method of
RICHARD B. RESNICK, M.D.
New York, New York

Definitions

Narcotic poisoning refers to an acute overdose of any drug that is included in the class of opioids. *Opioids* are the natural or synthetic compounds whose principal pharmacologic actions are morphine-like. They are sometimes referred to as *narcotic analgesics*. Their medical uses are primarily for relief of pain, coughing, and diarrhea.

Commonly prescribed opioids include the following:

Generic name:	*Common trade name:*
Codeine	
Dihydrocodeine	Paracodin
Heroin*	
Hydrocodone	Hycodan
Hydromorphone	Dilaudid
LAAM (l-alpha-acetylmethadol)*	
Levorphanol	Levo-Dromoran
Meperidine	Demerol
Methadone†	Dolophine
Metopon	Metopon
Morphine	
Oxycodone	Percodan
Oxymorphone	Numorphan
Opium	Pantopon
Paregoric	
Propoxyphene	Darvon

Diagnosis

Characteristic Signs. 1. Diminished alertness (ranging from light somnolence to a deep coma).

*Heroin and LAAM are Schedule I drugs and are not available by prescription. However, heroin is readily available through illicit channels and is the most commonly abused opiate. LAAM is undergoing clinical investigation as a maintenance medication for opiate-dependent patients who ingest it under program supervision only.

†Methadone products may be dispensed only by maintenance programs approved by the Food and Drug Administration and the designated State authority. Through diversion by some patients in maintenance programs, take-home doses of methadone have led to its easy availability and to the frequent occurrence of accidental overdose by children.

2. Depressed respiratory rate (as low as 2 to 4 breaths per minute or apnea).

3. Miosis (pupils are symmetrical in size and often pinpoint).

Note 1: Decreased alertness and depressed respiratory rate are also found in acute overdose from other central nervous system (CNS) depressants such as alcohol, sedatives, and hypnotic drugs. A mixed narcotic and non-narcotic sedative overdose may coexist.

Note 2: In the presence of severe anoxia, the pupils may be fully dilated and nonreactive to light. Miosis may be absent in meperidine overdose.

Associated Findings. 1. Hypotension, cyanosis, decreased body temperature, and flaccid muscles.

2. Needle or track marks along superficial veins in chronic heroin abusers.

3. Focal or generalized convulsions are common in cases of propoxyphene and meperidine poisoning.

4. A history of opiate abuse.

5. Exposure to available opiates, particularly in children.

6. Possession of needles, syringes or containers that contained opiates is highly suggestive of the diagnosis in patients showing the characteristic signs.

Treatment

Primary Treatment. 1. Maintain ventilation. (a) Remove manually or by suction any foreign matter obstructing airway patency. (b) Artificial respiration is given by mouth-to-mouth resuscitation until oropharyngeal or endotracheal intubation with Ambu bag respiration, using oxygen, can be accomplished.

2. Administer a narcotic antagonist. Naloxone (Narcan) is the drug of choice. Begin with 0.4 mg. (1 ml.) intravenously and repeat every 1 to 3 minutes until spontaneous respiration is restored to at least 10 breaths per minute. If intravenous administration is not immediately possible, administer the naloxone subcutaneously or sublingually (sublingual administration is not listed in the manufacturer's official directive).

Naloxone's duration of action (approximately 30 minutes) is considerably shorter than the duration of action of opiates. Therefore after there is improvement in respiratory rate, the physician must continue to administer naloxone until the opioid that caused the poisoning has been sufficiently metabolized so that it will no longer depress respiration. The preferred route for continued naloxone administration is intramuscular, as this will produce a longer-lasting effect. The time period for continuing the administration of naloxone can range from 4 hours for short-acting opioids, such as morphine, to 72 hours for LAAM.

In postoperative patients who have narcotic-induced respiratory depression, smaller doses of naloxone (0.1 to 0.2 mg.) are usually sufficient. Excessive dosage can cause reversal of analgesia.

In children and in neonates the initial dose of naloxone is 0.01 mg. per kg. of body weight. This dose is then repeated in accordance with the suggested guidelines for adults.

Caution: In a patient who is opiate dependent, the amount of naloxone that is given must be carefully titrated in order to avoid precipitating an acute opiate abstinence syndrome. The dosage of naloxone should be enough to restore spontaneous respirations, but not necessarily consciousness, without causing sweating, chills, tremor, agitation, piloerection, abdominal cramps, or vomiting.

If naloxone is not available, nalorphine (Nalline) or levallorphan (Lorfan) may be used similarly. Nalorphine, 5 to 10 mg. (1 to 2 ml.) every 3 to 5 minutes, or levallorphan, 0.5 to 1.0 mg. (0.5 to 1 ml.) every 10 to 15 minutes, is comparable in antagonist potency to naloxone, 0.4 mg. (1 ml.) every 1 to 3 minutes, for beginning therapy.

Caution: Nalorphine and levallorphan have morphine-like agonist effects and will, in the absence of opiates, produce respiratory depression and miosis. Their use therefore can confuse the diagnosis and aggravate the respiratory depression resulting from nonopioid drugs. They can also produce psychotomimetic side effects.

If the patient does not show a response to three doses of an antagonist, it suggests that the respiratory depression is due to causes other than opioid overdose. Additional doses of nalorphine or levallorphan should be given with extreme caution for the reasons noted above. These risks are not posed by additional doses of naloxone, as it is a "pure" antagonist (i.e., lacking in agonist effects).

Supportive Treatment. 1. Maintain venous patency with a continuous drip of intravenous fluids (glucose in water with supplemental electrolytes).

2. Monitor vital signs every 15 to 30 minutes and continue oxygen until consciousness is fully restored.

3. A urine sample should be analyzed immediately for drug content.

4. Institute specific therapy for shock, pulmonary edema, convulsions, urinary retention, pneumonia, or other complications.

Follow-up Treatment. The circumstances that led to the narcotic poisoning must be ascertained with appropriate follow-up recommendations:

1. An opiate-dependent individual should be referred to a drug abuse treatment facility in his community.

2. Psychiatric consultation is needed in cases of suicide attempt.

3. If a child has accidentally ingested an opiate, it is essential to provide the parents with

guidance and information so that they can take appropriate precautions to avoid a recurrence. If child neglect is suspected, referral to an appropriate mental health worker or community agency is recommended.

PSYCHONEUROSIS

method of
CHARLES E. WELLS, M.D.
Nashville, Tennessee

Psychoneurosis is the diagnostic rubric which designates a limited group of specific psychiatric disorders, each manifested by a set of discrete symptoms and signs. These disorders (obsessive-compulsive neurosis is an example) are rarely encountered in pure form by most general physicians; they are, in fact, uncommon even among the patients treated by psychiatrists. I, therefore, shall not confine my discussion of therapy to this limited group of somewhat rare disorders. Instead, I shall consider the broader spectrum of psychiatric disorders likely to be encountered with some frequency by all practitioners regardless of their areas of specialization. From a nosologic standpoint these disorders are most commonly diagnosed as *mixed psychoneuroses* and *character disorders*. Treatment of the psychoses will not be dealt with here.

Patients with mixed psychoneuroses and character disorders commonly present themselves to their physicians because of (1) symptoms (such as anxiety, depression, hypochondriasis) or behavioral patterns (such as phobias, compulsions) which patients recognize as outside the range of their usual experience or usual self (neurosis); (2) symptoms (such as anxiety, depression, anger, suspiciousness) sometimes but not always attributed by patients to behavioral patterns (repeated failures, social isolation, erratic employment, for example) which they interpret as a usual, normal, and ordinary part of the self (character disorder); (3) somatic symptoms, without evidence of physical disease, arising from either a neurosis or a character disorder; (4) symptoms of psychologic discomfort (especially depression, anger, and fear), arising in a setting of recognized or unrecognized physical illness; (5) somatic symptoms, arising in a setting of recognized physical disease, which are out of keeping in character or intensity with the physical disease; or (6) behavior sufficiently distressing to the family or associates that it results in patients being brought to the physician for help.

Patients who fall into groups 3, 4, or 5 above may cause considerable diagnostic puzzlement. When the physician suspects, however, that a patient's symptoms arise largely from psychiatric causes, it is important that this be explained early in the evaluative process and that the patient be led to understand that the treatment of psychologic distress is as accepted a part of the physician's role as is the treatment of physical distress.

No single treatment plan is appropriate for every patient coming to the physician with psychiatric dysfunction in the guises listed above. Selection and implementation of the appropriate treatment grow out of the patient evaluation. No attempt will be made here to discuss the complexities of patient evaluation. Rather, the elements in patient evaluation which specifically affect treatment choice will be discussed in the broader context of treatment planning.

Two aims are basic to all varieties of psychiatric treatment: (1) the development of a therapeutic alliance between therapist and patient, and (2) the relief of symptomatic distress.

All modes of psychiatric treatment depend on the construction of a therapeutic alliance. This means essentially that physician and patient must join forces to pool their resources in joint determination to reach an agreed goal, which commonly includes relief of distressing symptoms either as the primary goal or as one of an accepted set of objectives. Establishment of a therapeutic alliance, the sine qua non of effective therapy, is often easy, but it may at times be difficult or even impossible. It may develop in a single interview, or it may require months of prickly negotiation. A therapeutic alliance is especially difficult to achieve in those patients who fear placing trust in others or fear submission to others and in those who lack the capacity to develop strong object relations.

Secondly, symptomatic relief must be an acknowledged goal of treatment, though not necessarily the first or most important objective. Therapy neglecting this aim is doomed to failure. Sometimes a degree of symptomatic relief must be achieved before development of a therapeutic alliance can be started. For example, some relief of severe anxiety through use of anxiolytic agents may be required before an extremely anxious patient can begin to relate to the physician as a person.

The most common therapeutic modalities currently available for the treatment of psychiatric disorders are listed in Table 1, along with some indications for their specific use. Five varieties of

TABLE 1. **Spectrum of Treatment Modalities Available for Psychiatric Disorders**

	BEHAVIOR THERAPY	PHARMACOLOGIC THERAPY	DIRECTIVE THERAPY	SUPPORTIVE THERAPY	INSIGHT THERAPY
Therapist characteristics	Performed only by specialists	Performed by specialists and nonspecialists			Performed only by specialists
Symptom characteristics	Most effective in relief of discrete, limited symptoms				Most effective in relief of multiple, diffuse symptoms
Patient characteristics	Unlikely to tolerate increased discomfort and yet remain in treatment				Likely to tolerate increased discomfort and yet remain in treatment
	Needful of guidelines and rules				Tolerant of uncertainty
	Nonverbal				Verbal
	Unable to free-associate				Able to free-associate
	Not psychologically minded				Psychologically minded
	Not inquisitive about self				Inquisitive about self

treatment are listed, along with the suggestion that these modes form a spectrum with specific treatment applicabilities. At one end of the spectrum lie the behavior therapies (including biofeedback techniques); at the other end lie the insight therapies, which subsume the varieties of psychoanalytically oriented psychotherapies. Both behavior therapy and insight therapy should be performed by specialists; the specific techniques of their use will not be considered further here. When the general physician considers that one of these techniques is indicated, the physician usually refers the patient to an appropriate therapist. Between these two ends of the spectrum lie pharmacologic therapy, directive therapy, and supportive therapy, the three modalities discussed in most detail here.

Behavior Therapy and Insight Therapy

Some mention is needed of situations in which behavior therapy or insight therapy should be chosen as primary treatment modalities. Behavior therapy, as its name implies, aims primarily at behavioral change, with secondary reduction of the subjective distress that has resulted from the maladaptive behavior. Behavior therapy is most effective when the maladaptive pattern can be precisely defined and is limited. Examples of problems which might be approached effectively through behavioral techniques are an unreasonable fear of driving an automobile or a fear which inhibits speaking in public. The effectiveness of these techniques lessens as the targeted behavioral change loses definition. These techniques are often excellent for patients who are nonverbal, lack interest in the factors underlying their distress, and cannot formulate their aims other than in terms of symptom relief. The establishment of a therapeutic alliance is, however, no less important for the success of behavior therapy than for other treatment modalities.

At the other end of this proposed spectrum lie the insight therapies (or the psychoanalytically oriented psychotherapies). Insight therapy should not be attempted by the nonspecialist. In general, the recommendation for insight therapy is restricted to those patients who are verbal, are able to free-associate easily, are psychologically oriented, manifest an interest in seeking the origins of their own discomfort, and are keen for self-knowledge. Poor ego strength is generally a contraindication to this therapeutic modality. Insight therapy is most effective in patients with multifaceted problems (which might most appropriately be termed "problems in living").

The other three forms of treatment are the ones most important for the nonspecialist to master; they are equally important for the psychiatrist.

Pharmacologic Therapy

Psychotropic medications are never, of course, used alone; they are, however, not infrequently the primary therapeutic instrument. Except in clear-cut instances of depressive illness, medications are most useful in nonpsychotic patients (1) when the patient is unable or unwilling to make any connection between environmental pressures or psychologic conflicts and the emergence of distressing symptoms; (2) when the patient (or sometimes the physician) is unable to conceptualize and enter into a therapeutic relationship in which medications are not employed; or (3) in acute and subacute disorders with precisely delineated target symptoms such as anxiety, depression, or insomnia.

Psychotropic medications cannot be relied on to provide long-term relief, but they may be used effectively over long periods to help build and maintain a therapeutic relationship, especially in patients in whom development of a therapeutic alliance is difficult. The dangers of long-term pharmacologic therapy are many and well recognized, but at certain times and in certain patients their protracted use cannot be avoided. Medications are often used as ancillary therapeutic modalities in other forms of psychiatric treatment, but in these their role is clearly secondary.

Anxiolytic agents, antidepressants, and hypnotics are the classes of medications appropriate for these common psychiatric syndromes. Antipsychotic medications (major tranquilizers) are usually reserved for psychotic disorders.

Directive Therapy

In directive therapy, the physician openly assumes responsibility for directing the patient's behavior and for ordering the patient's environment. The tools used by the physician to influence the patient's actions include suggestion, advice, urging, and even exhortation. The effectiveness of any of these tools rests, of course, upon the patient's liking for, trust in, and desire to cooperate with the therapist. The physician's capacity for manipulating the environment depends on the cooperation of families, schools, employers, and social agencies. Directive therapy has over the years been given a bad name, the usual criticism being that it creates and perpetuates the patient's dependency and therefore fails to promote autonomy and self-sufficiency. Caution in the use of directive therapy is always in order, but undeniably it is useful in a limited group of patients—and in some patients it is the only practicable approach. Directive therapy should be reserved for patients with lifelong patterns of dependency coupled with poor ego strength. Even in these patients, the physician should strive to limit the extent of dependency and to foster whatever degree of individual responsibility is attainable for the person.

Supportive Therapy

Supportive psychotherapy is probably the most effective therapeutic instrument for the general physician's use in treating patients with mixed psychoneuroses and character disorders. Supportive psychotherapy is also a basic therapeutic instrument for the psychiatrist.

Supportive psychotherapy gains its treatment objectives through two parallel processes: (1) a sustaining and strengthening of the patient's usual coping and defensive mechanisms; and (2) a strong relationship between patient and therapist manifested by mutual respect and autonomy. Regression is generally avoided, and although some degree of dependency by the patient may be accepted, it is not to the extent often tolerated in directive therapy. Supportive therapy focuses on problems currently confronting the patient; its concern is with the here and now. Although some consideration of the genesis of the problems is not excluded, this type of treatment does not focus on earlier determinants or seek its results through understanding them.

Although education about the self is integral to all types of psychotherapy, education takes a particular form in supportive therapy. This is perhaps best described as being analogous to what transpires between a professional tennis coach and his pupil. A good tennis coach usually concentrates and capitalizes on the pupil's strengths, seeking to utilize these to achieve the best play possible. Certainly the good coach observes and points out the pupil's errors and faults of style, and certainly the coach tries to help the pupil avoid these—but the coach knows that too much emphasis on the player's faults and limitations can be counterproductive. Thus the coach leads the player to rely on his best strokes while avoiding his poorer ones. The coach also teaches not only the proper moves but when to make them. Thus strategy and planning occupy a significant portion of both coach and trainee's efforts. Only rarely, with sufficient cause and with trepidation, does the coach seek to remake a player's game.

The relationship between coach and pupil is just as important in the educative process as is the information transmitted. Through this relationship the player develops the willingness to look at faults and avoid them, the capacity to analyze the game and plan appropriate strategy, the devotion to hard work and at times discouraging practice, a commitment to trying new approaches and taking chances, and the strength to suffer defeats in the quest for an identified objective. For many players, these would be impossible without the relationship between coach and pupil.

These basic coaching principles are likely to be used whether the player is expert or novice, naturally talented or athletically inept, young or old. There is considerable scope for individualizing the quantity and the timing of the coaching instruction. Some pupils require only a few lessons confined to a single problem; others need a lengthy ongoing learning process; and still others return to the coach again and again to work on recurrent or successive problems.

The analogy with supportive therapy is close. In supportive therapy, the therapist seeks to capitalize on the patient's strengths; the therapist is oriented more to the "healthy" and adaptive aspects of the patient's functioning than to the "unhealthy" and maladaptive aspects. In learning as much as possible about the patient, the therapist tries to identify in particular the ways the patient has successfully coped with problems and pressures in the past. The therapist is familiar with those tasks which are common to all persons—schooling, social and sexual relationships, separation from parents and home, work, marriage, building a family, loss of parents and close friends, moving to a new locale, growing old—and the therapist learns which hurdles the patient successfully surmounted and how the patient did so. Failures and mistakes are not ignored, but neither are they allowed to dominate the field of vision. The patient and therapist agree to focus selectively on defined areas which involve significant problems in living and to work toward a solution (or at least improvement) in these. Supportive psychotherapy never aims to achieve personality reorganization. Rather, it involves study of ongoing day-to-day problems and development of strategies (perceptual and behavioral) for dealing with these more effectively and efficiently.

This therapeutic modality is applicable to a wide range of patients and problems. It can be used in patients with considerable ego strength and in those with significant ego defects, in patients with a pattern of successful problem solving or of repeated failures, in those with acute or with chronic problems, in the aged or in the young. In addition, the techniques of its application can be varied widely, from a single or few therapy sessions in an acute situation to many therapeutic interviews (or even a permanent ongoing therapeutic relationship) with chronic problems, from interviews as brief as 15 or 20 minutes to as long as 45 or 50 minutes, and from an individual relationship in which confidentiality is the rule to involvement with spouse, family, or even others close to the patient. Some patients may return to the therapist again and again at wide intervals for help with recurrent or differing problems.

The nature of the therapeutic relationship is just as important to the success of the therapy as is the material selected for consideration. The ideal relationship is not one of dependency of the patient on the therapist (though elements of dependency can seldom be avoided) but is rather a trusting willingness on the part of the patient to use the physician's therapeutic skills to achieve growth in mastering significant problems in living. The physician should be visualized as one who is both helpful and supportive, but not as one who looks *after* or does *for* the patient. It is both a friendly and a professional relationship in which independence and respect are preserved and valued.

Thus far, treatment has been discussed in terms of fitting the most appropriate therapeutic instrument to the patient's individual situation. It must be acknowledged in closing that treatment choices cannot always be made on such ideal bases. In fact, the type of treatment is often dictated by the time available for treatment and by social and economic forces existing in the life of both therapist and patient. These conditions often require compromise with the therapeutic ideal, but lack of consideration for these constraints often leads to failure and disappointment, in situations in which working within them might lead to effective even if not optimal results.

DELIRIUM

method of
WILLIAM H. WAINWRIGHT, M.D.
New York, New York

The delirious reactions, or acute brain syndromes, occur as a result of diffuse impairment of brain tissue function arising from a wide variety of underlying disorders. They are usually of sudden onset and relatively short duration, with islands of lucidity in periods of fear, confusion, disorientation, incoherence, illusions, hallucinations (most often visual), and restlessness. Certain aspects of the psychopathologic changes exhibited usually depend more upon the individual personality of the patient than upon the cause. The actual content of fearful dreams or hallucinations will reflect the inner life of the patient. Although the clinical picture may vary in intensity in the same patient from time to time, the acute brain syndrome usually progresses by stages of increasing severity of symptoms. It is essential that the physician be alert to the early symptoms, so that treatment may be instituted without delay.

Signs and Symptoms of Stages of Delirium

Stage I. The symptoms are bewilderment, restlessness, uneasiness, dull headache, sensitivity to noise and light, irritability, fearful dreams, slight difficulty in grasping, slight retention disorder, distractability, vivid past memories, and anxiety with rapid pulse, wet hands, and dilated pupils.

These symptoms of cognitive functioning (thinking, attention, memory, and perception) require vigorous treatment at this stage to prevent subsequent development of more serious problems.

Stage II. Hypnagogic hallucinations are recognized as imaginations and disappear when the eyes are open. Dreams hang on after the patient awakens. Clouding of consciousness, illusions, hallucinations, disorientation (aggravated by darkness), and *fear* are common.

This should be considered a medical and psychiatric emergency of the gravest nature.

Stage III. The neurologic symptoms, with slurred speech, ataxic movements, and indistinct mumbling, may be irreversible.

Stage IV. Stupor, in which partial arousal is possible, is followed by coma, in which there is total loss of consciousness and no voluntary movement.

Death may ensue.

Treatment of Delirium

1. Determination of cause and removal or modification of underlying cause. The causes to be investigated include infections, intoxications (alcohol, barbiturates, bromides, belladonna, alkaloids, adrenocortical compounds, hallucinogens), trauma (brain injury, eye surgery, open heart procedures), cerebral vascular disease, cerebral degenerative disease, convulsive disorders, metabolic disorders (thyroidism, diabetes, liver malfunction, uremia, electrolyte imbalance), and sleep or sensory deprivation.

2. Reassurance, with particular attention to the patient's assets, alleviation of fear, and reality orientation. Explain all procedures carefully. Allow no unnecessary procedures, and keep the staff as constant as possible. Each unfamiliar event or face will tend to confuse the patient. Have a close relative, friend, or staff member stay with the patient at all times. If the presence of a certain person seems to be disturbing, avoid having this person visit. Have familiar objects brought from home to help reassure the patient (such as a radio, so that he may listen to a favorite news program). Keep the room lighted at night to avoid disorientation, misidentification, and fear upon awakening.

3. Rest, by adequate use of chloral hydrate, 0.5 to 1.5 grams, or amobarbital (sodium Amytal), 0.2 to 0.4 gram. Prescribe barbiturates for sleep, not for sedation. Be cautious when using barbiturates with other medication for control of agitation.

4. Relaxation with phenothiazines for alleviation of fear. Chlorpromazine by mouth or intramuscularly is clinically effective. Start with 25 mg. intramuscularly; if no adverse reaction occurs, 50 to 75 mg. may be given intramuscularly every 4 hours. With favorable response switch to oral medication (50 to 200 mg. every 6 to 8 hours).

In case of severe liver damage, chlordiazepoxide is a satisfactory substitute in dosages of 50 to 100 mg. parenterally every 2 to 4 hours. Do not give more than 300 mg. in a 6 hour period. (See manufacturer's official brochure before exceeding 300 mg. in 24 hours.)

Haloperidol intramuscularly up to 5 mg. every hour may be used instead of chlorpromazine or chlordiazepoxide. When adequate control of excitement is reached, oral doses up to 40 mg. daily assure continuing relief.

The choice of drug used for the control of excitement should be that which is most familiar to the treating physician consistent with the patient's physical condition. Gradual reduction of medication over a 7 day period is usually sufficient if the underlying illness is controlled. Continue to keep the patient in a state of ease with meticulous nursing care. Repeated calm, consistent clarification of all procedures is necessary to avoid recurrent bewilderment or fear. Prolonged tub baths may be of help, but if the patient objects to them, do not force him. Eliminate disconcerting shadows, sounds, and movement. Reassure the patient gently and repeatedly if misinterpretation does occur. Do not argue with the patient, but attempt to distract him by changing the subject to a neutral topic or by activity consistent with physical condition.

5. Restriction, by protecting against self-injury (e.g., peg windows, keep razors locked up).

6. Restoration of adequate nourishment and hydration by addition of intravenous feeding if necessary, with special attention to electrolyte balance and vitamin supplements. Urge the patient to eat and drink at his convenience, not necessarily on the rigid hospital schedule. Arrange for the family to bring favorite foods from home.

7. The acute brain syndrome is generally transient and reversible. However, when recovery is incomplete (as in cerebral degenerative disease), there may be residuals of all symptoms on an intermittent or continuous basis. Supportive psychotherapy with emphasis on realistic future planning will be very helpful.

AFFECTIVE DISORDERS

method of
NANCY C. ANDREASEN, M.D.
Iowa City, Iowa

The affective disorders are perhaps the most common psychiatric disorders seen in medical practice. Because the symptoms of affective disorder mimic a variety of somatic illnesses, patients suffering from affective disorder may present themselves first to a primary care physician rather than a psychiatrist. Simple uncomplicated forms of affective disorder are relatively easy to treat, and consequently the primary care physician may choose to manage these himself rather than refer the patient to a psychiatrist.

Classification of Affective Disorders

As their name indicates, the affective disorders are characterized primarily by a disturbance in mood or affect. The disturbance may manifest itself as either elation or unhappiness, and the two clinical syndromes associated with these extremes are referred to as mania and depression. Most patients suffering from affective disorder experience only depression. A few patients experience mood swings between the two poles of affective disorder. These patients, who experience both mania and depression, are referred to as bipolar. Patients who experience depression only are sometimes referred to as unipolar. Unipolar disturbances are typically depressive. Unipolar mania is extremely rare, and most patients who present first with mania typically go on to experience the depressive pole at some later date. Consequently, most psychiatrists conceptualize a person who has suffered from mania only as being bipolar rather than unipolar when they plan management and treatment.

The manic syndrome is characterized primarily by elation or euphoria, although at times the mood may be irritable or expansive. Mania can be diagnosed when a patient manifests the characteristic disturbance in mood, in association with at least three or four other typical symptoms: insomnia (especially early morning awakening without any sensation of fatigue), increased energy, increased interest in a wide range of activities, excessive talkativeness or sociability, poor concentration, racing thoughts, pressure of speech, intrusiveness, and poor judgment. Some patients with mania experience a variety of grandiose delusions, such as the belief in a special mission or a special relationship with God. Because they feel so good, manics are notably resistant to seeking treatment unless they have experienced previous episodes of mania, which have heightened their awareness of its risks and complications. Because of his expansiveness and poor judgment, the manic may find himself in a variety of legal and social difficulties, such as foolish and inappropriate business or sexual ventures. Because of the heightened energy and activity, severe mania may be life-threatening, particularly in patients who have associated medical illnesses. Prior to the development of adequate treatment methods, approximately 15 per cent of all manics died from overactivity and exhaustion.

The depressive syndrome is characterized by a dysphoric mood, typically despondency but occasionally anxiety, in association with three or four other characteristic symptoms: decreased appetite, weight loss, insomnia, decreased energy, impaired concentration, guilt feelings, loss of interest or pleasure, and diurnal variation (characteristic changes in mood state throughout the day, with morning typically being worst and evening best). The depressive syndrome is an extremely common one. Depending on how it is defined, the estimated lifetime prevalence for depression is somewhere between 2 and 15 per cent. In terms of its phenomenologic appearance, the psychiatric illness "depression" exists on a continuum with the ubiquitous human experience of transient unhappiness. Consequently, the physician seeing a patient who presents with a phenomenologic syndrome suggestive of depression must attempt to determine whether he is seeing a treatable illness or a "normal" response to life stress. The distinction is an important one, because one of the somatic therapies for depression is appropriate for the former but not the latter.

In attempting to delineate those depressions more likely to respond to somatic treatment from those less likely, psychiatrists have divided depressions into a variety of dichotomous subtypes: endogenous versus reactive depression, psychotic versus neurotic depression, primary versus secondary depression, and "pure depression" versus "depressive spectrum disease." Each of these dichotomies stresses a particular characteristic of depression which may be helpful in predicting a response to treatment. The endogenous-reactive dichotomy emphasizes the importance of precipitating factors; an endogenous depression is one without any apparent precipitating factors and is more likely to respond to antidepressant medication than a reactive depression, which occurs in response to some stressful life event. In addition, endogenous depressions tend to have a characteristic symptom picture, including early morning awakening, weight loss, diurnal variation, and inability to experience happiness or pleasure. The psychotic-neurotic dichotomy stresses severity and chronicity; a psychotic depression is severe, incapacitating, and typically has a relatively clear onset and offset, whereas a neurotic depression is milder, not incapacitating, and typically chronic. The primary-secondary dichotomy stresses the existence of another psychiatric illness prior to the development of depressive symptoms; a primary depression is one which occurs in a person who has had no previous psychiatric illness, whereas a secondary depression occurs in a person who has had a prior psychiatric illness, typically alcoholism, hysteria, or antisocial personality. Finally, the "pure depressive"–"depressive spectrum" dichotomy emphasizes the importance of family history of psychiatric illness; a pure depression is one occurring in a person who has no family history of psychiatric illness or a family history of depression only, whereas depressive spectrum disease occurs in a person who has a family history of a disease other than depression, such as hysteria, alcoholism, or antisocial personality. Endogenous, psychotic, primary, or "pure" depressions are all more likely to respond to tricyclic antidepressants.

The factors suggesting a good response to pharmacotherapy are summarized in Table 1. It should be emphasized, however, that these factors

TABLE 1. Factors in Depression Suggesting a Good Response to Pharmacotherapy

1. Endogenous phenomenology
   a. Terminal insomnia
   b. Diurnal variation
   c. Nonresponsivity of mood
   d. Weight loss
2. Absence of precipitating factors
3. Family history of depression
4. Relatively clear or acute onset of symptoms
5. Previous good response to pharmacotherapy
6. No previous psychiatric symptoms (excluding previous depressions)

are guidelines only, and that each individual case must be carefully evaluated. The severity of symptoms, degree of incapacity, and risk for complications such as suicide must all be weighed, and in many instances a trial of medication may be appropriate even in patients whose symptoms appear to be reactive or chronic. No matter what treatment plan is decided upon, each patient should be carefully re-evaluated weekly or bimonthly and the appropriateness of the treatment plan reassessed.

Course and Complications

Mania. The first episode of mania is usually during early adult life. The course tends to be episodic, with periods of illness being followed by periods of complete remission. The natural history of mania is such that most episodes remit spontaneously within weeks or months, and consequently treatment of mania tends only to shorten the duration of the episode. The complications of mania are primarily social: marital discord, divorce, business difficulties, financial extravagance, sexual indiscretions, and alcohol abuse. These complications tend to result from the manic's euphoria, irritability, or poor judgment. A manic syndrome can rapidly switch to a depression, with the risk for suicide being heightened when the patient becomes remorsefully aware of his previous behavior.

Depression. Suicide is the most serious complication of depression. Approximately 15 per cent of all hospitalized patients suffering from depression die by suicide. Several factors are suggestive of an increase in suicidal risk: age over 40, history of alcohol or drug abuse, being divorced or living alone, history of prior suicide attempt, and expression of suicidal ideation (particularly when detailed plans have been formulated).

Suicidal risk should always be carefully evaluated in any patient suffering from depression, beginning with a direct inquiry as to whether the patient has considered taking his life. If the patient is a risk for suicide, he should be treated as an inpatient rather than an outpatient in order to minimize the risk. Evidence also suggests that depressed patients treated with electroconvulsive therapy (ECT) have a lower incidence of suicide than those treated with tricyclic antidepressants. Because of the risk for suicide, some precautions should be used when prescribing tricyclic antidepressants for outpatients. Tricyclic antidepressants may be lethal in relatively small overdoses, with death having been reported secondary to overdoses ranging from 500 to 5000 mg. Consequently, some patients intending only to make a suicidal gesture may miscalculate and ingest a lethal amount. These drugs should be prescribed in small amounts, particularly to people living alone. Whether or not suicidal thoughts have occurred should be discussed openly with each depressed patient and a promise obtained from the patient that he or she will contact the physician prior to making any suicide attempt.

Although suicide is the most serious complication of depression, other social and personal complications may also occur. Decreased energy, poor concentration, and lack of interest may cause poor performance at work or in school. Apathy and decreased sexual interest may lead to marital discord. The depressive symptoms may also initiate problems with drug and alcohol abuse. Some patients may begin to take amphetamines or other stimulants in an effort to increase their energy. Other patients may attempt to treat their sleep disturbance by taking sedative hypnotics or alcohol at night. Eventually the patient may become dependent on any of these various types of drugs.

Treatment of Depression

Four types of treatment are used for depression: (1) tricyclic antidepressants; (2) monamine oxidase inhibitors (MAOIs); (3) electroconvulsive therapy (ECT); and (4) psychotherapy. Ordinarily these are used in the order listed. Occasionally several of these treatments may be used concurrently.

Tricyclic Antidepressants. Most patients suffering from depression should be treated first with a tricyclic antidepressant. Approximately 70 per cent of all depressions will show improvement with tricyclics. The family of tricyclic antidepressants share the common feature of diminishing depressive symptomatology, but they vary in their side effects. Some are significantly more sedating than others. Since some depressions are complicated by agitation or psychomotor retardation, the clinician will often wish to select an antidepressant on the basis of its degree of sedation in order to treat the agitation or retardation. Although the side effects of tricyclics occur immediately, the therapeutic action does not occur for approximately 3 weeks. Some patients will feel somewhat better immediately, however, because of the sedating or energizing side effects of the tricyclics. The generic and trade names and usual doses of some common tricyclic antidepressants are listed in Table 2. They are ordered in terms of their sedative side effects, with those listed first being most sedating and those listed last the least sedating. At present amitriptyline and imipramine are the most widely used.

Because the side effects of tricyclic antidepressants are unpleasant and because of the lag in

TABLE 2. **Usual Doses of Commonly Used Tricyclic Antidepressants**

GENERIC NAME	TRADE NAME	DAILY DOSAGE RANGE	USUAL DAILY DOSE
Doxepin	Sinequan	75–200 mg.	150 mg.
Amitriptyline	Elavil	75–200 mg.	150 mg.
Imipramine	Tofranil	75–200 mg.	150 mg.
Nortriptyline	Aventyl	30–100 mg.	75 mg.
Desipramine	Norpramin	75–200 mg.	150 mg.
Protriptyline	Vivactil	10–40 mg.	30 mg.

therapeutic response, noncompliance can be a significant problem with the tricyclic antidepressants. The patient should be instructed that he may well feel worse before he begins to feel better. Common side effects such as dry mouth or sedation should be explained to him, and he should be told that he may not begin to feel a lifting of his depressive symptomatology for 2 or 3 weeks, although some patients feel better more quickly. The patient should be urged to bear with whatever unpleasant side effects he feels for at least 4 weeks in order to give the tricyclics a fair trial. To further reduce noncompliance, initial dosages should be small. For example, the physician may prescribe a starting dose of 50 mg. of imipramine. The dosage may then be titrated upward by 25 mg. every 2 days until the usual therapeutic dose is reached. Outpatients suffering from depression will usually be able to continue working and feel relatively less discomfort from side effects when medication is managed this way. For inpatients the initial dose may be larger (e.g., 75 to 100 mg.), and the upward titration achieved more rapidly. To further minimize noncompliance, tricyclic antidepressants are usually given in a single bedtime dose. This concentrates more of the side effects during the period when the patient is sleeping and, in the case of the more sedating tricyclics, may immediately relieve the patient's complaints of insomnia. It may not be possible to give the more energizing tricyclics, such as desipramine hydrochloride (Norpramine) or protriptyline (Vivactil), in a single bedtime dose, because they may exacerbate the patient's sleep disturbance. Although in rare instances it may be necessary to change to another tricyclic after a few days because of severe problems with side effects (usually the amount of sedation or stimulation), in most instances it is best to use a single tricyclic for a period of at least 3 weeks before switching to either another tricyclic or another form of treatment.

The tricyclic antidepressants have many side effects which may pose problems for both patient and physician. Common anticholinergic side effects include dry mouth, thirst, constipation (paralytic ileus), urinary retention, blurred vision (decreased accommodation), impotence, and palpitations. Cardiovascular side effects include palpitations, tachycardia, orthostatic hypotension, and electrocardiographic (ECG) changes (T-wave depression, prolonged QT interval, ST segment depression). Allergic reactions, including agranulocytosis and intrahepatic biliary obstruction and jaundice, have also been reported. Because of their anticholinergic and cardiovascular side effects, tricyclics are usually contraindicated in patients with glaucoma or cardiac disease. Doxepin (Sinequan) has relatively few cardiovascular side effects and may be prescribed for patients with a history of cardiac disease.

The tricyclics interact with a variety of other drugs. They inhibit the effect of antihypertensives such as guanethidine by preventing the uptake of guanethidine into the adrenergic neuron. They interact with the monamine oxidase inhibitors (MAOIs) to produce excessive central and peripheral sympathetic stimulation. Ordinarily tricyclics should not be used in conjunction with either guanethidine or MAOIs. Some drugs, such as barbiturates, increase the metabolism of the tricyclics. Other drugs, such as phenothiazines or glucocorticosteroids, inhibit tricyclic metabolism.

Approximately 30 per cent of patients treated with tricyclics will not respond. If the depression is felt to be relatively mild and the complications are not significant and severe, then the clinician will usually elect a trial of either MAOIs or psychotherapy. If the depression and its complications are considered significant and severe, however, then hospitalization and treatment with electroconvulsive therapy (ECT) is indicated. Occasionally the clinician may prefer a trial of another tricyclic instead.

The patient who responds well to tricyclics should usually be kept on medication for a period of 6 months. If the patient has not had a history of recurrent episodes, then the tricyclics should be slowly discontinued. Most patients experience mild withdrawal symptoms, such as insomnia and restlessness, if the tricyclics are discontinued abruptly. Consequently they should be discontinued in increments of 25 to 50 mg. per week. The patient should be warned to contact the physician if depressive symptoms begin to recur when the tricyclics are being discontinued. There is some evidence that patients with recurrent depressions may benefit either from maintenance tricyclics or from maintenance lithium. Because evidence for the efficacy of these two forms of maintenance treatment is not overwhelming, the potential benefit and potential risks should be carefully weighed.

Monamine Oxidase Inhibitors. The MAOIs provide less effective treatment for depression, but some patients may respond well to them, particularly patients with milder forms of depression. The trade and generic names and usual dosages of some common MAOIs appear in Table 3. Of these, tranylcypromine (Parnate) is perhaps the most widely used and most effective, although it also tends to have more severe side effects. Perhaps because it is structurally related to the amphetamines, it tends to be energizing and stimulating.

As in the case of tricyclics, the therapeutic effect does not occur until approximately 3 weeks after the onset of treatment. Side effects and risks of treatment with MAOIs are more significant and severe than with the tricyclics. The MAOIs interact with a variety of commonly used substances to produce a hypertensive crisis. These include cheese, fermented wines, amphetamines, and narcotic analgesics. The MAOIs also interact with tricyclic antidepressants, as discussed above, and with oral hypoglycemics and insulin, so that their hypoglycemic response is enhanced and prolonged. Because the complications of the various interactions may be life-threatening, patients should be warned about them carefully and thoroughly. (The physician should carefully review the Physician's Desk Reference [PDR] for further details before prescribing a specific MAOI.) Like the tricyclics, the MAOIs are also dangerous substances for overdose, with death having been reported when from 170 to 750 mg. has been ingested.

In addition to the aforementioned interactions, a variety of side effects may also occur. These include headache, insomnia, irritability, excitability, restlessness, anxiety, psychomotor stimulation, orthostatic hypotension, peripheral neuropathy, and hepatocellular jaundice. These drugs should be avoided in patients with a history of cardiovascular or liver disease. Hyperreflexia is a useful indicator that the upper dosage range has been reached.

If a therapeutic response to the MAOIs occurs, the physician should then reduce the dosage by approximately one half to a maintenance level, because of the various risks and side effects of these drugs. As in the case of the tricyclics, the physician should usually maintain the patient on an MAOI for about 6 months and then gradually discontinue the medication.

Electroconvulsive Therapy. Electroconvulsive therapy (ECT) is probably the most effective treatment for depression. When compared with tricyclic antidepressants as well as all other forms of treatment for depression, electroconvulsive therapy leads to a significantly lower mortality rate during the years subsequent to the depressive episode. Although electroconvulsive therapy has been reported to have a higher relapse rate than tricyclic antidepressants, this finding probably results from the fact that only more severe depressions are treated with electroconvulsive therapy. Although its efficacy as a treatment for depression is clear and unquestioned, it is ordinarily used only in patients who are suicidal, are incapacitated, or have not responded to a 4 week trial of tricyclics. A minority of clinicians consider it the first treatment of choice for all forms of depression. Disadvantages of ECT include confusion, amnesia, recent memory loss, the use of hexobarbital and succinylcholine for anesthesia, and patient apprehensiveness. It is a safer form of treatment than tricyclics for patients with cardiovascular disease or pregnant women. Brain tumors and recent cerebrovascular accidents (CVAs) are the only absolute contraindications, and ECT should also be used with discretion in patients who have had a recent myocardial infarction.

Prior to the administration of the ECT, patients should be given a careful medical evaluation. This should include a complete physical examination, SMA 6 and 12, ECG, chest film, skull films, and views of the cervical and thoracic spine. If the patient shows evidence of significant degenerative bone and joint disease, particular care should be given to providing adequate muscular

TABLE 3. **Usual Doses of Commonly Used MAOIs**

GENERIC NAME	TRADE NAME	DAILY DOSAGE RANGE	USUAL MAINTENANCE DOSE
Tranylcypromine	Parnate	10–30 mg.	20 mg.
Phenelzine	Nardil	15–75 mg.	30 mg.
Isocarboxazid	Marplan	10–30 mg.	20 mg.

relaxation during the convulsions. Patients with evidence of conductive defect on the ECG should be monitored with a continuous ECG during their first ECT if the conductive defects are considered significant. A cardiologist or orthopedic surgeon should be consulted in such instances.

Electroconvulsive therapy should be given only after adequate patient preparation and with adequate modification. Patients should not be given anything by mouth for at least 8 hours prior to the treatment. One mg. of atropine should be given subcutaneously 30 minutes before the treatment in order to reduce secretions. Just prior to the treatment, the patient is sedated with hexabarbital (Brevital) given intravenously at a rate of 10 mg. per 5 seconds until the patient is asleep (usually after 60 to 70 mg.). Patient weight and possible habituation to alcohol, tranquilizers, or sedatives are factors which determine the appropriate dose. Succinylcholine (Anectine) is used to produce muscular relaxation during the convulsion. The usual dose is 0.3 mg. per kg., although this amount may be modified upward or downward depending on the patient's muscle mass. Because these medications produce temporary respiratory arrest, adequate supportive equipment to manage a variety of respiratory and cardiac complications is required. Some clinicians prefer to give ECT with the assistance of an anesthesiologist. The convulsion is produced 45 to 60 seconds after administration of succinylcholine by applying electrodes over the anterior portion of the temporal bone bilaterally and using a shock of 150 volts for a duration of 0.5 second. The usual course of ECT is eight treatments given at the rate of three per week. Because of the resulting amnesia and confusion, ECT should be given only to inpatients. The patients should remain in the hospital 1 to 2 weeks after the last treatment so that the amnesia and confusion can clear adequately. The amnesia is ordinarily completely gone after 1 month. In order to prevent a risk of relapse after ECT, some clinicians choose to place the patient on maintenance tricyclics after the series of ECTs has been completed.

Psychotherapy. Supportive psychotherapy is frequently helpful for patients whose depressive symptoms are in part triggered by situational problems. Supportive therapy may be used either to assist them in coping with these problems or to help them discover ways to alter their environment. Although supportive therapy is sometimes considered more appropriate for patients with mild situational depression, some patients with more severe depression may also need supportive therapy to assist them in coping with difficult life situations. Some patients may experience depressive symptoms as a result of specific "cognitive sets." That is, they may typically react to situations with self-criticism, self-doubt, and self-blame. Cognitive psychotherapy may be used to help them explore and modify these self-denigrating and depression-evoking attitudes. Such therapy may be the treatment of choice in patients with chronic mild depressive symptoms.

Treatment of Mania

The treatment of mania has been dramatically altered in recent years through the discovery of the usefulness of lithium salts both therapeutically and prophylactically. Lithium is currently the mainstay of treatment for mania, although phenothiazines or butyrophenones may also be useful during the acute phase.

Lithium. Lithium is usually used through the acute phase of mania either alone or in conjunction with another drug. Studies have suggested that lithium alone is preferable to a phenothiazine such as chlorpromazine in manic patients who are relatively less agitated. On the other hand, chlorpromazine should be used either alone or in conjunction with lithium in the highly agitated patient. Lithium tends to have a higher compliance rate than phenothiazines because the patient feels less sluggish and fatigued and has fewer side effects, so it should be used alone when possible. Full remission of psychotic symptomatology does not occur in patients on lithium for approximately 1 week, however, and consequently a phenothiazine is often necessary in the severely disturbed patient in order to control agitation and other behavioral symptoms.

Lithium dosage during the acute phase is usually 1800 mg. per day, although a range from 600 to 4000 mg. may be required to produce adequate blood levels. Lithium dosages are monitored by blood levels at least every other day during the acute phase, and a range of 0.9 to 1.4 mEq. per liter is considered to be an adequate blood level. Rarely patients may show toxic symptoms when the blood level is in this range, and in this situation the toxic symptoms should be used as a guideline for reducing dosage rather than the blood level. After the mania "breaks" (i.e., the manic symptoms disappear relatively abruptly), the patient's tolerance for lithium tends to decrease abruptly, and the dosage should be reduced to approximately half the therapeutic dose in order to maintain blood levels between 0.7 and 1.2 mEq. per liter. Lithium dosages are ordinarily given three times a day, and a typical schedule for the initiation of lithium treatment would be as follows: day 1, 300 mg. three times daily; day 2, 600 mg. three times daily; day 3, 1500 to 2400 mg. of lithium per day, depending on blood level achieved on previous dosages. Blood levels are measured in the morning prior to the ingestion of the first lithium dose.

Lithium is eliminated completely by the kidney. Fifty per cent is cleared in 24 hours and 90 per cent in 48 hours. Consequently blood levels tend to fluctuate rapidly in response to changes in dosage. Prior to beginning a patient on lithium, the physician should do a careful physical examination and obtain an SMA 18, T_4, and electrocardiogram in order to establish normal renal function and have baseline indices of liver, thyroid, and cardiac functioning.

Lithium may have a wide variety of adverse effects, ranging from minor intolerance to life-threatening toxicity. Some symptoms of lithium intolerance may be mildly uncomfortable for the patient. These include transient nausea, abdominal discomfort, diarrhea, thirst, polyuria, muscle weakness, and hand tremor. Most of these occur only during the early days of lithium therapy and tend to subside after a few days to weeks. Nevertheless, these symptoms should not be treated lightly, because a few of them may be prodromal symptoms of significant lithium toxicity. Consequently, the patient should be informed of these various symptoms of lithium intolerance and urged to report them to the physician.

The onset of lithium poisoning is usually preceded by a variety of prodromal symptoms during several days prior to the more severe effects: drowsiness, tremor, vomiting, diarrhea, and ataxia. When toxicity sets in, the patient shows symptoms of impaired consciousness, seizures, and coma. These symptoms usually occur at blood levels greater than 1.4 mEq. per liter, but some have been reported even within the therapeutic dose range. Consequently, patients with blood levels in the higher ranges should be followed quite closely. In nearly all instances, the symptoms of lithium poisoning have been reversible, but a few cases of irreversible central nervous system toxicity have been reported. When such symptoms of lithium poisoning occur, the drug should be discontinued immediately, and renal excretion may be increased by the use of mannitol.

Lithium also has a variety of endocrine and metabolic effects. Lithium ingestion often results in a decrease in T_4, and some patients may develop a goiter and become hypothyroid. Patients may also show a decrease in glucose tolerance and elevation in growth hormone. A syndrome resembling diabetes insipidus occasionally occurs in patients treated with lithium. When these metabolic or endocrine effects occur, the clinician must weigh the need for lithium against the risks of the specific side effect. If the patient has had severe recurrent mania which has been well controlled only with lithium, the clinician will usually elect to continue the lithium and treat or manage the endocrine symptomatology. If the indications for lithium are not strong and clear, however, the drug should be discontinued, and the endocrine and metabolic symptoms will usually abate. Lithium usually causes changes in the ECG which are not clinically significant in a patient with a previously normal ECG. Hepatotoxicity has also been reported.

Lithium interacts with several drugs. Interaction with thiazide diuretics leads to lithium retention and consequently will result in increased serum lithium levels. Although lithium may be used in conjunction with thiazide diuretics, it should be used cautiously and with careful monitoring of serum lithium levels. Lithium has been reported to interact with haloperidol to produce an organic brain syndrome, which in several instances has been based on irreversible brain damage. Although the mechanism for this interaction is unknown, the simultaneous use of lithium and haloperidol should be avoided.

Phenothiazines and Butyrophenones. These medications are ordinarily used only during the acute phase of mania. Haloperidol, in dosages ranging from 3 mg. per day to 15 mg. per day, is particularly useful, although its use with lithium is currently contraindicated. The more sedating phenothiazines, such as chlorpromazine (Thorazine), are also highly effective treatments for the acute phase of mania. Because they can be safely used in conjunction with lithium, they are at present the treatment of choice during the acute phase for those patients who do not respond to lithium alone. The initial starting dose of chlorpromazine is usually 100 mg. two or three times daily. The dosages are then titrated upward over several days to a total ranging from 300 to 1000 mg. per day. This dosage can usually be decreased rapidly within a week or two, and the phenothiazine is usually totally discontinued once maintenance lithium is underway.

Electroconvulsive Therapy. Very occasionally a manic patient will not respond to either antipsychotic medication or lithium. Most of these patients will respond well to electroconvulsive therapy. It is given in the same way as has been described for depression. Electroconvulsive therapy may also be indicated even prior to a trial of antipsychotics or lithium for the patient who is so severely agitated that his mania is considered life-threatening or for the pregnant patient. ECT may also present a lower risk for some patients with cardiovascular disease than does either phenothiazine treatment or relatively prolonged manic symptoms.

Maintenance Lithium. The use of maintenance lithium to prevent recurrent mania has been a significant breakthrough in the treatment of affective disorders during recent years. A number of studies have repeatedly shown that it significantly reduces the risk for recurrence. Maintenance lithium is indicated for those patients who have had two or more episodes of mania requiring hospitalization. Clinical judgment must be used to decide whether patients should be placed on maintenance lithium after their first episode. As in the case of acute mania, the blood level is used as a guideline in determining dosage. Maintenance dosages are usually 300 mg. three or four times daily, and a blood level ranging from 0.5 to 1.2 mEq. per liter is usually considered appropriate. Patients who experience mild gastrointestinal upset on maintenance lithium should take their medication with meals or milk. Problems with lithium side effects or lithium toxicity are rare with maintenance lithium. A few patients may complain that lithium makes them less creative or prevents them from going as fast as they would like. Such patients may resist complying with maintenance lithium. Most will find that the mild reduction in activity is not as harmful as the potentially disastrous effects of recurrent mania.

SCHIZOPHRENIA

method of
STEPHEN FLECK, M.D.
New Haven, Connecticut

Introduction

Schizophrenia is a pervasive personality disorder characterized by defective reality relatedness and social disabilities, a faulty sense of identity, and perceptual disorders associated with idiosyncratic thinking, all of which seem related to deficiencies in the structure and dynamics of the families in which schizophrenics grow up. These basic psychologic aberrations are manifested clinically by elaborate symptoms and socially unacceptable behavior, but the condition may be latent. Despite many claims that there is a clearly defined biochemical basis for schizophrenia and a vast research literature on this subject, the mechanisms identified so far in schizophrenic patients remain relatively isolated findings whose role in the development of schizophrenia remains unclear. These factors, be they chromosomal, bioaminic, or enzymatic, cannot account for the clinical state, and their correction as such could not meet schizophrenics' treatment needs in terms of either personality changes or social habilitation. Schizophrenia is best considered a psychosocial deficiency disease for which aberrations in the neuropsychologic matrix could be responsible, but malfunctioning family environments in which these patients grow up account for many of their symptoms. Two thirds of acute schizophrenics recovered in intensive therapeutic environments before psychoactive drugs were available, reexperiencing emotional growth and (re)integrating a sense of identity, by learning or relearning to use symbols and interaction modes characteristic of the nonschizophrenic world.

The treatment of schizophrenia, therefore, should consist of a comprehensive therapeutic-educational process, although often this treatment cannot be undertaken until disturbances in arousal mechanisms, excitement, and anxiety have been ameliorated or brought under control through psychoactive drugs. The patients' families or spouses also need therapeutic attention. Unfortunately, most schizophrenics are not treated in this comprehensive fashion because of shortage or lack of skilled manpower in most hospitals and a dearth of appropriate community services. Moreover, limitations of funds, especially of insurance coverage for private hospitals or general hospital services, often dictate abbreviated treatment periods regardless of treatment indications, and the majority of third-party payers also fail to provide for transitional programs, i.e., day or night hospitalizations, or for other rehabilitative needs. It is deplorable that these deficiencies are often rationalized away by arguments that not enough is known about schizophrenia and its etiology to provide rational treatment, which indeed is extensive and expensive, or that drug-induced amelioration of undesirable behaviors constitutes adequate treatment.

The treatment of chronically disabled schizophrenics, who occupy about one third of the beds in governmental mental hospitals, will not be considered here, but they deserve humane care and institutional programs affording them maximum activity within safe limits dictated by their continued disturbance. Much of this chronicity is now preventable by the active comprehensive treatment of acutely ill schizophrenic patients, although they may require hospitalization more than once.

The typical acute schizophrenic patient today is a young adult or adolescent, and very few hospital patients over 30 years of age are diagnosed for the first time as being schizophrenic. To the extent that epidemiologic data in the mental health field can be relied upon, there is no hard evidence that the overall incidence of schizophrenia has changed, or is changing. However, one caveat is in order. An excess incidence of schizophrenia in family members of schizophrenics cannot be doubted no matter how transmitted. Because many more schizophrenics live in the community than in hospitals, sex education and contraceptive advice and supplies must be provided for all patients prior to discharge from hospitals or as a part of outpatient management. Patients' social disabilities need not preclude sexual intercourse, especially for those who are married.

Establishing therapeutic contact with acute schizophrenics may be very difficult and even impossible if patients are very disturbed, be they excited and combative or mute and withdrawn. Although many schizophrenics can be treated as outpatients, and many more get along outside hospitals at least intermittently, either with chemotherapy only or without any treatment, the treatment of overtly schizophrenic people begins in the hospital, or at least in a day hospital. Only an overview of the many facets and complexities of the therapeutic, educational, and socializing programs can be presented. These will apply to independent small psychiatric hospitals and to active treatment units in large mental hospitals, in general hospitals, or in mental health centers.

Facilities and Staffing

Because the treatment of schizophrenics is primarily psychologic and interpersonal, a therapeutic environment geared to these tasks must be provided around the clock. This requires a professional staff organized in special ways, a hierarachy of interpersonal programs, drugs, wet pack facilities, and, once in a great while, electric shock apparatus.

The professional staff should number about 20 for that many patients and 25 to 30 for 40 to 50 patients. Fifty patients (not necessarily all schizophrenics) is maximal for an efficient unit treatment program. At least 10 per cent of the staff should be experienced psychiatrists, and one half of the staff should be experienced nurses or senior psychiatric aides. The remainder of the staff consists of social workers, psychologists, and recreational and activities workers and teachers. If residents in training and other trainees are part of the service, they can replace some of the professionals listed, but not completely lest education be jeopardized. Most trainees should be added to the staff figures, although they must be fully integrated into the program, which is enriched thereby. All staff is conceived here as "full time," having their primary work assignments in such a unit.

The organization of this staff as a team must provide for role flexibility and daily structured communication opportunities, staff meetings, patient-staff meetings, and other groupings. These meetings are in addition to trainees' teaching exercises and special or routine case conferences. Staff meetings must be democratic forums where professional role hierarchies are set aside so that information about patients and staff, families and visitors, and the communal interactions can be shared freely. Therapeutic endeavor must pervade the entire atmosphere, and not be limited to "therapy sessions" or other special encounters. In such a milieu all staff must be sophisticated in listening and observing on many levels so that they can respond helpfully to patients and share insights with colleagues. The treatment needs of psychotic patients and therapeutic opportunities cannot be scheduled, and a night duty nurse or aide must be as alert to therapeutic opportunities as the psychotherapist in his office.

Patients must be held responsible for as much of their individual and collective daily life as possible. The overriding principle is that patients should retain as much responsibility for themselves as is consistent with safety and therapeutic indications to be dependent and unburdened. They also should be encouraged to share in responsibilities for the ward community as much as they are capable of assuming. Ideally, these judgments are made jointly by patients and staff through combined committees and some form of patient governance. An integrated school program with teachers trained to guide emotionally disturbed youngsters should be available for young patients.

The physical facilities should provide adequate space for some privacy, although most patients do not need single rooms, and many derive benefits from one or more roommates. Single rooms should be available for some patients, especially those in need of continuous, individual, professional companionship. Sufficient office space should exist so that at least half the number of staff can carry out individual or small group treatments simultaneously. Space requirements also include a room where the entire community can meet, rooms for group meetings and for group or family therapy, a classroom, and recreational and activities areas, including some outdoor space. A gymnasium is no luxury. Also needed are dining and kitchen facilities. About 20,000 square feet will accommodate 50 patients as described, exclusive of hallways, outdoor space, or a gymnasium and business offices.

The annual budget for an appropriately appointed and staffed institution for 50 patients is in the range of $2,000,000 (including professional fees and amortization of a $3,000,000 plant), which means a daily rate of about $140.00 for each patient, or an annual expense rate of $50,000 per patient. These figures are cited because the federal government spends much less than that for patients in Veterans Administration Hospitals and most states spend still less. Thus the treatment of schizophrenic patients is very much tied to economic factors, and the disproportionately high accumulation of chronic schizophrenic patients in the lower socioeconomic classes, first documented by Hollingshead and Redlich in 1958, can therefore be attributed to poverty and the underfinancing of public institutions. However, because treatment experience has been accumulated largely with middle-class patients, it cannot be assumed a priori that the treatment modalities outlined here are applicable in detail across the social class boundaries, because sociodynamics, one of the important therapeutic variables, are class dependent.

The Role of Drug Treatment

The acute schizophrenic should be treated with phenothiazines or equivalent psychoactive drugs in dosages sufficient to make him comfortable in the hospital environment. This means that he can tolerate some contact with professional personnel and also with at least a few patients. During the early phase of hospitalization when either excitement or withdrawal is marked, "specialing," i.e., assigning a staff member for constant companionship, or having patients spell each other every hour or so as companions throughout the patient's waking period, is important. If severe agitation and excitement cannot be ameliorated by the combination of chemical restraint and selected companionship, wet packs are often effective and soothing. Once in a great while electric shock treatment is indicated to abort self-destructive and combative behavior not controllable by chemicals.

The introduction of phenothiazines has changed the treatment of schizophrenics so radically that chemotherapy is often presented as *the* treatment of schizophrenics. On the other hand, a precise delineation of drug effects is possible only in individual patients who are being studied carefully (and therefore treated intensively) by a psychotherapeutically sophisticated observer in a well-defined milieu. Drug studies rarely meet these criteria for evaluation because they are extraordinarily expensive in terms of experienced therapeutic and research manpower for a statistically adequate study sample. Phenothiazine medication will usually allay anxiety and excitement or help patients to become less withdrawn and adjust to, and interact to some extent with, others in the hospital environment.

The drug used most widely and safely is chlorpromazine (Thorazine), which is given orally in divided doses of from 200 to 800 mg. per day. For quick effects 25 to 50 mg. can be given intramuscularly. Another widely used phenothiazine is perphenazine (Trilafon), 16 to 48 mg. daily, up to 64 mg. if necessary. If phenothiazines are to be avoided or are ineffective, haloperidol (up to 1.5 mg. per day) is available, or molindone or loxapine.

There is no advantage of one drug over another except as established by clinical trials of about 1 month's duration. Intramuscular injection of fluphenazine enanthate (25 mg.) is available for patients who cannot be relied upon to take oral medication regularly. Hypotension is the most common side effect and must be guarded against, especially with intramuscular administration, but every organ and system can be affected adversely by these drugs, and although the mild side reaction can often be controlled by dose adjustments, changes in medications are also often indicated. Antiparkinsonism medication may be used if symptoms warrant it. Benztropine mesylate (Cogentin) in doses of 1 to 2 mg. is recommended to accompany each dose of a phenothiazine.

Reserpine is inferior to the phenothiazines, but if phenothiazines are poorly tolerated, reserpine can be useful. Its effects are delayed and are often preceded by increased excitement during the first weeks. It, too, has hypotensive properties and produces Parkinsonism, and has unwelcome depressive side effects. The dose is 1 to 5 mg. daily. In very agitated and excitable patients, lithium carbonate may be beneficial. Nine hundred to 1200 mg. will usually effect a therapeutic blood level of 0.8 to 1.2 mEq. per liter.

If depressive affect is judged to require drug treatment, the two most effective antidepressants are imipramine (Tofranil) and amitriptyline (Elavil) given in doses of from 75 to 150 mg. Imipramine can be given up to 200 mg. The side effects of these drugs are atropine-like but also include jaundice and some tremors, and hypotension. Other antidepressants are not recommended, and neither minor tranquilizers nor amphetamines should be given.

Laboratory control of all these medications should include blood studies and liver function tests every 10 days for the first 6 weeks and monthly thereafter.

Drug treatment may be continued indefinitely, even after discharge from the hospital. Dose reduction or discontinuation should be based on evidence of sustained improvement and personality growth observed through frequent psychotherapeutic contacts, or because of serious untoward drug reactions. Although drugs affect psychotherapeutic processes, they need not interfere, and without psychotherapy there is no reliable indication for changes in or cessation of medication. Patients who have relapsed repeatedly should be maintained on phenothiazines indefinitely. However, as the years have gone by with many patients on these medications, greater respect for tardive dyskinesia, a very unwelcome complication, has developed. The incidence is not insignificant, as was thought earlier; nor are the corneal changes in patients who have been on chlorpromazine for a very long time. The latter therefore should not be used chronically unless medication for psychotic symptoms is indicated and other drugs cannot be given.

Interpersonal Treatments

These consist of individual, family, and sociotherapy. After the patients can tolerate individualized companionship, they should be gradually introduced to the ward or milieu program. This may begin with some tangible activity in a workshop, structured recreation, or some activity program related to the ward organization and patient government. They should then be assigned to group therapy and also be included in therapeutic sessions with the family, if possible.

The dyadic treatment of schizophrenic patients is a most challenging and specialized psychotherapeutic task. It demands of the therapist an intensive personal investment in attention on more levels than in any other psychotherapeutic work. These patients' "inattention," their inability to maintain the interactional set, their quick shifts in mood, their unexpected and unexpectable associations and responses, and their sensitivity to those aspects of communication behavior which nonschizophrenics usually screen out of awareness command extraordinary efforts and alertness by the therapist to keep attuned to the patient. The therapist must be constantly prepared for switches from the idiosyncratic, from the symbolic and allegorical, to quite rational forms of verbal and nonverbal communication. The therapist must furthermore be circumspect lest failure to understand, or intended or inadvertent disagreement with the patient, be experienced by the patient as extremely discouraging and devastating.

The almost daily therapeutic encounters cannot be described here in detail but usually continue over weeks or months, and eventually and slowly, as patients gain in trust and in more realistic self-awareness, and interact more with the environment, they often become more depressed. Although antidepressant medications may be tried, especially because suicidal danger is often quite real, their effectiveness at this stage is not established. However, the depression indicates also the beginning of personality growth, and reliance on drugs must not replace psychotherapeutic work which aims at mastery of the depressive affect instead of avoidance or suppression of it. But overcoming depression is a labile process involving considerable mood swings and recurrent discouragement, and if destructive behavior ensues, therapy may also have to be more protective. Depression at this stage of treatment often reflects a more realistic appraisal by patients of their aloneness and of their interpersonal incompetencies, as well as a beginning awareness of separateness and the development of a sense of self. It is at this stage that group therapy and peer experience are particularly helpful and sociotherapeutic. Productive activity geared to the patient's ability and education must be available as an important source of increasing self-esteem.

"Group therapy" in the hospital differs from outpatient group therapy, because inpatients are together and interact with each other throughout the day. Moreover, patient groups on a ward should be in part "task-groups" with managerial responsibility for the group members and the community's daily life. Without such participant administration on the part of patients, sociotherapy is not likely to become substantive. Patient government and special patient committees are the other components of sociotherapy. Staff leadership and participation in work groups and in patient government should be minimal, but considerable in patient-management groups.

Family therapy with family units and with groups of families is an essential concurrent treatment modality on a once-to-twice-weekly schedule. At what stage in treatment the patient can be weaned from the hospital environment and become an outpatient is a complex issue which cannot be determined by psychologic factors only. The patient's life situation, the family's role in the illness and in treatment, and community facilities and attitudes enter into these considerations, in addition to the patient's readiness to work or study. Discharge of schizophrenic patients must be gradual, and usually should follow demonstration of satisfactory work or school adjustment while in the hospital. The patient's family should be prepared through concurrent therapeutic work throughout the hospital period to accept the patient back into a readjusted family environment, or, if indicated, to let the patient live away from the family. In brief, no plan for patients will work unless their families have been prepared and enabled to tolerate and cooperate with it. Discharge from the hospital may be to a halfway house to which every psychiatric hospital should have access, and individual treatment and often group therapy also must continue. If the hospital staff cannot assume this outpatient phase of treatment, individual treatment with the "outside" psychiatrist should begin before the formal discharge; the same principle applies to group therapy. Furthermore, special group programs to bridge the hospital-community gap have been found effective, especially if such groups are led by former patients who have mastered this transition themselves.

SECTION 16

Physical and Chemical Injuries

BURNS

method of
HUGO F. CARVAJAL, M.D.,
DONALD H. PARKS, M.D.,
and DUANE L. LARSON, M.D.
Galveston, Texas

Introduction

Burns are due to the effect of thermal injury upon skin and may be classified according to their depth.

First degree burns, such as sunburns, involve only the epithelium and manifest themselves as erythema. Second degree burns destroy the epithelium and part of the corium but spare dermal appendages from which re-epithelialization may occur. The skin appears red and denuded, blister formation is common, and the areas injured are usually painful. In third degree burns the entire thickness of the dermis is destroyed and re-epithelialization is limited to the periphery of the lesions.

Emergency Management

At the Scene. At the site of the accident, an adequate airway must be assured, smoldering clothing removed, cool water compresses and clean sheets applied, and rapid evacuation to an Emergency Room facility undertaken. Oxygen by mask should be applied en route. Chemical burns must be irrigated with copious amounts of tap water immediately. The priorities of medical procedures at the emergency facility are listed in Table 1.

At the Hospital. In essence, proper management should include, in order of importance, (1) assessment of the respiratory system; (2) brief physical examination to rule out associated injuries or pre-existing pathology; (3) adequate intravenous therapy to prevent shock, dehydration, and organ failure; (4) emptying of the stomach to prevent gastric dilatation, vomiting, and aspiration; (5) insertion of an indwelling urinary catheter; (6) cleansing, debridement, and dressing of the burn wound; and (7) administration of antibiotics, sedatives, and tetanus prophylaxis.

Installation of a large intravenous cannula, either by percutaneous technique or, if difficult, by long saphenous venous cutdown, is a major priority and must not be delayed. Parenteral therapy is recommended for all burns over 15 per cent in adults or 10 per cent in small children. An effective intravenous line must be assured before any long distance transport of the burn victim from a primary care facility is allowed.

EXTENT AND SEVERITY OF THE BURN. The patient's weight and length should be measured carefully, and the areas of total body surface and of the surface that is burned should be ascertained. Weight is measured before bed clothing, restraints, or dressings are applied and afterward as well. The wounds are cleansed and debrided (bullae left intact), their depth assessed, and the extent of the second and third degree burns estimated by using body proportion charts corrected for age (Fig. 1). This is particularly important in children, in whom body proportions vary significantly. In adults the rule of nines is still adequate. Circumferential third degree burns must be recognized and escharotomies performed to prevent ischemia of the extremities or respiratory embarrassment resulting from chest wall involvement.

MEDICATIONS. Although the risk of tetanus following burns is small, we continue to recommend tetanus prophylaxis in the form of tetanus

TABLE 1. **Priorities of Medical Procedures During the Emergency Phase**

PROCEDURE	INDICATION	COMMENT
1. Establish an adequate airway	Burns of the face, laryngeal edema, smoke inhalation	Avoid emergency tracheostomy
2. Examine for trauma to head, skeleton, or nervous system	Explosions	Remove clothing; radiologic examination helpful
3. Begin intravenous infusion	To prevent intravascular dehydration	Use isotonic fluids
4. Empty stomach through a nasogastric tube	To prevent gastric dilatation, vomiting, or aspiration	Antacids may be helpful
5. Insert an indwelling urinary catheter	To monitor hourly urine output	Use a closed drainage system
6. Examine the burn wound	To estimate depth and extent	Use burn charts corrected for use
7. Clean, debride, and dress the burn area	To minimize microbial colonization	Use topical antimicrobial therapy
8. Administer medications	To treat infections; to prevent tetanus; for sedation	Use intravenous route for sedation
9. Begin fluid, electrolyte, and protein administration	To replace antecedent deficits and concurrent losses	Use appropriate formulas to estimate requirements

toxoid (DPT for children less than 6 years of age and Td for older children and adults) if 5 years have elapsed since the last booster injection. Passive protection with tetanus immune globulin (TIG) is indicated only when the patient has had less than two previous injections of tetanus toxoid. The recommended dose for TIG is 250 to 500 units given intramuscularly. Penicillin prophylaxis in the form of a single dose of benzathine penicillin (1.2 million units intramuscularly) is also recommended to eradicate beta-hemolytic streptococci and prevent colonization of the wounds with this organism. Analgesia can be provided with meperidine hydrochloride (Demerol) given intravenously in doses of 20 mg. per square meter of body surface every 4 to 6 hours as needed. Other analgesics or sedatives can be used as well.

FLUID THERAPY FOR THE FIRST 24 HOURS. To accomplish the three major objectives of fluid therapy (Table 2), burn resuscitation programs should include the following: (1) The resuscitation formula should accurately predict fluid requirements for patients of different ages and sizes of burns. (2) The composition of replacement and maintenance fluids should closely approximate that of the fluids lost. (3) The adequacy of fluid resuscitation should be carefully monitored throughout the first 48 hours after the injury.

The use of the surface area method to estimate fluid requirements in burned patients has simplified their management for the first 24 to 48 hours. In essence the program relates fluid losses (edema and evaporation of water) and maintenance fluid requirements to body surface and surface area burned (square meters), rather than weight or percentage figures. This method allows standardization of fluid therapy for adults and children, and fluids are estimated as follows:

2000 ml. per square meter of body surface per 24 hours
plus
5000 ml. per square meter of body surface *burned* per 24 hours

According to the Galveston formula, half of the first 24 hour requirements is administered during the first 8 hours and the other half during the subsequent 16 hours.

With the exception of antacids (15 to 20 ml. per square meter of body surface every 2 hours) given in an attempt to decrease the incidence of stress ulcer, the patient should receive no fluids or

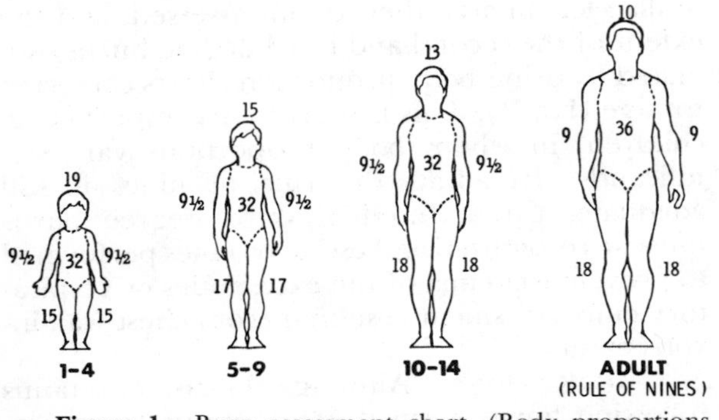

Figure 1. Burn assessment chart. (Body proportions have been modified from Lund, C. C., and Browder, N. C.: Surg. Gynec. Obstet., *79*:352–358, 1944.)

TABLE 2. **Objectives of Fluid Resuscitation Therapy in Burned Patients**

1. Correction of antecedent fluid, electrolyte, and protein deficits
2. Replacement of concurrent losses and maintenance fluids
3. Prevention of edema formation

food by mouth during the first 24 hours after injury. The reason for this is that paralytic ileus, vomiting, and gastric dilatation are not uncommon following severe burns. Furthermore, intestinal absorption of water and sodium is unpredictable during this phase.

If a body surface nomogram is not available, an acceptable alternative is a fluid calculation based on 3 ml. per per cent burn per kilogram of body weight.

Hydrating Solutions. As a result of the burn injury, water, electrolytes, and proteins are lost from the intravascular compartment into the interstitial tissues. Furthermore, as the skin continuity is lost, water evaporates rapidly, the net result being volume contraction. If such losses are not replaced, variable degrees of hypovolemia, hyponatremia, hypoproteinemia, and acidosis will develop, depending upon the size of the injury. To prevent electrolyte imbalance, shock, and acidosis, replacement fluids should approximate the losses. In the process of fluid resuscitation, however, it is difficult to decide whether a patient needs more sodium, albumin, or free water for hydration, and these decisions are often made on an empirical basis. Thus it seems desirable to use a single solution for intravenous therapy. Although there are those who recommend hypertonic salt solution containing no protein for hydration, we believe that such therapy is unnecessary and may even be deleterious, as it may result in dangerous hypernatremia. Composite burn solutions can be tailored to the patient's needs, but for the present the following generalizations regarding resuscitation fluids for either adults or children seem valid: (1) The concentration of sodium should be isotonic or only slightly hypotonic (120 to 130 mEq. per liter). (2) Bicarbonate or lactate should be added to combat acidosis (20 mEq. per liter). This also facilitates the preparation of a more physiologic fluid mixture (sodium:chloride ratio of 3:2). (3) The concentration of albumin should not exceed 1.25 grams per 100 ml. (4) Adequate quantities of carbohydrates should be added to provide a protein-sparing effect (5 per cent glucose).

The addition of 12.5 grams of salt-poor albumin (50 ml. of a 25 per cent solution) to 950 ml. of Hartmann's solution (lactated Ringer's in 5 per cent dextrose and water) makes an ideal burn solution. Potassium is not added during the first 24 hours, because large amounts of K^+ are released from injured cells into extracellular fluids, and acidosis or renal failure may result in dangerous hyperkalemia. Once the latter two complications have been ruled out and the level of blood urea nitrogen has returned to normal, 20 to 30 mEq. of potassium phosphate can be added safely to each liter of intravenous fluid.

Monitoring the State of Hydration. If the objectives of fluid resuscitation (Table 2) are being accomplished, the patient should remain in fluid, electrolyte, and protein balance, and edema of injured and noninjured tissues should be kept to a minimum. In practice, however, this ideal state of homeostasis is seldom reached, and the patient is either mildly dehydrated or overhydrated and may disclose mild to moderate electrolyte or protein deficits. Although the surface area formula has proved to be highly accurate in predicting fluid needs, its product still represents only an estimate, and its efficacy must be ascertained on every patient treated. Proper use and interpretation of clinical and laboratory guides to fluid therapy are therefore essential. In patients with other types of trauma or fluid loss, the state of hydration can be assessed on the basis of appearance and turgor of the skin, mucous membranes, urine output, state of sensorium, eyeball pressure, peripheral circulation, and vital signs. In the burned patient, however, some of these variables lose their predictive value. Skin turgor cannot be used, because as the capillary permeability is enhanced the skin becomes edematous. Since the patients are often anxious and in pain, the mucous membranes are frequently dry as a result of hyperventilation. Hypersecretion of antidiuretic hormone, irrespective of intravascular volume changes, leads to oliguria and a highly concentrated urine. If sedatives or analgesics are administered, the sensorium may be clouded regardless of the state of hydration. Peripheral circulation, as determined by venous capillary filling of the nail beds, can be used only if the extremity is not burned and circumferential burns proximal to the site of testing have not occurred, or the tourniquet effect resulting from the burn has been relieved by escharotomies. Changes in vital signs may be due to other factors such as fever or hypothermia, pain, apprehension, or medications. A fall in blood pressure usually occurs too late to be of value for precise fluid adjustment, a drop in volume of 10 to 12 per cent being necessary before a concomitant fall in blood pressure occurs. Table 3 lists clinical and laboratory guides to resuscitation therapy.

The single best variable is the general appearance of the patient. The hematocrit is also of value, as it provides an index of hemoconcentration, which reflects plasma loss at the beginning of therapy and progressive hemodilution as the state of hydration improves.

Although the aforementioned variables can still give a general idea of the patient's condition and perhaps the state of hydration, physicians must recognize the limitations of the signs they are monitoring and be aware that any variable by itself

TABLE 3. **Clinical and Laboratory Guides to Resuscitation Therapy**

- Vital signs
  - Pulse
  - Respiration
  - Temperature
  - Blood pressure
- Physical examination
  - General appearance
  - State of sensorium
  - Peripheral circulation (venous capillary filling)
  - Body weight
- Laboratory data
  - Hematocrit value
  - Blood, urine, urea
  - Serum and urine osmolality
  - Blood pH, Po_2, Pco_2
  - Serum and urine electrolytes
  - Urine specific gravity
- Fluid losses
  - Gastric losses
  - Hourly urine volume

can be misleading, that trends have greater value than single determinations, and that as many indicators as possible should be correlated before a decision is made to increase or decrease the quantities of fluid to be administered. Urine output should be evaluated in the light of other variables, and no attempts should be made to attain excessive urine volumes.

FLUID THERAPY FOR THE SECOND AND SUBSEQUENT DAYS. During the second day the administration of antacid should be discontinued and homogenized milk feedings begun. Total fluid requirements during the second and subsequent days may be estimated on the following bases:

1500 ml. per square meter of body surface
per 24 hours
plus
4000 ml. per square meter of body surface
burned per 24 hours

As oral fluid therapy is initiated and increasing quantities of milk are given, the intravenous fluids (composite solution) are simultaneously decreased in order to maintain a constant total hourly fluid intake.

Ideally, by the end of 48 hours, oral fluid administration will have replaced intravenous therapy. From the second day on, milk may be given every 1 to 2 hours either by mouth or through a nasogastric tube until the time of discharge. The milk program not only reduces the incidence of stress ulcers but also helps meet the excessive calorie demands of the burned patient. However, since the concentration of sodium in milk is low (25 mEq. per liter), sodium supplementation in the form of sodium chloride tablets or elixir (125 to 150 mEq. per square meter per day) needs to be given. In the elderly, an increasing serum potassium may be associated with a large intake of milk; thus a decrease in the quantity of milk administered is necessary.

NUTRITION. Trauma usually increases basal energy expenditures. In burns this is accentuated by the calories spent in the evaporation of water from the wounds. Evaporative water losses may be estimated as 3500 to 4000 ml. per square meter of burn area, and the caloric expenditure may be calculated by multiplying the evaporative water loss by 0.576, the number of calories required to evaporate 1 ml. of water. A simple method to estimate calorie requirements in burn patients is as follows:

1800 kcal. per square meter of body surface
per 24 hours
plus
2200 kcal. per square meter of body surface
burned per 24 hours

The increased calorie demands are usually met by oral feedings of milk (0.66 cal. per ml.) and a well balanced diet, but occasionally nasogastric feedings may be necessary.

BLOOD AND ALBUMIN REQUIREMENTS. The loss of albumin in the form of burn exudate continues beyond the first 24 hours until the wounds are covered. In order to prevent edema, serum albumin levels should be maintained above 2 grams per 100 ml. Ordinarily, this can be accomplished with the infusion of 100 to 150 grams of salt-poor albumin per square meter of body surface burned per week (two or three divided doses). Albumin infusions are better tolerated when given over a 12 hour period and in concentrations no greater than 5 grams per 100 ml. of diluent. Fresh frozen plasma provides an ideal source of this albumin.

Blood lost as a direct result of the injury or complications thereof needs to be replaced during the second to fifth day after the burn, depending on the severity of the trauma. Except in the patient actively bleeding or disclosing severe concomitant hypoproteinemia, packed cell transfusions are safer and better tolerated than whole blood. In most cases packed cells in the amount of 10 ml. per kg. of body weight, given over 3 to 4 hour periods, are sufficient to compensate for blood loss.

Management of the Burn Wound

Once the condition of the patient has been stabilized and resuscitative measures are well underway, the wounds should be cleansed and debrided in a tub bath containing povidone-iodine (Betadine) (10 parts per 1,000,000) or sodium hypochlorite (Clorox) in concentrations of 1:120. A whirlpool system prevents the hypochlorite solution from becoming oxidized in contact with living matter. The wounds are then rinsed and dried, and the need for escharotomies is assessed (see below). Following this procedure, the wounds are covered with fine mesh gauze impregnated with an antibacterial cream (e.g., silver sulfadiazine cream [Silvadene]) and held in place with elastic net (Hyginet).

Tub baths are repeated daily with reapplication of the silver sulfadiazine unless specific indications exist to alter either the frequency of dressing change or the topical antibiotic.

Escharotomy. Escharotomy implies an incision through third or, occasionally, deep second degree burned integument to relieve the tourniquet effect of the hard, unyielding eschar in circumferential burns. These usually involve the extremities, but other anatomic sites must be assessed, such as the chest or upper abdomen, where the heavy eschar may compromise excursion of the chest wall. It is important to realize that electrical trauma presents a far different pathophysiologic injury to the soft tissues, particularly muscle around bone, which swell rapidly, producing tremendous pressures within fascial compartments and rendering all structures in those compartments ischemic. Bone in this case acts as a resistor to the flow of current releasing heat. Fasciotomy as well as escharotomy is necessary to adequately release the underlying structures.

No anesthetic, analgesia, or special equipment is needed to perform an escharotomy. The incision should be carried from normal proximal tissue on the extremity, for example, to the fingertips if all tissues are involved. The release of constricting burn eschar on the chest should be made up the anterior axillary line from the region of the twelfth rib and curved medially toward the sternal notch. Transverse release should be done at the level of the costal margin.

Escharotomy often results in delayed hemorrhage as the blood supply is restored, so the patient must be watched closely for 1 to 2 hours after the procedure to verify hemostasis. The incision is then dressed with topical antimicrobial cream and a light dressing applied.

Burn Excision. The availability of good anesthesia, blood for transfusion, and skilled burn team personnel allows for an aggressive surgical approach to the eschar in many cases.

Tangential excision is a method of obtaining rapid eschar removal by excising shavings of eschar until pinpoint deep dermal bleeding is obtained and then immediately autografting this surface. The technique is carried out on the third to fifth postburn day, is used in deep second degree burns as estimated by the appearance and insensitivity, and should be limited to 20 to 25 per cent of the body surface. Thin split-skin grafts in sheets are applied to the exposed surface and ideally should be left exposed to allow personnel to evacuate hematomas that may form beneath the graft. The advantages of tangential excision include rapid closure of the burn wound, shortened hospital stay, and decreased incidence of hypertrophic scar.

Tangential debridement is a technique using dermatome knives and excising necrotic burn tissue in an effort to reduce bulk of the eschar. It is employed when the eschar is several days old, soft, and necrotic, or in extensive burns in conjunction with daily hydrotherapy. The objective is to remove the dead tissue which serves as a pabulum for bacterial proliferation. By tangentially debriding wounds early, appearance of a graftable granulation bed is hastened and, again, the morbid period is shortened.

Tangential debridement must be carried out in conjunction with hydrotherapy and topical antimicrobial drugs, and bloody oozing should be expected and may require frequent transfusion.

Excision of burn wounds to fascia may be indicated for massive burns over 60 per cent of the body surface area or in wounds in which bacterial invasion of the relatively ischemic subcutaneous fat is occurring. In the former group, excision over 20 to 25 per cent of the body, with immediate grafting on the exposed fascia with autograft meshed 3:1 and covered with a biologic dressing such as amnion, quickly reduces the mass of burn tissue and provides an excellent chance for rapid closure of a portion of the wound. The fascial plane is relatively avascular, and the epithelium from the mesh usually coalesces by about 10 days postgrafting. While the meshed grafts are taking, tangential debridement of the other burned areas is carried out every second or third day, so that by 7 to 10 days all eschar will have been removed.

When burn wound sepsis intervenes, implying invasion of viable tissue beneath burn eschar with organisms greater than 10^5 per gram of tissue, then neither topical nor parenteral antimicrobial therapy can hope to control and eradicate the organisms. Consequently, a surgical excisional approach to fascia is indicated and should be done as an emergency procedure in the presence of massive systemic antimicrobial therapy. This antimicrobial therapy consists of gentamicin in a dose of 6 mg. per kg. and methicillin in doses of 200 mg. per kg. as a recommended first line of defense. Antibiotic choice must be altered as sensitivities dictate.

Skin Grafting. Successful grafting of full-thickness losses requires autograft (except in the case of identical twins). Grafts are obtained with an air-driven dermatome and generally should be 10 to 12 thousandths of an inch thick. The scalp provides an excellent donor site, particularly in massive burns in which buttocks and thighs may not be available. The scalp may be cropped repeatedly about every 7 to 10 days with no damage to hair growth.

Meshed grafting allows an increased area of coverage with a smaller donor site but does leave a cosmetically unattractive area in most cases.

Anesthesia. Ketamine provides the anesthetic agent of choice in burn patients and is safe and effective, but one must avoid any narcotic drugs or irritation to the larynx with this type of anesthesia.

Late Complications of Burns

Hypertrophic scar and scar contracture comprise the major disabling features of the healed burn wound.

Pregrafting Phase. Prior to grafting of the burn patient, thermoplastic splints are prescribed, retaining affected elbows or knees in extension, the neck in extension, arms abducted, ankles at 90 degrees, and hands allowing slight wrist extension, metacarpophalangeal flexion, and interphalangeal extension with thumb abduction and flexion.

Grafting. During the grafting phase, splints may be ill-advised owing to their abrasive nature; so here, careful patient positioning is adhered to, again placing the joints as described.

Postgrafting. Once grafts are stable, splinting is again rigidly imposed, and a program of constant, controlled pressure is instituted, based on the pathophysiologic studies demonstrating prevention of contractures and suppression of hypertrophic scar. In the early postgrafting period, splints as described are worn continuously except for periods of supervised activity and bathing. Elastic wraps are also worn 24 hours a day except for bathing; once the patient has been discharged and his weight has stabilized, elasticized garments are prescribed and again worn 24 hours a day.

Hypertrophic scars and severe contractures usually become apparent at 3 months, and scar activity may persist for up to 1 to 2 years. It has been shown that the pressure phenomenon hastens the onset of scar maturity as indicated by flattening, softening, and blanching of the raised, firm, red, hypertrophic scar. Splints are effective in overcoming the shortening effect of voluntary muscles and scar myofibroblasts, which will tend to shorten a wound until an equal and opposite force is met. The splint provides that force which will retain major joints in an ideal position.

DISTURBANCES DUE TO COLD

method of
E. E. HEDBLOM, CAPTAIN, MC, USN (RET.)
Brunswick, Maine

Temperature and moisture govern the type of cold weather injury; wind, moisture, and length of exposure govern the rate of development and severity. Preventive measures are included, for as Rear Admiral William Mills, Jr., MC,USNR,* of Anchorage, Alaska, says: "The best treatment of a frozen foot is its prevention."

Chilblains

This mildest of cold dry injuries occurs with repeated prolonged exposure of dry bare skin to temperatures from the low 60°s F. down to freezing. Common in the bare knees and cheeks of children, acute pornio is red and swollen, may be tender, and usually itches. Between periods of reexposure the skin is red and rough. There is no loss of tissue in untreated patients.

Treatment. 1. Wind-resistant clothing to prevent bare skin exposure to cold.

2. Animal or fish-fat ointments allay itching and skin breaks.

Frostbite (Superficial Dry Freezing)

To clarify the literature's confusing "degrees of frostbite" and to designate what should be immediately thawed in the field, I define *frostbite* as frosting of the skin (little deeper than sunburn) which always precedes a freezing injury. When thawed, tender redness will be followed by branny desquamation or, if more severe, by blisters and sheet desquamation. It is common following brief exposures to extreme cold. Below 23°F. (−5°C.), the speed of contraction depends on temperature, duration, and mode of exposure. "Instant" frostbite occurs with exposure of bare skin to supercooled metal, liquids (fuels, solvents, alcohol), and sudden blasts of cold air. Accompany-

*First physician to document treatment of freezing injuries with minimal or no tissue loss.

ing this condition per se there is rarely a remarkable lowering of general body temperature.

Frostbite is dangerous on the feet and annoying about the face and hands. Onset is signaled by a sudden blanching of the skin of the nose, ear, or cheek, which may be subjectively noted as a momentary tingling or "ping." Face muscles won't work. The "buddy system," by which men watch each other's faces for telltale yellow-white spots, minimizes skin loss by early detection. The skin is anesthetic. In severe cold, when face, hands, or feet *stop* hurting, *investigate immediately!* Unthawed frostbitten skin is cold, frosty, and crisp, but it moves freely over subcutaneous joints or cartilage. Thawed frostbite may be indistinguishable from thawed freezing injury.

Prevention of Frostbite. FACE. A moderately stiff, 4 to 5 inch deep tunnel in front of the facial aperture of parkas protects the face from winds except 60° dead ahead. The tunnel should contain a malleable wire at the outer aperture so that the opening may be shaped. Face masks are needed for high winds or propeller blast. A muffler or long heavy wool stocking covering cheeks, nose, and chin will work for short exposures.

HANDS. Shearling-lined leather gloves or mittens are most satisfactory. Avoid wetting hands with fluids that freeze below 32°F. (0°C.). Touching very cold metal with moist bare hands results in the skin sticking to the metal, often causing mechanical loss of tissue as well as quick frostbite.

FEET. Footgear *must* be roomy enough to permit easy flexion and extension of the toes to increase circulation and delay frostbite, particularly in cases of forced immobility or injury concomitant to trail or plane operations. Boots or galoshes worn over ordinary shoes are to be avoided, for feet freeze because tightly laced shoes restrict circulation already compromised by cold and shock.

Treatment of Frostbite. Thaw *immediately* lest it progress to a freezing injury. The face and ears are thawed in the field by placing a warm hand over the spot until it hurts again. Fingers are best treated, if the parka has sufficiently large sleeves, by drawing the arm inside and warming the hand in the opposite armpit. (Axillary warming through zipper front coats allows excessive loss of "core" temperature from the exposed thorax and, under survival conditions, predisposes to general hypothermia.) Frostbitten feet are best thawed on the warm belly under the parka of a companion (the height of brotherly love and the hallmark of a true trailmate). If alone, warm the heel in one cupped hand and the toes in the other hand.

Chemical heating pads and pocket warmers are rarely available or working when needed. Placed on bare skin without insulation, they may cause burns. Under *no* conditions should frostbite be thawed by rubbing, with or without snow or slush!

Freezing Injury (Deep Frostbite)

When ice crystals form in tissues deep to the skin and its immediate subcutaneous tissues, an extremity is *frozen.* This is the "third and fourth degree frostbite" of the literature which cannot be clinically distinguished before or during treatment, and as treatment is the same for both, why quibble about degree? Freezing occurs most critically in the feet, occasionally in the hands and ears.

Unthawed it is painless. The skin has a pallid yellow color and will not roll over bony prominences. Members may be solid or "wooden," but are never brittle. When the patient is brought indoors, the skin will collect droplets of moisture from the atmosphere like a cocktail glass. Blisters appear in 12 to 36 hours. Unless rapidly rewarmed, red-violet discoloration appears spontaneously on the first to fifth day. Skin and nails usually blacken in 10 to 14 days and will slough usually within 60 to 72 days. There is always some degree of subcutaneous fat atrophy distal to the line of demarcation of the injury, although skin and nails usually completely regenerate. With the best treatment there is usually some loss of digital joint motion.

Residual hypesthesias, paresthesias, and sensitivity to cold in recovered extremities are probably caused by *anoxic injury* to the parasympathetics from *wet* cold exposure suffered prior to freezing (sweat or environmental water in the boot). These sequelae may be more severe in frozen extremities which have not been rapidly rewarmed on initial treatment.

Prevention of Freezing. 1. Prevent frostbite or thaw it immediately (see previous discussion).

2. Maintain "core" temperature with adequate clothing, shelter, fluids, and nutrition.

3. Avoid alcohol in the cold. It promotes rapid cooling from peripheral vascular dilatation (the subjective "warm" feeling). More important, alcoholic euphoria makes a person careless, decreasing self-control, judgment, perception, and ambition to fight the cold—all of which are necessary for survival.

4. Avoid fatigue, for, like alcohol, overexertion induces neglect as well as lack of strength for preventive measures.

Treatment of Freezing Injuries. FIELD FIRST AID. 1. Raise the patient's *core* temperature (see Hypothermia).

2. There must be *no* constriction to circulation above or over the frozen area. Immobilize concomitant fractures and dislocations loosely and

without traction, for the snug bandages necessary for traction jeopardize circulation and increase freezing damage. For the same reason, avoid pneumatic splints.

3. *Never* thaw a *frozen* extremity until arrival at a facility with water, heat, power, and equipment for sterile bed care where extremities can be *rapidly* rewarmed, for the following reasons: (a) If thawed and *refrozen*, loss of digits and perhaps a hand or foot is the invariable outcome from early gangrene. (b) The swollen, edematous, painful thawed extremity is more subject to infection during transportation than if left frozen, and *infection* is the chief reason for loss of tissue. (c) A man with a frozen foot is *not* a stretcher patient unless he suffers concomitant serious injury. (Under survival conditions, keeping one leg frozen, Peter Freuchen walked miles and days for help, knowing that when the leg thawed he would be helpless.) (d) A stretcher patient requires at least two men to carry him or pull him on sled or toboggan; and an ambulance, truck, or helicopter will haul only four to six stretcher patients, but it will take three to four times that many ambulatory patients. (e) Quick thaw of freezing injury in warm water is a *specific* therapy which minimizes ultimate tissue loss and sequelae. Rather than thaw in the field, it is preferable to keep an extremity frozen 2 to 4 more hours to enable rapid rewarming with immediate hospital care.

4. If the frozen member has thawed spontaneously or has been thawed by a well-intentioned friend, bandage is loosely in a voluminous cotton-wool bandage to prevent further trauma during sleeping bag stretcher transportation.

5. *No alcohol,* vasodilators, anticoagulants, or massage.

HOSPITAL TREATMENT. 1. Raise the patient's core temperature.

2. Routinely and vigorously treat shock with elevation of feet, warmth, oxygen, and intravenous plasma or dextran. Patients, particularly those with concomitant injuries, often go into *profound shock* when entering a facility where it's warm.

3. If still frozen, *rapidly rewarm* in tub or water bath with pump or paddle, open-top washing machine, or whirlpool bath. A safe temperature is midway between "warm" 102°F. (39°C.) and "hot" 116°F. (47°C.) to the normal elbow. Mills and his associates in Alaska have successfully used 100 to 112°F. (38 to 44°C.). Thawing may take 20 to 30 minutes but it should be continued until all paleness of the digital tips has turned pink to burgundy red, and *no longer*. These patients may require protective measures, opiates, and sometimes force to bring first thawing to the proper end, for it's *damned painful*. *Never* use dry heat, for this may superimpose a burn on the already insulted tissues. If thawed on admission, *do not rewarm*.

4. Tetanus booster on admission.

5. Physiotherapy (*most* important!). (a) Half hour whirlpool water bath 90 to 98°F. (32 to 36.7°C.), containing a mild detergent or soap, every 8 hours, until healing or spontaneous amputation takes place. (b) Immediate active (*not* passive) joint motion, particularly during hydrotherapy. This usually requires supervision and encouragement to overcome the patient's discomfort or laziness. (c) Buerger's exercises 20 to 30 minutes every 4 hours during the day.

6. Surgical care.

a. Until the skin is dry and without blebs (2 to 3 weeks), all attendants *must* use sterile isolation technique with masks, gowns, gloves, and bedsheets to minimize secondary infection. Open treatment of the elevated member under a cradle is recommended, without dressings, bandages, or ointment. Sterile cotton between toes or fingers minimizes maceration.

b. Blisters invariably complicate freezing injuries. Early clear blisters down to the tips of the digits are a good sign. Higher and particularly blood-filled blisters indicate that a digit may be lost. *Leave all unbroken blebs alone!* For the first 2 to 3 weeks, debridement is strictly limited to trimming gross skin flaps loosened in hydrotherapy. When the wound is dry and uninfected, circumferential eschars interfering with circulation or joint flexion may be slit laterally or dorsally. Trust the whirlpool to atraumatically and aseptically debride all blisters and local infection.

c. *No amputation for at least 3 months* or until after autogenous amputation, unless overwhelming infection or concurrent injury requires it! Delay minimizes tissue loss and ultimately reduces hospitalization time by providing healthier tissues for necessary repairs or skin grafts. Color of skin or line of demarcation is *not* indicative of end result. Skin can always be replaced; a prematurely amputated digit, hand, foot, or leg cannot!

d. Split thickness or pedicle skin grafts when denuded granulating areas are ready.

e. *Sympathectomy*. Recovered *dry* frozen injuries are usually relatively painless. After 6 months, if concurrent disabling *wet* cold sequelae are improved by sympathetic block, sympathectomy may be performed.

7. Broad-spectrum antibiotics are administered only with evidence of deep infection or cellulitis.

8. Psychiatric measures. During the first 3 months, pleasant environment, frequent visits, encouragement, and occupational therapy are mandatory. Opiates should be avoided after initial thawing because patients are easily addicted. They

often persuade surgeons to amputate because of depression over a black foot or finger. Meprobamate may be indicated during the first 90 days. (The physician may need therapy himself during this period, for his urge to do something surgical makes him the patient's and his own worst enemy!)

9. I have found that ascorbic acid, 100 mg. diphenhydramine, 50 mg., nicotinic acid, 50 mg., and zinc sulfate, 50 mg., every 4 hours, promotes epithelization (as do vitamin E, 10 to 50 I.U., and vitamin A, 25,000 to 50,000 I.U., daily).

10. Smoking is discouraged.

11. *No* anticoagulants except aspirin, 648 mg. every 4 hours, given primarily to alleviate the discomfort of active joint motion; theoretically it might assist in restoring capillary circulation. *No* vasodilators, high intensity sound, or diathermy.

12. Weight bearing is allowed only after some cornification of the new epithelium.

Immersion Foot (Trench Foot or Bomb Shelter Foot)

This results from wet cooling of an extremity for hours or days at temperatures of 68°F. (20°C.) down to freezing. Dependency or immobility of the extremity predisposes. Sailors in sea water and soldiers with wet feet in trench or foxhole suffer the same condition. Nerve, muscle, and blood vessel injury caused by cooling and anoxia is the common factor. General body chilling and venous stasis are causative factors.

In the first stage of *ischemia* the foot is cold, swollen, waxy, and mottled, with cyanotic, burgundy to blue splotches. It is resilient to palpation, in contradistinction to the unthawed frozen foot. Skin is sodden and friable. Anesthesia and loss of deep proprioception make walking difficult.

The second, *hyperemic* stage lasts days to weeks. The feet are red, swollen, and hot; blisters form; infection and gangrene are common. "Recovered" immersion feet often have edema, deep pain, superficial burning, cold sensitivity, and hyperhidrosis, which may last for months to years.

Prevention of Immersion Foot. 1. Avoid rubber (nonbreathing) footgear when weather conditions permit.

2. Dry the feet and change *wool* socks when feet get sweaty or wet (every 3 to 4 hours, at least).

3. Periodic elevation, air drying, fire warming, and massage promote circulation.

4. Avoid tight or constricting clothing.

Treatment of Immersion Foot. This differs from the treatment of frostbite in the following particulars:

1. Hydrotherapy is indicated only for debridement of blebs, ulcers, and infection, should they occur.

2. Vasodilation and circulation should be assisted within hours by (a) sympathetic block, (b) heparinization until the feet have normal vascular response and are relatively painless, and (c) an ounce (30 ml.) of hard liquor every hour (2 oz. [60 ml.] every 2 hours during sleeping hours) the first 10 to 20 days.

3. Drugs for relief of pain are more often necessary, but should be used minimally and discontinued as soon as possible.

4. Massive vitamin B complex therapy is certainly indicated.

In a military environment such as Korea where winter days were in the 40°F. range and temperatures at night were below freezing, *or* in uniform subfreezing temperatures in which men wear watertight thermal boots and their feet are usually bathed in their own perspiration, cold injuries are usually mixed wet and dry cold. If it is suspected that an immersion foot may also have been *frozen once*, therapy directed toward the frozen foot regimen will probably produce the best end result.

General Hypothermia (Dry Cold)

In subfreezing weather over twice as many die from carbon monixide poisoning as from freezing, and most hypothermic ("exposure") deaths occur in the 30 to 50°F. range.

In brief physiologic review, like an internal combustion engine, man burns fuel (food) to produce heat. Asleep, body curled in the fetal position (engine idling), the minimal human fire (basal metabolic rate [BMR]) must maintain a "core" (rectal) temperature of 95°F. (35°C.) or above to be self-sustaining. Reduced oxygen (e.g., altitude, emphysema, asphyxia) or food, faulty blood circulation (dehydration or poor physical conditioning), fatigue, narcosis, injury, illness, or shock—singly or in combination—diminishes the BMR.

At environmental temperatures less than 68°F. (20°C.), man's survival depends on his insulation (clothing, shelter, body fat), ratio of body surface to volume, BMR, food fuel reserves, knowledge of basal survival techniques, and the will to survive.

To conserve body fuel it must be realized that the skeletal muscle contraction of light work doubles or trebles the BMR. Hard work multiplies it by 30 to 40, and usually results in sweating. Skin wet with sweat or outdoor moisture suffers *very rapid* heat loss, worsened by increasing winds.

When core temperature sinks below 95°F. (35°C.), there is uncontrollable shivering and poor muscular coordination. Heart rate, blood pressure, respiration, and BMR are diminished; speech and thinking are impaired, and there may be amnesia. At 86°F. (30°C.) respirations are quite slow, atrial arrhythmias begin, and behavior will be irrational with hallucinations and apathy. By 78 to 80°F. (25.5 to 27°C.) the subject will be unconscious and areflexic. Atrial and then ventricular fibrillation with cardiac arrest usually occur around 77°F. (25°C.), but one patient survived a 61°F. (16°C.) core temperature.

Those who have come close describe freezing to death in dry cold as a fairly pleasant way to go. Extreme fatigue (only the fatigued sleep through the violent shivering), weakness, and joint stiffness are followed by a feeling of warmth, comfort, and an overpowering sleepiness. Unconsciousness and death follow painlessly.

Prevention. 1. Conserve body fuel with adequate water and wind-*resistant* clothing.

2. On the trail take frequent brief rests.

3. At *first* fatigue or shivering, find or make shelter to keep dry and out of the wind.

4. After fuel is gathered and fire built, spend as much time as possible curled up in a sleeping bag.

5. Maintain hydration and avoid *alcohol*.

Treatment. Same as that of immersion hypothermia (see below).

Immersion Hypothermia (Acute, Wet Cold)

Sea water freezes at 28.6°F. (−2°C.). It may be assumed that most polar water with ice nearby is this cold. Man submerged in this water, depending on amounts and type of clothing worn, has his breath knocked out. After initial shivering the body goes into a position of spastic fetal flexion with hands and knees under the chin, and voluntary control of the muscles is lost. (The ungloved hand is useless in 1 to 5 minutes.) Loss of breathing is caused by spasticity of trunk musculature.

In water the nude body core temperature falls roughly 14 times faster than in still air at the same temperature. On first immersion there is reflex contraction of skin arterioles to save core temperature. This gives a fleeting increase in blood pressure and heart rate. Consciousness lasts 5 to 7 minutes; death occurs in 10 to 20 minutes.

At Dachau, exposure of the back of the head and neck to sea water at 29° to 30°F. was found to cause massive cerebral hemorrhage with death, so this part of the anatomy should be particularly protected.

In a few instances men have saved themselves by violent exertion as soon as they hit polar water and were able to swim some distance and pull themselves out on the ice or up a ladder. More have died, or would have without help, because of muscle spasm.

In water at 41°F. (5°C.) for 12 minutes it has been found that moderate work doubles the rate at which rectal temperature falls because of increased blood circulation and water heat convection. Working as hard as possible only slightly decreases the rate of temperature loss. In water at 59°F. (15°C.) conventional clothing reduces loss of temperature by about three fourths. If in a marine disaster at temperatures not causing the acute reactions, exert yourself as little as possible—you'll live longer. The obese are better insulated from loss of temperature (and slower to rewarm), responding in direct proportion to the thickness of their subcutaneous fat.

With a large number of subjects, as in shipwreck, treat those not breathing but alive and the unconscious first. Continuous pouring of water at 105 to 112°F. over those waiting for treatment will increase the number of survivors. After removal from the water, a paradoxical "after drop" in core temperature of up to 7°F. and lasting 20 or more minutes may occur following initial rewarming efforts. This is due to vasodilation increasing the return to the core of peripherally cooled blood.

Prevention. 1. Beware of thin ice (*think safety*)!

2. Immersion suits with waterproof gloves and boots for those in contact with wintry waters (and inflatable *covered* life rafts).

3. If you go in the drink in conventional clothing, get on land or safe ice *immediately*, roll in the snow to dry your soaked clothes, and then get on your feet and *keep in motion* to the nearest warm shelter. Your frozen outer clothing will be an excellent windbreak!

Treatment for Immersion or General Hypothermia. UNCONSCIOUS, NOT BREATHING. 1. Artificial respiration with oxygen, if available, keeping the patient as warm as possible with warm wet packs. If pulseless, give closed cardiac massage and try an intravenous bolus of 50 to 100 mg. of lidocaine and prayer.

2. Atrial fibrillation usually reverts spontaneously, although it may continue for 1 to 2 hours after body temperature has returned to normal.

3. In general (dry) hypothermia, dehydration is often acute, and warmed intravenous glucose, dextran, or both are indicated to expand blood volume.

4. Cold shock causes strychnine-like electroencephalographic patterns; hence, stimulants probably should not be used. A low serum sodium suggests adrenal failure, and hydrocortisone, 200 mg. intravenously, may be lifesaving.

UNCONSCIOUS, BREATHING. 1. Place in a tub or shower with water 105 to 112°F. (40 to 45°C.) or put naked in a warmed sleeping bag with a stripped trailmate, and *keep there* until the patient has stopped shivering.

2. When conscious, *if* the patient was not alcoholic on admission (and many are), 2 to 4 oz. (60 to 120 ml.) of hard liquor in a tall, hot, sugary

drink promotes quicker warming and a sense of well-being.

Pulmonary Chilling

During hyperventilation with strenuous exercise at very low temperatures, and particularly at altitude, man may cough up blood. This is *not* frostbite, because no tissue is frozen. Respiratory mucosal hyperemia causes it. Concurrently or as an aftermath, depending on time and temperature of exposure, altitude, and the patient, an asthmatic type of breathing may occur for hours up to a day or two.

Acute primary diaphragmitis, Hedblom's syndrome (Carl Arthur, Sr.), is a primary myositis and spasm of the diaphragm with referred shoulder and upper abdominal muscle pain caused by upper respiratory tract chilling or infection; it may last 1 to 2 weeks.

Pulmonary chilling may be prevented on the trail by slowing down and by utilizing parka hoods, face masks, or folded mufflers which allow rebreathing of warmed, humidified expired air.

Treatment of pulmonary chilling is symptomatic: humidification of quarters to 30 to 50 per cent humidity, bed rest, steam inhalations, oxygen as needed and if available, and forbearance from smoking until asthmatic breathing, hemoptysis, pain, and cough subside. (This is a really good time to quit smoking!)

DISTURBANCES DUE TO HEAT

method of
JOHN F. RYAN, M.D.
Boston, Massachusetts

Patients who present with excessive heat storage abnormalities can be classified into three categories: (1) heat cramps, (2) heat exhaustion, and (3) heat stroke. A differential diagnosis is made by symptoms. Heat cramps are the mildest form of the hyperthermic syndrome. Increased disturbances lead to a diagnosis of heat exhaustion, whereas the most severe situation is heat stroke. All are stages of the same heat storage dysfunction.

Heat cramps are characterized by localized muscle cramping. The treatment consists of rest in a cool environment and electrolyte determination and replacement either orally or parenterally, depending on whether the patient is vomiting.

Heat exhaustion is accompanied by water depletion and hypovolemia. The symptoms are severe headache, lassitude, vomiting, tachycardia, and hypotension. Treatment is similar to that of heat cramps, i.e., rehydration and rest.

Heat stroke is a medical emergency. The mortality of heat stroke has been reported as ranging from 17 to 70 per cent. It is recognizable by three signs: (1) neurologic abnormalities, (2) hyperthermia, and (3) hot dry skin, either pink or ashen in hue.

Rectal temperature has been reported usually in excess of 41°C. (105°F.). Core temperature is higher. Sweating is frequently, but not always, absent. Consumption coagulopathy associated with petechiae and gross hemorrhage has been reported.

Central nervous system symptoms are initially those of headache, dizziness, and confusion. These are followed by coma associated on occasion with such findings as convulsions, hemiplegia, decorticate posturing, or fecal incontinence. In fatal cases, cerebral edema has been present at autopsy.

High fever appears related to increased heat storage in the body caused by decreased radiation and convection related to a high ambient temperature. Evaporation by sweating is usually reduced also owing to a high relative humidity.

The hot dry skin owes its variation in color to peripheral perfusion. Pink color is present when perfusion through skin and skeletal muscle is increased. Ashen color usually represents low cardiac output and hypotension.

Treatment of heat stroke is aimed at reducing body temperature, maintaining or restoring a high cardiac output, and correcting any electrolyte derangement present.

Clothing should be removed, and an intravenous line, a central venous catheter, and a Foley catheter inserted. An electrocardiogram and suitable pulse detector (precordial stethoscope) should be monitored continuously. If the patient is unconscious, an arterial blood sample should be drawn. Oxygen administration, endotracheal intubation, and ventilation may be indicated by the clinical situation or by hypoxemia and/or hypoventilation noted in the arterial blood.

Cooling can be accomplished by administration of previously refrigerated Ringer's lactate and by ice bath immersion. Once the temperature is lowered to 38°C. (100°F.), cooling measures should be terminated to prevent inadvertent hypothermia. Rehydration will be accompanied by increased urinary output. If anuria occurs and persists despite hydration, electrolyte correction, and diuretic administration, then early dialysis should be considered.

A recently noted complication of anesthesia, malignant hyperthermia, is characterized by tachycardia, tachypnea, and dark blood in the surgical field; arrhythmias are common. Rigidity may follow succinylcholine administration during intubation, or it may or may not occur later in the syndrome. Fever is usually a later sign and commonly rises rapidly to 43 to 45°C. (110 to 113°F.). It is most important to stress the need for noting and diagnosing any unexplained sharp rise in pulse rate during anesthesia, especially when the more common causes of tachycardia are not present or have been eliminated from the differential diagnosis. The mortality rate is 58 per cent. Malignant hyperthermia occurs suddenly and unexpectedly, usually during an otherwise uneventful anesthesia and surgery. The cause appears to be related to an inability of calcium transfer from the sarcoplasm of muscle to its primary storage area, the sarcoplasmic reticulum. The increasing calcium concentration in muscle leads to a marked increase in aerobic and later anaerobic metabolism, causing a severe respiratory and metabolic acidosis. Later cellular membrane integrity is impaired, leading to hyperkalemia and high plasma levels of intracellular muscle constituents.

Treatment consists of stopping the anesthetic, administering 100 per cent oxygen, hyperventilation, correcting the acidosis, treating the hyperkalemia, cooling, procainamide therapy (an intravenous infusion of 15 mg. per kg. administered over 10 to 15 minutes is suggested; this agent has not been associated with the marked cardiac depression encountered with the larger doses of procaine hydrochloride), and maintaining urine output. Indices to be monitored include electrocardiogram, temperature, Foley catheter, arterial line, and central venous pressure line. Complications have been reported as consumption coagulopathy, renal failure, inadvertent hypothermia, pulmonary edema, hyperkalemia, muscle necrosis, and neurologic sequelae.

SPIDER BITES (BLACK WIDOW AND BROWN RECLUSE) AND SCORPION STINGS

method of
RICHARD S. BERGER, M.D.
New Brunswick, New Jersey

Spiders

Brown Recluse (and Other Loxosceles Spiders). These spiders are found throughout the United States, although bites are most commonly reported from the lower Ohio, Missouri, and Mississippi River basin. The bite of this arachnid produces a toxic reaction caused by an enzymatic venomous substance. If a small amount of venom is injected by the spider or if the patient is immune because of previous bites, only erythema and edema occur. In the more severe cases, the venom damages dermal blood vessels and produces hemorrhage, blanching (within 24 to 72 hours), and finally necrosis. Systemic symptoms, seen mainly in severe reactions, begin as early as 36 hours and include morbilliform rash, urticaria, fever, nausea and vomiting, and occasionally hemolysis or diffuse intravascular coagulation (DIC). Most deaths have been in small children, secondary to DIC.

Therapy depends on the severity of the reaction as determined by the progression of signs and symptoms in the first 12 to 24 hours. For minor, local urticarial reactions, antihistamines will control the symptoms. In patients with a more severe reaction with toxic systemic symptoms, systemic steroids (1 mg. per kg. of prednisone per day), bed rest, and close observation are required. Systemic steroids are also recommended for bites in areas of cosmetic concern and in areas of functional importance, such as fingers and genitals. Heparin therapy is recommended if signs of diffuse intravascular coagulation are present.

Presently, no satisfactory treatment is available to prevent the cutaneous necrosis. Although systemic and intralesional steroids (2.5 to 5 mg. per ml.) are used by many physicians, controlled studies in animals fail to show that steroids decrease the amount of necrosis.

Excision and repair of the area of necrosis should be delayed until the area of necrosis is well delineated and healing has begun.

Black Widow (Latrodectus Mactans). The neurotoxic effect of the spider's venom produces severe cramps, waves of pain, and a board-like abdomen, symptoms which mimic those of an acute abdomen. Systemic treatment with muscle relaxants (diazepam [Valium], 5 to 10 mg.) and intravenous calcium gluconate helps relieve the muscle spasm. Narcotics may be required for pain. A specific antivenin is available for high risk patients—i.e., small children, hypertensives, and the aged (over 60). It is administered intramuscularly after appropriate skin tests for allergy to normal horse serum are found to be negative.

Scorpions

In most areas of the United States, the sting from the scorpion causes only a painful local reaction similar to a bee sting. However, in the southwest, envenomation by *Centruroides sculpturatus* or *C. gertschi* produces neurotoxic symptoms rather than a local reaction and is potentially lethal.

Hyperesthesia or numbness spreads from the site to involve the whole extremity. Within 1 or 2 hours, malaise, restlessness, lacrimation, salivation, rhinorrhea, sweating, nausea, and vomiting appear. The patient passes from an agitated state into coma and finally convulsions. Cardiovascular signs may also develop. Again, the patients at risk are the very young, the aged, and the hypertensive.

Cool compresses and observation for 24 hours are all that is necessary for most scorpion stings. For *Centruroides sculpturatus* and *C. gertschi*, immediate treatment consists of placing a tourniquet proximal to the site of the sting and then cooling the area. Once the area is cool, the ligature is removed and the area is kept cool for 2 hours. The patient should be hospitalized. Specific antivenin, available in the poison centers in the Southwest region, is given if central nervous system or cardiovascular symptoms develop. Atropine (0.5 to 1 mg.) and phenobarbital (32 mg.) are given for symptomatic relief. Morphine or meperidine should be *avoided.*

PORTUGUESE MAN-OF-WAR (JELLYFISH) STINGS

method of
BRUCE W. HALSTEAD, M.D.
Colton, California

There are several hundred species of coelenterate jellyfishes capable of inflicting stings. The symptoms vary in nature from a mild skin irritation to death. One of the more severe coelenterate stingers is the Portuguese man-of-war, which in the strict sense of the term is not a jellyfish, but is a colonial hydroid. True jellyfishes are members of the class *Scyphozoa,* whereas the Portuguese man-of-war *(Physalia)* is a member of the class *Hydrozoa.* There are two species of *Physalia, P. physalis* of the tropical Atlantic Ocean and *P. utriculus* of the Indo-Pacific region. Both species are capable of inflicting extremely painful stings with their nematocyst apparatus.

The venom of *Physalia* is a highly labile protein complex having neurotoxic properties. The venom is readily destroyed by heating to 60°C., by drying, or by alcohol, ether, acetone, or most other organic solvents.

The clinical effects most commonly reported from the stings of *Physalia* are intense local pain extending along a pattern corresponding to the lymphatic drainage (i.e., axillary lymph nodes) and joint and muscle pain. The pain varies from moderate to severe, sharp, shooting, or throbbing, depending upon the description given by the patient. The pain has sometimes been described as similar to that of an electric shock. The usual lesion is a discontinuous line of small papules, each surrounded by a small zone of erythema. There may be well-defined linear welts or scattered areas of punctate whealing and redness. Whealing is prompt and rarely massive, and usually disappears within a few hours. The erythema may remain for about 24 hours. However, slow-healing skin ulcers may continue for a period of time. The intensity of the sting appears to vary, depending upon the length of time that the tentacle remains in contact with the sting. Lesions caused by the multiple-tentacled Atlantic species *P. physalis* are usually more extensive than those produced by the single-tentacled *P. utriculus.* The local effects may be accompanied by headache, malaise, primary shock, collapse, faintness, pallor, weakness, cyanosis, nervousness, hysteria, chills and fever, muscular cramps, abdominal rigidity, nausea, vomiting, respiratory distress, backache, throat constriction, collapse, coma, and so on. No authenticated deaths from *Physalia* stings have been reported.

Therapy

Prompt first-aid measures are of particular importance in *Physalia* stings, as well as in all other types of jellyfish stings, because as long as the tentacles adhere to the victim's skin they continue to discharge their venom. The following procedures are therefore recommended: (1) Remove adhering tentacles with the use of gloves, bathing towel, seaweed, gunny sack, dry sand, salt, sugar, or any dry powder. This should be done immediately. (2) Pour alcohol over the wounded areas as soon as possible. Rinse the skin off with salt water after at least 2 minutes have elapsed. Do not rub the wounded area with sand. (3) Apply a corticosteroid-analgesic balm, preferably by aerosol.

Priority of treatment must be governed by such problems as shock, respiratory arrest, cardiac complications, and skin reactions. For the most part treatment is symptomatic. There are no known specific antidotes. The application of compresses moistened with aromatic spirits of ammonia has been found to be effective. In the absence of all other medicinals, native islanders apply urine, with surprisingly good results.

The Commonwealth Serum Laboratories, Melbourne, Australia, have recently developed a jellyfish antivenin for the deadly sea wasp *(Chironex fleckeri).* The stings of this jellyfish are extremely painful, and may cause death. Although *Chironex* is an Australian jellyfish, there are closely related species inhabiting West Indian waters. Any victim who has received the first aid measures mentioned above and continues to have difficulty in breathing, swallowing, or speaking or continues to be in severe pain may require sea wasp antivenin. The antivenin is supplied in containers of 20,000 units. Complete instructions as to its use are supplied by the manufacturer.

ACUTE MISCELLANEOUS POISONING

method of
JAY M. ARENA, M.D.
Durham, North Carolina

The basic treatment for acute poisoning, whether drug or chemical, is mainly symptomatic and supportive. Overtreatment of the poisoned patient with large doses of nonspecific and questionably effective antidotes, stimulants, sedatives, and other therapeutic agents often does far more harm and damage than the poison itself. A calm attitude, with the judicious use of drugs, parenteral fluids, and electrolytes for homeostasis, and the maintenance of an adequate airway are far more effective than heroic measures, which usually are unnecessary. As a matter of fact, it is often difficult to tell whether recovery from an acute poisoning occurred because of or in spite of the treatment used. Remember: "Treat the patient, not the poison."

Severe Poisoning

1. Establish adequate airway by inserting an oropharyngeal or endotracheal tube. Often, however, extension of the head and forward displacement of the mandible are sufficient. The situation may require mouth-to-mouth breathing or mechanical respiratory equipment. Physiologic improvement of the patient's condition is often notable when tissues receive adequate oxygen.
2. Empty the stomach with a large nasogastric tube and analyze a sample of the contents. Assess the patient's general condition and obtain pertinent information.
3. Generally, legs and head are elevated to the level of the right atrium to allow venous drainage of the lower extremities and promote circulatory pooling in the head and thorax. Cardiac failure may necessitate alterations in position.
4. Elastic bandaging of the legs prevents venous stasis. Passive leg exercises are advisable if depression is extreme. The patient is turned from side to side every 2 hours to promote pulmonary drainage and reduce atelectasis.
5. Homeostasis is maintained by parenteral fluid according to blood electrolyte concentrations and urine output. An indwelling urethral catheter is placed in the bladder to permit accurate hourly measurement of output. When the kidney is not damaged, fluid therapy is aided by hourly measurement of urine specific gravity.
6. If oliguria is associated, electrocardiographic examination and frequent measurement of serum potassium are required.
7. Vital signs are recorded every 15 minutes or more frequently if values are labile or vasopressors are administered.
8. Drugs should be given only when specifically required. Rarely, such as in cyanide poisoning, is therapy with an antidote significantly urgent. Intensive supportive therapy reduces the need for medication.
9. Central nervous system stimulants should not be used to improve respiration. These drugs impart a false sense of security, and harmful reactions such as rebound depression or convulsions may occur. If the myocardium is hypoxic, epinephrine may induce fatal ventricular fibrillation.
10. Intravenous vasopressors such as phenylephrine, methoxamine, or other adrenergic drugs may be required if the patient has tachycardia above 110 pulse beats per minute, prolonged capillary filling time, pallor, or diaphoresis. Moderate hypotension as low as 80 mm. Hg does not necessitate vigorous therapy with vasopressors unless urinary output is depressed. Extremely potent agents, such as levarterenol bitartrate, are used for severe shock, but vasoconstrictors may significantly depress urinary output.

Oral Poisons

Attempt to remove the unabsorbed poison when the poison has been taken by mouth. Many poisons are in themselves emetics, but if vomiting does not occur spontaneously, it should be induced. However, emesis should not be attempted in caustic, corrosive, and petroleum-distillate poisoning, or if the patient is semiconscious or comatose.

In children emesis can best be induced by having them drink a glass of water or milk (never carbonated fluids), after which they should be gagged with the finger or the posterior pharynx stroked with a blunt object. Warm saline solution or mustard water as an emetic is impractical. An overdose of salt in a child could be dangerous (hypernatremia) and even fatal.

Syrup of ipecac (not the fluid extract) can be given in doses of 10 to 15 ml. and repeated in 15 to 30 minutes if emesis does not occur. For best results, 1 or 2 glasses of water* should be given after the administration of the syrup of ipecac, because emesis may not occur on an empty stomach. Activated charcoal should never be given simultaneously with ipecac, because it will absorb the ipecac and prevent its emetic effects. Recent studies indicating that induced vomiting

*Milk should not be used, as it will delay emesis.

empties the stomach of ingested poisons more effectively than does gastric lavage have produced increased enthusiasm for its use. Nevertheless, the ipecac that fails to effect vomiting either remains in the gastrointestinal tract as an irritant or is absorbed and exerts actions concomitantly with any toxins already present, and its cardiotoxic effects must be kept in mind. Syrup of ipecac or apomorphine should not be used when antiemetic drugs have been ingested, if more than an hour or two has elapsed. Gastric lavage would be safer and more effective.

If syrup of ipecac is not available, the mechanical method, gagging with fingers or spoon, is the safest and the most logical form of treatment in the home and should be tried first.

The use of table salt as a home emetic, particularly in children, should be discouraged. Fatal salt poisoning has occurred in children and adults from this obsolete method.

Apomorphine, 0.03 mg. per lb. (0.066 mg. per kg.), given subcutaneously, usually causes prompt vomiting. Since it is a respiratory depressant, it should not be given if the patient is comatose, if the respirations are slow or labored, or if the poisoning is by a respiratory depressant. Naloxone hydrochloride (Narcan) preferably, or other narcotic antagonists (see antidote chart, p. 890), will rapidly terminate the emetic effects of apomorphine and help to diminish the subsequent depression (their use, however, is not mandatory, and is often unnecessary). The combined proper use of these drugs for emptying the stomach in acute poisoning has already been shown to be effective and safe, both experimentally and clinically. The advantages are (1) rapid emesis with removal of all gastric contents, (2) no obstruction of lavage tubes, producing delays and incomplete emptying, and (3) reflux of contents (such as enteric-coated tablets) from the upper intestinal tract into the stomach.

Gastric Lavage. Gastric lavage is indicated within 3 hours after ingestion of a poison and even several hours later if large amounts of milk or food were taken beforehand or if enteric-coated or stomach emptying delaying drugs have been ingested. Gastric lavage is contraindicated after the ingestion of strong corrosive agents such as alkali (concentrated ammonia water, lye) or mineral acids (considered safe here if done within 30 minutes). Strychnine poisoning, because of the danger of producing a convulsion, and the ingestion of petroleum distillates (danger of aspiration pneumonia) are also contraindications. In semicomatose or comatose patients gastric lavage should be attempted only after an endotracheal tube with inflatable cuff has been inserted. Consult toxicology texts for specific instructions and techniques in performing a gastric lavage, especially in children.

General Rules. 1. Identify the poison.

2. Administer a specific antidote and a local antidote for residual poison not removed by evacuation of stomach contents.

3. Give an antagonist when available.

4. Administer symptomatic treatment as indicated.

5. When the nature of the poison is unknown, give activated charcoal. One to 2 tablespoonfuls to a 240 ml. (8 oz.) glass of water is suitable for oral use or lavage. The "universal antidote" is not effective and is not recommended.

6. In massive ingestions (suicidal attempts) when therapeutic results fail to reach expectations, rule out concretions in the stomach (x-ray or surgery if necessary). Give castor oil as a solvent and to hurry the material through the intestinal tract. Follow with activated charcoal.

Antidotes. Antidotes may be given to render the poison inert or to prevent its absorption by changing its physical nature (see Table 1, Therapeutic Agents).

Inhaled Poisons

Remove the victim from the gas atmosphere and apply artificial respiration if necessary.

Injected Poisons

Apply tourniquets central to the point of injection. If feasible, remove as much of the poison as possible by surgery and suction.

Absorbed Dermal Poisons

Flush skin with large quantities of water after all clothing has been removed.

Chemical Burns

Flush skin with water thoroughly and repeatedly. Consult ophthalmologist for eye care as soon as possible after thorough flushing. Do not use chemical antidotes in the eye.

Supportive Measures

Adequate amounts of fluids by mouth or parenterally are important, especially if poison is excreted by the kidney. (See articles on Parenteral Fluid Therapy, pp. 459 to 468). Use of blood transfusions, exchange blood transfusions (small children), and hemodialysis if an artificial kidney is available may be helpful. Lipid dialysis is a useful technique in the treatment of poisonings by glutethimide, pentobarbital, secobarbital, phenothiazines, camphor, and other lipid-soluble sub-

TABLE 1. **Therapeutic Agents***

TO NEUTRALIZE ACIDS†

1. Magnesia magma (milk of magnesia), 100 to 300 ml. (4 to 10 ounces)
2. Sodium bicarbonate (dilute solution)
3. Calcium hydroxide solution (lime water), 200 ml. (6⅔ ounces)
4. Aluminum hydroxide gel, 60 ml. (2 ounces)
5. Precipitated calcium carbonate (chalk), 100 grams (3⅓ ounces)
6. Wall plaster—crushed in water
7. Soap solution

TO NEUTRALIZE ALKALIS†

1. Vinegar (5% acetic acid), 100 to 200 ml.
2. Lemon juice, 100 to 200 ml.
3. Orange juice, 100 to 300 ml.
4. Dilute (0.5%) hydrochloric acid, 100 to 200 ml.

DEMULCENTS

1. Olive oil, 200 ml. (6⅔ ounces)
2. White of egg, 60 to 100 ml. (2 to 4 ounces)
3. Any vegetable oil, 200 ml. (6⅔ ounces)
4. Milk
5. Starch water
6. Liquid petrolatum (mineral oil)
7. Butter

EMETICS

1. Syrup of ipecac, 10 to 15 ml. repeated in 15 to 30 minutes if necessary (do not allow to remain in stomach)
2. Apomorphine, 6 mg. for adults, 1 or 2 mg. for children 1 to 2 years old, subcutaneously (0.03 mg./lb.). Respiratory depressant effect may be counteracted by Narcan, 0.01 mg./kg.
3. Household mustard or table salt used for emetic purposes should be discouraged. Fatal salt poisoning in children and adults has been documented.

STIMULANTS

1. Caffeine and sodium benzoate, 0.5 gram (7½ grains) subcutaneously
2. Coramine (nikethamide), 5 ml. intravenously or subcutaneously
3. Metrazol, 0.1 gram (1½ grains)
4. Black coffee by rectum

SEDATIVES

1. Phenobarbital, 0.03 to 0.1 gram (½ to 1½ grains)
2. Pentobarbital sodium, 0.1 gram (1½ grains)
3. Barbital sodium, 0.3 to 0.6 gram (5 to 10 grains) orally or subcutaneously
4. Chloral hydrate, 0.5 to 1 gram (7½ to 15 grains) orally
5. Sodium bromide, 0.3 to 1 gram (5 to 15 grains) orally
6. Paraldehyde, 3 to 15 ml. by mouth (double dose by rectum)

*From *Davison's Compleat Pediatrician,* 9th Edition, Lea and Febiger, Publisher.

†It is unlikely that serious exothermic effects will occur from the use of well diluted, mild neutralizing agents.

stances that cannot be effectively removed by hemodialysis using an aqueous dialysate. Peritoneal dialysis with its inexpensive disposal equipment and easy technique may also be indicated and is particularly valuable for use in children.

Shock

Therapy of shock requires careful consideration of the action of the poison ingested, the administration of vasopressor agents, steroids, the replacement of fluids, and transfusion of blood when needed.

COMMON POISONS AND THERAPY

(Modified from Arena, Jay M.: *Poisoning: Toxicology, Symptoms, Treatment,* 4th Edition, Springfield, Illinois, Charles C Thomas, Publisher; and *Davison's Compleat Pediatrician,* 9th Edition, Lea and Febiger, Publisher.)

1. Acetaldehyde

See Methaldehyde.

2. Acetaminophen

This compound with a half-life of 1 to 2 hours does not produce the gastrointestinal hemorrhagic or acid-base disturbance of acetylsalicylic acid, but it has a more subtle form of hepatic toxicity which can be serious. Treatment is symptomatic and supportive.

Oral methionine (Pedameth), 2.5 grams every 4 hours up to 10 grams, has recently been found effective in reducing the frequency and severity of acetaminophen-induced liver damage. (This use of methionine is not listed in the manufacturer's official directive.) Although this compound has few side effects and is of low toxicity, it does have the potential to aggravate a pre-existing hepatic disease, and therefore should only be given early (before 12 hours) after ingestion, before the likely acetaminophen hepatic effects take place.

N-acetylcysteine (Mucomyst), based on preliminary evaluation, appears to act as a glutathione substitute and to directly combine with the toxic acetaminophen metabolite. It is presently being recommended as the oral drug of choice (loading dose of 140 mg. per kg., followed by 70 mg. per kg. every 4 hours, for a total of 18 doses), if given within 12 hours after ingestion. (This use of N-acetylcysteine is not listed in the manufacturer's official directive.)

3. Acetanilid

Gastric lavage or emesis. Saline cathartic. Methylene blue for methemoglobinemia. Discontinue drugs in chronic poisoning or idiosyncrasies.

4. Acetic Acid (Glacial)

Magnesium oxide. Demulcents. For inhalation, treat pulmonary edema. Shock therapy.

5. Acetone

Gastric lavage or emesis. Analeptics and respiratory stimulants if necessary. Artificial respiration and oxygen.

6. Acetylsalicylic Acid (Aspirin)

See Salicylates.

7. Alkalis

Give milk and force water, followed by diluted vinegar or fruit juices by mouth. Do not use strong acids. Demulcents. Corticosteroids to prevent stricture. Esophageal dilation after fourth day. Broad-spectrum antibiotics.

8. Aminophylline

See Xanthines.

9. Ammonia (Ammonium Hydroxide)

See Alkalis. Force water.

Do not dilute with acids, because heat may be generated.

10. Amphetamine

Gastric lavage or emesis. Activated charcoal. Sedation or short-acting barbiturates with caution. Chlorpromazine (Thorazine), 1 to 2 mg. per kg. intramuscularly and repeat if necessary. Haloperidol (Haldol), 0.5 to 2.0 mg. three times daily, has been used effectively recently.

11. Amyl Acetate (Banana Oil, Pear Oil)

See Acetone.

12. Aniline and Derivatives (Dimethylaniline, Nitroaniline, Toluidine)

Gastric lavage or emesis. Artificial respiration and oxygen. For skin contact, thorough cleansing. Methylene blue for methemoglobinemia.

13. Antihistaminics

Gastric lavage or emesis. Activated charcoal. Saline cathartic. Do not use stimulants. Levarterenol for hypotension. Short-acting barbiturates with caution.

14. Antimony

Gastric lavage with 1 per cent sodium bicarbonate solution. Demulcents. BAL. Maintain fluid and electrolyte balance.

15. Antipyrine (Phenazone)

See Acetanilid.

16. ANTU (Alphanaphthylthiourea)

Gastric lavage or emesis. Saline cathartic. Oxygen. Avoid oils (more readily soluble).

17. Arsenic Trioxide (White Arsenic)

Gastric lavage or emesis. Thirty ml. tincture of ferric chloride and 30 grams of sodium carbonate in 120 ml. of water as antidote in lavage (remove precipitant). BAL. Shock therapy.

18. Arsine Gas

Move from environment. Exchange transfusion. BAL (ineffective). Industrial prevention with education, ventilation, etc.

19. Aspidium (Male Fern) Oleoresin

Gastric lavage or emesis. Activated charcoal. Saline cathartic. Demulcents. Short-acting barbiturates. Artificial respiration and oxygen. Avoid fats and oils.

20. Atropine

Gastric lavage with 4 per cent tannic acid solution or emesis. Pilocarpine or physostigmine for parasympathomimetic effects. Miotic for eyes. Oxygen. Small doses of barbiturates, chloral hydrate, or paraldehyde for delirium or convulsions. Cold packs or alcohol sponging. Indwelling catheter.

21. Barbiturates (Table 2)

There is no specific antidote for the barbiturates. In acute poisoning, current practices in most centers with much experience consider the immediate establishment of adequate pulmonary ventilation as well as control of shock of prime importance, whereas analeptics are considered subsidiary, if not actually contraindicated. The evidence indicates that the most favorable results are obtained by careful attention to respiratory and circulatory functions.

Forced diuresis by giving large amounts of fluids intravenously and also giving diuretics (Diamox or mercurials) reduces the need for vasopressor drugs, prevents renal complications and hyperthermia, and lessens crust formation in the respiratory tract. Contraindications are cardiac and renal disease. Pulmonary edema does not seem to be a serious hazard. Hemodialysis should be resorted to when indicated.

In addition to supportive measures, treatment for intoxication with this group of drugs should include forced diuresis with alkalinization of the urine. Dialysis need be considered only in the presence of renal function compromise. Alkalinization of the urine should be considered if intermediate or long-acting barbiturates have been ingested. The nonionized form of these drugs is highly lipid soluble and easily crosses the tubular membranes in the kidney; the ionized form is not lipid soluble and does not cross the

TABLE 2. **Treatment of Barbiturate Intoxication**

CONDITION	TREATMENT	GUIDES
Respiratory insufficiency	Airway, suction; endotracheal intubation, cuffed tube, lavage; humidified oxygen; mechanical ventilation, pressure- or volume-controlled ventilator	Arterial Po_2, O_2 saturation, Pco_2, pH, minute ventilation; x-ray film of chest; airway pressure
Hypovolemia	Albumin, 5% solution, 1 liter, then dextrose, 10% in sodium chloride 0.9 per cent solution; potassium chloride supplement, 40–120 mEq.	Central venous pressure, arterial pressure, urine output, and osmolality
Low urinary output	Fluid infusion: furosemide, 40 mg. I.V., or ethacrynic acid, 25 mg. I.V.	Urinary output and osmolality
Heart failure	Digoxin, 0.5 mg. I.V., followed by 1–4 doses of 0.25 mg. digoxin at 1–2 hour intervals	Central venous pressure, ECG
Pneumonia	Ampicillin sodium, 1 gram every 4 hours I.V.; methicillin sodium, 1 gram every 6 hours I.V.; chloramphenicol sodium succinate, 500 mg. every 6 hours I.V.; gentamicin sulfate, 0.75 mg./kg. every 6 hours I.M.	Sputum and blood culture, with antibiotic sensitivity; chloramphenicol after aspiration of gastric contents; gentamicin for gram-negative bacteria resistant to other antibiotics
Dialysis	Peritoneal; lipid; hemodialysis (preferred)	Barbiturate levels of 3.5 mg./100 ml. for short-acting drugs and 8–10 mg./100 ml. for long-acting agents; impaired hepatic and renal function

tubular membrane. Since alkalinization of the urine increases the ionized form of the intermediate and long-acting barbiturates, tubular reabsorption is decreased, resulting in more rapid clearance of the drug. Administration of intravenous sodium bicarbonate raises the urine pH to about 8.0, a point at which the ionized form of the intermediate and long-acting barbiturates is significantly increased.

The nonbarbiturate hypnotics include glutethimide and methyprylon. The history is of paramount importance in the diagnosis of overdoses with these agents. Physical signs are not specific and may be confused with signs of overdoses of other types of CNS depressants. If lethargy, mydriasis, hypotension, flaccid paralysis, and respiratory depression are present, intoxication with these drugs should be considered. Determination of serum and urine levels may also be helpful in confirming the diagnosis. Glutethimide also produces alternating periods of coma and relative alertness; this effect is due to the periodic increases in blood levels of glutethimide resulting from its excretion via the biliary tract with reabsorption into the circulation from the gastrointestinal tract. Lethal plasma levels of glutethimide and methyprylon are not known. The approximate fatal dose of glutethimide is 10 to 12 grams and that of methyprylon is greater than 6 grams. Supportive measures, forced diuresis, and dialysis are the most effective measures for treating overdoses of these drugs. Large doses of activated charcoal have also been shown to be beneficial.

Immediate gastric lavage with a solution of saline and activated charcoal. Continue lavage with isotonic saline until the return is clear. Use castor oil for instillation and withdrawal to increase solubility of sedatives and dissolve concretions. Ensure clear airway. Respiratory stimulants such as picrotoxin or pentylenetetrazol (Metrazol), administered in subconvulsive doses, are not often used in present-day therapy. Artificial respiration. Administration of 100 per cent oxygen. For circulatory depression and shock caused by depression of vasomotor center, as well as direct action on smooth muscle in blood vessel wall: pressor amines such as levarterenol (which acts directly on vascular smooth muscle). Intravenous hydrocortisone. Blood transfusions. Trendelenburg position. For water loss from skin and lungs, decrease in urine, electrolytes variable: adequate hydration with 5 to 10 per cent glucose in water to facilitate renal elimination of barbiturates. Use of electrolytes based on analysis of plasma. After the vital signs have been stabilized and adequate renal function has been ascertained, urea or Diamox-induced (forced) osmotic diuresis with alkalization of urine has proved to be effective and successful therapy in reducing mortality, severity of intoxication, and duration of treatment and hospital stay, and is now the treatment of choice in most centers. For hypostatic pneumonia resulting from hypotension and hypoventilation: prophylactic antibiotics. For depression of kidney function resulting from hypotension and central antidiuretic action of barbiturates: exchange transfusions (children). Intermittent peritoneal dialysis. Artificial kidney (lipid dialysis). For cerebral edema: mannitol or urea. (See also Narcotic Poisoning, pp. 851 to 853.)

TABLE 3. **Treatment of Convulsions Due to Poisoning***

DRUG	METHOD OF ADMINISTRATION AND DOSAGE	ADVANTAGES	DISADVANTAGES
Ether	Open drop	Dosage easily determined. Good minute-to-minute control. No sterile precautions	Difficult to give in presence of convulsion. Requires constant supervision by physician
Thiopental sodium (Pentothal sodium)	Give 2.5% sterile solution I.V. until convulsions are controlled. Maximum dose: 0.5 ml./kg.	Good minute-to-minute control. Can be given easily during convulsion	Doses larger than recommended may cause persistent respiratory depression. Requires sterile equipment and administration
Pentobarbital sodium (Nembutal sodium)	Give 5 mg./kg. gastric tube, rectally, or I.V. as sterile 2.5% solution at a rate not to exceed 1 ml./minute until convulsions are controlled	Good control of initial dose	No control of effects after drug has been given. Requires sterile precautions. May produce severe respiratory depression
Phenobarbital sodium	Give 1-2 mg./kg. I.M. or gastric tube and repeat as necessary at a 30 minute interval up to a maximum of 5 mg./kg.	Effects last 12–14 hours	Causes severe persistent respiratory depression in overdoses
Succinylcholine chloride	Give 10-50 mg. I.V. slowly and give artificial respiration during period of apnea. Repeat as necessary	Will control convulsions of any type. Effect lasts only 1-5 minutes. Circulation not ordinarily affected	Artificial respiration must be maintained during use. No antidote is available. Apnea may persist for several hours in some cases
Trimethadione (Tridione)	Give 1 gram I.V. slowly. Maximum dose: 5 grams	Little depression of respiration	Not effective in all types of convulsions
Tribromoethanol (Avertin)	Only by rectal instillation. 50-60 mg./kg. causes drowsiness, amnesia. 70-80 mg./kg. produces light unconsciousness and analgesia	Ease of administration and pleasant induction without mental distress and respiratory irritation	A nonvolatile anesthetic given by a route which prevents adequate control once it is administered. Contraindicated when renal or hepatic injury exists
Amobarbital sodium (Amytal)	Give 2% sterile solution. Dose range 0.4-0.8 gram	Immediate action and lasts 3-6 hours	Inhibits the cardiac action of the vagus. May produce severe respiratory depression
Diphenylhydantoin sodium (Dilantin)	Give slowly I.V. 150-250 mg. from Steri-Vial and repeat in 30 minutes with 100-150 mg. if necessary	Lack of marked hypnotic and narcotic activity	Solution is highly alkaline and perivenous infiltration may cause sloughing. Not always effective, and other anticonvulsants frequently must be used. Cardiac arrest has been reported after I.V. therapy
Paraldehyde	Give 5-15 ml. gastric tube, rectally or I.M.	Little depression of respiration. Effects last 12 hours	Harmful in presence of hepatic disease. Old and loosely stoppered solutions can break down to acetic acid and produce serious intoxication
Diazepam (Valium)	Give 2-5 mg. I.M. or I.V. Repeat in 2 hours if necessary	More effective for relieving muscle spasm associated with seizures	Hypotension and respiratory depression or muscular weakness may occur if used with barbiturates

*From *Davison's Compleat Pediatrician,* 9th edition, Lea and Febiger, Publisher.

TABLE 4. **Antidote Chart***

ANTIDOTE	DOSE	POISON	REACTION (ANTIDOTE) AND COMMENTS
Acids, weak Acetic acid, 1% Vinegar, 5% acetic acid (diluted 1:4 with water) Hydrochloric acid, 0.5%	100-200 ml.	Alkali, caustic	
Activated charcoal Darco G (Atlas Chem.) Nuchar C (W. Va. Pulp & Paper; Merck) Norit A (Amer. Norit Co.)	1-2 tbsp. to glass water or a mixture of soupy consistency	Effective for virtually all poisons (except cyanide), organic and inorganic compounds of large and small molecules	Broad spectrum of activity No reaction except staining
Alcohol, ethyl	I.V. as 5% sol. in bicarbonate or saline sol. P.O. as 3-4 oz. of whiskey (45%) every 4 hours for 1-3 days	Methyl alcohol Ethylene glycol	Metabolizes methyl alcohol and prevents formation of toxic formic acid; glycols into oxalates
Alkali, weak Magnesium oxide (preferred) Sodium bicarbonate	2.5% sol. (25 grams/liter) 5% sol. (50 grams/liter)	Acid, corrosive	Gastric distention from liberated carbon dioxide
Ammonium acetate	5 ml. in 500 ml. water	Formaldehyde (formalin)	Forms relatively harmless methenamine
Ammonium hydroxide	0.2% sol. Both are for gastric lavage		
Atropine sulfate	1-2 mg. I.M. and repeat in 30 minutes	Organic phosphate esters: Guthion, malathion, parathion, mushroom, TEPP, trithion, etc., other cholinesterase inhibitors	Atropinization
Antivenins	See circular for dosage instruction		
Specific			
Antivenin (*Crotalidae*) Polyvalent (Wyeth)		N. and S. Amer. snakebite venoms	
Antivenin (*Latrodectus mactans,* and *curacaviensis* (Merck, Sharp, & Dohme)		Black widow spider venom	
Antivenin (*Micrurus*) (Wyeth Laboratories and C. Amaral and Cia L.T.D.A. Cloria 34, PO Box 2123, São Paulo, Brazil)		Coral snake venom	
Nonspecific		Black widow spider venom	
Adult (may be used without antivenin, *for adult only*)			
Methocarbamol (Robaxin)	On diagnosis, 1 amp. (1 gram, 10 ml.) I.V. in 15 ml. isotonic saline sol. over 5 minute period or in I.V. drip. Follow in 12 hours with 2 tab. (1500 mg.) 3 times a day for 2 days		Muscle relaxant
Orphenadrine citrate (Norflex)	On diagnosis, 1 amp. (2 ml., 60 mg.) I.V. in 5 ml. isotonic saline sol. followed in 12 hours by 1 tab. (100 mg.) 2 times a day for 2 days		Muscle relaxant
Child Antivenin	Antivenin I.V. followed in 1 hour by methocarbamol 1 tab. (500 mg.) and 1 every 12 hours for 2 days		In children the antivenin should be used; this may be supplemented with the muscle relaxant when necessary
Bromobenzene	Adult: 1 gram Child: 0.25 gram (in lavage sol.)	Selenium	Nephrotoxic
Calcium EDTA or Versene (ethylenediamine tetra-acetate) [DPTA (diethylenetriamine pentaacetic acid), more promising analogue]	25-50 mg./kg. 2% sol. 2 times a day for 5 days 50 mg./kg., 20% sol. (0.5% procaine) I.M. daily for 5-7 days Repeat these courses after 2 day rest period	Cadmium Cobalt Copper Digitalis Iron Lead (combined therapy with BAL for encephalitis) Nickel, and other metals	Increases urinary potassium excretion Use sodium salt (Na EDTA) for digitalis in place of Ca EDTA which chelates Ca ion producing hypocalcemia and reduces synergistic action of the Ca and digitalis, converting dangerous arrhythmias to sinus arrhythmias (other specific therapy preferred) Oral EDTA should not be used until all lead has been removed or absorbed from the GI tract

*From *Davison's Compleat Pediatrician,* 9th edition, Lea and Febiger, Publisher.

TABLE 4. **Antidote Chart** (*Continued*)

ANTIDOTE	DOSE	POISON	REACTION (ANTIDOTE) AND COMMENTS
Calcium lactate	10% sol. (in lavage sol.)	Chlorinated hydrocarbons Fluoride Oxalates	
Calcium gluconate	10% sol. 5-10 ml. I.M. or I.V., may be repeated in 8-12 hours	Black widow spider and insect bites	Muscle relaxant Bradycardia Flushing Local necrosis from perivenous infiltration (methocarbamol, etc., also effective)
Chlorpromazine (Thorazine)	1-2 mg./kg. I.M.	Amphetamine*	Drowsiness Hypotension Neuromuscular (parkinsonian)
Copper sulfate	0.25–3.0 grams in glass of water	Phosphorus	Forms insoluble copper phosphide
Cyanide poison kit (Eli Lilly stock #M76)			
Amyl nitrite pearls Sodium nitrite	0.2 ml. (inhalation); follow with 3.0% sol. (10 ml.) in 2-4 minutes *and*	Cyanide	Hypotension
Sodium thiosulfate	25% sol. (50 ml.) in 10 min. through same needle and vein (repeat with ½ doses if necessary)	Iodine	Sodium thiosulfate used alone for iodine; forms harmless sodium iodide
Deferoxamine B (Desferal, Ciba) Desferal isolated from streptomyces pilosus	1-2 grams I.M. or I.V. (adults, repeat if necessary every 4-12 hours; also 5-10 grams via nasogastric tube following gastric lavage†	Iron Hemochromatosis	Diarrhea Hypotension
Dimercaprol (BAL)	*Severe intoxication* Day 1: 3.0 mg./kg. every 4 hours (6 injections) Day 2: Same Day 3: 3.0 mg./kg. every 6 hours (4 injections) Days 4-13 (or until recovery): 3.0 mg./kg. every 12 hours (2 injections) *Mild intoxication* Day 1: 2.5 mg./kg. every 4 hours (6 injections) Day 2: Same Day 3: 2.5 mg./kg. every 12 hours Days 4–13 (or until recovery): further 2.5 mg./kg. daily (1 injection)	Antimony Arsenic Bismuth Gold Mercury (acrodynia) Nickel Lead (combined therapy with EDTA for encephalitis) Contraindicated for iron	Flushing Myalgia Nausea and vomiting Nephrotoxic Hypotension Pulmonary edema Salivation and lacrimation Temperature elevation (especially in children)
Diphenhydramine hydrochloride (Benadryl)	10-50 mg. I.V. or I.M.	Phenothiazine tranquilizers (for extrapyramidal neuromuscular manifestations)	Atropine-like effect Drowsiness
Dithizon	10 mg./kg. twice a day P.O. with 100 ml. 10% glucose sol. for 5 days	Thallium	Diabetogenic Not available for therapeutic use. May be obtained through a chemical company
Household antidotes Milk Raw eggs Flour Starches		Arsenic Mercury and other heavy metals Same as above Iodine	These are useful and readily available antidotes that can be used in an emergency. All have demulcent properties
Hydrogen peroxide	3% sol. (10 ml. in 100 ml. water as lavage sol.)	Potassium permanganate Oxidizing agent for many other compounds	Irritation of mucous membranes Distention of abdomen from release of gas
Iodine, tincture	15 drops in 120 ml. water	Precipitant for: Lead Mercury Quinine Silver Strychnine	Precipitants must be thoroughly removed by gastric lavage
Magnesium sulfate	2.5% sol. for lavage	Precipitant for: Barium Lead	
Sodium sulfate	10% sol. I.M. and repeat in 30 minutes Also as catharsis for rapid elimination of toxic agent from GI tract	Hypervitaminosis D Hypercalcemia (glucocorticoid therapy preferable)	

*Recent reports have indicated that haloperidol (Haldol) is more effective in smaller doses than chlorpromazine for amphetamine intoxication.

†Some reports suggest that large oral doses of deferoxamine can be absorbed and result in systemic toxicity, and its oral use is being questioned.

TABLE 4. **Antidote Chart** (*Continued*)

ANTIDOTE	DOSE	POISON	REACTION (ANTIDOTE) AND COMMENTS
Methylene blue	I.V.: 1% sol. given slowly (2 mg./kg.) and repeat in 1 hour if necessary P.O.: 3-5 mg./kg. (action much slower)	Methemoglobinemia produced by over 100 drugs and chemicals: Acetanilid Aniline derivatives Chlorates Dinitrophenol Nitrites Pyridium, etc.	Perivenous infiltration can produce severe necrosis
Monoacetin (glyceryl monoacetate)	0.5 ml./kg. I.M. or in saline sol. I.V. Repeat as necessary	Sodium fluoroacetate "1080"	Not available commercially. If parenteral therapy not feasible, can give 100 ml. of monoacetin in water
Nalorphine (Nalline) or Levallorphan (Lorfan) or	Adult: 5-10 mg. I.M. or I.V. and repeat in ½ hour Child: 0.1-0.2 mg./kg. I.M. or I.V. and repeat in ½ hour. Adult: 0.5-1.0 mg. I.M. or I.V. Child: 0.02 mg. per kg. I.M. or I.V.	Codeine Demerol Dionin Heroin Methadone Morphine Pantopon	Withdrawal symptoms Depression effects in other than narcotic compounds
Naloxone (Narcan)	0. 01 mg. per kg. I.V., I.M., or S.C.	(For respiratory and cardiovascular depression)	Produces no respiratory depression, psychotomimetic effects, circulatory changes, or miosis
Penicillamine and its derivatives (Cuprimine)	1-5 grams P.O.	Mercury and other heavy metals	Fever Stupor Nausea and vomiting Myalgia Leukopenia, thrombocytopenia Nephrosis, reversible Optic axial neuritis, reversible Ineffective when severe vomiting is prominent
Petrolatum, liquid (mineral oil)			Solvent Demulcent
Physostigmine salicylate (Antilirium)	1–2 mg. I.M. or I.V.*	Atropine and related alkaloids; anticholinergic compounds; particularly effective for the cardiac arrhythmias and CNS toxic effects of the tricyclic antidepressant drugs Atropine and related alkaloids	Excess can produce diarrhea, bradycardia, hypersalivation, rhinorrhea, and cholinergic crisis; Rx with propantheline bromide (Pro-Banthine) preferable to atropine
Pilocarpine (not being marketed in tablet form in U. S.)	P.O.: 2-4 mg. I.M.: 0.25-0.5 mg.		Antagonizes the parasympathetic (mydriasis and dry mouth), not central, effects of atropine
Potassium permanganate	1:5,000 and 1:10,000 sol. for gastric lavage	Nicotine Physostigmine Quinine Strychnine Oxidizing agent for many alkaloids and organic poisons	Strong irritant and should not be used in strong dilutions or with any residual particles
Pralidoxime iodine (2-PAM iodine) Pralidoxime chloride (2-PAM chloride)	Adult: 1-2 grams Child: 25-50 mg./kg. I.M. or I.V. as 5% sol.	Organic phosphate esters Cholinesterase inhibition by any agent: chemical, drug, etc.	Diplopia Dizziness Headache
Protamine sulfate	1% sol. I.V. slowly (mg./mg.) to that of heparin	Heparin	Sensitivity effects
Sodium chloride	1 tsp. salt to 1 pt. water (approximately normal saline sol.) 6-12 grams P.O. in divided doses or in isotonic saline I.V.	Silver nitrate Bromides	Forms noncorrosive silver chloride Hypernatremia
Sodium formaldehyde sulfoxalate	5% in lavage sol. (preferably combined with 5% sodium bicarbonate)	Mercury salts	BAL therapy should follow gastric lavage
Sodium thiosulfate	P.O.: 2-3 grams or I.M.: 10 or 25% sol. Repeat in 3-4 hours	Iodine Cyanide	
Starch	80 grams/1000 ml. water	Iodine	

*Not approved by FDA for intravenous use in children.

TABLE 4. **Antidote Chart** (*Continued*)

ANTIDOTE	DOSE	POISON	REACTION (ANTIDOTE) AND COMMENTS
Tannic acid	4% in lavage sol. Never use in greater concentrations	Precipitates alkaloids, certain glucosides, and many metals	Hepatotoxic Tannates formed should not be allowed to remain in the stomach Because of its hepatotoxicity, should be used cautiously and in no greater than 4% sol.
Universal antidote (activated charcoal alone preferable)	Two parts pulverized charcoal (burned toast); One part magnesium oxide (milk of magnesia); One part tannic acid (strong tea sol.)	Obsolete for any use	Over-rated and ineffective. Can actually be harmful in that it may give false sense of security to those who use it
Vitamin K_1	25-150 mg. I.V. Rate not to exceed 10 mg./min.	Coumarin derivatives: Coumarin Marcoumar Warfarin, etc.	Bleeding Focal hemorrhages

22. *Barium* (Soluble Salts)

Gastric lavage with 2 to 5 per cent solution of either magnesium or sodium sulfate. Ten ml. of 10 per cent sodium sulfate intravenously, repeated in 30 minutes for serious symptoms. Artificial respiration and oxygen. Procainamide for ventricular arrhythmias. Potassium.

23. *Benadryl* (Diphenhydramine HCl)

See Antihistaminics.

24. *Benzene* (Benzol)

Gastric lavage or emesis. Artificial respiration and oxygen. Shock therapy. Blood transfusion if necessary. Avoid fats, oils, alcohol, and epinephrine or related drugs (these induce ventricular fibrillation).

25. *Benzene Hexachloride* (BHC)

Gastric lavage or emesis. Wash skin thoroughly. Short-acting barbiturates. Avoid fats, oils, and epinephrine.

26. *Benzine* (Petroleum Ether, Naphtha)

See Kerosene.

27. *Beryllium*

Calcium disodium edetate (edathamil). Corticosteroids for chemical pneumonitis. Excision of skin granulomas and ulcers. Prevention with education of beryllium-using workers or operators.

28. *Bismuth* (Soluble Compounds)

Gastric lavage or emesis. Activated charcoal. Saline cathartic. BAL. Discontinue medication at first sign of toxicity. Methylene blue for methemoglobinemia.

29. *Boric Acid* (Boracic Acid)

Gastric lavage or emesis. Saline cathartic. Shock and convulsive therapy. Peritoneal dialysis or exchange transfusion.

30. *Botulism*

See pages 26 to 29 and 895.

31. *Bromides*

Discontinue all sources of bromides. Six to 12 grams of sodium chloride in divided doses with 4 liters of water daily for 1 to 4 weeks (adult dose). Isotonic salt solution or ammonium chloride intravenously in more serious cases. Hemodialysis with artificial kidney.

32. *Cadmium*

Gastric lavage or emesis. Move patient from exposure. Saline cathartic. Calcium disodium edetate (edathamil). BAL contraindicated (BAL and cadmium combination is nephrotoxic). Artificial respiration and oxygen. Antibiotics and corticosteroids for chemical pneumonitis and pulmonary edema.

33. *Caffeine*

See Xanthines.

34. *Camphor*

Gastric lavage or emesis. Demulcents. Short-acting barbiturates. Artificial respiration and oxygen. Shock therapy. Avoid fats, oils, alcohol, and opiates.

35. Cantharidin (Spanish Fly, Russian Fly)

Gastric lavage (cautiously because of corrosive effects) or emesis. Demulcents. Therapy for shock. Short-acting barbiturates. Adequate fluids for diuresis. Avoid morphine because of respiratory depression.

36. Carbon Dioxide

Terminate exposure; move patient to fresh air. Artificial respiration and oxygen. Respiratory and blood pressure stimulants.

37. Carbon Disulfide

Gastric lavage or emesis, if ingested. Move from exposure. Artificial respiration and oxygen. Pulmonary edema and therapy for shock. Short-acting barbiturates. Prevention: maximum allowable concentration (MAC) must be observed at all times. For skin contact, wash thoroughly.

38. Carbon Monoxide

Move patient from exposure immediately. Artificial respiration and oxygen. Administration of 100 per cent oxygen in a pressure chamber, if available. Hypothermia. Blood transfusion or washed red blood cells given early. Chronic carbon monoxide poisoning and therapy are questionable.

39. Carbon Tetrachloride

Gastric lavage or emesis, if ingested. Move from source of exposure. Remove contaminated clothes. Artificial respiration and oxygen. Shock therapy with special emphasis on fluid and electrolytes in face of oliguria or anuria. Avoid fats, oils, alcohol, epinephrine, and related compounds. Prevention: use of less toxic chemicals such as methyl chloroform.

40. Chloral Hydrate

See Barbiturates.

41. Chlorates

Gastric lavage with care, or emesis. Demulcents. Shock therapy. Methylene blue for methemoglobinemia.

42. Chlordane

Gastric lavage or emesis. Short-acting barbiturates. For skin contamination, thorough washing of skin and removal of contaminated clothing. Avoid fats, oils, demulcents, and epinephrine, which should never be used in any halogenated insecticide poisoning.

43. Chlorinated Alkalis (Hypochlorites, Chlorine)

Careful gastric lavage or emesis for large amounts only. Diluted vinegar and fruit juices. Demulcents. Move from exposure and wash skin thoroughly. Antibiotics and corticosteroids for pulmonary edema and pneumonitis from chlorine inhalation. Oral magnesium oxide (paradoxical as it may sound) to prevent formation of irritating hypochlorous acid.

44. Chloroform

Gastric lavage or emesis. Demulcents. Artificial respiration and oxygen. Respiratory and cardiac stimulants. Ten per cent calcium gluconate intravenously (slowly).

45. Chlorothiazide (Diuril)

Discontinue use of drug. Correct fluid and electrolyte imbalance.

46. Chromium (Potassium Salt, Chromic Oxide)

Gastric lavage or emesis. Demulcents. One per cent aluminum acetate wet dressings for skin contamination. Ten per cent edetate (edathamil) ointment for skin ulcers. Remove from source of exposure whether it be from inhalation or skin contact.

47. Cocaine

Gastric lavage or emesis. Remove drug from skin or mucous membranes. Short-acting barbiturates. Artificial respiration and oxygen.

48. Codeine

Gastric lavage or emesis. Saline cathartic. Nalorphine (Nalline), levallorphan (Lorfan), or naloxone (Narcan). Artificial respiration and oxygen. Maintain body heat and fluid balance.

49. Colchicine

Gastric lavage or emesis. Saline cathartic. Artificial respiration and oxygen. Shock therapy. Discontinue or reduce dosages of drug at first sign of toxicity.

50. Copper

Gastric lavage or emesis if vomiting has not occurred. Demulcents. Shock therapy. Calcium disodium edetate (edathamil). Penicillamine derivatives.

51. Cosmetics

Deodorants (aluminum salts, titanium dioxide, antibacterial agents); depilatories (soluble sulfides or calcium thioglycolate): gastric lavage or emesis, if large amount ingested.

Hair tints and dyes: discontinue use if allergy develops.

52. *Curare*

Discontinue drug immediately. Endotracheal catheter and use a positive pressure artificial respirator with oxygen until muscle function returns. Neostigmine or edrophonium chloride. Cold packs or alcohol sponging for temperature elevation.

53. *Cyanides* (Hydrogen, Potassium, Sodium)

Gastric lavage or emesis, if ingested. See antidote chart for cyanide poison kit. Artificial respiration and oxygen. Remove contaminated clothing and wash skin thoroughly.

54. *DDT* (Chlorobenzene Insecticide, TDE, DFDT, DMC, Methoxychlor, Neotrane, Ovotran, Dilan, Dimite)

Gastric lavage or emesis. Saline cathartic. Short-acting barbiturates. Artificial respiration and oxygen. Remove contaminated clothing and wash skin thoroughly. Avoid fats, oils, demulcents, epinephrine, and related compounds.

55. *Demerol HCl* (Meperidine HCl)

See Morphine.

56. *Detergents* (Anionic and Nonionic Surfactants, Phosphate Salts, Sodium Sulfate and Carbonate, Fatty Acid Amides)

Unless taken in large quantities, no serious toxic symptoms other than gastrointestinal symptoms; at present causing havoc with public water supplies. Milk, eggwhites, mild soap solution by mouth.

57. *Diamthazole* (Asterol)*

Use as directed only or discontinue use. Should not be used in children under 6 years of age. Short-acting barbiturates.

58. *Dichlorohydrin*

See Carbon Tetrachloride.

59. *Dichlorophenoxyacetic Acid* (2,4-D; 2,4,5-T Esters or Salts)

Gastric lavage or emesis. Quinidine sulfate to relieve myotonia and suppress ventricular arrhythmias. Antipyretic for hyperpyrexia.

*This product was discontinued in the United States (1966), but is still available in Europe.

60. *Dieldrin*

See Chlordane (Indane Derivatives).

61. *Diethyltoluamide* (Dimethylphthalate, Indalone)

Gastric lavage or emesis. Demulcents. Short-acting barbiturates.

62. *Digitalis* (Purple Foxglove) (Digitoxin)

Discontinue use. Gastric lavage or emesis for accidental or suicidal ingestion. Artificial pacemaker. Potassium chloride, orally or intravenously, under electrocardiographic observation. Procainamide, quinidine, diphenylhydantoin (Dilantin), propranolol hydrochloride, lidocaine, or atropine.

63. *Dilantin Sodium*

See Diphenylhydantoin Scdium.

64. *Dimethyl Sulfate*

Move to fresh air; eyes, skin, and mucous membranes should be washed thoroughly with water. Weak alkali wet dressings for skin burns. Antibiotics and corticosteroids for pneumonitis. In contaminated areas deactivate by spraying with water or 5 per cent sodium hydroxide solution.

65. *Dinitro-ortho-cresol* (Dinitrophenol Derivatives)

Gastric lavage with sodium bicarbonate solution or emesis. For skin contamination wash thoroughly with weak alkaline solution. Oxygen and circulatory stimulants. Reduce temperature with cold packs or alcohol sponging. Maintain fluid and electrolyte balance.

66. *Dioxane*

See Acetone.

67. *Diphenhydramine HCl* (Benadryl HCl)

See Antihistaminics.

68. *Diphenylhydantoin Sodium, Phenytoin* (Dilantin Sodium)

Gastric lavage or emesis for ingestion. Discontinue use or reduce dosage.

69. *Dithiocarbamate* (Ferbam)

Discontinue use of spray. Avoid alcohol.

70. *Doriden*

See Barbiturates.

71. *Emetine* (Alkaloid of Ipecac)

Gastric lavage if emesis has not taken place.

Maintain fluid and electrolyte balance. Cautious digitalization. Cardiac pacemaker until EKG is normal and pulse regular.

72. *Ephedrine*

Gastric lavage or emesis. Activated charcoal. Short-acting barbiturates. Phentolamine (Regitine) early, to block hypertensive effects.

73. *Epinephrine* (Adrenalin)

See Ephedrine.

74. *Ergot Derivatives*

Gastric lavage or emesis. Activated charcoal, 1 to 2 tbsp. in water. Saline cathartic. Atropine sulfate for abdominal pain and spasm, 10 per cent solution of calcium gluconate for myalgia, and papaverine HCl or mecholyl as vascular antispasmodic. Short-acting barbiturates and artificial respiration and oxygen, if necessary.

75. *Essential (Volatile) Oils*

One hundred milliliters of castor oil, then remove by gastric lavage. Saline cathartic. Demulcents. Short-acting barbiturates. Artificial respiration and oxygen. Maintain fluid and electrolyte balance.

76. *Ether*

Artificial respiration and oxygen. Maintain adequate airway, blood pressure, and body temperature.

77. *Ethyl Alcohol (Pure)* (Whiskey = 40 to 50 per cent Alcohol; Wines = 10 to 20 per cent Alcohol; Beers = 2 to 6 per cent Alcohol)

Gastric lavage or emesis. Sodium bicarbonate, 1 tsp. to 1 pt. water, every 1 to 2 hours to prevent acidosis. Intravenous bicarbonate for acidosis. Caffeine and sodium benzoate or strong coffee. Hypertonic glucose or urea for cerebral edema. Intravenous glucose for hypoglycemia. Avoid depressant drugs (barbiturates interfere with enzymatic action of alcohol dehydrogenase) and potent respiratory stimulants.

78. *Ethylene Chlorohydrin* (Ethylene Dichloride)

Gastric lavage or emesis. Move from exposure. Artificial respiration and oxygen. Thorough washing for skin contact. Epinephrine or levarterenol for maintaining blood pressure.

79. *Ethylene Glycol* (Diethylene Glycol, Propylene Glycol)

Gastric lavage or emesis. Artificial respiration and oxygen. Ten per cent calcium gluconate intravenously to precipitate metabolic product, oxalic acid, and oxalates. Maintain body temperature, fluids, and electrolytes. Short-acting barbiturates. Dialysis. Oral and intravenous ethyl alcohol (see Methyl Alcohol).

80. *Ferrous Sulfate* (Copperas, Green Vitriol; Approximately 20 per cent Elemental Iron)

Clearance with suction and maintenance of open airways. Control of shock with available intravenous fluids, blood, plasma, and oxygen. Gastric lavage with concentrated solution of sodium bicarbonate, 5 per cent disodium phosphate, or milk until returning fluid is clear. Critically ill patients should receive calcium disodium edetate (edathamil) intravenously; if none given orally, intravenous dose should be 70 to 80 mg. per kg. per 24 hours in dextrose or isotonic saline solution in an 0.5 to 2 per cent concentration; if used orally (and rate of its absorption through a gut wall damaged by iron is not known), only half the aforementioned dose should be used intravenously, 35 to 40 mg. per kg. per 24 hours. Guided by the clinical picture and daily iron levels in serum, and, if measurements are available, by the urinary output of edetate (edathamil) and iron, intravenous and/or oral calcium disodium edetate (edathamil) is continued in a total daily dose of no more than 70 to 80 mg. per kg.; duration of treatment with this drug should not be, and need not be, longer than 5 days. Deferoxamine (Desferal), a chelating agent, has been demonstrated to be effective in the treatment of acute iron poisoning. Dosage recommended is 5 to 10 grams by mouth or nasogastric tube* and 1 to 2 grams intravenously (slowly to avoid hypotensive effects) or intramuscularly. Parenteral therapy can be repeated if serum iron levels remain high. Follow-up liver function tests and study of gastrointestinal tract with a radiopaque medium for strictures.

81. *Fluorides* (Fluorine, Hydrogen Fluoride, Fluorosilicates [insoluble])

Gastric lavage or emesis with lime water (0.15 per cent calcium hydroxide), calcium chloride solution (1 tsp. per 1000 ml. water), or milk. Ten per cent calcium gluconate intravenously or intramuscularly. Demulcents. For inhalation move to fresh air. Artificial respiration and oxygen. Prophylactic antibiotics and corticosteroids for pulmonary irritation and edema. Wash skin immediately and thoroughly with water and apply magnesium oxide paste with 20 per cent glycerin.

*There are some studies suggesting that large doses of deferoxamine can be absorbed and result in systemic toxicity, and its oral use is now being questioned.

82. *Fluoroacetate Sodium*

Gastric lavage or emesis. Saline cathartic. Ten per cent calcium gluconate or sodium glycerol monoacetate (Monacetin). Short-acting barbiturates. Procainamide for arrhythmia. For skin contact, wash thoroughly.

83. *Food Poisoning* (Botulism)
See also Foodborne Illness (pp. 26–29).

Types A and B polyvalent antitoxin (inadequately processed vegetables and meats) or Type E antitoxin (fish and marine products). Trivalent (A, B, E) antitoxin now available.* Maintain an airway. Parenteral fluids.

84. *Formaldehyde* (Formalin)

Gastric lavage with 0.1 per cent ammonia or 1 per cent ammonium carbonate solution. Saline cathartic. Combat shock or collapse; levarterenol if necessary.

85. *Glutethimide* (Doriden)
See Barbiturates.

86. *Gold*

Discontinue use of parenteral therapy. Dimercaprol (BAL). Antihistaminic therapy. Supportive therapy for renal and hematologic effects.

87. *Hydralazine* (Apresoline, Phthalazine Derivatives)

Gastric lavage or emesis. Discontinue use or reduce dosage. Maintain blood pressure.

88. *Hydrochloric Acid* (Muriatic Acid)

Do not use gastric lavage after 1 hour of ingestion. Neutralize acid with magnesium oxide, milk of magnesia, or lime water. Give demulcents. Maintain blood pressure, fluids, and electrolytes. Antibiotics and corticosteroids to prevent infection and strictures. Thorough washing of skin and application of magnesium oxide paste. Gastroscopy for determining corrosive injury to the stomach.

89. *Hydroquinone*

Gastric lavage or emesis. Saline cathartic. Methylene blue for methemoglobinemia.

90. *Hypochlorites* (Clorox, etc.)
See Chlorinated Alkalis.

*U.S. Communicable Disease Center, Atlanta, Georgia. Telephone number for day coverage is (404) 633-3753 (4, 5, 6); for night and weekends, (404) 633-2176.

91. *Iodine* (Iodoform, Iodides)

Give suspension of starch or flour or 1 to 5 per cent solution of sodium thiosulfate. If not available, use milk or egg whites. Follow by gastric lavage. Regulate fluids and electrolytes, depending on degree of renal involvement. Epinephrine, diphenhydramine (Benadryl), or hydrocortisone for anaphylactoid reaction.

92. *Isoniazid*

Prompt gastric lavage or emesis (symptoms appear within 30 minutes). Discontinue drug or reduce dosage. Pyridoxine, 200 to 400 mg. intravenously. Short-acting barbiturates intravenously for convulsions. Parenteral sodium bicarbonate for acidosis. Hemodialysis. Osmotic diuresis (mannitol, urea, furosemide, or ethacrynic acid) hastens excretion.

93. *Isopropyl Alcohol* (Rubbing Alcohol)
See Ethyl Alcohol.

94. *Kerosene* (Petroleum Distillates: Benzine, Gasoline, Naphtha, Mineral Seal Oil, etc.)

Prevent aspiration. Gastric lavage or emesis to be avoided. Fifty ml. of mineral or vegetable oil by mouth (if not forced). Oxygen and antibiotics. Corticosteroids for pulmonary edema and chemical or lipoid pneumonitis (particularly for mineral seal oil aspiration). Results are equivocal, yet since therapy is short range, it may benefit those with severe pulmonary distress and "shock" lung.

95. *Lead*

Gastric lavage with 1 per cent sodium sulfate solution, followed by saline cathartic for immediate ingestion. Calcium disodium edetate (edathamil) intravenously or intramuscularly for 5 days and repeat if necessary. Four per cent urea (30 per cent in severe cases) intravenously for encephalopathy with increased intracranial pressure: craniectomy may be necessary. Mannitol and/or adrenal corticosteroids are also used for this purpose and often preferred. Ten per cent solution of calcium gluconate or morphine for severe abdominal pain (colic). Early diagnosis and treatment are paramount in preventing death or serious sequelae in children. BAL combined with calcium disodium edetate (edathamil) therapy is more effective in lead encephalitis than use of edetate (edathamil) alone. Penicillamine (Cuprimine) as an oral chelating agent has recently been reported to be effective and may be used in adjunctive therapy as an investigational drug.

96. *Mace* (Anti-Riot Gas)
See Tear Gases.

97. *Manganese*

Remove from further exposure. Antibiotics and corticosteroids for pneumonitis. Calcium disodium edetate (edathamil) may be beneficial if given early. Antiparkinsonian drugs. Diphenhydramine (Benadryl), biperiden hydrochloride (Akineton), or methylphenidate hydrochloride (Ritalin).

98. *Marihuana*

Removal of drug exposure (characteristic "burnt rope" acrid odor on clothes and body). There are no withdrawal symptoms except with extreme cases of habituation.

99. *Meperidine HCl* (Demerol HCl)

See Morphine.

100. *Meprobamate* (Equanil, Miltown, etc.)

Gastric lavage or emesis. Saline cathartic. Artificial respiration and oxygen. Maintain blood pressure with methoxamine hydrochloride.

101. *Menthol*

See Phenol.

102. *Mercury Compounds*

Gastric lavage immediately with egg white solution or with 5 per cent sodium formaldehyde sulfoxylate; if unavailable, a 2 to 5 per cent solution of sodium bicarbonate may be used. Magnesium sulfate as cathartic (early only). BAL. Penicillamine derivatives (oral antidote). Maintain fluid and electrolyte balance and nutrition. Spironolactone (Aldactone) has prevented renal tubular necrosis in experimental animals (rats).

103. *Metaldehyde* (Changes to Acetaldehyde)

Gastric lavage or emesis. Demulcents. Short-acting barbiturates. Artificial respiration, oxygen, and antibiotics. Parenteral chlorpromazine and calcium gluconate.

104. *Methadone* (Dolophine)

See Morphine.

105. *Methyl Alcohol*

To prevent the formation of formic acid and formates, 10 ml. ethyl alcohol per hour can suppress the metabolism of methyl alcohol. In severe poisoning ethyl alcohol can be given intravenously in 5 per cent concentration in bicarbonate or saline solution and 3 to 4 oz. of whiskey (45 per cent alcohol) orally every 4 to 6 hours for 1 to 3 days. Combat acidosis. Hemodialysis is paramount in serious poisoning.

106. *Methyl Bromide* (Chloride, Iodide)

Move from exposure. Artificial respiration and oxygen. Epinephrine for bronchospasm; antibiotics and corticosteroids for pneumonitis. Prevention: safety dispensers for fumigant use.

107. *Methyl Salicylate* (Oil of Wintergreen)

See Salicylates. Gastric lavage, however, may be worthwhile, even several hours after ingestion, because methyl salicylate is poorly absorbed.

108. *Metrazol*

See Pentylenetetrazol.

109. *Morphine* (Codeine, Heroin, Propoxyphene [Darvon], Meperidine [Demerol], Dihydromorphinone [Dilaudid], Opium Alkaloids [Pantopon])

Gastric lavage (before loss of consciousness). Do not use syrup of ipecac or apomorphine. Activated charcoal. Saline cathartic. Delay absorption of intramuscular drug with tourniquet and cryotherapy. Maintain adequate airway, body temperature, fluids, and electrolytes. Give narcotic antagonists Nalline or Lorfan. Naloxone hydrochloride (Narcan) is preferable (see antidote chart, p. 890). Ephedrine for hypotension and bradycardia—methoxamine or phenylephrine if pulse is rapid. Doxapram hydrochloride (Dopram), 3 to 5 ml. intravenously, is the respiratory stimulant of choice, but it has short-lasting effects (3 to 5 minutes).

110. *Muscarine* (Some Mushrooms)

Artificial respiration with oxygen. Atropine, 1 to 2 mg. every hour until free of respiratory effects. PAM or Protopam chloride may be useful adjunct therapy. Gastric lavage or emesis if vomiting has not occurred. Thioctic acid, an investigational compound, has been reported to be effective in European trials.

111. *Naphthalene* (Mothballs, Repellents, etc., Paradichlorobenzene, Camphor)

Gastric lavage or emesis for ingestion. Give sodium bicarbonate every 4 hours to maintain alkaline urine and prevent renal blockage with acid hematin crystals. Blood transfusions as necessary. Short-acting barbiturates. Avoid use of milk, oils, or fatty meals. In prevention, these products should be kept out of hands and clothes of children (symptoms produced not only by ingestion but also by inhalation and transcutaneous absorption).

112. *Naphthol*

See Phenol.

113. Nickel (Nickel Carbonyl)

Remove from skin by thorough washing. Artificial respiration and oxygen. BAL. Antibiotics and corticosteroids for pneumonitis.

114. Nicotine

Gastric lavage or emesis. Activated charcoal. Short-acting barbiturates. Artificial respiration and oxygen; use of positive pressure resuscitator through period of respiratory failure may prevent death. Thorough washing of skin and removal of clothing will be necessary for skin contamination.

115. Nitrates, Nitrites

Gastric lavage or emesis. Saline cathartic. Methylene blue for methemoglobinemia. Maintain blood pressure with levarterenol. Short-acting barbiturates for convulsions.

116. Nitric Acid

Give large amounts of water. Neutralize with lime water, magnesia, etc. Gastric lavage cautiously if seen within the first half hour. Gastroscopy to detect caustic burns of the stomach. Demulcents. Morphine for pain, but avoid large doses and possible depression. Shock therapy. Corticosteroids to prevent stricture formation. For eye and skin contact wash thoroughly with water: *do not use chemical antidotes.*

117. Nitrobenzene

Gastric lavage or emesis. Artificial respiration and oxygen. Methylene blue, 1 per cent solution for methemoglobinemia. Avoid fats and oils.

118. Opium

See Morphine.

119. Oxalates

Gastric lavage with calcium lactate solution, 10 grams (2 tsp.) per 100 ml. Ten per cent calcium gluconate intravenously. Give milk and demulcents.

120. Paraldehyde

Gastric lavage or emesis. Artificial respiration and oxygen. Maintain body temperature, fluids, and electrolytes.

121. Paraquat

Induce vomiting with syrup of ipecac or perform gastric lavage if vomiting has not occurred. If lavage is performed, care must be taken, as paraquat may be corrosive to the esophagus.

Immediately following vomiting or lavage, give approximately 200 to 500 ml. of a 30 per cent aqueous suspension of an adsorbent clay (such as Robinson's bentonite U.S.P., or Robinson's fuller's earth U.S.P.) plus an effective dose of cathartic, e.g., magnesium sulfate, to remove paraquat from the entire gastrointestinal tract. Repeat as often as practical (every 2 to 4 hours for several days until paraquat can no longer be detected in blood, urine, or dialysate). If bentonite or fuller's earth is not immediately available, an adsorbent such as powdered activated charcoal should be used until better clays are obtained. Oxygen should be used sparingly and cautiously for dyspnea or cyanosis, because it may aggravate the lung lesions. Forced diuresis should be started as soon as possible to remove paraquat from the blood. If renal function is impaired, hemodialysis or peritoneal dialysis may be of value. Use of forced diuresis and hemodialysis together may aid in hastening the removal of paraquat. Monitor the patient's blood urea nitrogen (BUN) and serum creatinine levels, as these are early indicators of systemic poisoning and are useful to determine the patient's progress. Also, obtain daily chest x-rays, arterial oxygen partial pressure, pulmonary function studies, and chest auscultation. Obtain urine, blood, and dialysate samples initially and at least daily to monitor the elimination of paraquat.

For skin contamination, clothing should be removed and the skin thoroughly washed with soap and water for several minutes. If the eyes are involved, they should be irrigated immediately for 10 to 15 minutes and then seen by an ophthalmologist.

122. Parathion (Phosphate Ester Insecticides) (Malathion, Systox, EPN, Diazinon, Guthion, Trithion, TEPP, OMPA, Co-Ral, Phosdrin)

Prompt induction of emesis or gastric lavage with 5 per cent $NaHCO_3$ for ingestion only. Decontaminate by removal of all soiled clothes and thorough washing of skin. Maintain clear airway and respirations with laryngeal intubation and artificial respiration and oxygen. Atropine, 1 to 2 mg. intramuscularly or intravenously and repeat at 20 to 30 minute intervals, as soon as cyanosis has cleared (chance of ventricular fibrillation). Continue atropine until definite improvement occurs and is maintained (sometimes 2 or more days). The total dosage required may be phenomenal (over 1000 mg.). PAM (pralidoxime chloride), a cholinesterase reactivator as 5 per cent solution intravenously. Avoid narcotics, barbiturates, epinephrine, aminophylline, ether, and phenothiazine derivatives, because they further reduce cholinesterase activity and some are respiratory depressants.

123. *Pentachlorophenol*

Gastric lavage or emesis. Removal of contaminated clothing and thorough washing of skin. Short-acting barbiturates.

124. *Pentylenetetrazol* (Metrazol)

Delay absorption of intramuscular drug with tourniquet and cryotherapy. Gastric lavage or emesis for ingestion. Short-acting barbiturate for convulsions. Cold packs and alcohol sponging for hyperthermia.

125. *Permanganate, Potassium*

Thorough lavage of stomach with 3 per cent hydrogen peroxide (10 ml. in 100 ml. of water). Milk or demulcents. Combat collapse and shock.

126. *Phenacetin* (Acetophenetidin)

See Acetanilid.

127. *Phenol* (Derivatives) (Creosote, Guaiacol, Resorcinol, Thymol)

Careful gastric lavage, followed by 60 ml. of castor oil which dissolves phenol and hastens its removal. Activated charcoal. Maintain body temperature, fluids, electrolytes. For skin and mucous membranes, wash thoroughly and follow by application of castor oil or 10 per cent ethyl alcohol. Short-acting barbiturates for convulsions and antibiotics as prophylaxis in pulmonary edema.

128. *Phenolphthalein*

Gastric lavage or emesis. Activated charcoal. Castor oil if given early to hasten the drug through the intestinal tract, but no other solvents because they increase laxative action.

129. *Phenothiazine Derivatives*

Discontinue drug or reduce dosage. In blood dyscrasias or jaundice do not change to another derivative. Gastric lavage for ingestion of large doses. Antiparkinsonian drugs are rarely necessary. Injectable diphenhydramine hydrochloride (Benadryl) is effective in treatment of extrapyramidal symptoms. Biperiden (Akineton) parenterally or orally. Methylphenidate (Ritalin).

130. *Phosphoric Acid*

See Table 1.

131. *Phosphorus* (Red [Nonabsorbed, Nontoxic], Yellow [Volatile and Highly Toxic], Phosphine)

Thorough gastric lavage with potassium permanganate (1:5000) or 3 per cent hydrogen peroxide. Copper sulfate, 0.25 gram in glass of water, forms insoluble copper phosphide. One hundred ml. of mineral oil as a solvent (to prevent absorption and hasten elimination) and repeat in 2 hours. Maintain body temperature, fluids, and electrolytes. Give glucose, vitamin K, and 10 per cent calcium gluconate, if indicated. Exposure to phosphine must be terminated at once, and use of contaminated water for drinking or bathing should be forbidden.

132. *Physostigmine* (Eserine) (Pilocarpine, Neostigmine, Methacholine [Mecholyl], Muscarine)

Gastric lavage or emesis. Maintain artificial respiration until antidote (propantheline [Pro-Banthine], which is preferable to atropine) can be given; 30 mg. intramuscularly every 6 hours may be necessary throughout entire crisis. Maintain airway and remove pulmonary secretion (postural drainage).

133. *Picrotoxin*

Gastric lavage or emesis. Slow absorption of injected drug by application of cold and/or tourniquet. Short-acting barbiturate. Cold packs or alcohol sponging for hyperthermia.

134. *Procaine*

See Cocaine—but much less toxic.

135. *Pyrethrum* (Insect Flowers)

Gastric lavage or emesis unless kerosene is more suspected than pyrethrum. Demulcents. Short-acting barbiturates for convulsions.

136. *Pyribenzamine* (Tripelennamine)

See Antihistaminics.

137. *Quaternary Ammonium Compounds* (Cationic Detergents)

Gastric lavage with soapy water, milk or gelatin solution, or emesis. Demulcents or soapy solution. Maintain clear airway; artificial respiration and oxygen. Short-acting barbiturates for convulsions. Atropine recommended without good basis for its use. Avoid alcohol. Thoroughly wash with soap and water for excessive skin contacts.

138. *Quinine and Cinchona-like Compounds* (Quinidine, Synthetic Hydrocupreine Compounds [Optochin, Numoquin], Plasmochin, Chloroquine [Aralen], Quinacrine [Atabrine])

Gastric lavage or emesis. Discontinue use of

drug. Activated charcoal. Levarterenol for hypotension. Artificial respiration and oxygen.

139. Radiation Syndrome

Remove external clothing and wash clothing and entire body with soap and water. Fresh blood or platelet-enriched plasma. Bone marrow replacement. Antibiotics as prophylaxis for infections.

140. Rotenone

Gastric lavage or emesis if vomiting has not already occurred. Wash thoroughly for skin contact. Short-acting barbiturates. Avoid fats and oils.

141. Ryania

See Rotenone.

142. Sabadilla (Cevadilla)

Demulcents. Activated charcoal. Gastric lavage is usually unnecessary because vomiting occurs early.

143. Salicylate

I. Immediate (emesis or gastric lavage)
   A. Evaluation of severity of intoxication (extrapolation method of Done)
   B. Appraisal of status of dehydration
   C. Determination of acid-base imbalance. Test urine with Phenistix paper and Nitrazene paper
   D. Determination of electrolyte imbalance
   E. Draw blood for the following laboratory tests:
      1. Salicylate level
      2. CO_2-combining content
      3. Plasma CO_2 content
      4. pH
      5. Serum electrolytes

II. Pending laboratory report
   A. Start intravenous fluids (5 per cent glucose in ⅓ isotonic saline)
   B. If dehydration is severe, hydrating solution should be given at the rate of 8 ml. per $m.^2$ body surface per minute for 30 to 45 minutes
   C. After that time, slow down hydrating solution to 2 ml. per $m.^2$ per minute
   D. Correct bicarbonate and potassium deficits as indicated (average requirement: 5 mEq. $NaHCO_3$ per kg. and 2 mEq. K per kg. for 12 hours)
   E. In presence of clinical acidosis and acid urine, $NaHCO_3$ should be given in initial hydrating solution
   F. Cool water body sponging for hyperpyrexia

III. In life-threatening intoxication, consider exchange transfusion in young children, peritoneal dialysis with 5 per cent albumin solution (Albumisol), or dialysis with artificial kidney

IV. Administer vitamin K and B complex, the route of administration depending on the condition of the patient

V. Maintenance management
   A. Test each urine voided with Nitrazene paper
   B. Periodic (frequent) determination of:
      1. Blood CO_2-combining power
      2. Blood CO_2 content
      3. Blood pH

144. Santonin

Gastric lavage or emesis. Saline cathartic. Short-acting barbiturates. Avoid opiates.

145. Sea Nettle (Portuguese Man-of-War)

See separate article, p. 881.

146. Selenium

Move from occupational environment. Eliminate from diet. Bromobenzene solution, 0.25 to 1 gram in lavage.

147. Silver Nitrate

Dilute with isotonic saline solution (0.9 per cent = 1 tsp. salt per 1 pt. water) and thorough lavage of stomach; a relatively insoluble and noncorrosive silver chloride is formed in this reaction. Sodium sulfate cathartic (1 oz. per cup of water). Milk or demulcents. Shock therapy. Meperidine (Demerol) or codeine for pain.

148. Solanine

Gastric lavage or emesis. Activated charcoal. Pilocarpine. Artificial respiration and circulatory stimulants as necessary.

149. Squill (Red, White)

See Digitalis. Gastric lavage or emesis. Demulcents. Quinidine sulfate. Avoid epinephrine or other stimulants.

150. Strychnine

If symptoms have begun, avoid gastric lavage or emesis. Activated charcoal, followed by gastric lavage if asymptomatic. Short-acting barbiturates. Avoid stimuli and opiates. Artificial respiration and oxygen. Muscle relaxants: diazepam (Valium) is particularly effective.

151. Sulfides (Carbon Disulfide, Soluble Sulfides, Hydrogen Sulfide)

Move from exposure. Artificial respiration and oxygen. Remove swallowed poison by gastric lavage or emesis. Wash skin thoroughly for skin contact and use burn therapy. Antibiotics prevent secondary infection.

152. Sulfonamides

Gastric lavage or emesis for overdosage. Discontinue drug. Alkali and large intake of fluid if renal function is normal. Hemodialysis in severe poisoning.

153. Sulfur Dioxide

Move to fresh air. Artificial respiration and oxygen. Antibiotics and corticosteroids for pneumonitis.

154. Sulfuric Acid

See Hydrochloric Acid.

155. Tear Gases

The most commonly used preparations are chloracetophenone, ethylbromoacetate, bromoacetone, bromobenzyl cyanide, and bromomethylethylketone. *Alpha-chloroacetophenone,* even though called a "gas," is actually a fine powder. In commercial blast-dispersion cartridges, it is mixed half and half with silica anhydride, and a standard shotgun primer is used as a propellant. The mixture is an effective lacrimator in concentrations as low as 2 ppm. of air. It can cause extreme irritation and edema of the mucous membranes of the nose and eyes if discharged into the face, and temporary blindness may result. *Mace* contains recrystallized 2-chloroacetophenone (0.9 per cent 1,1,1-trichloroethane), solvents and propellants—Freon, kerosene, methylchloroform, 4.0 per cent.

The eyes should be irrigated for 15 minutes with isotonic saline solution or water, followed by an anti-flammatory eye ointment. For clothing and skin contamination the clothes should be removed and a thorough shower taken.

156. Tetrachloroethane

See Carbon Tetrachloride.

157. Thallium

Gastric lavage or emesis. For skin contamination, wash thoroughly. Activated charcoal twice a day, 1 to 2 tbs., and potassium chloride, 3 to 5 grams daily for 5 to 7 days. BAL. Dithizon (no preparations marketed for therapeutic use), 10 mg. per kg. twice a day for 5 days. Maintain body temperature, blood pressure, fluids, and electrolytes. Antibiotics for pneumonitis. Artane for tremors and ataxia.

158. Thiocyanates

Inorganic: Gastric lavage or emesis. Saline cathartic. Give 2 to 4 liters of fluid daily if renal function is normal. Hemodialysis or peritoneal dialysis, if necessary.

Organic (lauryl, ethyl, and methyl thiocyanate, lethane 60): See Cyanides for treatment.

159. Thiourea

Discontinue use of drug. Antibiotics and corticosteroids for bone marrow depression.

160. Thiram (Tetramethylthiuram Disulfide)

Gastric lavage or emesis. Wash thoroughly for skin contact and remove contaminated clothing. Avoid fats, oils, lipid solvents, and especially alcohol. Artificial respiration and oxygen.

161. Toxaphene

See DDT.

162. Trichloroethylene

See Carbon Tetrachloride.

163. Tricyclic (Dibenzazepine) Compounds

When a patient has convulsions, coma, signs of atropinism, and cardiac arrhythmias, one should strongly suspect tricyclic antidepressant poisoning specifically, and intoxication by other anticholinergic drugs and chemicals in general.

Treatment of intoxication from tricyclic antidepressant tranquilizers is supportive and symptomatic, with particular attention to the correction of cardiac arrhythmias and maintenance of blood pressure and respiration. Vital signs should be monitored continuously. EKG monitoring is advisable, and severely intoxicated patients should be treated in an intensive care unit. Cardiac arrhythmias may progress to cardiac arrest owing to ventricular fibrillation or asystole. Death may occur rapidly after a sudden drop of blood pressure and pulse rate. The use of defibrillators and internal or external pacemakers has been advocated. However, in one nonfatal case, an external DC defibrillator produced no alleviation of arrhythmias, and in a fatal case an external pacemaker was tried unsuccessfully. Although documentation is limited, some arrhythmias were controlled in individual patients by use of the parasympathomimetic drugs; physostigmine, drug of choice (readily crosses the blood-brain barrier, 1 mg. intravenously); pyridostigmine (Mestinon) and neostigmine (Prostigmin) or by the beta-adrenergic blocking agent, propranolol (Inderal). Since it is not possible to predict which patient will respond, it may be necessary to try more than one antiarrhythmic drug. Intravenous sodium diphenylhydantoin has had dramatic antiarrhythmic properties and may also be of value in preventing convulsions which occur frequently. Congestive heart failure is treated by digitalization. However, rapid digitalization should be avoided in a situation in which multiple ventricular ectopic beats are likely to occur. The administration of sodium bicarbonate* and potassium may aid in treating the cardiovascular effects. Convulsions may cause a dangerous increase in the cardiac workload. Agitation, tremors, and convulsions have been successfully treated with parenteral barbiturates. However, use of barbiturates is questionable if drugs that inhibit monoamine oxidase have also been taken by the patient in overdosage or in recent therapy. Also, barbiturates may increase respiratory depression, particularly in children. It is advisable to have equipment available for artificial ventilation and resuscitation. Diazepam (Valium) has been used as an alternative to barbiturates for controlling convulsions, and is considered the drug of choice by some. Hypotension and shock may be treated by intravenous fluids of glucose, saline solution, or plasma, and cautious administration of vasopressor agents such as levarterenol (l-norepinephrine; Levophed), phenylephrine, or metaraminol which will increase blood pressure without increasing heart rate. Any of these sympathomimetic drugs may induce cardiac arrhythmia and must therefore be used with caution. Other sympathomimetic drugs such as epinephrine and isoproterenol which stimulate the beta receptor sites of the heart should be avoided, because they cause additional increases in the heart rate and may lead to fatal ventricular fibrillation. Respiration must be maintained. Intratracheal artificial respiration is effective and the need for it should be anticipated. Patients should be observed for possible recurrence of respiratory distress after resumption of spontaneous breathing. Various methods have been attempted to hasten excretion of these drugs. They are absorbed quickly from the gastrointestinal tract and are largely bound to plasma proteins. In addition, they are rapidly accumulated in the body tissues, so that high serum concentrations do not occur. They are excreted in the urine largely as glucuronides of the demethylated and hydroxylated metabolites. They are also reportedly secreted into the stomach after absorption. Beneficial effects have been reported from use of exchange transfusion, repeated gastric lavage, and osmotic diuresis. Although evidence is equivocal as to the effectiveness of osmotic diuresis in removing significant amounts of these drugs, it is the general belief that diuresis is beneficial. Osmotic diuresis with mannitol has been employed in the treatment of a number of cases of intoxication with tricyclic antidepressant drugs. In one adult, only 5 per cent of the ingested dose of amitriptyline was recovered in the urine (as amitriptyline and its principal metabolites) after a 10 hour period of forced diuresis with mannitol. Since these drugs also promote urinary retention, catheterization should be considered if diuresis is attempted. Care must also be used to prevent overhydration leading to increased cardiac workload. Continuous or repeated gastric lavage has also been recommended to speed excretion. Although continuous gastric lavage was effectively employed in a child intoxicated with imipramine who exhibited coma, convulsions, and cardiac disturbances, it may be unwise to attempt during convulsive stages. Hemodialysis and peritoneal dialysis are not effective in removing significant amounts of these drugs.

In children the tricyclics are especially treacherous. When a verified ingestion occurs, it probably would be wise to hospitalize the child for monitoring for at least 24 hours, even though the patient may be asymptomatic at the time of admission.

*In one series sodium bicarbonate was the most clinically effective method of treatment of arrhythmias in children; experimental studies support this view.

164. *Tridione* (Trimethadione)

Gastric lavage or emesis for unusual ingestion. Discontinue drug or reduce dosage. Antibiotics and corticosteroids for bone marrow depression.

165. *Trinitrotoluene* (TNT)

Gastric lavage or emesis. Saline cathartic. Methylene blue for methemoglobinemia. Remove contaminated clothing and wash skin thoroughly. Short-acting barbiturates.

166. *Tri-ortho-cresyl Phosphate* ("Machine Oil")

Gastric lavage or emesis. Treat as for paralytic poliomyelitis with hydrotherapy, massage, and orthopedic care. Respirators or rocking bed until sufficient recovery occurs.

167. *Tripelennamine* (Pyribenzamine)

See Antihistaminics.

168. *Turpentine*

Gastric lavage or emesis. Demulcents. Saline cathartic. Stimulants for depression. Artificial respiration and oxygen if necessary.

169. Veratrum (Hellbore)

Gastric lavage or emesis. Activated charcoal. Saline cathartic. Atropine every hour to block reflex fall of blood pressure. Phentolamine hydrochloride or other sympathetic blocking agents should be given if hypertension present.

170. Vitamins (Vitamin A, Vitamin D, Vitamin K)

Discontinue use or reduce dosage. Symptomatic and supportive therapy as indicated for hypervitaminosis.

171. Warfarin (Coumadin, Panwarfin)

Gastric lavage or emesis. Vitamin K in adequate dosage. Transfusion of fresh blood if hemorrhage is severe.

172. Xanthines (Aminophylline, Theophylline, Theobromine, and Caffeine)

Gastric lavage or emesis. Antacids or demulcents. If suppository, remove by enema. Short-acting barbiturates. Oxygen.

173. Xylene (Benzene, Toluene, Cumene, and Mesitylene)

Cautious gastric lavage. Fifty ml. of mineral oil left in stomach. Saline cathartic. Artificial respiration and oxygen. Avoid digestible fats, oils, and epinephrine. Wash thoroughly for skin contact.

174. Zinc (Sulfate, Oxide, Phosphide [Releases Phosphine on contact with water; See Phosphine under Phosphorus])

Gastric lavage or emesis for ingestion. Move patient from source of inhalation. Artificial respiration and oxygen. Antibiotics and corticosteroids for "metal fume fever" and pneumonitis.

SECTION 17

Appendices and Index

TABLE OF METRIC AND APOTHECARIES' SYSTEMS

(Approved *approximate* dose equivalents are enclosed in parentheses. Use *exact* equivalents in calculations.)

Conversion Factors

METRIC	APOTHECARIES'
1 milligram (mg.)	1/64 grain
64.79 milligrams	1 grain (65 mg.)
1 gram	15.43 grains (15 grains)
1 cubic centimeter (cc.)	16 minims

METRIC	APOTHECARIES'
3.88 cubic centimeters or grams	1 dram (4 cc. or grams)
31.103 cubic centimeters or grams	1 ounce (30 cc. or grams)
473.167 cubic centimeters	1 pint (500 cc.)

WEIGHTS

METRIC		APOTHECARIES'
0.0001 gram	0.1 mg.	1/640 grain (1/600 grain)
0.0002 gram	0.2 mg.	1/320 grain (1/300 grain)
0.0003 gram	0.3 mg.	1/210 grain (1/200 grain)
0.0004 gram	0.4 mg.	1/150 grain
0.0005 gram	0.5 mg.	1/120 grain
0.0006 gram	0.6 mg.	1/100 grain
0.0007 gram	0.7 mg.	1/90 grain
0.0008 gram	0.8 mg.	1/80 grain
0.0009 gram	0.9 mg.	1/75 grain
0.001 gram	1 mg.	1/64 grain (1/60 grain)
0.0011 gram	1.1 mg.	1/60 grain
0.0013 gram	1.3 mg.	1/50 grain (1.2 mg.)
0.0014 gram	1.4 mg.	1/48 grain
0.0016 gram	1.6 mg.	1/40 grain (1.5 mg.)
0.0018 gram	1.8 mg.	1/36 grain
0.0020 gram	2 mg.	1/32 grain (1/30 grain)
0.0022 gram	2.2 mg.	1/30 grain
0.0026 gram	2.6 mg.	1/25 grain
0.003 gram	3 mg.	1/20 grain
0.004 gram	4 mg.	1/16 grain (1/15 grain)
0.005 gram	5 mg.	1/12 grain
0.006 gram	6 mg.	1/10 grain
0.007 gram	7 mg.	1/9 grain
0.008 gram	8 mg.	1/8 grain
0.009 gram	9 mg.	1/7 grain
0.01 gram	10 mg.	1/6 grain
0.013 gram	13 mg.	1/5 grain (12 mg.)
0.016 gram	16 mg.	1/4 grain (15 mg.)
0.02 gram	20 mg.	1/3 grain
0.025 gram	25 mg.	3/8 grain
0.03 gram	30 mg.	2/5 grain (1/2 grain)
0.032 gram	32 mg.	1/2 grain (30 mg.)
0.04 gram	40 mg.	3/5 grain (2/3 grain)
0.043 gram	43 mg.	2/3 grain (40 mg.)
0.05 gram	50 mg.	3/4 grain

METRIC		APOTHECARIES'
0.057 gram	57 mg.	7/8 grain
0.06 gram	60 mg.	9/10 grain (1 grain)
0.065 gram	65 mg.	1 grain (60 mg.)
0.07 gram	70 mg.	1-1/20 grains
0.08 gram	80 mg.	1-1/5 grains
0.09 gram	90 mg.	1-1/3 grains
0.097 gram	97 mg.	1-1/2 grains (0.1 gram)
0.12 gram	120 mg.	2 grains
0.2 gram	200 mg.	3 grains
0.24 gram	240 mg.	4 grains (0.25 gram)
0.3 gram	300 mg.	4-1/2 grains
0.33 gram	330 mg.	5 grains (0.3 gram)
0.4 gram	400 mg.	6 grains
0.45 gram	450 mg.	7 grains
0.5 gram	500 mg.	7-1/2 grains
0.53 gram	530 mg.	8 grains
0.6 gram	600 mg.	9 grains
0.65 gram	650 mg.	10 grains (0.6 gram)
0.73 gram	730 mg.	11 grains
0.80 gram	800 mg.	12 grains (0.75 gram)
0.86 gram	860 mg.	13 grains
0.93 gram	930 mg.	14 grains
1. gram	1000 mg.	15 grains
1.06 grams	1060 mg.	16 grains
1.13 grams	1130 mg.	17 grains
1.18 grams	1180 mg.	18 grains
1.26 grams	1260 mg.	19 grains
1.30 grams	1300 mg.	20 grains
1.50 grams	1500 mg.	22 grains
2 grams	2000 mg.	30 grains (1/2 dram)
4 grams		1 dram (60 grains)
5 grams		75 grains
8 grams		2 drams (7.5 grams)
10 grams		2-1/2 drams
15 grams		4 drams
30 grams		1 ounce

LIQUID MEASURES*

METRIC	APOTHECARIES'
0.03 cubic centimeter	1/2 minim
0.05 cubic centimeter	3/4 minim
0.06 cubic centimeter	1 minim
0.1 cubic centimeter	1-1/2 minims
0.2 cubic centimeter	3 minims
0.25 cubic centimeter	4 minims
0.3 cubic centimeter	5 minims
0.5 cubic centimeter	8 minims
0.6 cubic centimeter	10 minims
0.75 cubic centimeter	12 minims
1 cubic centimeter	15 minims
2 cubic centimeters	30 minims
3 cubic centimeters	45 minims
4 cubic centimeters	1 fluid dram
5 cubic centimeters	1-1/4 fluid drams

METRIC	APOTHECARIES'
8 cubic centimeters	2 fluid drams
10 cubic centimeters	2-1/2 fluid drams
15 cubic centimeters	4 fluid drams
20 cubic centimeters	5-1/2 fluid drams
25 cubic centimeters	5/6 fluid ounce
30 cubic centimeters	1 fluid ounce
50 cubic centimeters	1-3/4 fluid ounces
60 cubic centimeters	2 fluid ounces
100 cubic centimeters	3-1/2 fluid ounces
120 cubic centimeters	4 fluid ounces
200 cubic centimeters	7 fluid ounces
250 cubic centimeters	8 fluid ounces
360 cubic centimeters	12 fluid ounces
500 cubic centimeters	1 pint
1000 cubic centimeters	1 quart

* Note: A cubic centimeter (cc.) is the approximate equivalent of a milliliter (ml.). The terms are used interchangeably in general medicine.

TABLES OF HEIGHT AND WEIGHT FOR MEN AND WOMEN*

DESIRABLE WEIGHTS FOR MEN OF AGES 25 AND OVER

Weight in Pounds According to Frame (In Indoor Clothing)

HEIGHT (WITH SHOES ON) 1-INCH HEELS *Feet*	*Inches*	SMALL FRAME	MEDIUM FRAME	LARGE FRAME
5	2	112–120	118–129	126–141
5	3	115–123	121–133	129–144
5	4	118–126	124–136	132–148
5	5	121–129	127–139	135–152
5	6	124–133	130–143	138–156
5	7	128–137	134–147	142–161
5	8	132–141	138–152	147–166
5	9	136–145	142–156	151–170
5	10	140–150	146–160	155–174
5	11	144–154	150–165	159–179
6	0	148–158	154–170	164–184
6	1	152–162	158–175	168–189
6	2	156–167	162–180	173–194
6	3	160–171	167–185	178–199
6	4	164–175	172–190	182–204

* Courtesy of the Metropolitan Life Insurance Company.

DESIRABLE WEIGHTS FOR WOMEN OF AGES 25 AND OVER

Weight in Pounds According to Frame (In Indoor Clothing)

HEIGHT (WITH SHOES ON) 2-INCH HEELS *Feet*	*Inches*	SMALL FRAME	MEDIUM FRAME	LARGE FRAME
4	10	92– 98	96–107	104–119
4	11	94–101	98–110	106–122
5	0	96–104	101–113	109–125
5	1	99–107	104–116	112–128
5	2	102–110	107–119	115–131
5	3	105–113	110–122	118–134
5	4	108–116	113–126	121–138
5	5	111–119	116–130	125–142
5	6	114–123	120–135	129–146
5	7	118–127	124–139	133–150
5	8	122–131	128–143	137–154
5	9	126–135	132–147	141–158
5	10	130–140	136–151	145–163
5	11	134–144	140–155	149–168
6	0	138–148	144–159	153–173

For girls between 18 and 25, subtract 1 pound for each year under 25.

GLOSSARY OF AMERICAN DRUG NAMES AND INTERNATIONAL SYNONYMS *

United States Adopted Name	British Approved or International Nonproprietary Name
Acenocoumarol	Nicoumalone
Acetaminophen	Paracetamol
Acetarsone	Acetarsol
Actinomycin	Actinomycin C
Albuterol	Salbutamol
Ambuphylline	Bufylline
Aminitrozole	Acinitrazole
Amithizone	Thiacetazone
Amobarbital	Amylobarbitone
Amoxycillin	Amoxycilline
Amphecloral	Amfecloral
Anazoline	Anoxynaphthonate
Anisotropine	Octatropine
Anthralin	Dithranol
Antimony sodium gluconate	Sodium stibogluconate
Antipyrine	Phenazone
Arylam	Sevin
Asparaginase	Colaspase
Barbital	Barbitone
Bendazac	Bindazac
Bendroflumethiazide	Bendrofluazide
Benoxinate	Oxybuprocaine
Betazole	Ametazole
Biphenamine	Xenysalate
Bismuth subcarbonate	Bismuth oxycarbonate
Bromisovalum	Bromeval
Bunamiodyl	Buniodyl
Busulfan	Busulphan
Butabarbital	Secbutabarbitone
Butethal	Butobarbitone
Butyl aminobenzoate	Butesine
Calciferol	Ergosterol
Calcium benzoylpas	Calcium benzamidosalicylate
Carbachol	Carbamoylcholine
Carbenoxalone	Carbenoxolone
Chaulmoogra oil	Hydnocarpus oil
Chloroazodin	Chlorazodin
Chlorobutanol	Chlorbutol
Chloroguanide	Proguanil
Chlorophenothane	Dicophane
Chlorothen	Chloropyrilene
Colistimethate	Colistin methanesulphomethate
Corticotropin	Corticotrophin
Cosyntropin	Tetracosactrin
Cromolyn	Cromoglycate
Cyclobarbital	Cyclobarbitone
Cyclocumarol	Cyclocoumarol
Daunomycin	Rubidomycin
Deferoxamine	Desferrioxamine
Demeclocycline	Demethylchlortetracycline
Desoxycorticosterone	Deoxycortone
Dextroamphetamine	Dexamphetamine
Dibucaine	Cinchocaine
Dichloroisoproterenol	Dichloroisoprenaline
Dicumarol	Dicoumarol
Diethyl dithiolisophthalate	Ditophal
Diethylstilbestrol	Stilboestrol
Diiodohydroxyquin	Diiodohydroxyquinoline
Dinoprost tromethamine	Dinoprostone
Disodium-p-melaminylphenyl arsonate	Melarsen
Dromostanolone	Drostanolone
Dyphylline	Diprophylline
Echothiophate	Ecothiopate
Epinephrine	Adrenaline
Ergocalciferol	Calciferol
Ergonovine	Ergometrine
Estradiol	Oestradiol
Estrogen	Oestrogen
Ethenzamide	Etenzamide
Ethinyl estradiol	Ethinyloestradiol
Ethylaminobenzoate	Benzocaine
Ethylestrenol	Ethyloestrenol
Evans blue	Azovan blue
Fantridone	Fanthridone
Fibrinolysin, human	Plasmin
Floxacillin	Flucloxacillin
Flucloronide	Fluclorolone acetonide
Flurandrenolide	Flurandrenolone
Flurogestone	Flugestone
Fonazine	Dimethothiazine
Fructose	Levulose
Furosemide	Frusemide
Gestronorone	Gestronol
Glyburide	Glibenclamide
Glycobiarsol	Bismuth glycolylarsanilate
Glycopyrrolate	Glycopyrronium
Heptabarbital	Heptabarbitone
Hexacarbacholine	Carbolonium
Hexachlorophene	Hexachlorophane
Hexamarium	Distigmine
Hexestrol	Hexoestrol
Hexobarbital	Hexobarbitone
Hydralazine	Hydrallazine
Hydrocortisone	Cortisol
Hydroxypropyl methylcellulose	Hypromellose
Indigotindisulfonate sodium	Indigo carmine
Inositol niacinate	Inositol nicotinate
Iodochlorhydroxyquin	Clioquinol
Iodopyracet	Diodrast
Iothiouracil	Iodothiouracil
Isoflurophate	Dyflos
Isoproterenol	Isoprenaline
Isosorbide dinitrate	Sorbide nitrate
Leucovorin calcium	Calcium folinate
Lidocaine	Lignocaine
Mechlorethamine	Mustine
Meclizine	Meclozine
Melanotropin	Intermedin
Melphalan	Melfalan
Menadione	Menaphthone
Menotropins	Follicle-stimulating hormone
Meparfynol	Methylpentynol
Mepazine	Pecazine
Meperidine	Pethidine
Mephenytoin	Methoin
Mephobarbital	Methylphenobarbitone
Metaproterenol	Orciprenaline
Methabarbital	Methabarbitone
Methacholine	Acetylmethylcholine
Methandrostenolone	Methandienone
Methantheline	Methanthelinium
Methenamine hippurate	Hexamine hippurate
Methohexital	Methohexitone
Methopholine	Metofoline
Methscopolamine bromide	Hyoscine methobromide
Methylatropine nitrate	Atropine methyl nitrate
Methylergonovine	Methylergometrine
Methyprylon	Methylprylone
Mineral oil	Paraffin, liquid
Nequinate	Methyl benzoquate
Niacin	Nicotinic acid
Niacinamide	Nicotinamide
Nikethamide	Nicethamide
Nitroglycerin	Glyceryl trinitrate
Norepinephrine	Noradrenaline
Norethindrone	Norethisterone
Norethynodrel	Noretynodrel
Normeperidine	Norpethidine
Nylidrin	Buphenine
Ouabain	Strophanthin
Oxtriphylline	Choline theophyllinate

GLOSSARY OF AMERICAN DRUG NAMES AND INTERNATIONAL SYNONYMS* *(Continued)*

United States Adopted Name	British Approved or International Nonproprietary Name
Peanut oil	Arachis oil
Penicillin G	Benzylpenicillin
Pentobarbital	Pentobarbitone
Pentylenetetrazole	Leptazol
Phenobarbital	Phenobarbitone
Physostigmine	Eserine
Phytonadione	Phytomenadione
Polyethylene glycol	Macrogol
Progestin	Allylestrenol
Proparacaine	Proxymetacaine
Propoxyphene	Dextropropoxyphene
Pyrilamine	Mepyramine
Pyrvinium pamoate	Vipyrnium embonate
Quinacrine	Mepacrine
Riboflavin	Riboflavine
Rifampin	Rifampicin
Rolicyprine	Rolicypram
Scopolamine	Hyoscine
Secobarbital	Quinalbarbitone
Seperidol	Clofluperol
Sodium acetylhydroxyarsanilate	Orsanine
Solasulfone	Solapsone
Succinylcholine	Suxamethonium
Succinylsulfathiazole	Succinylsulphathiazole
Sulfacetamide	Sulphacetamide
Sulfadiazine	Sulphadiazine
Sulfadimethoxine	Sulphadimethoxine
Sulfaethidole	Sulphaethidole
Sulfalene	Sulfametopyrazine
Sulfameter	Sulphamethoxydiazine
Sulfamethazine	Sulfadimidine
Sulfamethizole	Sulphamethizole
Sulfamethoxazole	Sulphamethoxazole
Sulfamethoxypyridazine	Sulphamethoxypyridazine
Sulfamoxole	Sulphamoxole
Sulfaphenazole	Sulphaphenazole
Sulfaproxyline	Sulphaproxyline
Sulfasalazine	Sulphasalazine
Sulfasomizole	Sulphasomizole
Sulfathiazole	Sulphathiazole
Sulfinpyrazone	Sulphinpyrazone
Sulfisomidine	Sulphasomidine
Sulfisoxazole	Sulphafurazole
Sulfomyxin	Sulphomyxin
Tetracaine	Amethocaine
Tetramisole	Levamisole
Thiabendazole	Mintezol
Thialbarbital	Thialbarbitone
Thiamine	Aneurine
Thimerosal	Thiomersal
Thiopental	Thiopentone
Thyrotropin	Thyrotrophin
Thyroxin	Thyroxine
Tilidine	Tilidate
Triethylenemelamine	Tretamine
Triflupromazine	Flupromazine
Trihexyphenidyl	Benzhexol
Trimethadione	Troxidone
Trimethaphan	Trimetaphan
Trimethoprim-sulfamethoxazole	Co-trimoxazole
Troleandomycin	Triacetyloleandomycin
Tromethamine	Trometamol
Uracil mustard	Uramustine
Urethan	Urethane
Vinbarbital	Vinbarbitone
Vitamin A	Retinol

*Modified from Modell, W., Schild, H. O., and Wilson, A.: Applied Pharmacology (American edition). Philadelphia, W. B. Saunders Company, 1976.

LABORATORY REFERENCE VALUES OF CLINICAL IMPORTANCE

prepared by
REX B. CONN, M.D.
Atlanta, Georgia

THE INTERNATIONAL SYSTEM OF UNITS FOR LABORATORY MEASUREMENTS (LE SYSTÈME INTERNATIONAL D'UNITÉS)

Physicians are accustomed to receiving laboratory reports with measurements expressed in metric units such as the gram, liter, or milliliter; however, an extensive modification of the metric system has been adopted by clinical laboratories in many countries, and plans are being formulated to make a similar change in the United States. This adaptation is the International System of Units (Le Système International d'Unités), usually abbreviated S.I. Units. Whereas the metric system utilizes the centimeter, the gram, and the second as basic units, the International System uses the meter, the kilogram, and the second as well as four other basic units.

The overriding consideration for adopting the International System is that it will provide a common language among the various scientific disciplines throughout the world for unambiguous communication regarding all types of measurements. In the medical field, the advantages of conversion are that chemical relationships between various substances will become more readily apparent and there will be an international uniformity in laboratory reporting. The most serious disadvantage in making this conversion is that physicians will have to become accustomed to a new set of figures for almost all laboratory measurements. Because of this inconvenience, as well as a potential for serious misinterpretation of laboratory data, the conversion must be undertaken cautiously and only after a logical plan has been formulated and discussed. There appears to be little question, however, that the International System will be adopted in this country. Clinical laboratories in most western European countries, Canada, and Australia are already using S.I. Units, and American medical journals are adopting the practice of expressing measurements in both conventional and S.I. Units.

The International System

The International System is a coherent approach to all types of measurement which utilizes seven dimensionally independent basic quantities: mass, length, time, thermodynamic temperature, electric current, luminous intensity, and amount of substance. Each of these quantities is expressed in a clearly defined *basic unit* (Table 1).

Two or more basic units may be combined to provide *derived units* (Table 2) for expressing other measurements such as mass concentration (kilograms per cubic meter) and velocity (meters per second). Standardized prefixes (Table 3) for basic and derived units are used to express fractions or multiples of the basic units so that any measurement can be expressed in a value between 0.001 and 1000.

Medical Applications

The most profound change in laboratory reports will result from expressing concentration as amount per volume (moles per liter) rather than mass per volume (milligrams per 100 milliliters). The advantages in the former expression can be seen in the following:

Conventional Units

1.0 gram of hemoglobin
- Combines with 1.37 ml. of oxygen
- Contains 3.4 mg. of iron
- Forms 34.9 mg. of bilirubin

S.I. Units

1.0 mmol of hemoglobin
- Combines with 4.0 mmol of oxygen
- Contains 4.0 mmol of iron
- Forms 4.0 mmol of bilirubin

Chemical relationships between lactic acid and pyruvic acid and the glucose from which both are derived, as well as the relationship between bilirubin and the binding capacity of albumin, are other examples of chemical relationships that will be clarified by using the new system.

There are a number of laboratory and other medical measurements for which the S.I. Units appear to offer little advantage, and some which are disadvantageous because the change would require replacement or revision of instruments such as the sphygmomanometer. The cubic meter is the derived unit for volume; however, it is inappropriately large for medical measurements and the liter has been retained. Thermodynamic

TABLE 1. **Basic Units**

PROPERTY	BASIC UNIT	SYMBOL
Length	metre	m
Mass	kilogram	kg
Amount of substance	mole	mol
Time	second	s
Thermodynamic temperature	kelvin	K
Electric current	ampere	A
Luminous intensity	candela	cd

TABLE 2. **Derived Units**

DERIVED PROPERTY	DERIVED UNIT	SYMBOL
Area	square metre	m^2
Volume	cubic metre	m^3
	litre	l
Mass concentration	kilogram/cubic metre	kg/m^3
	gram/litre	g/l
Substance concentration	mole/cubic metre	mol/m^3
	mole/litre	mol/l
Temperature	degree Celsius	C = K − 273.15

temperature expressed in kelvins is not more informative for medical measurements. Since the Celsius degree is the same as the Kelvin degree, the Celsius scale will be used. Celsius rather than centigrade is the preferred term.

Selection of units for expressing enzyme activity presents certain difficulties. Literally dozens of different units have been used in expressing enzyme activity, and interlaboratory comparison of enzyme results is impossible unless the assay system is precisely defined. In 1964 the International Union of Biochemistry attempted to remedy the situation by proposing the International Unit for enzymes. This unit was defined as the amount of enzyme that will catalyze the conversion of 1 micromole of substrate per minute under standard conditions. Difficulties remain, however, as enzyme activity is affected by the temperature, pH, the type and amount of substrate, the presence of inhibitors, and other factors. Enzyme activity can be expressed in S.I. Units, and the katal has been proposed to express activities of all catalysts, including enzymes. The katal is that amount of enzyme which catalyzes a reaction rate of 1 mole per second. Thus adoption of the katal as the unit of enzyme activity would provide no more information than is obtained when results are expressed in International Units.

TABLE 3. **Standard Prefixes**

PREFIX	MULTIPLICATION FACTOR	SYMBOL
atto	10^{-18}	a
femto	10^{-15}	f
pico	10^{-12}	p
nano	10^{-9}	n
micro	10^{-6}	μ
milli	10^{-3}	m
centi	10^{-2}	c
deci	10^{-1}	d
deca	10^{1}	da
hecto	10^{2}	h
kilo	10^{3}	k
mega	10^{6}	M
giga	10^{9}	G
tera	10^{12}	T

Hydrogen ion concentration in blood is customarily expressed as pH, but in S.I. Units it would be expressed in nanomoles per liter. It appears unlikely that the very useful pH scale will be discarded.

Pressure measures, such as blood pressure and partial pressures of blood gases, would be expressed in S.I. Units, using the Pascal, a unit that can be derived from the basic units for mass, length, and time. This change probably will not be adopted in the early phases of the conversion to S.I. Units. Similarly, a proposed change in expressing osmolality in terms of the depression of freezing point is inappropriate, because osmolality may be calculated from vapor pressure as well as freezing point measurement.

Conventions

A number of conventions have been adopted to standardize usage of S.I. Units:

1. No periods are used after the symbol for a unit (kg not kg.), and it remains unchanged when used in the plural (70 kg not 70 kgs).
2. A half space rather than a comma is used to divide large numbers into groups of three (5 400 000 not 5,400,000).
3. Compound prefixes should be avoided (nanometer not millimicrometer).
4. Multiples and submultiples are used in steps of 10^3 or 10^{-3}.
5. The degree sign for the temperature scales is omitted (38 C not 38°C).
6. The preferred spelling is metre not meter, litre not liter.
7. Report of a measurement should include information on the system, the component, the kind of quantity, the numerical value, and the unit. For example: *System,* serum. *Component,* glucose. *Kind of quantity,* substance concentration. *Value,* 5.10. *Unit,* mmol/l.
8. The name of the component should be unambiguous; for example, "serum bilirubin" might refer to unconjugated bilirubin or to total bilirubin. For acids and bases, the maximally ionized form is used in naming the component; for example, lactate or urate rather than lactic acid or uric acid.

Tables of Reference Values

Tables accompanying this article indicate "normal values" for most of the commonly performed laboratory tests. The title of the tables has been changed from the "normal values" of previous years to "reference values" to conform to current usage. The reference value is given in conventional units, the conversion factor is indicated when appropriate, and the value in S.I. Units is calculated from these figures. Notes (pp. 924 and 925) are used to provide additional information.

REFERENCE VALUES IN HEMATOLOGY

	CONVENTIONAL UNITS		FACTOR	S.I. UNITS	NOTES
Acid hemolysis test (Ham)	No hemolysis		—	No hemolysis	
Alkaline phosphatase, leukocyte	Total score 14–100		—	Total score 14–100	
Carboxyhemoglobin	Up to 5% of total		0.01	0.05 of total	a
Cell counts					
Erythrocytes					
Males	4.6–6.2 million/cu. mm.		10^6	$4.6–6.2 \times 10^{12}/l$	
Females	4.2–5.4 million/cu. mm.			$4.2–5.4 \times 10^{12}/l$	
Children (varies with age)	4.5–5.1 million/cu. mm.			$4.5–5.1 \times 10^{12}/l$	
Leukocytes					
Total	4500–11,000/cu. mm.		10^6	$4.5–11.0 \times 10^9/l$	
Differential	*Percentage*	*Absolute*			
Myelocytes	0	0/cu. mm.	10^6	0/1	b
Band neutrophils	3–5	150–400/cu. mm.		$150–400 \times 10^6/l$	
Segmented neutrophils	54–62	3000–5800/cu. mm.		$3000–5800 \times 10^6/l$	
Lymphocytes	25–33	1500–3000/cu. mm.		$1500–3000 \times 10^6/l$	
Monocytes	3–7	300–500/cu. mm.		$300–500 \times 10^6/l$	
Eosinophils	1–3	50–250/cu. mm.		$50–250 \times 10^6/l$	
Basophils	0–0.75	15–50/cu. mm.		$15–50 \times 10^6/l$	
Platelets	150,000–350,000/cu. mm.		10^6	$150–350 \times 10^9/l$	
Reticulocytes	25,000–75,000/cu. mm. 0.5–1.5% of erythrocytes		10^6	$25–75 \times 10^9/l$	b
Coagulation tests					
Bleeding time (Duke)	1–5 min.		—	1–5 min	
Bleeding time (Ivy)	Less than 5 min.		—	Less than 5 min	
Clot retraction, qualitative	Begins in 30–60 min.		—	Begins in 30–60 min	
	Complete in 24 hrs.		—	Complete in 24 h	
Coagulation time (Lee-White)	5–15 min. (glass tubes)		—	5–15 min (glass tubes)	
	19–60 min. (siliconized tubes)		—	19–60 min (siliconized tubes)	
Fibrinogen	200–400 mg./100 ml.		0.0293	5.9–11.7 μmol/l	c
Fibrinolysins	0		—	0	
Partial thromboplastin time, activated (APTT)	35–45 sec.		—	35–45 s	
Prothrombin consumption	Over 80% consumed in 1 hr.		0.01	Over 0.80 consumed in 1 h	a
Prothrombin content	100% (calculated from prothrombin time)		0.01	1.0 (calculated from prothrombin time)	a
Prothrombin time (one stage)	12.0–14.0 sec.		—	12.0–14.0 s	
Thromboplastin generation test	Compared to normal control		—	Compared to normal control	
Tourniquet test	Ten or fewer petechiae in a 2.5 cm. circle after 5 min.		—	Ten or fewer petechiae in a 2.5 cm circle after 5 min	
Cold hemolysin test (Donath-Landsteiner)	No hemolysis		—	No hemolysis	

Component	Conventional units	Average	Factor	SI units	Average	Ref.
Corpuscular values of erythrocytes (values are for adults; in children, values vary with age)						
M.C.H. (mean corpuscular hemoglobin)	27–31 picogm.		0.0155	0.42–0.48 fmol		d
M.C.V. (mean corpuscular volume)	80–105 cu. micra		1.0	80–105 fl		
M.C.H.C. (mean corpuscular hemoglobin concentration)	32–36%		0.01	0.32–0.36		a
Haptoglobin (as hemoglobin binding capacity)	100–200 mg./100 ml.		0.155	16–31 μmol/l		d
Hematocrit						
Males	40–54 ml./100 ml.		0.01	0.40–0.54		a
Females	37–47 ml./100 ml.			0.37–0.47		
Newborn	49–54 ml./100 ml.			0.49–0.54		
Children (varies with age)	35–49 ml./100 ml.			0.35–0.49		
Hemoglobin						
Males	14.0–18.0 grams/100 ml.		0.155	2.17–2.79 mmol/l		d
Females	12.0–16.0 grams/100 ml.			1.86–2.48 mmol/l		
Newborn	16.5–19.5 grams/100 ml.			2.56–3.02 mmol/l		
Children (varies with age)	11.2–16.5 grams/100 ml.			1.74–2.56 mmol/l		
Hemoglobin, fetal	Less than 1% of total		0.01	Less than 0.01 of total		a
Hemoglobin A_2	1.5–3.0% of total		0.01	0.015–0.03 of total		a
Hemoglobin, plasma	0–5.0 mg./100 ml.		0.155	0–0.8 μmol/l		d
Methemoglobin	0–130 mg./100 ml.		0.155	4.7–20 μmol/l		e
Osmotic fragility of erythrocytes	Begins in 0.45–0.39% NaCl Complete in 0.33–0.30% NaCl		171	Begins in 77–67 mmol/l NaCl Complete in 56–51 mmol/l NaCl		
Sedimentation rate						
Wintrobe: Males	0–5 mm. in 1 hr.		—	0–5 mm/h		
Wintrobe: Females	0–15 mm. in 1 hr.		—	0–15 mm/h		
Westergren: Males	0–15 mm. in 1 hr.		—	0–15 mm/h		
Westergren: Females	0–20 mm. in 1 hr.		—	0–20 mm/h		
(May be slightly higher in children and during pregnancy)						
Bone marrow, differential cell count	*Range*	*Average*		*Range*	*Average*	
Myeloblasts	0.3–5.0%	2.0%	0.01	0.003–0.05	0.02	a
Promyelocytes	1.0–8.0%	5.0%		0.01–0.08	0.05	
Myelocytes: Neutrophilic	5.0–19.0%	12.0%		0.05–0.19	0.12	
Eosinophilic	0.5–3.0%	1.5%		0.005–0.03	0.015	
Basophilic	0.0–0.5%	0.3%		0.00–0.005	0.003	
Metamyelocytes	13.0–32.0%	22.0%		0.13–0.32	0.22	
Polymorphonuclear neutrophils	7.0–30.0%	20.0%		0.07–0.30	0.20	
Polymorphonuclear eosinophils	0.5–4.0%	2.0%		0.005–0.04	0.02	
Polymorphonuclear basophils	0.0–0.7%	0.2%		0.00–0.007	0.002	
Lymphocytes	3.0–17.0%	10.0%		0.03–0.17	0.10	
Plasma cells	0.0–2.0%	0.4%		0.00–0.02	0.004	
Monocytes	0.5–5.0%	2.0%		0.005–0.05	0.02	
Reticulum cells	0.1–2.0%	0.2%		0.001–0.02	0.002	
Megakaryocytes	0.3–3.0%	0.4%		0.003–0.03	0.004	
Pronormoblasts	1.0–8.0%	4.0%		0.01–0.08	0.04	
Normoblasts	7.0–32.0%	18.0%		0.07–0.32	0.18	

REFERENCE VALUES FOR BLOOD, PLASMA AND SERUM

(For some procedures the reference values may vary depending upon the method used)

	CONVENTIONAL UNITS	FACTOR	S.I. UNITS	NOTES
Acetoacetate plus acetone, serum				
Qualitative	Negative	—	Negative	
Quantitative	0.3–2.0 mg./100 ml.	10	3–20 mg/l	
Aldolase, serum	0–11 milliunits/ml. (I.U.) (30°)	1.0	0–11 units/l (30 C)	f
Alpha amino nitrogen, serum	3.0–5.5 mg./100 ml.	0.714	2.1–3.9 mmol/l	
Ammonia, blood	80–110 mcg./100 ml.	0.587	47–65 μmol/l	
Amylase, serum	Less than 160 Caraway units/100 ml.	—	Less than 160 Caraway units/dl	f
Ascorbic acid, blood	0.4–1.5 mg./100 ml.	56.8	23–85 μmol/l	
Bilirubin, serum				
Direct	0.1–0.4 mg./100 ml.	17.1	1.7–6.8 μmol/l	
Indirect	0.2–0.7 mg./100 ml. (Total minus direct)	17.1	3.4–12 μmol/l (Total minus direct)	
Total	0.3–1.1 mg./100 ml.	17.1	5.1–19 μmol/l	
Bromsulphalein (BSP) (Inject 5 mg./kg. body weight, draw sample at 45 min.)	Less than 5%	0.01	Less than 0.05	a
Calcium, serum	4.5–5.5 mEq./liter	0.50	2.25–2.75 mmol/l	
	9.0–11.0 mg./100 ml.	0.25	2.25–2.75 mmol/l	
	(Slightly higher in children)		(Slightly higher in children)	
	(Varies with protein concentration)		(Varies with protein concentration)	
Calcium, ionized, serum	2.1–2.6 mEq./liter	0.50	1.05–1.30 mmol/l	
	4.25–5.25 mg./100 ml.	0.25	1.05–1.30 mmol/l	
Carbon dioxide content, serum				
Adults	24–30 mEq./liter	1.0	24–30 mmol/l	
Infants	20–28 mEq./liter	1.0	20–28 mmol/l	
Carbon dioxide tension (P_{CO_2}), blood	35–45 mm. Hg	—	35–45 mm Hg	g
Carotene, serum	50–300 mcg./100 ml.	0.0186	0.93–5.58 μmol/l	
Ceruloplasmin, serum	23–44 mg./100 ml.	0.0662	1.5–2.9 μmol/l	h
Chloride, serum	96–106 mEq./liter	1.0	96–106 mmol/l	
Cholesterol, serum				
Total	150–250 mg./100 ml.	0.0259	3.9–6.5 mmol/l	
Esters	68–76% of total cholesterol	0.01	0.68–0.76 of total cholesterol	a
Cholinesterase				
Serum	0.5–1.3 pH units	—	0.5–1.3 pH units	f
Erythrocytes	0.5–1.0 pH unit	—	0.5–1.0 pH unit	f
Copper, serum				
Males	70–140 mcg./100 ml.	0.157	11–22 μmol/l	
Females	85–155 mcg./100 ml.	0.157	13–24 μmol/l	
Cortisol, plasma (8 A.M.)	6–16 mcg./100 ml.	27.6	170–440 nmol/l	
Creatine, serum	0.2–0.8 mg./100 ml.	76.3	15–61 μmol/l	

Creatine phosphokinase, serum				
Males	0–50 milliunits/ml. (I.U.) (30°)	1.0	0–50 units/l (30 C)	f
Females	0–30 milliunits/ml. (I.U.) (30°) (Oliver-Rosalki)	1.0	0–30 units/l (30 C) (Oliver-Rosalki)	f
Creatine phosphokinase isoenzymes, serum				
CPK-MM	Present	—	Present	
CPK-MB	Absent	—	Absent	
CPK-BB	Absent	—	Absent	
Creatinine, serum	0.7–1.5 mg./100 ml.	88.4	62–133 μmol/l	
Cryoglobulins, serum	0	—	0	
Fatty acids, total, serum	190–420 mg./100 ml.	0.0352	7–15 mmol/l	i
Fibrinogen, plasma	200–400 mg./100 ml.	0.0293	5.9–11.7 μmol/l	c
Folate, serum	5–21 nanogm./ml.	2.27	11–48 nmol/l	
Gastrin, serum	0–200 picogm./ml.	1.0	0–200 ng/l	
Glucose (fasting)				
Blood	60–100 mg./100 ml.	0.0555	3.33–5.55 mmol/l	
Plasma or serum	70–115 mg./100 ml.	0.0555	3.89–6.38 mmol/l	
Haptoglobin, serum	100–200 mg./100 ml. (As hemoglobin binding capacity)	0.155	16–31 μmol/l (As hemoglobin binding capacity)	d
Hydroxybutyric dehydrogenase, serum	0–180 milliunits/ml. (I.U.) (30°) (Rosalki-Wilkinson)	1.0	0–180 units/l (30 C) (Rosalki-Wilkinson)	f
	114–290 units/ml. (Wroblewski)	—	114–290 units/ml (Wroblewski)	f
17-Hydroxycorticosteroids, plasma	8–18 mcg./100 ml.	0.0276	0.22–0.50 μmol/l	j
Immunoglobins, serum				
IgG	550–1900 mg./100 ml.	0.01	5.5–19.0 g/l	
IgA	60–333 mg./100 ml.	0.01	0.60–3.3 g/l	
IgM	45–145 mg./100 ml. (Varies with age in children)	0.01	0.45–1.5 g/l (Varies with age in children)	
Insulin, plasma (fasting)	5–25 microunits/ml.	1.0	5–25 milliunits/l	
Iodine, protein bound, serum	3.5–8.0 mcg./100 ml.	0.0788	0.28–0.63 μmol/l	k
Iron, serum	75–175 mcg./100 ml.	0.179	13–31 μmol/l	
Iron binding capacity, serum				
Total	250–410 mcg./100 ml.	0.179	45–73 μmol/l	
Saturation	20–55%	0.01	0.20–0.55	a
17-Ketosteroids, plasma	25–125 mcg./100 ml.	0.0347	0.87–4.34 μmol/l	l
Lactate, blood, venous	0.6–1.8 mEq./liter	1.0	0.6–1.8 mmol/l	
Lactate dehydrogenase, serum	0–300 milliunits/ml. (I.U.) (30°) (Wroblewski modified)	1.0	0–300 units/l (30 C) (Wroblewski modified)	f
	150–450 units/ml. (Wroblewski)	—	150–450 units/ml (Wroblewski)	
	80–120 units/ml. (Wacker)	—	80–120 units/ml (Wacker)	
Lactate dehydrogenase isoenzymes, serum				
LDH_1	22–37% of total	0.01	0.22–0.37 of total	a
LDH_2	30–46% of total		0.30–0.46 of total	
LDH_3	14–29% of total		0.14–0.29 of total	
LDH_4	5–11% of total		0.05–0.11 of total	
LDH_5	2–11% of total		0.02–0.11 of total	
Leucine aminopeptidase, serum	14–40 milliunits/ml. (I.U.) (30°)	1.0	14–40 units/l (30 C)	f
Lipase, serum	0–1.5 units (Cherry-Crandall)	—	0–1.5 units (Cherry-Crandall)	f
Lipids, total, serum	450–850 mg./100 ml.	0.01	4.5–8.5 g/l	m

Table continued on the following page

REFERENCE VALUES FOR BLOOD, PLASMA AND SERUM (*Continued*)

(For some procedures the reference values may vary depending upon the method used)

	CONVENTIONAL UNITS	FACTOR	S.I. UNITS	NOTES
Magnesium, serum	1.5–2.5 mEq./liter	0.50	0.75–1.25 mmol/l	
	1.8–3.0 mg./100 ml.	0.411		
5′-Nucleotidase, serum	Less than 1.6 milliunits/ml. (30°)	1.0	Less than 1.6 units/l (30 C)	f
Nitrogen, nonprotein, serum	15–35 mg./100 ml.	0.714	10.7–25.0 mmol/l	
Osmolality, serum	285–295 mOsm./kg. serum water	—	285–295 mmol/kg serum water	n
Oxygen, blood				
Capacity	16–24 vol.% (varies with hemoglobin)	0.446	7.14–10.7 mmol/l (varies with hemoglobin)	o
Content — Arterial	15–23 vol.%	0.446	6.69–10.3 mmol/l	o
Content — Venous	10–16 vol.%	0.446	4.46–7.14 mmol/l	o
Saturation — Arterial	94–100% of capacity	0.01	0.94–1.00 of capacity	a
Saturation — Venous	60–85% of capacity	0.01	0.60–0.85 of capacity	a
Tension, pO_2 — Arterial	75–100 mm. Hg	—	75–100 mm Hg	g
pH, arterial, blood	7.35–7.45	—	7.35–7.45	p
Phenylalanine, serum	Less than 3 mg./100 ml.	0.0605	Less than 0.18 mmol/l	
Phosphatase, acid, serum	0–7.0 milliunits/ml. (I.U.) (30°)	1.0	0–7.0 units/l (30 C)	f
	1.0–5.0 units (King-Armstrong)	—	1.0–5.0 units (King-Armstrong)	
Phosphatase, alkaline, serum	10–32 milliunits/ml. (I.U.) (30°)	1.0	10–32 units/l (30 C)	f
	5.0–13.0 units (King-Armstrong)	—	5.0–13.0 units (King-Armstrong)	
	(Values are higher in children)		(Values are higher in children)	
Phosphate, inorganic, serum				
Adults	3.0–4.5 mg./100 ml.	0.323	1.0–1.5 mmol/l	
Children	4.0–7.0 mg./100 ml.		1.3–2.3 mmol/l	
Phospholipids, serum	6–12 mg./100 ml.	0.323	1.9–3.9 mmol/l	
	(As lipid phosphorus)		(As lipid phosphorus)	
Potassium, serum	3.5–5.0 mEq./liter	1.0	3.5–5.0 mmol/l	
Protein, serum				
Total	6.0–8.0 grams/100 ml.	10	60–80 g/l	m
Albumin	3.5–5.5 grams/100 ml.	10	35–55 g/l	q
		0.154	0.54–0.85 mmol/l	
Globulin	2.5–3.5 grams/100 ml.	10	25–35 g/l	
Electrophoresis				
Albumin	3.5–5.5 grams/100 ml.	10	35–55 g/l	q
	52–68% of total	0.01	0.52–0.68 of total	a
Globulin				
$Alpha_1$	0.2–0.4 gram/100 ml.	10	2–4 g/l	m
	2–5% of total	0.01	0.02–0.05 of total	a
$Alpha_2$	0.5–0.9 gram/100 ml.	10	5–9 g/l	m
	7–14% of total	0.01	0.07–0.14 of total	a
Beta	0.6–1.1 grams/100 ml.	10	6–11 g/l	m
	9–15% of total	0.01	0.09–0.15 of total	a
Gamma	0.7–1.7 grams/100 ml.	10	7–17 g/l	m
	11–21% of total	0.01	0.11–0.21 of total	a

Protoporphyrin, erythrocyte	27–61 mcg./100 ml. packed RBC	0.0178	0.48–1.09 μmol/l packed RBC	
Pyruvate, blood	0.01–0.11 mEq./liter	1.0	0.01–0.11 mmol/l	
Sodium, serum	136–145 mEq./liter	1.0	136–145 mmol/l	
Sulfates, inorganic, serum	0.8–1.2 mg./100 ml.	104	83–125 μmol/l	
Testosterone, plasma				
Males	275–875 nanogm./100 ml.	0.0347	9.5–30 nmol/l	
Females	23–75 nanogm./100 ml.	0.0347	0.8–2.6 nmol/l	
Pregnant	38–190 nanogm./100 ml.	0.0347	1.3–6.6 nmol/l	
Thyroid stimulating hormone (TSH), serum	0–7 microunits/ml.	1.0	0–7 milliunits/l	
Thyroxine, free, serum	1.0–2.1 nanogm./100 ml.	12.9	13–27 pmol/l	
Thyroxine (T_4), serum	4.4–9.9 mcg./100 ml.	12.9	57–128 nmol/l	
Thyroxine binding globulin (TBG), serum (as thyroxine)	10–26 mcg./100 ml.	12.9	129–335 nmol/l	
Tri-iodothyronine (T_3), serum	150–250 nanogm./100 ml.	0.0154	2.3–3.9 nmol/l	
Thyroxine iodine, serum	2.9–6.4 mcg./100 ml.	78.8	229–504 nmol/l	k
Transaminase, serum				
SGOT (aspartate aminotransferase)	0–19 milliunits/ml. (I.U.) (30°) (Karmen modified)	1.0	0–19 units/l (30 C) (Karmen modified)	f
	15–40 units/ml. (Karmen)		15–40 units/ml (Karmen)	
	18–40 units/ml. (Reitman-Frankel)		18–40 units/ml (Reitman-Frankel)	
SGPT (alanine aminotransferase)	0–17 milliunits/ml. (I.U.) (30°) (Karmen modified)	1.0	0–17 units/l (30 C) (Karmen modified)	f
	6–35 units/ml. (Karmen)		6–35 units/ml (Karmen)	
	5–35 units/ml. (Reitman-Frankel)		5–35 units/ml (Reitman-Frankel)	
Triglycerides, serum	40–150 mg./100 ml.	0.01	0.4–1.5 g/l	
		0.0114	0.45–1.71 mmol/l	r
Urate (serum)				
Males	2.5–8.0 mg./100 ml.	0.0595	0.15–0.48 mmol/l	
Females	1.5–7.0 mg./100 ml.	0.0595	0.09–0.42 mmol/l	
Urea				
Blood	21–43 mg./100 ml.	0.167	3.5–7.2 mmol/l	
Plasma or serum	24–49 mg./100 ml.	0.167	4.0–8.2 mmol/l	
Urea nitrogen				
Blood	10–20 mg./100 ml.	0.714	7.1–14.3 mmol/l	k
Plasma or serum	11–23 mg./100 ml.	0.714	7.9–16.4 mmol/l	
Vitamin A, serum	20–80 mcg./100 ml.	0.0349	0.70–2.8 μmol/l	
Vitamin B_{12}, serum	300–1000 picogm./ml.	0.738	220–740 pmol/l	

REFERENCE VALUES FOR URINE

(For some procedures the reference values may vary depending upon the method used)

	CONVENTIONAL UNITS	FACTOR	S.I. UNITS	NOTES
Acetone and acetoacetate, qualitative	Negative	—	Negative	
Addis count				
Erythrocytes	0–130,000/24 hrs.	—	0–130 000/24 h	
Leukocytes	0–650,000/24 hrs.	—	0–650 000/24 h	
Casts (hyaline)	0–2000/24 hrs.	—	0–2000/24 h	
Albumin				
Qualitative	Negative	—	Negative	
Quantitative	10–100 mg./24 hrs.	—	10–100 mg/24 h	q
		0.0154	0.15–1.5 μmol/24 h	
Aldosterone	3–20 mcg./24 hrs.	2.77	8.3–55 nmol/24 h	
Alpha amino nitrogen	50–200 mg./24 hrs.	0.0714	3.6–14.3 mmol/24 h	
Ammonia nitrogen	20–70 mEq./24 hrs.	1.0	20–70 mmol/24 h	
Amylase	35–260 Caraway units/hr.	—	35–260 Caraway units/h	f
Bilirubin, qualitative	Negative	—	Negative	
Calcium				
Low Ca diet	Less than 150 mg./24 hrs.	0.025	Less than 3.8 mmol/24 h	
Usual diet	Less than 250 mg./24 hrs.	0.025	Less than 6.3 mmol/24 h	
Catecholamines				
Epinephrine	Less than 10 mcg./24 hrs.	5.46	Less than 55 nmol/24 h	
Norepinephrine	Less than 100 mcg./24 hrs.	5.91	Less than 590 nmol/24 h	
Total free catecholamines	4–126 mcg./24 hrs.	5.91	24–745 nmol/24 h	s
Total metanephrines	0.1–1.6 mg./24 hrs.	5.07	0.5–8.1 μmol/24 h	t
Chloride	110–250 mEq./24 hrs. (Varies with intake)	1.0	110–250 mmol/24 h (Varies with intake)	
Chorionic gonadotropin	0	—	0	
Copper	0–50 mcg./24 hrs.	0.0157	0–0.80 μmol/24 h	
Creatine				
Males	0–40 mg./24 hrs.	0.00762	0–0.30 mmol/24 h	
Females	0–100 mg./24 hrs. (Higher in children and during pregnancy)	0.00762	0–0.76 mmol/24 h (Higher in children and during pregnancy)	
Creatinine	15–25 mg./kg. body weight/24 hrs.	0.00884	0.13–0.22 mmol·kg^{-1} body weight/24 h	
Creatinine clearance				
Males	110–150 ml./min.	—	110–150 ml/min	
Females	105–132 ml./min. (1.73 sq. meter surface area)	—	105–132 ml/min (1.73 m^2 surface area)	
Cystine or cysteine, qualitative	Negative	—	Negative	
Dehydroepiandrosterone	Less than 15% of total 17-keto-steroids	0.01	Less than 0.15 of total 17-keto-steroids	a
Delta aminolevulinic acid	1.3–7.0 mg./24 hrs.	7.63	10–53 μmol/24 h	

Estrogens				
Males				
Estrone	3–8 μg./24 hrs.	3.70	11–30 nmol/24 h	
Estradiol	0–6 μg./24 hrs.	3.67	0–22 nmol/24 h	
Estriol	1–11 μg./24 hrs.	3.47	3–38 nmol/24 h	
Total	4–25 μg./24 hrs.	3.60	14–90 nmol/24 h	u
Females				
Estrone	4–31 μg./24 hrs.	3.70	15–115 nmol/24 h	
Estradiol	0–14 μg./24 hrs.	3.67	0–51 nmol/24 h	
Estriol	0–72 μg./24 hrs.	3.47	0–250 nmol/24 h	
Total	5–100 μg./24 hrs. (Markedly increased during pregnancy)	3.60	18–360 nmol/24 h (Markedly increased during pregnancy)	u
Glucose (as reducing substance)	Less than 250 mg./24 hrs.	—	Less than 250 mg/24 h	
Gonadotropins, pituitary	10–50 mouse units/24 hrs.	—	10–50 mouse units/24 h	
Hemoglobin and myoglobin, qualitative	Negative	—	Negative	
Hemogentisic acid, qualitative	Negative	—	Negative	
17-Hydroxycorticosteroids				
Males	3–9 mg./24 hrs.	2.76	8.3–25 μmol/24 h	j
Females	2–8 mg./24 hrs.		5.5–22 μmol/24 h	
5-Hydroxyindoleacetic acid				
Qualitative	Negative	—	Negative	
Quantitative	Less than 9 mg./24 hrs.	5.23	Less than 47 μmol/24 h	
17-Ketosteroids				
Males	6–18 mg./24 hrs.	3.47	21–62 μmol/24 h	l
Females	4–13 mg./24 hrs. (Varies with age)		14–45 μmol/24 h (Varies with age)	
Magnesium	6.0–8.5 mEq./24 hrs.	0.5	3.0–4.3 mmol/24 h	
Metanephrines (see Catecholamines)				
Osmolality	38–1400 mOsm./kg. water	—	38–1400 mmol/kg water	n
pH	4.6–8.0, average 6.0 (Depends on diet)	—	4.6–8.0, average 6.0 (Depends on diet)	p
Phenosulfonphthalein excretion (PSP)	25% or more in 15 min. 40% or more in 30 min. 55% or more in 2 hrs. (After injection of 1 ml PSP intravenously)	0.01	0.25 or more in 15 min 0.40 or more in 30 min 0.55 or more in 2 h (After injection of 1 ml PSP intravenously)	a
Phenylpyruvic acid, qualitative	Negative	—	Negative	
Phosphorus	0.9–1.3 gm./24 hrs.	32.3	29–42 mmol/24 h	
Porphobilinogen				
Qualitative	Negative	—	Negative	
Quantitative	0–0.2 mg./100 ml. Less than 2.0 mg./24 hrs.	4.42	0–0.9 μmol/l Less than 9 μmol/24 h	
Porphyrins				
Coproporphyrin	50–250 mcg./24 hrs.	1.53	77–380 nmol/24 h	
Uroporphyrin	10–30 mcg./24 hrs.	1.20	12–36 nmol/24 h	
Potassium	25–100 mEq./24 hrs. (Varies with intake)	1.0	25–100 mmol/24 h (Varies with intake)	

Table continued on the following page

REFERENCE VALUES FOR URINE (*Continued*)

(For some procedures the reference values may vary depending upon the method used)

	CONVENTIONAL UNITS	FACTOR	S.I. UNITS	NOTES
Pregnanediol				
Males	0.4–1.4 mg./24 hrs.	3.12	1.2–4.4 μmol/24 h	
Females				
Proliferative phase	0.5–1.5 mg./24 hrs.		1.6–4.7 μmol/24 h	
Luteal phase	2.0–7.0 mg./24 hrs.		6.2–22 μmol/24 h	
Postmenopausal phase	0.2–1.0 mg./24 hrs.		0.6–3.1 μmol/24 h	
Pregnant 16 weeks	5–21 mg./24 hrs.		16–66 μmol/24 h	
Pregnant 20 weeks	6–26 mg./24 hrs.		19–81 μmol/24 h	
Pregnant 24 weeks	12–32 mg./24 hrs.		37–100 μmol/24 h	
Pregnant 28 weeks	19–51 mg./24 hrs.		59–159 μmol/24 h	
Pregnant 32 weeks	22–66 mg./24 hrs.		69–206 μmol/24 h	
Pregnant 36 weeks	23–77 mg./24 hrs.		72–240 μmol/24 h	
Pregnant 40 weeks	23–63 mg./24 hrs.		72–197 μmol/24 h	
Pregnanetriol	Less than 2.5 mg./24 hrs. in adults	2.97	Less than 7.4 μmol/24 h in adults	
Protein				
Qualitative	Negative	—	Negative	
Quantitative	10–150 mg./24 hrs.		10–150 mg/24 h	m
Sodium	130–260 mEq./24 hrs. (Varies with intake)	1.0	130–260 mmol/24 h (Varies with intake)	
Specific gravity	1.003–1.030	—	1.003–1.030	
Titratable acidity	20–40 mEq./24 hrs.	1.0	20–40 mmol/24 h	
Urate	200–500 mg./24 hrs. (With normal diet)	0.00595	1.2–3.0 mmol/24 h (With normal diet)	
Urobilinogen	Up to 1.0 Ehrlich unit/2 hrs. (1–3 P.M.)	—	Up to 1.0 Ehrlich unit/2 h (1–3 P.M.)	
	0–4.0 mg./24 hrs.	—	0–4.0 mg/24 h	
Vanillylmandelic acid (VMA) (4-hydroxy-3-methoxymandelic acid)	1–8 mg./24 hrs.	5.05	5–40 μmol/24 h	

REFERENCE VALUES FOR THERAPEUTIC DRUG MONITORING

	CONVENTIONAL UNITS	FACTOR	S.I. UNITS	NOTES
Carbamazepine, serum (Tegretol)	0 Therapeutic levels: 5.0–14.0 mg./liter	4.23	0 Therapeutic levels: 21–59 μmol/l	
Digoxin, serum With dose of 0.25 mg. per day	0 Therapeutic levels: 0.8–1.6 mcg./liter	1.28	0 Therapeutic levels: 1.0–2.3 nmol/l	

With dose of 0.5 mg. per day (Sample obtained 12 to 24 hrs. after last dose)	0.9–2.4 mcg./liter		1.2–3.1 nmol/l
Diphenylhydantoin, serum (Dilantin)	0 Therapeutic levels: 10–20 mg./liter Toxic levels: Above 20 mg./liter	3.65	0 Therapeutic levels: 37–73 μmol/l Toxic levels: Above 73 μmol/l
Ethosuximide, serum (Zarontin)	0 Therapeutic levels: 40–80 mg./liter	7.08	0 Therapeutic levels: 283–566 μmol/l
Lithium, serum	0 Therapeutic levels: 0.8–1.5 mEq./liter Toxic level: Above 2 mEq./liter	1.0	0 Therapeutic levels: 0.8–1.5 mmol/l Toxic level: Above 2 mmol/l
Phenobarbital, serum	0 Therapeutic levels: 10.0–25.0 mg./liter Toxic levels: Vary widely because of developed tolerance	4.31	0 Therapeutic levels: 43–108 μmol/l Toxic levels: Vary widely because of developed tolerance
Primidone, serum (Mysoline)	0 Therapeutic levels: 4.0–10.0 mg./liter	4.58	0 Therapeutic levels: 18–46 μmol/l
Procainamide, serum (Pronestyl)	0 Therapeutic levels: 4.0–8.0 mg./liter	4.24	0 Therapeutic levels: 17–34 μmol/l
Quinidine, serum	0 Therapeutic levels: 2.0–5.0 mg./liter Toxic levels: Over 10 mg./liter	3.08	0 Therapeutic levels: 6.2–15 μmol/l Toxic levels: Over 31 μmol/l
Salicylate, plasma	0 Therapeutic levels: 20–25 mg./100 ml. Toxic levels: Over 30 mg./100 ml. Death 45–75 mg./100 ml.	0.0555	0 Therapeutic levels: 1.0–1.4 mmol/l Toxic levels: Over 1.7 mmol/l Death 2.5–4.2 mmol/l
Theophylline, serum	0 Therapeutic levels: 5.0–20.0 mg./liter Toxic levels: Above 30.0 mg./liter	5.55	0 Therapeutic levels: 28–111 μmol/l Toxic levels: Above 167 μmol/l
Thiocyanate, serum (Metabolite of sodium nitroprusside)	0 Therapeutic levels: 80–120 mg./liter	0.0169	0 Therapeutic levels: 1.4–2.0 mmol/l

REFERENCE VALUES IN TOXICOLOGY

	CONVENTIONAL UNITS	FACTOR	S.I. UNITS	NOTES
Arsenic, blood	3.5–7.2 mcg./100 ml.	0.133	0.47–0.96 μmol/l	
Arsenic, urine	Less than 100 mcg./24 hrs.	0.0133	Less than 1.3 μmol/24 h	
Bromides, serum	0	1.0	0	
	Toxic levels:		Toxic levels:	
	Above 17 mEq./liter		Above 17 mmol/l	
Carbon monoxide, blood	Up to 5% saturation	—	Up to 0.05 saturation	a
	Symptoms occur with 20% saturation		Symptoms occur with 0.20 saturation	
Ethanol, blood	Less than 0.005%	217	Less than 1 mmol/l	
Marked intoxication	0.3–0.4%		65–87 mmol/l	
Alcoholic stupor	0.4–0.5%		87–109 mmol/l	
Coma	Above 0.5%		Above 109 mmol/l	
Lead, blood	0–40 mcg./100 ml.	0.0483	0–2 μmol/l	
Lead, urine	Less than 100 mcg./24 hrs.	0.00483	Less than 0.48 μmol/24 h	
Mercury, urine	Less than 10 mcg./24 hrs.	4.98	Less than 50 nmol/24 h	

REFERENCE VALUES FOR CEREBROSPINAL FLUID

	CONVENTIONAL UNITS	FACTOR	S.I. UNITS	NOTES
Cells	Fewer than 5/cu. mm.; all mononuclear	—	Fewer than 5/μl; all mononuclear	
Chloride	120–130 mEq./liter	1.0	120–130 mmol/l	
	(20 mEq./liter higher than serum)		(20 mmol/l higher than serum)	
Electrophoresis	Predominantly albumin	—	Predominantly albumin	
Glucose	50–75 mg./100 ml.	0.0555	2.8–4.2 mmol/l	
	(20 mg./100 ml. less than serum)		(1.1 mmol/l less than serum)	
IgG				
Children under 14	Less than 8% of total protein	—	Less than 0.08 of total protein	a,m
Adults	Less than 14% of total protein		Less than 0.14 of total protein	
Pressure	70–180 mm. water		70–180 mm water	g
Protein, total	15–45 mg./100 ml.	0.01	0.150–0.450 g/l	m
	(Higher, up to 70 mg./100 ml., in elderly adults and children)		(Higher, up to 0.70 g/l, in elderly adults and children)	

REFERENCE VALUES FOR GASTRIC ANALYSIS

	CONVENTIONAL UNITS	FACTOR	S.I. UNITS	NOTES
Basal gastric secretion (1 hour)				
Concentration	(Mean ± 1 S.D.)		(Mean ± 1 S.D.)	
Males	25.8 ± 1.8 mEq./liter	1.0	25.8 ± 1.8 mmol/l	
Females	20.3 ± 3.0 mEq./liter		20.3 ± 3.0 mmol/l	
Output	(Mean ± 1 S.D.)		(Mean ± 1 S.D.)	
Males	2.57 ± 0.16 mEq./hr.	1.0	2.57 ± 0.16 mmol/h	
Females	1.61 ± 0.18 mEq./hr.		1.61 ± 0.18 mmol/h	
After histamine stimulation				
Normal	Mean output 11.8 mEq./hr.	1.0	Mean output 11.8 mmol/h	
Duodenal ulcer	Mean output 15.2 mEq./hr.		Mean output 15.2 mmol/h	
After maximal histamine stimulation				
Normal	Mean output 22.6 mEq./hr.	1.0	Mean output 22.6 mmol/h	
Duodenal ulcer	Mean output 44.6 mEq./hr.		Mean output 44.6 mmol/h	
Diagnex blue (Squibb): Anacidity	0–0.3 mg. in 2 hrs.	1.0	0–0.3 mg in 2 h	
Doubtful	0.3–0.6 mg. in 2 hrs.		0.3–0.6 mg in 2 h	
Normal	Greater than 0.6 mg. in 2 hrs.		Greater than 0.6 mg in 2 h	
Volume, fasting stomach content	50–100 ml.	—	0.05–0.1 litre	
Emptying time	3–6 hrs.	—	3–6 h	
Color	Opalescent or colorless	—	Opalescent or colorless	
Specific gravity	1.006–1.009	—	1.006–1.009	
pH (adults)	0.9–1.5	—	0.9–1.5	p

GASTROINTESTINAL ABSORPTION TESTS

	CONVENTIONAL UNITS	FACTOR	S.I. UNITS	NOTES
d-Xylose absorption test	After an 8 hour fast, 10 ml./kg. body weight of a 0.05 solution of d-xylose is given by mouth. Nothing further by mouth is given until the test has been completed. All urine voided during the following 5 hours is pooled, and blood samples are taken at 0, 60, and 120 minutes. Normally 0.26 (range 0.16–0.33) of ingested xylose is excreted within 5 hours, and the serum xylose reaches a level between 25 and 40 mg./100 ml. after 1 hour and is maintained at this level for another 60 minutes.		No change	

Table continued on the following page

GASTROINTESTINAL ABSORPTION TESTS (*Continued*)

	CONVENTIONAL UNITS	FACTOR	S.I. UNITS	NOTES
Vitamin A absorption	A fasting blood specimen is obtained and 200,000 units of vitamin A in oil is given by mouth. Serum vitamin A level should rise to twice fasting level in 3 to 5 hours.		No change	

REFERENCE VALUES FOR FECES

	CONVENTIONAL UNITS	FACTOR	S.I. UNITS	NOTES
Bulk	100–200 grams/24 hrs.	—	100–200 g/24 h	
Dry matter	23–32 grams/24 hrs.	—	23–32 g/24 h	
Fat, total	Less than 6.0 grams/24 hrs.	—	Less than 6.0 g/24 h	
Nitrogen, total	Less than 2.0 grams/24 hrs.	—	Less than 2.0 g/24 h	
Urobilinogen	40–280 mg./24 hrs.	—	40–280 mg/24 h	
Water	Approximately 65%	0.01	Approximately 0.65	a

REFERENCE VALUES FOR SEMEN ANALYSIS

	CONVENTIONAL UNITS	FACTOR	S.I. UNITS	NOTES
Volume	2–5 ml.; usually 3–4 ml.	—	2–5 ml; usually 3–4 ml	
Liquefaction	Complete in 15 min.	—	Complete in 15 min	
pH	7.2–8.0; average 7.8	—	7.2–8.0; average 7.8	p
Leukocytes	Occasional or absent	—	Occasional or absent	
Count	60–150 million/ml.	—	60–150 million/ml	
	Below 60 million/ml. is abnormal	—	Below 60 million/ml is abnormal	
Motility	80% or more motile	—	0.80 or more motile	a
Morphology	80–90% normal forms	—	0.80–0.90 normal forms	a

REFERENCE VALUES FOR IMMUNOLOGIC PROCEDURES

	CONVENTIONAL UNITS	FACTOR	S.I. UNITS	NOTES
Syphilis serology (RPR and VDRL)	Negative		No change	
Mono screen	Negative		No change	
R.A. test (latex)	1:40 Negative 1:80–1:160 Doubtful 1:320 Positive		No change	
Rose test	1:10 Negative 1:20–1:40 Doubtful 1:80 Positive		No change	
Anti-streptolysin O titer	Normal up to 1:128. Single test usually has little significance. Rise in titer or persistently elevated titer is significant.		No change	
Anti-hyaluronidase titer	Less than 1:200. Significant if rising titer can be demonstrated at weekly intervals.		No change	
C-reactive protein	Negative		No change	
Anti-nuclear antibody	One specimen is sufficient, unless the result is inconsistent with the clinical impression. Most patients with active lupus have high ANA titers (160 or greater); some have lower titers (20–40). Patients with inactive lupus may have a negative test. Antinuclear antibodies are occasionally present in patients with no evidence of systemic lupus, usually in lower titers (20–40).		No change	
Febrile agglutinins	Titers of 1:80 or greater may be significant, particularly if subsequent samples show rise in titer.		No change	
Tularemia agglutinins	1:80 Negative 1:160 Doubtful 1:320 Positive		No change	
Proteus OX-19 agglutinins	Titers of 1:80 or greater may be significant, particularly if subsequent samples show rise in titer.		No change	
Complement fixation tests	Titers of 1:8 or less are usually not significant. Paired sera showing rise in titer of more than two tubes are usually considered significant.		No change	
C3 Test	80–140 mg./100 ml.	0.01	0.80–1.40 g/l	q
C4 Test	11–75 mg./100 ml.	0.01	0.11–0.75 g/l	

NOTES

a. Percentage is expressed as a decimal fraction.

b. Percentage may be expressed as a decimal fraction; however, when the result expressed is itself a variable fraction of another variable, the absolute value is more meaningful. There is no reason, other than custom, for expressing reticulocyte counts and differential leukocyte counts in percentages or decimal fractions rather than in absolute numbers.

c. Molecular weight of fibrinogen = 341,000.

d. Molecular weight of hemoglobin = 64,500. Because of disagreement as to whether the monomer or tetramer of hemoglobin should be used in the conversion, it has been recommended that the conventional grams per deciliter be retained. The tetramer is used in the table; values given should be multiplied by 4 to obtain concentration of the monomer.

e. Molecular weight of methemoglobin = 64,500. See note d above.

f. Enzyme units have not been changed in these tables because the proposed enzyme unit, the katal, has not been universally adopted (1 International Unit = 16.7 nkat).

g. It has been proposed that pressure be expressed in the Pascal (1 mm Hg = 0.133 kPa); however, this convention has not been universally accepted.

h. Molecular weight of ceruloplasmin = 151,000.

i. "Fatty acids" includes a mixture of different aliphatic acids of varying molecular weight. A mean molecular weight of 284 has been assumed in calculating the conversion factor.

mit direct correlation with hemoglobin content, which is possible when oxygen content and capacity are expressed in molar quantities. One millimole of hemoglobin combines with 4 millimoles of oxygen.

p. Hydrogen ion concentration in S.I. units would be expressed in nanomoles per liter; however, this change has not received general approval. Conversion can be calculated as antilog (−pH).

q. Albumin is expressed in grams per liter to be consistent with units used for other proteins. Concentration of albumin may be expressed in mmol/l also, an expression that permits assessment of binding capacity of albumin for substances such as bilirubin. Molecular weight of albumin is 65,000.

r. Most techniques for quantitating triglycerides measure the glycerol moiety, and the total mass is calculated using an average molecular weight. The factor given assumes a mean molecular weight of 875 for triglycerides.

s. Calculated as norepinephrine, molecular weight 169.18.

t. Calculated as metanephrine, molecular weight 197.23.

u. Conversion factor calculated from molecular weights of estrone, estradiol, and estriol in proportions of 2:1:2.

REFERENCES

1. Baron, D. N., Broughton, P. M. G., Cohen, M., Lansley, T. S., Lewis, S. M., and Shinton, N. K.: J. Clin. Path., *27*:590, 1974.

j. Based upon molecular weight of cortisol 362.47.

k. The practice of expressing concentration of an organic molecule in terms of one of its constituent elements originated when measurements included a heterogeneous class of compounds (nonprotein nitrogenous compounds, iodine-containing compounds bound to serum proteins). It was carried over to expressing measurements of specific substances (urea, thyroxine), but the practice should be discarded. For iodine and nitrogen 1 mole is taken as the monoatomic form, although they occur as diatomic molecules.

l. Based upon molecular weight of dehydroepiandrosterone 288.41.

m. Weight per volume is retained as the unit because of the heterogeneous nature of the material measured.

n. The proposal that osmolality be reported as freezing point depression using the millikelvin as the unit has not been received with universal enthusiasm. The milliosmole is not an S.I. unit, and the unit used here is the millimole.

o. Volumes per cent might be converted to a decimal fraction; however, this would not per-

2. Castleman, B., and McNeely, B. U.: New Eng. J. Med., *290*:39, 1974.
3. Davidsohn, I., and Henry, J. B.: Clinical Diagnosis by Laboratory Methods, 15th ed. Philadelphia, W. B. Saunders Co., 1974.
4. Dawson, R. M. C., Elliott, D. C., Elliott, W. H., and Jones, K. M.: Data for Biochemical Research, 2nd ed. New York and Oxford, Oxford University Press, 1969.
5. Department of Laboratory Medicine, The Johns Hopkins Hospital: Clinical Laboratory Handbook. Baltimore, 1976.
6. Dybkaer, R.: Amer. J. Clin. Path., *52*:637, 1969.
7. Henry, R. J., Cannon, D. C., and Winkleman, J. W.: Clinical Chemistry—Principles and Techniques, 2nd ed. New York, Harper & Row, 1974.
8. International Committee for Standardization in Hematology, International Federation of Clinical Chemistry and World Association of Pathology Societies: Clin. Chem., *19*:135, 1973.
9. Lehmann, H. P.: Amer. J. Clin. Path., *65*:2, 1976.
10. Miale, J. B.: Laboratory Medicine—Hematology, 4th ed. St. Louis, C. V. Mosby, 1972.
11. Page, C. H., and Vigoureux, P.: The International System of Units (S.I.). U. S. Department of Commerce, National Bureau of Standards, Special Publication 330, 1974.
12. Tietz, N. W.: Fundamentals of Clinical Chemistry, 2nd ed. Philadelphia, W. B. Saunders Co., 1976.
13. Wintrobe, M. D., Lee, G. R., Boggs, D. R., Bithell, T. C., Athens, J. W., and Foerster, J.: Clinical Hematology, 7th ed. Philadelphia, Lea & Febiger, 1974.
14. Young, D. S.: New Eng. J. Med., *292*:795, 1975.

Index